DAVIS'S Comprehensive Handbook of

Laboratory & Diagnostic Tests with Nursing Implications

Activate your FREE subscription today!

P9-DNE-016

You're two steps away from your **FREE** 1-year subscription to **www.LabDxTest.com**, powered by Unbound Medicine®.

unbound MEDICINE

1. Simply type the following address into your web browser:

www.LabDxTest.com/labs/ub/bookcode

2. Enter your unique, personal code printed on this page.

www.LabDxTest.com features all of the monographs from **Davis's Comprehensive Handbook of Laboratory & Diagnostic Tests with Nursing Implications** database! It's accessible from your desktop, laptop, or any mobile device with a web browser.

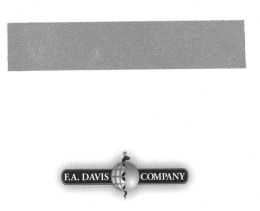

F.A. DAVIS COMPANY

Anne M. Van Leeuwen, MA, BS, MT (ASCP)

Debra Poelhuis-Leth, MS, RT (R) (M)

Mickey Lynn Bladh, RN, MSN

Davis's Comprehensive Handbook of

Laboratory & Diagnostic Tests—With Nursing Implications

Fourth Edition

 F. A. DAVIS COMPANY • Philadelphia

F.A. Davis Company
1915 Arch Street
Philadelphia, PA 19103

www.fadavis.com

Printed in the United States of America

Last digit indicates print number: 10 9 8 7 6 5 4 3 2 1

Publisher: Lisa B. Deitch
Art and Design Manager: Carolyn O'Brien
Managing Editor: David Orzechowski
Project Editor: Christina C. Burns

Library of Congress Cataloging-in-Publication Data

Van Leeuwen, Anne M.
 Davis's comprehensive handbook of laboratory and diagnostic tests : with nursing implications
  / Anne M. Van Leeuwen, Debra J. Poelhuis-Leth, Mickey L. Bladh. — 4th ed.
   p. ; cm.
 Comprehensive handbook of laboratory and diagnostic tests
 Includes bibliographical references and index.
 ISBN-13: 978-0-8036-2304-0
 ISBN-10: 0-8036-2304-6
 1. Diagnosis, Laboratory—Handbooks, manuals, etc. 2. Nursing—Handbooks, manuals, etc.
  I. Poelhuis-Leth, Debra J. II. Bladh, Mickey L. III. Title. IV. Title: Comprehensive handbook of
  laboratory and diagnostic tests.
 [DNLM: 1. Laboratory Techniques and Procedures—Handbooks. 2. Laboratory Techniques
  and Procedures—Nurses' Instruction. 3. Nursing Diagnosis—methods. 4. Diagnostic
  Techniques and Procedures—Handbooks. 5. Diagnostic Techniques and Procedures—
  Nurses' Instruction. QY 39]
 RB38.2.S37 2011
 616.07'5—dc22

                                       2010034840

Dedication

Inspiration springs from Passion. . . . Passion is born from unconstrained love, commitment, and a vision no one else can own.

Lynda, thank you—I could not have done this without your love, strong support, and belief in me. My gratitude to Mom, Dad, Adele, Gram . . . all my family and friends, for I am truly blessed by your humor and faith. A huge hug for my daughters, Sarah and Margaret—I love you very much. To my puppies, Maggie, Taylor, and Emma, for their endless and unconditional love. Many thanks to my friend and coauthor Debbie; to all the folks at F.A. Davis, especially Rob, Christina, Julia, Cynthia, and Frank for their guidance, support, and great ideas. My thanks and warm welcome to Mickey Bladh for her wonderful contributions to this fourth edition—and beyond. And, very special thanks to Lisa Deitch, publisher, for her friendship, excellent direction, and unwavering encouragement.

Anne M. Van Leeuwen, MA, BS, MT (ASCP)
Technical Supervisor, Yuma Operations
Sonora Quest Laboratories
Yuma, Arizona

To Bill, my husband, who always shows his support for my professional endeavors. To my beautiful children, Abbie and Andy, I love you both; please remember to always push yourselves to excel. Thanks, Mom and Dad, for always showing your pride in me and what I accomplish. Anne, Lisa, and Rob, your confidence, continued support, guidance, and assistance is always appreciated. A warm welcome to Mickey with her invaluable insights as part of our group. I look forward to our continued friendship.

Debra Poelhuis-Leth, MS, RT, (R) (M)
Director, Radiology Program
Montgomery County Community College
Pottstown, Pennsylvania

An eternity of searching would never have provided me with a man more loving and supportive than my husband, Eric. He is the sunshine in my soul, and I will be forever grateful for the blessing of his presence in my life. I am grateful to my five children, Eric, Anni, Phillip, Mari, and Melissa, for the privilege of being their mom; always remember that you are limited only by your imagination and willingness to try. To Anne and Deb, thanks so much for the opportunity to spread my wings, for your patience and guidance, and thanks to Lynda for the miracle of finding me. To all of those at F.A. Davis—Rob, Christina, and Lisa—you are the best. Lastly, to my beloved parents, thanks with hugs and kisses.

Mickey Lynn Bladh, RN, MSN
Coordinator, Nursing Education
Presbyterian Intercommunity Hospital
Whittier, California

About This Book

The authors would like to thank all the users of the previous editions for helping us identify what they like about this book as well as what might improve its value. We want to continue this dialogue. As writers, it is our desire to capture the interest of our readers, to provide essential information, and to continue to improve the presentation of the material in the book and ancillary products. We encourage our readers to provide feedback to the Web site and to the publisher's sales professionals. Your feedback helps us modify the material—to change with your changing needs. Several new monographs have been added: ductography, endoscopy sinus, fetoscopy, hysteroscopy, and sialography. Monographs have been expanded to include additional information; for example, we include new information about the gastric fluid analysis/gastric acid stimulation test, the use of pharmacogenetics to control the prothrombin time and international normalized ratio, and suggestions for patient teaching that reflect changes in standards of care, particularly with respect to cancer screening and the use of home test kits. Some monographs have been combined to consolidate similar tests, and a few less frequently used tests have been condensed into a mini-monograph format that highlights abbreviated test-specific facts, with the full monographs for those tests now resident on the DavisPlus Web site (http://davisplus.fadavis.com). The names of some test monographs have been changed to assist the reader in locating them more easily. For example, the tests that relate to the complete blood count have been renamed to begin with "Complete Blood Count, [test name]" (Complete Blood Count, Hemoglobin; Complete Blood Count, RBC Count; etc.), so they are grouped together alphabetically in the text; the individual tests are also listed separately under their own names in the index. All of these changes have been made in response to feedback from our readers.

The authors have taken care to enhance four areas in this new edition: pathophysiology that affects test results, patient safety, patient education, and integration of related laboratory and diagnostic testing. First, the Result section is now the Potential Diagnosis section and has been expanded to include an explanation of increased or decreased values, as many of you requested. We have included additional age-specific reference values for the geriatric population at the request of some of our readers. It should be mentioned that standardized information for the complexity of a geriatric population is difficult to document. Values may be increased or decreased in older adults due to the sole or combined effects of malnutrition, alcohol use, medications, and the presence of multiple chronic or acute diseases with or without muted symptoms. Second, the authors appreciate that nurses are the strongest patient advocates with a huge responsibility to protect the safety of their patients, and we have observed student nurses in clinical settings being interviewed by facility accreditation inspectors, so we have integrated a number of reminders that parallel The Joint Commission's national patient safety goals. The Pretest section reminds the nurse to positively identify the patient before providing care, treatment, or services. The Pretest section also addresses hand-off communication of critical information. The third area of emphasis is that each monograph coaches the student to focus on patient education and prepares the nurse to anticipate and respond to a patient's questions or concerns: describing the purpose of the procedure, addressing concerns about pain, understanding the implications of the test results, and describing postprocedural care. Various related Web sites for patient education are included throughout the book. And fourth, laboratory and diagnostic tests do not stand on their own—all the pieces fit together to form a picture. The section at the end of each monograph that lists related tests by modality has been changed to integrate both laboratory and diagnostic tests. The authors thought it might be more useful for a nurse to know what other tests might be ordered together—and all the related tests are listed alphabetically for ease of use.

Laboratory and diagnostic studies are essential components of a complete patient assessment. Examined in conjunction with an individual's history and physical examination, laboratory and diagnostic data provide clues about health status. Nurses are increasingly expected to integrate an understanding of laboratory and diagnostic procedures and expected outcomes in assessment, planning, implementation, and evaluation of nursing care. The data help develop and support nursing diagnoses, interventions, and outcomes.

Nurses may interface with laboratory and diagnostic testing on several levels, including:

- Interacting with patients and families of patients undergoing diagnostic tests or procedures and providing pretest, intratest, and post-test information and support
- Maintaining quality control to prevent or eliminate problems that may interfere with the accuracy and reliability of test results
- Ensuring completion of testing in a timely and accurate manner
- Collaborating with other health-care professionals in interpreting findings as they relate to planning and implementing total patient care
- Communicating significant alterations in test outcomes to appropriate health-care team members
- Coordinating interdisciplinary efforts

Whether the nurse's role at each level is direct or indirect, the underlying responsibility to the patient, family, and community remains the same.

This book is a reference for nurses, nursing students, and other health-care professionals. It is useful as a clinical tool as well as a supportive text to supplement clinical courses. It guides the nurse in planning what needs to be assessed, monitored, treated, and taught regarding pretest requirements, intratest procedures, and post-test care. It can be used by nursing students at all levels as a textbook in theory classes, integrating laboratory and diagnostic data as one aspect of nursing care; by practicing nurses to update information; and in clinical settings as a quick reference. Designed for use in academic and clinical settings, *Davis's Comprehensive Handbook of Laboratory and Diagnostic Tests—With Nursing Implications* provides a comprehensive reference that allows easy access to information about laboratory and diagnostic tests and procedures. A general overview of how all the tests and procedures included in this book relate to body systems can be found in tables at the end of the monographs. The tests and procedures are presented in this book in alphabetical order by their complete name, allowing the user to locate information quickly without having to first place tests in a specific category or body system. Each monograph is presented in a consistent format for easy identification of specific information at a glance. The following information is provided for each laboratory and diagnostic test:

- Each monograph is titled by the *test name*, given in its commonly used designation, and all monographs in the book are organized in alphabetical order.
- *Synonyms and Acronyms* for each test are listed where appropriate.
- The *Common* Use section includes a brief description of the purpose for the study.
- The *Specimen* section includes the amount of specimen usually collected and, where appropriate, the type of collection tube or container commonly recommended. Specimen requirements vary by laboratory. The amount of specimen collected is usually more than what is minimally required so that additional specimen is available, if needed, for repeat testing (quality-control failure, dilutions, or confirmation of unexpected results). In the case of diagnostic tests, the *type* of procedure (e.g., nuclear medicine, x-ray) is given.
- *Reference Values* for each monograph include age-specific and gender-specific variations, when indicated. It is important to consider the normal variation of laboratory values over the life span and across cultures; sometimes what might be considered an abnormal value in one circumstance is actually what is expected in another. Reference values for laboratory tests are given in conventional and standard international (SI) units. The factor used to convert conventional to SI units is also given. Because laboratory values can vary by method, each laboratory reference range is listed along with the associated methodology.
- The *Description* section includes the study's purpose and insight into how and why the test results can affect health.
- *Indications* are a list of what the test is used for in terms of assessment, evaluation, monitoring, screening, identifying, or assisting in the diagnosis of a clinical condition.
- The *Potential Diagnosis* section presents a list of conditions in which values may be increased or decreased and, in some cases, an explanation of variations that may be encountered.
- *Critical Findings* that may be life threatening or for which particular concern may be indicated are given along with age span considerations where applicable. This section also includes signs and symptoms associated with a critical value as well as possible nursing interventions.
- *Interfering Factors* are substances or circumstances that may influence the results of the test, rendering the results invalid or unreliable. Knowledge of interfering factors is an important aspect of quality assurance and includes pharmaceuticals, foods, natural and additive therapies, timing of test in relation to other tests or procedures, collection site, handling of specimen, and underlying patient conditions.
- The *Pretest* section addresses the need to:
  - Positively identify the patient using at least two unique identifiers before providing care, treatment, or services.

- Provide an explanation to the patient, in the simplest terms possible, of the purpose of the study.
- Obtain pertinent clinical, laboratory, dietary, and therapeutic history of the patient, especially as it pertains to comparison of previous test results, preparation for the test, and identification of potentially interfering factors.
- Explain the requirements and restrictions related to the procedure as well as what to expect; provide the education necessary for the patient to be properly informed.
- Anticipate and allay patient concerns or anxieties.
- Provide for patient safety.
- The *Intratest* section can be used in a quality-control assessment or as a guide to the nurse who may be called on to participate in specimen collection or perform preparatory procedures. It provides:
  - Specific directions for specimen collection and test performance
  - Important information such as patient sensation and expected duration of the procedure
  - Precautions to be taken by the nurse and patient
- The *Post-Test* section provides guidelines regarding:
  - Specific monitoring and therapeutic measures that should be performed after the procedure (e.g., maintaining bedrest, obtaining vital signs to compare with baseline values, signs and symptoms of complications)
  - Specific instructions for the patient and family, such as when to resume usual diet, medications, and activity
  - General nutritional guidelines related to excess or deficit as well as common food sources for dietary replacement
  - Indications for interventions from public health representatives or for special counseling related to test outcomes
  - Indications for follow-up testing that may be required within specific time frames
  - An alphabetical listing of related laboratory and/or diagnostic tests that is intended to provoke a deeper and broader investigation of multiple pieces of information; the tests provide data that, when combined, can form a more complete picture of health or illness
  - Reference to the specific body system tables of related laboratory and diagnostic tests that might bear on a patient's situation

Color and icons are used to facilitate locating critical information at a glance. On the inside front and back covers is a full-color chart describing tube tops used for various blood tests and their recommended order of draw.

The nursing process is evident throughout the laboratory and diagnostic monographs. Within each phase of the testing procedure, the nurse has certain roles and responsibilities. These should be evident in reading each monograph.

Information provided in the appendices includes a summary of specimen collection procedures and materials; a summary chart of transfusion reactions, their signs and symptoms, associated laboratory findings, and potential nursing interventions; an introduction to CLIA (Clinical Laboratory Improvement Amendments) with an explanation of the different levels of testing complexity; a summary chart that details suggested approaches to persons at various developmental stages to assist the provider in facilitating cooperation and understanding; a list of some of the herbs and nutraceuticals associated with adverse clinical reactions or drug interactions related to the affected body system; and guidelines for standard and universal precautions.

This book is also about teaching. Additional educationally supportive materials are provided for the instructor and student in an *Instructor's Guide,* available on the Instructor's Resource Disk (CD) and posted at DavisPlus (http://davisplus.fadavis.com). Organized by nursing curriculum, presentations and case studies with emphasis on laboratory and diagnostic test–related information and nursing implications have been developed for selected conditions and body systems; new to this edition is the sensory, obstetric, and nutrition coverage. Open-ended and NCLEX-type multiple-choice questions as well as suggested critical-thinking activities are provided. This supplemental material will aid the instructor in integrating laboratory and diagnostic materials in assessment and clinical courses and provide examples of activities to enhance student learning.

Newly developed for this fourth edition is a robust collection of online material for students and educators posted at the DavisPlus Web site (http://davisplus.fadavis.com):

- A searchable library of mini-monographs for all the active tests included in the text. The mini-monograph gives each test's full name, synonyms and acronyms, specimen type (laboratory tests) or area of application (diagnostic tests), reference ranges or contrast, and results.
- An archive of full monographs of retired tests that are referenced by mini-monographs in the text.
- Interactive drag-and-drop, quiz-show, flash card, and multiple-choice exercises.
- A printable file of critical values.
- A printable table of monograph template section titles matched to corresponding national patient safety goals.
- All the instructor and student material from the Instructor's Resource Disk.

The authors hope that the changes and additions made to the book and its CD and Web-based ancillaries will reward users with an expanded understanding of and appreciation for the place laboratory and diagnostic testing holds in the provision of high-quality nursing care and will make it easy for instructors to integrate this important content in their curricula.

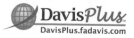
DavisPlus
DavisPlus.fadavis.com

Preface

Laboratory and diagnostic testing. The words themselves often conjure up cold and impersonal images of needles, specimens lined up in collection containers, and high-tech electronic equipment. But they do not stand alone. They are tied to, bound with, and tell of health or disease in the blood and tissue of a person. Laboratory and diagnostic studies augment the health-care provider's assessment of the quality of an individual's physical being. Test results guide the plans and interventions geared toward strengthening life's quality and endurance. Beyond the pounding noise of the MRI, the cold steel of the x-ray table, the sting of the needle, the invasive collection of fluids and tissue, and the probing and inspection is the gathering of evidence that supports the health-care provider's ability to discern the course of a disease and the progression of its treatment. Laboratory and diagnostic data must be viewed with thought and compassion, however, as well as with microscopes and machines. We must remember that behind the specimen and test result is the person from whom it came, a person who is someone's son, daughter, mother, father, husband, wife, friend.

This book is written to help health-care providers in their understanding and interpretation of laboratory and diagnostic procedures and their outcomes. Just as important, it is dedicated to all health-care professionals who experience the wonders in the science of laboratory and diagnostic testing, performed and interpreted in a caring and efficient manner.

Consultants

Connie J. Frisch, RN, MA
Nursing Instructor
Central Lakes College
Brainerd, Minnesota

Mary K. Gerepka, MS, APRN, BC
Instructor
Mountainside Hospital School of
    Nursing
Montclair, New Jersey

Peggy L. Hawkins, RN, MSN,
    PhD, BC
Professor of Nursing
Nursing Programs Director
College of Saint Mary
Omaha, Nebraska

Beth Langlois, RN, MSN, APRN, BC
CCU and Heart Failure Center
    Coordinator
Overlook Hospital, Atlantic Health
    System
Summit, New Jersey

Deborah Little, MSN, RN, CCRN,
    CNRN, APRN, BC
Faculty Instructor
Mountainside Hospital School of
    Nursing
Montclair, New Jersey

Brooke C. Martin, RN, MSN, CNM,
    ARNP
Associate Professor, Practical Nursing
    Program
Ivy Tech State College
Indianapolis, Indiana

Patricia A. Parsons, RN, MSN, MS
Director of Associate Degree Nursing
    Program
Riverland Community College
Austin, Minnesota

Contents

Acetylcholine Receptor Antibody

SYNONYM/ACRONYM: AChR (AChR-binding antibody, AChR-blocking antibody, and AChR-modulating antibody).

COMMON USE: To assist in confirming the diagnosis of myasthenia gravis.

SPECIMEN: Serum (1 mL) collected in a red-top tube.

REFERENCE VALUE: (Method: Radioimmunoassay) AChR binding antibody: Less than 0.4 nmol/L, AChR blocking antibody: Less than 15% blocking, and AChR modulating antibody: Less than 20% modulating.

DESCRIPTION: Normally when impulses travel down a nerve, the nerve ending releases a neurotransmitter called acetylcholine (ACh), which binds to receptor sites in the neuromuscular junction, eventually resulting in muscle contraction. Once the neuromuscular junction has been polarized, ACh is rapidly metabolized by the enzyme acetylcholinesterase. When present, AChR-binding antibodies can activate complement and create a complex of ACh, AChR-binding antibodies, and complement. This complex renders ACh unavailable for muscle receptor sites. If AChR binding antibodies are not detected, and myasthenia gravis (MG) is strongly suspected, AChR-blocking and AChR-modulating antibodies may be ordered. AChR-blocking antibodies impair or prevent ACh from attaching to receptor sites on the muscle membrane, resulting in poor muscle contraction. AChR-modulating antibodies destroy AChR sites, interfering with neuromuscular transmission. The lack of ACh bound to muscle receptor sites results in muscle weakness. Antibodies to AChR sites are present in 90% of patients with generalized MG and in 55% to 70% of patients who either have ocular forms of MG or are in remission. Approximately 10% to 15% of people with confirmed MG do not demonstrate detectable levels of AChR-binding, -blocking, or -modulating antibodies. MG is an acquired autoimmune disorder that can occur at any age. Its exact cause is unknown and seems to strike women between the ages of 20 and 40 years; men appear to be affected later in life than women. It can affect any voluntary muscle, but muscles that control eye, eyelid, facial movement, and swallowing are most frequently affected. Antibodies may not be detected in the first 6 to 12 months after the first appearance of symptoms. MG is a common complication associated with thymoma. The relationship between the thymus gland and MG is not completely understood. It is believed that miscommunication in the thymus gland directed at developing immune cells may trigger the development of autoantibodies responsible for MG. Remission after thymectomy is associated with a progressive decrease in antibody level. Other markers used in the study of MG include striational muscle antibodies, thyroglobulin, HLA-B8, and HLA-DR3. These antibodies are often undetectable in the early stages of MG.

1

INDICATIONS

- Confirm the presence but not the severity of MG
- Detect subclinical MG in the presence of thymoma
- Monitor the effectiveness of immunosuppressive therapy for MG
- Monitor the remission stage of MG

POTENTIAL DIAGNOSIS

Increased in

- Autoimmune liver disease
- Generalized MG *(Defective transmission of nerve impulses to muscles evidenced by muscle weakness. It occurs when normal communication between the nerve and muscle is interrupted at the neuromuscular junction. It is believed that miscommunication in the thymus gland directed at developing immune cells may trigger the development of autoantibodies responsible for MG.)*
- Lambert-Eaton myasthenic syndrome
- Primary lung cancer
- Thymoma associated with MG *(Defective transmission of nerve impulses to muscles evidenced by muscle weakness. It occurs when normal communication between the nerve and muscle is interrupted at the neuromuscular junction. It is believed that miscommunication in the thymus gland directed at developing immune cells may trigger the development of autoantibodies responsible for MG.)*

Decreased in

- Post-thymectomy *(The thymus gland produces the T lymphocytes responsible for cell-mediated immunity. T cells also help control B-cell development for the production of antibodies. T-cell response is directed at cells in the body that have been infected by bacteria, viruses, parasites, fungi, or protozoans. T cells also provide immune surveillance for cancerous cells. Removal of the thymus gland is strongly associated with a decrease in AChR antibody levels.)*

CRITICAL: N/A

INTERFERING FACTORS

- Drugs that may increase AChR levels include penicillamine (long-term use may cause a reversible syndrome that produces clinical, serological, and electrophysiological findings indistinguishable from MG).
- Biological false-positive results may be associated with amyotrophic lateral sclerosis, autoimmune hepatitis, Lambert-Eaton myasthenic syndrome, primary biliary cirrhosis, and encephalomyeloneuropathies associated with carcinoma of the lung.
- Immunosuppressive therapy is the recommended treatment for MG; prior immunosuppressive drug administration may result in negative test results.
- Recent radioactive scans or radiation within 1 wk of the test can interfere with test results when radioimmunoassay is the test method.

NURSING IMPLICATIONS AND PROCEDURE

PRETEST:

- Positively identify the patient using at least two unique identifiers before providing care, treatment, or services.
- *Patient Teaching:* Inform the patient that the test is used to identify antibodies responsible for decreased neuromuscular transmission and associated muscle weakness.
- Obtain a history of the patient's complaints, including a list of known allergens, especially allergies or sensitivities to latex, and any prior complications with general anesthesia.

- Obtain a history of the patient's musculoskeletal system, symptoms, and results of previously performed laboratory tests and diagnostic and surgical procedures.
- Note any recent procedures that can interfere with test results.
- Obtain a list of the patient's current medications, including herbs, nutritional supplements, and nutraceuticals (see Appendix F).
- Review the procedure with the patient. Inform the patient that specimen collection takes approximately 5 to 10 min. Address concerns about pain and explain that there may be some discomfort during the venipuncture.
- *Sensitivity to social and cultural issues*, as well as concern for modesty, is important in providing psychological support before, during, and after the procedure.
- There are no food, fluid, or medication restrictions unless by medical direction.

INTRATEST:

- If the patient has a history of allergic reaction to latex, avoid the use of equipment containing latex.
- Instruct the patient to cooperate fully and to follow directions. Direct the patient to breathe normally and to avoid unnecessary movement.
- Observe standard precautions, and follow the general guidelines in Appendix A. Positively identify the patient, and label the appropriate tubes with the corresponding patient demographics, date, and time of collection. Perform a venipuncture.
- Remove the needle and apply direct pressure with dry gauze to stop bleeding. Observe/assess venipuncture site for bleeding or hematoma formation and secure gauze with adhesive bandage.
- Promptly transport the specimen to the laboratory for processing and analysis.

POST-TEST:

- A report of the results will be sent to the requesting health-care provider (HCP), who will discuss the results with the patient.

- Recognize anxiety related to test results, and be appreciative of impaired activity related to lack of neuromuscular control, perceived loss of independence, and fear of shortened life expectancy. Discuss the implications of positive test results on the patient's lifestyle. It is important to note that a diagnosis of MG should be based on abnormal findings from two different diagnostic tests. These tests include AChR antibody assay, edrophonium test, repetitive nerve stimulation, and single-fiber electromyography. Thyrotoxicosis may occur in conjunction with MG; related thyroid testing may be indicated. MG patients may also produce antibodies that demonstrate reactivity in tests like ANA and RF that are not primarily associated with MG.
- Evaluate test results in relationship to future general anesthesia, especially regarding therapeutic management of MG with cholinesterase inhibitors. Succinylcholine-sensitive patients may be unable to metabolize the anesthetic quickly, resulting in prolonged or unrecoverable apnea.
- Provide teaching and information regarding the clinical implications of the test results as appropriate. Educate the patient regarding access to counseling services. Provide contact information, if desired, for the Myasthenia Gravis Foundation of America (www.myasthenia.org) and the Muscular Dystrophy Association (www.mdausa.org).
- Reinforce information given by the patient's HCP regarding further testing, treatment, or referral to another HCP. Answer any questions or address any concerns voiced by the patient or family.
- Depending on the results of this procedure, additional testing may be performed to evaluate or monitor progression of the disease process and determine the need for a change in therapy. If a diagnosis of MG is made, a computed tomography (CT) scan of the chest should be performed to rule out thymoma. Evaluate test results in

relation to the patient's symptoms and other tests performed.

RELATED MONOGRAPHS:

▶ Related tests include ANA, antithyro-globulin and antithyroid peroxidase antibodies, CT chest, myoglobin, pseudocholinesterase, RF, TSH, and total T$_4$.
▶ Refer to the Musculoskeletal System table at the end of the book for related tests by body system.

Acid Phosphatase, Prostatic

SYNONYM/ACRONYM: Prostatic acid phosphatase, *o*-phosphoric monoester phosphohydrolase, AcP, PAP.

COMMON USE: To assist in staging prostate cancer and document evidence of sexual intercourse through semen identification in alleged cases of rape and sexual abuse.

SPECIMEN: Serum (1 mL) collected in a red-top tube. A swab with vaginal secretions may be submitted in the appropriate transfer container. Other material such as clothing may be submitted for analysis. Consult the laboratory or emergency services department for the proper specimen collection instructions and containers.

REFERENCE VALUE: (Method: Spectrophotometric)

Conventional & SI Units
Less than 3.5 ng/mL

Values are elevated at birth, decrease by 6 mo, increase at approximately 10 yr through puberty, level off through adulthood, and may increase in advancing age.

POTENTIAL DIAGNOSIS

Increased in

AcP is released from any damaged cell in which it is stored, so diseases of the bone, prostate, and liver that cause cellular destruction demonstrate elevated AcP levels. Conditions that result in abnormal elevations of cells that contain AcP (e.g., leukemia, thrombocytosis) or conditions that result in rapid cellular destruction (sickle cell crisis) also reflect increased levels.

• Acute myelogenous leukemia
• After prostate surgery or biopsy
• Benign prostatic hypertrophy
• Liver disease
• Lysosomal storage diseases (Gaucher's disease and Niemann-Pick disease) *(AcP is stored in the lysosomes of blood cells, and increased levels are present in lysosomal storage diseases.)*
• Metastatic bone cancer
• Paget's disease
• Prostatic cancer
• Prostatic infarct
• Prostatitis
• Sickle cell crisis
• Thrombocytosis

Decreased in: N/A

CRITICAL FINDINGS: N/A

Find and print out the full monograph at DavisPlus (http://davisplus.fadavis .com, keyword Van Leeuwen).

Adrenal Gland Scan

SYNONYM/ACRONYM: Adrenal scintiscan.

COMMON USE: To assist in the diagnosis of Cushing's syndrome and differentiate between adrenal gland cancer and infection.

AREA OF APPLICATION: Adrenal gland.

CONTRAST: Intravenous radioactive NP-59 (iodomethyl-19-norcholesterol) or metaiodobenzylguanidine (MIBG).

DESCRIPTION: This nuclear medicine study evaluates function of the adrenal glands. The secretory function of the adrenal glands is controlled primarily by the anterior pituitary, which produces adrenocorticotropic hormone (ACTH). ACTH stimulates the adrenal cortex to produce cortisone and secrete aldosterone. Adrenal imaging is most useful in differentiation of hyperplasia versus adenoma in primary aldosteronism when computed tomography (CT) and magnetic resonance imaging (MRI) findings are equivocal. High concentrations of cholesterol (the precursor in the synthesis of adrenocorticosteroids, including aldosterone) are stored in the adrenal cortex. This allows the radionuclide, which attaches to the cholesterol, to be used in identifying pathology in the secretory function of the adrenal cortex. The uptake of the radionuclide occurs gradually over time; imaging is performed within 24 to 48 hr of injection of the radionuclide dose and continued daily for 3 to 5 days. Imaging reveals increased uptake, unilateral or bilateral uptake, or absence of uptake in the detection of pathological processes. Following prescanning treatment with corticosteroids, suppression studies can be done to differentiate the presence of tumor from hyperplasia of the glands.

INDICATIONS

- Aid in the diagnosis of Cushing's syndrome and aldosteronism
- Aid in the diagnosis of gland tissue destruction caused by infection, infarction, neoplasm, or suppression
- Aid in locating adrenergic tumors
- Determine adrenal suppressibility with prescan administration of corticosteroid to diagnose and localize adrenal adenoma, aldosteronomas, androgen excess, and low-renin hypertension
- Differentiate between asymmetric hyperplasia and asymmetry from aldosteronism with dexamethasone suppression test

POTENTIAL DIAGNOSIS

Normal findings in
- No evidence of tumors, infection, infarction, or suppression
- Normal bilateral uptake of radionuclide and secretory function of adrenal cortex

• Normal salivary glands and urinary bladder; vague shape of the liver and spleen sometimes seen

Abnormal findings in
• Adrenal gland suppression
• Adrenal infarction
• Adrenal tumor
• Hyperplasia
• Infection
• Pheochromocytoma

CRITICAL FINDINGS: N/A

INTERFERING FACTORS

This procedure is contraindicated for
• Patients who are pregnant or suspected of being pregnant unless the potential benefits of the procedure far outweigh the risks to the fetus and mother.

Factors that may impair clear imaging
• Retained barium from a previous radiological procedure.
• Inability of the patient to cooperate or remain still during the procedure because of age, significant pain, or mental status.

Other considerations
• Improper injection of the radionuclide may allow the tracer to seep deep into the muscle tissue, producing erroneous hot spots.
• Consultation with a health-care provider (HCP) should occur before the procedure for radiation safety concerns regarding younger patients or patients who are lactating.
• Risks associated with radiation overexposure can result from frequent x-ray or radionuclide procedures. Personnel working in the examination area should wear badges to record their radiation exposure level.

NURSING IMPLICATIONS AND PROCEDURE

PRETEST:

▶ Positively identify the patient using at least two unique identifiers before providing care, treatment, or services.

▶ *Patient Teaching:* Inform the patient this procedure can visualize and assess the function of the adrenal gland, which is located near the kidney.

▶ Obtain a history of the patient's complaints, including a list of known allergens.

▶ Obtain a history of the patient's endocrine system, symptoms, and results of previously performed laboratory tests and diagnostic and surgical procedures.

▶ All adrenal blood tests should be done before doing this test.

▶ Record the date of last menstrual period and determine the possibility of pregnancy in perimenopausal women.

▶ Obtain a list of the patient's current medications, including herbs, nutritional supplements, and nutraceuticals (see Appendix F).

▶ Review the procedure with the patient. Address concerns about pain and explain that there may be moments of discomfort and some pain experienced during the test. Inform the patient that the procedure is usually performed in a nuclear medicine department by a nuclear medicine technologist with support staff, and it takes approximately 60 to 120 min each day. Inform the patient the test usually involves a prolonged scanning schedule over a period of days.

▶ Administer saturated solution of potassium iodide (SSKI) 24 hr before the study to prevent thyroid uptake of the free radioactive iodine.

▶ *Sensitivity to social and cultural issues,* as well as concern for modesty, is important in providing psychological support before, during, and after the procedure.

▶ Explain that an IV line may be inserted to allow infusion of radionuclides or IV fluids.

There are no food, fluid, or medication restrictions unless by medical direction.

Instruct the patient to remove jewelry and other metallic objects from the area to be examined.

Make sure a written and informed consent has been signed prior to the procedure and before administering any medications.

INTRATEST:

Ensure that the patient has removed external metallic objects from the area to be examined prior to the procedure.

Have emergency equipment readily available.

Instruct the patient to void prior to the procedure and to change into the gown, robe, and foot coverings provided.

Insert an IV line, and inject the radionuclide IV on day 1; images are taken on days 1, 2, and 3. Imaging is done from the urinary bladder to the base of the skull to scan for a primary tumor. Each image takes 20 min, and total imaging time is 1 to 2 hr per day.

Instruct the patient to cooperate fully and to follow directions. Instruct the patient to remain still throughout the procedure because movement produces unreliable results.

Observe standard precautions, and follow the general guidelines in Appendix A.

POST-TEST:

A report of the results will be sent to the requesting HCP, who will discuss the results with the patient.

Unless contraindicated, advise the patient to drink increased amounts of fluids for 24 to 48 hr to eliminate the radionuclide from the body. Inform the patient that radionuclide is eliminated from the body within 24 to 48 hr.

No other radionuclide tests should be scheduled for 24 to 48 hr after this procedure.

Observe/assess the needle site for bleeding, hematoma formation, and inflammation.

Instruct the patient in the care and assessment of the injection site.

Instruct the patient to apply cold compresses to the puncture site as needed, to reduce discomfort or edema.

If a woman who is breastfeeding must have a nuclear scan, she should not breastfeed the infant until the radionuclide has been eliminated. This could take as long as 3 days. Instruct her to express the milk and discard it during the 3-day period to prevent cessation of milk production.

Instruct the patient to immediately flush the toilet and to meticulously wash hands with soap and water after each voiding for 48 hr after the procedure.

Instruct all caregivers to wear gloves when discarding urine for 48 hr after the procedure. Wash gloved hands with soap and water before removing gloves. Then wash ungloved hands after the gloves are removed.

Recognize anxiety related to test results. Discuss the implications of abnormal test results on the patient's lifestyle. Provide teaching and information regarding the clinical implications of the test results, as appropriate.

Reinforce information given by the patient's HCP regarding further testing, treatment, or referral to another HCP. Advise the patient that SSKI (120 mg/day) will be administered for 10 days after the injection of the radionuclide. Answer any questions or address any concerns voiced by the patient or family.

Depending on the results of this procedure, additional testing may be needed to evaluate or monitor progression of the disease process and determine the need for a change in therapy. Evaluate test results in relation to the patient's symptoms and other tests performed.

RELATED MONOGRAPHS:

Related tests include ACTH and challenge tests, aldosterone, angiography adrenal, catecholamines, CT abdomen, cortisol and challenge tests, HVA, MRI abdomen, metanephrines, potassium, renin, sodium, and VMA.

Refer to the Endocrine System table at the end of the book for related tests by body system.

Adrenocorticotropic Hormone
(and Challenge Tests)

SYNONYM/ACRONYM: Corticotropin, ACTH.

COMMON USE: To assist in the investigation of adrenocortical dysfunction using ACTH and cortisol levels in diagnosing disorders such as Addison's and Cushing's diseases.

SPECIMEN: Plasma (2 mL) from a lavender-top (EDTA) tube for adrenocorticotropic hormone (ACTH) and serum (1 mL) from a red-top tube for cortisol. Collect specimens in a prechilled heparinized plastic syringe, and carefully transfer into collection containers by gentle injection to avoid hemolysis. Alternatively, specimens can be collected in prechilled lavender- and red-top tubes. Tiger- and green-top (heparin) tubes are also acceptable for cortisol, but take care to use the same type of collection container for serial measurements. Immediately transport specimen, tightly capped and in an ice slurry, to the laboratory. The specimens should be immediately processed. Plasma for ACTH analysis should be transferred to a plastic container.

Procedure	Medication Administered, Adult Dosage	Recommended Collection Times
ACTH stimulation, rapid test	1 mg (low-dose protocol) cosyntropin IM	Three cortisol levels: baseline immediately before bolus, 30 min after bolus, and 60 min after bolus
Corticotropin-releasing hormone (CRH) stimulation	IV dose of 1 mg/kg ovine or human CRH	Eight cortisol and eight ACTH levels: baseline collected 15 min before injection, 0 min before injection, and then 5, 15, 30, 60, 120, and 180 min after injection
Dexamethasone suppression (overnight)	Oral dose of 1 mg dexamethasone (Decadron) at 11 p.m.	Collect cortisol at 8 a.m. on the morning after the dexamethasone dose
Metyrapone stimulation (overnight)	Oral dose of 30 mg/kg metyrapone with snack at midnight	Collect cortisol and ACTH at 8 a.m. on the morning after the metyrapone dose

IM = intramuscular, IV = intravenous.

REFERENCE VALUE: (Method: Immunochemiluminescent assay)

ACTH

Age	Conventional Units	SI Units (Conventional Units × 0.22)
Cord blood	50–570 pg/mL	11–125 pmol/L
Newborn	10–185 pg/mL	2–41 pmol/L
Adult supine specimen collected in morning	9–52 pg/mL	2–11 pmol/L
Women on oral contraceptives	5–29 pg/mL	1–6 pmol/L

ACTH Challenge Tests

ACTH (Cosyntropin) Stimulated, Rapid Test	Conventional Units	SI Units (Conventional Units × 27.6)
Baseline	Cortisol greater than 5 mcg/dL	Greater than 138 nmol/L
30- or 60-min response	Cortisol 18–20 mcg/dL or incremental increase of 7 mcg/dL over baseline value	496–552 nmol/L

Corticotropin-Releasing Hormone Stimulated	Conventional Units	SI Units (Conventional Units × 27.6)
	Cortisol peaks at greater than 20 mcg/dL within 30–60 minutes	Greater than 552 nmol/L

		SI Units (Conventional Units × 0.22)
	ACTH Increases twofold to fourfold within 30–60 min	Twofold to fourfold increase within 30–60 min

Dexamethasone Suppressed Overnight Test	Conventional Units	SI Units (Conventional Units × 27.6)
	Cortisol less than 1.8 mcg/dL next day	Less than 49.7 nmol/L

Metyrapone Stimulated Overnight Test	Conventional Units	SI Units (Conventional Units × 27.6)
	Cortisol less than 3 mcg/dL next day	Less than 83 nmol/L
		SI Units (Conventional Units × 0.22)
	ACTH greater than 75 pg/mL	Greater than 16.5 pmol/L
		SI Units (Conventional Units × 30)
	11-deoxycortisol greater than 70 ng/mL	Greater than 210 pmol/L

DESCRIPTION: Hypothalamic-releasing factor stimulates the release of adrenocorticotropin hormone (ACTH) from the anterior pituitary gland. ACTH stimulates adrenal cortex secretion of glucocorticoids, androgens, and, to a lesser degree, mineralocorticoids. Cortisol is the major glucocorticoid secreted by the adrenal cortex. ACTH and cortisol test results are evaluated together because a change in one normally causes a change in the other. ACTH secretion is stimulated by insulin, metyrapone, and vasopressin. It is decreased by dexamethasone. Cortisol excess from any source is termed *Cushing's syndrome.* Cortisol excess resulting from ACTH excess produced by the pituitary is termed *Cushing's disease.* ACTH levels exhibit a diurnal variation, peaking between 6 and 8 a.m. and reaching the lowest point between 6 and 11 p.m. Evening levels are generally one-half to two-thirds lower than morning levels. Cortisol levels also vary diurnally, with the lowest values occurring during the morning and peak levels occurring in the evening.

INDICATIONS
- Determine adequacy of replacement therapy in congenital adrenal hyperplasia
- Determine adrenocortical dysfunction
- Differentiate between increased ACTH release with decreased cortisol levels and decreased ACTH release with increased cortisol levels

POTENTIAL DIAGNOSIS

ACTH Result
Because ACTH and cortisol secretion exhibit diurnal variation with values being highest in the morning, a lack of change in values from morning to evening is clinically significant. Decreased concentrations of hormones secreted by the pituitary gland and its target organs are observed in hypopituitarism. In primary adrenal insufficiency (Addison's disease), because of adrenal gland destruction by tumor, infectious process, or immune reaction, ACTH levels are elevated while cortisol levels are decreased. Both ACTH and cortisol levels are

decreased in secondary adrenal insufficiency (i.e., secondary to pituitary insufficiency). Excess ACTH can be produced ectopically by various lung cancers such as oat-cell carcinoma and large-cell carcinoma of the lung and by benign bronchial carcinoid tumor.

Challenge Tests and Results

The ACTH (cosyntropin) stimulated rapid test directly evaluates adrenal gland function and indirectly evaluates pituitary gland and hypothalamus function. Cosyntropin is a synthetic form of ACTH. A baseline cortisol level is collected before the injection of cosyntropin. Specimens are subsequently collected at 30- and 60-min intervals. If the adrenal glands function normally, cortisol levels rise significantly after administration of cosyntropin.

The CRH stimulation test works as well as the dexamethasone suppression test (DST) in distinguishing Cushing's disease from conditions in which ACTH is secreted ectopically (e.g., tumors not located in the pituitary gland that secrete ACTH). Patients with pituitary tumors tend to respond to CRH stimulation, whereas those with ectopic tumors do not. Patients with adrenal insufficiency demonstrate one of three patterns depending on the underlying cause:

- Primary adrenal insufficiency— high baseline ACTH (in response to IV-administered ACTH) and low cortisol levels pre- and post-IV ACTH.
- Secondary adrenal insufficiency (pituitary)—low baseline ACTH that does not respond to ACTH stimulation. Cortisol levels do not increase after stimulation.

- Tertiary adrenal insufficiency (hypothalamic)—low baseline ACTH with an exaggerated and prolonged response to stimulation. Cortisol levels usually do not reach 20 mcg/dL.

The DST is useful in differentiating the causes of increased cortisol levels. Dexamethasone is a synthetic glucocorticoid that is 64 times more potent than cortisol. It works by negative feedback. It suppresses the release of ACTH in patients with a normal hypothalamus. A cortisol level less than 1.8 mcg/dL usually excludes Cushing's syndrome. With the DST, a baseline morning cortisol level is collected, and the patient is given a 1-mg dose of dexamethasone at bedtime. A second specimen is collected the following morning. If cortisol levels have not been suppressed, adrenal adenoma is suspected. The DST also produces abnormal results in the presence of certain psychiatric illnesses (e.g., endogenous depression).

The metyrapone stimulation test is used to distinguish corticotropin-dependent causes (pituitary Cushing's disease and ectopic Cushing's disease) from corticotropin-independent causes (e.g., carcinoma of the lung or thyroid) of increased cortisol levels. Metyrapone inhibits the conversion of 11-deoxycortisol to cortisol. Cortisol levels should decrease to less than 3 mcg/dL if normal pituitary stimulation by ACTH occurs after an oral dose of metyrapone. Specimen collection and administration of the medication are performed as with the overnight dexamethasone test.

Increased in

Overproduction of ACTH can occur as a direct result of either disease *(e.g., primary or ectopic tumor that secretes ACTH) or stimulation by physical or emotional stress, or it can be an indirect response to abnormalities in the complex feedback mechanisms involving the pituitary gland, hypothalamus, or adrenal glands.*

ACTH Increased In

- Addison's disease *(primary adrenocortical hypofunction)*
- Carcinoid syndrome
- Congenital adrenal hyperplasia
- Cushing's disease *(pituitary-dependent adrenal hyperplasia)*
- Depression
- Ectopic ACTH-producing tumors
- Menstruation
- Nelson's syndrome *(ACTH-producing pituitary tumors)*
- Non-insulin-dependent diabetes
- Pregnancy
- Sepsis
- Septic shock

Decreased in

Secondary adrenal insufficiency due to hypopituitarism (inadequate production by the pituitary) can result in decreased levels of ACTH. Conditions that result in overproduction or availability of high levels of cortisol can also result in decreased levels of ACTH.

ACTH Decreased in

- Adrenal adenoma
- Adrenal cancer
- Cushing's syndrome
- Exogenous steroid therapy

CRITICAL FINDINGS: N/A

INTERFERING FACTORS

- Drugs that may increase ACTH levels include insulin, metoclopramide, metyrapone, mifepristone (RU 486), and vasopressin.

- Drugs that may decrease ACTH levels include corticosteroids (e.g., dexamethasone) and pravastatin.
- Test results are affected by the time the test is done because ACTH levels vary diurnally, with the highest values occurring between 6 and 8 a.m. and the lowest values occurring at night. Samples should be collected at the same time of day, between 6 and 8 a.m.
- Excessive physical activity can produce elevated levels.
- ◆ The metyrapone stimulation test is contraindicated in patients with suspected adrenal insufficiency.
- ◆ Metyrapone may cause gastrointestinal distress and/or confusion. Administer oral dose of metyrapone with milk and snack.
- ◆ Rapid clearance of metyrapone, resulting in falsely increased cortisol levels, may occur if the patient is taking drugs that enhance steroid metabolism (e.g., phenytoin, rifampin, phenobarbital, mitotane, and corticosteroids). The requesting health-care provider (HCP) should be consulted prior to a metyrapone stimulation test regarding a decision to withhold these medications.

NURSING IMPLICATIONS AND PROCEDURE

PRETEST:

- Positively identify the patient using at least two unique identifiers before providing care, treatment, or services.
- *Patient Teaching:* Inform the patient this test can assist in evaluating the amount of hormone produced by the pituitary gland located at the base of the brain.
- Obtain a history of the patient's complaints, including a list of known allergens, especially allergies or sensitivities to latex.

- Obtain a history of the patient's endocrine system, symptoms, and results of previously performed laboratory tests and diagnostic and surgical procedures.
- Note any recent procedures that can interfere with test results.
- Obtain a list of the patient's current medications, especially drugs that enhance steroid metabolism, including herbs, nutritional supplements, and nutraceuticals (see Appendix F).
- Weigh patient and report weight to pharmacy for dosing of metyrapone (30 mg/kg body weight).
- Review the procedure with the patient. When ACTH hypersecretion is suspected, a second sample may be requested between 6 and 8 p.m. to determine if changes are the result of diurnal variation in ACTH levels. Inform the patient that more than one sample may be necessary to ensure accurate results, and samples are obtained at specific times to determine high and low levels of ACTH. Inform the patient that each specimen collection takes approximately 5 to 10 min. Address concerns about pain and explain that there may be some discomfort during the venipuncture.
- *Sensitivity to social and cultural issues,* as well as concern for modesty, is important in providing psychological support before, during, and after the procedure.
- There are no food, fluid, or medication restrictions unless by medical direction.
- Drugs that enhance steroid metabolism may be withheld by medical direction prior to metyrapone stimulation testing.
- Instruct the patient to refrain from strenuous exercise for 12 hr before the test and to remain in bed or at rest for 1 hr immediately before the test. Avoid smoking and alcohol use.
- Prepare an ice slurry in a cup or plastic bag to have on hand for immediate transport of the specimen to the laboratory.

- Have emergency equipment readily available in case of adverse reaction to metyrapone.
- If the patient has a history of allergic reaction to latex, avoid the use of equipment containing latex.
- Instruct the patient to cooperate fully and to follow directions. Direct the patient to breathe normally and to avoid unnecessary movement.
- Observe standard precautions, and follow the general guidelines in Appendix A. Positively identify the patient, and label the appropriate tubes with the corresponding patient demographics, date, and time of collection. Perform a venipuncture; collect the specimen in a prechilled plastic heparinized syringe or in prechilled collection containers as listed under the "Specimen" subheading.
- Adverse reactions to metyrapone include nausea and vomiting (N/V), abdominal pain, headache, dizziness, sedation, allergic rash, decreased white blood cell (WBC) count, and bone marrow depression. Signs and symptoms of overdose or acute adrenocortical insufficiency include cardiac arrhythmias, hypotension, dehydration, anxiety, confusion, weakness, impairment of consciousness, N/V, epigastric pain, diarrhea, hyponatremia, and hyperkalemia.
- Remove the needle and apply direct pressure with dry gauze to stop bleeding. Observe/assess venipuncture site for bleeding or hematoma formation and secure gauze with adhesive bandage.
- Promptly transport the specimen to the laboratory for processing and analysis. The tightly capped sample should be placed in an ice slurry immediately after collection. Information on the specimen label should be protected from water in the ice slurry by first placing the specimen in a protective plastic bag.

INTRATEST:

- Ensure that strenuous exercise was avoided for 12 hr before the test and that 1 hr of bedrest was taken immediately before the test. Samples should be collected between 6 and 8 a.m.

POST-TEST:

- A written report of the results will be sent to the requesting HCP, who will discuss the results with the patient.
- Instruct the patient to resume normal activity as directed by the HCP.

• Recognize anxiety related to test results, and offer support. Provide contact information, if desired, for the Cushing's Support and Research Foundation (www.csrf.net).

• Reinforce information given by the patient's HCP regarding further testing, treatment, or referral to another HCP. Answer any questions or address any concerns voiced by the patient or family.

• Depending on the results of this procedure, additional testing may be performed to evaluate or monitor progression of the disease process and determine the need for a change in therapy. If a diagnosis of Cushing's disease is made, pituitary computed tomography (CT) or magnetic resonance imaging (MRI) may be indicated prior to surgery. If a diagnosis of ectopic corticotropin syndrome is made, abdominal CT or MRI may be indicated prior to surgery. Evaluate test results in relation to the patient's symptoms and other tests performed.

RELATED MONOGRAPHS:

• Related tests include cortisol and challenge tests, CT abdomen, CT pituitary, MRI abdomen, MRI pituitary, TSH, and thyroxine.

• See the Endocrine System table at the end of the book for related tests by body system.

Alanine Aminotransferase

SYNONYM/ACRONYM: Serum glutamic pyruvic transaminase (SGPT), ALT.

COMMON USE: To assess liver function related to liver disease and/or damage.

SPECIMEN: Serum (1 mL) collected in a red- or tiger-top tube. Plasma (1 mL) collected in a green-top (heparin) tube is also acceptable.

REFERENCE VALUE: (Method: Spectrophotometry)

Age	Conventional & SI Units
Newborn–1 yr	13–45 units/L
2 yr–older adult	
Male	10–40 units/L
Female	7–35 units/L

Values may be slightly elevated in older adults due to the effects of medications and the presence of multiple chronic or acute diseases with or without muted symptoms.

DESCRIPTION: Alanine aminotransferase (ALT), formerly known as serum glutamic pyruvic transaminase (SGPT), is an enzyme produced by the liver. The highest concentration of ALT is found in liver cells; moderate amounts are found in kidney cells; and smaller amounts are found in heart, pancreas, spleen, skeletal muscle, and red blood cells. When liver damage occurs, serum levels of ALT rise to 50 times normal, making this a sensitive and useful test in evaluating liver injury.

INDICATIONS

- Compare serially with aspartate aminotransferase (AST) levels to track the course of liver disease
- Monitor liver damage resulting from hepatotoxic drugs
- Monitor response to treatment of liver disease, with tissue repair indicated by gradually declining levels

POTENTIAL DIAGNOSIS

Increased in

Related to release of ALT from damaged liver, kidney, heart, pancreas, red blood cells, or skeletal muscle cells.

- Acute pancreatitis
- AIDS (related to hepatitis B co-infection)
- Biliary tract obstruction
- Burns (severe)
- Chronic alcohol abuse
- Cirrhosis
- Fatty liver
- Hepatic carcinoma
- Hepatitis
- Infectious mononucleosis
- Muscle injury from intramuscular injections, trauma, infection, and seizures (recent)
- Muscular dystrophy
- Myocardial infarction
- Myositis
- Pancreatitis
- Pre-eclampsia
- Shock (severe)

Decreased in

- Pyridoxal phosphate deficiency *(related to a deficiency of pyridoxal phosphate that results in decreased production of ALT)*

CRITICAL FINDINGS: N/A

INTERFERING FACTORS

- Drugs that may increase ALT levels by causing cholestasis include anabolic steroids, dapsone, estrogens, ethionamide, icterogenin, mepazine, methandriol, oral contraceptives, oxymetholone, propoxyphene, sulfonylureas, and zidovudine.
- Drugs that may increase ALT levels by causing hepatocellular damage include acetaminophen (toxic), acetylsalicylic acid, anticonvulsants, asparaginase, carbutamide, cephalosporins, chloramphenicol, clofibrate, cytarabine, danazol, dinitrophenol, enflurane, erythromycin, ethambutol, ethionamide, ethotoin, florantyrone, foscarnet, gentamicin, gold salts, halothane, ibufenac, indomethacin, interleukin-2, isoniazid, lincomycin, low-molecular-weight heparin, metahexamide, metaxalone, methoxsalen, methyldopa, methylthiouracil, naproxen, nitrofurans, oral contraceptives, probenecid, procainamide, and tetracyclines.
- Drugs that may decrease ALT levels include cyclosporine, interferons, metronidazole (affects enzymatic test methods), and ursodiol.

NURSING IMPLICATIONS AND PROCEDURE

PRETEST:

- Positively identify the patient using at least two unique identifiers before providing care, treatment, or services.
- *Patient Teaching:* Inform the patient this test can assist with evaluation of liver function and help identify disease.
- Obtain a history of the patient's complaints, including a list of known allergens, especially allergies or sensitivities to latex.
- Obtain a history of the patient's hepatobiliary system, symptoms,

and results of previously performed laboratory tests and diagnostic and surgical procedures.

▶ Obtain a list of the patient's current medications including herbs, nutritional supplements, and nutraceuticals (see Appendix F).

▶ Review the procedure with the patient. Inform the patient that specimen collection takes approximately 5 to 10 min. Address concerns about pain and explain that there may be some discomfort during the venipuncture.

▶ *Sensitivity to social and cultural issues,* as well as concern for modesty, is important in providing psychological support before, during, and after the procedure.

▶ There are no food, fluid, or medication restrictions unless by medical direction.

INTRATEST:

▶ If the patient has a history of allergic reaction to latex, avoid the use of equipment containing latex.

▶ Instruct the patient to cooperate fully and to follow directions. Direct the patient to breathe normally and to avoid unnecessary movement.

▶ Observe standard precautions, and follow the general guidelines in Appendix A. Positively identify the patient, and label the appropriate tubes with the corresponding patient demographics, date, and time of collection. Perform a venipuncture.

▶ Remove the needle, and apply direct pressure with dry gauze to stop bleeding. Observe/assess venipuncture site for bleeding and hematoma formation and secure gauze with adhesive bandage.

▶ Promptly transport the specimen to the laboratory for processing and analysis.

POST-TEST:

▶ A written report of the results will be sent to the requesting health-care provider (HCP), who will discuss the results with the patient.

▶ Instruct the patient to resume usual diet, fluids, medications, or activity, as directed by the HCP.

▶ *Nutritional Considerations:* Increased ALT levels may be associated with liver disease. Dietary recommendations may be indicated and vary depending on the severity of the condition. A low-protein diet may be in order if the patient's liver has lost the ability to process the end products of protein metabolism. A diet of soft foods may be required if esophageal varices have developed. Ammonia levels may be used to determine whether protein should be added to or reduced from the diet. Patients should be encouraged to eat simple carbohydrates and emulsified fats (as in homogenized milk or eggs) rather than complex carbohydrates (e.g., starch, fiber, and glycogen [animal carbohydrates]) and complex fats, which require additional bile to emulsify them so that they can be used. The cirrhotic patient should be carefully observed for the development of ascites, in which case fluid and electrolyte balance requires strict attention.

▶ Reinforce information given by the patient's HCP regarding further testing, treatment, or referral to another HCP. Answer any questions or address any concerns voiced by the patient or family.

▶ Depending on the results of this procedure, additional testing may be performed to evaluate or monitor progression of the disease process and determine the need for a change in therapy. Evaluate test results in relation to the patient's symptoms and other tests performed.

RELATED MONOGRAPHS:

▶ Related tests include acetaminophen, ammonia, AST, bilirubin, biopsy liver, cholangiography percutaneous transhepatic, electrolytes, GGT, hepatitis antigens and antibodies, LDH, liver and spleen scan, and US liver.

▶ See the Hepatobiliary System table at the end of the book for related tests by body system.

Albumin and Albumin/Globulin Ratio

SYNONYM/ACRONYM: Alb, A/G ratio.

COMMON USE: To assess liver or kidney function and nutritional status.

SPECIMEN: Serum (1 mL) collected in a red- or tiger-top tube. Plasma (1 mL) collected in a green-top (heparin) tube is also acceptable.

REFERENCE VALUE: (Method: Spectrophotometry) Normally the albumin/globulin (A/G) ratio is greater than 1.

Age	Conventional Units	SI Units (Conventional Units × 10)
Newborn–11 mo	2.9–5.5 g/dL	29–55 g/L
1–40 yr	3.7–5.1 g/dL	37–51 g/L
41–60 yr	3.4–4.8 g/dL	34–48 g/L
61–90 yr	3.2–4.6 g/dL	32–46 g/L
Greater than 90 yr	2.9–4.5 g/dL	29–45 g/L

DESCRIPTION: Most of the body's total protein is a combination of albumin and globulins. Albumin, the protein present in the highest concentrations, is the main transport protein in the body. Albumin also significantly affects plasma oncotic pressure, which regulates the distribution of body fluid between blood vessels, tissues, and cells. Albumin is synthesized in the liver. Low levels of albumin may be the result of either inadequate intake, inadequate production, or excessive loss. Albumin levels are more useful as an indicator of chronic deficiency than of short-term deficiency.

Albumin levels are affected by posture. Results from specimens collected in an upright posture are higher than results from specimens collected in a supine position.

The albumin/globulin (A/G) ratio is useful in the evaluation of liver and kidney disease. The ratio is calculated using the following formula:

albumin/(total protein – albumin)

where globulin is the difference between the total protein value and the albumin value. For example, with a total protein of 7 g/dL and albumin of 4 g/dL, the A/G ratio is calculated as 4/(7 – 4) or 4/3 = 1.33. A reversal in the ratio, where globulin exceeds albumin (i.e., ratio less than 1.0), is clinically significant.

INDICATIONS
- Assess nutritional status of hospitalized patients, especially geriatric patients
- Evaluate chronic illness
- Evaluate liver disease

POTENTIAL DIAGNOSIS

Increased in
Any condition that results in a decrease of plasma water (e.g., dehydration); look for increase in hemoglobin and hematocrit. Decreases in the volume of intravascular liquid automatically result in concentration of the components present in the remaining liquid, as reflected by an elevated albumin level.
• Hyperinfusion of albumin

Decreased in
• *Insufficient intake:*
  Malabsorption *(related to lack of amino acids available for protein synthesis)*
  Malnutrition *(related to insufficient dietary source of amino acids required for protein synthesis)*
• *Decreased synthesis by the liver:*
  Acute and chronic liver disease (e.g., alcoholism, cirrhosis, hepatitis) *(evidenced by a decrease in normal liver function; the liver is the body's site of protein synthesis)*
  Genetic analbuminemia *(related to genetic inability of liver to synthesize albumin)*
• *Inflammation and chronic diseases result in production of acute-phase reactant and other globulin proteins; the increase in globulins causes a corresponding decrease in albumin:*
  Amyloidosis
  Bacterial infections
  Monoclonal gammopathies (e.g., multiple myeloma, Waldenström's macroglobulinemia)
  Neoplasm
  Parasitic infestations
  Peptic ulcer
  Prolonged immobilization
  Rheumatic diseases
  Severe skin disease

• *Increased loss over body surface:*
  Burns *(evidenced by loss of interstitial fluid albumin)*
  Enteropathies (e.g., gluten sensitivity, Crohn's disease, ulcerative colitis, Whipple's disease) *(evidenced by sensitivity to ingested substances or related to inadequate absorption from intestinal loss)*
  Fistula (gastrointestinal or lymphatic) *(related to loss of sequestered albumin from general circulation)*
  Hemorrhage *(related to fluid loss)*
  Kidney disease *(related to loss from damaged renal tubules)*
  Pre-eclampsia *(evidenced by excessive renal loss)*
  Rapid hydration or overhydration *(evidenced by dilution effect)*
  Repeated thoracentesis or paracentesis *(related to removal of albumin in accumulated third-space fluid)*
• *Increased catabolism:*
  Cushing's disease *(related to excessive cortisol induced protein metabolism)*
  Thyroid dysfunction *(related to overproduction of albumin binding thyroid hormones)*
• *Increased blood volume (hypervolemia):*
  Congestive heart failure *(evidenced by dilution effect)*
  Pre-eclampsia *(related to fluid retention)*
  Pregnancy *(evidenced by increased circulatory volume from placenta and fetus)*

CRITICAL FINDINGS: N/A

INTERFERING FACTORS
• Drugs that may increase albumin levels include carbamazepine, furosemide, phenobarbital, and prednisolone.
• Drugs that may decrease albumin levels include acetaminophen

(poisoning), amiodarone, asparaginase, dextran, estrogens, ibuprofen, interleukin-2, methotrexate, methyldopa, niacin, nitrofurantoin, oral contraceptives, phenytoin, prednisone, and valproic acid.

• Availability of administered drugs is affected by variations in albumin levels.

NURSING IMPLICATIONS AND PROCEDURE

PRETEST:

▸ Positively identify the patient using at least two unique identifiers before providing care, treatment, or services.

▸ *Patient Teaching:* Inform the patient this test can assist with evaluation of liver and kidney function, as well as chronic disease.

▸ Obtain a history of the patient's complaints, including a list of known allergens, especially allergies or sensitivities to latex.

▸ Obtain a history of the patient's gastrointestinal, genitourinary, and hepatobiliary systems; symptoms; and results of previously performed laboratory tests and diagnostic and surgical procedures.

▸ Obtain a list of the patient's current medications including herbs, nutritional supplements, and nutraceuticals (see Appendix F).

▸ Review the procedure with the patient. Inform the patient that specimen collection takes approximately 5 to 10 min. Address concerns about pain and explain that there may be some discomfort during the venipuncture.

▸ *Sensitivity to social and cultural issues,* as well as concern for modesty, is important in providing psychological support before, during, and after the procedure.

▸ There are no food, fluid, or medication restrictions unless by medical direction.

INTRATEST:

▸ If the patient has a history of allergic reaction to latex, avoid the use of equipment containing latex.

▸ Instruct the patient to cooperate fully and to follow directions. Direct the patient to breathe normally and to avoid unnecessary movement.

▸ Observe standard precautions, and follow the general guidelines in Appendix A. Positively identify the patient, and label the appropriate tubes with the corresponding patient demographics, date, and time of collection. Perform a venipuncture.

▸ Remove the needle and apply direct pressure with dry gauze to stop bleeding. Observe/assess venipuncture site for bleeding or hematoma formation and secure gauze with adhesive bandage.

▸ Promptly transport the specimen to the laboratory for processing and analysis.

POST-TEST:

▸ A written report of the results will be sent to the requesting health-care provider (HCP), who will discuss the results with the patient.

▸ *Nutritional Considerations:* Dietary recommendations may be indicated and will vary depending on the severity of the condition. Ammonia levels may be used to determine whether protein should be added to or reduced from the diet.

▸ Reinforce information given by the patient's HCP regarding further testing, treatment, or referral to another HCP. Answer any questions or address any concerns voiced by the patient or family.

▸ Depending on the results of this procedure, additional testing may be performed to evaluate or monitor progression of the disease process and determine the need for a change in therapy. Evaluate test results in relation to the patient's symptoms and other tests performed.

RELATED MONOGRAPHS:

▶ Related tests include ALT, ALP, ammonia, anti–smooth muscle antibodies, AST, bilirubin, biopsy liver, CBC hematocrit, CBC hemoglobin, CT biliary tract and liver, GGT, hepatitis antibodies and antigens, KUB studies, laparoscopy abdominal, liver scan, MRI abdomen, osmolality, potassium, prealbumin, protein total and fractions, radiofrequency ablation liver, sodium, and US liver.

▶ See the Gastrointestinal, Genitourinary, and Hepatobiliary systems tables at the end of the book for related tests by body system.

Aldolase

SYNONYM/ACRONYM: ALD.

COMMON USE: To assist in the diagnosis of muscle-wasting diseases such as muscular dystrophy or other diseases causing muscle and cellular damage such as hepatitis and cirrhosis of the liver.

SPECIMEN: Serum (1 mL) collected in a red- or tiger-top tube.

REFERENCE VALUE: (Method: Spectrophotometry)

Age	Conventional & SI Units
Newborn–2 yr	3.4–11.8 units/L
25 mo–16 yr	1.2–8.8 units/L
Adult	Less than 7.4 units/L

POTENTIAL DIAGNOSIS

Increased in

ALD is released from any damaged cell in which it is stored, so diseases of skeletal muscle, cardiac muscle, pancreas, and liver that cause cellular destruction demonstrate elevated ALD levels.

- Carcinoma (lung, breast, and genitourinary tract and metastasis to liver)
- Dermatomyositis
- Duchenne's muscular dystrophy
- Hepatitis (acute viral or toxic)
- Limb girdle muscular dystrophy
- Myocardial infarction
- Pancreatitis (acute)
- Polymyositis
- Severe crush injuries
- Tetanus
- Trichinosis *(related to myositis)*

Decreased in

- Hereditary fructose intolerance *(evidenced by hereditary deficiency of the aldolase B enzyme)*
- *Late stages of muscle-wasting diseases in which muscle mass has significantly diminished*

CRITICAL FINDINGS: N/A

Find and print out the full monograph at DavisPlus (http://davisplus.fadavis.com, keyword Van Leeuwen).

Aldosterone

SYNONYM/ACRONYM: N/A.

COMMON USE: To assist in the diagnosis of primary hyperaldosteronism disorders such as Conn's syndrome and Addison's disease. Blood levels fluctuate with dehydration and fluid overload. This test can be used in evaluation of hypertension.

SPECIMEN: Serum (1 mL) collected in a red- or tiger-top tube. Plasma (1 mL) collected in a green-top (heparin) or lavender-top (EDTA) tube is also acceptable.

REFERENCE VALUE: (Method: Radioimmunoassay)

Age	Conventional Units	SI Units (Conventional Units × 0.0277)
Cord blood	40–200 ng/dL	1.11–5.54 nmol/L
3 days–1 wk	7–184 ng/dL	0.19–5.10 nmol/L
1 mo–1 yr	5–90 ng/dL	0.14–2.49 nmol/L
13–23 mo	7–54 ng/dL	0.19–1.50 nmol/L
2–10 yr		
Supine	3–35 ng/dL	0.08–0.97 nmol/L
Upright	5–80 ng/dL	0.14–2.22 nmol/L
11–15 yr		
Supine	2–22 ng/dL	0.06–0.61 nmol/L
Upright	4–48 ng/dL	0.11–1.33 nmol/L
Adult		
Supine	3–16 ng/dL	0.08–0.44 nmol/L
Upright	7–30 ng/dL	0.19–0.83 nmol/L

These values reflect a normal-sodium diet. Values for a low-sodium diet are three to five times higher.

DESCRIPTION: Aldosterone is a mineralocorticoid secreted by the zona glomerulosa of the adrenal cortex in response to decreased serum sodium, decreased blood volume, and increased serum potassium. When needed, aldosterone also acts to increase sodium reabsorption in the renal tubules, resulting in potassium excretion and increased water retention, blood volume, and blood pressure. Changes in renal blood flow trigger or suppress release of renin from the glomeruli. The presence of circulating renin stimulates the liver to produce angiotensin I. Angiotensin I is converted by the lung and kidney into angiotensin II, a potent trigger for the release of aldosterone. Aldosterone and the renin-angiotensin system work together to regulate sodium and potassium levels. This test is of little diagnostic value in differentiating primary and secondary aldosteronism unless plasma renin activity is measured simultaneously (see monograph titled

"Renin"). A variety of factors influence serum aldosterone levels, including sodium intake, certain medications, and activity. Secretion of aldosterone is also affected by ACTH, a pituitary hormone that primarily stimulates secretion of glucocorticoids and minimally affects secretion of mineralocorticosteroids. Patients with serum potassium less than 3.6 mEq/L and 24-hour urine potassium greater than 40 mEq/L fit the general criteria to test for aldosteronism. Renin is low in primary aldosteronism and high in secondary aldosteronism. A ratio of plasma aldosterone to plasma renin activity greater than 50 is significant. Ratios greater than 20 obtained after unchallenged screening may indicate the need for further evaluation with a sodium-loading protocol. A captopril protocol can be substituted for patients who may not tolerate the sodium-loading protocol.

INDICATIONS
- Evaluate hypertension of unknown cause, especially with hypokalemia not induced by diuretics
- Investigate suspected hyperaldosteronism, as indicated by elevated levels
- Investigate suspected hypoaldosteronism, as indicated by decreased levels

POTENTIAL DIAGNOSIS

Increased in

Increased With Decreased Renin Levels

Primary hyperaldosteronism (evidenced by overproduction related to abnormal adrenal gland function):
- Adenomas (Conn's syndrome)
- Bilateral hyperplasia of the aldosterone-secreting zona glomerulosa cells

Increased With Increased Renin Levels

Secondary hyperaldosteronism (related to conditions that increase renin levels, which then stimulate aldosterone secretion):
- Bartter's syndrome *(related to excessive loss of potassium by the kidneys, leading to release of renin and subsequent release of aldosterone)*
- Cardiac failure *(related to diluted concentration of sodium by increased blood volume)*
- Chronic obstructive pulmonary disease
- Cirrhosis with ascites formation *(related to diluted concentration of sodium by increased blood volume)*
- Diuretic abuse *(related to direct stimulation of aldosterone secretion)*
- Hypovolemia *secondary to hemorrhage and transudation*
- Laxative abuse *(related to direct stimulation of aldosterone secretion)*
- Nephrotic syndrome *(related to excessive renal protein loss, development of decreased oncotic pressure, fluid retention, and diluted concentration of sodium)*
- Starvation (after 10 days) *(related to diluted concentration of sodium by development of edema)*
- Thermal stress *(related to direct stimulation of aldosterone secretion)*
- Toxemia of pregnancy *(related to diluted concentration of sodium by increased blood volume evidenced by edema; placental corticotropin-releasing hormone stimulates production of maternal adrenal hormones that can also contribute to edema)*

Decreased in

Without Hypertension
- Addison's disease *(related to lack of function in the adrenal cortex)*
- Hypoaldosteronism *secondary to renin deficiency*
- Isolated aldosterone deficiency

With Hypertension
- Acute alcohol intoxication *(related to toxic effects of alcohol on adrenal gland function and therefore secretion of aldosterone)*
- Diabetes *(related to impaired conversion of prerenin to renin by damaged kidneys, resulting in decreased aldosterone)*
- Excess secretion of deoxycorticosterone *(related to suppression of ACTH production by cortisol, which in turn affects aldosterone secretion)*
- Turner's syndrome (25% of cases) *(related to congenital adrenal hyperplasia resulting in underproduction of aldosterone and overproduction of androgens)*

CRITICAL FINDINGS: N/A

INTERFERING FACTORS
- Drugs that may increase aldosterone levels include amiloride, ammonium chloride, angiotensin, angiotensin II, dobutamine, dopamine, endralazine, fenoldopam, hydralazine, hydrochlorothiazide, laxatives (abuse), metoclopramide, nifedipine, opiates, potassium, spironolactone, and zacopride.
- Drugs that may decrease aldosterone levels include atenolol, captopril, carvedilol, cilazapril, enalapril, fadrozole, glycyrrhiza (licorice), ibopamine, indomethacin, lisinopril, nicardipine, NSAIDs, perindopril, ranitidine, saline, sinorphan, and verapamil. Prolonged heparin therapy also decreases aldosterone levels.
- Upright body posture, stress, strenuous exercise, and late pregnancy can lead to increased levels.
- Recent radioactive scans or radiation within 1 wk before the test can interfere with test results when radioimmunoassay is the test method.
- Diet can significantly affect results. A low-sodium diet can increase serum aldosterone, whereas a high-sodium diet can decrease levels. Decreased serum sodium and elevated serum potassium increase aldosterone secretion. Elevated serum sodium and decreased serum potassium suppress aldosterone secretion.

NURSING IMPLICATIONS AND PROCEDURE

PRETEST:
- Positively identify the patient using at least two unique identifiers before providing care, treatment, or services.
- *Patient Teaching:* Inform the patient this test evaluates dehydration and can assist in identification of the causes of muscle weakness or high blood pressure.
- Obtain a history of the patient's complaints, including a list of known allergens, especially allergies or sensitivities to latex.
- Obtain a history of known or suspected fluid or electrolyte imbalance, hypertension, renal function, or stage of pregnancy. Note the amount of sodium ingested in the diet over the past 2 wk.
- Obtain a history of the patient's endocrine and genitourinary systems, symptoms, and results of previously performed laboratory tests and diagnostic and surgical procedures.

- Note any recent procedures that can interfere with test results.
- Obtain a list of the patient's current medications, including herbs, nutritional supplements, and nutraceuticals (see Appendix F).
- Review the procedure with the patient. Inform the patient that specimen collection takes approximately 5 to 10 min. Inform the patient that multiple specimens may be required. Address concerns about pain and explain that there may be some discomfort during the venipuncture.
- *Sensitivity to social and cultural issues,* as well as concern for modesty, is important in providing psychological support before, during, and after the procedure.
- Inform the patient that the required position, supine/lying down or upright/sitting up, must be maintained for 2 hr before specimen collection. Some health-care providers (HCPs) may also order administration of furosemide (40 to 80 mg) upon arising.
- The patient should be on a normal-sodium diet (1 to 2 g of sodium per day) for 2 to 4 wk before the test. Protocols may vary among facilities.
- Under medical direction, the patient should avoid diuretics, antihypertensive drugs and herbals, and cyclic progestogens and estrogens for 2 to 4 wk before the test.

INTRATEST:

- Ensure that the patient has complied with dietary, medication, and pretesting preparations regarding activity.
- If the patient has a history of allergic reaction to latex, avoid the use of equipment containing latex.
- Instruct the patient to cooperate fully and to follow directions. Direct the patient to breathe normally and to avoid unnecessary movement.
- Observe standard precautions, and follow the general guidelines in Appendix A. Positively identify the patient, and label the appropriate tubes with the corresponding patient demographics, date, time of collection, patient position (upright or supine), and exact source of specimen (peripheral versus arterial). Perform a venipuncture after the patient has been in the upright (sitting or

standing) position for 2 hr. If a supine specimen is requested on an inpatient, the specimen should be collected early in the morning before rising.
- Remove the needle, and apply direct pressure with dry gauze to stop bleeding. Observe/assess venipuncture site for bleeding or hematoma formation and secure gauze with adhesive bandage.
- Promptly transport the specimen on ice to the laboratory for processing and analysis.

POST-TEST:

- A written report of the results will be sent to the requesting HCP, who will discuss the results with the patient.
- Instruct the patient to resume usual diet, medication, and activity as directed by the HCP.
- Instruct the patient to notify the HCP of any signs and symptoms of dehydration or fluid overload related to elevated aldosterone levels or compromised sodium regulatory mechanisms.
- *Nutritional Considerations:* Aldosterone levels are involved in the regulation of body fluid volume. Educate patients about the importance of proper water balance. Although there is no recommended dietary allowance (RDA) for water, adults need 1 mL/kcal per day. Infants need more water because their basal metabolic heat production is much higher than in adults. Tap water may also contain other nutrients. Water-softening systems replace minerals (e.g., calcium, magnesium, iron) with sodium, so caution should be used if a low-sodium diet is prescribed.
- *Nutritional Considerations:* Because aldosterone levels have an effect on sodium levels, some consideration may be given to dietary adjustment if sodium allowances need to be regulated. In 2004, the Institute of Medicine's Food and Nutrition Board established 2,300 mg as the recommended maximum daily intake of dietary sodium for adults; 1,900 mg/day for children. Educate patients with low sodium levels that the major source of dietary sodium is table salt. Many foods, such as milk and other dairy products, are also good sources of dietary sodium.

Most other dietary sodium is available through consumption of processed foods. Patients who need to follow low-sodium diets should avoid beverages such as colas, ginger ale, Gatorade, lemon-lime sodas, and root beer. Many over-the-counter medications, including antacids, laxatives, analgesics, sedatives, and antitussives, contain significant amounts of sodium. The best advice is to emphasize the importance of reading all food, beverage, and medicine labels. In 2004, the Institute of Medicine's Food and Nutrition Board established 4.7 g as the recommended maximum daily intake of dietary potassium for adults; 3.8 g/day for children. Potassium is present in all plant and animal cells, making dietary replacement simple. An HCP or nutritionist should be consulted before considering the use of salt substitutes.

▶ Reinforce information given by the patient's HCP regarding further testing, treatment, or referral to another HCP. Answer any questions or address any concerns voiced by the patient or family.

▶ Depending on the results of this procedure, additional testing may be performed to evaluate or monitor progression of the disease process and determine the need for a change in therapy. Evaluate test results in relation to the patient's symptoms and other tests performed.

RELATED MONOGRAPHS:

▶ Related tests include adrenal gland scan, biopsy kidney, BUN, catecholamines, cortisol, creatinine, glucose, magnesium, osmolality, potassium, protein urine, renin, sodium, and UA.

▶ See the Endocrine and Genitourinary systems tables at the end of the book for related tests by body system.

Alkaline Phosphatase and Isoenzymes

SYNONYM/ACRONYM: Alk Phos, ALP and fractionation, heat-stabile ALP.

COMMON USE: To assist in the diagnosis of liver cancer and cirrhosis, or bone cancer and bone fracture.

SPECIMEN: Serum (1 mL) collected in a red- or tiger-top tube. Plasma (1 mL) collected in a green-top (heparin) tube is also acceptable.

REFERENCE VALUE: (Method: Spectrophotometry for total alkaline phosphatase, inhibition/electrophoresis for fractionation)

Total ALP	Conventional & SI Units	Bone Fraction	Liver Fraction
1–5 yr			
Male	56–350 units/L	39–308 units/L	Less than 8–101 units/L
Female	73–378 units/L	56–300 units/L	Less than 8–53 units/L
6–7 yr			
Male	70–364 units/L	50–319 units/L	Less than 8–76 units/L
Female	73–378 units/L	56–300 units/L	Less than 8–53 units/L

(table continues on page 26)

Total ALP	Conventional & SI Units	Bone Fraction	Liver Fraction
8 yr			
Male	70–364 units/L	50–258 units/L	Less than 8–62 units/L
Female	98–448 units/L	78–353 units/L	Less than 8–62 units/L
9–12 yr			
Male	112–476 units/L	78–339 units/L	Less than 8–81 units/L
Female	98–448 units/L	78–353 units/L	Less than 8–62 units/L
13 yr			
Male	112–476 units/L	78–389 units/L	Less than 8–48 units/L
Female	56–350 units/L	28–252 units/L	Less than 8–50 units/L
14 yr			
Male	112–476 units/L	78–389 units/L	Less than 8–48 units/L
Female	56–266 units/L	31–190 units/L	Less than 8–48 units/L
15 yr			
Male	70–378 units/L	48–311 units/L	Less than 8–39 units/L
Female	42–168 units/L	20–115 units/L	Less than 8–53 units/L
16 yr			
Male	70–378 units/L	48–311 units/L	Less than 8–39 units/L
Female	28–126 units/L	14–87 units/L	Less than 8–50 units/L
17 yr			
Male	56–238 units/L	34–190 units/L	Less than 8–39 units/L
Female	28–126 units/L	17–84 units/L	Less than 8–53 units/L
18 yr			
Male	56–182 units/L	34–146 units/L	Less than 8–39 units/L
Female	28–126 units/L	17–84 units/L	Less than 8–53 units/L
19 yr			
Male	42–154 units/L	25–123 units/L	Less than 8–39 units/L
Female	28–126 units/L	17–84 units/L	Less than 8–53 units/L
20 yr			
Male	45–138 units/L	25–73 units/L	Less than 8–48 units/L
Female	33–118 units/L	17–56 units/L	Less than 8–50 units/L
Adult			
Male	35–142 units/L	11–73 units/L	0–93 units/L
Female	25–125 units/L	11–73 units/L	0–93 units/L

Values may be slightly elevated in older adults.

DESCRIPTION: Alkaline phosphatase (ALP) is an enzyme found in the liver; in Kupffer cells lining the biliary tract; and in bones, intestines, and placenta. Additional sources of ALP include the proximal tubules of the kidneys, pulmonary alveolar cells, germ cells, vascular bed, lactating mammary glands, and granulocytes of circulating blood. ALP is referred to as alkaline because it functions optimally at a pH of 9.0. This test is most useful for determining the presence of liver or bone disease.

Isoelectric focusing methods can identify 12 isoenzymes of ALP. Certain cancers produce small amounts of distinctive Regan and Nagao ALP isoenzymes. Elevations in three main

ALP isoenzymes, however, are of clinical significance: ALP_1 of liver origin, ALP_2 of bone origin, and ALP_3 of intestinal origin (normal elevations are present in Lewis antibody positive individuals with blood types O and B). ALP levels vary by age and gender. Values in children are higher than in adults because of the level of bone growth and development. An immunoassay method is available for measuring bone-specific ALP as an indicator of increased bone turnover and estrogen deficiency in postmenopausal women.

INDICATIONS

- Evaluate signs and symptoms of various disorders associated with elevated ALP levels, such as biliary obstruction, hepatobiliary disease, and bone disease, including malignant processes
- Differentiate obstructive hepatobiliary tract disorders from hepatocellular disease; greater elevations of ALP are seen in the former
- Determine effects of renal disease on bone metabolism
- Determine bone growth or destruction in children with abnormal growth patterns

POTENTIAL DIAGNOSIS

Increased in
Related to release of alkaline phosphatase from damaged bone, biliary tract, and liver cells

- Liver disease:
  Biliary atresia
  Biliary obstruction (acute cholecystitis, cholelithiasis, intrahepatic cholestasis of pregnancy, primary biliary cirrhosis)
  Cancer
  Chronic active hepatitis
  Cirrhosis
  Diabetes (diabetic hepatic lipidosis)
  Extrahepatic duct obstruction

  Granulomatous or infiltrative liver diseases (sarcoidosis, amyloidosis, TB)
  Infectious mononucleosis
  Intrahepatic biliary hypoplasia
  Toxic hepatitis
  Viral hepatitis

- Bone disease:
  Healing fractures
  Metabolic bone diseases (rickets, osteomalacia)
  Metastatic tumors in bone
  Osteogenic sarcoma
  Osteoporosis
  Paget's disease (osteitis deformans)

- Other conditions:
  Advanced pregnancy *(related to additional sources: placental tissue and new fetal bone growth; marked decline is seen with placental insufficiency and imminent fetal demise)*
  Cancer of the breast, colon, gallbladder, lung, or pancreas
  Congestive heart failure
  Familial hyperphosphatemia
  Hyperparathyroidism
  Perforated bowel
  Pneumonia
  Pulmonary and myocardial infarctions
  Pulmonary embolism
  Ulcerative colitis

Decreased in

- Anemia (severe)
- Celiac disease
- Folic acid deficiency
- HIV-1 infection
- Hypervitaminosis D
- Hypophosphatasia *(related to insufficient phosphorus source for ALP production; congenital and rare)*
- Hypothyroidism (characteristic in infantile and juvenile cases)
- Nutritional deficiency of zinc or magnesium
- Pernicious anemia
- Scurvy *(related to vitamin C deficiency)*
- Whipple's disease
- Zollinger-Ellison syndrome

CRITICAL FINDINGS: N/A

INTERFERING FACTORS

- Drugs that may increase ALP levels by causing cholestasis include anabolic steroids, erythromycin, ethionamide, gold salts, imipramine, interleukin-2, isocarboxazid, nitrofurans, oral contraceptives, phenothiazines, sulfonamides, and tolbutamide.
- Drugs that may increase ALP levels by causing hepatocellular damage include acetaminophen (toxic), amiodarone, anticonvulsants, arsenicals, asparaginase, bromocriptine, captopril, cephalosporins, chloramphenicol, enflurane, ethionamide, foscarnet, gentamicin, indomethacin, lincomycin, methyldopa, naproxen, nitrofurans, probenecid, procainamide, progesterone, ranitidine, tobramycin, tolcapone, and verapamil.
- Drugs that may cause an overall decrease in ALP levels include alendronate, azathioprine, calcitriol, clofibrate, estrogens with estrogen replacement therapy, and ursodiol.
- Hemolyzed specimens may cause falsely elevated results.
- Elevations of ALP may occur if the patient is nonfasting, usually 2 to 4 hr after a fatty meal, and especially if the patient is a Lewis-positive secretor of blood group B or O.

NURSING IMPLICATIONS AND PROCEDURE

PRETEST:

- Positively identify the patient using at least two unique identifiers before providing care, treatment, or services.
- *Patient Teaching:* Inform the patient this test can assist with determining the presence of liver or bone disease.
- Obtain a history of the patient's complaints, including a list of known allergens, especially allergies or sensitivities to latex.
- Obtain a history of the patient's hepatobiliary and musculoskeletal systems, symptoms, and results of previously performed laboratory tests and diagnostic and surgical procedures.
- Obtain a list of the patient's current medications, including herbs, nutritional supplements, and nutraceuticals (see Appendix F).
- Review the procedure with the patient. Inform the patient that specimen collection takes approximately 5 to 10 min. Address concerns about pain and explain that there may be some discomfort during the venipuncture.
- *Sensitivity to social and cultural issues,* as well as concern for modesty, is important in providing psychological support before, during, and after the procedure.
- There are no food, fluid, or medication restrictions unless by medical direction.

INTRATEST:

- If the patient has a history of allergic reaction to latex, avoid the use of equipment containing latex.
- Instruct the patient to cooperate fully and to follow directions. Direct the patient to breathe normally and to avoid unnecessary movement.
- Observe standard precautions, and follow the general guidelines in Appendix A. Positively identify the patient, and label the appropriate tubes with the corresponding patient demographics, date, and time of collection. Perform a venipuncture.
- Remove the needle and apply direct pressure with dry gauze to stop bleeding. Observe/assess venipuncture site for bleeding and hematoma formation and secure gauze with adhesive bandage.
- Promptly transport the specimen to the laboratory for processing and analysis.

POST-TEST:

- A written report of the results will be sent to the requesting health-care provider (HCP), who will discuss the results with the patient.
- *Nutritional Considerations:* Increased ALP levels may be associated with liver disease. Dietary recommendations may be indicated and vary depending on the severity of the condition. A low-protein diet may be in order if the patient's liver has lost the ability to process the end products of protein metabolism. A diet of soft foods may be required if esophageal varices have developed. Ammonia levels may be used to determine whether protein should be added to or reduced from the diet. Patients should be encouraged to eat simple carbohydrates and emulsified fats (as in homogenized milk or eggs) rather than complex carbohydrates (e.g., starch, fiber, and glycogen [animal carbohydrates]) and complex fats, which require additional bile to emulsify them so that they can be used. The cirrhotic patient should be carefully observed for the development of ascites, in which case fluid and electrolyte balance requires strict attention.
- Reinforce information given by the patient's HCP regarding further testing, treatment, or referral to another HCP. Answer any questions or address any concerns voiced by the patient or family.
- Depending on the results of this procedure, additional testing may be performed to evaluate or monitor progression of the disease process and determine the need for a change in therapy. Evaluate test results in relation to the patient's symptoms and other tests performed.

RELATED MONOGRAPHS:

- Related tests include acetaminophen, ALT, albumin, ammonia, anti-DNA antibodies, AMA/ASMA, ANA, α_1-antitrypsin, α_1-antitrypsin phenotyping, AST, bilirubin, biopsy bone, biopsy liver, bone scan, BMD, calcium, ceruloplasmin, collagen cross-linked telopeptides, C3 and C4, complements, copper, ERCP, GGT, hepatitis antigens and antibodies, hepatobiliary scan, KUB studies, magnesium, MRI abdomen, osteocalcin, PTH, phosphorus, potassium, protein, protein electrophoresis, PT/INR, salicylate, sodium, US liver, vitamin D, and zinc.
- See the Hepatobiliary and Musculoskeletal systems tables at the end of the book for related tests by body system.

Allergen-Specific Immunoglobulin E

SYNONYM/ACRONYM: Allergen profile, radioallergosorbent test (RAST).

COMMON USE: To assist in the identification of environmental allergens responsible for causing allergic reactions.

SPECIMEN: Serum (2 mL per group of six allergens, 0.5 mL for each additional individual allergen) collected in a red- or tiger-top tube.

REFERENCE VALUE: (Method: Radioimmunoassay)

RAST Scoring Method	Specific IgE	Alternate Scoring Method (ASM): Increasing Levels of Allergy Sensitivity	
Specific IgE Antibody Level	*International Units/L*	*ASM Class*	*ASM % Reference*
Absent or undetectable	Less than 0.35	0	Less than 70
Low	0.35–0.70	1	70–109
Moderate	0.71–3.50	2	110–219
High	3.51–17.50	3	220–599
Very high	Greater than 17.50	4	600–1,999
		5	2,000–5,999
		6	Greater than 5,999

DESCRIPTION: Allergen-specific immunoglobulin E (IgE) or a radioallergosorbent test (RAST) is generally requested for groups of allergens commonly known to incite an allergic response in the affected individual. The test is based on the use of a radiolabeled anti-IgE reagent to detect IgE in the patient's serum, produced in response to specific allergens. The panels include allergens such as animal dander, antibiotics, dust, foods, grasses, insects, trees, mites, molds, venom, and weeds. Allergen testing is useful for evaluating the cause of hay fever, extrinsic asthma, atopic eczema, respiratory allergies, and potentially fatal reactions to insect venom, penicillin, and other drugs or chemicals. RAST is an alternative to skin test anergy and provocation procedures, which can be inconvenient, painful, and potentially hazardous to patients.

INDICATIONS

- Evaluate patients who refuse to submit to skin testing or who have generalized dermatitis or other dermatopathic conditions
- Monitor response to desensitization procedures
- Test for allergens when skin testing is inappropriate, such as in infants
- Test for allergens when there is a known history of allergic reaction to skin testing
- Test for specific allergic sensitivity before initiating immunotherapy or desensitization shots
- Test for specific allergic sensitivity when skin testing is unreliable (patients taking long-acting antihistamines may have false-negative skin test)

POTENTIAL DIAGNOSIS

Different scoring systems are used in the interpretation of RAST results.

Increased in
Related to production of IgE, the antibody that primarily responds to conditions that stimulate an allergic response
- Allergic rhinitis
- Anaphylaxis
- Asthma (exogenous)
- Atopic dermatitis
- *Echinococcus* infection
- Eczema
- Hay fever
- Hookworm infection
- Latex allergy
- Schistosomiasis
- Visceral larva migrans

Decreased in
- Asthma (endogenous)
- Pregnancy
- Radiation therapy

CRITICAL FINDINGS: N/A

INTERFERING FACTORS
- Recent radioactive scans or radiation within 1 wk of the test can interfere with test results when radioimmunoassay is the test method.

NURSING IMPLICATIONS AND PROCEDURE

PRETEST:

- Positively identify the patient using at least two unique identifiers before providing care, treatment, or services.
- *Patient Teaching:* Inform the patient this test can assist in identification of causal factors related to allergic reaction.
- Obtain a history of the patient's complaints, including a list of known allergens, especially allergies or sensitivities to latex.
- Obtain a history of the patient's immune and respiratory systems, symptoms, and results of previously performed laboratory tests and diagnostic and surgical procedures.
- Note any recent procedures that can interfere with test results.
- Obtain a list of the patient's current medications, including herbs, nutritional supplements, and nutraceuticals (see Appendix F).
- Review the procedure with the patient. Inform the patient that specimen collection takes approximately 5 to 10 min. Address concerns about pain and explain that there may be some discomfort during the venipuncture.
- There are no food, fluid, or medication restrictions unless by medical direction.

INTRATEST:

- If the patient has a history of allergic reaction to latex, avoid the use of equipment containing latex.
- Instruct the patient to cooperate fully and to follow directions. Direct the patient to breathe normally and to avoid unnecessary movement.
- Observe standard precautions, and follow the general guidelines in Appendix A. Positively identify the patient, and label the appropriate tubes with the corresponding patient demographics, date, and time of collection. Indicate the specific allergen group to be tested on the specimen requisition. Perform a venipuncture.
- Remove the needle and apply direct pressure with dry gauze to stop bleeding. Observe/assess venipuncture site for bleeding and hematoma formation and secure gauze with adhesive bandage.
- Promptly transport the specimen to the laboratory for processing and analysis.

POST-TEST:

- A written report of the results will be sent to the requesting health-care provider (HCP), who will discuss the results with the patient.
- *Nutritional Considerations:* should be given to diet if food allergies are present. Lifestyle adjustments may be necessary depending on the specific allergens identified.
- Administer antibiotic therapy if ordered. Remind the patient of the importance of completing the entire course of antibiotic therapy, even if signs and symptoms disappear before completion of therapy.
- Reinforce information given by the patient's HCP regarding further testing, treatment, or referral to another HCP. Answer any questions or address any concerns voiced by the patient or family.
- Depending on the results of this procedure, additional testing may be performed to evaluate or monitor progression of the disease process and determine the need for a change in therapy. Evaluate test results in relation to the patient's symptoms and other tests performed.

RELATED MONOGRAPHS:

- Related tests include arterial/alveolar oxygen ratio, blood gases, complete blood count, eosinophil count, fecal analysis, hypersensitivity pneumonitis, IgE, and PFT.
- See the Immune and Respiratory systems tables at the end of the book for related tests by body system.

Alveolar/Arterial Gradient and Arterial/Alveolar Oxygen Ratio

SYNONYM/ACRONYM: Alveolar-arterial difference, A/a gradient, a/A ratio.

COMMON USE: To assist in assessing oxygen delivery and diagnosing causes of hypoxemia such as pulmonary edema, acute respiratory distress syndrome, and pulmonary fibrosis.

SPECIMEN: Arterial blood (1 mL) collected in a heparinized syringe. Specimen should be transported tightly capped and in an ice slurry.

REFERENCE VALUE: (Method: Selective electrodes that measure P_{O_2} and P_{CO_2})

Alveolar/arterial gradient	Less than 10 mm Hg at rest (room air)
	20–30 mm Hg at maximum exercise activity (room air)
Arterial/alveolar oxygen ratio	Greater than 0.75 (75%)

DESCRIPTION: A test of the ability of oxygen to diffuse from the alveoli into the lungs is of use when assessing a patient's level of oxygenation. This test can help identify the cause of hypoxemia (low oxygen levels in the blood) and intrapulmonary shunting that might result from one of the following three situations: ventilated alveoli without perfusion, unventilated alveoli with perfusion, or collapse of alveoli and associated blood vessels. Information regarding the alveolar/arterial (A/a) gradient can be estimated indirectly using the partial pressure of oxygen (P_{O_2}) (obtained from blood gas analysis) in a simple mathematical formula:

A/a gradient = P_{O_2} in alveolar air (estimated from the alveolar gas equation) – P_{O_2} in arterial blood (measured from a blood gas)

An estimate of alveolar P_{O_2} is accomplished by subtracting the water vapor pressure from the barometric pressure, multiplying the resulting pressure by the fraction of inspired oxygen (F_{IO_2}; percentage of oxygen the patient is breathing), and subtracting this from 1.25 times the arterial partial pressure of carbon dioxide (P_{CO_2}). The gradient is obtained by subtracting the patient's arterial P_{O_2} from the calculated alveolar P_{O_2}:

Alveolar P_{O_2} = [(barometric pressure – water vapor pressure) × F_{IO_2}] – [1.25 × P_{CO_2}]

The arterial/alveolar (a/A) ratio reflects the percentage of alveolar

Po_2 that is contained in arterial Po_2. It is calculated by dividing the arterial Po_2 by the alveolar Po_2

$$a/A = Pao_2/Pao_2$$

The A/a gradient increases as the concentration of oxygen the patient inspires increases. If the gradient is abnormally high, either there is a problem with the ability of oxygen to pass across the alveolar membrane or oxygenated blood is being mixed with nonoxygenated blood. The a/A ratio is not dependent on Fio_2; it does not increase with a corresponding increase in inhaled oxygen. For patients on a mechanical ventilator with a changing Fio_2, the a/A ratio can be used to determine if oxygen diffusion is improving.

INDICATIONS
- Assess intrapulmonary or coronary artery shunting
- Assist in identifying the cause of hypoxemia

POTENTIAL DIAGNOSIS

Increased in
- Acute respiratory distress syndrome (ARDS) *(related to thickened edematous alveoli)*
- Atelectasis *(related to mixing oxygenated and unoxygenated blood)*
- Arterial-venous shunts *(related to mixing oxygenated and unoxygenated blood)*
- Bronchospasm *(related to decrease in the diameter of the airway)*
- Chronic obstructive pulmonary disease *(related to decrease in the elasticity of lung tissue)*
- Congenital cardiac septal defects *(related to mixing oxygenated and unoxygenated blood)*
- Underventilated alveoli *(related to mucus plugs)*
- Pneumothorax *(related to collapsed lung, shunted air, and subsequent decrease in arterial oxygen levels)*
- Pulmonary edema *(related to thickened edematous alveoli)*
- Pulmonary embolus *(related to obstruction of blood flow to alveoli)*
- Pulmonary fibrosis *(related to thickened edematous alveoli)*

CRITICAL FINDINGS: N/A

INTERFERING FACTORS
- Specimens should be collected before administration of oxygen therapy or antihistamines.
- The patient's temperature should be noted and reported to the laboratory if significantly elevated or depressed so that measured values can be corrected to actual body temperature.
- Exposure of sample to room air affects test results.
- Values normally increase with increasing age (see monograph titled "Blood Gases").
- ◆ Samples for A/a gradient evaluation are obtained by arterial puncture, which carries a risk of bleeding, especially in patients with bleeding disorders or who are taking medications for a bleeding disorder.
- Prompt and proper specimen processing, storage, and analysis are important to achieve accurate results. Specimens should always be transported to the laboratory as quickly as possible after collection. Delay in transport of the sample or transportation without ice may affect test results.

A

NURSING IMPLICATIONS AND PROCEDURE

PRETEST:

- Positively identify the patient using at least two unique identifiers before providing care, treatment, or services.
- *Patient Teaching:* Inform the patient this test can help to assess respiratory status and identify the cause of the respiratory problems.
- Obtain a history of the patient's complaints, including a list of known allergens, especially allergies or sensitivities to latex or anesthetics.
- Obtain a history of the patient's cardiovascular and respiratory systems, especially any bleeding disorders and other symptoms, as well as results of previously performed laboratory tests and diagnostic and surgical procedures.
- Note any recent procedures that can interfere with test results.
- Obtain a list of the patient's current medications, including anticoagulants, aspirin and other salicylates, herbs, nutritional supplements, and nutraceuticals (see Appendix F). Note the last time and dose of medication taken.
- Indicate the type of oxygen, mode of oxygen delivery, and delivery rate as part of the test requisition process. Wait 30 min after a change in type or mode of oxygen delivery or rate for specimen collection.
- Review the procedure with the patient, and advise rest for 30 min before specimen collection. Address concerns about pain and explain that an arterial puncture may be painful. The site may be anesthetized with 1% to 2% lidocaine before puncture. Inform the patient that specimen collection usually takes 10 to 15 min. The person collecting the specimen should be notified beforehand if the patient is receiving anticoagulant therapy or taking aspirin or other natural products that may prolong bleeding from the puncture site.
- If the sample is to be collected by radial artery puncture, perform an Allen test before puncture to ensure that the patient has adequate collateral circulation to the hand. The modified Allen test is performed as follows: extend the patient's wrist over a rolled towel. Ask the patient to make a fist with the hand extended over the towel. Use the second and third fingers to locate the pulses of the ulnar and radial arteries on the palmar surface of the wrist. (The thumb should not be used to locate these arteries because it has a pulse.) Compress both arteries, and ask the patient to open and close the fist several times until the palm turns pale. Release pressure on the ulnar artery only. Color should return to the palm within 5 sec if the ulnar artery is functioning. This is a positive Allen test, and blood gases may be drawn from the radial artery site. The Allen test should then be performed on the opposite hand. The hand to which color is restored fastest has better circulation and should be selected for specimen collection.
- *Sensitivity to social and cultural issues,* as well as concern for modesty, is important in providing psychological support before, during, and after the procedure.
- There are no food, fluid, or medication restrictions unless by medical direction.
- Prepare an ice slurry in a cup or plastic bag to have ready for immediate transport of the specimen to the laboratory.

INTRATEST:

- If the patient has a history of allergic reaction to latex, avoid the use of equipment containing latex.
- Instruct the patient to cooperate fully and to follow directions. Direct the patient to breathe normally and to avoid unnecessary movement.
- Observe standard precautions, and follow the general guidelines in Appendix A. Positively identify the patient, and label the appropriate tubes with the corresponding patient demographics, date, and time of collection.
- Perform an arterial puncture, and collect the specimen in an air-free heparinized syringe. There is no demonstrable difference in results between samples collected in plastic syringes and samples collected in glass syringes. It is very important that no room air be

introduced into the collection container, because the gases in the room and in the sample will begin equilibrating immediately. The end of the syringe must be stoppered immediately after the needle is withdrawn from the puncture site. Apply a pressure dressing over the puncture site. Samples should be mixed by gentle rolling of the syringe to ensure proper mixing of the heparin with the sample, which will prevent the formation of small clots leading to rejection of the sample. The tightly capped sample should be placed in an ice slurry immediately after collection. Information on the specimen label should be protected from water in the ice slurry by first placing the specimen in a protective plastic bag. Promptly transport the specimen to the laboratory for processing and analysis.

POST-TEST:

▶ A written report of the results will be sent to the requesting health-care provider (HCP), who will discuss the results with the patient.

▶ Pressure should be applied to the puncture site for at least 5 min in the unanticoagulated patient and for at least 15 min in a patient receiving anticoagulant therapy. Observe/assess puncture site for bleeding or hematoma formation. Apply pressure bandage.

▶ Teach the patient breathing exercises to assist with the appropriate exchange of oxygen and carbon dioxide.

▶ Administer oxygen, if appropriate.

▶ Teach the patient how to properly use incentive spirometry or nebulizer, if ordered.

▶ Intervene appropriately for hypoxia and ventilatory disturbances.

▶ Reinforce information given by the patient's HCP regarding further testing, treatment, or referral to another HCP. Answer any questions or addess any concerns voiced by the patient or family.

▶ Depending on the results of this procedure, additional testing may be performed to evaluate or monitor progression of the disease process and determine the need for a change in therapy. Evaluate test results in relation to the patient's symptoms and other tests performed.

RELATED MONOGRAPHS:

▶ Related tests include allergen-specific IgE, α_1-antitrypsin, α_1-antitrypsin phenotyping, blood gases, chest x-ray, D-dimer, echocardiography, eosinophil count, fibrinogen, hypersensitivity pneumonitis, IgE, potassium, PFT, and sodium.

▶ See the Cardiovascular and Respiratory systems tables at the end of the book for related tests by body system.

Alzheimer's Disease Markers

SYNONYM/ACRONYM: CSF tau protein and β-amyloid-42, AD.

COMMON USE: To assist in diagnosing Alzheimer's disease and in monitoring the effectiveness of therapy.

SPECIMEN: Cerebrospinal fluid (CSF) (1 to 2 mL) collected in a plain plastic conical tube.

REFERENCE VALUE: (Method: Enzyme-linked immunosorbent assay) Simultaneous tau protein and β-amyloid-42 measurements in CSF are used in conjunction as biochemical markers of Alzheimer's disease (AD). Scientific studies indicate that a combination of elevated tau protein and decreased β-amyloid-42 protein levels are consistent with the presence of AD. Values are highly dependent on the reagents and standards used in the assay. Ranges vary among laboratories; the testing laboratory should be consulted for interpretation of results.

DESCRIPTION: AD is the most common cause of dementia in the elderly population. AD is a disorder of the central nervous system (CNS) that results in progressive and profound memory loss followed by loss of cognitive abilities and death. It may follow years of progressive formation of amyloid plaques and brain tangles, or it may appear as an early-onset form of the disease. Two recognized pathologic features of AD are neurofibrillary tangles and amyloid plaques found in the brain. Abnormal forms of the microtubule-associated tau protein are the main component of the classic neurofibrillary tangles found in patients with AD. Tau protein concentration is believed to reflect the number of neurofibrillary tangles and may be an indication of the severity of the disease. β-amyloid-42 is a free-floating protein normally present in CSF. It is believed to accumulate in the CNS of patients with AD, causing the formation of amyloid plaques on brain tissue. The result is that these patients have lower CSF values compared to age-matched healthy control participants. Recent research utilizing bio-barcode technology is investigating an association between increased levels of amyloid-beta-derived diffusable ligand (ADDL) in CSF and progression of AD. There is also an association between a gene that codes for the production of Apo E4 and development of late-onset AD.

INDICATIONS

- Assist in establishing a diagnosis of AD

POTENTIAL DIAGNOSIS

Decreased in

β-Amyloid-42 is decreased in up to 50% of healthy control participants.

- AD (related to accumulation in the brain with a corresponding decrease in CSF)
- Creutzfeldt-Jakob disease

Increased in

Tau protein is increased in AD.

- AD

CRITICAL FINDINGS: N/A

INTERFERING FACTORS

- Some patients with AD may have normal levels of tau protein because of an insufficient number of neurofibrillary tangles.

NURSING IMPLICATIONS AND PROCEDURE

PRETEST:

- Positively identify the patient using at least two unique identifiers before providing care, treatment, or services.
- *Patient Teaching:* Inform the patient this test can assist in diagnosing AD and/or evaluate the effectiveness of medication used to treat AD.
- Obtain a history of the patient's complaints, including a list of known allergens, especially allergies or sensitivities to latex or anesthetics.
- Obtain a history of the patient's neurological system, symptoms, and results of previously performed laboratory tests and diagnostic and surgical procedures.

A

Obtain a list of the patient's current medications, including herbs, nutritional supplements, and nutraceuticals (see Appendix F).

Review the procedure with the patient. Inform the patient that the procedure will be performed by a health-care provider (HCP) trained to perform the procedure and takes approximately 20 min. Address concerns about pain and explain that there may be some discomfort during the lumbar puncture. Inform the patient that a stinging sensation may be felt as the local anesthetic is injected. Instruct the patient to report any pain or other sensations that may require repositioning of the spinal needle.

Inform the patient that the position required for the lumbar puncture may be awkward but that someone will assist. Stress the importance of remaining still and breathing normally throughout the procedure.

Sensitivity to social and cultural issues, as well as concern for modesty, is important in providing psychological support before, during, and after the procedure.

There are no food, fluid, or medication restrictions unless by medical direction.

Make sure a written and informed consent has been signed prior to the procedure and before administering any medications.

INTRATEST:

If the patient has a history of allergic reaction to latex, avoid the use of equipment containing latex.

Instruct the patient to cooperate fully and to follow directions. Direct the patient to breathe normally and to avoid unnecessary movement.

Observe standard precautions, and follow the general guidelines in Appendix A. Positively identify the patient, and label the appropriate tubes with the corresponding patient demographics, date, and time of collection.

Record baseline vital signs, and assess neurologic status. Protocols may vary among facilities.

To perform a lumbar puncture, position the patient in the knee-chest position at the side of the bed. Provide pillows to support the spine or for the patient to grasp. The sitting position is an alternative. In this position, the patient must bend the neck and chest to the knees.

Prepare the site (usually between L3 and L4 or L4 and L5) with povidone-iodine, and drape the area.

A local anesthetic is injected. Using sterile technique, the HCP inserts the spinal needle through the spinous processes of the vertebrae and into the subarachnoid space. The stylet is removed. CSF drips from the needle if it is properly placed.

Attach the stopcock and manometer, and measure initial CSF pressure. Normal pressure for an adult in the lateral recumbent position is 90 to 180 mm H_2O. These values depend on the body position and are different in a horizontal or sitting position.

If the initial pressure is elevated, the HCP may perform Queckenstedt's test. To perform this test, apply pressure to the jugular vein for about 10 sec. CSF pressure usually rises in response to the occlusion, then rapidly returns to normal within 10 sec after the pressure is released. Sluggish response may indicate CSF obstruction.

Obtain CSF, and place in specimen tubes. Take a final pressure reading, and remove the needle. Clean the puncture site with an antiseptic solution, and apply a small bandage.

Promptly transport the specimen to the laboratory for processing and analysis.

POST-TEST:

A written report of the results will be sent to the requesting HCP, who will discuss the results with the patient.

After lumbar puncture, monitor vital signs and neurologic status every 15 min for 1 hr, then every 2 hr for 4 hr, and as ordered. Take the temperature every 4 hr for 24 hr. Compare with baseline values. Protocols may vary among facilities.

Administer fluids, if permitted, to replace lost CSF and help prevent or relieve headache, which is a side effect of lumbar puncture.

Observe/assess the puncture site for leakage, and frequently monitor body

A

signs, such as temperature and blood pressure.

- Position the patient flat, either on the back or abdomen, although some HCPs allow 30 degrees of elevation. Maintain this position for 8 hr. Changing position is acceptable as long as the body remains horizontal.
- Observe/assess the patient for neurological changes, such as altered level of consciousness, change in pupils, reports of tingling or numbness, and irritability.
- Recognize anxiety related to test results, and be supportive of perceived loss of independence and fear of shortened life expectancy. Discuss the implications of abnormal test results on the patient's lifestyle. Provide teaching and information regarding the clinical implications of the test results, as appropriate. Educate the patient and family members regarding access to counseling and other supportive services. Provide contact information

if desired, for the Alzheimer's Association (www.alz.org).

- Reinforce information given by the patient's HCP regarding further testing, treatment, or referral to another HCP. Answer any questions or address any concerns voiced by the patient or family.
- Depending on the results of this procedure, additional testing may be performed to evaluate or monitor progression of the disease process and determine the need for a change in therapy. Evaluate test results in relation to the patient's symptoms and other tests performed.

RELATED MONOGRAPHS:

- Related tests include evoked brain potentials, MRI brain, and PET scan brain.
- See the Musculoskeletal System table at the end of the book for related tests by body system.

Amino Acid Screen, Blood

SYNONYM/ACRONYM: N/A.

COMMON USE: To assist in diagnosing congenital metabolic disorders in infants, typically cystinosis, cystic fibrosis, and unexplained mental retardation.

SPECIMEN: Plasma (1 mL) collected in a green-top (heparin) tube.

REFERENCE VALUE: (Method: Chromatography) There are numerous amino acids. The following table includes those most frequently screened. All units are micromoles per deciliter (micromol/dL).

Age	Alanine	β-Alanine	Anserine	α-Amino-adipic Acid	α-Amino-N-butyric Acid
Premature	212–504	0	—	0	14–52
Newborn–1 mo	131–710	0–10	0	0	8–24
2 mo–18 yr	143–547	0–7	0	0	3–31
Adult	177–583	0–12	0	0–6	5–41

Age	γ-Amino-butyric Acid	γ-Aminoiso-butyric Acid	Arginine	Aspara-gine	Aspartic Acid
Premature	0	0	34–96	90–295	24–50
Newborn–1 mo	0–2	0	6–140	29–132	20–129
2 mo–18 yr	0	0	10–140	21–112	0–24
Adult	0	0	15–128	35–74	1–25

Age	Carnosine	Citrulline	Cysta-thionine	Cystine	Ethanol-amine
Premature	—	20–87	5–10	15–70	—
Newborn–1 mo	0–19	10–45	0–3	17–98	0–115
2 mo–18 yr	0	3–46	0–5	5–45	0–7
Adult	0	12–55	0–3	5–82	0–153

Age	Glutamic Acid	Glutamine	Glycine	Histidine	Homo-cystine
Premature	107–276	248–850	298–602	72–134	3–20
Newborn–1 mo	62–620	376–709	232–740	30–138	00
2 mo–18 yr	5–150	246–1182	81–436	41–125	0–5
Adult	10–131	205–756	151–490	72–124	0

Age	Hydroxy-lysine	Hydroxy-proline	Isoleucine	Leucine	Lysine
Premature	0	0–80	23–85	151–220	128–255
Newborn–1 mo	0–7	0–91	26–91	48–160	92–325
2 mo–18 yr	0–7	0–63	22–107	47–216	48–284
Adult	0	0–53	30–108	72–201	116–296

Age	Methio-nine	1-Methyl-histidine	3-Methyl-histidine	Ornithine	Phenyl-alanine
Premature	37–91	4–28	5–33	77–212	98–213
Newborn–1 mo	10–60	0–43	0–5	48–211	38–137
2 mo–18 yr	7–47	0–44	0–5	10–163	31–91
Adult	10–42	0–39	0–8	48–195	35–85

Age	Phospho-etha-nolamine	Phospho-serine	Proline	Sarcosine	Serine
Premature	5–35	10–45	92–310	0	127–248
Newborn–1 mo	3–27	7–47	110–417	0–625	99–395
2 mo–18 yr	0–69	1–30	52–369	0–9	58–186
Adult	0–40	2–14	97–329	0	58–181

(*table continues on page 40*)

Age	Taurine	Threonine	Tryptophan	Tyrosine	Valine
Premature	151–411	150–330	28–136	147–420	99–220
Newborn– 1 mo	46–492	90–329	0–60	55–147	86–190
2 mo–18 yr	10–170	24–226	0–71	22–115	64–321
Adult	54–210	60–225	10–140	34–112	119–336

DESCRIPTION: Amino acids are required for the production of proteins, enzymes, coenzymes, hormones, nucleic acids used to form DNA, pigments such as hemoglobin, and neurotransmitters. Testing for specific aminoacidopathies is generally performed on infants after an initial screening test with abnormal results. All 50 states have neonatal screening programs. Tests included in the screening profile vary among states. Certain congenital enzyme deficiencies interfere with normal amino acid metabolism and cause excessive accumulation of or deficiencies in amino acid levels. The major genetic disorders include phenylketonuria (PKU), tyrosinuria, and alcaptonuria, a defect in the phenylalanine-tyrosine conversion pathway. Accumulation of phenylalanine, in infants lacking the enzyme phenylalanine hydroxylase, results in progressive mental retardation. Renal aminoaciduria is also associated with conditions marked by defective tubular reabsorption from congenital disorders, such as hereditary fructose intolerance, cystinuria, and Hartnup's disease. Early diagnosis and treatment of certain aminoacidopathies can prevent mental retardation, reduced growth rates, and various unexplained symptoms. In most cases when plasma levels are elevated, urine levels are also elevated. Amino acid quantitation from plasma specimens is more informative, less variable, and less prone to analytic interference than from urine specimens. Urine specimens may be required to assist in the identification of disorders involving defective renal transport, where elevated levels are only manifested in the urine. Values are age-dependent. Amino acid concentrations demonstrate a significant circadian rhythm with values being lowest in the morning and highest in midafternoon.

INDICATIONS

- Assist in the detection of noninherited disorders evidenced by elevated amino acid levels
- Detect congenital errors of amino acid metabolism

POTENTIAL DIAGNOSIS

Increased in

Increased amino acid accumulation (total amino acids) occurs when a specific enzyme deficiency prevents its catabolism, with liver disease, or when there is impaired clearance by the kidneys:

Aminoacidopathies *(usually related to an inherited disorder; specific amino acids are implicated)*

Burns *(related to increased protein turnover)*

Diabetes *(related to gluconeogenesis, where protein is broken down as a means to generate glucose)*

Fructose intolerance *(related to hereditary enzyme deficiency)*

Malabsorption *(related to lack of transport and opportunity for catabolism)*

Renal failure (acute or chronic) *(related to impaired clearance)*

Reye's syndrome *(related to liver damage)*

Severe liver damage *(related to decreased production of amino acids by the liver)*

Shock *(related to increased protein turnover from tissue death and decreased deamination due to impaired liver function)*

Decreased in

Decreased (total amino acids) in conditions that result in increased renal excretion or insufficient protein intake or synthesis:

Adrenocortical hyperfunction *(related to excess cortisol, which assists in conversion of amino acids into glucose)*

Carcinoid syndrome *(related to increased consumption of amino acids, especially tryptophan, to form serotonin)*

Fever *(related to increased consumption)*

Glomerulonephritis *(related to increased renal excretion)*

Hartnup's disease *(related to increased renal excretion)*

Huntington's chorea *(related to increased consumption due to muscle tremors; possible insufficient intake)*

Malnutrition *(related to insufficient intake)*

Nephrotic syndrome *(related to increased renal excretion)*

Pancreatitis (acute) *(related to increased consumption as part of the inflammatory process and increased ureagenesis)*

Polycystic kidney disease *(related to increased renal excretion)*

Rheumatoid arthritis *(related to insufficient intake evidenced by lack of appetite)*

CRITICAL FINDINGS: N/A

INTERFERING FACTORS

- Drugs that may increase plasma amino acid levels include amino acids, bismuth salts, glucocorticoids, levarterenol, and 11-oxysteroids.
- Drugs that may decrease plasma amino acid levels include diethylstilbestrol, epinephrine, insulin, and progesterone.
- Amino acids exhibit a strong circadian rhythm; values are highest in the afternoon and lowest in the morning. Protein intake does not influence diurnal variation but significantly affects absolute concentrations.
- Failure to follow dietary restrictions before the procedure may cause the procedure to be canceled or repeated.

NURSING IMPLICATIONS AND PROCEDURE

PRETEST:

- Positively identify the patient using at least two unique identifiers before providing care, treatment, or services.
- *Patient Teaching:* Inform the parent/caregiver this test can assist in identification of inborn infant disorders.
- Obtain a history of the patient's complaints, including a list of known allergens, especially allergies or sensitivities to latex.
- Obtain a history of the patient's genitourinary and hepatobiliary systems, the patient's and parents' reproductive system as it relates to genetic disease, the patient's symptoms, and results of previously performed laboratory tests and diagnostic and surgical procedures.
- Obtain a list of the patient's current medications, including herbs, nutritional supplements, and nutraceuticals (see Appendix F).
- Review the procedure with the patient (and/or caregiver). Inform the patient (and/or caregiver) that specimen collection takes approximately 5 to 10 min. Address concerns about pain

A

and explain that there may be some discomfort during the venipuncture.

‣ *Sensitivity to social and cultural issues,* is important in providing psychological support before, during, and after the procedure.

‣ Instruct the patient to fast for 12 hr prior to the procedure.

‣ There are no fluid or medication restrictions unless by medical direction.

INTRATEST:

‣ Ensure that the patient has complied with dietary and other pretesting preparations; assure that food has been restricted for at least 12 hr prior to the procedure.

‣ If the patient has a history of allergic reaction to latex, avoid the use of equipment containing latex.

‣ Instruct the patient (and/or caregiver) to cooperate fully and to follow directions. Direct the patient to breathe normally and to avoid unnecessary movement. The caregiver may assist in preventing unnecessary movement.

‣ Observe standard precautions, and follow the general guidelines in Appendix A. Positively identify the patient, and label the appropriate tubes with the corresponding patient demographics, date, and time of collection. Perform a venipuncture.

‣ Remove the needle and apply direct pressure with dry gauze to stop bleeding. Observe/assess venipuncture site for bleeding or hematoma formation and secure gauze with adhesive bandage.

‣ Promptly transport the specimen to the laboratory for processing and analysis.

POST-TEST:

‣ A report of the results will be sent to the requesting health-care provider (HCP), who will discuss the results with the patient (and/or caregiver).

‣ Instruct the patient to resume usual diet as directed by the HCP.

‣ *Nutritional Considerations:* Instruct the patient (and/or caregiver) in special dietary modifications, as appropriate to treat deficiency, or refer caregiver to a qualified nutritionist. Amino acids are classified as essential (i.e., must be present simultaneously in sufficient quantities); conditionally or acquired essential (i.e., under certain stressful conditions, they become essential); and nonessential (i.e., can be produced by the body, when needed, if diet does not provide them). Essential amino acids include lysine, threonine, histidine, isoleucine, methionine, phenylalanine, tryptophan, and valine. Conditionally essential amino acids include cysteine, tyrosine, arginine, citrulline, taurine, and carnitine. Nonessential amino acids include alanine, glutamic acid, aspartic acid, glycine, serine, proline, glutamine, and asparagine. A high intake of specific amino acids can cause other amino acids to become essential.

‣ Recognize anxiety related to test results, and be supportive of perceived loss of independence and fear of shortened life expectancy. Discuss the implications of abnormal test results on the patient's lifestyle. Provide teaching and information regarding the clinical implications of the test results, as appropriate. Educate the patient (and/or caregiver) regarding access to genetic or other counseling services. Provide contact information, if desired, for the March of Dimes (www.marchofdimes.com) or the state department of health newborn screening program.

‣ Reinforce information given by the patien's HCP regarding further testing, treatment, or referral to another HCP. Answer any questions or address any concerns voiced by the patient or family.

‣ Depending on the results of this procedure, additional testing may be performed to evaluate or monitor progression of the disease process and determine the need for a change in therapy. Evaluate test results in relation to the patient's symptoms and other tests performed.

RELATED MONOGRAPHS:

‣ Related tests include ammonia and urine amino acid screen.

‣ See the Genitourinary, Hepatobiliary, and Reproductive systems tables at the end of the book for related tests by body system.

Amino Acid Screen, Urine

SYNONYM/ACRONYM: N/A.

COMMON USE: To assist in diagnosing congenital metabolic disorders in infants, typically cystinosis, phenylketonuria, and unexplained mental retardation.

SPECIMEN: Urine (10 mL) from a random or timed specimen collected in a clean plastic collection container with hydrochloric acid as a preservative.

REFERENCE VALUE: (Method: Chromatography) There are numerous amino acids. The following table includes those most frequently screened. All units are nanomoles per milligram (nmol/mg) creatinine.

Age	Alanine	β-Alanine	Anserine	α-Amino-adipic Acid	α-Amino-N-butyric Acid
Premature	1,320–4,040	1,020–3,500	–	70–460	50–710
Newborn–1 mo	982–3,055	25–288	0–3	0–180	8–65
2 mo–2 yr	767–6,090	0–297	0–5	45–268	30–136
2–18 yr	231–915	0–65	0	2–88	0–77
Adult	240–670	0–130	0	40–110	0–90

Age	γ-Amino-butyric Acid	β-Aminoiso-butyric Acid	Arginine	Asparagine	Aspartic Acid
Premature	20–260	50–470	190–820	1,350–5,250	580–1,520
Newborn–1 mo	0–15	421–3,133	35–214	185–1,550	336–810
2 mo–2 yr	0–105	802–4,160	38–165	252–1,280	230–685
2–18 yr	15–30	291–1,482	31–109	72–332	0–120
Adult	15–30	10–510	10–90	99–470	60–240

Age	Carnosine	Citrulline	Cystathionine	Cystine	Ethanolamine
Newborn–1 mo	97–665	27–181	16–147	212–668	840–3,400
2 mo–2 yr	203–635	22–180	33–470	68–710	0–2,230
2–18 yr	72–402	10–99	0–26	25–125	0–530
Adult	10–90	8–50	20–50	43–210	0–520

Age	Glutamic Acid	Glutamine	Glycine	Histidine	Homocystine
Premature	380–3,760	520–1,700	7,840–23,600	1,240–7,240	580–2,230

(*table continues on page 44*)

Age	Glutamic Acid	Glutamine	Glycine	Histidine	Homocystine
Newborn–1 mo	70–1,058	393–1,042	5,749–16,423	908–2,528	0–88
2 mo–2 yr	54–590	670–1,562	3,023–11,148	815–7,090	6–67
2–18 yr	0–176	369–1,014	897–4,500	644–2,430	0–32
Adult	39–330	190–510	730–4,160	460–1,430	0–32

Age	Hydroxylysine	Hydroxyproline	Isoleucine	Leucine	Lysine
Premature	–	560–5,640	250–640	190–790	1,860–15,460
Newborn–1 mo	10–125	40–440	125–390	78–195	270–1,850
2 mo–2 yr	0–97	0–4,010	38–342	70–570	189–850
2–18 yr	40–102	0–3,300	10–126	30–500	153–634
Adult	40–90	0–26	16–180	30–150	145–634

Age	Methionine	1-Methylhistidine	3-Methylhistidine	Ornithine	Phenylalanine
Premature	500–1,230	170–880	420–1,340	260–3,350	920–2,280
Newborn–1 mo	342–880	96–499	189–680	118–554	91–457
2 mo–2 yr	174–1,090	106–1,275	147–391	55–364	175–1,340
2–18 yr	16–114	170–1,688	182–365	31–91	61–314
Adult	38–210	170–1,680	160–520	20–80	51–250

Age	Phosphoethanolamine	Phosphoserine	Proline	Sarcosine	Serine
Premature	80–340	500–1,690	1,350–10,460	0	1,680–6,000
Newborn–1 mo	0–155	150–339	370–2,323	0–56	1,444–3,661
2 mo–2 yr	108–533	112–304	254–2,195	30–358	845–3,190
2–18 yr	18–150	70–138	0	0–26	362–1,100
Adult	20–100	40–510	0	0–80	240–670

Age	Taurine	Threonine	Tryptophan	Tyrosine	Valine
Premature	5,190–23,620	840–5,700	0	1,090–6,780	180–890
Newborn–1 mo	1,650–6,220	445–1,122	0	220–1,650	113–369
2 mo–2 yr	545–3,790	252–1,528	0–93	333–1,550	99–316
2–18 yr	639–1,866	121–389	0–108	122–517	58–143
Adult	380–1,850	130–370	0–70	90–290	27–260

DESCRIPTION: Amino acids are required for the production of proteins, enzymes, coenzymes, hormones, nucleic acids used to form DNA, pigments such as hemoglobin, and neurotransmitters. Testing for specific aminoacidopathies is generally performed on infants after an initial screening test with abnormal results. All 50 states have neonatal screening programs. Tests included in the screening profile vary among states. Certain congenital enzyme deficiencies interfere with normal amino acid metabolism and cause excessive accumulation of or deficiencies in amino acid levels. The major genetic disorders include phenylketonuria, tyrosinuria, and alcaptonuria, a defect in the phenylalanine-tyrosine conversion pathway. Renal aminoaciduria is also associated with conditions marked by defective tubular reabsorption from congenital disorders, such as hereditary fructose intolerance, cystinuria, and Hartnup's disease. Early diagnosis and treatment of certain aminoacidopathies can prevent mental retardation, reduced growth rates, and various unexplained symptoms. In most cases when plasma levels are elevated, urine levels are also elevated. Amino acid quantitations from plasma specimens are more informative, less variable, and less prone to analytic interference than from urine specimens. Urine specimens may be required to assist in the identification of disorders involving defective renal transport, where elevated levels are only manifested in the urine. Values are age dependent. Abnormal results on a random sample should be followed up with a timed collection. Amino acid concentrations demonstrate a significant circadian rhythm with values being lowest in the morning and highest in midafternoon.

INDICATIONS
- Assist in the detection of noninherited disorders evidenced by elevated amino acid levels
- Screen for congenital errors of amino acid metabolism

POTENTIAL DIAGNOSIS

Increased in
Increased amino acid accumulation (total amino acids) occurs when a specific enzyme deficiency prevents its catabolism or when there is impaired clearance by the kidneys:
- Primary causes *(inherited):*
  Aminoaciduria (specific)
  Cystinosis *(may be masked because of decreased glomerular filtration rate, so values may be in normal range)*
  Fanconi's syndrome
  Fructose intolerance
  Galactosemia
  Hartnup's disease
  Lactose intolerance
  Lowe's syndrome
  Maple syrup urine disease
  Tyrosinemia type I
  Tyrosinosis
  Wilson's disease
- Secondary causes *(noninherited):*
  Acute leukemia
  Chronic renal failure *(reduced glomerular filtration rate)*
  Chronic renal failure
  Diabetic ketosis
  Epilepsy *(transient increase related to disturbed renal function during grand mal seizure)*
  Folic acid deficiency
  Hyperparathyroidism
  Liver necrosis and cirrhosis
  Multiple myeloma

Muscular dystrophy (progressive)
Osteomalacia *(secondary to parathyroid hormone excess)*
Pernicious anemia
Thalassemia major
Vitamin deficiency *(B, C, and D; vitamin D–deficiency rickets, vitamin D–resistant rickets)*
Viral hepatitis *(related to the degree of hepatic involvement)*

Decreased in: N/A

CRITICAL FINDINGS: N/A

INTERFERING FACTORS
- Drugs that may increase urine amino acid levels include acetylsalicylic acid, bismuth, cisplatin, corticotropin, hydrocortisone, insulin, streptozocin, tetracycline, triamcinolone, and valproic acid.
- Numerous drugs may affect the test method and falsely increase urine amino acid levels.
- Drugs that may decrease urine amino acid levels include insulin.
- Amino acids exhibit a strong circadian rhythm; values are highest in the afternoon and lowest in the morning. Protein intake does not influence diurnal variation but significantly affects absolute concentrations.
- Dilute urine (specific gravity less than 1.010) should be rejected for analysis.
- Failure to follow dietary restrictions before the procedure may cause the procedure to be canceled or repeated.

NURSING IMPLICATIONS AND PROCEDURE

PRETEST:
- Positively identify the patient using at least two unique identifiers before providing care, treatment, or services.
- *Patient Teaching:* Inform the parent this test can assist in identification of inborn infant disorders.

- Obtain a history of the patient's complaints, including a list of known allergens, especially allergies or sensitivities to latex.
- Obtain a history of the patient's genitourinary and hepatobiliary systems, the patient's and parents' reproductive system as it relates to genetic disease, the patient's symptoms, and results of previously performed laboratory tests and diagnostic and surgical procedures.
- Obtain a list of the patient's current medications, including herbs, nutritional supplements, and nutraceuticals (see Appendix F).
- Review the procedure with the patient (and/or caregiver). Inform the patient and caregiver that random urine specimen collection takes approximately 5 min. Address concerns about pain and explain that no pain will be experienced during the test.
- *Sensitivity to social and cultural issues,* is important in providing psychological support before, during, and after the procedure.
- Instruct the patient to fast for 12 hr prior to the procedure.
- There are no fluid or medication restrictions unless by medical direction.
- Instruct the patient to avoid excessive exercise and stress during the 24-hr collection of urine.
- Review the procedure with the patient (and/or caregiver). Provide a nonmetallic urinal, bedpan, or toilet-mounted collection device.
- If a timed collection is requested, inform the patient that all urine collected over a 24-hr period must be saved; if a preservative has been added to the container, instruct the patient not to discard the preservative. Instruct the patient not to void directly into the laboratory collection container. Instruct the patient to avoid defecating in the collection device and to keep toilet tissue out of the collection device to prevent contamination of the specimen. Place a sign in the bathroom to remind the patient to save all urine.
- Instruct the patient to void all urine into the collection device and pour the urine into the laboratory collection container. Alternatively, the specimen can be left in the collection device for a health care staff member to add to the laboratory collection container.

A

▸ Ensure that the patient has complied with dietary and other pretesting preparations; assure that food has been restricted for at least 12 hr prior to the procedure.

▸ Observe standard precautions, and follow the general guidelines in Appendix A. Positively identify the patient, and label the appropriate specimen container with the corresponding patient demographics, date, and time of collection. Include on the timed specimen label the amount of urine and test start and stop times.

▸ Promptly transport the specimen to the laboratory for processing and analysis.

Random Specimen (collect in early morning)

▸ *Infant:* Clean and dry the genital area, attach the collection device securely to prevent leakage, and observe for voiding. Remove collection device carefully from the skin to prevent irritation. Transfer the urine into a specimen container. For dipstick method, place dipstick or reagent pad into the urine specimen or on the diaper saturated with urine. Remove, compare with color chart, and record results.

▸ *Adult:* Instruct the patient to obtain a clean-catch specimen as described in Appendix A. If an indwelling catheter is in place, it may be necessary to clamp off the catheter for 15 to 30 min before specimen collection. Cleanse specimen port with antiseptic swab, and then aspirate 5 mL of urine with a 21- to 25-gauge needle and syringe. Transfer urine to a properly labeled plastic container.

Timed Specimen

▸ Obtain a clean 3-L urine specimen container, toilet-mounted collection device, and plastic bag (for transport of the specimen container). The specimen must be refrigerated or kept on ice throughout the entire collection period. If an indwelling urinary catheter is in place, the drainage bag must be kept on ice.

▸ Begin the test between 6 and 8 a.m. if possible. Collect first voiding and discard. Record the time the specimen was discarded as the beginning of the timed collection period. The next morning, ask the patient to void at the same time the collection was started, and add this last voiding to the container. Urinary output should be recorded throughout the collection time.

▸ If an indwelling catheter is in place, replace the tubing and container system at the start of the collection time. Keep the container system on ice during the collection period, or empty the urine into a larger container periodically during the collection period; monitor to ensure continued drainage, and conclude the test the next morning at the same hour the collection started.

▸ At the conclusion of the test, compare the quantity of urine with the urinary output record for the collection. If the specimen contains less than what was recorded as output, some urine may have been discarded, invalidating the test.

▸ A written report of the results will be sent to the requesting health-care provider (HCP), who will discuss the results with the patient (and/or caregiver).

▸ Instruct the patient to resume usual diet as directed by the HCP.

▸ *Nutritional Considerations:* Instruct the patient (and/or caregiver) in special dietary modifications, as appropriate to treat deficiency, or refer caregiver to a qualified nutritionist. Amino acids are classified as essential (i.e., must be present simultaneously in sufficient quantities); conditionally or acquired essential (i.e., under certain stressful conditions, they become essential); and nonessential (i.e., can be produced by the body, when needed, if diet does not provide them). Essential amino acids include lysine, threonine, histidine, isoleucine, methionine, phenylalanine, tryptophan, and valine. Conditionally essential amino acids include cysteine, tyrosine, arginine, citrulline, taurine, and carnitine. Nonessential amino acids include alanine, glutamic acid, aspartic acid, glycine, serine, proline, glutamine, and asparagine. A high intake of specific amino acids can cause other amino acids to become essential.

▶ Recognize anxiety related to test results, and be supportive of perceived loss of independence and fear of shortened life expectancy. Discuss the implications of abnormal test results on the patient's lifestyle. Provide teaching and information regarding the clinical implications of the test results, as appropriate. Educate the patient (and/or caregiver) regarding access to genetic or other counseling services. Provide contact information, if desired, for the March of Dimes (www.marchofdimes.com) or your state department of health's newborn screening program.

▶ Reinforce information given by the patient's HCP regarding further testing, treatment, or referral to another HCP. Answer any questions or address any concerns voiced by the patient or family.

▶ Depending on the results of this procedure, additional testing may be performed to evaluate or monitor progression of the disease process and determine the need for a change in therapy. Evaluate test results in relation to the patient's symptoms and other tests performed.

RELATED MONOGRAPHS:

▶ Related tests include ammonia and amino acid screen blood.
▶ See the Genitourinary, Hepatobiliary, and Reproductive systems tables at the end of the book for related tests by body system.

δ-Aminolevulinic Acid

SYNONYM/ACRONYM: δ-ALA.

COMMON USE: To assist in diagnosing lead poisoning in children, or porphyria, a disorder that disrupts heme synthesis, primarily affecting the liver.

SPECIMEN: Urine (25 mL) from a timed specimen collected in a dark plastic container with glacial acetic acid as a preservative.

REFERENCE VALUE: (Method: Spectrophotometry)

Conventional Units	SI Units (Conventional Units × 7.626)
1.5–7.5 mg/24 hr	11.4–57.2 micromol/24 hr

DESCRIPTION: δ-Aminolevulinic acid (δ-ALA) is involved in the formation of porphyrins, which ultimately leads to hemoglobin synthesis. Toxins including alcohol, lead, and other heavy metals can inhibit porphyrin synthesis. Accumulated δ-ALA is excreted in urine. Symptoms of the acute phase of intermittent porphyrias include abdominal pain, nausea, vomiting, neuromuscular signs and symptoms, constipation, and occasionally psychotic behavior. Hemolytic anemia may also exhibit during the acute phase.

δ-ALA is a test of choice in the diagnosis of acute intermittent porphyria. Although lead poisoning can cause increased urinary excretion, the measurement of δ-ALA is not useful to indicate lead toxicity because it is not detectable in the urine until the blood lead level approaches and exceeds 40 mcg/dL, the level at which children should be evaluated to determine the need for chelation therapy.

INDICATIONS
• Assist in the diagnosis of porphyrias

POTENTIAL DIAGNOSIS

Increased in
Related to inhibition of the enzymes involved in porphyrin synthesis; results in accumulation of δ-ALA and is evidenced by exposure to medications, toxins, diet, or infection that can precipitate an attack
• Acute porphyrias
• Aminolevulinic acid dehydrase deficiency *(related to the inability to convert δ-ALA to porphobilinogen, leading to accumulation of δ-ALA)*
• Hereditary tyrosinemia
• Lead poisoning

Decreased in: N/A

CRITICAL FINDINGS

Conventional Units	SI Units (Conventional Units × 7.62)
Greater than 20 mg/24 hr	Greater then 152.5 micromol/24 hr

Note and immediately report to the health-care provider (HCP) abnormal results and associated symptoms.

INTERFERING FACTORS
• Drugs that may increase δ-ALA levels include penicillins.
• Cimetidine may decrease δ-ALA levels.
• Numerous drugs are suspected as potential initiators of attacks of acute porphyria, but those classified as unsafe for high-risk individuals include aminopyrine, apronalide, barbiturates, chlordiazepoxide, chlorpropamide, diazepam, dichloralphenazone, ergot preparations, glutethimide, griseofulvin, hydantoin derivatives, isopropyl dipyrone, meprobamate, methyldopa, methylsulfonal, methyprylone, oral contraceptives, pentazocine, phenytoin, progestogens, succinimide, sulfomethane, and tolbutamide.

NURSING IMPLICATIONS AND PROCEDURE

PRETEST:
▶ Positively identify the patient using at least two unique identifiers before providing care, treatment, or services.
▶ *Patient Teaching:* Inform the parent/patient this test can assist with identification of poisoning from lead or other toxins.
▶ Obtain a history of the patient's complaints, including a list of known allergens, especially allergies or sensitivities to latex.
▶ Obtain a history of the patient's hematopoietic system, symptoms, and results of previously performed laboratory tests and diagnostic and surgical procedures.
▶ Obtain a list of the patient's current medications, including herbs, nutritional supplements, and nutraceuticals (see Appendix F).
▶ Review the procedure with the patient. Provide a nonmetallic urinal, bedpan, or toilet-mounted collection device. Address concerns about pain and explain that there should be no discomfort during the procedure.

A

Usually a 24-hr time frame for urine collection is ordered. Inform the patient that all urine must be saved during that 24-hr period. Instruct the patient not to void directly into the laboratory collection container. Instruct the patient to avoid defecating in the collection device and to keep toilet tissue out of the collection device to prevent contamination of the specimen. Place a sign in the bathroom to remind the patient to save all urine.

Instruct the patient to void all urine into the collection device and then to pour the urine into the laboratory collection container. Alternatively, the specimen can be left in the collection device for a health care staff member to add to the laboratory collection container.

Sensitivity to social and cultural issues, as well as concern for modesty, is important in providing psychological support before, during, and after the procedure.

There are no food, fluid, or medication restrictions unless by medical direction.

INTRATEST:

If the patient has a history of allergic reaction to latex, avoid the use of equipment containing latex.

Instruct the patient to cooperate fully and to follow directions.

Observe standard precautions, and follow the general guidelines in Appendix A. Positively identify the patient, and label the appropriate collection container with the corresponding patient demographics, date, and time of collection.

Timed Specimen

Obtain a clean 3-L urine specimen container, toilet-mounted collection device, and plastic bag (for transport of the specimen container). The specimen must be refrigerated or kept on ice throughout the entire collection period. If an indwelling urinary catheter is in place, the drainage bag must be kept on ice.

Begin the test between 6 and 8 a.m. if possible. Collect first voiding and discard. Record the time the specimen was discarded as the beginning of the timed collection period. The next morning, ask the patient to void at the same time the collection was started, and add this last voiding to the container. Urinary output should be recorded throughout the collection time.

If an indwelling catheter is in place, replace the tubing and container system at the start of the collection time. Keep the container system on ice during the collection period, or empty the urine into a larger container periodically during the collection period. Monitor to ensure continued drainage, and conclude the test the next morning at the same hour the collection was begun.

At the conclusion of the test, compare the quantity of urine with the urinary output record for the collection. If the specimen contains less than what was recorded as output, some urine may have been discarded, invalidating the test.

Include on the specimen collection container's label the amount of urine as well as test start and stop times. Note the ingestion of any medications that may affect test results.

Promptly transport the specimen to the laboratory for processing and analysis.

POST-TEST:

A written report of the results will be sent to the requesting HCP, who will discuss the results with the patient.

Recognize anxiety related to test results. Discuss the implications of abnormal test results on the patient's lifestyle. Provide teaching and information regarding the clinical implications of the test results, as appropriate.

Reinforce information given by the patient's HCP regarding further

testing, treatment, or referral to another HCP. Answer any questions or address any concerns voiced by the patient or family.
▶ Depending on the results of this procedure, additional testing may be performed to evaluate or monitor progression of the disease process and determine the need for a change in therapy. Evaluate test results in relation to the patient's symptoms and other tests performed.

RELATED MONOGRAPHS:
▶ Related tests include CBC, erythrocyte protoporphyrin (free), lead, and porphyrins urine.
▶ See the Hematopoietic System table at the end of the book for related tests by body system.

Ammonia

SYNONYM/ACRONYM: NH_3.

COMMON USE: To assist in diagnosing liver disease such as hepatitis and cirrhosis. Assists in evaluating the effectiveness of treatment modalities. Specifically used to assist in diagnosing infant Reye's syndrome.

SPECIMEN: Plasma (1 mL) collected in completely filled lavender- (EDTA) or green-top (Na or Li heparin) tube. Specimen should be transported tightly capped and in an ice slurry.

REFERENCE VALUE: (Method: Spectrophotometry)

Age	Conventional Units	SI Units (Conventional Units × 0.714)
Newborn	90–150 mcg/dL	64–107 micromol/L
Adult male	27–102 mcg/dL	19–73 micromol/L
Adult female	19–87 mcg/dL	14–62 micromol/L

DESCRIPTION: Blood ammonia (NH_3) comes from two sources: deamination of amino acids during protein metabolism and degradation of proteins by colon bacteria. The liver converts ammonia in the portal blood to urea, which is excreted by the kidneys. When liver function is severely compromised, especially in situations in which decreased hepatocellular function is combined with impaired portal blood flow, ammonia levels rise. Ammonia is potentially toxic to the central nervous system.

INDICATIONS
• Evaluate advanced liver disease or other disorders associated with altered serum ammonia levels
• Identify impending hepatic encephalopathy with known liver disease

Access additional resources at davisplus.fadavis.com

- Monitor the effectiveness of treatment for hepatic encephalopathy, indicated by declining levels
- Monitor patients receiving hyperalimentation therapy

POTENTIAL DIAGNOSIS

Increased in

- Gastrointestinal hemorrhage *(related to decreased blood volume, which prevents ammonia from reaching the liver to be metabolized)*
- Genitourinary tract infection with distention and stasis *(related to decreased renal excretion; levels accumulate in the blood)*
- Hepatic coma *(related to insufficient functioning liver cells to metabolize ammonia; levels accumulate in the blood)*
- Inborn enzyme deficiency *(evidenced by inability to metabolize ammonia)*
- Liver failure, late cirrhosis *(related to insufficient functioning liver cells to metabolize ammonia)*
- Reye's syndrome *(related to insufficient functioning liver cells to metabolize ammonia)*
- Total parenteral nutrition *(related to ammonia generated from protein metabolism)*

Decreased in: N/A

CRITICAL FINDINGS: N/A

INTERFERING FACTORS

- Drugs that may increase ammonia levels include asparaginase, chlorthiazide, chlorthalidone, fibrin hydrolysate, furosemide, hydroflumethiazide, isoniazid, levoglutamide, mercurial diuretics, oral resins, thiazides, and valproic acid.
- Drugs/organisms that may decrease ammonia levels include diphenhydramine, kanamycin, monoamine oxidase inhibitors,

neomycin, tetracycline, and *Lactobacillus acidophilus*.
- Hemolysis falsely increases ammonia levels because intracellular ammonia levels are three times higher than plasma.
- Prompt and proper specimen processing, storage, and analysis are important to achieve accurate results. The specimen should be collected on ice; the collection tube should be filled completely and then kept tightly stoppered. Ammonia increases rapidly in the collected specimen, so analysis should be performed within 20 min of collection.

NURSING IMPLICATIONS AND PROCEDURE

PRETEST:

▶ Positively identify the patient using at least two unique identifiers before providing care, treatment, or services.
▶ *Patient Teaching:* Inform the patient this test can assist with the evaluation of liver function related to processing protein waste. May be used to assist in diagnosis of Reye's syndrome in infants.
▶ Obtain a history of the patient's complaints, including a list of known allergens, especially allergies or sensitivities to latex.
▶ Obtain a history of the patient's gastrointestinal, genitourinary, and hepatobiliary systems; symptoms; and results of previously performed laboratory tests and diagnostic and surgical procedures.
▶ Obtain a list of the patient's current medications, including herbs, nutritional supplements, and nutraceuticals (see Appendix F).
▶ Review the procedure with the patient. Inform the patient that specimen collection takes approximately 5 to 10 min. Address concerns about pain and explain that there may be some discomfort during the venipuncture.

Sensitivity to social and cultural issues, as well as concern for modesty, is important in providing psychological support before, during, and after the procedure.

▶ There are no food, fluid, or medication restrictions unless by medical direction.

INTRATEST:

▶ If the patient has a history of allergic reaction to latex, avoid the use of equipment containing latex.

▶ Instruct the patient to cooperate fully and to follow directions. Direct the patient to breathe normally and to avoid unnecessary movement.

▶ Observe standard precautions, and follow the general guidelines in Appendix A. Positively identify the patient, and label the appropriate tubes with the corresponding patient demographics, date, and time of collection. Perform a venipuncture.

▶ Remove the needle and apply direct pressure with dry gauze to stop bleeding. Observe/assess the veni-puncture site for bleeding or hematoma formation and secure the gauze with adhesive bandage.

▶ Promptly transport the specimen to the laboratory for processing and analysis. The tightly capped sample should be placed in an ice slurry imme-diately after collection. Information on the specimen label should be protected from water in the ice slurry by first placing the specimen in a protective plastic bag.

POST-TEST:

▶ A report of the results will be sent to the requesting health-care provider (HCP), who will discuss the results with the patient.

▶ *Nutritional Considerations:* Increased ammonia levels may be associated with liver disease. Dietary recommen-dations may be indicated, depending on the severity of the condition. A low-protein diet may be in order if the patient's liver has lost the ability

to process the end products of protein metabolism. A diet of soft foods may be required if esophageal varices have developed. Ammonia levels may be used to determine whether protein should be added to or reduced from the diet. Patients should be encouraged to eat simple carbohydrates and emulsified fats (as in homogenized milk or eggs) rather than complex carbohydrates (e.g., starch, fiber, and glycogen [animal carbohydrates]) and complex fats, which would require additional bile to emulsify them so that they could be used. The cirrhotic patient should be carefully observed for the development of ascites, in which case fluid and electrolyte balance requires strict attention.

▶ Reinforce information given by the patient's HCP regarding further testing, treatment, or referral to another HCP. Answer any questions or address any concerns voiced by the patient or family.

▶ Depending on the results of this procedure, additional testing may be performed to evaluate or monitor pro-gression of the disease process and determine the need for a change in therapy. Evaluate test results in relation to the patient's symptoms and other tests performed.

RELATED MONOGRAPHS:

▶ Related tests include ALT, albumin, analgesic and antipyretic drugs (acetaminophen and salicylates), anion gap, AST, bilirubin, biopsy liver, blood gases, BUN, blood calcium, CBC, CT biliary tract and liver, CT pelvis, cystometry, cystoscopy, EGD, electrolytes, GI blood loss scan, glucose, IVP, MRI pelvis, ketones, lactic acid, Mecke's scan, osmolality, protein, PT/INR, uric acid, and US pelvis.

▶ See the Gastrointestinal, Genitourinary, and Hepatobiliary systems tables at the end of the book for related tests by body system.

A

Amniotic Fluid Analysis

SYNONYM/ACRONYM: N/A.

COMMON USE: To assist in identification of fetal gender, genetic disorders such as hemophilia, chromosomal disorders such as Down syndrome, anatomical abnormalities such as spina bifida, and hereditary metabolic disorders such as cystic fibrosis.

SPECIMEN: Amniotic fluid (10 to 20 mL) collected in a clean amber glass or plastic container.

REFERENCE VALUE: (Method: Macroscopic observation of fluid for color and appearance, immunochemiluminometric assay [ICMA] for α_1-fetoprotein, electrophoresis for acetylcholinesterase, spectrophotometry for creatinine and bilirubin, chromatography for lecithin/sphingomyelin [L/S] ratio and phosphatidylglycerol, tissue culture for chromosome analysis, dipstick for leukocyte esterase, and automated cell counter for white blood cell count and lamellar bodies)

Test	Reference Value
Color	Colorless to pale yellow
Appearance	Clear
α_1-Fetoprotein	Less than 2.0 MoM*
Acetylcholinesterase	Absent
Creatinine	1.8–4.0 mg/dL at term
Bilirubin	Less than 0.075 mg/dL in early pregnancy
	Less than 0.025 mg/dL at term
L/S ratio	Greater than 2:1 at term
Phosphatidylglycerol	Present at term
Chromosome analysis	Normal karyotype
White blood cell count	None seen
Leukocyte esterase	Negative
Lamellar bodies	30,000–50,000 platelet equivalents

*MoM = multiples of the median.

DESCRIPTION: Amniotic fluid is formed in the membranous sac that surrounds the fetus. The total volume of fluid at term is 500 to 2,500 mL. In amniocentesis, fluid is obtained by ultrasound-guided needle aspiration from the amniotic sac. This procedure is generally performed between 14 and 16 weeks' gestation for accurate interpretation of test results, but it also can be done between 26 and 35 weeks' gestation if fetal distress is suspected.

Amniotic fluid is tested to identify genetic and neural tube defects, hemolytic diseases of the newborn, fetal infection, fetal renal malfunction, or maturity of the fetal lungs (see monograph titled "Lecithin/Sphingomyelin Ratio"). Several rapid tests are also used to differentiate amniotic fluid from other body fluids in a vaginal specimen when premature rupture of membranes (PROM) is suspected. A vaginal swab obtained from the posterior vaginal pool can be used to perform a rapid, waived procedure to aid in the assessment of PROM. Nitrazine paper impregnated with an indicator dye will produce a color change indicative of vaginal pH. Normal vaginal pH is acidic (4.5 to 6.0) and the color of the paper will not change. Amniotic fluid has an alkaline pH (7.1 to 7.3) and the paper will turn a blue color. False-positive results occur in the presence of semen, blood, alkaline urine, vaginal infection, or if the patient is receiving antibiotics. The amniotic fluid crystallization or Fern test is based on the observation of a fern pattern when amniotic fluid is placed on a glass slide and allowed to air dry. The fern pattern is due to the protein and sodium chloride content of the amniotic fluid. False-positive results occur in the presence of blood urine or cervical mucus. Both of these tests can produce false-negative results if only a small amount of fluid is leaked. The reliability of results is also significantly diminished with the passage of time (greater than 24 hr). AmniSure is an immunoassay that can be performed on a vaginal swab sample. It is a rapid test that detects placental alpha microglobulin-1 protein (PAMG-1), which is found in high concentrations in amniotic fluid. AmniSure does not demonstrate the high frequency of false-positive and false-negative results inherent with the pH and fern tests.

INDICATIONS

- Assist in the diagnosis of (in utero) metabolic disorders, such as cystic fibrosis, or errors of lipid, carbohydrate, or amino acid metabolism
- Detect infection secondary to ruptured membranes
- Detect fetal ventral wall defects
- Determine fetal maturity when preterm delivery is being considered; fetal maturity is indicated by an L/S ratio of 2:1 or greater (see monograph titled "Lecithin/Sphingomyelin Ratio")
- Determine fetal gender when the mother is a known carrier of a sex-linked abnormal gene that could be transmitted to male offspring, such as hemophilia or Duchenne's muscular dystrophy
- Determine the presence of fetal distress in late-stage pregnancy
- Evaluate fetus in families with a history of genetic disorders, such as Down syndrome, Tay-Sachs disease, chromosome or enzyme anomalies, or inherited hemoglobinopathies
- Evaluate fetus in mothers of advanced maternal age (some of the aforementioned tests are routinely requested in mothers age 35 and older)
- Evaluate fetus in mothers with a history of miscarriage or stillbirth
- Evaluate known or suspected hemolytic disease involving the fetus in an Rh-sensitized pregnancy, indicated by rising bilirubin levels,

especially after the 30th week of gestation

- Evaluate suspected neural tube defects, such as spina bifida or myelomeningocele, as indicated by elevated α_1-fetoprotein (see monograph titled "α_1-Fetoprotein" for information related to triple-marker testing)

POTENTIAL DIAGNOSIS

- Yellow, green, red, or brown fluid *indicates the presence of bilirubin, blood (fetal or maternal), or meconium, which indicate fetal distress or death, hemolytic disease, or growth retardation.*
- Elevated bilirubin levels *indicate fetal hemolytic disease or intestinal obstruction. Measurement of bilirubin is not usually performed before 20 to 24 weeks' gestation because no action can be taken before then. The severity of hemolytic disease is graded by optical density (OD) zones: A value of 0.28 to 0.46 OD at 28 to 31 weeks' gestation indicates mild hemolytic disease, which probably will not affect the fetus; 0.47 to 0.90 OD indicates a moderate effect on the fetus; and 0.91 to 1.0 OD indicates a significant effect on the fetus. A trend of increasing values with serial measurements may indicate the need for intrauterine transfusion or early delivery, depending on the fetal age. After 32 to 33 weeks' gestation, early delivery is preferred over intrauterine transfusion, because early delivery is more effective in providing the required care to the neonate.*
- Creatinine concentration greater than 2.0 mg/dL *indicates fetal maturity (at 36 to 37 wk) if maternal creatinine is also within the expected range. This value should be interpreted in conjunction with other parameters evaluated in amniotic fluid and especially with the L/S ratio, because normal lung development depends on normal kidney development.*
- An L/S ratio less than 2:1 and absence of phosphatidylglycerol at term *indicate fetal lung immaturity and possible respiratory distress syndrome. The expected L/S ratio for the fetus of an insulin-dependent diabetic mother is higher (3.5:1). (See monograph titled "Lecithin/Sphingomyelin Ratio.")*
- *Lamellar bodies are specialized alveolar cells in which lung surfactant is stored.* They are approximately the size of platelets. Their presence in sufficient quantities is an indicator of fetal lung maturity.
- Elevated α_1-fetoprotein levels and presence of acetylcholinesterase *indicate a neural tube defect (see monograph titled "α_1-Fetoprotein"). Elevation of acetylcholinesterase is also indicative of ventral wall defects.*
- Abnormal karyotype *indicates genetic abnormality (e.g., Tay-Sachs disease, mental retardation, chromosome or enzyme anomalies, and inherited hemoglobinopathies).* (See monograph titled "Chromosome Analysis, Blood.")
- Elevated white blood cell count and positive leukocyte esterase *are indicators of infection.*

CRITICAL FINDINGS: N/A

INTERFERING FACTORS

- Bilirubin may be falsely elevated if maternal hemoglobin or meconium is present in the sample; fetal acidosis may also lead to falsely elevated bilirubin levels.
- Bilirubin may be falsely decreased if the sample is exposed to light

or if amniotic fluid volume is excessive.

- Maternal serum creatinine should be measured simultaneously for comparison with amniotic fluid creatinine for proper interpretation. Even in circumstances in which the maternal serum value is normal, the results of the amniotic fluid creatinine may be misleading. A high fluid creatinine value in the fetus of a diabetic mother may reflect the increased muscle mass of a larger fetus. If the fetus is big, the creatinine may be high, and the fetus may still have immature kidneys.
- Contamination of the sample with blood or meconium or complications in pregnancy may yield inaccurate L/S ratios.
- α_1-Fetoprotein and acetylcholinesterase may be falsely elevated if the sample is contaminated with fetal blood.
- Karyotyping cannot be performed under the following conditions: (1) failure to promptly deliver samples for chromosomal analysis to the laboratory performing the test or (2) improper incubation of the sample, which causes cell death.
- Amniocentesis is contraindicated in women with a history of premature labor or incompetent cervix. It is also contraindicated in the presence of placenta previa or abruptio placentae.

NURSING IMPLICATIONS AND PROCEDURE

PRETEST:

- Positively identify the patient using at least two unique identifiers before providing care, treatment, or services.
- *Patient Teaching:* Inform the parent this procedure/test can assist in providing a sample of fluid that will allow for evaluation of fetal well being.

- Obtain a history of the patient's complaints, including a list of known allergens, especially allergies or sensitivities to latex or anesthetics.
- Obtain a history of the patient's reproductive system, previous pregnancies, symptoms, and results of previously performed laboratory tests and diagnostic and surgical procedures. Include any family history of genetic disorders such as cystic fibrosis, Duchenne's muscular dystrophy, hemophilia, sickle cell disease, Tay-Sachs disease, thalassemia, and trisomy 21. Obtain maternal Rh type. If Rh-negative, check for prior sensitization. A standard dose of $Rh_1(D)$ immune globulin Rhogam IM or Rhophylac IM or IV is indicated after amniocentesis; repeat doses should be considered if repeated amniocentesis is performed.
- Note any recent procedures that can interfere with test results.
- Record the date of the last menstrual period and determine the pregnancy weeks' gestation and expected delivery date.
- Obtain a list of the patient's current medications, including herbs, nutritional supplements, and nutraceuticals (see Appendix F).
- Review the procedure with the patient. Warn the patient that normal results do not guarantee a normal fetus. Assure the patient that precautions to avoid injury to the fetus will be taken by localizing the fetus with ultrasound. Address concerns about pain and explain that during the transabdominal procedure, any discomfort associated with a needle biopsy will be minimized with local anesthetics. If the patient is less than 20 weeks' gestation, instruct her to drink extra fluids 1 hr before the test and to refrain from urination. The full bladder assists in raising the uterus up and out of the way to provide better visualization during the ultrasound procedure. Patients who are at 20 weeks' gestation or beyond do not need to drink extra fluids and should void before the test, because an empty bladder is less likely to be accidentally punctured during specimen collection. Encourage relaxation and controlled breathing during the procedure to aid in

reducing any mild discomfort. Inform the patient that specimen collection is performed by a health-care provider (HCP) specializing in this procedure and usually takes approximately 20 to 30 min to complete.

▶ *Sensitivity to social and cultural issues,* as well as concern for modesty, is important in providing psychological support before, during, and after the procedure.

▶ There are no food, fluid, or medication restrictions unless by medical direction.

▶ *Make sure a written and informed consent has been signed prior to the procedure and before administering any medications.*

INTRATEST:

▶ Ensure that the patient has a full bladder before the procedure if gestation is 20 wk or less; have patient void before the procedure if gestation is 21 wk or more.

▶ Positively identify the patient, and label the appropriate collection containers with the corresponding patient demographics, date, time of collection, and site location.

▶ Have patient remove clothes below the waist. Assist the patient to a supine position on the examination table with the abdomen exposed. Drape the patient's legs, leaving the abdomen exposed. Raise her head or legs slightly to promote comfort and to relax the abdominal muscles. If the uterus is large, place a pillow or rolled blanket under the patient's right side to prevent hypertension caused by great-vessel compression. Instruct the patient to cooperate fully and to follow directions. Direct the patient to breathe normally and to avoid unnecessary movement during the local anesthetic and the procedure.

▶ Record maternal and fetal baseline vital signs, and continue to monitor throughout the procedure. Monitor for uterine contractions. Monitor fetal vital signs using ultrasound. Protocols may vary among facilities.

▶ Have emergency equipment readily available.

▶ Observe standard precautions, and follow the general guidelines in Appendix A.

▶ Assess the position of the amniotic fluid, fetus, and placenta using ultrasound.

▶ Assemble the necessary equipment, including an amniocentesis tray with solution for skin preparation, local anesthetic, 10- or 20-mL syringe, needles of various sizes (including a 22-gauge, 5-in. spinal needle), sterile drapes, sterile gloves, and foil-covered or amber-colored specimen collection containers.

▶ Cleanse suprapubic area with an antiseptic solution, and protect with sterile drapes. A local anesthetic is injected. Explain that this may cause a stinging sensation.

▶ A 22-gauge, 5-in. spinal needle is inserted through the abdominal and uterine walls. Explain that a sensation of pressure may be experienced when the needle is inserted. Explain to the patient how to use focused and controlled breathing for relaxation during the procedure.

▶ After the fluid is collected and the needle is withdrawn, apply slight pressure to the site. If there is no evidence of bleeding or other drainage, apply a sterile adhesive bandage to the site.

▶ Monitor the patient for complications related to the procedure (e.g., premature labor, allergic reaction, anaphylaxis).

POST-TEST:

▶ A report of the results will be sent to the requesting HCP, who will discuss the results with the patient.

▶ After the procedure, fetal heart rate and maternal life signs (i.e., heart rate, blood pressure, pulse, and respiration) should be compared with baseline values and closely monitored every 15 min for 30 to 60 min after the amniocentesis procedure. Protocols may vary among facilities.

▶ Observe/assess for delayed allergic reactions, such as rash, urticaria, tachycardia, hyperpnea, hypertension, palpitations, nausea, or vomiting. Immediately report symptoms to the appropriate HCP.

▶ Observe/assess the amniocentesis site for bleeding, inflammation, or hematoma formation.

- Instruct the patient in the care and assessment of the amniocentesis site.
- Instruct the patient to report any redness, edema, bleeding, or pain at the amniocentesis site.
- Instruct the patient to expect mild cramping, leakage of small amounts of amniotic fluid, and vaginal spotting for up to 2 days following the procedure. Instruct the patient to report moderate to severe abdominal pain or cramps, change in fetal activity, increased or prolonged leaking of amniotic fluid from abdominal needle site, vaginal bleeding that is heavier than spotting, and either chills or fever.
- Instruct the patient to rest until all symptoms have disappeared before resuming normal levels of activity.
- Administer standard RhoGAM dose to maternal Rh-negative patients to prevent maternal Rh sensitization should the fetus be Rh-positive.
- Recognize anxiety related to test results. Discuss the implications of abnormal test results on the patient's lifestyle. Provide teaching and information regarding the clinical implications of the test results, as appropriate. Encourage the family to seek appropriate counseling if concerned with pregnancy termination and to seek genetic counseling if a chromosomal abnormality is determined. Decisions regarding elective abortion should take place in the presence of both parents. Provide a nonjudgmental, nonthreatening atmosphere for discussing the risks and difficulties of delivering and raising a developmentally challenged infant as well as for exploring other options

(termination of pregnancy or adoption). It is also important to discuss problems the mother and father may experience (guilt, depression, anger) if fetal abnormalities are detected.
- Reinforce information given by the patient's HCP regarding further testing, treatment, or referral to another HCP. Inform the patient that it may be 2 to 4 wk before all results are available. Answer any questions or address any concerns voiced by the patient or family.
- Instruct the patient in the use of any ordered medications. Explain the importance of adhering to the therapy regimen. As appropriate, instruct the patient in significant side effects and systemic reactions associated with the prescribed medication. Encourage her to review corresponding literature provided by a pharmacist.
- Depending on the results of this procedure, additional testing may be performed to evaluate or monitor progression of the disease process and determine the need for a change in therapy. Evaluate test results in relation to the patient's symptoms and other tests performed.

RELATED MONOGRAPHS:
- Related tests include α_1-fetoprotein, antibodies anticardiolipin, blood groups and antibodies, chromosome analysis, fetal fibronectin, Kleihauer-Betke test, L/S ratio, lupus anticoagulant antibodies, and US biophysical profile obstetric.
- Refer to the Reproductive System table at the end of the book for related tests by body system.

Amylase

SYNONYM/ACRONYM: N/A.

COMMON USE: To assist in diagnosis and evaluation of the treatment modalities used for pancreatitis.

SPECIMEN: Serum (1 mL) collected in a red- or tiger-top tube. Plasma (1 mL) collected in a green-top (heparin) tube is also acceptable.

REFERENCE VALUE: (Method: Spectrophotometry)

Conventional & SI Units
30–110 units/L

Values may be slightly elevated in older adults due to the effects of medications and the presence of multiple chronic or acute diseases with or without muted symptoms.

DESCRIPTION: Amylase, a digestive enzyme, splits starch into disaccharides. Although many cells (e.g., liver, small intestine, ovaries, skeletal muscles) have amylase activity, circulating amylase is derived from the parotid glands and the pancreas. Amylase is a sensitive indicator of pancreatic acinar cell damage and pancreatic obstruction. Newborns and children up to 2 years old have little measurable serum amylase. In the early years of life, most of this enzyme is produced by the salivary glands. Amylase can be separated into pancreatic (P_1, P_2, P_3) and salivary (S_1, S_2, S_3) isoenzymes. Isoenzyme patterns are useful in identifying the organ source. Requests for amylase isoenzymes are rare because of the expense of the procedure and limited clinical utility of the result. Isoenzyme analysis is primarily used to assess decreasing pancreatic function in children 5 years and older who have been diagnosed with cystic fibrosis and who may be candidates for enzyme replacement. Cyst fluid amylase levels with isoenzyme analysis is useful in differentiating pancreatic neoplasms (low enzyme concentration) and pseudocysts (high enzyme concentration). Lipase is usually ordered in conjunction with amylase because lipase is more sensitive and specific to conditions affecting pancreatic function.

INDICATIONS
- Assist in the diagnosis of early acute pancreatitis; serum amylase begins to rise within 6 to 24 hr after onset and returns to normal in 2 to 7 days
- Assist in the diagnosis of macroamylasemia, a disorder seen in alcoholism, malabsorption syndrome, and other digestive problems
- Assist in the diagnosis of pancreatic duct obstruction, which causes serum amylase levels to remain elevated
- Detect blunt trauma or inadvertent surgical trauma to the pancreas
- Differentiate between acute pancreatitis and other causes of abdominal pain that require surgery

POTENTIAL DIAGNOSIS

Increased in
Amylase is released from any damaged cell in which it is stored, so conditions that affect the pancreas and parotid glands and cause cellular destruction demonstrate elevated amylase levels.
- Acute appendicitis *(related to enzyme release from damaged pancreatic tissue)*
- Administration of some drugs (e.g., morphine) is known to increase amylase levels *(related to increased biliary tract pressure as evidenced by effect of narcotic analgesic drugs)*

- Afferent loop syndrome *(related to impaired pancreatic duct flow)*
- Aortic aneurysm *(elevated amylase levels following rupture are associated with a poor prognosis; both S and P subtypes have been identified following rupture. The causes for elevation are mixed and difficult to state as a generalization)*
- Abdominal trauma *(related to release of enzyme from damaged pancreatic tissue)*
- Alcoholism *(related to increased secretion; salivary origin most likely)*
- Biliary tract disease *(related to impaired pancreatic duct flow)*
- Burns and traumatic shock
- Carcinoma of the head of the pancreas (advanced) *(related to enzyme release from damaged pancreatic tissue)*
- Common bile duct obstruction, common bile duct stones *(related to impaired pancreatic duct flow)*
- Diabetic ketoacidosis *(related to increased secretion; salivary origin most likely)*
- Duodenal obstruction *(accumulation in the blood as evidenced by leakage from the gut)*
- Ectopic pregnancy *(related to ectopic enzyme production by the fallopian tubes)*
- Extrapancreatic tumors (especially esophagus, lung, ovary)
- Gastric resection *(accumulation in the blood as evidenced by leakage from the gut)*
- Hyperlipidemias (etiology is unclear, but there is a distinct association with amylasemia)
- Hyperparathyroidism (etiology is unclear, but there is a distinct association with amylasemia)
- Intestinal obstruction *(related to impaired pancreatic duct flow)*

- Intestinal infarction *(related to impaired pancreatic duct flow)*
- Macroamylasemia *(related to decreased ability of renal glomeruli to filter large molecules as evidenced by accumulation in the blood)*
- Mumps *(related to increased secretion from inflamed tissue; salivary origin most likely)*
- Pancreatic ascites *(related to release of pancreatic fluid into the abdomen and subsequent absorption into the circulation)*
- Pancreatic cyst and pseudocyst *(related to release of pancreatic fluid into the abdomen and subsequent absorption into the circulation)*
- Pancreatitis *(related to enzyme release from damaged pancreatic tissue)*
- Parotitis *(related to increased secretion from inflamed tissue; salivary origin most likely)*
- Perforated peptic ulcer whether the pancreas is involved or not *(related to enzyme release from damaged pancreatic tissue; involvement of the pancreas may be unnoticed upon gross examination yet be present as indicated by elevated enzyme levels)*
- Peritonitis *(accumulation in the blood as evidenced by leakage from the gut)*
- Postoperative period *(related to complications of the surgical procedure)*
- Pregnancy *(related to increased secretion; salivary origin most likely related to hyperemesis or hyperlipidemia induced pancreatitis related to increased estrogen levels)*
- Renal disease *(related to decreased renal excretion as evidenced by accumulation in blood)*

- Some tumors of the lung and ovaries *(related to ectopic enzyme production)*
- Tumor of the pancreas or adjacent area *(related to release of enzyme from damaged pancreatic tissue)*

Decreased in

- Hepatic disease (severe) *(may be due to lack of amino acid production necessary for enzyme manufacture)*
- Pancreatectomy
- Pancreatic insufficiency

CRITICAL FINDINGS: N/A

INTERFERING FACTORS

- Drugs and substances that may increase amylase levels include acetaminophen, aminosalicylic acid, amoxapine, asparaginase, azathioprine, bethanechol, calcitriol, cholinergics, chlorthalidone, clozapine, codeine, corticosteroids, corticotropin, desipramine, dexamethasone, diazoxide, felbamate, fentanyl, fluvastatin, glucocorticoids, hydantoin derivatives, hydrochlorothiazide, hydroflumethiazide, meperidine, mercaptopurine, methacholine, methyclothiazide, metolazone, minocycline, morphine, nitrofurantoin, opium alkaloids, pegaspargase, pentazocine, potassium iodide, prednisone, procyclidine, tetracycline, thiazide diuretics, valproic acid, zalcitabine, and zidovudine.
- Drugs that may decrease amylase levels include anabolic steroids, citrates, and fluorides.

NURSING IMPLICATIONS AND PROCEDURE

PRETEST:

▸ Positively identify the patient using at least two unique identifiers before providing care, treatment, or services.

▸ *Patient Teaching:* Inform the patient this test can assist in evaluating pancreatic health and/or the effectiveness of medical treatment for pancreatitis.
▸ Obtain a history of the patient's complaints, including a list of known allergens, especially allergies or sensitivities to latex.
▸ Obtain a history of the patient's gastrointestinal and hepatobiliary systems, symptoms, and results of previously performed laboratory tests and diagnostic and surgical procedures.
▸ Obtain a list of the patient's current medications, including herbs, nutritional supplements, and nutraceuticals (see Appendix F).
▸ Review the procedure with the patient. Inform the patient that specimen collection takes approximately 5 to 10 min. Address concerns about pain and explain that there may be some discomfort during the venipuncture.
▸ *Sensitivity to social and cultural issues,* as well as concern for modesty, is important in providing psychological support before, during, and after the procedure.
▸ There are no food, fluid, or medication restrictions unless by medical direction.

INTRATEST:

▸ If the patient has a history of allergic reaction to latex, avoid the use of equipment containing latex.
▸ Instruct the patient to cooperate fully and to follow directions. Direct the patient to breathe normally and to avoid unnecessary movement.
▸ Observe standard precautions, and follow the general guidelines in Appendix A. Positively identify the patient, and label the appropriate tubes with the corresponding patient demographics, date, and time of collection. Perform a venipuncture.
▸ Remove the needle and apply direct pressure with dry gauze to stop bleeding. Observe/assess venipuncture site for bleeding or hematoma formation and secure gauze with adhesive bandage.
▸ Promptly transport the specimen to the laboratory for processing and analysis.

POST-TEST:

- A report of the results will be sent to the requesting health-care provider (HCP), who will discuss the results with the patient.
- *Nutritional Considerations:* Increased amylase levels may be associated with gastrointestinal disease or alcoholism. Small, frequent meals work best for patients with gastrointestinal disorders. Consideration should be given to dietary alterations in the case of gastrointestinal disorders. Usually after acute symptoms subside and bowel sounds return, patients are given a clear liquid diet, progressing to a low-fat, high-carbohydrate diet. Vitamin B_{12} may be ordered for parenteral administration to patients with decreased levels, especially if their disease prevents adequate absorption of the vitamin. The alcoholic patient should be encouraged to avoid alcohol and to seek appropriate counseling for substance abuse.
- Reinforce information given by the patient's HCP regarding further testing, treatment, or referral to another HCP. Answer any questions or address any concerns voiced by the patient or family.
- Depending on the results of this procedure, additional testing may be performed to evaluate or monitor progression of the disease process and determine the need for a change in therapy. Evaluate test results in relation to the patient's symptoms and other tests performed.

RELATED MONOGRAPHS:

- Related tests include ALT, ALP, AST, bilirubin, cancer antigens, calcium, C-peptide, CBC WBC count and differential, CT pancreas, ERCP, fecal fat, GGT, lipase, magnesium, MRI pancreas, mumps serology, peritoneal fluid analysis, triglycerides, and US pancreas.
- See the Gastrointestinal and Hepatobiliary systems tables at the end of the book for related tests by body system.

Analgesic and Antipyretic Drugs: Acetaminophen, Acetylsalicylic Acid

SYNONYM/ACRONYM: *Acetaminophen* (Acephen, Aceta, Apacet, APAP 500, Aspirin Free Anacin, Banesin, Cetaphen, Dapa, Datril, Dorcol, Exocrine, FeverALL, Genapap, Genebs, Halenol, Little Fevers, Liquiprin, Mapap, Myapap, Nortemp, Pain Eze, Panadol, Paracetamol, Redutemp, Ridenol, Silapap, Tempra, Tylenol, Ty-Pap, Uni-Ace, Valorin); *Acetylsalicylic acid* (salicylate, aspirin, Anacin, Aspergum, Bufferin, Easprin, Ecotrin, Empirin, Measurin, Synalgos, ZORprin, ASA).

COMMON USE: To assist in monitoring therapeutic drug levels and detect toxic levels of acetaminophen and salicylate in suspected overdose and drug abuse.

SPECIMEN: Serum (1 mL) collected in a red-top tube.

REFERENCE VALUE: (Method: Immunoassay)

Drug	Therapeutic Dose*	SI Units	Half-Life	Volume of Distribution	Protein Binding	Excretion
(SI = Conventional Units × 6.62)						
Acetamino-phen	10–30 mcg/mL	66–199 micromol/L	1–3 hr	0.95 L/kg	20%–50%	85%–95% hepatic, metabo-lites, renal
(SI = Conventional Units × 0.073)						
Salicylate	15–20 mg/dL	1.1–1.4 mmol/L	2–3 hr	0.1–0.3 L/kg	90%–95%	1° hepatic, metabo-lites, renal

*Conventional units.

DESCRIPTION: Acetaminophen is used for headache, fever, and pain relief, especially for individuals unable to take salicylate products or who have bleeding conditions. It is the analgesic of choice for children less than 13 yr old; salicylates are avoided in this age group because of the association between aspirin and Reye's syndrome. Acetaminophen is rapidly absorbed from the gastro-intestinal tract and reaches peak concentration within 30 to 60 min after administration of a therapeu-tic dose. It can be a silent killer because, by the time symptoms of intoxication appear 24 to 48 hr after ingestion, the antidote is inef-fective. Acetylsalicylic acid (ASA) is also used for headache, fever, and pain relief. Some patients with cardiovascular disease take small prophylactic doses. The main site of toxicity for both drugs is the liver, particularly in the presence of liver disease or decreased drug metabolism and excretion.

Many factors must be consid-ered in interpreting drug levels, including patient age, patient weight, interacting medications, electrolyte balance, protein levels, water balance, conditions that affect absorption and excretion, and the ingestion of substances (e.g., foods, herbals, vitamins, and minerals) that can potentiate or inhibit the intended target concentration.

INDICATIONS
- Suspected overdose
- Suspected toxicity
- Therapeutic monitoring

POTENTIAL DIAGNOSIS

Increased in
- Acetaminophen
  Alcoholic cirrhosis *(related to inability of damaged liver to metabolize the drug)*
  Liver disease *(related to inability of damaged liver to metabolize the drug)*
  Toxicity
- ASA
  Toxicity

Decreased in
- Noncompliance with therapeutic regimen

CRITICAL FINDINGS

Note: The adverse effects of subtherapeutic levels are also important. Care should be taken to investigate signs and symptoms of too little and too much medication. Note and immediately report to the health-care practitioner (HCP) any critically increased or subtherapeutic values and related symptoms.

Acetaminophen: Greater Than 150 mcg/mL (4 hr postingestion); Greater Than 50 mcg/mL (12 hr postingestion)

Signs and symptoms of acetaminophen intoxication occur in stages over a period of time. In stage I (0 to 24 hr after ingestion), symptoms may include gastrointestinal irritation, pallor, lethargy, diaphoresis, metabolic acidosis, and possibly coma. In stage II (24 to 48 hr after ingestion), signs and symptoms may include right upper quadrant abdominal pain; elevated liver enzymes, aspartate aminotransferase (AST), and alanine aminotransferase (ALT); and possible decreased renal function. In stage III (72 to 96 hr after ingestion), signs and symptoms may include nausea, vomiting, jaundice, confusion, coagulation disorders, continued elevation of AST and ALT, decreased renal function, and coma. Intervention may include gastrointestinal decontamination (stomach pumping) if the patient presents within 6 hr of ingestion or administration of *N*-acetylcysteine (Mucomyst) in the case of an acute intoxication in which the patient presents more than 6 hr after ingestion.

ASA: Greater Than 50 mg/dL

Signs and symptoms of salicylate intoxication include ketosis, convulsions, dizziness, nausea, vomiting, hyperactivity, hyperglycemia, hyperpnea, hyperthermia, respiratory arrest, and tinnitus. Possible interventions include administration of activated charcoal as vomiting ceases, alkalinization of the urine with bicarbonate, and a single dose of vitamin K (for rare instances of hypoprothrombinemia).

INTERFERING FACTORS

- Blood drawn in serum separator tubes (gel tubes).
- Contraindicated in patients with liver disease, and caution advised in patients with renal impairment.
- Drugs that may increase acetaminophen levels include diflunisal, metoclopramide, and probenecid.
- Drugs that may decrease acetaminophen levels include carbamazepine, cholestyramine, iron, oral contraceptives, and propantheline.
- Drugs that increase ASA levels include choline magnesium trisalicylate, cimetidine, furosemide, and sulfinpyrazone.
- Drugs and substances that decrease ASA levels include activated charcoal, antacids (aluminum hydroxide), corticosteroids, and iron.

NURSING IMPLICATIONS AND PROCEDURE

PRETEST:

- Positively identify the patient using at least two unique identifiers before providing care, treatment, or services.
- *Patient Teaching:* Inform the patient this test can assist with evaluation of how much medication is in his or her system.
- Obtain a complete history of the time and amount of drug ingested by the patient.

A

▶ Obtain a history of the patient's complaints, including a list of known allergens, especially allergies or sensitivities to latex.

▶ Review results of previously performed laboratory tests and diagnostic and surgical procedures.

▶ These medications are metabolized and excreted by the kidneys and liver. Obtain a history of the patient's genitourinary and hepatobiliary systems, symptoms, and results of previously performed laboratory tests and diagnostic and surgical procedures.

▶ Obtain a list of the patient's current medications, including herbs, nutritional supplements, and nutraceuticals (see Appendix F).

▶ Review the procedure with the patient. Inform the patient that specimen collection takes approximately 5 to 10 min. Address concerns about pain and explain that there may be some discomfort during the venipuncture.

▶ *Sensitivity to social and cultural issues,* as well as concern for modesty, is important in providing psychological support before, during, and after the procedure.

▶ There are no food, fluid, or medication restrictions unless by medical direction.

INTRATEST:

▶ If the patient has a history of allergic reaction to latex, avoid the use of equipment containing latex.

▶ Instruct the patient to cooperate fully and to follow directions. Direct the patient to breathe normally and to avoid unnecessary movement.

▶ Observe standard precautions, and follow the general guidelines in Appendix A. Positively identify the patient, and label the appropriate tubes with the corresponding patient demographics, date, and time of collection, noting the last dose of medication taken. Perform a venipuncture.

▶ Remove the needle and apply direct pressure with dry gauze to stop the bleeding. Observe/assess the venipuncture site for bleeding and hematoma formation and secure gauze with adhesive bandage.

▶ Promptly transport the specimen to the laboratory for processing and analysis.

POST-TEST:

▶ A report of the results will be sent to the requesting HCP, who will discuss the results with the patient.

▶ *Nutritional Considerations:* include avoidance of alcohol consumption.

▶ Reinforce information given by the patient's HCP regarding further testing, treatment, or referral to another HCP. Explain to the patient the importance of following the medication regimen and instructions regarding food and drug interactions. Answer any questions or address any concerns voiced by the patient or family.

▶ Instruct the patient to be prepared to provide the pharmacist with a list of other medications he or she is already taking in the event that the requesting HCP prescribes a medication.

▶ Depending on the results of this procedure, additional testing may be performed to evaluate or monitor progression of the disease process and determine the need for a change in therapy. Evaluate test results in relation to the patient's symptoms and other tests performed.

RELATED MONOGRAPHS:

▶ Related tests include ALT, AST, bilirubin, biopsy liver, BUN, CBC, creatinine, electrolytes, glucose, lactic acid, aPTT, and PT/INR.

▶ See the Genitourinary and Hepatobiliary systems tables at the end of the book for related tests by body system.

Angiography, Abdomen

SYNONYM/ACRONYM: Abdominal angiogram, abdominal arteriography.

COMMON USE: Visualize and assess abdominal organs/structure for tumor, infection, or aneurysm.

AREA OF APPLICATION: Abdomen.

CONTRAST: Intravenous iodine based.

DESCRIPTION: Angiography allows x-ray visualization of the large and small arteries, veins, and associated branches of the abdominal vasculature and organ parenchyma after contrast medium injection. This visualization is accomplished by the injection of contrast medium through a catheter, which most commonly has been inserted into the femoral artery and advanced through the iliac artery and aorta into the organ-specific artery. Images of the organ under study and associated vessels are displayed on a monitor and recorded or stored electronically for future viewing and evaluation. Patterns of circulation, organ function, and changes in vessel wall appearance can be viewed to help diagnose the presence of vascular abnormalities, aneurysm, tumor, trauma, or lesions. The catheter used to administer the contrast medium to confirm the diagnosis of organ lesions may be used to deliver chemotherapeutic drugs or different types of materials used to stop bleeding. Catheters with attached inflatable balloons and wire mesh stents are used to widen areas of stenosis and to keep vessels open, frequently replacing surgery. Angiography is one of the definitive tests for organ disease and may be used to evaluate chronic disease and organ failure, treat arterial stenosis, differentiate a vascular cyst from hypervascular cancers, and evaluate the effectiveness of medical or surgical treatment.

INDICATIONS
- Aid in angioplasty, atherectomy, or stent placement
- Allow infusion of thrombolytic drugs into an occluded artery
- Detect arterial occlusion, which may be evidenced by a transection of the artery caused by trauma or penetrating injury
- Detect artery stenosis, evidenced by vessel dilation, collateral vessels, or increased vascular pressure
- Detect nonmalignant tumors before surgical resection
- Detect thrombosis, arteriovenous fistula, aneurysms, or emboli in abdominal vessels
- Detect tumors and arterial supply, extent of venous invasion, and tumor vascularity
- Differentiate between tumors and cysts

- Evaluate organ transplantation for function or organ rejection
- Evaluate placement of a shunt or stent
- Evaluate tumor vascularity before surgery or embolization
- Evaluate the vascular system of prospective organ donors before surgery

POTENTIAL DIAGNOSIS

Normal findings in
- Normal structure, function, and patency of abdominal organ vessels
- Contrast medium normally circulates throughout abdomen symmetrically and without interruption
- No evidence of obstruction, variations in number and size of vessels, malformations, cysts, or tumors

Abnormal findings in
- Abscess or inflammation
- Arterial aneurysm
- Arterial stenosis, dysplasia, or organ infarction
- Arteriovenous fistula or other abnormalities
- Congenital anomalies
- Cysts or tumors
- Trauma causing tears or other disruption

CRITICAL FINDINGS
- Abscess
- Aneurysm

It is essential that critical diagnoses be communicated immediately to the appropriate health-care provider (HCP). A listing of these diagnoses varies among facilities. Note and immediately report to the HCP abnormal results and related symptoms.

INTERFERING FACTORS

This procedure is contraindicated for
- Patients with allergies to shellfish or iodinated contrast medium. The contrast medium used may cause a life-threatening allergic reaction. Patients with a known hypersensitivity to contrast medium may benefit from premedication with corticosteroids or the use of nonionic contrast medium.
- Patients with bleeding disorders.
- Patients who are pregnant or suspected of being pregnant, unless the potential benefits of the procedure far outweigh the risk of radiation exposure to the fetus.
- Elderly and compromised patients who are chronically dehydrated before the test, because of their risk of contrast-induced renal failure.
- Patients who are in renal failure.

Factors that may impair clear imaging
- Gas or feces in the gastrointestinal tract resulting from inadequate cleansing or failure to restrict food intake before the study.
- Retained barium from a previous radiological procedure.
- Metallic objects within the examination field (e.g., jewelry, body rings), which may inhibit organ visualization and can produce unclear images.
- Inability of the patient to cooperate or remain still during the procedure because of age, significant pain, or mental status.

Other considerations
- Consultation with an HCP should occur before the procedure for radiation safety concerns regarding younger patients or patients who are lactating.
- Risks associated with radiation overexposure can result from frequent x-ray procedures. Personnel in the room with the patient should wear a protective lead apron, stand behind a shield,

or leave the area while the examination is being done. Personnel working in the examination area should wear badges to record their level of radiation exposure.

- Failure to follow dietary restrictions and other pretesting preparations may cause the procedure to be canceled or repeated.

NURSING IMPLICATIONS AND PROCEDURE

PRETEST:

▶ Positively identify the patient using at least two unique identifiers before providing care, treatment, or services.

▶ *Patient Teaching:* Inform the patient this procedure can assist with the evaluation of abdominal organs.

▶ Obtain a history of the patient's complaints, including a list of known allergens, especially allergies or sensitivities to latex, iodine, seafood, contrast medium, or anesthetics.

▶ Obtain a history of the patient's cardiovascular system, symptoms, and results of previously performed laboratory tests and diagnostic and surgical procedures. Ensure results of coagulation testing are obtained and recorded prior to the procedure; BUN and creatinine results are also needed because contrast medium is to be used.

▶ Note any recent procedures that can interfere with test results, including examinations using iodine-based contrast medium or barium. Ensure that barium studies were performed more than 4 days before angiography.

▶ Record the date of the last menstrual period and determine the possibility of pregnancy in perimenopausal women.

▶ Obtain a list of the patient's current medications, including anticoagulants, aspirin and other salicylates, herbs, nutritional supplements, and nutraceuticals, especially those known to affect coagulation (see Appendix F). Such products should be discontinued by medical direction for the appropriate number of days prior to a surgical procedure. Note the last time and dose of medication taken.

▶ If contrast medium is scheduled to be used, patients receiving metformin (Glucophage) for non-insulin-dependent (type 2) diabetes should discontinue the drug on the day of the test and continue to withhold it for 48 hr after the test. Failure to do so may result in lactic acidosis.

▶ Review the procedure with the patient. Address concerns about pain and explain that there may be moments of discomfort and some pain experienced during the test. Inform the patient that the procedure is usually performed in a radiology or vascular suite by an HCP and takes approximately 30 to 60 min.

▶ *Sensitivity to social and cultural issues,* as well as concern for modesty, is important in providing psychological support before, during, and after the procedure.

▶ Explain that an IV line may be inserted to allow infusion of IV fluids, contrast medium, dye, or sedatives. Usually normal saline is infused.

▶ Inform the patient that a burning and flushing sensation may be felt throughout the body during injection of the contrast medium. After injection of the contrast medium, the patient may experience an urge to cough, flushing, nausea, or a salty or metallic taste.

▶ Instruct the patient to remove jewelry and other metallic objects from the area to be examined.

▶ Instruct the patient to fast and restrict fluids for 2 to 4 hr prior to the procedure. Protocols may vary among facilities.

▶ This procedure may be terminated if chest pain, severe cardiac arrhythmias, or signs of a cerebrovascular accident occur.

▶ *Make sure a written and informed consent has been signed prior to the procedure and before administering any medications.*

INTRATEST:

▶ Ensure the patient has complied with dietary and fluid restrictions for 2 to 4 hr prior to the procedure.

▶ Ensure the patient has removed all external metallic objects from the area to be examined.

If the patient has a history of allergic reactions to any substance or drug, administer ordered prophylactic steroids or antihistamines before the procedure. Use nonionic contrast medium for the procedure.

Have emergency equipment readily available.

Instruct the patient to void prior to the procedure and to change into the gown, robe, and foot coverings provided.

Instruct the patient to cooperate fully and to follow directions. Instruct the patient to remain still throughout the procedure because movement produces unreliable results.

Record baseline vital signs, and assess neurological status. Protocols may vary among facilities.

Observe standard precautions, and follow the general guidelines in Appendix A.

Establish an IV fluid line for the injection of emergency drugs and of sedatives.

Administer an antianxiety agent, as ordered, if the patient has claustrophobia. Administer a sedative to a child or to an uncooperative adult, as ordered.

Place electrocardiographic electrodes on the patient for cardiac monitoring. Establish a baseline rhythm; determine if the patient has ventricular arrhythmias.

Using a pen, mark the site of the patient's peripheral pulses before angiography; this allows for quicker and more consistent assessment of the pulses after the procedure.

Place the patient in the supine position on an examination table. Cleanse the selected area, and cover with a sterile drape.

A local anesthetic is injected at the site, and a small incision is made or a needle inserted under fluoroscopy.

The contrast medium is injected, and a rapid series of images is taken during and after the filling of the vessels to be examined. Delayed images may be taken to examine the vessels after a time and to monitor the venous phase of the procedure.

Instruct the patient to inhale deeply and hold his or her breathe while the images are taken, and then to exhale after the images are taken.

Instruct the patient to take slow, deep breaths if nausea occurs during the procedure.

Monitor the patient for complications related to the procedure (e.g., allergic reaction, anaphylaxis, bronchospasm).

The needle or catheter is removed, and a pressure dressing is applied over the puncture site.

Observe/assess the needle/catheter insertion site for bleeding, inflammation, or hematoma formation.

POST-TEST:

A report of the examination will be sent to the requesting HCP, who will discuss the results with the patient.

Instruct the patient to resume usual diet, fluids, medications, or activity, as directed by the HCP. Renal function should be assessed before metformin is resumed.

Monitor vital signs and neurological status every 15 min for 1 hr, then every 2 hr for 4 hr, and as ordered. Take temperature every 4 hr for 24 hr. Monitor intake and output at least every 8 hr. Compare with baseline values. Protocols may vary among facilities.

Observe for delayed allergic reactions, such as rash, urticaria, tachycardia, hyperpnea, hypertension, palpitations, nausea, or vomiting.

Instruct the patient to immediately report symptoms such as fast heart rate, difficulty breathing, skin rash, itching, chest pain, persistent right shoulder pain, or abdominal pain. Immediately report symptoms to the appropriate HCP.

Assess extremities for signs of ischemia or absence of distal pulse caused by a catheter-induced thrombus.

Observe/assess the needle/catheter insertion site for bleeding, inflammation, or hematoma formation.

Instruct the patient in the care and assessment of the site.

Instruct the patient to apply cold compresses to the puncture site as needed, to reduce discomfort or edema.

- Instruct the patient to maintain bedrest for 4 to 6 hr after the procedure or as ordered.
- Recognize anxiety related to test results, and be supportive of perceived loss of independent function. Discuss the implications of abnormal test results on the patient's lifestyle. Provide teaching and information regarding the clinical implications of the test results, as appropriate.
- Reinforce information given by the patient's HCP regarding further testing, treatment, or referral to another HCP. Answer any questions or address any concerns voiced by the patient or family.
- Depending on the results of this procedure, additional testing may be performed to evaluate or monitor progression of the disease process and determine the need for a change in therapy. Evaluate test results in relation to the patient's symptoms and other tests performed.

RELATED MONOGRAPHS:

- Related tests include angiography renal, BUN, CT abdomen, CT angiography, CT brain, CT spleen, CT thoracic, creatinine, KUB, MRA, MRI abdomen, MRI brain, MRI chest, MRI pelvis, aPTT, PT/INR, renogram, and US lower extremity.
- See the Cardiovascular System table at the end of the book for related tests by body system.

Angiography, Adrenal

SYNONYM/ACRONYM: Adrenal angiogram, adrenal arteriography.

COMMON USE: To visualize and assess the adrenal gland for cancer or other tumors or masses.

AREA OF APPLICATION: Adrenal gland.

CONTRAST: Intravenous iodine based.

DESCRIPTION: Adrenal angiography evaluates adrenal dysfunction by allowing x-ray visualization of the large and small arteries of the adrenal gland vasculature and parenchyma. This visualization is accomplished by the injection of contrast medium through a catheter that has been inserted into the femoral artery for viewing the artery (arteriography) or into the femoral vein for viewing the veins (venography). After the catheter is in place, a blood sample may be taken from the vein of each gland to assess cortisol levels in determining a diagnosis of Cushing's syndrome or the presence of pheochromocytoma. After injection of the contrast medium through the catheter, images of the adrenal glands and associated vessels surrounding the adrenal tissue are displayed on a monitor and are recorded on film or electronically. Patterns of circulation, adrenal function, and changes in vessel wall appearance can be viewed to help diagnose the presence of vascular abnormalities, trauma, or lesions. This definitive test for adrenal disease may be used to evaluate chronic adrenal disease, evaluate arterial or venous stenosis, differentiate an adrenal cyst from adrenal tumors, and evaluate medical therapy or surgery of the adrenal glands.

INDICATIONS

• Assist in the infusion of thrombolytic drugs into an occluded artery
• Assist with the collection of blood samples from the vein for laboratory analysis
• Detect adrenal hyperplasia
• Detect and determine the location of adrenal tumors evidenced by arterial supply, extent of venous invasion, and tumor vascularity
• Detect arterial occlusion, evidenced by a transection of the artery caused by trauma or a penetrating injury
• Detect arterial stenosis, evidenced by vessel dilation, collateral vessels, or increased vascular pressure
• Detect nonmalignant tumors before surgical resection
• Detect thrombosis, arteriovenous fistula, aneurysms, or emboli in vessels
• Differentiate between adrenal tumors and adrenal cysts
• Evaluate tumor vascularity before surgery or embolization
• Perform angioplasty, perform atherectomy, or place a stent

POTENTIAL DIAGNOSIS

Normal findings in

• Normal structure, function, and patency of adrenal vessels
• Contrast medium circulating throughout the adrenal gland symmetrically and without interruption

• No evidence of obstruction, variations in number and size of vessels and organs, malformations, cysts, or tumors

Abnormal findings in

• Adrenal adenoma
• Adrenal carcinoma
• Bilateral adrenal hyperplasia
• Pheochromocytoma

CRITICAL FINDINGS: N/A

INTERFERING FACTORS

This procedure is contraindicated for

• Patients with allergies to shellfish or iodinated dye. The contrast medium used may cause a life-threatening allergic reaction. Patients with a known hypersensitivity to contrast medium may benefit from premedication with corticosteroids or the use of nonionic contrast medium.
• Patients with bleeding disorders.
• Patients who are pregnant or suspected of being pregnant, unless the potential benefits of the procedure far outweigh the risks to the fetus and mother.
• Elderly and other patients who are chronically dehydrated before the test, because of their risk of contrast-induced renal failure.
• Patients who are in renal failure.

Factors that may impair clear imaging

• Gas or feces in the gastrointestinal tract resulting from inadequate cleansing or failure to restrict food intake before the study.
• Retained barium from a previous radiological procedure.
• Metallic objects within the examination field (e.g., jewelry, body rings), which may inhibit organ visualization and can produce unclear images.

- Inability of the patient to cooperate or remain still during the procedure because of age, significant pain, or mental status.

Other considerations

- Consultation with a health-care provider (HCP) should occur before the procedure for radiation safety concerns regarding younger patients or patients who are lactating.
- Risks associated with radiation overexposure can result from frequent x-ray procedures. Personnel in the examination room with the patient should wear a protective lead apron, stand behind a shield, or leave the area while the examination is being done. Personnel working in the examination area should wear badges to record their level of radiation exposure.
- Failure to follow dietary restrictions and other pretesting preparations may cause the procedure to be canceled or repeated.

NURSING IMPLICATIONS AND PROCEDURE

PRETEST:

▶ Positively identify the patient using at least two unique identifiers before providing care, treatment, or services.

▶ *Patient Teaching:* Inform the patient this procedure can assist with evaluation of the adrenal gland (located near the kidney).

▶ Obtain a history of the patient's complaints, including a list of known allergens (especially allergies or sensitivities to latex, iodine, seafood, anesthetics, or contrast medium).

▶ Obtain a history of the patient's endocrine system, symptoms, and results of previously performed laboratory tests and diagnostic and surgical procedures. Ensure results of coagulation testing are obtained and recorded prior to the procedure; BUN and creatinine results are also needed if contrast medium is to be used.

▶ Note any recent procedures that can interfere with test results, including examinations using iodine-based contrast medium or barium. Ensure that barium studies were performed more than 4 days before angiography.

▶ Record the date of the last menstrual period and determine the possibility of pregnancy in perimenopausal women.

▶ Obtain a list of the patient's current medications, including anticoagulants, aspirin and other salicylates, herbs, nutritional supplements, and nutraceuticals, especially those known to affect coagulation (see Appendix F). Such products should be discontinued by medical direction for the appropriate number of days prior to a surgical procedure. Note the last time and dose of medication taken.

▶ If contrast medium is scheduled to be used, patients receiving metformin (Glucophage) for non-insulin-dependent (type 2) diabetes should discontinue the drug on the day of the test and continue to withhold it for 48 hr after the test. Failure to do so may result in lactic acidosis.

▶ Review the procedure with the patient. Address concerns about pain and explain that there may be moments of discomfort and some pain experienced during the test. Inform the patient that the procedure is usually performed in a radiology or vascular suite by an HCP and takes approximately 30 to 60 min.

▶ *Sensitivity to social and cultural issues,* as well as concern for modesty, is important in providing psychological support before, during, and after the procedure.

▶ Explain that an IV line may be inserted to allow infusion of IV fluids, contrast medium, dye, or sedatives. Usually normal saline is infused.

▶ Inform the patient that a burning and flushing sensation may be felt throughout the body during injection of the contrast medium. After injection of the contrast medium, the patient may experience an urge to cough, flushing, nausea, or a salty or metallic taste.

◆ Instruct the patient to remove jewelry and other metallic objects from the area to be examined.

◆ Instruct the patient to fast and restrict fluids for 2 to 4 hr prior to the procedure. Protocols may vary among facilities.

◆ This procedure may be terminated if chest pain, severe cardiac arrhythmias, or signs of a cerebrovascular accident occur.

◆ *Make sure a written and informed consent has been signed prior to the procedure and before administering any medications.*

INTRATEST:

◆ Ensure the patient has complied with dietary, fluid, and medication restrictions and pretesting preparations.

◆ Ensure the patient has removed all external metallic objects from the area to be examined.

◆ If the patient has a history of allergic reactions to any substance or drug, administer ordered prophylactic steroids or antihistamines before the procedure. Use nonionic contrast medium for the procedure.

◆ Have emergency equipment readily available.

◆ Instruct the patient to void prior to the procedure and to change into the gown, robe, and foot coverings provided.

◆ Instruct the patient to cooperate fully and to follow directions. Instruct the patient to remain still throughout the procedure because movement produces unreliable results.

◆ Record baseline vital signs, and continue to monitor throughout the procedure. Protocols may vary among facilities.

◆ Observe standard precautions, and follow the general guidelines in Appendix A.

◆ Establish an IV fluid line for the injection of emergency drugs and of sedatives.

◆ Administer an antianxiety agent, as ordered, if the patient has claustrophobia. Administer a sedative to a child or to an uncooperative adult, as ordered.

◆ Place electrocardiographic electrodes on the patient for cardiac monitoring.

Establish a baseline rhythm; determine if the patient has ventricular arrhythmias.

◆ Using a pen, mark the site of the patient's peripheral pulses before angiography; this allows for quicker and more consistent assessment of the pulses after the procedure.

◆ Place the patient in the supine position on an examination table. Cleanse the selected area, and cover with a sterile drape.

◆ A local anesthetic is injected at the site, and a small incision is made or a needle inserted under fluoroscopy.

◆ The contrast medium is injected, and a rapid series of images is taken during and after the filling of the vessels to be examined. Delayed images may be taken to examine the vessels after a time and to monitor the venous phase of the procedure.

◆ Instruct the patient to inhale deeply and hold his or her breathe while the x-ray images are taken, and then to exhale after the images are taken.

◆ Instruct the patient to take slow, deep breaths if nausea occurs during the procedure.

◆ Monitor the patient for complications related to the procedure (e.g., allergic reaction, anaphylaxis, bronchospasm).

◆ The needle or catheter is removed, and a pressure dressing is applied over the puncture site.

◆ Observe/assess the needle/catheter insertion site for bleeding, inflammation, or hematoma formation.

POST-TEST:

◆ A report of the examination will be sent to the requesting HCP, who will discuss the results with the patient.

◆ Instruct the patient to resume usual diet, fluids, medications, or activity, as directed by the HCP. Renal function should be assessed before metformin is resumed.

◆ Monitor vital signs and neurological status every 15 min for 1 hr, then every 2 hr for 4 hr, and as ordered. Take temperature every 4 hr for 24 hr. Monitor intake and output at least every 8 hr. Compare with baseline values. Protocols may vary among facilities.

- Observe for delayed allergic reactions, such as rash, urticaria, tachycardia, hyperpnea, hypertension, palpitations, nausea, or vomiting.
- Instruct the patient to immediately report symptoms such as fast heart rate, difficulty breathing, skin rash, itching, chest pain, persistent right shoulder pain, or abdominal pain. Immediately report symptoms to the appropriate HCP.
- Assess extremities for signs of ischemia or absence of distal pulse caused by a catheter-induced thrombus.
- Observe/assess the needle/catheter insertion site for bleeding, inflammation, or hematoma formation.
- Instruct the patient in the care and assessment of the site.
- Instruct the patient to apply cold compresses to the puncture site as needed, to reduce discomfort or edema.
- Instruct the patient to maintain bed rest for 4 to 6 hr after the procedure or as ordered.
- Recognize anxiety related to test results, and be supportive of perceived loss of independent function. Discuss the implications of abnormal test

results on the patient's lifestyle. Provide teaching and information regarding the clinical implications of the test results, as appropriate.
- Reinforce information given by the patient's HCP regarding further testing, treatment, or referral to another HCP. Answer any questions or address any concerns voiced by the patient or family.
- Depending on the results of this procedure, additional testing may be performed to evaluate or monitor progression of the disease process and determine the need for a change in therapy. Evaluate test results in relation to the patient's symptoms and other tests performed.

RELATED MONOGRAPHS:

- Related tests include ACTH and challenge tests, adrenal gland scan, BUN, catecholamines, cortisol and challenge tests, creatinine, CT abdomen, HVA, KUB study, metanephrines, MRI abdomen, aPTT, PT/INR, renin, and VMA.
- Refer to the Endocrine System table at the end of the book for related tests by body system.

Angiography, Carotid

SYNONYM/ACRONYM: Carotid angiogram, carotid arteriography.

COMMON USE: To visualize and assess the carotid arteries and surrounding tissues for abscess, tumors, aneurysm, and evaluate for atherosclerotic disease related to stroke risk.

AREA OF APPLICATION: Neck/cervical area.

CONTRAST: Intravenous iodine based.

DESCRIPTION: The test evaluates blood vessels in the neck carrying arterial blood. This visualization is accomplished by the injection of contrast material through a catheter that has been inserted into the femoral artery for viewing the artery (arteriography). The angiographic catheter is a long tube about the size of a strand of spaghetti. After the injection of contrast media through the catheter, x-ray images of the carotid artery and associated vessels in surrounding tissue are displayed on a monitor and are recorded on film or electronically. The x-ray equipment is mounted on a C-shaped bed with the x-ray device beneath the table on which the patient lies. Over the patient is an image intensifier that receives the x-rays after they pass through the patient. Patterns of circulation or changes in vessel wall appearance can be viewed to help diagnose the presence of vascular abnormalities, disease, narrowing, enlargement, blockage, trauma, or lesions. This definitive test for arterial disease may be used to evaluate chronic vascular disease, arterial or venous stenosis, and medical therapy or surgery of the vasculature. Catheter angiography still is used in patients who may undergo surgery, angioplasty, or stent placement.

INDICATIONS

- Aid in angioplasty, atherectomy, or stent placement
- Allow infusion of thrombolytic drugs into an occluded artery
- Detect arterial occlusion, which may be evidenced by a transection of the artery caused by trauma or penetrating injury
- Detect artery stenosis, evidenced by vessel dilation, collateral vessels, or increased vascular pressure
- Detect nonmalignant tumors before surgical resection
- Detect tumors and arterial supply, extent of venous invasion, and tumor vascularity
- Detect thrombosis, arteriovenous fistula, aneurysms, or emboli in vessels

- Evaluate placement of a stent
- Differentiate between tumors and cysts
- Evaluate tumor vascularity before surgery or embolization
- Evaluate the vascular system of prospective organ donors before surgery

POTENTIAL DIAGNOSIS

Normal findings in

- Normal structure, function and patency of carotid arteries
- Contrast medium normally circulates throughout neck symmetrically and without interruption
- No evidence of obstruction, variations in number and size of vessels, malformations, cysts, or tumors

Abnormal findings in

- Abscess or inflammation
- Arterial aneurysm
- Arterial stenosis or dysplasia
- Aneurysms
- Arteriovenous fistula or other abnormalities
- Congenital anomalies
- Cysts or tumors
- Trauma causing tears or other disruption
- Vascular blockage or other disruption

CRITICAL FINDINGS: N/A

INTERFERING FACTORS

This procedure is contraindicated for

- Patients with allergies to shellfish or iodinated contrast medium. The contrast medium used may cause a life-threatening allergic reaction. Patients with a known hypersensitivity to contrast medium may benefit from premedication with corticosteroids or the use of nonionic contrast medium.

- Patients with bleeding disorders.
- Patients who are pregnant or suspected of being pregnant, unless the potential benefits of the procedure far outweigh the risk of radiation exposure to the fetus.
- ❖ Elderly and compromised patients who are chronically dehydrated before the test, because of their risk of contrast-induced renal failure.
- ❖ Patients who are in renal failure.

Factors that may impair clear imaging

- Gas or feces in the gastrointestinal tract resulting from inadequate cleansing or failure to restrict food intake before the study.
- Retained barium from a previous radiological procedure.
- Metallic objects within the examination field (e.g., jewelry, body rings), which may inhibit organ visualization and can produce unclear images.
- Inability of the patient to cooperate or remain still during the procedure because of age, significant pain, or mental status.

Other considerations

- Consultation with a health-care provider (HCP) should occur before the procedure for radiation safety concerns regarding younger patients or patients who are lactating.
- Risks associated with radiation overexposure can result from frequent x-ray procedures. Personnel in the room with the patient should wear a protective lead apron, stand behind a shield, or leave the area while the examination is being done. Personnel working in the examination area should wear badges to record their level of radiation exposure.

- Failure to follow dietary restrictions and other pretesting preparations may cause the procedure to be canceled or repeated.

NURSING IMPLICATIONS AND PROCEDURE

PRETEST:

▶ Positively identify the patient using at least two unique identifiers before providing care, treatment, or services.

▶ *Patient Teaching:* Inform the patient this procedure can assist with evaluation of the cardiovascular system.

▶ Obtain a history of the patient's complaints, including a list of known allergens, especially allergies or sensitivities to latex, iodine, seafood, contrast medium, anesthetics, or contrast medium.

▶ Obtain a history of the patient's cardiovascular system, symptoms, and results of previously performed laboratory tests and diagnostic and surgical procedures. Ensure results of coagulation testing are obtained and recorded prior to the procedure; BUN and creatinine results are also needed since contrast medium is to be used.

▶ Note any recent procedures that can interfere with test results, including examinations using iodine-based contrast medium or barium. Ensure that barium studies were performed more than 4 days before angiography.

▶ Record the date of the last menstrual period and determine the possibility of pregnancy in perimenopausal women.

▶ Obtain a list of the patient's current medications, including anticoagulants, aspirin and other salicylates, herbs, nutritional supplements, and nutraceuticals, especially those known to affect coagulation (see Appendix F). Such products should be discontinued by medical direction for the appropriate number of days prior to a surgical procedure. Note the last time and dose of medication taken.

If contrast medium is scheduled to be used, patients receiving metformin (Glucophage) for non-insulin-dependent (type 2) diabetes should discontinue the drug on the day of the test and continue to withhold it for 48 hr after the test. Failure to do so may result in lactic acidosis.

Review the procedure with the patient. Address concerns about pain and explain that there may be moments of discomfort and some pain experienced during the test. Inform the patient that the procedure is usually performed in a radiology or vascular suite by an HCP and takes approximately 30 to 60 min.

Sensitivity to social and cultural issues, as well as concern for modesty, is important in providing psychological support before, during, and after the procedure.

Explain that an IV line may be inserted to allow infusion of IV fluids, contrast medium, dye, or sedatives. Usually normal saline is infused.

Inform the patient that a burning and flushing sensation may be felt throughout the body during injection of the contrast medium. After injection of the contrast medium, the patient may experience an urge to cough, flushing, nausea, or a salty or metallic taste.

Instruct the patient to remove jewelry and other metallic objects from the area to be examined.

Instruct the patient to fast and restrict fluids for 2 to 4 hr prior to the procedure. Protocols may vary among facilities.

This procedure may be terminated if chest pain, severe cardiac arrhythmias, or signs of a cerebrovascular accident occur.

Make sure a written and informed consent has been signed prior to the procedure and before administering any medications.

INTRATEST:

Ensure the patient has complied with dietary, fluid, and medication restrictions and pretesting preparations.

Ensure the patient has removed all external metallic objects from the area to be examined.

If the patient has a history of allergic reactions to any substance or drug, administer ordered prophylactic steroids or antihistamines before the procedure. Use nonionic contrast medium for the procedure.

Have emergency equipment readily available.

Instruct the patient to void prior to the procedure and to change into the gown, robe, and foot coverings provided.

Instruct the patient to cooperate fully and to follow directions. Instruct the patient to remain still throughout the procedure because movement produces unreliable results.

Record baseline vital signs, and assess neurological status. Protocols may vary among facilities.

Observe standard precautions, and follow the general guidelines in Appendix A.

Establish an IV fluid line for the injection of emergency drugs and sedatives.

Administer an antianxiety agent, as ordered, if the patient has claustrophobia. Administer a sedative to a child or to an uncooperative adult, as ordered.

Place electrocardiographic electrodes on the patient for cardiac monitoring. Establish a baseline rhythm; determine if the patient has ventricular arrhythmias.

Using a pen, mark the site of the patient's peripheral pulses before angiography; this allows for quicker and more consistent assessment of the pulses after the procedure.

Place the patient in the supine position on an examination table. Cleanse the selected area, and cover with a sterile drape.

A local anesthetic is injected at the site, and a small incision is made or a needle is inserted under fluoroscopy.

The contrast medium is injected, and a rapid series of images is taken during and after the filling of the vessels to be examined. Delayed images may be taken to examine the vessels after a time and to monitor the venous phase of the procedure.

‣ Instruct the patient to inhale deeply and hold his or her breath while the images are taken, and then to exhale after the images are taken.

‣ Instruct the patient to take slow, deep breaths if nausea occurs during the procedure.

‣ Monitor the patient for complications related to the procedure (e.g., allergic reaction, anaphylaxis, bronchospasm).

‣ The needle or catheter is removed, and a pressure dressing is applied over the puncture site.

‣ Observe/assess the needle/catheter insertion site for bleeding, inflammation, or hematoma formation.

POST-TEST:

‣ A report of the examination will be sent to the requesting HCP, who will discuss the results with the patient.

‣ Instruct the patient to resume usual diet, fluids, medications, or activity, as directed by the HCP. Renal function should be assessed before metformin is resumed.

‣ Monitor vital signs and neurological status every 15 min for 1 hr, then every 2 hr for 4 hr, and as ordered. Take temperature every 4 hr for 24 hr. Monitor intake and output at least every 8 hr. Compare with baseline values. Protocols may vary from facility to facility.

‣ Observe for delayed allergic reactions, such as rash, urticaria, tachycardia, hyperpnea, hypertension, palpitations, nausea, or vomiting.

‣ Instruct the patient to immediately report symptoms such as fast heart rate, difficulty breathing, skin rash, itching, chest pain, persistent right shoulder pain, or abdominal pain. Immediately report symptoms to the appropriate HCP.

‣ Assess extremities for signs of ischemia or absence of distal pulse caused by a catheter-induced thrombus.

‣ Observe/assess the needle/catheter insertion site for bleeding, inflammation, or hematoma formation.

‣ Instruct the patient in the care and assessment of the site.

‣ Instruct the patient to apply cold compresses to the puncture site as needed, to reduce discomfort or edema.

‣ Instruct the patient to maintain bedrest for 4 to 6 hr after the procedure or as ordered.

‣ Recognize anxiety related to test results, and be supportive of perceived loss of independent function. Discuss the implications of abnormal test results on the patient's lifestyle. Provide teaching and information regarding the clinical implications of the test results, as appropriate.

‣ Reinforce information given by the patient's HCP regarding further testing, treatment, or referral to another HCP. Answer any questions or address any concerns voiced by the patient or family.

‣ Instruct the patient in the use of any ordered medications. Explain the importance of adhering to the therapy regimen. As appropriate, instruct the patient in significant side effects and systemic reactions associated with the prescribed medication. Encourage him or her to review corresponding literature provided by a pharmacist.

‣ Depending on the results of this procedure, additional testing may be performed to evaluate or monitor progression of the disease process and determine the need for a change in therapy. Evaluate test results in relation to the patient's symptoms and other tests performed.

RELATED MONOGRAPHS:

‣ Related tests include angiography abdomen, BUN, CT angiography, CT brain, creatinine, ECG, exercise stress test, MRA, MRI brain, PT/INR, plethysmography, US arterial Doppler lower extremities, and US peripheral Doppler.

‣ See the Cardiovascular System table at the end of the book for related tests by body system.

A

Angiography, Coronary

SYNONYM/ACRONYM: Angiography of heart, angiocardiography, cardiac angiography, cardiac catheterization, cineangiocardiography, coronary angiography, coronary arteriography.

COMMON USE: To visualize and assess the heart and surrounding structure for abnormalities, defects, aneurysm, and tumors.

AREA OF APPLICATION: Heart.

CONTRAST: Intravenous iodine based.

DESCRIPTION: Angiography allows x-ray visualization of the heart, aorta, inferior vena cava, pulmonary artery and vein, and coronary arteries after injection of contrast medium. Contrast medium is injected through a catheter, which has been inserted into a peripheral vein for a right heart catheterization or an artery for a left heart catheterization; through the same catheter, cardiac pressures are recorded. Images of the heart and associated vessels are displayed on a monitor and are recorded on film or electronically. Patterns of circulation, cardiac output, cardiac functions, and changes in vessel wall appearance can be viewed to help diagnose the presence of vascular abnormalities or lesions. Pulmonary artery abnormalities are seen with right heart views, and coronary artery and thoracic aorta abnormalities are seen with left heart views. Coronary angiography is a definitive test for coronary artery disease, and it is useful for evaluating other types of cardiac abnormalities.

INDICATIONS

- Allow infusion of thrombolytic drugs into an occluded coronary
- Detect narrowing of coronary vessels or abnormalities of the great vessels in patients with angina, syncope, abnormal electrocardiogram, hypercholesteremia with chest pain, and persistent chest pain after revascularization
- Evaluate cardiac muscle function
- Evaluate cardiac valvular and septal defects
- Evaluate disease associated with the aortic arch
- Evaluate previous cardiac surgery or other interventional procedures
- Evaluate ventricular aneurysms
- Monitor pulmonary pressures and cardiac output
- Perform angioplasty, perform atherectomy, or place a stent
- Quantify the severity of atherosclerotic, occlusive coronary artery disease

POTENTIAL DIAGNOSIS

Normal findings in
- Normal great vessels and coronary arteries

Abnormal findings in
- Aortic atherosclerosis
- Aortic dissection

A

- Aortitis
- Aneurysms
- Cardiomyopathy
- Congenital anomalies
- Coronary artery atherosclerosis and degree of obstruction
- Graft occlusion
- Pulmonary artery abnormalities
- Septal defects
- Trauma causing tears or other disruption
- Tumors
- Valvular disease

CRITICAL FINDINGS
- Aneurysm
- Aortic dissection

It is essential that critical diagnoses be communicated immediately to the appropriate health-care provider (HCP). A listing of these diagnoses varies among facilities. Note and immediately report to the HCP abnormal results and related symptoms.

INTERFERING FACTORS

This procedure is contraindicated for

- ✳ Patients with allergies to shellfish or iodinated contrast medium. The contrast medium used may cause a life-threatening allergic reaction. Patients with a known hypersensitivity to contrast medium may benefit from premedication with corticosteroids or the use of nonionic contrast medium.
- Patients with bleeding disorders.
- Patients who are pregnant or suspected of being pregnant, unless the potential benefits of the procedure far outweigh the risk of radiation exposure to the fetus.
- ✳ Elderly and compromised patients who are chronically dehydrated before the test, because of their risk of contrast-induced renal failure.
- ✳ Patients who are in renal failure.

Factors that may impair clear imaging

- Gas or feces in the gastrointestinal tract resulting from inadequate cleansing or failure to restrict food intake before the study.
- Retained barium from a previous radiological procedure.
- Metallic objects within the examination field (e.g., jewelry, body rings), which may inhibit organ visualization and can produce unclear images.
- Inability of the patient to cooperate or remain still during the procedure because of age, significant pain, or mental status.

Other considerations

- Consultation with an HCP should occur before the procedure for radiation safety concerns regarding younger patients or patients who are lactating.
- Risks associated with radiation overexposure can result from frequent x-ray procedures. Personnel in the room with the patient should wear a protective lead apron, stand behind a shield, or leave the area while the examination is being done. Personnel working in the examination area should wear badges to record their level of radiation exposure.
- Failure to follow dietary restrictions and other pretesting preparations may cause the procedure to be canceled or repeated.

NURSING IMPLICATIONS AND PROCEDURE

PRETEST:
▸ Positively identify the patient using at least two unique identifiers before providing care, treatment, or services.
▸ *Patient Teaching:* Inform the patient this procedure can assist with assessment

A

of cardiac function and check for heart disease.

▶ Obtain a history of the patient's complaints, including a list of known allergens (especially allergies or sensitivities to latex, iodine, seafood, anesthetics or contrast medium).

▶ Obtain a history of results of the patient's cardiovascular system, symptoms, and results of previously performed laboratory tests and diagnostic and surgical procedures. Ensure results of coagulation testing are obtained and recorded prior to the procedure; BUN and creatinine results are also needed if contrast medium is to be used.

▶ Note any recent procedures that can interfere with test results, including examinations using iodine-based contrast medium or barium. Ensure that barium studies were performed more than 4 days before angiography.

▶ Record the date of last menstrual period and determine the possibility of pregnancy in perimenopausal women.

▶ Obtain a list of the patient's current medications, including anticoagulants, aspirin and other salicylates, herbs, nutritional supplements, and nutraceuticals, especially those known to affect coagulation (see Appendix F). Such products should be discontinued by medical direction for the appropriate number of days prior to a surgical procedure. Note the last time and dose of medication taken.

▶ If contrast medium is scheduled to be used, patients receiving metformin (Glucophage) for non-insulin dependent (type 2) diabetes should be instructed as ordered to discontinue the drug on the day of the test and continue to withhold it for 48 hr after the test. Failure to do so may result in lactic acidosis.

▶ Review the procedure with the patient. Address concerns about pain and explain that there may be moments of discomfort and some pain experienced during the test. Inform the patient that the procedure is usually performed in a radiology or vascular suite by an HCP and takes approximately 30 to 60 min.

▶ *Sensitivity to social and cultural issues,* as well as concern for modesty, is important in providing psychological support before, during, and after the procedure.

▶ Explain that an IV line may be inserted to allow infusion of IV fluids, anesthetics, or sedatives. Usually normal saline is infused.

▶ Inform the patient that a burning and flushing sensation may be felt throughout the body during injection of the contrast medium. After injection of the contrast medium, the patient may experience an urge to cough, flushing, nausea, or a salty or metallic taste.

▶ Instruct the patient to remove jewelry and other metallic objects from the area to be examined.

▶ Instruct the patient to fast and restrict fluids for 2 to 4 hr prior to the procedure. Protocols may vary among facilities.

▶ This procedure may be terminated if chest pain, severe cardiac arrhythmias, or signs of a cerebrovascular accident occur.

▶ *Make sure a written and informed consent has been signed prior to the procedure and before administering any medications.*

INTRATEST:

▶ Ensure the patient has complied with dietary and fluid restrictions for 2 to 4 hr prior to the procedure.

▶ Ensure that the patient has removed external metallic objects from the area to be examined prior to the procedure.

▶ If the patient has a history of allergic reactions to any substance or drug, administer ordered prophylactic steroids or antihistamines before the procedure. Use nonionic contrast medium for the procedure.

▶ Have emergency equipment readily available.

▶ Instruct the patient to void prior to the procedure and to change into the gown, robe, and foot coverings provided.

▶ Instruct the patient to cooperate fully and to follow directions. Instruct the patient to remain still throughout the procedure because movement produces unreliable results.

▶ Record baseline vital signs, and continue to monitor throughout the procedure. Protocols may vary among facilities.

▶ Observe standard precautions, and follow the general guidelines in Appendix A.

- Establish an IV fluid line for the injection of emergency drugs and of sedatives.
- Administer an antianxiety agent, as ordered, if the patient has claustrophobia. Administer a sedative to a child or to an uncooperative adult, as ordered.
- Place electrocardiographic electrodes on the patient for cardiac monitoring. Establish a baseline rhythm; determine if the patient has ventricular arrhythmias.
- Using a pen, mark the site of the patient's peripheral pulses before angiography; this allows for quicker and more consistent assessment of the pulses after the procedure.
- Place the patient in the supine position on an examination table. Cleanse the selected area, and cover with a sterile drape.
- A local anesthetic is injected at the site, and a small incision is made or a needle is inserted under fluoroscopy.
- The contrast medium is injected, and a rapid series of images is taken during and after the filling of the vessels to be examined. Delayed images may be taken to examine the vessels after a time and to monitor the venous phase of the procedure.
- Instruct the patient to inhale deeply and hold his or her breath while the x-ray images are taken, and then to exhale after the images are taken.
- Instruct the patient to take slow, deep breaths if nausea occurs during the procedure.
- Monitor the patient for complications related to the procedure (e.g., allergic reaction, anaphylaxis, bronchospasm).
- The needle or catheter is removed, and a pressure dressing is applied over the puncture site.
- Observe/assess the needle/catheter insertion site for bleeding, inflammation, or hematoma formation.

POST-TEST:

- A report of the results will be sent to the requesting HCP, who will discuss the results with the patient.
- Instruct the patient to resume usual diet, fluids, medications, or activity as directed by the HCP. Renal function should be assessed before metformin is resumed.

- Monitor vital signs and neurological status every 15 min for 1 hr, then every 2 hr for 4 hr, and then as ordered by the HCP. Take temperature every 4 hr for 24 hr. Monitor intake and output at least every 8 hr. Compare with baseline values. Protocols may vary from facility to facility.
- Observe for delayed allergic reactions, such as rash, urticaria, tachycardia, hyperpnea, hypertension, palpitations, nausea, or vomiting.
- Instruct the patient to immediately report symptoms such as fast heart rate, difficulty breathing, skin rash, itching, chest pain, persistent right shoulder pain, or abdominal pain. Immediately report symptoms to the appropriate HCP.
- Assess extremities for signs of ischemia or absence of distal pulse caused by a catheter-induced thrombus.
- Observe/assess the needle/catheter insertion site for bleeding, inflammation, or hematoma formation.
- Instruct the patient in the care and assessment of the site and to observe for bleeding, hematoma formation, bile leakage, and inflammation. Any pleuritic pain, persistent right shoulder pain, or abdominal pain should be reported to the appropriate HCP.
- Instruct the patient to apply cold compresses to the puncture site as needed, to reduce discomfort or edema.
- Instruct the patient to maintain bedrest for 4 to 6 hr after the procedure or as ordered.
- *Nutritional Considerations:* A low-fat, low-cholesterol, and low-sodium diet should be consumed to reduce current disease processes and/or decrease risk of hypertension and coronary artery disease.
- Recognize anxiety related to test results. Discuss the implications of abnormal test results on the patient's lifestyle. Provide teaching and information regarding the clinical implications of the test results, as appropriate.
- Reinforce information given by the patient's HCP regarding further testing, treatment, or referral to another HCP. Answer any questions or address any concerns voiced by the patient or family.

A

▶ Instruct the patient in the use of any ordered medications. Explain the importance of adhering to the therapy regimen. As appropriate, instruct the patient in significant side effects and systemic reactions associated with the prescribed medication. Encourage him or her to review corresponding literature provided by a pharmacist.

▶ Depending on the results of this procedure, additional testing may be needed to evaluate or monitor progression of the disease process and determine the need for a change in therapy. Evaluate test results in relation to the patient's symptoms and other tests performed.

RELATED MONOGRAPHS:

▶ Related tests include angiography carotid, blood pool imaging, BNP, BUN, chest x-ray, CT abdomen, CT angiography, CT biliary tract and liver, CT cardiac scoring, CT spleen, CT thoracic, CK, creatinine, CRP, electrocardiography, electrocardiography transesophageal, Holter monitor, homocysteine, MR angiography, MRI abdomen, MRI chest, myocardial perfusion heart scan, plethysmography, aPTT, PT/INR, troponin, and US arterial Doppler carotid.

▶ Refer to the Cardiovascular System table at the end of the book for related tests by body system.

Angiography, Pulmonary

SYNONYM/ACRONYM: Pulmonary angiography, pulmonary arteriography.

COMMON USE: To visualize and assess the lungs and surrounding structure for abscess, tumor, cancer, defects, tuberculosis, and pulmonary embolism.

AREA OF APPLICATION: Pulmonary vasculature.

CONTRAST: Intravenous iodine based.

DESCRIPTION: Pulmonary angiography allows x-ray visualization of the pulmonary vasculature after injection of an iodinated contrast medium into the pulmonary artery or a branch of this great vessel. Contrast medium is injected through a catheter that has been inserted into the vascular system, usually through the femoral vein. It is one of the definitive tests for pulmonary embolism, but it is also useful for evaluating other types of pulmonary vascular abnormalities. It is definitive for peripheral pulmonary artery stenosis, anomalous pulmonary venous drainage, and pulmonary fistulae. Hemodynamic measurements during pulmonary angiography can assist in the diagnosis of pulmonary hypertension and cor pulmonale.

INDICATIONS

• Detect acute pulmonary embolism

• Detect arteriovenous malformations or aneurysms

• Detect tumors; aneurysms; congenital defects; vascular changes associated with emphysema, blebs, and bullae; and heart abnormalities

- Determine the cause of recurrent or severe hemoptysis
- Evaluate pulmonary circulation

POTENTIAL DIAGNOSIS

Normal findings in
- Normal pulmonary vasculature; radiopaque iodine contrast medium should circulate symmetrically and without interruption through the pulmonary circulatory system.

Abnormal findings in
- Aneurysms
- Arterial hypoplasia or stenosis
- Arteriovenous malformations
- Bleeding caused by tuberculosis, bronchiectasis, sarcoidosis, or aspergilloma
- Inflammatory diseases
- Pulmonary embolism (PE) acute or chronic
- Pulmonary sequestration
- Tumors

CRITICAL FINDINGS
- PE

It is essential that critical diagnoses be communicated immediately to the appropriate health-care provider (HCP). A listing of these diagnoses varies among facilities. Note and immediately report to the HCP abnormal results and related symptoms.

INTERFERING FACTORS

This procedure is contraindicated for
- Patients with allergies to shellfish or iodinated contrast medium. The contrast medium used may cause a life-threatening allergic reaction. Patients with a known hypersensitivity to contrast medium may benefit from premedication with corticosteroids or the use of nonionic contrast medium.
- Patients with bleeding disorders.
- Patients who are pregnant or suspected of being pregnant, unless the potential benefits of the procedure far outweigh the risks to the fetus and mother.
- Elderly and other patients who are chronically dehydrated before the test, because of their risk of contrast-induced renal failure.
- Patients who are in renal failure.

Factors that may impair clear imaging
- Retained barium from a previous radiological procedure.
- Metallic objects within the examination field (e.g., jewelry, body rings), which may inhibit organ visualization and can produce unclear images.
- Inability of the patient to cooperate or remain still during the procedure because of age, significant pain, or mental status.

Other considerations
- Consultation with an HCP should occur before the procedure for radiation safety concerns regarding younger patients or patients who are lactating.
- Risks associated with radiation overexposure can result from frequent x-ray procedures. Personnel in the room with the patient should wear a protective lead apron, stand behind a shield, or leave the area while the examination is being done. Personnel working in the examination area should wear badges to record their level of radiation exposure.
- Failure to follow dietary restrictions and other pretesting preparations may cause the procedure to be canceled or repeated.

A

NURSING IMPLICATIONS AND PROCEDURE

PRETEST:

▶ Positively identify the patient using at least two unique identifiers before providing care, treatment, or services.

▶ *Patient Teaching:* Inform the patient this procedure can assist with assessment of lung function and check for disease.

▶ Obtain a history of the patient's complaints, including a list of known allergens, especially allergies or sensitivities to latex, iodine, seafood, contrast medium, or anesthetics.

▶ Obtain a history of the patient's cardiovascular and respiratory systems, symptoms, and results of previously performed laboratory tests and diagnostic and surgical procedures. Ensure results of coagulation testing are obtained and recorded prior to the procedure; BUN and creatinine results are also needed if contrast medium is to be used.

▶ Note any recent procedures that can interfere with test results, including examinations using iodine-based contrast medium or barium. Ensure that barium studies were performed more than 4 days before angiography.

▶ Record the date of the last menstrual period and determine the possibility of pregnancy in perimenopausal women.

▶ Obtain a list of the patient's current medications, including anticoagulants, aspirin and other salicylates, herbs, nutritional supplements, and nutraceuticals, especially those known to affect coagulation (see Appendix F). Such products should be discontinued by medical direction for the appropriate number of days prior to a surgical procedure. Note the last time and dose of medication taken.

▶ If contrast medium is scheduled to be used, patients receiving metformin (Glucophage) for non-insulin-dependent (type 2) diabetes should discontinue the drug on the day of the test and continue to withhold it for 48 hr after the test. Failure to do so may result in lactic acidosis.

▶ Review the procedure with the patient. Address concerns about pain and explain that there may be moments of discomfort and some pain experienced during the test. Inform the patient that the procedure is usually performed in a radiology or vascular suite by an HCP and takes approximately 30 to 60 min.

▶ *Sensitivity to social and cultural issues,* as well as concern for modesty, is important in providing psychological support before, during, and after the procedure.

▶ Explain that an IV line may be inserted to allow infusion of IV fluids, contrast medium, or sedatives. Usually normal saline is infused.

▶ Inform the patient that a burning and flushing sensation may be felt throughout the body during injection of the contrast medium. After injection of the contrast medium, the patient may experience an urge to cough, flushing, nausea, or a salty or metallic taste.

▶ Instruct the patient to remove jewelry and other metallic objects from the area to be examined.

▶ Instruct the patient to fast and restrict fluids for 2 to 4 hr prior to the procedure. Protocols may vary among facilities.

▶ This procedure may be terminated if chest pain, severe cardiac arrhythmias, or signs of a cerebrovascular accident occur.

▶ *Make sure a written and informed consent has been signed prior to the procedure and before administering any medications.*

INTRATEST:

▶ Ensure the patient has complied with dietary, fluid, and medication restrictions and pretesting preparations for 2 to 4 hr prior to the procedure.

▶ Ensure the patient has removed all external metallic objects from the area to be examined.

▶ If the patient has a history of allergic reactions to any substance or drug, administer ordered prophylactic steroids or antihistamines before the procedure. Use nonionic contrast medium for the procedure.

▶ Have emergency equipment readily available.

▶ Instruct the patient to void prior to the procedure and to change into the gown, robe, and foot coverings provided.

Instruct the patient to cooperate fully and to follow directions. Instruct the patient to remain still throughout the procedure because movement produces unreliable results.

Record baseline vital signs, and continue to monitor throughout the procedure. Protocols may vary among facilities.

Observe standard precautions, and follow the general guidelines in Appendix A.

Establish an IV fluid line for the injection of emergency drugs and of sedatives.

Administer an antianxiety agent, as ordered, if the patient has claustrophobia. Administer a sedative to a child or to an uncooperative adult, as ordered.

Place electrocardiographic electrodes on the patient for cardiac monitoring. Establish a baseline rhythm; determine if the patient has ventricular arrhythmias.

Using a pen, mark the site of the patients peripheral pulses before angiography; this allows for quicker and more consistent assessment of the pulses after the procedure.

Place the patient in the supine position on an examination table. Cleanse the selected area, and cover with a sterile drape.

A local anesthetic is injected at the site, and a small incision is made or a needle is inserted under fluoroscopy.

The contrast medium is injected, and a rapid series of images is taken during and after the filling of the vessels to be examined.

Instruct the patient to inhale deeply and hold his or her breath while the images are taken, and then to exhale after the images are taken.

Instruct the patient to take slow, deep breaths if nausea occurs during the procedure.

Monitor the patient for complications related to the procedure (e.g., allergic reaction, anaphylaxis, bronchospasm).

The needle or catheter is removed, and a pressure dressing is applied over the puncture site.

Observe/assess the needle/catheter insertion site for bleeding, inflammation, or hematoma formation.

POST-TEST:

A report of the examination will be sent to the requesting HCP, who will discuss the results with the patient.

Instruct the patient to resume usual diet, fluids, medications, or activity, as directed by the HCP. Renal function should be assessed before metformin is resumed.

Monitor vital signs and neurological status every 15 min for 1 hr, then every 2 hr for 4 hr, and as ordered. Take the temperature every 4 hr for 24 hr. Monitor intake and output at least every 8 hr. Compare with baseline values. Protocols may vary from facility to facility.

Observe for delayed allergic reactions, such as rash, urticaria, tachycardia, hyperpnea, hypertension, palpitations, nausea, or vomiting.

Instruct the patient to immediately report symptoms such as fast heart rate, difficulty breathing, skin rash, itching, chest pain, persistent right shoulder pain, or abdominal pain. Immediately report symptoms to the appropriate HCP.

Assess extremities for signs of ischemia or absence of distal pulse caused by a catheter-induced thrombus.

Observe/assess the needle/catheter insertion site for bleeding, inflammation, or hematoma formation.

Instruct the patient in the care and assessment of the site.

Instruct the patient to apply cold compresses to the puncture site as needed, to reduce discomfort or edema.

Instruct the patient to maintain bedrest for 4 to 6 hr after the procedure or as ordered.

Recognize anxiety related to test results, and be supportive of perceived loss of independent function. Discuss the implications of abnormal test results on the patient's lifestyle. Provide teaching and information regarding the clinical implications of the test results, as appropriate.

Reinforce information given by the patient's HCP regarding further testing, treatment, or referral to another HCP. Answer any questions or address any concerns voiced by the patient or family.

Depending on the results of this procedure, additional testing may be performed to evaluate or monitor

progression of the disease process and determine the need for a change in therapy. Evaluate test results in relation to the patient's symptoms and other tests performed.

RELATED MONOGRAPHS:

▶ Related tests include alveolar/arterial gradient, blood gases, BUN, chest x-ray, creatinine, CT angiography, CT thoracic, ECG, FDP, lactic acid, lung perfusion scan, lung ventilation scan, MRA, MRI chest, aPTT, and PT/INR.

▶ Refer to the Cardiovascular and Respiratory systems tables at the end of the book for related tests by body system.

Angiography, Renal

SYNONYM/ACRONYM: Renal angiogram, renal arteriography.

COMMON USE: To visualize and assess the kidneys and surrounding structure for tumor, cancer, absent kidney, and level of renal disease.

AREA OF APPLICATION: Kidney.

CONTRAST: Intravenous iodine based.

DESCRIPTION: Renal angiography allows x-ray visualization of the large and small arteries of the renal vasculature and parenchyma or the renal veins and their branches. Contrast medium is injected through a catheter that has been inserted into the femoral artery or vein and advanced through the iliac artery and aorta into the renal artery or the inferior vena cava into the renal vein. Images of the kidneys and associated vessels are displayed on a monitor and recorded on film or electronically. Patterns of circulation, renal function, or changes in vessel wall appearance can be viewed to help diagnose the presence of vascular abnormalities, trauma, or lesions. This definitive test for renal disease may be used to evaluate chronic renal disease, renal failure, and renal artery stenosis; differentiate a vascular renal cyst from hypervascular renal cancers; and evaluate renal transplant donors, recipients, and the kidney after transplantation.

INDICATIONS

• Aid in angioplasty, atherectomy, or stent placement
• Allow infusion of thrombolytic drugs into an occluded artery
• Assist with the collection of blood samples from renal vein for renin analysis
• Detect arterial occlusion as evidenced by a transection of the renal artery caused by trauma or a penetrating injury
• Detect nonmalignant tumors before surgical resection
• Detect renal artery stenosis as evidenced by vessel dilation, collateral vessels, or increased renovascular pressure

- Detect renal tumors as evidenced by arterial supply, extent of venous invasion, and tumor vascularity
- Detect small kidney or absence of a kidney
- Detect thrombosis, arteriovenous fistulae, aneurysms, or emboli in renal vessels
- Differentiate between renal tumors and renal cysts
- Evaluate placement of a stent
- Evaluate postoperative renal transplantation for function or organ rejection
- Evaluate renal function in chronic renal failure or end-stage renal disease or hydronephrosis
- Evaluate the renal vascular system of prospective kidney donors before surgery
- Evaluate tumor vascularity before surgery or embolization

POTENTIAL DIAGNOSIS

Normal findings in
- Normal structure, function, and patency of renal vessels
- Contrast medium circulating throughout the kidneys symmetrically and without interruption
- No evidence of obstruction, variations in number and size of vessels and organs, malformations, cysts, or tumors

Abnormal findings in
- Abscess or inflammation
- Arterial stenosis, dysplasia, or infarction
- Arteriovenous fistula or other abnormalities
- Congenital anomalies
- Intrarenal hematoma
- Renal artery aneurysm
- Renal cysts or tumors
- Trauma causing tears or other disruption

CRITICAL FINDINGS: N/A

INTERFERING FACTORS

This procedure is contraindicated for
- ✦ Patients with allergies to shellfish or iodinated contrast medium. The contrast medium used may cause a life-threatening allergic reaction. Patients with a known hypersensitivity to contrast medium may benefit from premedication with corticosteroids or the use of nonionic contrast medium.
- Patients with bleeding disorders.
- Patients who are pregnant or suspected of being pregnant, unless the potential benefits of the procedure far outweigh the risks to the fetus and mother.
- ✦ Elderly and other patients who are chronically dehydrated before the test, because of their risk of contrast-induced renal failure.
- ✦ Patients who are in renal failure.

Factors that may impair clear imaging
- Gas or feces in the gastrointestinal tract resulting from inadequate cleansing or failure to restrict food intake before the study.
- Retained barium from a previous radiological procedure.
- Metallic objects within the examination field (e.g., jewelry, body rings), which may inhibit organ visualization and can produce unclear images.
- Inability of the patient to cooperate or remain still during the procedure because of age, significant pain, or mental status.

Other considerations
- Consultation with a health-care provider (HCP) should occur before the procedure for radiation safety concerns regarding younger patients or patients who are lactating.
- Risks associated with radiation overexposure can result from

A

frequent x-ray procedures. Personnel in the room with the patient should wear a protective lead apron, stand behind a shield, or leave the area while the examination is being done. Personnel working in the examination area should wear badges to record their level of radiation exposure.

• Failure to follow dietary restrictions and other pretesting preparations may cause the procedure to be canceled or repeated.

NURSING IMPLICATIONS AND PROCEDURE

PRETEST:

‣ Positively identify the patient using at least two unique identifiers before providing care, treatment, or services.

‣ *Patient Teaching:* Inform the patient this procedure can assist in assessment of kidney function and check for disease.

‣ Obtain a history of the patient's complaints, including a list of known allergens (especially allergies or sensitivities to latex, iodine, seafood, anesthetics or contrast medium).

‣ Obtain a history of the patient's genitourinary system, symptoms, and results of previously performed laboratory tests and diagnostic and surgical procedures. Ensure results of coagulation testing are obtained and recorded prior to the procedure; BUN and creatinine results are also needed since contrast medium is to be used.

‣ Note any recent procedures that can interfere with test results, including examinations using iodine-based contrast medium or barium. Ensure that barium studies were performed more than 4 days before angiography.

‣ Record the date of the last menstrual period and determine the possibility of pregnancy in perimenopausal women.

‣ Obtain a list of the patient's current medications, including anticoagulants, aspirin and other salicylates, herbs, nutritional supplements, and nutraceuticals (see Appendix F). Such

products should be discontinued by medical direction for the appropriate number of days prior to a surgical procedure. Note the last time and dose of medication taken.

‣ If contrast medium is scheduled to be used, patients receiving metformin (Glucophage) for non-insulin-dependent (type 2) diabetes should discontinue the drug on the day of the test and continue to withhold it for 48 hr after the test. Failure to do so may result in lactic acidosis.

‣ Review the procedure with the patient. Address concerns about pain and explain that there may be moments of discomfort and some pain experienced during the test. Inform the patient that the procedure is usually performed in a radiology or vascular suite by an HCP and takes approximately 30 to 60 min.

‣ *Sensitivity to social and cultural issues,* as well as concern for modesty, is important in providing psychological support before, during, and after the procedure.

‣ Explain that an IV line may be inserted to allow infusion of IV fluids, contrast medium, or sedatives. Usually normal saline is infused.

‣ Inform the patient that a burning and flushing sensation may be felt throughout the body during injection of the contrast medium. After injection of the contrast medium, the patient may experience an urge to cough, flushing, nausea, or a salty or metallic taste.

‣ Instruct the patient to remove jewelry, and other metallic objects from the area to be examined.

‣ Instruct the patient to fast and restrict fluids for 2 to 4 hr prior to the procedure. Protocols may vary among facilities.

‣ This procedure may be terminated if chest pain, severe cardiac arrhythmias, or signs of a cerebrovascular accident occur.

‣ *Make sure a written and informed consent has been signed prior to the procedure and before administering any medications.*

A

- Ensure the patient has complied with dietary, fluid, and medication restrictions for 2 to 4 hr prior to the procedure.
- Ensure the patient has removed all external metallic objects from the area to be examined.
- If the patient has a history of allergic reactions to any substance or drug, administer ordered prophylactic steroids or antihistamines before the procedure. Use nonionic contrast medium for the procedure.
- Have emergency equipment readily available.
- Instruct the patient to void prior to the procedure and to change into the gown, robe, and foot coverings provided.
- Instruct the patient to cooperate fully and to follow directions. Instruct the patient to remain still throughout the procedure because movement produces unreliable results.
- Record baseline vital signs, and continue to monitor throughout the procedure. Protocols may vary among facilities.
- Observe standard precautions, and follow the general guidelines in Appendix A.
- Establish an IV fluid line for the injection of emergency drugs or of sedatives.
- Administer an antianxiety agent, as ordered, if the patient has claustrophobia. Administer a sedative to a child or to an uncooperative adult, as ordered.
- Place electrocardiographic electrodes on the patient for cardiac monitoring. Establish a baseline rhythm; determine if the patient has ventricular arrhythmias.
- Using a pen, mark the site of the patient's peripheral pulses before angiography; this allows for quicker and more consistent assessment of the pulses after the procedure.
- Place the patient in the supine position on an exam table. Cleanse the selected area, and cover with a sterile drape.
- A local anesthetic is injected at the site, and a small incision is made or a needle is inserted under fluoroscopy.
- The contrast medium is injected, and a rapid series of images is taken during and after the filling of the vessels to be examined. Delayed images may be taken to examine the vessels after a time and to monitor the venous phase of the procedure.

- Instruct the patient to inhale deeply and hold his or her breath while the images are taken, and then to exhale after the images are taken.
- Instruct the patient to take slow, deep breaths if nausea occurs during the procedure.
- Monitor the patient for complications related to the procedure (e.g., allergic reaction, anaphylaxis, bronchospasm).
- The needle or catheter is removed, and a pressure dressing is applied over the puncture site.
- Observe/assess the needle/catheter insertion site for bleeding, inflammation, or hematoma formation.

- A report of the examination will be sent to the requesting HCP, who will discuss the results with the patient.
- Instruct the patient to resume usual diet, fluids, medications, or activity, as directed by the HCP. Renal function should be assessed before metformin is resumed.
- Monitor vital signs and neurological status every 15 min for 1 hr, then every 2 hr for 4 hr, and as ordered. Take temperature every 4 hr for 24 hr. Monitor intake and output at least every 8 hr. Compare with baseline values. Protocols may vary among facilities.
- Observe for delayed allergic reactions, such as rash, urticaria, tachycardia, hyperpnea, hypertension, palpitations, nausea, or vomiting.
- Instruct the patient to immediately report symptoms such as fast heart rate, difficulty breathing, skin rash, itching, chest pain, persistent right shoulder pain, or abdominal pain. Immediately report symptoms to the appropriate HCP.
- Assess extremities for signs of ischemia or absence of distal pulse caused by a catheter-induced thrombus.
- Observe/assess the needle/catheter insertion site for bleeding, inflammation, or hematoma formation.
- Instruct the patient in the care and assessment of the site.
- Instruct the patient to apply cold compresses to the puncture site as needed, to reduce discomfort or edema.

‣ Instruct the patient to maintain bedrest for 4 to 6 hr after the procedure or as ordered.

‣ Recognize anxiety related to test results, and be supportive of perceived loss of independent function. Discuss the implications of abnormal test results on the patient's lifestyle. Provide teaching and information regarding the clinical implications of the test results, as appropriate.

‣ Reinforce information given by the patient's HCP regarding further testing, treatment, or referral to another HCP. Answer any questions or address any concerns voiced by the patient or family.

‣ Depending on the results of this procedure, additional testing may be needed to evaluate or monitor progression of the disease process and determine the need for a change in therapy. Evaluate test results in relation to the patient's symptoms and other tests performed.

RELATED MONOGRAPHS:

‣ Related tests include biopsy kidney, BUN, creatinine, CT abdomen, CT angiography, culture urine, cytology urine, KUB study, IVP, MRA, MRI abdomen, aPTT, PT/INR, renin, renogram, US kidney, and UA.

‣ Refer to the Genitourinary System table at the end of the book for related tests by body system.

Angiotensin-Converting Enzyme

SYNONYM/ACRONYM: Angiotensin I-converting enzyme (ACE).

COMMON USE: To assist in diagnosing, evaluating treatment, and monitoring the progression of sarcoidosis, a granulomatous disease that primarily affects the lungs.

SPECIMEN: Serum (1 mL) collected in a red- or tiger-top tube.

REFERENCE VALUE: (Method: Spectrophotometry)

Age	Conventional Units	SI Units (Conventional Units × 0.017)
0–2 yr	5–83 units/L	0.09–1.41 microKat/L
3–7 yr	8–76 units/L	0.14–1.29 microKat/L
8–14 yr	6–89 units/L	0.10–1.51 microKat/L
Greater than 14 yr	12–68 units/L	0.20–1.16 microKat/L

POTENTIAL DIAGNOSIS
Increased in
• Bronchitis (acute and chronic) *(related to release of ACE from damaged pulmonary tissue)*
• Connective tissue disease *(related to release of ACE from scarred and damaged pulmonary tissue)*
• Gaucher's disease *(related to release of ACE from damaged pulmonary tissue; Gaucher's disease is due to the hereditary deficiency of an enzyme that results in accumulation of a fatty substance that damages pulmonary tissue)*
• Hansen's disease (leprosy)

- Histoplasmosis and other fungal diseases
- Hyperthyroidism (untreated) *(related to possible involvement of thyroid hormones in regulation of ACE)*
- Pulmonary fibrosis *(related to release of ACE from damaged pulmonary tissue)*
- Rheumatoid arthritis *(related to development of interstitial lung disease, pulmonary fibrosis, and release of ACE from damaged pulmonary tissue)*

- Sarcoidosis *(related to release of ACE from damaged pulmonary tissue)*

Decreased in
- Advanced pulmonary carcinoma *(related to lack of functional cells to produce ACE)*
- The period following corticosteroid therapy for sarcoidosis *(evidenced by cessation of effective therapy)*

CRITICAL FINDINGS: N/A

Find and print out the full monograph at DavisPlus (http://davisplus.fadavis .com, keyword Van Leeuwen).

Anion Gap

SYNONYM/ACRONYM: Agap.

COMMON USE: To assist in diagnosing metabolic disorders that result in metabolic acidosis and electrolyte imbalance such as severe dehydration.

SPECIMEN: Serum (1 mL) for electrolytes collected in a red- or tiger-top tube. Plasma (1 mL) collected in a green-top (heparin) tube is also acceptable.

REFERENCE VALUE: (Method: Anion gap is derived mathematically from the direct measurement of sodium, chloride, and total carbon dioxide.) There are differences between serum and plasma values for some electrolytes. The reference ranges listed are based on serum values.

Age	Conventional Units	SI Units (Conventional Units × 1)
Child or adult	8–16 mEq/L	8–16 mmol/L

DESCRIPTION: The anion gap is used most frequently as a clinical indicator of metabolic acidosis. The most common causes of an increased gap are lactic acidosis and ketoacidosis.

The concept of estimating electrolyte disturbances in the extracellular fluid is based on the principle of electrical neutrality. The formula includes the major cation (sodium) and anions (chloride and bicarbonate) found in extracellular fluid. The anion gap is calculated as follows:

$$anion\ gap = sodium - (chloride + HCO_3^-)$$

Because bicarbonate (HCO_3^-) is not directly measured on most chemistry analyzers, it is estimated by substitution of the total carbon dioxide (Tco_2) value in the calculation. Some laboratories may include potassium in the calculation of the anion gap. Calculations including potassium can be invalidated because minor amounts of hemolysis can contribute significant levels of potassium leaked into the serum as a result of cell rupture. The anion gap is also widely used as a laboratory quality-control measure because low gaps usually indicate a reagent, calibration, or instrument error.

INDICATIONS
- Evaluate metabolic acidosis
- Indicate the presence of a disturbance in electrolyte balance
- Indicate the need for laboratory instrument recalibration or review of electrolyte reagent preparation and stability

POTENTIAL DIAGNOSIS

Increased in
Metabolic acidosis that results from the accumulation of unmeasured anionic substances like proteins, phosphorus, sulfates, ketoacids, or other organic acid waste products of metabolism
- Dehydration (severe)
- Ketoacidosis *caused by starvation, high-protein/low-carbohydrate diet, diabetes, and alcoholism*

- Lactic acidosis *(shock, excessive exercise, some malignancies)*
- Poisoning (salicylate, methanol, ethylene glycol, or paraldehyde)
- Renal failure
- Uremia

Decreased in
Conditions that result in metabolic alkalosis
- Chronic vomiting or gastric suction *(related to alkalosis due to net loss of acid)*
- Excess alkali ingestion
- Hypergammaglobulinemia *(related to an increase in measurable anions relative to the excessive production of unmeasured cationic M proteins)*
- Hypoalbuminemia *(related to decreased levels of unmeasured anionic proteins relative to stable and measurable cation concentrations)*
- Hyponatremia *(related to net loss of cations)*
Significant acidosis or alkalosis can result from increased levels of unmeasured cations like ionized calcium and magnesium or unmeasured anions like proteins, phosphorus, sulfates, or other organic acids, the effects of which may not be accurately reflected by the calculated anion gap.

CRITICAL FINDINGS: N/A

INTERFERING FACTORS
- Drugs that can increase or decrease the anion gap include those listed in the individual electrolyte (i.e., sodium, chloride, calcium, magnesium, and total carbon dioxide), total protein, lactic acid, and phosphorus monographs.
- Specimens should never be collected above an IV line because of the potential for dilution when the specimen and the IV solution combine in the collection container,

falsely decreasing the result. There is also the potential of contaminating the sample with the substance of interest if it is present in the IV solution, falsely increasing the result.

NURSING IMPLICATIONS AND PROCEDURE

PRETEST:

▶ Positively identify the patient using at least two unique identifiers before providing care, treatment, or services.
▶ *Patient Teaching:* Inform the patient this test can assist in the evaluation of electrolyte balance.
▶ Obtain a history of the patient's complaints, including a list of known allergens, especially allergies or sensitivities to latex.
▶ Obtain a history of the patient's cardiovascular, endocrine, gastrointestinal, genitourinary, hematopoietic, immune, and respiratory systems; symptoms; and results of previously performed laboratory tests and diagnostic and surgical procedures.
▶ Obtain a list of the patient's current medications, including herbs, nutritional supplements, and nutraceuticals (see Appendix F).
▶ Review the procedure with the patient. Inform the patient that specimen collection takes approximately 5 to 10 min. Address concerns about pain and explain that there may be some discomfort during the venipuncture.
▶ *Sensitivity to social and cultural issues,* as well as concern for modesty, is important in providing psychological support before, during, and after the procedure.
▶ There are no food, fluid, or medication restrictions unless by medical direction.

INTRATEST:

▶ If the patient has a history of allergic reaction to latex, avoid the use of equipment containing latex.
▶ Instruct the patient to cooperate fully and to follow directions. Direct the patient to breathe normally and to avoid unnecessary movement.

▶ Observe standard precautions, and follow the general guidelines in Appendix A. Positively identify the patient, and label the appropriate tubes with the corresponding patient demographics, date, and time of collection. Perform a venipuncture.
▶ Remove the needle and apply direct pressure with dry gauze to stop bleeding. Observe/assess venipuncture site for bleeding and hematoma formation and secure gauze with adhesive bandage.
▶ Promptly transport the specimen to the laboratory for processing and analysis.

POST-TEST:

▶ A report of the results will be sent to the requesting health-care provider (HCP), who will discuss the results with the patient.
▶ *Nutritional Considerations:* Specific dietary considerations are listed in the monographs on individual electrolytes (i.e., sodium, chloride, calcium, magnesium, and potassium), total protein, and phosphorus.
▶ *Nutritional Considerations:* The anion gap can be used to indicate the presence of dehydration. Evaluate the patient for signs and symptoms of dehydration. Dehydration is a significant and common finding in geriatric patients.
▶ Reinforce information given by the patient's HCP regarding further testing, treatment, or referral to another HCP. Answer any questions or address any concerns voiced by the patient or family.
▶ Depending on the results of this procedure, additional testing may be performed to evaluate or monitor progression of the disease process and determine the need for a change in therapy. Evaluate test results in relation to the patient's symptoms and other tests performed.

RELATED MONOGRAPHS:

▶ Related tests include albumin, blood gases, BUN, creatinine, electrolytes, ethanol (drugs of abuse), glucose, ketones, lactic acid, osmolality, protein and fractions, salicylate, and UA.
▶ See the Cardiovascular, Endocrine, Gastrointestinal, Genitourinary, Hematopoietic, Immune, and Respiratory systems tables at the end of the book for related tests by body system.

Antiarrhythmic Drugs: Digoxin, Disopyramide, Flecainide, Lidocaine, Procainamide, Quinidine

SYNONYM/ACRONYM: *Digoxin* (Digitek, Lanoxicaps, Lanoxin); *disopyramide* (Norpace, Norpace CR); *flecainide* (flecainide acetate, Tambocor); *lidocaine* (Xylocaine); *procainamide* (Procanbid, Pronestyl, Pronestyl SR); *quinidine* (Quinidex Extentabs, quinidine sulface SR, quinidine gluconate SR).

COMMON USE: To evaluate specific drugs for subtherapeutic, therapeutic, or toxic levels in treatment of heart failure and cardiac arrhythmias.

SPECIMEN: Serum (1 mL) collected in a red-top tube.

Drug	Route of Administration	Recommended Collection Time
Digoxin	Oral	Trough: 12–24 hr after dose Never draw peak samples
Disopyramide	Oral	Trough: immediately before next dose Peak: 2–5 hr after dose
Flecainide	Oral	Trough: immediately before next dose Peak: 3 hr after dose
Lidocaine	IV	15 min, 1 hr, then every 24 hr
Procainamide	IV	15 min; 2, 6, 12 hr; then every 24 hr
Procainamide	Oral	Trough: immediately before next dose Peak: 75 min after dose
Quinidine sulfate	Oral	Trough: immediately before next dose Peak: 1 hr after dose
Quinidine gluconate	Oral	Trough: immediately before next dose Peak: 5 hr after dose
Quinidine polygalacturonate	Oral	Trough: immediately before next dose Peak: 2 hr after dose

REFERENCE VALUE: (Method: Immunoassay)

Drug (Indication)	Therapeutic Dose*	SI Units	Half-Life (hr)	Volume of Distribution (L/kg)	Protein Binding (%)	Excretion
(SI = Conventional Units × 1.28)						
Digoxin	0.5–2.0 ng/mL	0.6–2.6 nmol/L	20–60	7	20–30	1° renal
(SI = Conventional Units × 2.95)						
Disopyramide (atrial arrhythmias)	2.8–3.2 mcg/mL	8.3–9.4 micromol/L	4–10	0.7–0.9	20–60	1° renal
Disopyramide (ventricular arrhythmias)	3.3–5.0 mcg/mL	9.7–15.0 micromol/L				1° renal
(SI = Conventional Units × 2.41)						
Flecainide	0.2–1.0 mcg/mL	0.5–2.4 micromol/L	7–19	5–13	40–50	1° renal
(SI = Conventional Units × 4.27)						
Lidocaine	1.5–5.0 mcg/mL	6.4–21.4 micromol/L	1.5–2	1–1.5	60–80	1° hepatic
(SI = Conventional Units × 4.23)						
Procainamide	4–10 mcg/mL	17–42 micromol/L	2–6	2–4	10–20	1° renal
(SI = Conventional Units × 3.61)						
Procainamide + N-acetyl procainamide	10–30 mcg/mL	36–108 micromol/L	8			1° renal
(SI = Conventional Units × 3.08)						
Quinidine	2–5 mcg/mL	6–15 micromol/L	6–8	2–3	70–90	Renal and hepatic

*Conventional units.

A

DESCRIPTION: Cardiac glycosides are used in the prophylactic management and treatment of heart failure and ventricular and atrial arrhythmias. Because these drugs have narrow therapeutic windows, they must be monitored closely. The signs and symptoms of toxicity are often difficult to distinguish from those of cardiac disease. Patients with toxic levels may show gastrointestinal, ocular, and central nervous system effects and disturbances in potassium balance.

Many factors must be considered in effective dosing and monitoring of therapeutic drugs, including patient age, patient weight, interacting medications, electrolyte balance, protein levels, water balance, conditions that affect absorption and excretion, and the ingestion of substances (e.g., foods, herbals, vitamins, and minerals) that can either potentiate or inhibit the intended target concentration. Peak and trough collection times should be documented carefully in relation to the time of medication administration.

IMPORTANT NOTE

This information must be communicated clearly and accurately to avoid misunderstanding of the dose time in relation to the collection time. Miscommunication between the individual administering the medication and the individual collecting the specimen is the most frequent cause of subtherapeutic levels, toxic levels, and misleading information used in the calculation of future doses.

INDICATIONS

- Assist in the diagnosis and prevention of toxicity
- Monitor compliance with therapeutic regimen
- Monitor patients who have a pacemaker, who have impaired renal or hepatic function, or who are taking interacting drugs

POTENTIAL DIAGNOSIS

Level	Result
Normal levels	Therapeutic effect
Subtherapeutic levels	Adjust dose as indicated
Toxic levels	Adjust dose as indicated
Digoxin	Renal impairment, CHF,* elderly patients
Disopyramide	Renal impairment
Flecainide	Renal impairment, CHF
Lidocaine	Hepatic impairment, CHF
Procainamide	Renal impairment
Quinidine	Renal and hepatic impairment, CHF, elderly patients

*CHF = congestive heart failure.

A

CRITICAL FINDINGS

Adverse effects of subtherapeutic levels are important. Care should be taken to investigate the signs and symptoms of too little and too much medication. Note and immediately report to the health-care provider (HCP) any critically increased or subtherapeutic values and related symptoms.

Digoxin: Greater Than 2.5 ng/mL

Signs and symptoms of digoxin toxicity include arrhythmias, anorexia, hyperkalemia, nausea, vomiting, diarrhea, changes in mental status, and visual disturbances (objects appear yellow or have halos around them). Possible interventions include discontinuing the medication, continuous electrocardiographic (ECG) monitoring (prolonged P-R interval, widening QRS interval, lengthening Q-Tc interval, and atrioventricular block), transcutaneous pacing, administration of activated charcoal (if the patient has a gag reflex and central nervous system function), support and treatment of electrolyte disturbance, and administration of Digibind (digoxin immune Fab). The amount of Digibind given depends on the level of digoxin to be neutralized. Digoxin levels must be measured before the administration of Digibind. Digoxin levels should not be measured for several days after administration of Digibind in patients with normal renal function (1 wk or longer in patients with decreased renal function). Digibind cross-reacts in the digoxin assay and may provide misleading elevations or decreases in values depending on the particular assay in use by the laboratory.

Disopyramide: Greater Than 7 mcg/mL

Signs and symptoms of disopyramide toxicity include prolonged Q-T interval, ventricular tachycardia, hypotension, and heart failure. Possible interventions include discontinuing the medication, airway support, and ECG and blood pressure monitoring.

Flecainide: Greater Than 1 mcg/mL

Signs and symptoms of flecainide toxicity include exaggerated pharmacological effects resulting in arrhythmia. Possible interventions include discontinuing the medication as well as continuous ECG, respiratory, and blood pressure monitoring.

Lidocaine: Greater Than 6 mcg/mL

Signs and symptoms of lidocaine toxicity include slurred speech, central nervous system depression, cardiovascular depression, convulsions, muscle twitches, and possible coma. Possible interventions include continuous ECG monitoring, airway support, and seizure precautions.

Procainamide: Greater Than 12 mcg/mL; Procainamide + N-Acetyl Procainamide: Greater Than 30 mcg/mL

The active metabolite of procainamide is N-acetyl procainamide (NAPA). Signs and symptoms of procainamide toxicity include torsade de pointes (ventricular tachycardia), nausea, vomiting, agranulocytosis, and hepatic disturbances. Possible interventions include airway protection, emesis, gastric lavage, and administration of sodium lactate.

Quinidine: Greater Than 8 mcg/mL

Signs and symptoms of quinidine toxicity include ataxia, nausea, vomiting, diarrhea, respiratory system depression, hypotension, syncope, anuria, arrhythmias (heart block, widening of QRS and Q-T intervals), asystole, hallucinations, paresthesia, and irritability. Possible interventions include airway support, emesis, gastric lavage, administration of activated charcoal, administration of sodium lactate, and temporary transcutaneous or transvenous pacemaker.

INTERFERING FACTORS

- Blood drawn in serum separator tubes (gel tubes).
- Contraindicated in patients with liver disease, and caution advised in patients with renal impairment.
- Drugs that may increase digoxin levels or increase risk of toxicity include amiodarone, amphotericin B, diclofenac, diltiazem, erythromycin, ibuprofen, indomethacin, nifedipine, nisoldipine, propafenone, propantheline, quinidine, spironolactone, tetracycline, tiapamil, troleandomycin, and verapamil.
- Drugs that may decrease digoxin levels include albuterol, aluminum hydroxide (antacids), carbamazepine, cholestyramine, colestipol, digoxin immune Fab, hydralazine, hydroxychloroquine, iron, kaolin-pectin, magnesium hydroxide, magnesium trisilicate, metoclopramide, neomycin, nitroprusside, paroxetine, phenytoin, rifabutin, sulfasalazine, and ticlopidine.
- Drugs that may increase disopyramide levels or increase risk of toxicity include amiodarone, atenolol, ritonavir, and troleandomycin.
- Drugs that may decrease disopyramide levels include phenobarbital, phenytoin, rifabutin, and rifampin.
- Drugs that may increase flecainide levels or increase risk of toxicity include amiodarone and cimetidine.
- Drugs that may decrease flecainide levels include carbamazepine, charcoal, phenobarbital, and phenytoin.
- Drugs that may increase lidocaine levels or increase risk of toxicity

include β-blockers, cimetidine, metoprolol, nadolol, propranolol, and ritonavir.
- Drugs that may decrease lidocaine levels include phenytoin.
- Drugs that may increase procainamide levels or increase risk of toxicity include amiodarone, cimetidine, quinidine, ranitidine, and trimethoprim.
- Drugs that may increase quinidine levels or increase risk of toxicity include acetazolamide, amiodarone, cimetidine, itraconazole, mibefradil, nifedipine, nisoldipine, quinidine, ranitidine, thiazide diuretics, and verapamil.
- Drugs that may decrease quinidine levels include kaolin-pectin, ketoconazole, phenobarbital, phenytoin, rifabutin, and rifampin.
- Digitoxin cross-reacts with digoxin; results are falsely elevated if digoxin is measured when the patient is taking digitoxin.
- Digitalis-like immunoreactive substances are found in the serum of some patients who are not taking digoxin, causing false-positive results. Patients whose serum contain digitalis-like immunoreactive substances usually have a condition related to salt and fluid retention, such as renal failure, hepatic failure, low-renin hypertension, and pregnancy.
- Unexpectedly low digoxin levels may be found in patients with thyroid disease.
- Disopyramide may cause a decrease in glucose levels. It may also potentiate the anticoagulating effects of warfarin.
- Long-term administration of procainamide can cause false-positive antinuclear antibody results and development of a lupuslike syndrome in some patients.
- Quinidine may potentiate the effects of neuromuscular blocking medications and warfarin anticoagulants.

- Concomitant administration of quinidine and digoxin can rapidly raise digoxin to toxic levels. If both drugs are to be given together, the digoxin level should be measured before the first dose of quinidine and again in 4 to 6 days.

NURSING IMPLICATIONS AND PROCEDURE

PRETEST:

▶ Positively identify the patient using at least two unique identifiers before providing care, treatment, or services.

▶ *Patient Teaching:* Inform the patient this test can assist in monitoring for subtherapeutic, therapeutic, or toxic drug levels.

▶ Obtain a history of the patient's complaints, including a list of known allergens, especially allergies or sensitivities to latex.

▶ Obtain a history of the patient's cardiovascular system, symptoms, and results of previously performed laboratory tests and diagnostic and surgical procedures.

▶ These medications are metabolized and excreted by the kidneys and liver.

▶ Obtain a list of the patient's current medications, including herbs, nutritional supplements, and nutraceuticals (see Appendix F). Note the last time and dose of medication taken.

▶ Review the procedure with the patient. Inform the patient that specimen collection takes approximately 5 to 10 min. Address concerns about pain and explain that there may be some discomfort during the venipuncture.

▶ *Sensitivity to social and cultural issues,* as well as concern for modesty, is important in providing psychological support before, during, and after the procedure.

▶ There are no food, fluid, or medication restrictions unless by medical direction.

INTRATEST:

▶ If the patient has a history of allergic reaction to latex, avoid the use of equipment containing latex.

▶ Instruct the patient to cooperate fully and to follow directions. Direct the patient to breathe normally and to avoid unnecessary movement.

▶ Observe standard precautions, and follow the general guidelines in Appendix A. Consider recommended collection time in relation to the dosing schedule. Positively identify the patient, and label the appropriate tubes with the corresponding patient demographics, date, and time of collection, noting the last dose of medication taken. Perform a venipuncture.

▶ Remove the needle and apply direct pressure with dry gauze to stop bleeding. Observe/assess venipuncture site for bleeding or hematoma formation and secure gauze with adhesive bandage.

▶ Promptly transport the specimen to the laboratory for processing and analysis.

POST-TEST:

▶ A report of the results will be sent to the requesting HCP, who will discuss the results with the patient.

▶ *Nutritional Considerations:* include avoidance of alcohol consumption.

▶ Reinforce information given by the patient's HCP regarding further testing, treatment, or referral to another HCP. Explain to the patient the importance of following the medication regimen and instructions regarding drug interactions. Instruct the patient to immediately report any unusual sensations (e.g., dizziness, changes in vision, loss of appetite, nausea, vomiting, diarrhea, weakness, or irregular heartbeat) to his or her HCP. Instruct the patient not to take medicine within 1 hr of food high in fiber. Answer any questions or address any concerns voiced by the patient or family.

▶ Instruct the patient to be prepared to provide the pharmacist with a list of other medications he or she is already taking in the event that the requesting HCP prescribes a medication.

▶ Depending on the results of this procedure, additional testing may be performed to evaluate or monitor progression of the disease process and determine the need for a change in therapy. Testing for aspirin responsiveness/resistance may be a consideration for patients, especially women, on low-dose aspirin therapy. Evaluate test results in relation to the patient's symptoms and other tests performed.

RELATED MONOGRAPHS:

▶ Related tests include ALT, albumin, ALP, apolipoprotein A and B, atrial natriuretic peptide, BNP, blood gases, BUN, CRP, calcium, calcium ionized, cholesterol (total, HDL, and LDL), CBC platelet count, CK and isoenzymes, creatinine, glucose, glycated hemoglobin, homocysteine, ketones, LDH and isoenzymes, magnesium, myoglobin, potassium, triglycerides, and troponin.

▶ See the Cardiovascular System table at the end of the book for related tests by body system.

Antibiotic Drugs—Aminoglycosides: Amikacin, Gentamicin, Tobramycin; Tricyclic Glycopeptide: Vancomycin

SYNONYM/ACRONYM: *Amikacin* (Amikin); *gentamicin* (Garamycin, Genoptic, Gentacidin, Gentafair, Gentak, Gentamar, Gentrasul, G-myticin, Oco-Mycin, Spectro-Genta); *tobramycin* (Nebcin, Tobrex); *vancomycin* (Lyphocin, Vancocin, Vancoled).

COMMON USE: To evaluate specific drugs for subtherapeutic, therapeutic, or toxic levels in treatment of infection.

SPECIMEN: Serum (1 mL) collected in a red-top tube.

Drug	Route of Administration	Recommended Collection Time*
Amikacin	IV, IM	Trough: immediately before next dose Peak: 30 min after the end of a 30-min IV infusion
Gentamicin	IV, IM	Trough: immediately before next dose Peak: 30 min after the end of a 30-min IV infusion
Tobramycin	IV, IM	Trough: immediately before next dose Peak: 30 min after the end of a 30-min IV infusion
Tricyclic glycopeptide and vancomycin	IV, PO	Trough: immediately before next dose Peak: 30–60 min after the end of a 60-min IV infusion

*Usually after fifth dose if given every 8 hr or third dose if given every 12 hr.
IM = intramuscular; IV = intravenous; PO = by mouth.

REFERENCE VALUE: (Method: Immunoassay)

Drug	Therapeutic Dose*	SI Units	Half-Life (hr)	Distribution (L/kg)	Volume of Binding (%)	Protein Excretion
(SI = Conventional Units × 1.71) Amikacin						
Peak	20–30 mcg/mL	34–51 micromol/L	4–8	0.4–1.3	50	1° renal
Trough	1–8 mcg/mL	2–14 micromol/L				
(SI = Conventional Units × 2.09) Gentamicin (Standard dosing)						
Peak	6–10 mcg/mL	12–21 micromol/L	4–8	0.4–1.3	50	1° renal
Trough	0.5–1.5 mcg/mL	1–3 micromol/L				
(SI = Conventional Units × 2.09) Tobramycin						
Peak	6–10 mcg/mL	13–21 micromol/L	4–8	0.4–1.3	50	1° renal
Trough	0.5–1.5 mcg/mL	1–3 micromol/L				
(SI = Conventional Units × 0.69) Vancomycin						
Peak	30–40 mcg/mL	21–28 micromol/L	4–8	0.4–1.3	50	1° renal
Trough	5–10 mcg/mL	3–7 micromol/L				

*Conventional units.

DESCRIPTION: The aminoglycoside antibiotics amikacin, gentamicin, and tobramycin are used against many gram-negative (*Acinetobacter, Citrobacter, Enterobacter, Escherichia coli, Klebsiella, Proteus, Providencia, Pseudomonas, Raoultella, Salmonella, Serratia, Shigella,* and *Stenotrophomonas*) and some gram-positive (*Staphylococcus aureus*) pathogenic microorganisms. Aminoglycosides are poorly absorbed through the gastrointestinal tract and are most frequently administered IV.

Vancomycin is a tricyclic glycopeptide antibiotic used against many gram-positive microorganisms, such as staphylococci, *Streptococcus pneumoniae*, group A β-hemolytic streptococci, enterococci, *Corynebacterium*, and *Clostridium*. Vancomycin has also been used in an oral form for the treatment of pseudomembranous colitis resulting from *Clostridium difficile* infection. This approach is less frequently used because of the emergence of vancomycin-resistant enterococci (VRE).

Many factors must be considered in effective dosing and monitoring of therapeutic drugs, including patient age, patient weight, interacting medications, electrolyte balance, protein levels, water balance, conditions that affect absorption and excretion, and ingestion of substances (e.g., foods, herbals, vitamins, and minerals) that can either potentiate or inhibit the intended target concentration. The most serious side effects of the aminoglycosides and vancomycin are nephrotoxicity and irreversible ototoxicity (uncommon). Peak and trough collection times should be documented carefully in relation to the time of medication administration. Creatinine levels should be monitored every 2 to 3 days to detect renal impairment due to toxic drug levels.

IMPORTANT NOTE
This information must be clearly and accurately communicated to avoid misunderstanding of the dose time in relation to the collection time. Miscommunication between the individual administering the medication and the individual collecting the specimen is the most frequent cause of subtherapeutic levels, toxic levels, and misleading information used in the calculation of future doses. Some pharmacies use a computerized pharmacokinetics approach to dosing that eliminates the need to be concerned about peak and trough collections; random specimens are adequate.

INDICATIONS
- Assist in the diagnosis and prevention of toxicity
- Monitor renal dialysis patients or patients with rapidly changing renal function
- Monitor therapeutic regimen

POTENTIAL DIAGNOSIS

Level	Result
Normal levels	Therapeutic effect
Subtherapeutic levels	Adjust dose as indicated
Toxic levels	Adjust dose as indicated

Level	Result
Amikacin	Renal, hearing impairment
Gentamicin	Renal, hearing impairment
Tobramycin	Renal, hearing impairment
Vancomycin	Renal, hearing impairment

CRITICAL FINDINGS

The adverse effects of subtherapeutic levels are important. Care should be taken to investigate signs and symptoms of too little and too much medication. Note and immediately report to the health-care provider (HCP) any critically increased or subtherapeutic values and related symptoms.

Signs and symptoms of toxic levels of these antibiotics are similar and include loss of hearing and decreased renal function. The most important intervention is accurate therapeutic drug monitoring so the medication can be discontinued before irreversible damage is done.

Drug Name	Toxic Levels
Amikacin	Peak greater than 30 mcg/mL, trough greater than 8 mcg/mL
Gentamicin	Peak greater than 12 mcg/mL, trough greater than 2 mcg/mL
Tobramycin	Peak greater than 12 mcg/mL, trough greater than 2 mcg/mL
Vancomycin	Peak greater than 80 mcg/mL, trough greater than 20 mcg/mL

INTERFERING FACTORS

- Blood drawn in serum separator tubes (gel tubes).
- Contraindicated in patients with liver disease, and caution advised in patients with renal impairment.
- Drugs that may decrease aminoglycoside efficacy include penicillins (e.g., carbenicillin, piperacillin).
- Obtain a culture before and after the first dose of aminoglycosides.
- The risks of ototoxicity and nephrotoxicity are increased by the concomitant administration of aminoglycosides.

NURSING IMPLICATIONS AND PROCEDURE

PRETEST:

▶ Positively identify the patient using at least two unique identifiers before providing care, treatment, or services.

▶ *Patient Teaching:* Inform the patient this test can assist in monitoring for subtherapeutic, therapeutic, or toxic drug levels used in treatment of infection.

▶ Obtain a history of the patient's complaints, including a list of known allergens, especially allergies or sensitivities to latex.

▶ Obtain a history of the patient's immune system, symptoms, and results of previously performed laboratory tests and diagnostic and surgical procedures.

▶ Nephrotoxicity is a risk associated with administration of aminoglycosides. Obtain a history of the patient's genitourinary system, symptoms, and results of previously performed laboratory tests and diagnostic and surgical procedures.

▶ Ototoxicity is a risk associated with administration of aminoglycosides. Obtain a history of the patient's known or suspected hearing loss, including type and cause; ear conditions with treatment regimens; ear surgery; and other tests and procedures to assess and diagnose auditory deficit.

- Obtain a list of the patient's current medications, including herbs, nutritional supplements, and nutraceuticals (see Appendix F). Note the last time and dose of medication taken.
- Review the procedure with the patient. Inform the patient that specimen collection takes approximately 5 to 10 min. Address concerns about pain and explain that there may be some discomfort during the venipuncture.
- Obtain a culture, if ordered, before the first dose of aminoglycosides.
- *Sensitivity to social and cultural issues,* as well as concern for modesty, is important in providing psychological support before, during, and after the procedure.
- There are no food, fluid, or medication restrictions unless by medical direction.

INTRATEST:

- If the patient has a history of allergic reaction to latex, avoid the use of equipment containing latex.
- Instruct the patient to cooperate fully and to follow directions. Direct the patient to breathe normally and to avoid unnecessary movement.
- Observe standard precautions, and follow the general guidelines in Appendix A. Consider recommended collection time in relation to the dosing schedule. Positively identify the patient and label the appropriate tubes with the corresponding patient demographics, date, and time of collection, noting the last dose of medication taken. Perform a venipuncture.
- Remove the needle and apply direct pressure with dry gauze to stop bleeding. Observe/assess venipuncture site for bleeding or hematoma formation and secure gauze with adhesive bandage.
- Promptly transport the specimen to the laboratory for processing and analysis.

POST-TEST:

- A report of the results will be sent to the requesting HCP, who will discuss the results with the patient.
- Instruct the patient receiving aminoglycosides to immediately report any unusual symptoms (e.g., hearing loss, decreased urinary output) to his or her HCP.
- *Nutritional Considerations:* include avoidance of alcohol consumption.
- Administer antibiotic therapy if ordered. Remind the patient of the importance of completing the entire course of antibiotic therapy, even if signs and symptoms disappear before completion of therapy.
- Reinforce information given by the patient's HCP regarding further testing, treatment, or referral to another HCP. Explain to the patient the importance of following the medication regimen and instructions regarding food and drug interactions. Answer any questions or address any concerns voiced by the patient or family.
- Instruct the patient to be prepared to provide the pharmacist with a list of other medications he or she is already taking in the event that the requesting HCP prescribes a medication.
- Depending on the results of this procedure, additional testing may be performed to evaluate or monitor progression of the disease process and determine the need for a change in therapy. Evaluate test results in relation to the patient's symptoms and other tests performed.

RELATED MONOGRAPHS:

- Related tests include albumin, audiometry hearing loss, BUN, creatinine, creatinine clearance, cultures bacterial (ear, eye, skin, wound, blood, stool, sputum, urine), otoscopy, potassium, spondee speech recognition test, tuning fork tests, and UA.
- See the Auditory, Genitourinary, and Immune systems tables at the end of the book for related tests by body system.

Antibodies, Anti-Cyclic Citrullinated Peptide

SYNONYM/ACRONYM: Anti-CCP antibodies.

COMMON USE: To assist in diagnosing and monitoring rheumatoid arthritis.

SPECIMEN: Serum (1 mL) collected in a red- or tiger-top tube.

REFERENCE VALUE: IgG Ab (Method: Immunoassay, enzyme-linked immunosorbent assay [ELISA])

Negative	Less than 20 units
Weak positive	20–39 units
Moderate positive	40–59 units
Strong positive	60 units or greater

DESCRIPTION: Rheumatoid arthritis (RA) is a chronic, systemic autoimmune disease that damages the joints. Inflammation caused by autoimmune responses can affect other organs and body systems. The current American Academy of Rheumatology criteria state that a patient must have four of seven criteria to be diagnosed with RA: morning stiffness, arthritis of three or more joint areas, arthritis of hand joints, symmetric arthritis, rheumatoid nodules, abnormal amounts of rheumatoid factor, and radiographic changes. The study of RA is complex, and it is believed that multiple genes may be involved in the manifestation of RA. Scientific research has revealed an unusual peptide conversion from arginine to citrulline that results in formation of antibodies whose presence provides the basis for this test. Studies show that detection of antibodies formed against citrullinated peptides is specific and sensitive in detecting RA in both early and established disease. Anti-CCP assays have 96% specificity and 78% sensitivity for RA, compared to the traditional IgM rheumatoid factor (RF) marker with a specificity of 60% to 80% and sensitivity of 75% to 80% for RA. Anti-CCP antibodies are being used as a marker for erosive disease in RA, and the antibodies have been detected in healthy patients years before the onset of RA symptoms and diagnosed disease. Some studies have shown that as many as 40% of patients seronegative for RF are anti-CCP positive. The combined presence of RF and anti-CCP has a 99.5% specificity for RA. Women are two to three times more likely than men to develop RA. While RA is most likely to affect people aged 35 to 50, it can affect all ages.

INDICATIONS

- Assist in the diagnosis of RA in both symptomatic and asymptomatic individuals
- Assist in the identification of erosive disease in RA
- Assist in the diagnostic prediction of RA development in undifferentiated arthritis

POTENTIAL DIAGNOSIS

Increased in

- RA *(The immune system produces antibodies that attack the joint tissues. Inflammation of the synovium, membrane that lines the joint, begins a process called synovitis. If untreated, the synovitis can expand beyond the joint tissue to surrounding ligaments, tissues, nerves, and blood vessels.)*

Decreased in: N/A

CRITICAL FINDINGS: N/A

INTERFERING FACTORS: N/A

NURSING IMPLICATIONS AND PROCEDURE

PRETEST:

- *Patient Teaching:* Inform the patient this test can assist in identifying the cause of joint inflammation.
- Obtain a history of the patient's complaints, including a list of known allergens, especially allergies or sensitivities to latex.
- Obtain a history of the patient's immune and musculoskeletal systems, symptoms, and results of previously performed laboratory tests and diagnostic and surgical procedures.
- Obtain a list of the patient's current medications, including herbs, nutritional supplements, and nutraceuticals (see Appendix F).
- Review the procedure with the patient. Inform the patient that specimen

collection takes approximately 5 to 10 min. Address concerns about pain and explain that there may be some discomfort during the venipuncture.

- *Sensitivity to social and cultural issues,* as well as concern for modesty, is important in providing psychological support before, during, and after the procedure.
- There are no food, fluid, or medication restrictions unless by medical direction.

INTRATEST:

- If the patient has a history of allergic reaction to latex, avoid the use of equipment containing latex.
- Instruct the patient to cooperate fully and to follow directions. Direct the patient to breathe normally and to avoid unnecessary movement.
- Observe standard precautions, and follow the general guidelines in Appendix A. Positively identify the patient, and label the appropriate tubes with the corresponding patient demographics, date, and time of collection. Perform a venipuncture.
- Remove the needle and apply direct pressure with dry gauze to stop bleeding. Observe/assess venipuncture site for bleeding or hematoma formation and secure gauze with adhesive bandage.
- Promptly transport the specimen to the laboratory for processing and analysis.

POST-TEST:

- A report of the results will be sent to the requesting health-care provider (HCP), who will discuss the results with the patient.
- Recognize anxiety related to test results, and be supportive of impaired activity related to anticipated chronic pain resulting from joint inflammation, impairment in mobility, muscular deformity, and perceived loss of independence. Discuss the implications of abnormal test results on the patient's lifestyle. Provide teaching and information regarding the clinical implications of the test results as appropriate. Explain the importance of physical activity in the treatment plan. Educate the patient regarding access

A

to physical therapy, occupational therapy, and counseling services. Provide contact information, if desired, for the Arthritis Foundation (www.arthritis .org). Encourage the patient to take medications as ordered. Treatment with disease-modifying antirheumatic drugs (DMARDs) and biologic response modifiers may take as long as 2 to 3 mo to demonstrate their effects.
- Reinforce information given by the patient's HCP regarding further testing, treatment, or referral to another HCP. Answer any questions or address any concerns voiced by the patient or family.

- Depending on the results of this procedure, additional testing may be performed to evaluate or monitor progression of the disease process and determine the need for a change in therapy.

RELATED MONOGRAPHS:
- Related tests include ANA, arthroscopy, BMD, bone scan, CBC, CRP, ESR, MRI musculoskeletal, radiography bone, RF, synovial fluid analysis, and uric acid.
- Refer to the Immune and Musculoskeletal systems tables at the end of the book for related tests by body system.

Antibodies, Anti-Glomerular Basement Membrane

SYNONYM/ACRONYM: Goodpasture's antibody, anti-GBM.

COMMON USE: To assist in differentiating Goodpasture's syndrome (an autoimmune disease) from renal dysfunction.

SPECIMEN: Serum (1 mL) collected in a red- or tiger-top tube. Lung or kidney tissue also may be submitted for testing. Refer to related biopsy monographs for specimen-collection instructions.

REFERENCE VALUE: (Method: Enzyme immunoassay) Less than 3 units/mL = negative.

DESCRIPTION: Glomerulonephritis or inflammation of the kidney is initiated by an immune response, usually to an infection. It can be classified as either antibody-mediated or cell-mediated glomerulonephritis. Goodpasture's syndrome is a rare hypersensitivity condition characterized by the presence of circulating anti-glomerular basement membrane antibodies (GBM) in the blood and the deposition of immunoglobulin and complement in renal basement membrane tissue. Severe and progressive glomerulonephritis can lead to the development of pulmonary hemorrhage and idiopathic pulmonary hemosiderosis. The presence of anti-GBM antibodies can also be demonstrated in renal biopsy tissue cells of affected patients. Autoantibodies may also be directed to act against lung tissue in Goodpasture's syndrome.

A

INDICATIONS

- Differentiate glomerulonephritis caused by anti-GBM from glomerulonephritis from other causes
- Monitor therapy for glomerulonephritis caused by anti-GBM

POTENTIAL DIAGNOSIS

Increased in
- Glomerulonephritis *(evidenced by the presence of anti-GBM antibodies)*
- Goodpasture's syndrome *(related to nephritis of autoimmune origin)*
- Idiopathic pulmonary hemosiderosis

Decreased in: N/A

CRITICAL FINDINGS: N/A

INTERFERING FACTORS: N/A

NURSING IMPLICATIONS AND PROCEDURE

PRETEST:

- Positively identify the patient using at least two unique identifiers before providing care, treatment, or services.
- *Patient Teaching:* Inform the patient this test can assist in diagnosing a disease that can affect the kidneys or lungs.
- Obtain a history of the patient's complaints, including a list of known allergens, especially allergies or sensitivities to latex.
- Obtain a history of the patient's genitourinary, immune, and respiratory systems; symptoms; and results of previously performed laboratory tests and diagnostic and surgical procedures.
- Obtain a list of the patient's current medications, including herbs, nutritional supplements, and nutraceuticals (see Appendix F).

- Review the procedure with the patient. Inform the patient that specimen collection takes approximately 5 to 10 min. Address concerns about pain and explain that there may be some discomfort during the venipuncture.
- *Sensitivity to social and cultural issues,* as well as concern for modesty, is important in providing psychological support before, during, and after the procedure.
- There are no food, fluid, or medication restrictions unless by medical direction.

INTRATEST:

- If the patient has a history of allergic reaction to latex, avoid the use of equipment containing latex.
- Instruct the patient to cooperate fully and to follow directions. Direct the patient to breathe normally and to avoid unnecessary movement.
- Observe standard precautions, and follow the general guidelines in Appendix A. Positively identify the patient, and label the appropriate tubes with the corresponding patient demographics, date, and time of collection. Perform a venipuncture.
- Remove the needle and apply direct pressure with dry gauze to stop bleeding. Observe/assess venipuncture site for bleeding or hematoma formation and secure gauze with adhesive bandage.
- Promptly transport the specimen to the laboratory for processing and analysis.

POST-TEST:

- A report of the results will be sent to the requesting health-care provider (HCP), who will discuss the results with the patient.
- Recognize anxiety related to test results, and be supportive of perceived loss of independence and fear of shortened life expectancy. Discuss the implications of abnormal test results on the patient's lifestyle. Provide teaching and information regarding the clinical implications of the test results, as appropriate. Educate the patient regarding access to counseling services.

▸ Reinforce information given by the patient's HCP regarding further testing, treatment, or referral to another HCP. Answer any questions or address any concerns voiced by the patient or family.

▸ Depending on the results of this procedure, additional testing may be performed to evaluate or monitor progression of the disease process and determine the need for a change in therapy. Evaluate test results in relation to the patient's symptoms and other tests performed.

RELATED MONOGRAPHS:

▸ Related tests include ANCA, biopsy kidney, biopsy lung, IVP, renogram, US kidney, and UA.

▸ See the Genitourinary, Immune, and Respiratory systems tables at the end of the book for related tests by body system.

Antibodies, Antimitochondrial and Antismooth Muscle

SYNONYM/ACRONYM: AMA, ASMA, Actin antibody (ASMA).

COMMON USE: To assist in the differential diagnosis of chronic liver disease, typically biliary cirrhosis.

SPECIMEN: Serum (1 mL) collected in a red-top tube.

REFERENCE VALUE: (Method: Indirect fluorescent antibody):
AMA Negative: Titer less than 1:20.
ASMA Negative: Titer less than 1:20.

DESCRIPTION: Primary biliary cirrhosis (PBC) is a disease in which the small bile ducts of the liver are destroyed by an inflammatory process. Antimitochondrial antibodies are found in 90% of patients with PBC. Mitochondrial M2 antibody has a higher degree of specificity than any of the other three types of detectable mitochondrial antibodies (M1, M5, M6) for PBC. PBC is identified most frequently in women aged 35 to 60. Testing is useful in the differential diagnosis of chronic liver disease because antimitochondrial antibodies are rarely detected in extrahepatic biliary obstruction, various forms of hepatitis, and cirrhosis. Antismooth muscle antibodies are autoantibodies found in high titers in the sera of patients with autoimmune diseases of the liver and bile duct. Smooth muscle antibodies are directed against the F-actin subunits present in all smooth muscle fibers and are therefore not organ specific. Simultaneous testing for antimitochondrial antibodies can be useful in the differential diagnosis of chronic liver disease.

INDICATIONS

AMA

- Assist in the diagnosis of PBC
- Assist in the differential diagnosis of chronic liver disease

ASMA

- Differential diagnosis of liver disease

POTENTIAL DIAGNOSIS

Increased in

The exact cause of PBC is unknown. There is a high degree of correlation between the presence of AMA and ASMA with PBC, and PBC therefore is thought to be an autoimmune disease. The antibodies have been identified in the sera of patients with other autoimmune diseases.

AMA

- Hepatitis (alcoholic, viral)
- PBC
- Rheumatoid arthritis (occasionally)
- Systemic lupus erythematosus (occasionally)
- Thyroid disease (occasionally)

ASMA

- Autoimmune hepatitis
- Chronic active viral hepatitis
- Infectious mononucleosis
- PBC
- Primary sclerosing cholangitis

Decreased in: N/A

CRITICAL FINDINGS: N/A

INTERFERING FACTORS

- Drugs and substances that may increase AMA levels include labetalol (liver damage).
- Drugs and substances that may decrease AMA levels include cyclosporine and ursodiol.

NURSING IMPLICATIONS AND PROCEDURE

PRETEST:

- Positively identify the patient using at least two unique identifiers before providing care, treatment, or services.
- *Patient Teaching:* Inform the patient this test can assist in the diagnosis of liver disease.
- Obtain a history of the patient's complaints, including a list of known allergens, especially allergies or sensitivities to latex.
- Obtain a history of the patient's hepatobiliary and immune systems, symptoms, and results of previously performed laboratory tests and diagnostic and surgical procedures.
- Obtain a list of the patient's current medications, including herbs, nutritional supplements, and nutraceuticals (see Appendix F).
- Review the procedure with the patient. Inform the patient that specimen collection takes approximately 5 to 10 min. Address concerns about pain and explain that there may be some discomfort during the venipuncture.
- *Sensitivity to social and cultural issues,* as well as concern for modesty, is important in providing psychological support before, during, and after the procedure.
- There are no food, fluid, or medication restrictions unless by medical direction.

INTRATEST:

- If the patient has a history of allergic reaction to latex, avoid the use of equipment containing latex.
- Instruct the patient to cooperate fully and to follow directions. Direct the patient to breathe normally and to avoid unnecessary movement.
- Observe standard precautions, and follow the general guidelines in Appendix A. Positively identify the patient, and label the appropriate tubes

with the corresponding patient demographics, date, and time of collection. Perform a venipuncture.
- Remove the needle and apply direct pressure with dry gauze to stop bleeding. Observe/assess venipuncture site for bleeding or hematoma formation and secure gauze with adhesive bandage.
- Promptly transport the specimen to the laboratory for processing and analysis.

POST-TEST:

- A report of the results will be sent to the requesting health-care provider (HCP), who will discuss the results with the patient.
- *Nutritional Considerations:* The presence of antimitochondrial or antismooth muscle antibodies may be associated with liver disease. Dietary recommendations may be indicated and vary depending on the severity of the condition. A low-protein diet may be in order if the liver cannot process the end products of protein metabolism. A diet of soft foods may be required if esophageal varices have developed. Ammonia levels may be used to determine whether protein should be added to or reduced from the diet. Patients should be encouraged to eat simple carbohydrates and emulsified fats

(as in homogenized milk or eggs) rather than complex carbohydrates (e.g., starch, fiber, and glycogen [animal carbohydrates]) and complex fats, which require additional bile to emulsify them so that they can be used. Observe the cirrhotic patient carefully for the development of ascites; if ascites develops, pay strict attention to fluid and electrolyte balance.
- Reinforce information given by the patient's HCP regarding further testing, treatment, or referral to another HCP. Answer any questions or address any concerns voiced by the patient or family.
- Depending on the results of this procedure, additional testing may be performed to evaluate or monitor progression of the disease process and determine the need for a change in therapy. Evaluate test results in relation to the patient's symptoms and other tests performed.

RELATED MONOGRAPHS:

- Related tests include albumin, ALP, ammonia, ANCA, ANA, bilirubin, biopsy liver, electrolytes, and GGT.
- See the Hepatobiliary and Immune systems tables at the end of the book for related tests by body system.

Antibodies, Antineutrophilic Cytoplasmic

SYNONYM/ACRONYM: Cytoplasmic antineutrophil cytoplasmic antibody (c-ANCA), perinuclear antineutrophil cytoplasmic antibody (p-ANCA).

COMMON USE: To assist in diagnosing and monitoring the effectiveness of therapeutic interventions for Wegener's syndrome.

SPECIMEN: Serum (1 mL) collected in a red-top tube.

REFERENCE VALUE: (Method: Indirect immunofluorescence) Negative.

A

DESCRIPTION: Antineutrophil cytoplasmic autoantibodies (ANCA) are associated with vasculitis and glomerulonephritis. There are two types of cytoplasmic neutrophil antibodies, identified by their cellular staining characteristics. c-ANCA (cytoplasmic) is specific for proteinase 3 in neutrophils and monocytes and is found in the sera of patients with Wegener's granulomatosis (WG). Wegener's syndrome includes granulomatous inflammation of the upper and lower respiratory tract and vasculitis. Systemic necrotizing vasculitis is an inflammation of the blood vessels. p-ANCA (perinuclear) is specific for myeloperoxidase, elastase, and lactoferrin, as well as other enzymes in neutrophils. p-ANCA is present in the sera of patients with pauci-immune necrotizing glomerulonephritis.

INDICATIONS
- Assist in the diagnosis of WG and its variants
- Differential diagnosis of ulcerative colitis
- Distinguish between biliary cirrhosis and sclerosing cholangitis
- Distinguish between vasculitic disease and the effects of therapy

POTENTIAL DIAGNOSIS

Increased in
The exact mechanism by which ANCA are developed is unknown. One theory suggests colonization with bacteria capable of expressing microbial superantigens. It is thought that the superantigens may stimulate a strong cellular autoimmune response in genetically susceptible individuals. Another theory suggests the immune system may be stimulated by an accumulation of the antigenic targets of ANCA due to ineffective destruction of old neutrophils or ineffective removal of neutrophil cell fragments containing proteinase, myeloperoxidase, elastase, lactoferrin, or other proteins.

- c-ANCA
  WG and its variants
- p-ANCA
  Alveolar hemorrhage
  Angiitis and polyangiitis
  Autoimmune liver disease
  Capillaritis
  Churg-Strauss syndrome
  Crescentic glomerulonephritis
  Felty's syndrome
  Glomerulonephritis
  Inflammatory bowel disease
  Leukocytoclastic skin vasculitis
  Microscopic polyarteritis
  Rheumatoid arthritis
  Vasculitis

Decreased in: N/A

CRITICAL FINDINGS: N/A

INTERFERING FACTORS: N/A

NURSING IMPLICATIONS AND PROCEDURE

PRETEST:
- Positively identify the patient using at least two unique identifiers before providing care, treatment, or services.
- *Patient Teaching:* Inform the patient this test can assist in identifying the cause of inflammatory activity.

- Obtain a history of the patient's complaints, including a list of known allergens, especially allergies or sensitivities to latex.
- Obtain a history of the patient's gastrointestinal, genitourinary, hepatobiliary, immune, and musculoskeletal systems; symptoms; and results of previously performed laboratory tests and diagnostic and surgical procedures.
- Obtain a list of the patient's current medications, including herbs, nutritional supplements, and nutraceuticals (see Appendix F).
- Review the procedure with the patient. Inform the patient that specimen collection takes approximately 5 to 10 min. Address concerns about pain and explain that there may be some discomfort during the venipuncture.
- There are no food, fluid, or medication restrictions unless by medical direction.

INTRATEST:

- If the patient has a history of allergic reaction to latex, avoid the use of equipment containing latex.
- Instruct the patient to cooperate fully and to follow directions. Direct the patient to breathe normally and to avoid unnecessary movement.
- Observe standard precautions, and follow the general guidelines in Appendix A. Positively identify the patient, and label the appropriate tubes with the corresponding patient demographics, date, and time of collection. Perform a venipuncture.
- Remove the needle and apply direct pressure with dry gauze to stop bleeding. Observe/assess venipuncture site for bleeding or hematoma formation and secure the gauze with adhesive bandage.

- Promptly transport the specimen to the laboratory for processing and analysis.

POST-TEST:

- A report of the results will be sent to the requesting health-care provider (HCP), who will discuss the results with the patient.
- Recognize anxiety related to test results, and be supportive of perceived loss of independence and fear of shortened life expectancy. Discuss the implications of abnormal test results on the patient's lifestyle. Provide teaching and information regarding the clinical implications of the test results, as appropriate. Educate the patient regarding access to counseling services.
- Reinforce information given by the patient's HCP regarding further testing, treatment, or referral to another HCP. Answer any questions or address any concerns voiced by the patient or family.
- Depending on the results of this procedure, additional testing may be performed to evaluate or monitor progression of the disease process and determine the need for a change in therapy. Evaluate test results in relation to the patient's symptoms and other tests performed.

RELATED MONOGRAPHS:

- Related tests include antibodies anti-glomerular basement membrane, antibodies AMA/ASMA, antibodies ANA, biopsy kidney, eosinophil count, and RF.
- See the Gastrointestinal, Genitourinary, Hepatobiliary, Immune, and Musculoskeletal systems tables at the end of the book for related tests by body system.

A

Antibodies, Antinuclear, Anti-DNA, Anticentromere, Antiextractable Nuclear Antigen, Anti-Jo, and Antiscleroderma

SYNONYM/ACRONYM: Antinuclear antibodies (ANA), anti-DNA (anti-ds DNA), antiextractable nuclear antigens (anti-ENA, ribonucleoprotein [RNP], Smith [Sm], SS-A/Ro, SS-B/La), anti-Jo (antihistidyl transfer RNA [tRNA] synthase), and antiscleroderma (progressive systemic sclerosis [PSS] antibody, Scl-70 antibody, topoisomerase I antibody).

COMMON USE: To diagnose multiple systemic autoimmune disorders; primarily used for diagnosis of systemic lupus erythematosus (SLE).

SPECIMEN: Serum (3 mL) collected in a red-top tube.

REFERENCE VALUE: (Method: Indirect fluorescent antibody for ANA and anticentromere; enzyme-linked immunosorbent assay [ELISA] for anti-DNA; immunodiffusion for ENA and Scl-70; immunoassay for Jo-1).

ANA and anticentromere:Titer of 1:40 or less. Anti-ENA, Jo-1, and anti-Scl-70: Negative. Reference ranges for Jo-1 vary widely due to differences in methods and the testing laboratory should be consulted directly.

Anti-DNA

Negative	Less than 24 international units
Borderline	25–30 international units
Positive	31–200 international units
Strong positive	Greater than 200 international units

DESCRIPTION: Antinuclear antibodies (ANA) are autoantibodies mainly located in the nucleus of affected cells. The presence of ANA indicates SLE, related collagen vascular diseases, and immune complex diseases. Antibodies against cellular DNA are strongly associated with SLE. Anticentromere antibodies are a subset of ANA. Their presence is strongly associated with CREST syndrome (*c*alcinosis, *R*aynaud's phenomenon, *e*sophageal dysfunction, *s*clerodactyly, and *t*elangiectasia). Women are much more likely than men to be diagnosed with SLE. Jo-1 is an autoantibody found in the sera of some ANA-positive patients. Compared to the presence of other autoantibodies, the presence of Jo-1 suggests a more aggressive course and a higher risk of mortality. The clinical effects of this autoantibody include acute onset fever, dry and crackled skin on the hands, Raynaud's phenomenon, and arthritis. The extractable nuclear antigens (ENAs) include ribonucleoprotein (RNP), Smith (Sm), SS-A/Ro, and SS-B/La antigens. ENAs and antibodies to them are found in various combinations in individuals with combinations of overlapping rheumatological symptoms. The American College of Rheumatology issued a list of 11 signs and/or symptoms in 1982 to assist in differentiating lupus from similar diseases. The patient should have four or more of these to establish suspicion of lupus; the symptoms do not have to manifest at the same time: malar rash (rash over the cheeks), discoid rash (red raised patches), photosensitivity (exposure resulting in development of or increase in skin rash), oral ulcers, nonerosive arthritis involving two or more peripheral joints, pleuritis or pericarditis, renal disorder (as evidenced by excessive protein in urine or the presence of casts in the urine), neurological disorder (seizures or psychosis in the absence of drugs known to cause these effects), hematological disorder (hemolytic anemia, leukopenia, lymphopenia, thrombocytopenia where the leukopenia or lymphopenia occurs on more than two occasions and the thrombocytopenia occurs in the absence of drugs known to cause it), positive ANA in the absence of a drug known to induce lupus, or immunological disorder (evidenced by positive anti-ds DNA, positive anti-Sm, positive antiphospholipid such as anticardiolipin antibody or a false-positive VDRL syphilis test).

INDICATIONS

- Assist in the diagnosis and evaluation of SLE
- Assist in the diagnosis and evaluation of suspected immune disorders, such as rheumatoid arthritis, systemic sclerosis, polymyositis, Raynaud's syndrome, scleroderma, Sjögren's syndrome, and mixed connective tissue disease
- Assist in the diagnosis and evaluation of idiopathic inflammatory myopathies

POTENTIAL DIAGNOSIS

ANA Pattern*	Associated Antibody	Associated Condition
Rim and/or homogeneous	Double-stranded DNA	SLE
	Single- or double-stranded DNA	
Homogeneous	Histones	SLE
Speckled	Sm (Smith) antibody	SLE, mixed connective tissue disease, Raynaud's scleroderma, Sjögren's syndrome
	RNP*	Mixed connective tissue disease, various rheumatoid conditions
	SS-B/La, SS-A/Ro	Various rheumatoid conditions

(table continues on page 118)

ANA Pattern*	Associated Antibody	Associated Condition
Diffuse speckled with positive mitotic figures	Centromere	PSS with CREST, Raynaud's
Nucleolar	Nucleolar, RNP	Scleroderma, CREST

*ANA patterns are helpful in that certain conditions are frequently associated with specific patterns. RNP = ribonucleoprotein.

Increased in

- Anti-Jo-1 *is associated with dermatomyositis, idiopathic inflammatory myopathies, and polymyositis*
- ANA *is associated with drug-induced lupus erythematosus*
- ANA *is associated with lupoid hepatitis*
- ANA *is associated with mixed connective tissue disease*
- ANA *is associated with polymyositis*
- ANA *is associated with progressive systemic sclerosis*
- ANA *is associated with Raynaud's syndrome*
- ANA *is associated with rheumatoid arthritis*
- ANA *is associated with Sjögren's syndrome*
- ANA *and anti-DNA are associated with SLE*
- Anti-RNP *is associated with mixed connective tissue disease*
- Anti-Scl 70 *is associated with progressive systemic sclerosis and scleroderma*
- Anti-SS-A and anti-SS-B *are helpful in antinuclear antibody (ANA)–negative cases of SLE*
- Anti-SS-A/ANA–positive, anti-SS-B–negative patients *are likely to have nephritis*
- Anti-SS-A/anti-SS-B–positive sera *are found in patients with neonatal lupus*
- Anti-SS-A–positive patients *may also have antibodies associated with antiphospholipid syndrome*
- Anti-SS-A/La *is associated with primary Sjögren's syndrome*
- Anti-SS-A/Ro *is a predictor of congenital heart block in neonates born to mothers with SLE*
- Anti-SS-A/Ro–positive patients *have photosensitivity*

Decreased in: N/A

CRITICAL FINDINGS: N/A

INTERFERING FACTORS

- Drugs that may cause positive ANA results include acebutolol (diabetics), anticonvulsants (increases with concomitant administration of multiple antiepileptic drugs), carbamazepine, chlorpromazine, ethosuximide, hydralazine, isoniazid, methyldopa, oxyphenisatin, penicillins, phenytoin, primidone, procainamide, quinidine, and trimethadione.
- A patient can have lupus and test ANA-negative.
- Inability of the patient to cooperate or remain still during the procedure because of age, significant pain, or mental status may interfere with the test results.

NURSING IMPLICATIONS AND PROCEDURE

PRETEST:

- Positively identify the patient using at least two unique identifiers before providing care, treatment, or services.

A

- **Patient Teaching:** Inform the patient this test can assist in evaluating immune system function.
- Obtain a history of the patient's complaints, including a list of known allergens, especially allergies or sensitivities to latex.
- Obtain a history of the patient's immune and musculoskeletal systems, symptoms, and results of previously performed laboratory tests and diagnostic and surgical procedures.
- Obtain a list of the patient's current medications, including herbs, nutritional supplements, and nutraceuticals (see Appendix F).
- Review the procedure with the patient. Inform the patient that specimen collection takes approximately 5 to 10 min. Address concerns about pain and explain that there may be some discomfort during the venipuncture.
- **Sensitivity to social and cultural issues,** as well as concern for modesty, is important in providing psychological support before, during, and after the procedure.
- There are no food, fluid, or medication restrictions unless by medical direction.

INTRATEST:

- If the patient has a history of allergic reaction to latex, avoid the use of equipment containing latex.
- Instruct the patient to cooperate fully and to follow directions. Direct the patient to breathe normally and to avoid unnecessary movement.
- Observe standard precautions, and follow the general guidelines in Appendix A. Positively identify the patient, and label the appropriate tubes with the corresponding patient demographics, date, and time of collection. Perform a venipuncture.
- Remove the needle and apply direct pressure with dry gauze to stop bleeding. Observe/assess venipuncture site for bleeding or hematoma formation and secure gauze with adhesive bandage.
- Promptly transport the specimen to the laboratory for processing and analysis.

POST-TEST:

- A report of the results will be sent to the requesting health-care provider (HCP), who will discuss the results with the patient.
- Recognize anxiety related to test results, and be supportive of perceived loss of independence and fear of shortened life expectancy. Collagen and connective tissue diseases are chronic and, as such, they must be addressed on a continuous basis. Discuss the implications of abnormal test results on the patient's lifestyle. Provide teaching and information regarding the clinical implications of the test results, as appropriate. Educate the patient regarding access to counseling services. Provide contact information, if desired, for the Lupus Foundation of America (www.lupus.org) or for the Arthritis Foundation (www.arthritis.org).
- Educate the patient, as appropriate, regarding the importance of preventing infection, which is a significant cause of death in immunosuppressed individuals.
- Reinforce information given by the patient's HCP regarding further testing, treatment, or referral to another HCP. Answer any questions or address any concerns voiced by the patient or family.
- Depending on the results of this procedure, additional testing may be performed to evaluate or monitor progression of the disease process and determine the need for a change in therapy. Evaluate test results in relation to the patient's symptoms and other tests performed.

RELATED MONOGRAPHS:

- Related tests include antibodies anticyclic citrullinated peptide, arthroscopy, biopsy kidney, biopsy skin, BMD, bone scan, chest x-ray, complement C3 and C4, complement total, CRP, ESR, EMG, MRI musculoskeletal, procainamide, radiography bone, RF, and synovial fluid analysis.
- See the Immune and Musculoskeletal systems tables at the end of the book for related tests by body system.

A

Antibodies, Antisperm

SYNONYM/ACRONYM: Infertility screen.

COMMON USE: To evaluate testicular fertility and identify causes of infertility such as congenital defects, cancer, and torsion.

SPECIMEN: Serum (1 mL) collected in a red-top tube.

REFERENCE VALUE: (Method: Immunoassay)

Result	Sperm Bound by Immunobead (%)
Negative	0–15
Weak positive	16–30
Moderate positive	31–50
Strong positive	51–100

immunobead sperm antibody test used to identify antibodies directly attached to the sperm. Semen and cervical mucus can also be tested for antisperm antibodies.

DESCRIPTION: Normally sperm develop in the seminiferous tubules of the testes separated from circulating blood by the blood-testes barrier. Any situation that disrupts this barrier can expose sperm to detection by immune response cells in the blood and subsequent antibody formation against the sperm. Antisperm antibodies attach to the head, midpiece, or tail of the sperm, impairing motility and ability to penetrate the cervical mucosa. The antibodies can also cause clumping of sperm, which may be noted on a semen analysis. A major cause of infertility in men is blocked efferent testicular ducts. Reabsorption of sperm from the blocked ducts may also result in development of sperm antibodies. Another more specific and sophisticated method than measurement of circulating antibodies is the

INDICATIONS
- Evaluation of infertility

POTENTIAL DIAGNOSIS

Increased in
Conditions that affect the integrity of the blood-testes barrier can result in antibody formation.
- Blocked testicular efferent duct *(related to absorption of sperm by blocked vas deferens)*
- Congenital absence of the vas deferens *(related to absorption of sperm by blocked vas deferens)*
- Cryptorchidism *(related to disruption in the integrity of the blood-testes barrier)*
- Infection (orchitis, prostatitis) *(related to disruption in the integrity of the blood-testes barrier)*
- Inguinal hernia repair prior to puberty *(related to disruption in the integrity of the blood-testes barrier)*
- Testicular biopsy *(related to disruption in the integrity of the blood-testes barrier)*
- Testicular cancer *(related to disruption in the integrity of the blood-testes barrier)*

- Testicular torsion *(related to disruption in the integrity of the blood-testes barrier)*
- Varicocele *(related to disruption in the integrity of the blood-testes barrier)*
- Vasectomy *(related to absorption of sperm by blocked vas deferens)*
- Vasectomy reversal *(related to interaction between sperm and autoantibodies developed after vasectomy)*

Decreased in: N/A

CRITICAL FINDINGS: N/A

INTERFERING FACTORS
- The patient should not ejaculate for 3 to 4 days before specimen collection if semen will be evaluated.
- Sperm antibodies have been detected in pregnant women and in women with primary infertility.

NURSING IMPLICATIONS AND PROCEDURE

PRETEST:
- Positively identify the patient using at least two unique identifiers before providing care, treatment, or services.
- *Patient Teaching:* Inform the patient this test can assist in the evaluation of infertility and provide guidance through assistive reproductive techniques.
- Obtain a history of the patient's complaints, including a list of known allergens, especially allergies or sensitivities to latex.
- Obtain a history of the patient's reproductive system, symptoms, and results of previously performed laboratory tests and diagnostic and surgical procedures.
- Obtain a list of the patient's current medications, including herbs, nutritional supplements, and nutraceuticals (see Appendix F).
- Review the procedure with the patient. Inform the patient that specimen collection takes approximately 5 to 10 min

and that additional specimens may be required. Address concerns about pain and explain that there may be some discomfort during the venipuncture.
- *Sensitivity to social and cultural issues,* as well as concern for modesty, is important in providing psychological support before, during, and after the procedure.
- There are no food, fluid, or medication restrictions unless by medical direction.

INTRATEST:
- If the patient has a history of allergic reaction to latex, avoid the use of equipment containing latex.
- Instruct the patient to cooperate fully and to follow directions. Direct the patient to breathe normally and to avoid unnecessary movement.
- Observe standard precautions, and follow the general guidelines in Appendix A. Positively identify the patient, and label the appropriate tubes with the corresponding patient demographics, date, and time of collection. Perform a venipuncture.
- Remove the needle and apply direct pressure with dry gauze to stop bleeding. Observe/assess venipuncture site for bleeding or hematoma formation and secure gauze with adhesive bandage.
- Promptly transport the specimen to the laboratory for processing and analysis.

POST-TEST:
- A report of the results will be sent to the requesting health-care provider (HCP), who will discuss the results with the patient.
- Recognize anxiety related to test results. Discuss the implications of abnormal test results on the patient's lifestyle. Educate the patient regarding access to counseling services. Provide a supportive, nonjudgmental environment when assisting a patient through the process of fertility testing. Educate the patient regarding access to counseling services, as appropriate.
- Reinforce information given by the patient's HCP regarding further

A

testing, treatment, or referral to another HCP. Answer any questions or address any concerns voiced by the patient or family.

▶ Depending on the results of this procedure, additional testing may be performed to evaluate or monitor progression of the disease process and determine the need for a change in therapy. Evaluate test results in relation to the patient's symptoms and other tests performed.

RELATED MONOGRAPHS:

▶ Related tests include HCG, LH, progesterone, semen analysis, testosterone, and US scrotal.

▶ See the Reproductive System tables at the end of the book for related tests by body system.

Antibodies, Antistreptolysin O

SYNONYM/ACRONYM: Streptozyme, ASO.

COMMON USE: To assist in the diagnosis of streptococcal infection.

SPECIMEN: Serum (1 mL) collected in a red-top tube.

REFERENCE VALUE: (Method: Immunoturbidometric) Adult: Less than 200 international units/mL; 17 yr and younger: Less than 150 international units/mL.

DESCRIPTION: Group A β-hemolytic streptococci secrete the enzyme streptolysin O, which can destroy red blood cells. The enzyme acts as an antigen and stimulates the immune system to develop streptolysin O antibodies. These antistreptolysin O (ASO) antibodies occur within 1 wk after the onset of a streptococcal infection and peak 2 to 3 wk later. Detection of the antibody over several weeks strongly suggests exposure to group A β-hemolytic streptococci. The ASO titer usually returns to preinfection levels within 6 to 12 mo, assuming reinfection has not occurred. Up to 95% of patients with acute glomerulonephritis and up to 85% of patients with rheumatic fever demonstrate a rise in titer. ASO titer may not become elevated in some patients who experience sequelae involving the skin or kidneys, and the antideoxyribonuclease-B, streptococcal test may a better test for these patients.

INDICATIONS

• Assist in establishing a diagnosis of streptococcal infection
• Evaluate patients with streptococcal infections for the development of acute rheumatic fever or nephritis
• Monitor response to therapy in streptococcal illnesses

POTENTIAL DIAGNOSIS

Increased in
Presence of antibodies, especially a rise in titer, is indicative of exposure.
• Endocarditis
• Glomerulonephritis

- Rheumatic fever
- Scarlet fever

Decreased in: N/A

CRITICAL FINDINGS: N/A

INTERFERING FACTORS
- Drugs that may decrease ASO titers include antibiotics and corticosteroids because therapy suppresses antibody response.
- False-positive ASO titers can be caused by elevated levels of serum β-lipoprotein (observed in liver disease).

NURSING IMPLICATIONS AND PROCEDURE

PRETEST:
- Positively identify the patient using at least two unique identifiers before providing care, treatment, or services.
- *Patient Teaching:* Inform the patient this test can assist in documenting exposure to streptococcal bacteria.
- Obtain a history of the patient's complaints, including a list of known allergens, especially allergies or sensitivities to latex.
- Obtain a history of the patient's immune system, symptoms, and results of previously performed laboratory tests and diagnostic and surgical procedures.
- Obtain a list of the patient's current medications, including herbs, nutritional supplements, and nutraceuticals (see Appendix F).
- Review the procedure with the patient. Inform the patient that specimen collection takes approximately 5 to 10 min. Address concerns about pain and explain that there may be some discomfort during the venipuncture.
- *Sensitivity to social and cultural issues,* as well as concern for modesty, is important in providing psychological support before, during, and after the procedure.
- There are no food, fluid, or medication restrictions unless by medical direction.

INTRATEST:
- If the patient has a history of allergic reaction to latex, avoid the use of equipment containing latex.
- Instruct the patient to cooperate fully and to follow directions. Direct the patient to breathe normally and to avoid unnecessary movement.
- Observe standard precautions, and follow the general guidelines in Appendix A. Positively identify the patient, and label the appropriate tubes with the corresponding patient demographics, date, and time of collection. Perform a venipuncture.
- Remove the needle and apply direct pressure with dry gauze to stop bleeding. Observe/assess venipuncture site for bleeding or hematoma formation and secure gauze with adhesive bandage.
- Promptly transport the specimen to the laboratory for processing and analysis.

POST-TEST:
- A report of the results will be sent to the requesting health-care provider (HCP), who will discuss the results with the patient.
- Administer antibiotics as ordered. Remind the patient of the importance of completing the entire course of antibiotic therapy even if signs and symptoms disappear before completion of therapy.
- Reinforce information given by the patient's HCP regarding further testing, treatment, or referral to another HCP. Answer any questions or address any concerns voiced by the patient or family.
- Depending on the results of this procedure, additional testing may be performed to evaluate or monitor progression of the disease process and determine the need for a change in therapy. Evaluate test results in relation to the patient's symptoms and other tests performed.

RELATED MONOGRAPHS:
- Related tests include culture throat, group A streptococcal screen, and antideoxyribonuclease-B streptococcal.
- See the Immune System table at the end of the book for related tests by body system.

Antibodies, Antithyroglobulin and Antithyroid Peroxidase

SYNONYM/ACRONYM: Thyroid antibodies, antithyroid peroxidase antibodies (thyroid peroxidase [TPO] antibodies were previously called thyroid antimicrosomal antibodies).

COMMON USE: To assist in the diagnosis of hypothyroid and hyperthyroid disease.

SPECIMEN: Serum (1 mL) collected in a red-top tube.

REFERENCE VALUE: (Method: Immunoassay)

Antibody	Conventional Units
Antithyroglobulin antibody	Less than 20 international units/mL
Antiperoxidase antibody	Less than 35 international units/mL

DESCRIPTION: Thyroid antibodies are mainly immunoglobulin G-type antibodies. Antithyroid peroxidase antibodies (anti-TPO antibodies) bind with microsomal antigens on cells lining the microsomal membrane of thyroid tissue. They are thought to destroy thyroid tissue as a result of stimulation by lymphocytic killer cells. These antibodies are present in hypothyroid and hyperthyroid conditions. Anti-TPO antibodies are present in Hashimoto's autoimmune thyroiditis, a major cause of hypothyroidism. Hypothyroidism in women of childbearing age is a significant concern because of the deleterious effects of insufficient thyroxine levels on fetal brain development. Anti-TPO antibodies are also demonstrable in Graves' disease, a major cause of hyperthyroidism. Graves' disease is the most common type of thyrotoxicosis in women of childbearing age, impairing fertility and increasing risk of miscarriage to 26%. Transplacental passage of anti-TPO antibodies in pregnant patients may affect the developing fetus or lead to thyroid disease in the neonate. Mild depression is more common in postpartum women with anti-TPO antibodies. Antithyroglobulin antibodies are autoantibodies directed against thyroglobulin. The function of these antibodies is unclear. Both tests are normally requested together.

INDICATIONS
• Assist in confirming suspected inflammation of thyroid gland
• Assist in the diagnosis of suspected hypothyroidism caused by thyroid tissue destruction
• Assist in the diagnosis of suspected thyroid autoimmunity in patients with other autoimmune disorders

POTENTIAL DIAGNOSIS

Increased in

The presence of these antibodies differentiates the autoimmune origin of these disorders from non-autoimmune causes, which may influence treatment decisions.

- Autoimmune disorders
- Graves' disease
- Goiter
- Hashimoto's thyroiditis
- Idiopathic myxedema
- Pernicious anemia
- Thyroid carcinoma

Decreased in: N/A

CRITICAL FINDINGS: N/A

INTERFERING FACTORS

- Lithium may increase thyroid antibody levels.

NURSING IMPLICATIONS AND PROCEDURE

PRETEST:

- Positively identify the patient using at least two unique identifiers before providing care, treatment, or services.
- *Patient Teaching:* Inform the patient this test can assist in evaluating thyroid gland function.
- Obtain a history of the patient's complaints, including a list of known allergens, especially allergies or sensitivities to latex.
- Obtain a history of the patient's endocrine and immune systems, symptoms, and results of previously performed laboratory tests and diagnostic and surgical procedures.
- Obtain a list of the patient's current medications, including herbs, nutritional supplements, and nutraceuticals (see Appendix F).
- Note any recent procedures that can interfere with test results.
- Review the procedure with the patient. Inform the patient that specimen collection takes approximately 5 to 10 min. Address concerns about pain and explain that there may be some discomfort during the venipuncture.
- There are no food, fluid, or medication restrictions unless by medical direction.

INTRATEST:

- If the patient has a history of allergic reaction to latex, avoid the use of equipment containing latex.
- Instruct the patient to cooperate fully and to follow directions. Direct the patient to breathe normally and to avoid unnecessary movement.
- Observe standard precautions, and follow the general guidelines in Appendix A. Positively identify the patient, and label the appropriate tubes with the corresponding patient demographics, date, and time of collection. Perform a venipuncture.
- Remove the needle and apply direct pressure with dry gauze to stop bleeding. Observe/assess venipuncture site for bleeding or hematoma formation and secure gauze with adhesive bandage.
- Promptly transport the specimen to the laboratory for processing and analysis.

POST-TEST:

- A report of the results will be sent to the requesting health-care provider (HCP), who will discuss the results with the patient.
- Reinforce information given by the patient's HCP regarding further testing, treatment, or referral to another HCP. Answer any questions or address any concerns voiced by the patient or family.
- Depending on the results of this procedure, additional testing may be performed to evaluate or monitor progression of the disease process and determine the need for a change in therapy. Evaluate test results in relation to the patient's symptoms and other tests performed.

RELATED MONOGRAPHS:

- Related tests include biopsy thyroid, CBC, FT₃, FT₄, RAIU, T4, thyroid scan, thyroglobulin, TSH, TT3, and US thyroid.
- See the Endocrine and Immune systems tables at the end of the book for related tests by body system.

Antibodies, Cardiolipin, Immunoglobulin G, and Immunoglobulin M

SYNONYM/ACRONYM: Antiphospholipid antibody, lupus anticoagulant, LA, ACA.

COMMON USE: To detect the presence of antiphospholipid antibodies, which can lead to the development of blood vessel problems and complications including stroke, heart attack, and miscarriage.

SPECIMEN: Serum (1 mL) collected in a red-top tube.

REFERENCE VALUE: (Method: Immunoassay, enzyme-linked immunosorbent assay [ELISA])

IgG (GPL = 1 unit IgG phospholipid)	IgM (MPL = 1 unit IgM phospholipid)
Negative: 0–10 GPL	Negative: 0–9 MPL
Indeterminate: 11–19 GPL	Indeterminate: 10–19 MPL
Low-medium positive: 20–80 GPL	Low-medium positive: 20–80 MPL
Positive: Greater than 80 GPL	Greater than 80 MPL

DESCRIPTION: Cardiolipin antibody (ACA) is one of several identified antiphospholipid antibodies. ACAs are of IgG, IgM, and IgA subtypes, which react with proteins in the blood that are bound to phospholipid and interfere with normal blood vessel function. The two primary types of problems they cause are narrowing and irregularity of the blood vessels and blood clots in the blood vessels. ACAs are found in individuals with lupus erythematosus, lupus-related conditions, infectious diseases, drug reactions, and sometimes fetal loss. ACAs are often found in association with lupus anticoagulant. Increased antiphospholipid antibody levels have been found in pregnant women with lupus who have had miscarriages. The combination of noninflamma- tory thrombosis of blood vessels, low platelet count, and history of miscarriage is termed *antiphospholipid antibody syndrome* and is documented by a medium or high level of IgG or IgM on two or more occasions, tested 6 or more weeks apart.

INDICATIONS
• Assist in the diagnosis of antiphospholipid antibody syndrome

POTENTIAL DIAGNOSIS

Increased in
While ACAs are observed in specific diseases, the exact mechanism of these antibodies in disease is unclear. In fact, the production of ACA can be induced by bacterial, treponemal, and viral infections. Development of ACA under this

circumstance is transient and not associated with an increased risk of antiphospholipid antibody syndrome. Patients who initially demonstrate positive ACA levels should be retested after 6 to 8 wk to rule out transient antibodies that are usually of no clinical significance.

- Antiphospholipid antibody syndrome
- Chorea
- Drug reactions
- Epilepsy
- Infectious diseases
- Mitral valve endocarditis
- Patients with lupuslike symptoms (often antinuclear antibody–negative)
- Placental infarction
- Recurrent fetal loss (strong association with two or more occurrences)
- Recurrent venous and arterial thromboses

Decreased in: N/A

CRITICAL FINDINGS: N/A

INTERFERING FACTORS

- Drugs that may increase anticardiolipin antibody levels include chlorpromazine, penicillin, procainamide, phenytoin, and quinidine.
- Cardiolipin antibody is partially cross-reactive with syphilis reagin antibody and lupus anticoagulant. False-positive rapid plasma reagin results may occur.

NURSING IMPLICATIONS AND PROCEDURE

PRETEST:

- Positively identify the patient using at least two unique identifiers before providing care, treatment, or services.
- *Patient Teaching:* Inform the patient this test can assist in evaluating the amount of potentially harmful circulating antibodies.

- Obtain a history of the patient's complaints, including a list of known allergens, especially allergies or sensitivities to latex.
- Obtain a history of the patient's hematopoietic, immune, and reproductive systems; symptoms; and results of previously performed laboratory tests and diagnostic and surgical procedures.
- Obtain a list of the patient's current medications, including herbs, nutritional supplements, and nutraceuticals (see Appendix F).
- Review the procedure with the patient. Inform the patient that specimen collection takes approximately 5 to 10 min. Address concerns about pain and explain that there may be some discomfort during the venipuncture.
- *Sensitivity to social and cultural issues,* as well as concern for modesty, is important in providing psychological support before, during, and after the procedure.
- There are no food, fluid, or medication restrictions unless by medical direction.

INTRATEST:

- If the patient has a history of allergic reaction to latex, avoid the use of equipment containing latex.
- Instruct the patient to cooperate fully and to follow directions. Direct the patient to breathe normally and to avoid unnecessary movement.
- Observe standard precautions, and follow the general guidelines in Appendix A. Positively identify the patient, and label the appropriate tubes with the corresponding patient demographics, date, and time of collection. Perform a venipuncture.
- Remove the needle and apply direct pressure with dry gauze to stop bleeding. Observe/assess venipuncture site for bleeding or hematoma formation and secure gauze with adhesive bandage.
- Promptly transport the specimen to the laboratory for processing and analysis.

POST-TEST:

- A report of the results will be sent to the requesting health-care provider (HCP), who will discuss the results with the patient.

◆ Recognize anxiety related to test results, and be supportive of fear of shortened life expectancy. Discuss the implications of abnormal test results on the patient's lifestyle. Provide teaching and information regarding the clinical implications of the test results, as appropriate. Educate the patient regarding access to counseling services. Provide contact information, if desired, for the Lupus Foundation of America (www.lupus.org).

◆ Reinforce information given by the patient's HCP regarding further testing, treatment, or referral to another HCP. Answer any questions or address any concerns voiced by the patient or family.

◆ Depending on the results of this procedure, additional testing may be performed to evaluate or monitor progression of the disease process and determine the need for a change in therapy. Evaluate test results in relation to the patient's symptoms and other tests performed.

RELATED MONOGRAPHS:

◆ Related tests include ANA, CBC, CBC platelet count, fibrinogen, lupus anticoagulant antibodies, protein C, protein S, and syphilis serology.

◆ See the Hematopoietic, Immune, and Reproductive systems tables at the end of the book for related tests by body system.

Antibodies, Gliadin
(Immunoglobulin G and Immunoglobulin A)

SYNONYM/ACRONYM: Endomysial antibodies (EMA), gliadin (IgG and IgA) antibodies.

COMMON USE: To assist in the diagnosis and monitoring of gluten-sensitive enteropathies that may damage intestinal mucosa.

SPECIMEN: Serum (1 mL) collected in a red-top tube.

REFERENCE VALUE: (Method: Immunoassay)

IgA and IgG Gliadin Antibody	Conventional Units
Age	
0–2 yr	Less than 50 units/mL
2 yr–adult	Less than 25 units/mL

DESCRIPTION: Gliadin is a water-soluble protein found in the gluten of wheat, rye, oats, and barley. The intestinal mucosa of certain individuals does not digest gluten, allowing a toxic buildup of gliadin and intestinal inflammation. The inflammatory response interferes with intestinal absorption of nutrients and damages the intestinal mucosa. In severe cases, intestinal mucosa can be lost. Immunoglobulin G (IgG) and immunoglobulin A (IgA) gliadin antibodies are detectable in the serum of patients with gluten-sensitive enteropathy. Endomysial tissue transglutaminase (tTG) and deaminated gliadin peptides (DGP) are two other serological tests commonly used to investigate gluten-sensitive enteropathies. Gliadin IgA tests are the most sensitive for celiac disease (CD). However, it is also recognized that a significant percentage of patients with CD are also IgA deficient, meaning false-negative IgA results may be misleading in some cases. Estimates of up to 98% of individuals susceptible to CD carry either the DQ2 or DQ8 HLA cell surface receptors, which initiate formation of antibodies to gliadin. While it appears there is a strong association between CD and these gene markers, up to 40% of individuals without CD also carry the DQ2 or DQ8 markers. Molecular testing is available to establish the absence or presence of these susceptibility markers. CD is an inherited condition with significant impact on quality of life for the affected individual. The use of serological markers is useful in disease monitoring because research has established a relationship between amount of gluten in the diet and degree of intestinal damage as reflected by the level of detectable antibodies. CD shares an association with a number of other conditions such as type 1 diabetes, Down's syndrome, and Turner's syndrome.

INDICATIONS

- Assist in the diagnosis of asymptomatic gluten-sensitive enteropathy in some patients with dermatitis herpetiformis
- Assist in the diagnosis of gluten-sensitive enteropathies
- Assist in the diagnosis of nontropical sprue
- Monitor dietary compliance of patients with gluten-sensitive enteropathies

POTENTIAL DIAGNOSIS

Increased in
Evidenced by the combination of detectable gliadin or endomysial antibodies and improvement with a gluten-free diet.
- Asymptomatic gluten-sensitive enteropathy
- Celiac disease
- Dermatitis herpetiformis *(etiology of this skin manifestation is unknown, but there is an association related to gluten-sensitive enteropathy)*
- Nontropical sprue

Decreased in
- IgA deficiency *(related to an inability to produce IgA and evidenced by decreased IgA levels and false-negative IgA gliadin tests)*
- Children under the age of 18 mo *(related to immature immune system and low production of IgA)*

CRITICAL FINDINGS: N/A

INTERFERING FACTORS
- Conditions other than gluten-sensitive enteropathy can result in elevated antibody levels without corresponding histological evidence. These conditions include Crohn's disease, postinfection

malabsorption, and food protein intolerance.

• A negative IgA gliadin result, especially with a positive IgG gliadin result in an untreated patient, does not rule out active gluten-sensitive enteropathy.

NURSING IMPLICATIONS AND PROCEDURE

PRETEST:

▶ Positively identify the patient using at least two unique identifiers before providing care, treatment, or services.

▶ *Patient Teaching:* Inform the patient this test can assist with evaluating the ability to digest gluten foods such as wheat, rye, and oats.

▶ Obtain a history of the patient's complaints, including a list of known allergens, especially allergies or sensitivities to latex.

▶ Obtain a history of the patient's gastrointestinal and immune systems, symptoms, and results of previously performed laboratory tests and diagnostic and surgical procedures.

▶ Obtain a list of foods and the patient's current medications, including herbs, nutritional supplements, and nutraceuticals (see Appendix F).

▶ Review the procedure with the patient. Inform the patient that specimen collection takes approximately 5 to 10 min. Address concerns about pain and explain that there may be some discomfort during the venipuncture.

▶ *Sensitivity to social and cultural issues,* as well as concern for modesty, is important in providing psychological support before, during, and after the procedure.

▶ There are no food, fluid, or medication restrictions unless by medical direction.

INTRATEST:

▶ If the patient has a history of allergic reaction to latex, avoid the use of equipment containing latex.

▶ Instruct the patient to cooperate fully and to follow directions. Direct the patient to breathe normally and to avoid unnecessary movement.

▶ Observe standard precautions, and follow the general guidelines in Appendix A. Positively identify the patient, and label the appropriate tubes with the corresponding patient demographics, date, and time of collection. Perform a venipuncture.

▶ Remove the needle and apply direct pressure with dry gauze to stop bleeding. Observe/assess venipuncture site for bleeding or hematoma formation and secure gauze with adhesive bandage.

▶ Promptly transport the specimen to the laboratory for processing and analysis.

POST-TEST:

▶ A report of the results will be sent to the requesting health-care provider (HCP), who will discuss the results with the patient.

▶ *Nutritional Considerations:* Encourage the patient with abnormal findings to consult with a qualified nutritionist to plan a gluten-free diet. This dietary planning is complex because patients are often malnourished and have other related nutritional problems.

▶ Recognize anxiety related to test results, and offer support. Discuss the implications of abnormal test results on the patient's lifestyle. Provide teaching and information regarding the clinical implications of the test results, as appropriate. Educate the patient regarding access to appropriate counseling services. Provide contact information, if desired, for the Celiac Disease Foundation (www.celiac.org) or Children's Digestive Health and Nutrition Foundation (www.cdhnf.org).

▶ Reinforce information given by the patient's HCP regarding further testing, treatment, or referral to another HCP. Answer any questions or address any concerns voiced by the patient or family.

▶ Depending on the results of this procedure, additional testing may be performed to evaluate or monitor

progression of the disease process and determine the need for a change in therapy. Evaluate test results in relation to the patient's symptoms and other tests performed.

RELATED MONOGRAPHS:

▶ Related tests include albumin, biopsy intestine, biopsy skin, calcium,

capsule endoscopy, colonoscopy, D-xylose tolerance test, electrolytes, fecal analysis, fecal fat, folic acid, immunoglobulins (IgA), iron, and lactose tolerance test.

▶ See the Gastrointestinal and Immune systems tables at the end of the book for related tests by body system.

Anticonvulsant Drugs: Carbamazepine, Ethosuximide, Phenobarbital, Phenytoin, Primidone, Valproic Acid

SYNONYM/ACRONYM: *Carbamazepine* (Carbamazepinum, Carbategretal, Carbatrol, Carbazep, CBZ, Epitol, Tegretol, Tegretol XR); *ethosuximide* (Suxinutin, Zarontin, Zartalin); *phenobarbital* (Barbita, Comizial, Fenilcal, Gardenal, Phenemal, Phenemalum, Phenobarb, Phenobarbitone, Phenylethylmalonylurea, Solfoton, Stental Extentabs); *phenytoin* (Antisacer, Dilantin, Dintoina, Diphenylan Sodium, Diphenylhydantoin, Ditan, Epanutin, Epinat, Fenitoina, Fenytoin, Fosphenytoin); *primidone* (Desoxyphenobarbital, Hexamidinum, Majsolin, Mylepsin, Mysoline, Primaclone, Prysolin); *valproic acid* (Depacon, Depakene, Depakote, Depakote XR, Depamide, Dipropylacetic Acid, Divalproex Sodium, Epilim, Ergenyl, Leptilan, 2-Propylpentanoic Acid, 2-Propylvaleric Acid, Valkote, Valproate Semisodium, Valproate Sodium).

COMMON USE: To monitor specific drugs for subtherapeutic, therapeutic, or toxic levels in evaluation of treatment.

SPECIMEN: Serum (1 mL) collected in a red-top tube.

Drug*	Route of Administration
Carbamazepine	Oral
Ethosuximide	Oral
Phenobarbital	Oral
Phenytoin	Oral
Primidone	Oral
Valproic Acid	Oral

*Recommended collection time = trough: immediately before next dose (at steady state) or at a consistent sampling time.

REFERENCE VALUE: (Method: Immunoassay)

Drug	Therapeutic Dose*	SI Units	Half-Life (hr)	Volume of Distribution (L/kg)	Protein Binding (%)	Excretion
(SI = Conventional Units × 4.23) Carbamazepine	4–12 mcg/mL	17–51 micromol/L	15–40	0.8–1.8	60–80	Hepatic
(SI = Conventional Units × 7.08) Ethosuximide	40–100 mcg/mL	283–708 micromol/L	25–70	0.7	0–5	Renal
(SI = Conventional Units × 4.31) Phenobarbital	Adult: 15–40 mcg/mL Child: 15–30 mcg/mL	Adult: 65–172 micromol/L Child: 65–129 micromol/L	Adult: 50–140 Child: 40–70	0.5–1.0 L/kg	40–50	80% Hepatic 20% Renal
(SI = Conventional Units × 3.96) Phenytoin	10–20 mcg/mL	40–79 micromol/L	20–40	0.6–0.7	85–95	Hepatic
(SI = Conventional Units × 4.58) Primidone	Adult: 5–12 mcg/mL Child: 7–10 mcg/mL	Adult: 23–55 micromol/L Child: 32–46 micromol/L	4–12	0.5–1.0	0–20	Hepatic
(SI = Conventional Units × 6.93) Valproic acid	50–120 mcg/mL	347–832 micromol/L	8–15	0.1–0.5	85–95	Hepatic

*Conventional units.

DESCRIPTION: Anticonvulsants are used to reduce the frequency and severity of seizures for patients with epilepsy. Carbamazepine is also used for controlling neurogenic pain in trigeminal neuralgia and diabetic neuropathy and for treating for bipolar disease and other neurological and psychiatric conditions. Valproic acid is also used for some psychiatric conditions like bipolar disease and for prevention of migraine headache.

Many factors must be considered in effective dosing and monitoring of therapeutic drugs, including patient age, patient weight, interacting medications, electrolyte balance, protein levels, water balance, conditions that affect absorption and excretion, and the ingestion of substances (e.g., foods, herbals, vitamins, and minerals) that can either potentiate or inhibit the intended target concentration.

Peak and trough collection times should be documented carefully in relation to the time of medication administration.

IMPORTANT NOTE

This information must be clearly and accurately communicated to avoid misunderstanding of the dose time in relation to the collection time. Miscommunication between the individual administering the medication and the individual collecting the specimen is the most frequent cause of subtherapeutic levels, toxic levels, and misleading information used in calculation of future doses.

INDICATIONS

- Assist in the diagnosis of and prevention of toxicity
- Evaluate overdose, especially in combination with ethanol
- Monitor compliance with therapeutic regimen

POTENTIAL DIAGNOSIS

Level	Response
Normal levels	Therapeutic effect
Subtherapeutic levels	Adjust dose as indicated
Toxic levels	Adjust dose as indicated
Carbamazepine	Hepatic impairment
Ethosuximide	Hepatic impairment
Phenobarbital	Hepatic impairment
Phenytoin	Hepatic impairment
Primidone	Hepatic impairment
Valproic acid	Hepatic impairment

CRITICAL FINDINGS

It is important to note the adverse effects of toxic and subtherapeutic levels. Care must be taken to investigate signs and symptoms of not enough medication and too much medication. Note and immediately report to the health-care provider (HCP) any critically increased or subtherapeutic values and related symptoms.

A

Carbamazepine: Greater Than 20 mcg/mL

Signs and symptoms of carbamazepine toxicity include respiratory depression, seizures, leukopenia, hyponatremia, hypotension, stupor, and possible coma. Possible interventions include gastric lavage (contraindicated if ileus is present); airway protection; administration of fluids and vasopressors for hypotension; treatment of seizures with diazepam, phenobarbital, or phenytoin; cardiac monitoring; monitoring of vital signs; and discontinuing the medication. Emetics are contraindicated.

Ethosuximide: Greater Than 200 mcg/mL

Signs and symptoms of ethosuximide toxicity include nausea, vomiting, and lethargy. Possible interventions include administration of activated charcoal, administration of saline cathartic and gastric lavage (contraindicated if ileus is present), airway protection, hourly assessment of neurologic function, and discontinuing the medication.

Phenobarbital: Greater Than 60 mcg/mL

Signs and symptoms of phenobarbital toxicity include cold, clammy skin; ataxia; central nervous system (CNS) depression; hypothermia; hypotension; cyanosis; Cheyne-Stokes respiration; tachycardia; possible coma; and possible renal impairment. Possible interventions include gastric lavage, administration of activated charcoal with cathartic, airway protection, possible intubation and mechanical ventilation (especially during gastric lavage if there is no gag reflex), monitoring for hypotension, and discontinuing the medication.

Phenytoin (adults): Greater Than 40 mcg/mL

Signs and symptoms of phenytoin toxicity include double vision, nystagmus, lethargy, CNS depression, and possible coma. Possible interventions include airway support, electrocardiographic monitoring, administration of activated charcoal, gastric lavage with warm saline or tap water, administration of saline or sorbitol cathartic, and discontinuing the medication.

Primidone: Greater Than 24 mcg/mL

Signs and symptoms of primidone toxicity include ataxia, anemia, CNS depression, lethargy, somnolence, vertigo, and visual disturbances. Possible interventions include airway protection, treatment of anemia with vitamin B_{12} and folate, and discontinuing the medication.

Valproic Acid: Greater Than 200 mcg/mL

Signs and symptoms of valproic acid toxicity include loss of appetite, mental changes, numbness, tingling, and weakness. Possible interventions include administration of activated charcoal and naloxone and discontinuing the medication.

INTERFERING FACTORS

- Blood drawn in serum separator tubes (gel tubes).
- Contraindicated in patients with liver disease, and caution advised in patients with renal impairment.
- Drugs that may increase carbamazepine levels or increase risk of toxicity include acetazolamide, azithromycin, bepridil, cimetidine, danazol, diltiazem, erythromycin, felodipine, fluoxetine, flurithromycin, fluvoxamine, gemfibrozil, isoniazid, itraconazole, josamycin,

ketoconazole, loratadine, macrolides, niacinamide, nicardipine, nifedipine, nimodipine, nisoldipine, propoxyphene, ritonavir, terfenadine, troleandomycin, valproic acid, verapamil, and viloxazine.

- Drugs that may decrease carbamazepine levels include phenobarbital, phenytoin, and primidone.
- Carbamazepine may affect other body chemistries as seen by a decrease in calcium, sodium, T_3, T_4 levels, and WBC count and increase in ALT, alkaline phosphatase, ammonia, AST, and bilirubin levels.
- Drugs that may increase ethosuximide levels include isoniazid, ritonavir, and valproic acid.
- Drugs that may decrease ethosuximide levels include phenobarbital, phenytoin, and primidone.
- Drugs that may increase phenobarbital levels or increase risk of toxicity include barbital drugs, furosemide, primidone, salicylates, and valproic acid.
- Phenobarbital may affect the metabolism of other drugs, increasing their effectiveness, such as β-blockers, chloramphenicol, corticosteroids, doxycycline, griseofulvin, haloperidol, methylphenidate, phenothiazines, phenylbutazone, propoxyphene, quinidine, theophylline, tricyclic antidepressants, and valproic acid.
- Phenobarbital may affect the metabolism of other drugs, decreasing their effectiveness, such as chloramphenicol, cyclosporine, ethosuximide, oral anticoagulants, oral contraceptives, phenytoin, theophylline, vitamin D, and vitamin K.
- Phenobarbital is an active metabolite of primidone, and both drug levels should be monitored while the patient is receiving primidone

to avoid either toxic or subtherapeutic levels of both medications.
- Phenobarbital may affect other body chemistries as seen by a decrease in bilirubin and calcium levels and increase in alkaline phosphatase, ammonia, and gamma glutamyl transferase levels.
- Drugs that may increase phenytoin levels or increase the risk of phenytoin toxicity include amiodarone, azapropazone, carbamazepine, chloramphenicol, cimetidine, disulfiram, ethanol, fluconazole, halothane, ibuprofen, imipramine, levodopa, metronidazole, miconazole, nifedipine, phenylbutazone, sulfonamides, trazodone, tricyclic antidepressants, and trimethoprim. Small changes in formulation (i.e., changes in brand) also may increase phenytoin levels or increase the risk of phenytoin toxicity.
- Drugs that may decrease phenytoin levels include bleomycin, carbamazepine, cisplatin, disulfiram, folic acid, intravenous fluids containing glucose, nitrofurantoin, oxacillin, rifampin, salicylates, and vinblastine.
- Primidone decreases the effectiveness of carbamazepine, ethosuximide, felbamate, lamotrigine, oral anticoagulants, oxcarbazepine, topiramate, and valproate.
- Primidone may affect other body chemistries as seen by a decrease in calcium levels and increase in alkaline phosphatase levels.
- Drugs that may increase valproic acid levels or increase risk of toxicity include dicumarol, phenylbutazone, and high doses of salicylate.
- Drugs that may decrease valproic acid levels include carbamazepine, phenobarbital, phenytoin, and primidone.

A

NURSING IMPLICATIONS AND PROCEDURE

PRETEST:

▶ Positively identify the patient using at least two unique identifiers before providing care, treatment, or services.

▶ *Patient Teaching:* Inform the patient this test can assist with monitoring for subtherapeutic, therapeutic, or toxic drug levels.

▶ Obtain a history of the patient's complaints, including a list of known allergens, especially allergies or sensitivities to latex.

▶ These medications are metabolized and excreted by the kidneys and liver. Obtain a history of the patient's genitourinary and hepatobiliary systems, symptoms, and results of previously performed laboratory tests and diagnostic and surgical procedures.

▶ Obtain a list of the patient's current medications, including herbs, nutritional supplements, and nutraceuticals (see Appendix F). Note the last time and dose of medication taken.

▶ Review the procedure with the patient. Inform the patient that specimen collection takes approximately 5 to 10 min. Address concerns about pain and explain that there may be some discomfort during the venipuncture.

▶ *Sensitivity to social and cultural issues,* as well as concern for modesty, is important in providing psychological support before, during, and after the procedure.

▶ There are no food, fluid, or medication restrictions unless by medical direction.

INTRATEST:

▶ If the patient has a history of allergic reaction to latex, avoid the use of equipment containing latex.

▶ Direct the patient to breathe normally and to avoid unnecessary movement.

▶ Observe standard precautions, and follow the general guidelines in Appendix A.

Consider recommended collection time in relation to dosing schedule. Positively identify the patient, and label the appropriate tubes with the corresponding patient demographics, date, and time of collection, noting the last dose of medication taken. Perform a venipuncture.

▶ Remove the needle and apply direct pressure with dry gauze to stop bleeding. Observe/assess venipuncture site for bleeding or hematoma formation and secure gauze with adhesive bandage.

▶ Promptly transport the specimen to the laboratory for processing and analysis.

POST-TEST:

▶ A report of the results will be sent to the requesting HCP, who will discuss the results with the patient.

▶ *Nutritional Considerations:* Antiepileptic drugs antagonize folic acid, and there is a corresponding slight increase in the incidence of fetal malformations in children of epileptic mothers. Women of childbearing age who are taking carbamazepine, phenobarbital, phenytoin, primadone, and/or valproic acid should also be prescribed supplemental folic acid to reduce the incidence of neural tube defects. Neonates born to epileptic mothers taking antiseizure medications during pregnancy may experience a temporary drug-induced deficiency of vitamin K–dependent coagulation factors. This can be avoided by administration of vitamin K to the mother in the last few weeks of pregnancy and to the infant at birth.

▶ Reinforce information given by the patient's HCP regarding further testing, treatment, or referral to another HCP. Explain to the patient the importance of following the medication regimen and instructions regarding drug interactions. Instruct the patient to immediately report any unusual sensations (e.g., ataxia, dizziness, dyspnea, lethargy, rash, tremors, mental changes, weakness, or visual disturbances) to his or her HCP. Answer any questions

or address any concerns voiced by the patient or family.
▶ Instruct the patient to be prepared to provide the pharmacist with a list of other medications he or she is already taking in the event that the requesting HCP prescribes a medication.
▶ Depending on the results of this procedure, additional testing may be performed to evaluate or monitor progression of the disease process and determine the need for a change in therapy.

Evaluate test results in relation to the patient's symptoms and other tests performed.

RELATED MONOGRAPHS:
▶ Related tests include ALT, albumin, AST, bilirubin, BUN, CBC, creatinine, electrolytes, GGT, and protein blood total and fractions.
▶ See the Genitourinary and Hepatobiliary systems tables at the end of the book for related tests by body system.

Antideoxyribonuclease-B, Streptococcal

SYNONYM/ACRONYM: ADNase-B, AntiDNase-B titer, antistreptococcal DNase-B titer, streptodornase.

COMMON USE: To assist in assessment of the cause of recent infection, such as streptococcal exposure, by identification of antibodies.

SPECIMEN: Serum (1 mL) collected in a red-top tube.

REFERENCE VALUE: (Method: Spectrophotometry)

Age	Normal Results
Preschoolers	Less than 61 units
School-age children	Less than 171 units
Adults	Less than 86 units

DESCRIPTION: The presence of streptococcal deoxyribonuclease (DNase)-B antibodies is an indicator of recent group A, beta hemolytic streptococcal infection, especially if a rise in antibody titer can be shown. This test is more sensitive than the antistreptolysin O test. Anti-DNase B titers rise more slowly than ASO titers, peaking 4 to 8 wk after infection. They also decline much more slowly, remaining elevated for several months. A rise in titer of two or more dilution increments between acute and convalescent specimens is clinically significant.

INDICATIONS
• Investigate the presence of streptococcal antibodies as a source of recent infection

A

POTENTIAL DIAGNOSIS

Increased in
Presence of antibodies, especially a rise in titer, is indicative of exposure.
- Post streptococcal glomerulo-nephritis
- Rheumatic fever
- Streptococcal infections (systemic)

Decreased in: N/A

CRITICAL FINDINGS: N/A

INTERFERING FACTORS: N/A

NURSING IMPLICATIONS AND PROCEDURE

PRETEST:

- Positively identify the patient using at least two unique identifiers before providing care, treatment, or services.
- *Patient Teaching:* Inform the patient this test can assist in documenting recent streptococcal infection.
- Obtain a history of the patient's complaints, including a list of known allergens, especially allergies or sensitivities to latex.
- Obtain a history of the patient's immune system, symptoms, and results of previously performed laboratory tests and diagnostic and surgical procedures.
- Obtain a list of the patient's current medications, including herbs, nutritional supplements, and nutraceuticals (see Appendix F).
- Review the procedure with the patient. Inform the patient that specimen collection takes approximately 5 to 10 min. Address concerns about pain and explain that there may be some discomfort during the venipuncture.
- *Sensitivity to social and cultural issues,* as well as concern for modesty, is important in providing psychological support before, during, and after the procedure.
- There are no food, fluid, or medication restrictions unless by medical direction.

INTRATEST:

- If the patient has a history of allergic reaction to latex, avoid the use of equipment containing latex.
- Instruct the patient to cooperate fully and to follow directions. Direct the patient to breathe normally and to avoid unnecessary movement.
- Observe standard precautions, and follow the general guidelines in Appendix A. Positively identify the patient, and label the appropriate tubes with the corresponding patient demographics, date, and time of collection. Perform a venipuncture.
- Remove the needle and apply direct pressure with dry gauze to stop bleeding. Observe/assess venipuncture site for bleeding or hematoma formation and secure gauze with adhesive bandage.
- Promptly transport the specimen to the laboratory for processing and analysis.

POST-TEST:

- A report of the results will be sent to the requesting health-care provider (HCP), who will discuss the results with the patient.
- Administer analgesics and antibiotics if ordered. Remind the patient of the importance of completing the entire course of antibiotic therapy, even if signs and symptoms disappear before completion of therapy.
- Reinforce information given by the patient's HCP regarding further testing, treatment, or referral to another HCP. Inform the patient that a convalescent specimen may be requested in 7 to 10 days. Answer any questions or address any concerns voiced by the patient or family.
- Depending on the results of this procedure, additional testing may

be performed to evaluate or monitor progression of the disease process and determine the need for a change in therapy. Evaluate test results in relation to the patient's symptoms and other tests performed.

RELATED MONOGRAPHS:

- Related tests include antibodies antistreptolysin O, culture throat, and group A streptococcal screen.
- See the Immune System table at the end of the book for related tests by body system.

Antidepressant Drugs (Cyclic): Amitriptyline, Nortriptyline, Doxepin, Imipramine, Desipramine

SYNONYM/ACRONYM: *Cyclic antidepressants: amitriptyline* (Elavil, Endep, Etrafon, Limbitrol, Triavil); *nortriptyline* (Allegron, Aventyl HCL, Nortrilen, Norval, Pamelor); *doxepin* (Adapin, Co-Dax, Novoxapin, Sinequan, Triadapin); *imipramine* (Berkomine, Dimipressin, Iprogen, Janimine, Pentofrane, Presamine, SK-Pramine, Tofranil PM); *desipramine* (Norpramin).

COMMON USE: To monitor subtherapeutic, therapeutic, or toxic drug levels in evaluation of effective treatment modalities.

SPECIMEN: Serum (1 mL) collected in a red-top tube.

Drug	Route of Administration	Recommended Collection Time
Amitriptyline	Oral	Trough: immediately before next dose (at steady state)
Nortripyline	Oral	Trough: immediately before next dose (at steady state)
Doxepin	Oral	Trough: immediately before next dose (at steady state)
Imipramine	Oral	Trough: immediately before next dose (at steady state)
Desipramine	Oral	Trough: immediately before next dose (at steady state)

REFERENCE VALUE: (Method: Chromatography for amitriptyline, nortriptyline, and doxepin; immunoassay for imipramine and desipramine)

Drug	Therapeutic Dose*	SI Units	Half-Life (h)	Volume of Distribution (L/kg)	Protein Binding (%)	Excretion
(SI = Conventional Units × 3.61) Amitriptyline, alone	80–200 ng/mL	289–722 nmol/L	20–40	10–36	85–95	Hepatic
(SI = Conventional Units × 3.8) Nortriptyline, alone	50–150 ng/mL	190–570 nmol/L	20–60	15–23	90–95	Hepatic
(SI = Conventional Units × 3.58) Combined doxepin and desmethyldoxepin	150–250 ng/mL	540–900 nmol/L	10–25	10–30	75–85	Hepatic
(SI = Conventional Units × 3.57) Combined imipramine and desipramine	100–300 ng/mL	350–1,070 nmol/L	6–18	9–23	60–95	Hepatic

*Conventional units.

DESCRIPTION: Cyclic antidepressants are used in the treatment of major depression. They have also been used effectively to treat bipolar disorder, panic disorder, attention deficit-hyperactivity disorder (ADHD), obsessive-compulsive disorder (OCD), enuresis, eating disorders (bulimia nervosa in particular), nicotine dependence (tobacco), and cocaine dependence. Numerous drug interactions occur with the cyclic antidepressants.

Many factors must be considered in effective dosing and monitoring of therapeutic drugs, including patient age, patient weight, interacting medications, electrolyte balance, protein levels, water balance, conditions that affect absorption and excretion, and the ingestion of substances (e.g., foods, herbals, vitamins, and minerals) that can either potentiate or inhibit the intended target concentration. Trough collection times should be documented carefully in relation to the time of medication administration.

IMPORTANT NOTE

This information must be clearly and accurately communicated to avoid misunderstanding of the dose time in relation to the collection time. Miscommunication between the individual administering the medication and the individual collecting the specimen is the most frequent cause of subtherapeutic levels, toxic levels, and misleading information used in calculation of future doses.

INDICATIONS

- Assist in the diagnosis and prevention of toxicity
- Evaluate overdose, especially in combination with ethanol (*Note:* Doxepin abuse is unusual.)
- Monitor compliance with therapeutic regimen

POTENTIAL DIAGNOSIS

Level	Response
Normal levels	Therapeutic effect
Subtherapeutic levels	Adjust dose as indicated
Toxic levels	Adjust dose as indicated
Amitriptyline	Hepatic impairment
Nortriptyline	Hepatic impairment
Doxepin	Hepatic impairment
Imipramine	Hepatic impairment
Desipramine	Hepatic impairment

CRITICAL FINDINGS

It is important to note the adverse effects of toxic and subtherapeutic levels of antidepressants. Care must be taken to investigate signs and symptoms of too little and too much medication. Note and immediately report to the health-care provider (HCP) any critically increased or subtherapeutic values and related symptoms.

Cyclic antidepressants
- Amitriptyline: Greater than 500 ng/mL
- Nortriptyline: Greater than 500 ng/mL
- Combined amitriptyline and nortriptyline: greater than 500 ng/mL
- Combined doxepin and desmethyl-doxepin: greater than 500 ng/mL
- Combined desipramine and imipramine: greater than 500 ng/mL

Signs and symptoms of cyclic antidepressant toxicity include agitation, drowsiness, hallucinations, confusion, seizures, arrhythmias, hyperthermia, flushing, dilation of the pupils, and possible coma. Possible interventions include administration of activated charcoal; emesis; gastric lavage with saline; administration of physostigmine to counteract seizures, hypertension, or respiratory depression; administration of bicarbonate, propranolol, lidocaine, or phenytoin to counteract arrhythmias; and electrocardiographic monitoring.

INTERFERING FACTORS
- Blood drawn in serum separator tubes (gel tubes).
- Contraindicated in patients with liver disease, and caution advised in patients with renal impairment.
- Cyclic antidepressants may potentiate the effects of oral anticoagulants.

NURSING IMPLICATIONS AND PROCEDURE

PRETEST:
- Positively identify the patient using at least two unique identifiers before providing care, treatment, or services.
- *Patient Teaching:* Inform the patient this test can assist in monitoring subtherapeutic, therapeutic, or toxic drug levels.
- Obtain a history of the patient's complaints, including a list of known allergens, especially allergies or sensitivities to latex.
- These medications are metabolized and excreted by the kidneys and liver. Obtain a history of the patient's genitourinary and hepatobiliary systems, symptoms, and results of previously performed laboratory tests and diagnostic and surgical procedures.
- Obtain a list of the patient's current medications, including herbs, nutritional supplements, and nutraceuticals (see Appendix F). Note the last time and dose of medication taken.
- Review the procedure with the patient. Inform the patient that specimen collection takes approximately 5 to 10 min. Address concerns about pain and explain that there may be some discomfort during the venipuncture.
- *Sensitivity to social and cultural issues,* as well as concern for modesty, is important in providing psychological support before, during, and after the procedure.
- There are no food, fluid, or medication restrictions unless by medical direction.

INTRATEST:
- If the patient has a history of allergic reaction to latex, avoid the use of equipment containing latex.
- Instruct the patient to cooperate fully and to follow directions. Direct the patient to breathe normally and to avoid unnecessary movement.
- Observe standard precautions, and follow the general guidelines in Appendix A. Consider recommended collection time in relation to dosing schedule. Positively identify the patient, and label the appropriate tubes with the corresponding patient demographics, date, and time of collection, noting the last dose of medication taken. Perform a venipuncture.
- Remove the needle and apply direct pressure with dry gauze to stop bleeding. Observe/assess venipuncture site for bleeding or hematoma formation and secure gauze with adhesive bandage.
- Promptly transport the specimen to the laboratory for processing and analysis.

A

▶ A report of the results will be sent to the requesting HCP, who will discuss the results with the patient.

▶ *Nutritional Considerations:* include avoidance of alcohol consumption.

▶ Reinforce information given by the patient's HCP regarding further testing, treatment, or referral to another HCP. Explain to the patient the importance of following the medication regimen and instructions regarding drug interactions. Instruct the patient to immediately report any unusual sensations (e.g., severe headache, vomiting, sweating, visual disturbances) to his or her HCP. Blood pressure should be monitored regularly. Answer any questions or address any concerns voiced by the patient or family.

▶ Instruct the patient to be prepared to provide the pharmacist with a list of other medications he or she is already taking in the event that the requesting HCP prescribes a medication.

▶ Depending on the results of this procedure, additional testing may be performed to evaluate or monitor progression of the disease process and determine the need for a change in therapy. Evaluate test results in relation to the patient's symptoms and other tests performed.

RELATED MONOGRAPHS:

▶ Related tests include ALT, albumin, AST, bilirubin, BUN, creatinine, CBC, electrolytes, GGT, and protein blood total and fractions.

▶ See the Genitourinary and Hepatobiliary systems tables at the end of the book for related tests by body system.

Antidiuretic Hormone

SYNONYM/ACRONYM: Vasopressin, arginine vasopressin hormone, ADH.

COMMON USE: To evaluate disorders that affect urine concentration related to fluctuations of ADH secretion, such as diabetes insipidus.

SPECIMEN: Plasma (1 mL) collected in a lavender-top (EDTA) tube.

REFERENCE VALUE: (Method: Radioimmunoassay) Normally hydrated adults: 0 to 5 pg/mL; normally hydrated children (1 day to 18 yr): 0.5 to 1.7.

Age	Antidiuretic Hormone	SI Units (Conventional Units × 0.926)
Neonates	Less than 1.5 pg/mL	Less than 1.4 pmol/L
1 day–18 yr	0.5–1.5 pg/mL	Less than 0.5–1.4 pmol/L
Adult	0–5 pg/mL	0–4.6 pmol/L

RECOMMENDATION

This test should be ordered and interpreted with results of a serum osmolality.

A

Serum Osmolality*	Antidiuretic Hormone	SI Units (Conventional Units × 0.926)
270–280 mOsm/kg	Less than 1.5 pg/mL	Less than 1.4 pmol/L
280–285 mOsm/kg	Less than 2.5 pg/mL	Less than 2.3 pmol/L
285–290 mOsm/kg	1–5 pg/mL	0.9–4.6 pmol/L
290–295 mOsm/kg	2–7 pg/mL	1.9–6.5 pmol/L
295–300 mOsm/kg	4–12 pg/mL	3.7–11.1 pmol/L

*Conventional units.

DESCRIPTION: Antidiuretic hormone (ADH) is formed by the hypothalamus and stored in the posterior pituitary gland. ADH is released in response to increased serum osmolality or decreased blood volume. When the hormone is active, water is reabsorbed by the kidneys into the circulating plasma instead of being excreted, and small amounts of concentrated urine are produced; in its absence, large amounts of dilute urine are produced. Although a 1% change in serum osmolality stimulates ADH secretion, blood volume must decrease by approximately 10% for ADH secretion to be induced. Psychogenic stimuli, such as stress, pain, and anxiety, may also stimulate ADH release, but the mechanism is unclear.

INDICATIONS
- Assist in the diagnosis of known or suspected malignancy associated with syndrome of inappropriate ADH secretion (SIADH), such as oat cell lung cancer, thymoma, lymphoma, leukemia, pancreatic carcinoma, prostate gland carcinoma, and intestinal carcinoma; elevated ADH levels indicate the presence of this syndrome
- Assist in the diagnosis of known or suspected pulmonary conditions associated with SIADH, such as tuberculosis, pneumonia, and positive-pressure mechanical ventilation
- Detect central nervous system trauma, surgery, or disease that may lead to impaired ADH secretion
- Differentiate neurogenic (central) diabetes insipidus from nephrogenic diabetes insipidus by decreased ADH levels in neurogenic diabetes insipidus or elevated levels in nephrogenic diabetes insipidus if normal feedback mechanisms are intact
- Evaluate polyuria or altered serum osmolality to identify possible alterations in ADH secretion as the cause

POTENTIAL DIAGNOSIS

Increased in
- Acute intermittent porphyria *(speculated to be related to the release of ADH from damaged cells in the hypothalamus and effect of hypovolemia; the mechanisms are unclear)*
- Brain tumor *(related to ADH production from the tumor or release from damaged cells in an adjacent affected area)*
- Disorders involving the central nervous system, thyroid gland, and adrenal gland *(numerous conditions influence the release of ADH)*
- Ectopic production *(related to ADH production from a systemic neoplasm)*

- Guillain-Barré syndrome *(relationship to SIADH is unclear)*
- Hypovolemia *(potent instigator of ADH release)*
- Nephrogenic diabetes insipidus *(related to lack of renal system response to ADH stimulation; evidenced by increased secretion of ADH)*
- Pain, stress, or exercise *(all are potent instigators of ADH release)*
- Pneumonia *(related to SIADH)*
- Pulmonary tuberculosis *(related to SIADH)*
- SIADH *(numerous conditions influence the release of ADH)*
- Tuberculous meningitis *(related to SIADH)*

Decreased in

Decreased production or secretion of ADH in response to changes in blood volume or pressure

- Hypervolemia *(related to increased blood volume, which inhibits secretion of ADH)*
- Nephrotic syndrome *(related to destruction of pituitary cells that secrete ADH)*
- Pituitary (central) diabetes insipidus *(related to destruction of pituitary cells that secrete ADH)*
- Pituitary surgery *(related to destruction or removal of pituitary cells that secrete ADH)*
- Psychogenic polydipsia *(evidenced by decreased osmolality, which inhibits secretion of ADH)*

CRITICAL FINDINGS

Effective treatment of SIADH depends on identifying and resolving the cause of increased ADH production. Signs and symptoms of SIADH are the same as those for hyponatremia, including irritability, tremors, muscle spasms, convulsions, and neurologic changes. The patient has enough sodium, but it is diluted in excess retained water.

INTERFERING FACTORS

- Drugs that may increase ADH levels include cisplatin, ether, furosemide, hydrochlorothiazide, lithium, methyclothiazide, and polythiazide.
- Drugs that may decrease ADH levels include chlorpromazine, clonidine, demeclocycline, ethanol, and phenytoin.
- Recent radioactive scans or radiation within 1 week before the test can interfere with test results when radioimmunoassay is the test method.
- ADH exhibits diurnal variation, with highest levels of secretion occurring at night; first morning collection is recommended.
- ADH secretion is also affected by posture, with higher levels measured while upright.

NURSING IMPLICATIONS AND PROCEDURE

PRETEST:

▶ Positively identify the patient using at least two unique identifiers before providing care, treatment, or services.
▶ *Patient Teaching:* Inform the patient this test can assist in providing information about effective urine concentration.
▶ Obtain a history of the patient's complaints, including a list of known allergens, especially allergies or sensitivities to latex.
▶ Obtain a history of the patient's endocrine and genitourinary systems, symptoms, and results of previously performed laboratory tests and diagnostic and surgical procedures.
▶ Note any recent procedures that can interfere with test results.
▶ Obtain a list of the patient's current medications, including herbs, nutritional supplements, and nutraceuticals (see Appendix F).
▶ Review the procedure with the patient. Inform the patient that specimen collection takes approximately 5 to 10 min. Address concerns about pain and explain that there

A

may be some discomfort during the venipuncture.

▶ *Sensitivity to social and cultural issues*, as well as concern for modesty, is important in providing psychological support before, during, and after the procedure.

▶ There are no food, fluid, or medication restrictions unless by medical direction.

▶ Prepare an ice slurry in a cup or plastic bag to have ready for immediate transport of the specimen to the laboratory. Prechill the lavender-top tube in the ice slurry.

INTRATEST:

▶ If the patient has a history of allergic reaction to latex, avoid the use of equipment containing latex.

▶ Instruct the patient to cooperate fully and to follow directions. The patient should be encouraged to be calm and in a sitting position for specimen collection. Direct the patient to breathe normally and to avoid unnecessary movement.

▶ Observe standard precautions, and follow the general guidelines in Appendix A. Positively identify the patient, and label the appropriate tubes with the corresponding patient demographics, date, and time of collection. Perform a venipuncture.

▶ Remove the needle and apply direct pressure with dry gauze to stop bleeding. Observe/assess venipuncture site for bleeding or hematoma formation and secure gauze with adhesive bandage.

▶ The sample should be placed in an ice slurry immediately after collection. Information on the specimen label should be protected from water in the ice slurry by first placing the specimen in a protective plastic bag. Promptly transport the specimen to the laboratory for processing and analysis.

POST-TEST:

▶ A report of the results will be sent to the requesting health-care provider (HCP), who will discuss the results with the patient.

▶ Reinforce information given by the patient's HCP regarding further testing, treatment, or referral to another HCP. Inform the patient, as appropriate, that treatment may include diuretic therapy and fluid restriction to successfully eliminate the excess water. Answer any questions or address any concerns voiced by the patient or family.

▶ Depending on the results of this procedure, additional testing may be performed to evaluate or monitor progression of the disease process and determine the need for a change in therapy. Evaluate test results in relation to the patient's symptoms and other tests performed.

RELATED MONOGRAPHS:

▶ Related tests include BUN, chest x-ray, chloride, osmolality, phosphorus, potassium, sodium, TSH, uric acid, and UA.

▶ See the Endocrine and Genitourinary systems tables at the end of the book for related tests by body system.

Antipsychotic Drugs and Antimanic Drugs: Haloperidol, Lithium

SYNONYM/ACRONYM: *Antipsychotic drugs: haloperidol* (Dozic, Fortunan, Haldol, Haldol Decanoate, Haloneural, Serenace); *antimanic drugs: lithium* (Cibalith-S, Eskalith, Lithane, Lithobid, Lithonate, Lithotabs, PFI-Lith, Phasal).

COMMON USE: To assist in monitoring subtherapuetic, therapeutic, or toxic drug levels related to medical interventions.

SPECIMEN: Serum (1 mL) collected in a red-top tube.

Drug	Route of Administration	Recommended Collection Time
Haloperidol	Oral	Peak: 3–6 hr
Lithium	Oral	Trough: at least 12 hr after last dose; steady state occurs at 90–120 hr

REFERENCE VALUE: (Method: Chromatography for haloperidol; ion-selective electrode for lithium)

Drug	Therapeutic Dose*	SI Units	Half-Life (hr)	Volume of Distribution (L/kg)	Protein Binding (%)	Excretion
(SI = Conventional Units × 2)						
Haloperidol	5–20 ng/mL	10–40 nmo/L	15–40	18–30	90	Hepatic
(SI = Conventional Units × 1)						
Lithium	0.6–1.4 mEq/L	0.6–1.4 mmol/L	18–24	0.7–1.0	0	Renal

*Conventional units.

DESCRIPTION: Haloperidol is an antipsychotic tranquilizer used for treatment of acute and chronic psychotic disorders, Tourette's syndrome, and hyperactive children with severe behavioral problems. Frequent monitoring is important due to the unstable relationship between dosage and circulating steady-state concentration. Lithium is used in the treatment of manic depression. Daily monitoring of lithium levels is important until the proper dosage is achieved. Lithium is cleared and reabsorbed by the kidney. Clearance is increased when sodium levels are increased and decreased in conditions associated with low sodium levels; therefore, patients receiving lithium therapy should try to maintain a balanced daily intake of sodium. Lithium levels affect other organ systems. A high incidence of pulmonary complications is associated with lithium toxicity. Lithium can also affect cardiac conduction, producing T-wave depressions. These electrocardiographic (ECG) changes are usually insignificant and reversible and are seen in 10% to 20% of patients on lithium therapy. Chronic lithium therapy has been shown to result in enlargement of the thyroid gland in a small percentage of patients.

Many factors must be considered in effective dosing and monitoring of therapeutic drugs, including patient age, patient weight, interacting medications, electrolyte balance,

A

protein levels, water balance, conditions that affect absorption and excretion, and the ingestion of substances (e.g., foods, herbals, vitamins, and minerals) that can either potentiate or inhibit the intended target concentration. Peak collection times should be documented carefully in relation to the time of medication administration.

IMPORTANT NOTE: This information must be clearly and accurately communicated to avoid misunderstanding of the dose time in relation to the collection time. Miscommunication between the individual administering the medication and the individual collecting the specimen is the most frequent cause of subtherapeutic levels, toxic levels, and misleading information used in calculation of future doses.

INDICATIONS
- Assist in the diagnosis and prevention of toxicity
- Monitor compliance with therapeutic regimen

POTENTIAL DIAGNOSIS

Level	Response
Normal levels	Therapeutic effect
Subtherapeutic levels	Adjust dose as indicated
Toxic levels	Adjust dose as indicated
Haloperidol	Hepatic impairment
Lithium	Renal impairment

CRITICAL FINDINGS

It is important to note the adverse effects of toxic and subtherapeutic levels. Care must be taken to investigate signs and symptoms of not enough medication and too much medication. Note and immediately report to the health-care provider (HCP) any critically increased or subtherapeutic values and related symptoms.

Haloperidol: Greater Than 42 ng/mL

Signs and symptoms of haloperidol toxicity include hypotension, myocardial depression, respiratory depression, and extrapyramidal neuromuscular reactions. Possible interventions include emesis (contraindicated in the absence of gag reflex or central nervous system depression or excitation) and gastric lavage followed by administration of activated charcoal.

Lithium: Greater Than 2 mEq/L

Signs and symptoms of lithium toxicity include ataxia, coarse tremors, muscle rigidity, vomiting, diarrhea, confusion, convulsions, stupor, T-wave flattening, loss of consciousness, and possible coma. Possible interventions include administration of activated charcoal, gastric lavage, and administration of intravenous fluids with diuresis.

INTERFERING FACTORS
- Blood drawn in serum separator tubes (gel tubes).
- Contraindicated in patients with liver disease, and caution advised in patients with renal impairment.

- Haloperidol may increase levels of tricyclic antidepressants and increase the risk of lithium toxicity.
- Drugs that may increase lithium levels include angiotensin-converting enzyme inhibitors, some NSAIDs, and thiazide diuretics.
- Drugs and substances that may decrease lithium levels include acetazolamide, osmotic diuretics, theophylline, and caffeine.

NURSING IMPLICATIONS AND PROCEDURE

PRETEST:

- Positively identify the patient using at least two unique identifiers before providing care, treatment, or services.
- *Patient Teaching:* Inform the patient this test can assist in monitoring subtherapeutic, therapeutic, or toxic drug levels.
- Obtain a history of the patient's complaints, including a list of known allergens, especially allergies or sensitivities to latex.
- These medications are metabolized and excreted by the kidneys and liver. Obtain a history of the patient's genitourinary and hepatobiliary systems, symptoms, and results of previously performed laboratory tests and diagnostic and surgical procedures.
- Obtain a list of the patient's current medications, including herbs, nutritional supplements, and nutraceuticals (see Appendix F). Note the last time and dose of medication taken.
- Review the procedure with the patient. Inform the patient that specimen collection takes approximately 5 to 10 min. Address concerns about pain and explain that there may be some discomfort during the venipuncture.
- *Sensitivity to social and cultural issues*, as well as concern for modesty, is important in providing psychological

support before, during, and after the procedure.
- There are no food, fluid, or medication restrictions unless by medical direction.

INTRATEST:

- If the patient has a history of allergic reaction to latex, avoid the use of equipment containing latex.
- Instruct the patient to cooperate fully and to follow directions. Direct the patient to breathe normally and to avoid unnecessary movement.
- Observe standard precautions, and follow the general guidelines in Appendix A. Consider recommended collection time in relation to dosing schedule. Positively identify the patient, and label the appropriate tubes with the corresponding patient demographics, date, and time of collection, noting the last dose of medication taken. Perform a venipuncture.
- Remove the needle and apply direct pressure with dry gauze to stop bleeding. Observe/assess venipuncture site for bleeding or hematoma formation and secure gauze with adhesive bandage.
- Promptly transport the specimen to the laboratory for processing and analysis.

POST-TEST:

- A report of the results will be sent to the requesting HCP, who will discuss the results with the patient.
- *Nutritional Considerations* include avoidance of alcohol consumption.
- Reinforce information given by the patient's HCP regarding further testing, treatment, or referral to another HCP. Explain to the patient the importance of following the medication regimen and instructions regarding drug interactions.
- Instruct the patient receiving haloperidol to immediately report any unusual symptoms (e.g., arrhythmias, blurred vision, dry eyes, repetitive uncontrolled movements) to his or

her HCP. Instruct the patient receiving lithium to immediately report any unusual symptoms (e.g., anorexia, nausea, vomiting, diarrhea, dizziness, drowsiness, dysarthria, tremor, muscle twitching, visual disturbances) to his or her HCP. Answer any questions or address any concerns voiced by the patient or family.

♦ Instruct the patient to be prepared to provide the pharmacist with a list of other medications he or she is already taking in the event that the requesting HCP prescribes a medication.

♦ Depending on the results of this procedure, additional testing may be performed to evaluate or monitor progression of the disease process and determine the need for a change in therapy. Evaluate test results in relation to the patient's symptoms and other tests performed.

RELATED MONOGRAPHS:

♦ Related laboratory tests include albumin, BUN, calcium, creatinine, ECG, glucose, magnesium, osmolality urine, potassium, sodium, T_4, and TSH.

♦ See the Genitourinary and Hepatobiliary systems tables at the end of the book for related tests by body system.

Antithrombin III

SYNONYM/ACRONYM: Heparin cofactor assay, AT-III.

COMMON USE: To assist in diagnosing heparin resistance or disorders resulting from a hypercoagulable state such as thrombus.

SPECIMEN: Plasma (1 mL) collected in a completely filled blue-top (3.2% sodium citrate) tube. If the patient's hematocrit exceeds 55%, the volume of citrate in the collection tube must be adjusted.

REFERENCE VALUE: (Method: Radioimmunodiffusion)

	Conventional Units	SI Units (Conventional Units × 10)
Immunological assay	21–30 mg/dL	210–300 mg/L

	Conventional Units	SI Units (Conventional Units × 10)
Functional assay		
Neonate	39–87% of standard	0.39–0.87
6 mo–adult	85–115% of standard	0.85–1.15

DESCRIPTION: Antithrombin III (AT-III) can inhibit thrombin (factor IIa) and factors IX, X, XI, and XII. It is a heparin cofactor, produced by the liver, interacting with heparin and thrombin.

AT-III acts to increase the rate at which thrombin is neutralized or inhibited, and it decreases the total quantity of thrombin inhibited. Patients with low levels of AT-III show some level of resistance to heparin therapy and are at risk for venous thrombosis. AT III deficiency can be acquired (most common) or congenital.

INDICATIONS
• Investigate tendency for thrombosis

POTENTIAL DIAGNOSIS

Increased in
• Acute hepatitis
• Renal transplantation *(Some studies have demonstrated high levels of AT III in proximal tubule epithelial cells at the time of renal transplant. The exact relationship between the kidneys and AT III levels is unknown. It is believed the kidneys may play a role in main-taining plasma levels of AT III as evidenced by the correlation between renal disease and low AT III levels.)*
• Vitamin K deficiency *(decreased consumption related to impaired coagulation factor function)*

Decreased in
• Carcinoma *(related to decreased synthesis)*
• Chronic liver failure *(related to decreased synthesis)*
• Cirrhosis *(related to decreased synthesis)*
• Congenital deficiency
• Disseminated intravascular coagulation *(related to increased consumption)*
• Liver transplantation or partial hepatectomy *(related to decreased synthesis)*
• Nephrotic syndrome *(related to increased protein loss)*
• Pulmonary embolism *(related to increased consumption)*
• Venous thrombosis *(related to increased consumption)*

CRITICAL FINDINGS: N/A

INTERFERING FACTORS
• Drugs that may increase AT-III levels include anabolic steroids, gemfibrozil, and warfarin (Coumadin).
• Drugs that may decrease AT-III levels include asparaginase, estrogens, heparin, and oral contraceptives.
• Hematocrit greater than 55% may cause falsely prolonged results because of anticoagulant excess relative to plasma volume.
• Incompletely filled collection tubes, specimens contaminated with heparin, clotted specimens, or unprocessed specimens not delivered to the laboratory within 1 to 2 hr of collection should be rejected.
• Placement of the tourniquet for longer than 1 min can result in venous stasis and changes in the concentration of the plasma pro-teins to be measured. Platelet activation may also occur under these conditions, resulting in erroneous measurements.

NURSING IMPLICATIONS AND PROCEDURE

PRETEST:

▶ Positively identify the patient using at least two unique identifiers before providing care, treatment, or services.
▶ *Patient Teaching:* Inform the patient this test can assist in diagnosing clotting disorders.
▶ Obtain a history of the patient's complaints, including a list of known allergens, especially allergies or sensi-tivities to latex.
▶ Obtain a history of the patient's hematopoietic system, symptoms, and results of previously performed labora-tory tests and diagnostic and surgical procedures.

A

▶ Obtain a list of the patient's current medications, including herbs, nutritional supplements, and nutraceuticals (see Appendix F).
▶ Review the procedure with the patient. Inform the patient that specimen collection takes approximately 5 to 10 min. Address concerns about pain and explain that there may be some discomfort during the venipuncture.
▶ *Sensitivity to social and cultural issues,* as well as concern for modesty, is important in providing psychological support before, during, and after the procedure.
▶ There are no food, fluid, or medication restrictions unless by medical direction.

INTRATEST:

▶ If the patient has a history of allergic reaction to latex, avoid the use of equipment containing latex.
▶ Instruct the patient to cooperate fully and to follow directions. Direct the patient to breathe normally and to avoid unnecessary movement.
▶ Observe standard precautions, and follow the general guidelines in Appendix A. Positively identify the patient, and label the appropriate tubes with the corresponding patient demographics, date, and time of collection. Perform a venipuncture. Fill tube completely. *Important note:* Two different concentrations of sodium citrate preservative are currently added to blue-top tubes for coagulation studies: 3.2% and 3.8%. The Clinical and Laboratory Standards Institute/CLSI (formerly the National Committee for Clinical Laboratory Standards/NCCLS) guideline for sodium citrate is 3.2%. Laboratories establish reference ranges for coagulation testing based on numerous factors, including sodium citrate concentration, test equipment, and test reagents. It is important to ask the laboratory which concentration it recommends, because each concentration will have its own specific reference range. When multiple specimens are

drawn, the blue-top tube should be collected after sterile (i.e., blood culture) tubes. Otherwise, when using a standard vacutainer system, the blue top is the first tube collected. When a butterfly is used, due to the added tubing, an extra red-top tube should be collected before the blue-top tube to ensure complete filling of the blue-top tube.
▶ Remove the needle and apply direct pressure with dry gauze to stop bleeding. Observe/assess venipuncture site for bleeding or hematoma formation and secure gauze with adhesive bandage.
▶ Promptly transport the specimen to the laboratory for processing and analysis. The CLSI recommendation for processed and unprocessed samples stored in unopened tubes is that testing should be completed within 1 to 4 hr of collection. If the patient has a known hematocrit above 55%, adjust the amount of anticoagulant in the collection tube before drawing the blood according to the CLSI guidelines:

$$\text{Anticoagulant vol. [x]} = (100 - \text{hematocrit})/(595 - \text{hematocrit}) \times \text{total vol. of anticoagulated blood required}$$

Example:

$$\text{Patient hematocrit} = 60\%$$
$$= [(100 - 60)/(595 - 60) \times 5.0]$$
$$= 0.37 \text{ mL sodium citrate for a 5-mL standard drawing tube}$$

POST-TEST:

▶ A report of the results will be sent to the requesting health-care provider (HCP), who will discuss the results with the patient.
▶ Reinforce information given by the patient's HCP regarding further testing, treatment, or referral to another HCP. Answer any questions or address any concerns voiced by the patient or family.
▶ Depending on the results of this procedure, additional testing may be performed to evaluate or monitor progression of the disease process and determine the need for a change in therapy. Evaluate test results in relation to the

patient's symptoms and other tests performed.

- Related tests include antibodies cardiolipin, echocardiography, lung

perfusion scan, aPTT, protein C, protein S, venography lower extremities, and vitamin K.
- See the Hematopoietic System table at the end of the book for related tests by body system.

A

α_1-Antitrypsin and α_1-Antitrypsin Phenotyping

SYNONYM/ACRONYM: α_1-antitrypsin: A_1AT, α_1-AT, AAT; α_1-antitrypsin phenotyping: A_1AT phenotype, α_1-AT phenotype, AAT phenotype, Pi phenotype.

COMMON USE: To assist in the identification of chronic obstructive pulmonary disease (COPD) and liver disease associated with α_1-antitrypsin (α_1-AT) deficiency.

SPECIMEN: Serum (1 mL) for α_1-AT and serum (2 mL) for α_1-AT phenotyping collected in a red- or tiger-top tube.

REFERENCE VALUE: (Method: Rate nephelometry for α_1-AT, isoelectric focusing/high-resolution electrophoresis for α_1-AT phenotyping)

α_1-Antitrypsin

Age	Conventional Units	SI Units (Conventional Units × 0.01)
0–1 mo	124–348 mg/dL	1.24–3.48 g/L
2–6 mo	111–297 mg/dL	1.11–2.97 g/L
7 mo–2 yr	95–251 mg/dL	0.95–2.51 g/L
3–19 yr	110–279 mg/dL	1.10–2.79 g/L
Adult	126–226 mg/dL	1.26–2.26 g/L

α_1-Antitrypsin Phenotyping

There are three major protease inhibitor phenotypes:

- MM—Normal
- SS—Intermediate; heterozygous
- ZZ—Markedly abnormal; homozygous

The total level of measurable α_1-AT varies with genotype. The effects of α_1-AT deficiency depend on the patient's personal habits but are most severe in patients who smoke tobacco.

DESCRIPTION: α_1-AT is the main glycoprotein produced by the liver. Its inhibitory function is directed against proteolytic enzymes, such as trypsin, elastin, and plasmin, released by alveolar macrophages and bacteria. In the absence of α_1-AT, functional tissue is

A

destroyed by proteolytic enzymes and replaced with excessive connective tissue. Emphysema develops at an earlier age in α_1-AT–deficient emphysema patients than in other emphysema patients. α_1-AT deficiency is passed on as an autosomal recessive trait. Inherited deficiencies are associated early in life with development of lung and liver disorders. In the pediatric population, the ZZ phenotype usually presents as liver disease, cholestasis, and cirrhosis. Greater than 80% of ZZ-deficient individuals ultimately develop chronic lung or liver disease. It is important to identify inherited deficiencies early in life. Typically, α_1-AT–deficient patients have circulating levels less than 50 mg/dL. Patients who have α_1-AT values less than 140 mg/dL should be phenotyped.

Elevated levels are found in normal individuals when an inflammatory process, such as rheumatoid arthritis, bacterial infection, neoplasm, or vasculitis, is present. Decreased levels are found in affected patients with COPD and in children with cirrhosis of the liver. Deficiency of this enzyme is the most common cause of liver disease in the pediatric population. Decreased α_1-AT levels also may be elevated into the normal range in heterozygous α_1-AT–deficient patients during concurrent infection, pregnancy, estrogen therapy, steroid therapy, cancer, and postoperative periods. Homozygous α_1-AT–deficient patients do not show such an elevation.

INDICATIONS
- Assist in establishing a diagnosis of COPD
- Assist in establishing a diagnosis of liver disease
- Detect hereditary absence or deficiency of α_1-AT

POTENTIAL DIAGNOSIS

Increased in
- Acute and chronic inflammatory conditions *(related to rapid, nonspecific response to inflammation)*
- Carcinomas *(related to rapid, nonspecific response to inflammation)*
- Estrogen therapy
- Postoperative recovery *(related to rapid, nonspecific response to inflammation or stress)*
- Pregnancy *(related to rapid, nonspecific response to stress)*
- Steroid therapy
- Stress (extreme physical) *(related to rapid, nonspecific response to stress)*

Decreased in
- COPD *(related to malnutrition and evidenced by decreased protein synthesis)*
- Homozygous α_1-AT–deficient patients *(related to decreased protein synthesis)*
- Liver disease (severe) *(related to decreased protein synthesis)*
- Liver cirrhosis (child) *(related to decreased protein synthesis)*
- Malnutrition *(related to insufficient protein intake)*
- Nephrotic syndrome *(related to increased protein loss from diminished renal function)*

CRITICAL FINDINGS: N/A

INTERFERING FACTORS
- α_1-AT is an acute-phase reactant protein, and any inflammatory process elevates levels. If a serum C-reactive protein is performed simultaneously and is positive,

A

the patient should be retested for α_1-AT in 10 to 14 days.
- Rheumatoid factor causes false-positive elevations.
- Drugs that may increase serum α_1-AT levels include aminocaproic acid, estrogen therapy, oral contraceptives (high-dose preparations), oxymetholone, streptokinase, tamoxifen, and typhoid vaccine.

NURSING IMPLICATIONS AND PROCEDURE

PRETEST:

▶ Positively identify the patient using at least two unique identifiers before providing care, treatment, or services.

▶ *Patient Teaching:* Inform the patient this test can assist in identifying lung and liver disease.

▶ Obtain a history of the patient's complaints, including a list of known allergens, especially allergies or sensitivities to latex.

▶ Obtain a history of the patient's hepatobiliary and respiratory systems, symptoms, and results of previously performed laboratory tests and diagnostic and surgical procedures.

▶ Obtain a list of the patient's current medications, including herbs, nutritional supplements, and nutraceuticals (see Appendix F). Oral contraceptives should be withheld 24 hr before the specimen is collected, although this restriction should first be confirmed with the health-care provider (HCP) ordering the test.

▶ Review the procedure with the patient. Inform the patient that specimen collection takes approximately 5 to 10 min. Address concerns about pain and explain to the patient that there may be some discomfort during the venipuncture.

▶ *Sensitivity to social and cultural issues*, as well as concern for modesty, is important in providing psychological support before, during, and after the procedure.

▶ There are no food, fluid, or medication restrictions unless by medical direction.

INTRATEST:

▶ If the patient has a history of allergic reaction to latex, avoid the use of equipment containing latex.

▶ Instruct the patient to cooperate fully and to follow directions. Direct the patient to breathe normally and to avoid unnecessary movement.

▶ Observe standard precautions, and follow the general guidelines in Appendix A. Positively identify the patient, and label the appropriate tubes with the corresponding patient demographics, date, and time of collection. Perform a venipuncture.

▶ Remove the needle and apply direct pressure with dry gauze to stop bleeding. Observe/assess venipuncture site for bleeding or hematoma formation and secure gauze with adhesive bandage.

▶ Promptly transport the specimen to the laboratory for processing and analysis.

POST-TEST:

▶ A report of the results will be sent to the requesting HCP, who will discuss the results with the patient.

▶ Instruct the patient to resume usual medication as directed by the HCP.

▶ *Nutritional Considerations:* Malnutrition is commonly seen in α_1-AT–deficient patients with severe respiratory disease for many reasons, including fatigue, lack of appetite, and gastrointestinal distress. Research has estimated that the daily caloric intake required for respiration in patients with COPD is 10 times higher than that required in normal individuals. Inadequate nutrition can result in hypophosphatemia, especially in the respirator-dependent patient. During periods of starvation, phosphorus leaves the intracellular space and moves outside the tissue, resulting in dangerously decreased phosphorus levels. Adequate intake of vitamins A and C is important to prevent pulmonary infection and to decrease the extent of lung tissue damage. The importance of following the prescribed diet should be stressed to the patient and caregiver.

Nutritional Considerations: Water balance must be closely monitored in α_1-AT–deficient patients with COPD. Fluid retention can lead to pulmonary edema.

Educate the patient with abnormal findings in preventive measures for protection of the lungs (e.g., avoid contact with persons who have respiratory or other infections; avoid the use of tobacco; avoid areas having highly polluted air; and avoid work environments with hazards such as fumes, dust, and other respiratory pollutants).

Instruct the affected patient in deep breathing and pursed-lip breathing to enhance breathing patterns as appropriate. Inform the patient of smoking cessation programs, as appropriate.

Recognize anxiety related to test results, and be supportive of fear of shortened life expectancy. Discuss the implications of abnormal test results on the patient's lifestyle. Provide teaching and information regarding the clinical implications of the test results, as appropriate. Because decreased α_1-AT can be an inherited disorder, it may be appropriate to recommend resources for genetic counseling if levels less than 140 mg/dL are reported. It may also be appropriate to inform the patient that α_1-AT phenotype testing can be performed on family members to determine the homozygous or heterozygous nature of the deficiency.

Reinforce information given by the patient's HCP regarding further testing, treatment, or referral to another HCP. Inform the patient of the importance of medical follow-up, and suggest ongoing support resources to assist the patient in coping with chronic illness and possible early death. Answer any questions or address any concerns voiced by the patient or family.

Depending on the results of this procedure, additional testing may be performed to evaluate or monitor progression of the disease process and determine the need for a change in therapy. Evaluate test results in relation to the patient's symptoms and other tests performed.

RELATED MONOGRAPHS:

Related tests include ACE, anion gap, arterial/alveolar oxygen ratio, biopsy lung, blood gases, blood pool imaging, bronchoscopy, electrolytes, lung perfusion scan, lung ventilation scan, osmolality, PET heart, phosphorus, PFTs, plethysmography, and pulse oximetry if COPD is suspected. ALT, albumin, ALP, ammonia, bilirubin and fractions, biopsy liver, cholangiography percutaneous transhepatic, cholangiography postop, CT biliary tract and liver, ERCP, GGT, hepatobiliary scan, liver and spleen scan, protein and fractions, PT/INR, and US liver if liver disease is suspected.

See the Hepatobiliary and Respiratory systems tables at the end of the book for related tests by body system.

Apolipoprotein A and B

SYNONYM/ACRONYM: Apo A (Apo A1) and Apo B (Apo B100).

COMMON USE: To identify levels of circulating lipoprotein to evaluate the risk of coronary artery disease.

SPECIMEN: Serum (1 mL) collected in a red- or tiger-top tube or plasma collected in a green- (heparin) or lavender-top (EDTA) tube.

REFERENCE VALUE: (Method: Immunonephelometry)

Apolipoprotein A

Age	Conventional Units	SI Units (Conventional Units × 0.01)
Newborn		
Male	41–93 mg/dL	0.41–0.93 g/L
Female	38–106 mg/dL	0.38–1.06 g/L
6 mo–4 yr		
Male	67–163 mg/dL	0.67–1.63 g/L
Female	60–148 mg/dL	0.60–1.48 g/L
Adult		
Male	81–166 mg/dL	0.81–1.66 g/L
Female	80–214 mg/dL	0.80–2.14 g/L

Apolipoprotein B

Age	Conventional Units	SI Units (Conventional Units × 0.01)
Newborn–5 yr	11–31 mg/dL	0.11–0.31 g/L
5–17 yr		
Male	47–139 mg/dL	0.47–1.39 g/L
Female	41–96 mg/dL	0.41–0.96 g/L
Adult		
Male	46–174 mg/dL	0.46–1.74 g/L
Female	46–142 mg/dL	0.46–1.42 g/L

DESCRIPTION: Apolipoproteins assist in the regulation of lipid metabolism by activating and inhibiting enzymes required for this process. The apolipoproteins also help keep lipids in solution as they circulate in the blood and direct the lipids toward the correct target organs and tissues in the body. A number of types

A

of apolipoproteins have been identified (A, B, C, D, E, H, J), each of which contain subgroups. Apolipoprotein A (Apo A), the major component of high-density lipoprotein (HDL), is synthesized in the liver and intestines. Apo A-I activates the enzyme lecithin-cholesterol acyltransferase (LCAT), whereas Apo A-II inhibits LCAT. It is believed that Apo A measurements may be more important than HDL cholesterol measurements as a predictor of coronary artery disease (CAD). There is an inverse relationship between Apo A levels and risk for developing CAD. Because of difficulties with method standardization, the above-listed reference ranges should be used as a rough guide in assessing abnormal conditions. Values for African Americans are 5 to 10 mg/dL higher than values for whites. Apolipoprotein B (Apo B), the major component of the low-density lipoproteins (chylomicrons, low-density lipoprotein [LDL], and very-low-density lipoprotein), is synthesized in the liver and intestines.

INDICATIONS
• Evaluation for risk of CAD

POTENTIAL DIAGNOSIS
Apolipoproteins are the protein portion of lipoproteins. Their function is to transport and to assist in cell surface receptor recognition and cellular absorption of lipoproteins to be used as energy. While studies of the exact role of

apolipoproteins in health and disease continue, there is a very strong association between Apo A and HDL "good" cholesterol and Apo B and LDL "bad" cholesterol.

Apolipoprotein A

Increased in
• Familial hyper-α-lipoproteinemia
• Pregnancy
• Weight reduction

Decreased in
• Abetalipoproteinemia
• Cholestasis
• Chronic renal failure
• Coronary artery disease
• Diabetes (uncontrolled)
• Diet high in carbohydrates or polyunsaturated fats
• Familial deficiencies of related enzymes and lipoproteins (e.g., Tangier's disease)
• Hemodialysis
• Hepatocellular disorders
• Hypertriglyceridemia
• Nephrotic syndrome
• Premature coronary heart disease
• Smoking

Apolipoprotein B

Increased in
• Anorexia nervosa
• Biliary obstruction
• Coronary artery disease
• Cushing's syndrome
• Diabetes
• Dysglobulinemia
• Emotional stress
• Hemodialysis
• Hepatic disease
• Hepatic obstruction
• Hyperlipoproteinemias
• Hypothyroidism
• Infantile hypercalcemia
• Nephrotic syndrome
• Porphyria
• Pregnancy
• Premature CAD

- Renal failure
- Werner's syndrome

Decreased in
- Acute stress (burns, illness)
- Chronic anemias
- Chronic pulmonary disease
- Familial deficiencies of related enzymes and lipoproteins (e.g., Tangier's disease)
- Hyperthyroidism
- Inflammatory joint disease
- Intestinal malabsorption
- α-Lipoprotein deficiency (Tangier's disease)
- Malnutrition
- Myeloma
- Reye's syndrome
- Weight reduction

CRITICAL FINDINGS: N/A

INTERFERING FACTORS
- Drugs and substances that may increase Apo A levels include anticonvulsants, beclobrate, bezafibrate, ciprofibrate, estrogens, furosemide, lovastatin, pravastatin, prednisolone, simvastatin, and ethanol (abuse).
- Drugs that may decrease Apo A levels include androgens, β-blockers, diuretics, and probucol.
- Drugs that may increase Apo B levels include amiodarone, androgens, β-blockers, catecholamines, cyclosporine, diuretics, ethanol (abuse), etretinate, glucogenic corticosteroids, oral contraceptives, and phenobarbital.
- Drugs that may decrease Apo B levels include beclobrate, captopril, cholestyramine, fibrates, ketanserin, lovastatin, niacin, nifedipine, pravastatin, prazosin, probucol, and simvastatin.
- Failure to follow dietary restrictions before the procedure may cause the procedure to be canceled or repeated.

NURSING IMPLICATIONS AND PROCEDURE

PRETEST:
- Positively identify the patient using at least two unique identifiers before providing care, treatment, or services.
- *Patient Teaching:* Inform the patient this test can assist in assessing and monitoring risk for coronary artery (heart) disease.
- Obtain a history of the patient's complaints, including a list of known allergens, especially allergies or sensitivities to latex.
- Obtain a history of the patient's cardiovascular system, symptoms, and results of previously performed laboratory tests and diagnostic and surgical procedures.
- Obtain a list of the patient's current medication, including herbs, nutritional supplements, and nutraceuticals (see Appendix F).
- Review the procedure with the patient. Inform the patient that specimen collection takes approximately 5 to 10 min. Address concerns about pain and explain that there may be some discomfort during the venipuncture.
- *Sensitivity to social and cultural issues,* as well as concern for modesty, is important in providing psychological support before, during, and after the procedure.
- The patient should abstain from food for 6 to 12 hr before specimen collection.
- There are no fluid or medication restrictions unless by medical direction.

INTRATEST:
- Ensure that the patient has complied with dietary or activity restrictions, and pretesting preparations; assure that food has been restricted for at least 6 to 12 hr prior to the procedure.
- If the patient has a history of allergic reaction to latex, avoid the use of equipment containing latex.
- Instruct the patient to cooperate fully and to follow directions. Direct the patient to breathe normally and to avoid unnecessary movement.

A

- Observe standard precautions, and follow the general guidelines in Appendix A. Positively identify the patient, and label the appropriate tubes with the corresponding patient demographics, date, and time of collection. Perform a venipuncture.
- Remove the needle and apply direct pressure with dry gauze to stop bleeding. Observe/assess venipuncture site for bleeding or hematoma formation and secure gauze with adhesive bandage.
- Promptly transport the specimen to the laboratory for processing and analysis.

POST-TEST:

- A report of the results will be sent to the requesting health-care provider (HCP), who will discuss the results with the patient.
- Instruct the patient to resume usual diet as directed by the HCP.
- *Nutritional Considerations:* Decreased Apo A and/or increased Apo B levels may be associated with CAD. The American Heart Association and National Heart, Lung, and Blood Institute (NHBLI) recommend nutritional therapy for individuals identified to be at high risk for developing CAD or individuals who have specific risk factors and/or existing medical conditions (e.g., elevated LDL cholesterol levels, other lipid disorders, insulin-dependent diabetes, insulin resistance, or metabolic syndrome). If overweight, the patient should be encouraged to achieve a normal weight. The NHLBI's National Cholesterol Education Program (NCEP) revised its dietary guidelines for reducing CAD in 2001. Guidelines for the Therapeutic Lifestyle Changes (TLC) diet are outlined in the Third Report of the Expert Panel on Detection, Evaluation, and Treatment of High Blood Cholesterol in Adults (Adult Treatment Panel III [ATP III]). The TLC diet emphasizes a reduction in foods high in saturated fats and cholesterol. Red meats, eggs, and dairy products are the major sources of saturated fats and cholesterol. If triglycerides also are elevated, the patient should be advised to eliminate or reduce alcohol and simple carbohydrates from the diet. The TLC approach also includes the use of plant stanols or sterols and increased dissolved fiber as an option for lowering LDL cholesterol levels; nutritional recommendations for daily total caloric intake; recommendations for allowable percentage of calories derived from fat (saturated and unsaturated), carbohydrates, protein, and cholesterol; as well as recommendations for daily expenditure of energy.

- *Nutritional Considerations:* Overweight patients with high blood pressure should be encouraged to achieve a normal weight. Other changeable risk factors warranting patient education include strategies to safely decrease sodium intake, increase physical activity, decrease alcohol consumption, eliminate tobacco use, and decrease cholesterol levels.

- *Social and Cultural Considerations:* Numerous studies point to the prevalence of excess body weight in American children and adolescents. Experts estimate that obesity is present in 25% of the population ages 6 to 11. The medical, social, and emotional consequences of excess body weight are significant. Special attention should be given to instructing the child and caregiver regarding health risks and weight-control education.

- Recognize anxiety related to test results, and be supportive of fear of shortened life expectancy. Discuss the implications of abnormal test results on the patient's lifestyle. Provide teaching and information regarding the clinical implications of the test results, as appropriate. Educate the patient regarding access to counseling services. Provide contact information, if desired, for the American Heart Association (www.americanheart.org) or the NHLBI (www.nhlbi.nih.gov).

- Reinforce information given by the patient's HCP regarding further testing, treatment, or referral to another HCP. Answer any questions or address any concerns voiced by the patient or family.

- Depending on the results of this procedure, additional testing may be performed to evaluate or monitor

A

progression of the disease process and determine the need for a change in therapy. Evaluate test results in relation to the patient's symptoms and other tests performed.

RELATED MONOGRAPHS:

▶ Related tests include antiarrhythmic drugs, AST, ANP, BNP, blood gases, CRP, calcium and ionized calcium, cholesterol (total, HDL, and LDL), CK and isoenzymes, CT scoring, echocardiography, glucose, glycated hemoglobin, Holter monitor, homocysteine, ketones, LDH and isoenzymes, lipoprotein electrophoresis, magnesium, MRI chest, myocardial infarct scan, myocardial perfusion heart scan, myoglobin, PET heart, potassium, triglycerides, and troponin.

▶ See the Cardiovascular System table at the end of the book for related tests by body system.

Arthrogram

SYNONYM/ACRONYM: Joint study.

COMMON USE: To assess and identify the cause of persistent joint pain and monitor the progression of joint disease.

AREA OF APPLICATION: Shoulder, elbow, wrist, hip, knee, ankle, temporomandibular joint.

CONTRAST: Iodinated or gadolinium.

DESCRIPTION: An arthrogram evaluates the cartilage, ligaments, and bony structures that compose a joint. After local anesthesia is administered to the area of interest, a fluoroscopically guided small-gauge needle is inserted into the joint space. Fluid in the joint space is aspirated and sent to the laboratory for analysis. Contrast medium is inserted into the joint space to outline the soft tissue structures and the contour of the joint. After brief exercise of the joint, radiographs or magnetic resonance images (MRIs) are obtained. Arthrograms are used primarily for assessment of persistent, unexplained joint discomfort.

INDICATIONS
• Evaluate pain, swelling, or dysfunction of a joint
• Monitor disease progression

POTENTIAL DIAGNOSIS

Normal findings in
• Normal bursae, menisci, ligaments, and articular cartilage of the joint (note: the cartilaginous surfaces and menisci should be smooth, without evidence of erosion, tears, or disintegration)

Abnormal findings in
• Arthritis
• Cysts
• Diseases of the cartilage (chondromalacia)
• Injury to the ligaments
• Joint derangement

- Meniscal tears or laceration
- Muscle tears
- Osteochondral fractures
- Osteochondritis dissecans
- Synovial tumor
- Synovitis

CRITICAL FINDINGS: N/A

INTERFERING FACTORS

This procedure is contraindicated for
- Patients with allergies to shellfish or iodinated dye. The contrast medium used may cause a life-threatening allergic reaction. Patients with a known hypersensitivity to the medium may benefit from premedication with corticosteroids or the use of a nonionic contrast medium.
- Patients with metal in their body, such as shrapnel or ferrous metal in the eye.
- Patients with cardiac pacemakers, because the pacemaker can be deactivated by MRI.
- Use of gadolinium-based contrast agents (GBCAs) is contraindicated in patients with acute or chronic severe renal insufficiency (glomerular filtration rate less than 30 mL/min/1.73 m^2). Patients should be screened for renal dysfunction prior to administration. The use of GBCAs should be avoided in these patients unless the benefits of the studies outweigh the risks and if essential diagnostic information is not available using non–contrast-enhanced diagnostic studies.
- Patients who are pregnant or suspected of being pregnant, unless the potential benefits of the procedure far outweigh the risks to the fetus and mother.
- Patients with bleeding disorders, active arthritis, or joint infections.

Factors that may impair clear imaging
- Metallic objects within the examination field which may inhibit organ visualization and can produce unclear images
- Inability of the patient to cooperate or remain still during the procedure because of age, significant pain, or mental status

Other considerations
- Consultation with a health-care provider (HCP) should occur before the procedure for radiation safety concerns regarding younger patients or patients who are lactating.
- Risks associated with radiation overexposure can result from frequent x-ray procedures. Personnel in the examination room with the patient should wear a protective lead apron, stand behind a shield, or leave the area while the examination is being done. Personnel working in the examination area should wear badges to record their level of radiation exposure.

NURSING IMPLICATIONS AND PROCEDURE

PRETEST:
▶ Positively identify the patient using at least two unique identifiers before providing care, treatment, or services.
▶ *Patient Teaching:* Inform the patient this procedure can assist in assessing the joint being examined.
▶ Obtain a history of the patient's complaints, including a list of known allergens, especially allergies or sensitivities to latex, iodine, seafood, contrast medium, anesthetics and dyes.
▶ Obtain a history of the patient's musculoskeletal system, symptoms, and previously performed laboratory tests and diagnostic and surgical procedures. Ensure that the results of blood tests are obtained and recorded before the

procedure, especially coagulation tests, BUN, and creatinine, if contrast medium is to be used. Obtain a history of renal dysfunction if the use of GBCA is anticipated.

▶ Ensure the results of BUN, creatinine, and eGFR (estimated glomerular filtration rate) are obtained if GBCA is to be used.

▶ Record the date of the last menstrual period and determine the possibility of pregnancy in perimenopausal women.

▶ Obtain a list of the patient's current medications, including anticoagulants, aspirin and other salicylates, herbs, nutritional supplements, and nutraceuticals (see Appendix F). Such products should be discontinued by medical direction for the appropriate number of days prior to a surgical procedure. Note the last time and dose of medication taken.

▶ Review the procedure with the patient. Address concerns about pain and explain that there may be moments of discomfort and some pain experienced during the test. Inform the patient that the procedure is usually performed in the radiology department by an HCP and takes approximately 30 to 60 min.

▶ *Sensitivity to social and cultural issues,* as well as concern for modesty, is important in providing psychological support before, during, and after the procedure.

▶ There are no food, fluid, or medication restrictions unless by medical direction.

▶ *Make sure a written and informed consent has been signed prior to the procedure and before administering any medications.*

INTRATEST:

▶ Ensure that the patient has removed all external metallic objects prior to the procedure.

▶ If the patient has a history of allergic reactions to any substance or drug, administer ordered prophylactic steroids or antihistamines before the procedure.

▶ Have emergency equipment readily available.

▶ Instruct the patient to void prior to the procedure and to change into the gown, robe, and foot coverings provided.

▶ Observe standard precautions and follow the general guidelines in Appendix A. Instruct the patient to cooperate fully and to follow directions.

▶ Place the patient on the table in a supine position.

▶ The skin surrounding the joint is aseptically cleaned and anesthetized.

▶ A small-gauge needle is inserted into the joint space.

▶ Any fluid in the space is aspirated and sent to the laboratory for analysis.

▶ Contrast medium is inserted into the joint space with fluoroscopic guidance.

▶ The needle is removed, and the joint is exercised to help distribute the contrast medium.

▶ X-rays or MRIs are taken of the joint.

▶ Instruct the patient to cooperate fully and to follow directions. Instruct the patient to remain still throughout the procedure because movement produces unreliable results.

▶ During x-ray imaging, lead protection is placed over the gonads to prevent their irradiation.

▶ If MRI images are taken, supply earplugs to the patient to block out the loud, banging sounds that occur during the test. Instruct the patient to communicate with the technologist during the examination via a microphone within the scanner.

POST-TEST:

▶ A report of the examination will be sent to the requesting HCP, who will discuss the results with the patient.

▶ Observe/assess the joint for swelling after the test. Apply ice as needed.

▶ Instruct the patient to use a mild analgesic (aspirin, acetaminophen), as ordered, if there is discomfort.

▶ Advise the patient to avoid strenuous activity until approved by the HCP.

▶ Instruct the patient to notify the HCP if fever, increased pain, drainage, warmth, edema, or swelling of the joint occurs.

▶ Inform the patient that noises from the joint after the procedure are common and should disappear 24 to 48 hr after the procedure.

▶ Recognize anxiety related to test results. Discuss the implications of abnormal test results on the patient's lifestyle. Provide teaching and information regarding the clinical implications of the test results, as appropriate.

▶ Reinforce information given by the patient's HCP regarding further testing, treatment, or referral to another HCP. Answer any questions or address any concerns voiced by the patient or family.

▶ Depending on the results of this procedure, additional testing may be needed to evaluate or monitor progression of the disease process and determine the need for a change in therapy. Evaluate test results in relation to the patient's symptoms and other tests performed.

RELATED MONOGRAPHS:

▶ Related tests include antibodies anticyclic citrullinated peptide, ANA, arthroscopy, BMD, bone scan, BUN, CBC, CRP, creatinine, ESR, MRI musculoskeletal, PT/INR, radiography bone, RF, synovial fluid analysis, and uric acid.

▶ Refer to the Musculoskeletal System table at the end of the book for related tests by body system.

Arthroscopy

SYNONYM/ACRONYM: N/A.

COMMON USE: To obtain direct visualization of a specific joint to aid in diagnosis of joint disease.

AREA OF APPLICATION: Joints.

CONTRAST: None.

DESCRIPTION: Arthroscopy provides direct visualization of a joint through the use of a fiberoptic endoscope. The arthroscope has a light, fiberoptics, and lenses; it connects to a monitor, and the images are recorded for future study and comparison. This procedure is used for inspection of joint structures, performance of a biopsy, and surgical repairs to the joint. Meniscus removal, spur removal, and ligamentous repair are some of the surgical procedures that may be performed. This procedure is most commonly performed to diagnose athletic injuries and acute or chronic joint disorders. Because arthroscopy allows

direct visualization, degenerative processes can be accurately differentiated from injuries. A local anesthetic allows the arthroscope to be inserted through the skin with minimal discomfort. This procedure may also be done under a spinal or general anesthetic, especially if surgery is anticipated.

INDICATIONS

• Detect torn ligament or tendon
• Evaluate joint pain and damaged cartilage
• Evaluate meniscal, patellar, condylar, extrasynovial, and synovial injuries or diseases of the knee
• Evaluate the extent of arthritis

- Evaluate the presence of gout
- Monitor effectiveness of therapy
- Remove loose objects

POTENTIAL DIAGNOSIS

Normal findings in
- Normal muscle, ligament, cartilage, synovial, and tendon structures of the joint

Abnormal findings in
- Arthritis
- Chondromalacia
- Cysts
- Degenerative joint changes
- Ganglion or Baker's cyst
- Gout or pseudogout
- Joint tumors
- Loose bodies
- Meniscal disease
- Osteoarthritis
- Osteochondritis
- Rheumatoid arthritis
- Subluxation, fracture, or dislocation
- Synovitis
- Torn cartilage
- Torn ligament
- Torn rotator cuff
- Trapped synovium

CRITICAL FINDINGS: N/A

INTERFERING FACTORS

This procedure is contraindicated for
- Patients with bleeding disorders, active arthritis, or cardiac conditions.
- Patients with joint infection or skin infection near proposed arthroscopic site.
- Patients who have had an arthrogram within the last 14 days.

Factors that may impair clear imaging
- Inability of the patient to cooperate or remain still during the procedure because of age, significant pain, or mental status.

- Fibrous ankylosis of the joint preventing effective use of the arthroscope.
- Joints with flexion of less than 50°.

Other considerations
- Failure to follow dietary restrictions before the procedure may cause the procedure to be canceled or repeated.

NURSING IMPLICATIONS AND PROCEDURE

PRETEST:

- Positively identify the patient using at least two unique identifiers before providing care, treatment, or services.
- *Patient Teaching:* Inform the patient this procedure can assist in assessing the joint being examined.
- Obtain a history of the patient's complaints, including a list of known allergens, especially allergies or sensitivities to latex and anesthetics.
- Obtain a history of the patient's musculoskeletal system, symptoms, and results of previously performed laboratory tests and diagnostic and surgical procedures.
- Record the date of the last menstrual period and determine the possibility of pregnancy in perimenopausal women.
- Obtain a list of the patient's current medications including anticoagulants, aspirin and other salicylates, herbs, nutritional supplements, and nutraceuticals (see Appendix F). Such products should be discontinued by medical direction for the appropriate number of days prior to a surgical procedure. Note the last time and dose of medication taken.
- Review the procedure with the patient. Address concerns about pain, and explain that some discomfort and pain may be experienced during the test. Inform the patient that the procedure is performed by a health-care provider (HCP), usually in the radiology department, and takes approximately 30 to 60 min.

- Explain that a preprocedure sedative may be administered to promote relaxation, as ordered.
- Crutch walking should be taught before the procedure if it is anticipated postoperatively.
- The joint area and areas 5 to 6 in. above and below the joint are shaved and prepared for the procedure.
- *Sensitivity to social and cultural issues,* as well as concern for modesty, is important in providing psychological support before, during, and after the procedure.
- Instruct the patient to refrain from food and fluids for 6 to 8 hr before the test. Protocols may vary among facilities.
- *Make sure a written and informed consent has been signed prior to the procedure and before administering any medications.*

INTRATEST:

- Ensure the patient has complied with food and fluid restrictions for at least 6 to 8 hr prior to the procedure.
- Resuscitation equipment and patient monitoring equipment must be available.
- Instruct the patient to void prior to the procedure and to change into the gown, robe, and foot coverings provided.
- The extremity is scrubbed, elevated, and wrapped with an elastic bandage from the distal portion of the extremity to the proximal portion to drain as much blood from the limb as possible.
- A pneumatic tourniquet placed around the proximal portion of the limb is inflated, and the elastic bandage is removed.
- As an alternative to a tourniquet, a mixture of lidocaine with epinephrine and sterile normal saline may be instilled into the joint to help reduce bleeding.
- The joint is placed in a 45° angle, and a local anesthetic is administered.
- A small incision is made in the skin in the lateral or medial aspect of the joint.
- The arthroscope is inserted into the joint spaces. The joint is manipulated as it is visualized. Added puncture sites

may be needed to provide a full view of the joint.
- Biopsy or treatment can be performed at this time, and photographs should be taken for future reference.
- After inspection, specimens may be obtained for cytological and microbiological study. All specimens are placed in appropriate containers, labeled with the corresponding patient demographics, date and time of collection, site location, and promptly sent to the laboratory.
- The joint is irrigated, and the arthroscope is removed. Manual pressure is applied to the joint to remove remaining irrigation solution.
- The incision sites are sutured, and a pressure dressing is applied.
- Sterile gloves and gowns are worn throughout the procedure.

POST-TEST:

- A report of the results will be sent to the requesting HCP, who will discuss the results with the patient.
- Advise the patient to avoid strenuous activity involving the joint until approved by the HCP.
- Instruct the patient to resume normal diet and medications, as directed by the HCP.
- Monitor the patient's circulation and sensations in the joint area.
- Instruct the patient to immediately report symptoms such as fever, excessive bleeding, difficulty breathing, incision site redness, swelling, and tenderness.
- Instruct the patient to elevate the joint when sitting and to avoid overbending of the joint to reduce swelling.
- Instruct the patient to take an analgesic for joint discomfort after the procedure; ice bags may be used to reduce postprocedure swelling.
- Inform the patient to shower after 48 hr but to avoid a tub bath until after his or her appointment with the HCP.
- Recognize anxiety related to test results. Discuss the implications of abnormal test results on the patient's lifestyle. Provide teaching and

information regarding the clinical implications of the test results, as appropriate.

» Reinforce information given by the patient's HCP regarding further testing, treatment, or referral to another HCP. Answer any questions or address any concerns voiced by the patient or family.

» Depending on the results of this procedure, additional testing may be needed to evaluate or monitor progression of the disease process and determine the need for a change in therapy. Evaluate test results in relation to the patient's symptoms and other tests performed.

RELATED MONOGRAPHS:

» Related tests include anti-cyclic citrullinated peptide, ANA, arthrogram, BMD, bone scan, CBC, CRP, ESR, MRI musculoskeletal, radiography of the bone, RF, synovial fluid analysis, and uric acid.

» Refer to the Musculoskeletal System table at the end of the book for related tests by body system.

Aspartate Aminotransferase

SYNONYM/ACRONYM: Serum glutamic-oxaloacetic transaminase, AST, SGOT.

COMMON USE: An indicator of cellular damage in liver disease, such as hepatitis or cirrhosis, and in heart disease, such as myocardial infarction.

SPECIMEN: Serum (1 mL) collected in a red- or tiger-top tube.

REFERENCE VALUE: (Method: Spectrophotometry, enzymatic at 37°C)

Age	Conventional Units	SI Units (Conventional Units × 0.017)
Newborn	25–75 units/L	0.43–1.28 micro kat/L
10 days–23 mo	15–60 units/L	0.26–1.02 micro kat/L
2–3 yr	10–56 units/L	0.17–0.95 micro kat/L
4–6 yr	20–39 units/L	0.34–0.66 micro kat/L
7–19 yr	12–32 units/L	0.20–0.54 micro kat/L
20–49 yr		
Male	20–40 units/L	0.34–0.68 micro kat/L
Female	15–30 units/L	0.26–0.51 micro kat/L
Greater than 50 yr (older adult)		
Male	10–35 units/L	0.17–0.60 micro kat/L
Greater than 45 yr (older adult)		
Female	10–35 units/L	0.17–0.60 micro kat/L

Values may be slightly elevated in older adults due to the effects of medications and the presence of multiple chronic or acute diseases with or without muted symptoms.

DESCRIPTION: Aspartate aminotransferase (AST) is an enzyme that catalyzes the reversible transfer of an amino group between aspartate and α-ketoglutaric acid. It was formerly known as serum glutamic-oxaloacetic transaminase (SGOT). AST exists in large amounts in liver and myocardial cells and in smaller but significant amounts in skeletal muscle, kidneys, pancreas, red blood cells, and the brain. Serum AST rises when there is cellular damage to the tissues where the enzyme is found. AST values greater than 500 units/L are usually associated with hepatitis and other hepatocellular diseases in an acute phase. AST levels are very elevated at birth, decrease with age to adulthood, and increase slightly in elderly adults. *Note*: Measurement of AST in evaluation of myocardial infarction has been replaced by more sensitive tests, such as creatine kinase–MB fraction (CK-MB) and troponin.

INDICATIONS
- Assist in the diagnosis of disorders or injuries involving the tissues where AST is normally found
- Assist (formerly) in the diagnosis of myocardial infarction (*Note*: AST rises within 6 to 8 hr, peaks at 24 to 48 hr, and declines to normal within 72 to 96 hr of a myocardial infarction if no further cardiac damage occurs)
- Compare serially with alanine aminotransferase levels to track the course of hepatitis
- Monitor response to therapy with potentially hepatotoxic or nephrotoxic drugs
- Monitor response to treatment for various disorders in which AST may be elevated, with tissue repair indicated by declining levels

POTENTIAL DIAGNOSIS

Increased in
AST is released from any damaged cell in which it is stored, so conditions that affect the liver, kidneys, heart, pancreas, red blood cells, or skeletal muscle, and cause cellular destruction demonstrate elevated AST levels.

Significantly Increased in (greater than five times normal levels)
- Acute hepatitis *(AST is very elevated in acute viral hepatitis)*
- Acute hepatocellular disease *(especially related to chemical toxicity or drug overdose; moderate doses of acetaminophen have initiated severe hepatocellular disease in alcoholics)*
- Acute pancreatitis
- Shock

Moderately Increased in (three to five times normal levels)
- Alcohol abuse (chronic)
- Biliary tract obstruction
- Cardiac arrhythmias
- Cardiac catheterization, angioplasty, or surgery
- Cirrhosis
- Chronic hepatitis
- Congestive heart failure
- Infectious mononucleosis
- Liver tumors
- Muscle diseases (e.g., dermatomyositis, dystrophy, gangrene, polymyositis, trichinosis)
- Myocardial infarct
- Reye's syndrome
- Trauma *(related to injury or surgery of liver, head, and other sites where AST is found)*

Slightly Increased in (two to three times normal)

- Cerebrovascular accident
- Cirrhosis, fatty liver *(related to obesity, diabetes, jejunoileal bypass, administration of total parenteral nutrition)*
- Delirium tremens
- Hemolytic anemia
- Pericarditis
- Pulmonary infarction

Decreased in

- Hemodialysis *(presumed to be related to a corresponding deficiency of vitamin B_6 observed in hemodialysis patients)*
- Uremia *(related to a build up of toxins which modify the activity of coenzymes required for transaminase activity)*
- Vitamin B_6 deficiency *(related to the lack of vitamin B_6, a required cofactor for the transaminases)*

CRITICAL FINDINGS: N/A

INTERFERING FACTORS

- Drugs that may increase AST levels by causing cholestasis include amitriptyline, anabolic steroids, androgens, benzodiazepines, chlorothiazide, chlorpropamide, dapsone, erythromycin, estrogens, ethionamide, gold salts, imipramine, mercaptopurine, nitrofurans, oral contraceptives, penicillins, phenothiazines, progesterone, propoxyphene, sulfonamides, tamoxifen, and tolbutamide.
- Drugs that may increase AST levels by causing hepatocellular damage include acetaminophen, acetylsalicylic acid, allopurinol, amiodarone, anabolic steroids, anticonvulsants, asparaginase, azithromycin, bromocriptine, captopril, cephalosporins, chloramphenicol, clindamycin, clofibrate, danazol, enflurane, ethambutol, ethionamide,

fenofibrate, fluconazole, fluoroquinolones, foscarnet, gentamicin, indomethacin, interferon, interleukin-2, levamisole, levodopa, lincomycin, low-molecular-weight heparin, methyldopa, monoamine oxidase inhibitors, naproxen, nifedipine, nitrofurans, oral contraceptives, probenecid, procainamide, quinine, ranitidine, retinol, ritodrine, sulfonylureas, tetracyclines, tobramycin, and verapamil.
- Drugs that may decrease AST levels include allopurinol, cyclosporine, interferon alpha, naltrexone, progesterone, trifluoperazine, and ursodiol.
- Hemolysis falsely increases AST values.
- Hemodialysis falsely decreases AST values.

NURSING IMPLICATIONS AND PROCEDURE

PRETEST:

- Positively identify the patient using at least two unique identifiers before providing care, treatment, or services.
- *Patient Teaching:* Inform the patient this test can assist in assessing liver function.
- Obtain a history of the patient's complaints, including a list of known allergens, especially allergies or sensitivities to latex.
- Obtain a history of the patient's cardiovascular and hepatobiliary systems, symptoms, and results of previously performed laboratory tests and diagnostic and surgical procedures.
- Obtain a list of the patient's current medications, including herbs, nutritional supplements, and nutraceuticals (see Appendix F).
- Review the procedure with the patient. Inform the patient that specimen

collection takes approximately 5 to 10 min. Address concerns about pain, and explain to the patient that there may be some discomfort during the venipuncture.

▶ *Sensitivity to social and cultural issues,* as well as concern for modesty, is important in providing psychological support before, during, and after the procedure.

▶ There are no food, fluid, or medication restrictions unless by medical direction.

INTRATEST:

▶ If the patient has a history of allergic reaction to latex, avoid the use of equipment containing latex.

▶ Instruct the patient to cooperate fully and to follow directions. Direct the patient to breathe normally and to avoid unnecessary movement.

▶ Observe standard precautions, and follow the general guidelines in Appendix A. Positively identify the patient, and label the appropriate tubes with the corresponding patient demographics, date, and time of collection. Perform a venipuncture.

▶ Remove the needle and apply direct pressure with dry gauze to stop bleeding. Observe/assess venipuncture site for bleeding or hematoma formation and secure gauze with adhesive bandage.

▶ Promptly transport the specimen to the laboratory for processing and analysis.

POST-TEST:

▶ A report of the results will be sent to the requesting health-care provider (HCP), who will discuss the results with the patient.

▶ *Nutritional Considerations:* Increased AST levels may be associated with liver disease. Dietary recommendations may be indicated and will vary depending on the condition and its severity. Currently, there are no specific medications that can be given to cure hepatitis, but elimination of alcohol ingestion and a diet optimized for convalescence are commonly

included in the treatment plan. A high-calorie, high-protein, moderate-fat diet with a high fluid intake is often recommended for patients with hepatitis. Treatment of cirrhosis is different; a low-protein diet may be in order if the patient's liver can no longer process the end products of protein metabolism. A diet of soft foods may be required if esophageal varices have developed. Ammonia levels may be used to determine whether protein should be added to or reduced from the diet. Patients should be encouraged to eat simple carbohydrates and emulsified fats (as in homogenized milk or eggs) rather than complex carbohydrates (e.g., starch, fiber, and glycogen [animal carbohydrates]) and complex fats, which require additional bile to emulsify them so that they can be used. The cirrhotic patient should be observed carefully for the development of ascites, in which case fluid and electrolyte balance requires strict attention.

▶ *Nutritional Considerations:* Increased AST levels may be associated with coronary artery disease (CAD). The American Heart Association and National Heart, Lung, and Blood Institute (NHBLI) recommend nutritional therapy for individuals identified to be at high risk for developing CAD or individuals who have specific risk factors and/or existing medical conditions (e.g., elevated low-density lipoprotein LDL cholesterol levels, other lipid disorders, insulin-dependent diabetes, insulin resistance, or metabolic syndrome). If overweight, the patient should be encouraged to achieve a normal weight. The NHLBI's National Cholesterol Education Program (NCEP) revised its dietary guidelines for reducing CAD in 2001. Guidelines for the Therapeutic Lifestyle Changes (TLC) diet are outlined in the Third Report of the Expert Panel on Detection, Evaluation, and Treatment of High Blood Cholesterol in Adults (Adult Treatment Panel III [ATP III]). The TLC diet emphasizes a reduction in foods high in saturated fats and cholesterol. Red meats, eggs, and dairy products are the major sources of saturated fats and cholesterol. If triglycerides also are elevated, the patient should be advised to eliminate or reduce alcohol and simple carbohydrates from the diet. The TLC approach also includes the use of plant stanols or sterols and increased dissolved fiber as an option for lowering LDL cholesterol levels; nutritional recommendations for daily total caloric intake; recommendations for allowable percentage of calories derived from fat (saturated and unsaturated), carbohydrates, protein, and cholesterol; as well as recommendations for daily expenditure of energy.

▶ *Nutritional Considerations:* Overweight patients with high blood pressure should be encouraged to achieve a normal weight. Other changeable risk factors warranting patient education include strategies to safely decrease sodium intake, increase physical activity, decrease alcohol consumption, eliminate tobacco use, and decrease cholesterol levels.

▶ *Social and Cultural Considerations:* Numerous studies point to the prevalence of excess body weight in American children and adolescents. Experts estimate that obesity is present in 25% of the population ages 6 to 11. The medical, social, and emotional consequences of excess body weight are significant. Special attention should be given to instructing the child and caregiver regarding health risks and weight-control education.

▶ Recognize anxiety related to test results, and be supportive of fear of shortened life expectancy. Discuss the implications of abnormal test results on the patient's lifestyle. Provide teaching and information regarding the clinical implications of the test results, as appropriate. Educate the patient regarding access to counseling services. Provide contact information, if desired, for the American Heart Association (www.americanheart.org) or the NHLBI (www.nhlbi.nih.gov).

▶ Instruct the patient to immediately report chest pain and changes in breathing pattern to the HCP.

▶ Reinforce information given by the patient's HCP regarding further testing, treatment, or referral to another HCP. Answer any questions or address any concerns voiced by the patient or family.

▶ Depending on the results of this procedure, additional testing may be performed to evaluate or monitor progression of the disease process and determine the need for a change in therapy. Evaluate test results in relation to the patient's symptoms and other tests performed.

RELATED MONOGRAPHS:

▶ Related tests include acetaminophen, ALT, albumin, ALP, ammonia, AMA/ASMA, α_1-antitrypsin/phenotyping, bilirubin and fractions, biopsy liver, cholangiography percutaneous transhepatic, cholangiography post-op, CT biliary tract and liver, ERCP, ethanol, ferritin, GGT, hepatitis antigens and antibodies, hepatobiliary scan, iron/total iron-binding capacity, liver and spleen scan, protein and fractions, PT/INR, and US liver if liver disease is suspected; and antiarrhythmic drugs, apolipoprotein A and B, ANP, BNP, blood gases, CRP, calcium/ionized calcium, CT scoring, cholesterol (total, HDL, and LDL), CK, echocardiography, Holter monitor, homocysteine, LDH, MRI chest, myocardial infarct scan, myocardial perfusion heart scan, myoglobin, PET heart, potassium, triglycerides, and troponin if myocardial infarction is suspected.

▶ See the Cardiovascular and Hepatobiliary systems tables at the end of the book for related tests by body system.

A

Atrial Natriuretic Peptide

SYNONYM/ACRONYM: Atrial natriuretic hormone, atrial natriuretic factor, ANF, ANH.

COMMON USE: To assist in diagnosing and monitoring congestive heart failure (CHF) and to differentiate CHF from other causes of dyspnea.

SPECIMEN: Plasma (1 mL) collected in a chilled, lavender-top tube. Specimen should be transported tightly capped and in an ice slurry.

REFERENCE VALUE: (Method: Radioimmunoassay)

Conventional Units	SI Units (Conventional Units × 1)
20–77 pg/mL	20–77 ng/L

POTENTIAL DIAGNOSIS

Increased in
ANP is secreted in response to increased hemodynamic load caused by physiological stimuli as with atrial stretch or endocrine stimuli from the aldosterone/renin system.

- Asymptomatic cardiac volume overload
- CHF
- Elevated cardiac filling pressure
- Paroxysmal atrial tachycardia

Decreased in: N/A

CRITICAL FINDINGS: N/A

Find and print out the full monograph at DavisPlus (http://davisplus.fadavis.com, keyword Van Leeuwen).

Audiometry, Hearing Loss

SYNONYM/ACRONYM: N/A.

COMMON USE: To evaluate hearing loss in school-age children but can be used for all ages.

AREA OF APPLICATION: Ears.

CONTRAST: N/A.

DESCRIPTION: Tests to estimate hearing ability can be performed on patients of any age (e.g., at birth before discharge from a hospital or birthing center, as part of a school screening program, or as adults if indicated). Hearing loss audiometry includes quantitative testing for a hearing deficit. An audiometer is used to measure and record thresholds of hearing by air conduction and bone conduction tests. The test results determine if hearing loss is conductive, sensorineural, or a combination of both. An elevated air-conduction threshold with a normal bone-conduction threshold indicates a conductive hearing loss. An equally elevated threshold for both air and bone conduction indicates a sensorineural hearing loss. An elevated threshold of air conduction that is greater than an elevated threshold of bone conduction indicates a composite of both types of hearing loss. A conductive hearing loss is caused by an abnormality in the external auditory canal or middle ear, and a sensorineural hearing loss by an abnormality in the inner ear or of the VIII (auditory) nerve. Sensorineural hearing loss can be further differentiated clinically by sensory (cochlear) or neural (VIII nerve) lesions. Sensorineural hearing loss is permanent. Additional information for comparing and differentiating between conductive and sensorineural hearing loss can be obtained from hearing loss tuning fork tests.

INDICATIONS

- Determine the need for a type of hearing aid and evaluate its effectiveness
- Determine the type and extent of hearing loss and if further radiological, audiological, or vestibular procedures are needed to identify the cause
- Evaluate communication disabilities and plan for rehabilitation interventions
- Evaluate degree and extent of preoperative and postoperative hearing loss following stapedectomy in patients with otosclerosis
- Screen for hearing loss in infants and children and determine the need for a referral to an audiologist

POTENTIAL DIAGNOSIS

ASHA Category	Pure Tone Averages
Normal range or no impairment	−10–15 dB*
Slight loss	16–25 dB
Mild loss	26–40 dB
Moderate loss	41–55 dB
Moderately severe loss	56–70 dB
Severe loss	71–90 dB
Profound loss	Greater than 91 dB

*dB = decibel.

A

Normal findings in
- Normal pure tone average of −10 to 15 dB for infants, children, or adults

Abnormal findings in
- Causes of conductive hearing loss

Impacted cerumen

Obstruction of external ear canal *(related to presence of a foreign body)*

Otitis externa *(related to infection in ear canal)*

Otitis media *(related to poor eustachian tube function or infection)*

Otitis media serus *(related to fluid in middle ear due to allergies or a cold)*

Otosclerosis

- Causes of sensorineural hearing loss

Congenital damage or malformations of the inner ear

Meniere's disease

Ototoxic drugs *(aminoglycosides, e.g., gentamicin or tobramycin; salicylates, e.g., aspirin)*

Presbyacusis *(gradual hearing loss experienced in advancing age)*

Serious infections *(meningitis, measles, mumps, other viral, syphilis)*

Trauma to the inner ear *(related to exposure to noise in excess of 90 dB or as a result of physical trauma)*

Tumor *(e.g., acoustic neuroma, cerebellopontine angle tumor, meningioma)*

Vascular disorders

CRITICAL FINDINGS: N/A

INTERFERING FACTORS

Factors that may impair the results of the examination
- Inability of the patient to cooperate or remain still during the procedure because of age, language barriers, significant pain, or mental status may interfere with the test results.
- Noisy environment or extraneous movements can affect results.
- Tinnitus or other sensations can cause abnormal responses.
- Improper earphone fit or audiometer calibration can affect results.
- Failure to follow pretesting preparations before the procedure may cause the procedure to be canceled or repeated.

NURSING IMPLICATIONS AND PROCEDURE

PRETEST:

- Positively identify the patient using at least two unique identifiers before providing care, treatment, or services.
- *Patient Teaching:* Inform the patient/caregiver this procedure can assist in detecting hearing loss.
- Obtain a history of the patient's complaints, including a list of known allergens.
- Obtain a history of the patient's known or suspected hearing loss, including type and cause; ear conditions with treatment regimens; ear surgery; and other tests and procedures to assess and diagnose auditory deficit.
- Obtain a history of the patient's symptoms and results of previously performed laboratory tests and diagnostic and surgical procedures.
- Obtain a list of the patient's current medications, including herbs, nutritional supplements, and nutraceuticals (see Appendix F).
- Review the procedure with the patient. Address concerns about pain and explain that no discomfort will be experienced during the test. Inform the patient that an audiologist or health-care provider (HCP) specializing in this procedure performs the test in a quiet, soundproof room, and that the test can take up 20 min to evaluate both ears. Explain that each ear will be tested separately by using earphones and/or a device placed behind the ear to deliver sounds of varying intensities. Address concerns about claustrophobia, as appropriate. Explain and demonstrate to the patient how to communicate with the audiologist and how to exit from the room.

Sensitivity to social and cultural issues, as well as concern for modesty, is important in providing psychological support before, during, and after the procedure.

• There are no food, fluid, or medication restrictions unless by medical direction.

• Ensure that the external auditory canal is clear of impacted cerumen.

• *Make sure a written and informed consent has been signed prior to the procedure and before administering any medications.*

INTRATEST:

• Instruct the patient to cooperate fully and to follow directions. Instruct the patient to remain still during the procedure because movement produces unreliable results.

• Perform otoscopy examination to ensure that the external ear canal is free from any obstruction (see monograph titled "Otoscopy").

• Test for closure of the canal from the pressure of the earphones by compressing the tragus. Tendency for the canal to close (often the case in children and elderly patients) can be corrected by the careful insertion of a small stiff plastic tube into the anterior canal.

• Place the patient in a sitting position in comfortable proximity to the audiometer in a soundproof room. The ear not being tested is masked to prevent crossover of test tones, and the earphones are positioned on the head and over the ear canals. Infants and children may be tested using earphones that are inserted into the ear, unless contraindicated. An oscillating probe may be placed over the mastoid process behind the ear or on the forehead if bone conduction testing is to be performed as part of the hearing assessment.

• Start the test by providing a trial tone of 15 to 20 dB above the expected threshold to the ear for 1 to 2 sec to familiarize the patient with the sounds. Instruct the patient to press the button each time a tone is heard, no matter how loudly or faintly it is perceived. If no response is indicated, the level is increased until a response is obtained and then raised in 10-dB increments or until the audiometer's limit is reached for the test frequency. The test results are plotted on a graph called an audiogram using symbols that indicate the ear tested and responses using earphones (air conduction) or oscillator (bone conduction).

Air Conduction

• Air conduction is tested first by starting at 1,000 Hz and gradually decreasing the intensity 10 dB at a time until the patient no longer presses the button, indicating that the tone is no longer heard. The intensity is then increased 5 dB at a time until the tone is heard again. This is repeated until the same response is achieved at a 50% response rate at the same hertz level. The threshold is derived from the lowest decibel level at which the patient correctly identifies three out of six responses to a tone at that hertz level. The test is continued for each ear, testing the better ear first, with tones delivered at 1,000 Hz; 2,000 Hz; 4,000 Hz; and 8,000 Hz, and then again at 1,000 Hz; 500 Hz; and 250 Hz to determine a second threshold. Results are recorded on a graph called an audiogram. Averaging the air conduction thresholds at the 500-Hz; 1,000-Hz; and 2,000-Hz levels reveals the degree of hearing loss and is called the pure tone average (PTA).

Bone Conduction

• Bone conduction testing is performed in a similar manner to air conduction testing. The raised and lowered tones are delivered as in air conduction using 250 Hz; 500 Hz; 1,000 Hz; 2,000 Hz; and 4,000 Hz to determine the thresholds. An analysis of thresholds for air and bone conduction tones is done to determine the type of hearing loss (conductive, sensorineural, or mixed).

• In children between 6 mo and 2 yr of age, minimal response levels can be determined by behavioral responses to test tone. In the child 2 yr and older, play audiometry that requires the child to perform a task or raise a hand in response to a specific tone is performed. In children 12 yr and older, the child is asked to follow directions in identifying objects; response to speech of specific intensities can be used to evaluate hearing loss that is affected by speech frequencies.

POST-TEST:

- A report of the results will be sent to the requesting HCP, who will discuss the results with the patient.
- Instruct the patient to resume usual activity, as directed by the HCP.
- Recognize anxiety related to test results, and be supportive of impaired activity related to hearing loss or perceived loss of independence. Discuss the implications of abnormal test results on the patient's lifestyle. Provide teaching and information regarding the clinical implications of the test results, as appropriate. Educate the patient regarding access to counseling services. Provide contact information, if desired, for the American Speech-Language-Hearing Association (www.asha.org) or for assistive technology at ABLEDATA (sponsored by the National Institute on Disability and Rehabilitation Research, www.abledata.com).
- Reinforce information given by the patient's HCP regarding further testing, treatment, or referral to another HCP. As appropriate, instruct the patient in the use, cleaning, and storing of a hearing aid. Answer any questions or address any concerns voiced by the patient or family.
- Depending on the results of this procedure, additional testing may be performed to evaluate or monitor progression of the disease process and determine the need for a change in therapy. Evaluate test results in relation to the patient's symptoms and other tests performed.

RELATED MONOGRAPHS:

- Related tests include analgesic and antipyretic drugs, antibiotic drugs, cultures bacterial (ear), evoked brain potential studies for hearing loss, gram stain, otoscopy, spondee speech reception threshold, and tuning fork tests (Webber, Rinne).
- Refer to the table of tests associated with the Auditory System at the end of the book.

β₂-Microglobulin, Blood and Urine

SYNONYM/ACRONYM: β_2-M, BMG.

COMMON USE: To assist in diagnosing malignancy such as lymphoma, leukemia, or multiple myeloma. Also valuable in assessing for chronic severe inflammatory and renal diseases.

SPECIMEN: Serum (1 mL) collected in a red-top tube or 5 mL urine from a timed collection in a clean plastic container with 1 N NaOH as a preservative.

REFERENCE VALUE: (Method: Immunochemiluminometric assay)

Sample	Conventional Units
Serum	
Newborn	1.6–4.8 mg/L
Adult	0.6–2.4 mg/L
Urine	0–300 mcg/L

DESCRIPTION: β_2-Microglobulin (BMG) is an amino acid peptide component of human leukocyte antigen (HLA) complexes. BMG is on the surface of most cells and is therefore a useful indicator of cell death or unusually high levels of cell production. BMG is a small protein and is readily reabsorbed by kidneys with normal function. BMG increases in inflammatory conditions and when lymphocyte turnover increases, such as in lymphocytic leukemia or when T-lymphocyte helper (OKT4) cells are attacked by HIV. Serum BMG becomes elevated with malfunctioning glomeruli but decreases with malfunctioning tubules because it is metabolized by the renal tubules. Conversely, urine BMG decreases with malfunctioning glomeruli but becomes elevated with malfunctioning tubules.

INDICATIONS

- Detect aminoglycoside toxicity
- Detect chronic lymphocytic leukemia, multiple myeloma, lung cancer, hepatoma, or breast cancer

- Detect HIV infection (*Note:* levels do not correlate with stages of infection)
- Evaluate renal disease to differentiate glomerular from tubular dysfunction
- Monitor antiretroviral therapy

POTENTIAL DIAGNOSIS

Increased in

- AIDS *(related to increased lymphocyte turnover)*
- Aminoglycoside toxicity *(related to renal damage; urine BMG becomes elevated before creatinine)*
- Amyloidosis *(related to chronic inflammatory conditions associated with increased BMG and other acute-phase reactant proteins)*
- Autoimmune disorders *(related to increased lymphocyte turnover)*
- Breast cancer *(related to increased lymphocyte turnover; serum BMG indicates tumor growth rate, size, and response to treatment)*
- Crohn's disease *(related to chronic inflammatory conditions associated with increased BMG and other acute-phase reactant proteins)*
- Felty's syndrome *(related to chronic inflammatory conditions associated with increased BMG and other acute-phase reactant proteins)*
- Hepatitis *(related to increased lymphocyte turnover in response to viral infection)*
- Hepatoma *(related to increased lymphocyte turnover; serum BMG*

indicates tumor growth rate, size, and response to treatment)
- Hyperthyroidism *(related to increased lymphocyte turnover in immune thyroid disease)*
- Leukemia (chronic lymphocytic) *(related to increased lymphocyte turnover; serum BMG indicates tumor growth rate, size, and response to treatment)*
- Lung cancer *(related to increased lymphocyte turnover; serum BMG indicates tumor growth rate, size, and response to treatment)*
- Lymphoma *(related to increased lymphocyte turnover; serum BMG indicates tumor growth rate, size, and response to treatment)*
- Multiple myeloma *(related to increased lymphocyte turnover)*
- Poisoning with heavy metals, such as mercury or cadmium *(related to renal damage that decreases BMG absorption)*
- Renal dialysis *(related to ability of renal tubule to reabsorb BMG)*
- Renal disease (glomerular): serum only *(related to ability of renal tubule to reabsorb BMG)*
- Renal disease (tubular): urine only *(related to ability of renal tubule to reabsorb BMG)*
- Sarcoidosis
- Systemic lupus erythematosus *(related to chronic inflammatory conditions associated with increased BMG and other acute phase reactant proteins)*
- Vasculitis *(related to chronic inflammatory conditions associated with increased BMG and other acute phase reactant proteins)*
- Viral infections (e.g., cytomegalovirus) *(related to increased lymphocyte turnover)*

Decreased in
- Renal disease (glomerular): urine only
- Renal disease (tubular): serum only
- Response to zidovudine (AZT) *(related to decreased viral replication and lymphocyte destruction)*

CRITICAL FINDINGS: N/A

INTERFERING FACTORS
- Drugs and proteins that may increase serum BMG levels include cyclosporin A, gentamicin, and interferon alfa.
- Drugs that may decrease serum BMG levels include zidovudine.
- Drugs that may increase urine BMG levels include azathioprine, cisplatin, cyclosporin A, furosemide, gentamicin, iodixanol, iopentol, mannitol, nifedipine, sisomicin, and tobramycin.
- Urinary BMG is unstable at pH less than 5.5.

NURSING IMPLICATIONS AND PROCEDURE

PRETEST:
- Positively identify the patient using at least two unique identifiers before providing care, treatment, or services.
- *Patient Teaching:* Inform the patient that the test is used to evaluate renal disease, AIDS, and certain malignancies.
- Obtain a history of the patient's complaints, including a list of known allergies, especially allergies or sensitivities to latex.
- Obtain a history of the patient's genitourinary and immune systems, symptoms, and results of previously performed laboratory tests and diagnostic and surgical procedures.
- Note any recent procedures that can interfere with test results.
- Obtain a list of the patient's current medications, including herbs, nutritional supplements, and nutraceuticals (see Appendix F).
- *Sensitivity to social and cultural issues,* as well as concern for modesty, is important in providing psychological support before, during, and after the procedure.
- There are no food, fluid, or medication restrictions unless by medical direction.

Blood

- Review the procedure with the patient. Inform the patient that specimen collection takes approximately 5 to 10 min. Address concerns about pain and explain that there may be some discomfort during the venipuncture.

Urine

- Review the procedure with the patient. Provide a nonmetallic urinal, bedpan, or toilet-mounted collection device.
- Usually a 24-hr urine collection is ordered. Inform the patient that all urine over a 24-hr period must be saved; instruct the patient to avoid defecating in the collection device and to keep toilet tissue out of the collection device to prevent contamination of the specimen. Place a sign in the bathroom as a reminder to save all urine.
- Instruct the patient to void all urine into the collection device and then pour the urine into the laboratory collection container. Alternatively, the specimen can be left in the collection device for a health care staff member to add to the laboratory collection container.

INTRATEST:

- Instruct the patient to cooperate fully and to follow directions. Direct the patient to breathe normally and to avoid unnecessary movement during the venipuncture.
- Observe standard precautions, and follow the general guidelines in Appendix A. Positively identify the patient, and label the appropriate tubes or collection containers with the corresponding patient demographics, date, and time of collection.

Blood

- If the patient has a history of allergic reaction to latex, avoid the use of equipment containing latex.
- Perform a venipuncture.
- Remove the needle and apply direct pressure with dry gauze to stop bleeding. Observe/assess venipuncture site for bleeding or hematoma formation and secure gauze with adhesive bandage.

Urine

- Obtain a clean 3-L urine specimen container, toilet-mounted collection device, and plastic bag (for transport of the specimen container). The specimen must be refrigerated or kept on ice throughout the entire collection period. If an indwelling urinary catheter is in place, the drainage bag must be kept on ice.
- If possible, begin the test between 6 and 8 a.m. Collect first voiding and discard. Record the time the specimen was discarded as the beginning of the timed collection period. At the same time the next morning, ask the patient to void and add this last voiding to the container. Urinary output should be recorded throughout the collection time.
- If an indwelling catheter is in place, replace the tubing and container system at the start of the collection time. Keep the container system on ice during the collection period, or empty the urine into a larger container periodically during the collection period; monitor to ensure continued drainage, and conclude the test the next morning at the same hour the collection started.
- At the conclusion of the test, compare the quantity of urine with the urinary output record for the collection. If the specimen contains less than what was recorded as output, some urine may have been discarded, thus invalidating the test.

Blood or Urine

- Promptly transport the specimen to the laboratory for processing and analysis. Include on the urine specimen label the amount of urine and ingestion of any medications that can affect test results.

POST-TEST:

- A report of the results will be sent to the requesting health-care provider (HCP), who will discuss the results with the patient.
- Educate the patient regarding the risk of infection related to immunosuppressed inflammatory response and fatigue related to decreased energy production.

Nutritional Considerations: Stress the importance of good nutrition, and suggest that the patient meet with a nutritional specialist. Also, stress the importance of following the care plan for medications and follow-up visits.

Social and Cultural Considerations: Recognize anxiety related to test results, and be supportive of impaired activity related to weakness, perceived loss of independence, and fear of shortened life expectancy. Discuss the implications of abnormal test results on the patient's lifestyle. Provide teaching and information regarding the clinical implications of the test results, as appropriate. Educate the patient regarding access to counseling services. Provide contact information, if desired, for AIDS information provided by the National Institutes of Health (www.aidsinfo.nih.gov).

Social and Cultural Considerations: Counsel the patient, as appropriate, regarding risk of transmission and proper prophylaxis, and reinforce the importance of strict adherence to the treatment regimen.

Social and Cultural Considerations: Offer support, as appropriate, to patients who may be the victims of rape or sexual assault. Educate the patient regarding access to counseling services. Provide a nonjudgmental, nonthreatening atmosphere for a discussion during which risks of sexually transmitted diseases are explained. It is also important to discuss problems the patient may experience (e.g., guilt, depression, anger).

Reinforce information given by the patient's HCP regarding further testing, treatment, or referral to another HCP. Inform the patient that retesting may be necessary. Answer any questions or address any concerns voiced by the patient or family.

Depending on the results of this procedure, additional testing may be performed to evaluate or monitor progression of the disease process and determine the need for a change in therapy. Evaluate test results in relation to the patient's symptoms and other tests performed.

RELATED MONOGRAPHS:

Related tests include antibiotic drugs, ANA, barium enema, biopsy (bone marrow, biopsy breast, biopsy liver, biopsy lung, biopsy lymph node), BUN, capsule endoscopy, CD4/CD8 enumeration, colonoscopy, CRP, cancer antigens, CBC, creatinine, cultures (mycobacteria, sputum, viral), cytology sputum, CMV, ESR, gallium scan, GGT, hepatitis antigens and antibodies (A, B, C), HIV-1/HIV-2 serology, immunofixation electrophoresis, immunoglobulins (A, G, and M), liver and spleen scan, lymphangiogram, MRI breast, mammogram, microalbumin, osmolality, protein total and fractions, renogram, RF, stereotactic breast biopsy, TB tests, US (breast, liver, lymph node), and UA.

Refer to the Genitourinary and Immune systems tables at the end of the book for related tests by body system.

Barium Enema

SYNONYM/ACRONYM: Air-contrast barium enema, double-contrast barium enema, lower GI series, BE.

COMMON USE: To assist in diagnosing bowel disease in the colon such as tumors and polyps.

AREA OF APPLICATION: Colon.

CONTRAST: Barium sulfate, air, iodine mixture.

DESCRIPTION: This radiological examination of the colon, distal small bowel, and occasionally the appendix follows instillation of barium using a rectal tube inserted into the rectum or an existing ostomy. The patient must retain the barium while a series of radiographs are obtained. Visualization can be improved by using air or barium as the contrast medium (double-contrast study). A combination of x-ray and fluoroscopy techniques is used to complete the study. This test is especially useful in the evaluation of patients experiencing lower abdominal pain, changes in bowel habits, or the passage of stools containing blood or mucus, and for visualizing polyps, diverticula, and tumors. A barium enema may be therapeutic; it may reduce an obstruction caused by intussusception, or telescoping of the intestine. Barium enema should be performed before an upper gastrointestinal (GI) study or barium swallow.

INDICATIONS

- Determine the cause of rectal bleeding, blood, pus, or mucus in feces
- Evaluate suspected inflammatory process, congenital anomaly, motility disorder, or structural change
- Evaluate unexplained weight loss, anemia, or a change in bowel pattern
- Identify and locate benign or malignant polyps or tumors

POTENTIAL DIAGNOSIS

Normal findings in
- Normal size, filling, shape, position, and motility of the colon
- Normal filling of the appendix and terminal ileum

Abnormal findings in
- Appendicitis
- Colorectal cancer
- Congenital anomalies
- Crohn's disease
- Diverticular disease
- Fistulas
- Gastroenteritis
- Granulomatous colitis
- Hirschsprung's disease
- Intussusception
- Perforation of the colon
- Polyps
- Sarcoma
- Sigmoid torsion
- Sigmoid volvulus
- Stenosis
- Tumors
- Ulcerative colitis

CRITICAL FINDINGS: N/A

INTERFERING FACTORS

This procedure is contraindicated for
- Patients with allergies to shellfish or iodinated dye, when iodinated contrast medium is used. The contrast medium, when used, may cause life-threatening allergic reaction. Patients with a known hypersensitivity to contrast medium may benefit from premedication with corticosteroids or the use of nonionic contrast medium.
- Patients who are pregnant or suspected of being pregnant, unless the potential benefits of the procedure far outweigh the risks to the fetus and mother.
- Patients with intestinal obstruction, acute ulcerative colitis, acute diverticulitis, megacolon, or suspected rupture of the colon.

Factors that may impair clear imaging
- Gas or feces in the GI tract resulting from inadequate cleansing or failure to restrict food intake before the study.

B

- Retained barium from a previous radiological procedure.
- Metallic objects within the examination field (e.g., jewelry, body rings).
- Improper adjustment of the radiographic equipment to accommodate obese or thin patients.
- Incorrect patient positioning, which may produce poor visualization of the area to be examined.
- Inability of the patient to cooperate or remain still during the procedure because of age, significant pain, or mental status.
- Spasm of the colon, which can mimic the radiographic signs of cancer. (*Note:* The use of intravenous glucagon minimizes spasm.)
- Inability of the patient to tolerate introduction of or retention of barium, air, or both in the bowel.

Other considerations
- Complications of the procedure may include hemorrhage and cardiac arrhythmias.
- The procedure may be terminated if chest pain or severe cardiac arrhythmias occur.
- Failure to follow dietary restrictions and other pretesting preparations may cause the procedure to be canceled or repeated.
- Consultation with a health-care provider (HCP) should occur before the procedure for radiation safety concerns regarding younger patients or patients who are lactating.
- Risks associated with radiation overexposure can result from frequent x-ray procedures. Personnel in the room with the patient should wear a protective lead apron, stand behind a shield, or leave the area while the examination is being done. Personnel working in the area during the examination should wear badges to record their level of radiation exposure.

NURSING IMPLICATIONS AND PROCEDURE

PRETEST:

- Positively identify the patient using at least two unique identifiers before providing care, treatment, or services.
- *Patient Teaching:* Inform the patient this procedure can assist in assessing the colon.
- Obtain a history of the patient's complaints, including a list of known allergens, especially allergies or sensitivities to latex, iodine, seafood, anesthetics, or contrast mediums.
- Obtain a history of the patient's gastrointestinal system, symptoms, and results of previously performed laboratory tests and diagnostic and surgical procedures.
- Verify that this procedure is performed before an upper GI study or barium swallow.
- Record the date of the last menstrual period and determine the possibility of pregnancy in perimenopausal women.
- Obtain a list of the patient's current medications including anticoagulants, aspirin and other salicylates, herbs, nutritional supplements, and nutraceuticals (see Appendix F). Note the last time and dose of medication taken.
- Review the procedure with the patient. Address concerns about pain and explain that there may be moments of discomfort and some pain experienced during the test. Inform the patient that the procedure is performed in a radiology department, by an HCP specializing in this procedure, with support staff, and takes approximately 30 min.
- *Sensitivity to social and cultural issues,* as well as concern for modesty, is important in providing psychological support before, during, and after the procedure.
- Patients with a colostomy will be ordered special preparations and colostomy irrigation.
- Inform the patient that a laxative and cleansing enema may be needed the day before the procedure, with cleansing enemas on the morning of the procedure, depending on the institution's policy.

- Instruct the patient to remove all metallic objects from the area of the procedure.
- Instruct the patient to eat a low-residue diet for several days before the procedure and to consume only clear liquids the evening before the test. The patient should fast and restrict fluids for 8 hr prior to the procedure. Protocols may vary among facilities.

INTRATEST:

- Ensure the patient has complied with dietary, fluid, and medication restrictions and pretesting preparations.
- Ensure the patient has removed all external metallic objects from the area to be examined.
- Assess for completion of bowel preparation according to the institution's procedure.
- Have emergency equipment readily available.
- Instruct the patient to void prior to the procedure and to change into the gown, robe, and foot coverings provided.
- Instruct the patient to cooperate fully and to follow directions. Instruct the patient to remain still throughout the procedure because movement produces unreliable results.
- Observe standard precautions, and follow the general guidelines in Appendix A.
- Place the patient in the supine position on an examination table and take an initial image.
- Instruct the patient to lie on his or her left side (Sims' position). A rectal tube is inserted into the anus and an attached balloon is inflated after it is situated against the anal sphincter.
- Barium is instilled into the colon by gravity, and its movement through the colon is observed by fluoroscopy.
- For patients with a colostomy, an indwelling urinary catheter is inserted into the stoma and barium is administered.
- Images are taken with the patient in different positions to aid in the diagnosis.
- If a double-contrast barium enema has been ordered, air is then instilled in the intestine and additional images are taken.
- The patient is helped to the bathroom to expel the barium or placed on a bedpan if unable to ambulate.
- After expulsion of the barium, a postevacuation image is taken of the colon.

POST-TEST:

- A report of the examination will be sent to the requesting HCP, who will discuss the results with the patient.
- Instruct the patient to resume usual diet, medications, or activity, as directed by the HCP.
- Instruct the patient to take a mild laxative and increase fluid intake (four 8-oz glasses) to aid in elimination of barium, unless contraindicated.
- Carefully monitor the patient for fatigue and fluid and electrolyte imbalance.
- Instruct the patient that stools will be white or light in color for 2 to 3 days. If the patient is unable to eliminate the barium, or if stools do not return to normal color, the patient should notify the HCP.
- Advise patients with a colostomy that tap water colostomy irrigation may aid in barium removal.
- Recognize anxiety related to test results. Discuss the implications of abnormal test results on the patient's lifestyle. Provide teaching and information regarding the clinical implications of the test results, as appropriate.
- Reinforce information given by the patient's HCP regarding further testing, treatment, or referral to another HCP. Decisions regarding the need for and frequency of occult blood testing, colonoscopy, or other cancer screening procedures should be made after consultation between the patient and HCP. The most current guidelines for colon cancer screening of the general population as well as individuals with increased risk are available from the American Cancer Society (www.cancer .org) and the American College of Gastroenterology (www.gi.org). Answer any questions or address any concerns voiced by the patient or family.
- Depending on the results of this procedure, additional testing may be performed to evaluate or monitor progression of the disease process and determine the need for a change in therapy. Evaluate test results in relation

to the patient's symptoms and other tests performed.

RELATED MONOGRAPHS:

▶ Related tests include cancer antigens, colonoscopy, colposcopy, CT abdomen, fecal analysis, MRI abdomen, PET pelvis, and proctosigmoidoscopy.
▶ Refer to the Gastrointestinal System table at the end of the book for related tests by body system.

Barium Swallow

SYNONYM/ACRONYM: Esophagram, video swallow, esophagus x-ray, swallowing function, esophagraphy.

COMMON USE: To assist in diagnosing disease of the esophagus such as stricture and tumor.

AREA OF APPLICATION: Esophagus.

CONTRAST: Barium sulfate, water-soluble iodinated contrast.

DESCRIPTION: This radiological examination of the esophagus evaluates motion and anatomic structures of the esophageal lumen by recording images of the lumen while the patient swallows a barium solution of milkshake consistency and chalky taste. The procedure uses fluoroscopic and cineradiographic techniques. The barium swallow is often performed as part of an upper gastrointestinal (GI) series or cardiac series and is indicated for patients with a history of dysphagia and gastric reflux. The study may identify reflux of the barium from the stomach back into the esophagus. Muscular abnormalities such as achalasia, as well as diffuse esophageal spasm, can be easily detected with this procedure.

INDICATIONS

• Confirm the integrity of esophageal anastomoses in the postoperative patient
• Detect esophageal reflux, tracheoesophageal fistulas, and varices
• Determine the cause of dysphagia or heartburn
• Determine the type and location of foreign bodies within the pharynx and esophagus
• Evaluate suspected esophageal motility disorders
• Evaluate suspected polyps, strictures, Zenker's diverticula, tumor, or inflammation

POTENTIAL DIAGNOSIS

Normal findings in
• Normal peristalsis through the esophagus into the stomach with normal size, filling, patency, and shape of the esophagus

Abnormal findings in
- Achalasia
- Acute or chronic esophagitis
- Benign or malignant tumors
- Chalasia
- Diverticula
- Esophageal ulcers
- Esophageal varices
- Hiatal hernia
- Perforation of the esophagus
- Strictures or polyps

CRITICAL FINDINGS: N/A

INTERFERING FACTORS

This procedure is contraindicated for
- Patients who are pregnant or suspected of being pregnant, unless the potential benefits of the procedure far outweigh the risks to the fetus and mother.
- Patients with intestinal obstruction or suspected esophageal rupture, unless water-soluble iodinated contrast medium is used.
- Patients with suspected tracheoesophageal fistula, unless barium is used.

Factors that may impair clear imaging
- Metallic objects within the examination field.
- Improper adjustment of the radiographic equipment to accommodate obese or thin patients, which can cause overexposure or underexposure.
- Incorrect patient positioning, which may produce poor visualization of the area to be examined.
- Inability of the patient to cooperate or remain still during the procedure because of age, significant pain, or mental status.

Other considerations
- Failure to follow dietary restrictions and other pretesting preparations may cause the procedure to be canceled or repeated.
- A potential complication of a barium swallow is barium-induced fecal impaction.
- Ensure that the procedure is done after cholangiography and barium enema.
- Consultation with a health-care provider (HCP) should occur before the procedure for radiation safety concerns regarding younger patients or patients who are lactating.
- Risks associated with radiation overexposure can result from frequent x-ray procedures. Personnel in the room with the patient should wear a protective lead apron, stand behind a shield, or leave the area while the examination is being done. Personnel working in the examination area should wear badges to record their level of radiation exposure.

NURSING IMPLICATIONS AND PROCEDURE

PRETEST:
▶ Positively identify the patient using at least two unique identifiers before providing care, treatment, or services.
▶ *Patient Teaching:* Inform the patient this procedure can assist in assessing the esophagus.
▶ Obtain a history of the patient's complaints, including a list of known allergens, especially allergies or sensitivities to latex, iodine, seafood, anesthetics, or contrast medium.
▶ Obtain a history of the patient's gastrointestinal system, symptoms, and results of previously performed laboratory tests and diagnostic and surgical procedures.
▶ Ensure that this procedure is performed before an upper GI study or video swallow.
▶ Record the date of the last menstrual period and determine the possibility of pregnancy in perimenopausal women.

B

▶ Obtain a list of the patient's current medications, including herbs, nutritional supplements, and nutraceuticals (see Appendix F).

▶ Explain to the patient that some pain may be experienced during the test, and there may be moments of discomfort. Review the procedure with the patient and explain the need to swallow a barium contrast medium. Inform the patient that the procedure is performed in a radiology department by a HCP and takes approximately 15 to 30 min.

▶ *Sensitivity to social and cultural issues,* as well as concern for modesty, is important in providing psychological support before, during, and after the procedure.

▶ Instruct the patient to remove all external metallic objects from the area to be examined.

▶ Instruct the patient to fast and restrict fluids for 8 hr prior to the procedure. Protocols may vary among facilities.

INTRATEST:

▶ Ensure the patient has complied with dietary and fluid restrictions for 8 hr prior to the procedure.

▶ Ensure the patient has removed all external metallic objects from the area to be examined.

▶ Instruct the patient to void prior to the procedure and to change into the gown, robe, and foot coverings provided.

▶ Instruct the patient to cooperate and follow directions. Instruct the patient to remain still throughout the procedure because movement produces unreliable results.

▶ Observe standard precautions, and follow the general guidelines in Appendix A.

▶ Instruct the patient to stand in front of the x-ray fluoroscopy screen. Place the patient supine on the radiographic table if he or she is unable to stand.

▶ An initial image is taken, and the patient is asked to swallow a barium solution with or without a straw.

▶ Multiple images at different angles may be taken.

▶ The patient may be asked to drink additional barium to complete the study. Swallowing the additional barium evaluates the passage of barium from the esophagus into the stomach.

POST-TEST:

▶ A report of the results will be sent to the requesting HCP, who will discuss the results with the patient.

▶ Instruct the patient to resume usual diet, fluids, medications, and activity, as directed by the HCP.

▶ Carefully monitor the patient for fatigue and fluid and electrolyte imbalance.

▶ Instruct the patient to take a mild laxative and increase fluid intake (four 8-oz glasses) to aid in elimination of barium, unless contraindicated.

▶ Instruct the patient that stools will be white or light in color for 2 to 3 days. If the patient is unable to eliminate the barium, or if stools do not return to normal color, the patient should notify the requesting HCP.

▶ Recognize anxiety related to test results. Discuss the implications of abnormal test results on the patient's lifestyle. Provide teaching and information regarding the clinical implications of the test results, as appropriate.

▶ Reinforce information given by the patient's HCP regarding further testing, treatment, or referral to another HCP. Answer any questions or address any concerns voiced by the patient or family.

▶ Depending on the results of this procedure, additional testing may be performed to evaluate or monitor progression of the disease process and determine the need for a change in therapy. Evaluate test results in relation to the patient's symptoms and other tests performed.

RELATED MONOGRAPHS:

▶ Related tests include capsule endoscopy, chest x-ray, CT thoracic, endoscopy, esophageal manometry, gastroesophageal reflux scan, MRI chest, and thyroid scan.

▶ Refer to the Gastrointestinal System table at the end of the book for related tests by body system.

Bilirubin and Bilirubin Fractions

SYNONYM/ACRONYM: Conjugated/direct bilirubin, unconjugated/indirect bilirubin, delta bilirubin, TBil.

COMMON USE: A multipurpose lab test that acts as an indicator for various diseases of the liver or for disease that affects the liver.

SPECIMEN: Serum (1 mL) collected in a red- or tiger-top tube. Plasma (1 mL) collected in green-top (heparin) tube or in a heparinized microtainer is also acceptable. Protect sample from direct light.

REFERENCE VALUE: (Method: Spectrophotometry) Total bilirubin levels in infants should decrease to adult levels by day 10 as the development of the hepatic circulatory system matures. Values in breastfed infants may take longer to reach normal adult levels. Values in premature infants may initially be higher than in full-term infants and also take longer to decrease to normal levels.

Bilirubin	Conventional Units	SI Units (Conventional Units × 17.1)
Total bilirubin		
Newborn–1 day	1.4–8.7 mg/dL	24–149 micromol/L
1–2 days	3.4–11.5 mg/dL	58–97 micromol/L
3–5 days	1.5–12.0 mg/dL	26–205 micromol/L
1 mo–older adult	0.3–1.2 mg/dL	5–21 micromol/L
Unconjugated bilirubin	Less than 1.1 mg/dL	Less than 19 micromol/L
Conjugated bilirubin	Less than 0.3 mg/dL	Less than 5 micromol/L
Delta bilirubin	Less than 0.2 mg/dL	Less than 3 micromol/L

DESCRIPTION: Bilirubin is a by-product of heme catabolism from aged red blood cells (RBCs). Bilirubin is primarily produced in the liver, spleen, and bone marrow. Total bilirubin is the sum of unconjugated or indirect bilirubin, monoglucuronide and diglucuronide, conjugated or direct bilirubin, and albumin-bound delta bilirubin. Unconjugated bilirubin is carried to the liver by albumin, where it becomes conjugated. In the small intestine, conjugated bilirubin converts to urobilinogen and then to urobilin. Urobilin is then excreted in the feces. Increases in bilirubin levels can result from prehepatic, hepatic, and/or posthepatic conditions, making fractionation useful in determining the cause of the increase in total bilirubin levels. Delta bilirubin has a longer half-life than the other bilirubin fractions and therefore remains elevated during convalescence after the other fractions have decreased to normal levels. Delta bilirubin can be calculated using the formula:

Delta bilirubin = Total bilirubin − (Indirect bilirubin + Direct bilirubin)

When bilirubin concentration increases, the yellowish pigment deposits in skin and sclera. This increase in yellow pigmentation is termed *jaundice* or *icterus*. Bilirubin levels can also be checked using noninvasive methods. Defects in bilirubin excretion can be identified in a routine urinalysis. Hyperbilirubinemia in neonates can be reliably evaluated using transcutaneous measurement devices.

INDICATIONS

- Assist in the differential diagnosis of obstructive jaundice
- Assist in the evaluation of liver and biliary disease
- Monitor the effects of drug reactions on liver function
- Monitor the effects of phototherapy on jaundiced newborns
- Monitor jaundice in newborn patients

POTENTIAL DIAGNOSIS

Increased in

- Prehepatic (hemolytic) jaundice *(related to excessive amounts of heme released from RBC destruction. Heme is catabolized to bilirubin in concentrations that exceed the liver's conjugation capacity, and indirect bilirubin accumulates)*

Erythroblastosis fetalis
Hematoma
Hemolytic anemias
Pernicious anemia
Physiological jaundice of the newborn
The post blood transfusion period, when a number of units are rapidly infused or in the case of a delayed transfusion reaction
RBC enzyme abnormalities (i.e., glucose-6-phosphate dehydrogenase, pyruvate kinase, spherocytosis)

- Hepatic jaundice *(related to bilirubin conjugation failure)*
Crigler-Najjar syndrome
- Hepatic jaundice *(related to disturbance in bilirubin transport)*
Dubin-Johnson syndrome *(related to preconjugation transport failure)*
Gilbert's syndrome *(related to postconjugation transport failure)*
- Hepatic jaundice *(evidenced by liver damage or necrosis that interferes with excretion into bile ducts either by physical obstruction or drug inhibition and bilirubin accumulates)*
Alcoholism
Cholangitis
Cholecystitis
Cholestatic drug reactions
Cirrhosis
Hepatitis
Hepatocellular damage
Infectious mononucleosis
- Posthepatic jaundice *(evidenced by blockage that interferes with excretion into bile ducts, resulting in accumulated bilirubin)*
Advanced tumors of the liver
Biliary obstruction
- Other conditions
Anorexia or starvation *(related to liver damage)*
Hypothyroidism *(related to effect on the liver whereby hepatic enzyme activity for formation of conjugated or direct bilirubin is enhanced in combination with decreased flow of bile and*

secretion of bile acids; results in
accumulation of direct bilirubin)
Premature or breastfed infants
(evidenced by diminished hepatic
function of the liver in premature
infants; related to inability of neonate
to feed in sufficient quantity.
Insufficient breast milk intake results in
weight loss, decreased stool formation,
and decreased elimination of bilirubin)

Decreased in: N/A

CRITICAL FINDINGS
• Greater than 15 mg/dL

Note and immediately report to the health-care provider (HCP) any critically increased values and related symptoms.

Sustained hyperbilirubinemia can result in brain damage. Kernicterus refers to the deposition of bilirubin in the basal ganglia and brainstem nuclei. There is no exact level of bilirubin that puts infants at risk for developing kernicterus. Symptoms of kernicterus in infants include lethargy, poor feeding, upward deviation of the eyes, and seizures. Intervention for infants may include early frequent feedings to stimulate gastrointestinal motility, phototherapy, and exchange transfusion.

INTERFERING FACTORS
• Drugs that may increase bilirubin levels by causing cholestasis include anabolic steroids, androgens, butaperazine, chlorothiazide, chlorpromazine, chlorpropamide, cinchophen, dapsone, dienestrol, erythromycin, estrogens, ethionamide, gold salts, hydrochlorothiazide, icterogenin, imipramine, iproniazid, isocarboxazid, isoniazid, meprobamate, mercaptopurine, meropenem, methandriol, nitrofurans, norethandrolone, nortriptyline, oleandomycin, oral contraceptives, penicillins, phenothiazines, prochlorperazine, progesterone, promazine, promethazine, propoxyphene, protriptyline, sulfonamides, tacrolimus, thiouracil, tolazamide, tolbutamide, thiacetazone, trifluoperazine, and trimeprazine.
• Drugs that may increase bilirubin levels by causing hepatocellular damage include acetaminophen (toxic), acetylsalicylic acid, allopurinol, aminothiazole, anabolic steroids, asparaginase, azathioprine, azithromycin, carbamazepine, carbutamide, chloramphenicol, clindamycin, clofibrate, chlorambucil, chloramphenicol, chlordane, chloroform, chlorzoxazone, clonidine, colchicine, coumarin, cyclophosphamide, cyclopropane, cycloserine, cyclosporine, dactinomycin, danazol, desipramine, dexfenfluramine, diazepam, diethylstilbestrol, dinitrophenol, enflurane, ethambutol, ethionamide, ethoxazene, factor IX complex, felbamate, flavaspidic acid, flucytosine, fusidic acid, gentamicin, glycopyrrolate, guanoxan, haloperidol, halothane, hycanthone, hydroxyacetamide, ibuprofen, interferon, interleukin-2, isoniazid, kanamycin, labetalol, levamisole, lincomycin, melphalan, mesoridazine, metahexamide, metaxalone, methotrexate, methoxsalen, methyldopa, nitrofurans, oral contraceptives, oxamniquine, oxyphenisatin, pemoline, penicillin, perphenazine, phenazopyridine, phenelzine, phenindione, pheniprazine, phenothiazines, piroxicam, probenecid, procainamide, pyrazinamide, quinine, sulfonylureas, thiothixene, timolol, tobramycin, tolcapone, tretinoin, trimethadione, urethan, and verapamil.
• Drugs that may increase bilirubin levels by causing hemolysis include aminopyrine, amphotericin B, carbamazepine, cephaloridine,

cephalothin, chloroquine, dimercaprol, dipyrone, furadaltone, furazolidone, mefenamic acid, melphalan, mephenytoin, methylene blue, nitrofurans, nitrofurazone, pamaquine, penicillins, pentaquine, phenylhydrazine, piperazine, pipobroman, primaquine, procainamide, quinacrine, quinidine, quinine, stibophen, streptomycin, sulfonamides, triethylenemelamine, tyrothricin, and vitamin K.

• Drugs that may decrease bilirubin levels include anticonvulsants, barbiturates (newborns), chlorophenothane, cyclosporine, flumecinolone (newborns), and salicylates.

• Bilirubin is light sensitive. Therefore, the collection container should be suitably covered to protect the specimen from light between the time of collection and analysis.

NURSING IMPLICATIONS AND PROCEDURE

PRETEST:

▶ Positively identify the patient using at least two unique identifiers before providing care, treatment, or services.
▶ *Patient Teaching:* Inform the patient this test can assist in assessing liver function.
▶ Obtain a history of the patient's complaints, including a list of known allergens, especially allergies or sensitivities to latex.
▶ Obtain a history of the patient's hepatobiliary system, symptoms, and results of previously performed laboratory tests and diagnostic and surgical procedures.
▶ Obtain a list of the patient's current medication, including herbs, nutritional supplements, and nutraceuticals (see Appendix F).
▶ Review the procedure with the patient. Inform the patient that specimen collection takes approximately 5 to 10 min. Address concerns about pain and explain that there may be some discomfort during the venipuncture.

▶ *Sensitivity to social and cultural issues,* as well as concern for modesty, is important in providing psychological support before, during, and after the procedure.
▶ There are no food, fluid, or medication restrictions unless by medical direction.

INTRATEST:

▶ If the patient has a history of allergic reaction to latex, avoid the use of equipment containing latex.
▶ Instruct the patient to cooperate fully and to follow directions. Direct the patient to breathe normally and to avoid unnecessary movement.
▶ Observe standard precautions, and follow the general guidelines in Appendix A. Positively identify the patient, and label the appropriate tubes with the corresponding patient demographics, date, and time of collection. Perform a venipuncture.
▶ Remove the needle and apply direct pressure with dry gauze to stop bleeding. Observe/assess venipuncture site for bleeding or hematoma formation and secure gauze with adhesive bandage.
▶ Protect the specimen from light and promptly transport the specimen to the laboratory for processing and analysis.

POST-TEST:

▶ A report of the results will be sent to the requesting HCP, who will discuss the results with the patient.
▶ *Nutritional Considerations:* Increased bilirubin levels may be associated with liver disease. Dietary recommendations may be indicated depending on the condition and severity of the condition. Currently, for example, there are no specific medications that can be given to cure hepatitis, but elimination of alcohol consumption and a diet optimized for convalescence are commonly included in the treatment plan. A high-calorie, high-protein, moderate-fat diet with a high fluid intake is often recommended for the patient with hepatitis. Treatment of cirrhosis is different because a low-protein diet may be in order if the patient's liver has lost the ability to process the end products of protein metabolism. A diet of soft foods

may also be required if esophageal varices have developed. Ammonia levels may be used to determine whether protein should be added to or reduced from the diet. Patients should be encouraged to eat simple carbohydrates and emulsified fats (as in homogenized milk or eggs) rather than complex carbohydrates (e.g., starch, fiber, and glycogen [animal carbohydrates]) and complex fats, which require additional bile to emulsify them so that they can be used. The cirrhotic patient should be carefully observed for the development of ascites, in which case fluid and electrolyte balance requires strict attention. The alcoholic patient should be encouraged to avoid alcohol and also to seek appropriate counseling for substance abuse.

▶ Intervention for hyperbilirubinemia in the neonatal patient may include early frequent feedings (to stimulate gastrointestinal motility), phototherapy, and exchange transfusion.

▶ Reinforce information given by the patient's HCP regarding further testing, treatment, or referral to another HCP.

Answer any questions or address any concerns voiced by the patient or family.

▶ Depending on the results of this procedure, additional testing may be performed to evaluate or monitor progression of the disease process and determine the need for a change in therapy. Evaluate test results in relation to the patient's symptoms and other tests performed.

RELATED MONOGRAPHS:

▶ Related tests include ALT, albumin, ALP, ammonia, amylase, AMA/ASMA, α_1-antitrypsin/phenotyping, AST, biopsy liver, cholesterol, coagulation factor assays, CBC, cholangiography percutaneous transhepatic, cholangiography post-op, CT biliary tract and liver, copper, ERCP, GGT, hepatobiliary scan, hepatitis serologies, infectious mononucleosis screen, lipase, liver and spleen scan, protein total and fractions, PT/INR, US liver, and UA.

▶ See the Hepatobiliary System table at the end of the book for related tests by body system.

Biopsy, Bladder

SYNONYM/ACRONYM: N/A.

COMMON USE: To assist in diagnosing bladder cancer.

SPECIMEN: Bladder tissue or cells.

REFERENCE VALUE: (Method: Macroscopic and microscopic examination of tissue) No abnormal tissue or cells.

DESCRIPTION: Biopsy is the excision of a sample of tissue that can be analyzed microscopically to determine cell morphology and the presence of tissue abnormalities. This test is used to assist in confirming the diagnosis of cancer when clinical symptoms or other diagnostic findings are suspicious.

A urologist performs a biopsy of the bladder during cystoscopic examination. The procedure is usually carried out under general anesthesia. After the bladder is filled with saline for irrigation, the bladder and urethra are examined by direct and lighted visualization using a cystoscope. A sample of suspicious bladder tissue is then excised and examined macroscopically and microscopically to determine the presence of cell morphology and tissue abnormalities.

INDICATIONS
• Assist in confirmation of malignant lesions of the bladder or ureter, especially if tumor is seen by radiological examination
• Assist in the evaluation of cases in which symptoms such as hematuria persist after previous treatment (e.g., removal of polyps or kidney stones)
• Monitor existing recurrent benign lesions for malignant changes

POTENTIAL DIAGNOSIS
• Positive findings in neoplasm of the bladder or ureter

CRITICAL FINDINGS
• Assessment of clear margins after tissue excision
• Classification or grading of tumor
• Identification of malignancy

It is essential that critical diagnoses be communicated immediately to the requesting health-care provider (HCP). A listing of these diagnoses varies among facilities.

INTERFERING FACTORS
• This test is contraindicated in patients with an acute infection of the bladder, urethra, or prostate.
• ✦ This procedure is contraindicated in patients with bleeding disorders.
• Failure to follow dietary restrictions before the procedure may cause the procedure to be canceled or repeated.

NURSING IMPLICATIONS AND PROCEDURE

PRETEST:
▶ Positively identify the patient using at least two unique identifiers before providing care, treatment, or services.
▶ *Patient Teaching:* Inform the patient this procedure can assist in establishing a diagnosis of bladder disease.
▶ Obtain a history of the patient's complaints, including a list of known allergens, especially allergies or sensitivities to latex or anesthetics.
▶ Obtain a history of the patient's genitourinary system, any bleeding disorders or other symptoms, and results of previously performed laboratory tests and diagnostic and surgical procedures.
▶ Record the date of the last menstrual period and determine the possibility of pregnancy in perimenopausal women.
▶ Note any recent procedures that can interfere with test results.
▶ Obtain a list of the patient's current medications including anticoagulants, aspirin and other salicylates, herbs, nutritional supplements, and nutraceuticals (see Appendix F). Such products should be discontinued by medical direction for the appropriate number of days prior to a surgical procedure.
▶ Review the procedure with the patient. Inform the patient that it may be necessary to remove hair from the site before the procedure. Inform the patient that back pain and burning or pressure in the genital area may

be experienced after the procedure. Prophylactic antibiotics may be administered before the procedure in certain cases. Address concerns about pain and explain that a general anesthesia will be administered prior to the biopsy. Explain that no pain will be experienced during the biopsy. Inform the patient that the biopsy is performed under sterile conditions by an HCP specializing in this procedure. The procedure usually takes about 30 to 45 min to complete.

▶ *Sensitivity to social and cultural issues,* as well as concern for modesty, is important in providing psychological support before, during, and after the procedure.

▶ Explain that an IV line will be inserted to allow infusion of IV fluids, antibiotics, anesthetics, and analgesics.

▶ Instruct the patient that nothing should be taken by mouth for 6 to 8 hr prior to a general anesthetic, or that only clear liquids may be taken for 8 hr prior to the procedure if local anesthesia is to be used. Protocols may vary among facilities.

▶ *Make sure a written and informed consent has been signed prior to the procedure and before administering any medications.*

INTRATEST:

▶ Ensure that the patient has complied with dietary restrictions; ensure that food has been restricted for at least 6 to 8 hr prior to the procedure.

▶ Ensure that anticoagulant therapy has been withheld for the appropriate number of days prior to the procedure. Number of days to withhold medication is dependent on the type of anticoagulant. Notify the HCP if patient anticoagulant therapy has not been withheld.

▶ Have emergency equipment readily available.

▶ Have the patient void before the procedure.

▶ Observe standard precautions, and follow the general guidelines in Appendix A. Positively identify the patient, and label the appropriate collection containers with the corresponding patient demographics, date and time of collection, and site location.

▶ Assist the patient to a comfortable position, and direct the patient to breathe normally during the beginning of the general anesthetic.

▶ Record baseline vital signs, and continue to monitor throughout the procedure. Protocols may vary among facilities.

Cystoscopy

▶ After administration of general anesthesia, place the patient in a lithotomy position on the examination table (with the feet up in stirrups). Drape the patient's legs. Clean the external genitalia with a suitable antiseptic solution and drape the area with sterile towels.

▶ Once the cystoscope is inserted, the bladder is irrigated with saline. A tissue sample is removed using a cytology brush or biopsy forceps. Catheters may be used to obtain samples from the ureter.

Open Biopsy

▶ After administration of general anesthesia and surgical preparation are completed, an incision is made, suspicious areas are located, and tissue samples are collected.

General

▶ Monitor the patient for complications related to the procedure (e.g., allergic reaction, anaphylaxis).

▶ Place tissue samples in properly labeled specimen container containing formalin solution, and promptly transport the specimen to the laboratory for processing and analysis.

POST-TEST:

▶ A report of the results will be sent to the requesting HCP, who will discuss the results with the patient.

▶ Instruct the patient to resume preoperative diet, as directed by the HCP. Assess the patient's ability to swallow before allowing the patient to attempt liquids or solid foods.

▶ Monitor vital signs and neurological status every 15 min for 1 hr, then every 2 hr for 4 hr, and then as ordered by the HCP. Monitor temperature every 4 hr for 24 hr. Monitor intake and output at least every 8 hr. Compare with baseline values. Notify the HCP if temperature is elevated. Protocols may vary among facilities.

▶ Instruct the patient on intake and output recording and provide appropriate measuring containers.

▶ Encourage fluid intake of 3,000 mL in 24 hr unless contraindicated.

▶ Observe for delayed allergic reactions, such as rash, urticaria, tachycardia, hyperpnea, hypertension, palpitations, nausea, or vomiting.

▶ Instruct the patient to immediately report pain, chills, or fever. Assess for infection, hemorrhage, or perforation of the bladder.

▶ Inform the patient that blood may be seen in the urine after the first or second postprocedural voiding.

▶ Instruct the patient to report any further changes in urinary pattern, volume, or appearance.

Open Biopsy

▶ Observe/assess the biopsy site for bleeding, inflammation, or hematoma formation.

▶ Instruct the patient in the care and assessment of the site.

▶ Instruct the patient to report any redness, edema, bleeding, or pain at the biopsy site.

General

▶ Assess for nausea, pain, and bladder spasms. Administer antiemetic, analgesic, and antispasmodic medications as needed and as directed by the HCP.

▶ Administer antibiotic therapy if ordered. Remind the patient of the importance of completing the entire course of antibiotic therapy, even if signs and symptoms disappear before completion of therapy.

▶ Recognize anxiety related to test results. Discuss the implications of abnormal test results on the patient's lifestyle. Provide teaching and information regarding the clinical implications of the test results, as appropriate. Educate the patient regarding access to counseling services.

▶ Reinforce information given by the patient's HCP regarding further testing, treatment, or referral to another HCP. Answer any questions or address any concerns voiced by the patient or family.

▶ Instruct the patient in the use of any ordered medications. Explain the importance of adhering to the therapy regimen. As appropriate, instruct the patient in significant side effects and systemic reactions associated with the prescribed medication. Encourage him or her to review corresponding literature provided by a pharmacist.

▶ Depending on the results of this procedure, additional testing may be performed to evaluate or monitor progression of the disease process and determine the need for a change in therapy. Evaluate test results in relation to the patient's symptoms and other tests performed.

RELATED MONOGRAPHS:

▶ Related tests include calculus kidney stone panel, cystometry, cystoscopy, cystourethrography voiding, IVP, KUB studies, MRI bladder, US bladder, UA, and urine bladder cancer markers.

▶ Refer to the Genitourinary System table at the end of the book for related tests by body system.

Biopsy, Bone

SYNONYM/ACRONYM: N/A.

COMMON USE: To assist in diagnosing bone cancer.

SPECIMEN: Bone tissue.

REFERENCE VALUE: (Method: Microscopic study of bone samples) No abnormal tissue or cells.

DESCRIPTION: Biopsy is the excision of a sample of tissue that can be analyzed microscopically to determine cell morphology and the presence of tissue abnormalities. This test is used to assist in confirming the diagnosis of cancer when clinical symptoms or x-rays are suspicious. After surgical incision to reveal the affected area, bone biopsy is obtained. An alternative collection method is needle biopsy in which a plug of bone is removed using a special serrated needle.

It is essential that critical diagnoses be communicated immediately to the requesting health-care provider (HCP). A listing of these diagnoses varies among facilities.

INTERFERING FACTORS

- This procedure is contraindicated in patients with bleeding disorders.
- Failure to follow dietary restrictions before the procedure may cause the procedure to be canceled or repeated.

INDICATIONS

- Differentiation of a benign from a malignant bone lesion
- Radiographic evidence of a bone lesion

POTENTIAL DIAGNOSIS

Abnormal findings in

- Ewing's sarcoma
- Multiple myeloma
- Osteoma
- Osteosarcoma

CRITICAL FINDINGS

- Classification or grading of tumor
- Identification of malignancy

NURSING IMPLICATIONS AND PROCEDURE

PRETEST:

- Positively identify the patient using at least two unique identifiers before providing care, treatment, or services.
- *Patient Teaching:* Inform the patient this procedure can assist to establish a diagnosis of bone disease.
- Obtain a history of the patient's complaints, including a list of known allergens, especially allergies or sensitivities to latex or anesthetics.
- Obtain a history of the patient's immune and musculoskeletal systems, especially any bleeding disorders and other symptoms, and results of previously performed laboratory

tests and diagnostic and surgical procedures.

▶ Record the date of the last menstrual period and determine the possibility of pregnancy in perimenopausal women.

▶ Note any recent procedures that can interfere with test results.

▶ Obtain a list of the patient's current medications, including anticoagulants, aspirin and other salicylates, herbs, nutritional supplements, and nutraceuticals (see Appendix F). Such products should be discontinued by medical direction for the appropriate number of days prior to a surgical procedure.

▶ Review the procedure with the patient. Inform the patient that it may be necessary to remove hair from the site before the procedure. Address concerns about pain and explain that a sedative and/or analgesia will be administered to promote relaxation and reduce discomfort prior to the percutaneous biopsy; general anesthesia will be administered prior to the open biopsy. Explain to the patient that no pain will be experienced during the test when general anesthesia is used but that any discomfort with a needle biopsy will be minimized with local anesthetics and systemic analgesics. Inform the patient that the biopsy is performed under sterile conditions by an HCP specializing in this procedure. The surgical procedure usually takes about 30 min to complete, and sutures may be necessary to close the site. A needle biopsy usually takes about 20 min to complete.

▶ *Sensitivity to social and cultural issues,* as well as concern for modesty, is important in providing psychological support before, during, and after the procedure.

▶ Explain that an IV line will be inserted to allow infusion of IV fluids, anesthetics, analgesics, or IV sedation.

Open Biopsy

▶ Instruct the patient that nothing should be taken by mouth for 6 to 8 hr prior to a general anesthetic. Protocols may vary among facilities.

Needle Biopsy

▶ Instruct the patient that nothing should be taken by mouth for at least 4 hr prior to the procedure to reduce the risk of nausea and vomiting. Protocols may vary among facilities.

General

▶ *Make sure a written and informed consent has been signed prior to the procedure and before administering any medications.*

INTRATEST:

▶ Ensure that the patient has complied with dietary restrictions; ensure that food has been restricted for at least 4 to 8 hr depending on the anesthetic chosen for the procedure.

▶ Ensure that anticoagulant therapy has been withheld for the appropriate number of days prior to the procedure. Number of days to withhold medication is dependent on the type of anticoagulant. Notify the HCP if patient anticoagulant therapy has not been withheld.

▶ Have emergency equipment readily available.

▶ Have the patient void before the procedure.

▶ Observe standard precautions, and follow the general guidelines in Appendix A. Positively identify the patient, and label the appropriate collection containers with the corresponding patient demographics, date and time of collection, and site location.

▶ Assist the patient to the desired position depending on the test site to be used, and direct the patient to breathe normally during the beginning of the general anesthetic. Instruct the patient to cooperate fully and to follow directions. For the patient undergoing local anesthesia, direct him or her to breathe normally and to avoid unnecessary movement during the procedure.

▶ Record baseline vital signs, and continue to monitor throughout the procedure. Protocols may vary among facilities.

▶ After the administration of general or local anesthesia, shave and cleanse the site with an antiseptic solution, and drape the area with sterile towels.

Open Biopsy

▶ After administration of general anesthesia and surgical preparation are completed, an incision is made, suspicious area(s) are located, and tissue samples are collected.

Needle Biopsy
- Instruct the patient to take slow, deep breaths when the local anesthetic is injected. Protect the site with sterile drapes. A small incision is made and the biopsy needle is inserted to remove the specimen. Pressure is applied to the site for 3 to 5 min, then a sterile pressure dressing is applied.

General
- Monitor the patient for complications related to the procedure (e.g., allergic reaction, anaphylaxis).
- Place tissue samples in properly labeled specimen container containing formalin solution, and promptly transport the specimen to the laboratory for processing and analysis.

POST-TEST:
- A report of the examination will be sent to the requesting HCP, who will discuss the results with the patient.
- Instruct the patient to resume preoperative diet, as directed by the HCP. Assess the patient's ability to swallow before allowing the patient to attempt liquids or solid foods.
- Monitor vital signs and neurological status every 15 min for 1 hr, then every 2 hr for 4 hr, and then as ordered by the HCP. Monitor temperature every 4 hr for 24 hr. Monitor intake and output at least every 8 hr. Compare with baseline values. Notify the HCP if temperature is elevated. Protocols may vary among facilities.
- Observe/assess for delayed allergic reactions, such as rash, urticaria, tachycardia, hyperpnea, hypertension, palpitations, nausea, or vomiting.
- Observe/assess the biopsy site for bleeding, inflammation, or hematoma formation.
- Instruct the patient in the care and assessment of the site.
- Instruct the patient to report any redness, edema, bleeding, or pain at the biopsy site. Instruct the patient to immediately report chills or fever.

- Assess for nausea and pain. Administer antiemetic and analgesic medications as needed and as directed by the HCP.
- Administer antibiotic therapy if ordered. Remind the patient of the importance of completing the entire course of antibiotic therapy, even if signs and symptoms disappear before completion of therapy.
- Recognize anxiety related to test results. Discuss the implications of abnormal test results on the patient's lifestyle. Provide teaching and information regarding the clinical implications of the test results, as appropriate. Educate the patient regarding access to counseling services.
- Reinforce information given by the patient's HCP regarding further testing, treatment, or referral to another HCP. Inform the patient of a follow-up appointment for removal of sutures, if indicated. Answer any questions or address any concerns voiced by the patient or family.
- Instruct the patient in the use of any ordered medications. Explain the importance of adhering to the therapy regimen. As appropriate, instruct the patient in significant side effects and systemic reactions associated with the prescribed medication. Encourage him or her to review corresponding literature provided by a pharmacist.
- Depending on the results of this procedure, additional testing may be performed to evaluate or monitor progression of the disease process and determine the need for a change in therapy. Evaluate test results in relation to the patient's symptoms and other tests performed.

RELATED MONOGRAPHS:
- Related tests include ALP, biopsy bone marrow, bone scan, calcium, CBC, cortisol, immunofixation electrophoresis, immunoglobulins (A, G, and M), β_2-microglobulin, MRI musculoskeletal, PTH, phosphorus, total protein and fractions, UA, and vitamin D.
- See the Immune and Musculoskeletal systems tables at the end of the book for related tests by body system.

Biopsy, Bone Marrow

SYNONYM/ACRONYM: N/A.

COMMON USE: To assist in diagnosing hematological diseases and in identifying and staging cancers such as leukemia.

SPECIMEN: Bone marrow aspirate, bone core biopsy, marrow and peripheral smears.

REFERENCE VALUE: (Method: Microscopic study of bone and bone marrow samples, flow cytometry) Reference ranges are subject to many variables, and therefore the laboratory should be consulted for their specific interpretation. Some generalities may be commented on regarding findings as follows:

- Ratio of marrow fat to cellular elements is related to age, with the amount of fat increasing with increasing age.
- Normal cellularity, cellular distribution, presence of megakaryocytes, and absence of fibrosis or tumor cells.
- The myeloid-to-erythrocyte ratio (M:E) is 2:1 to 4:1 in adults. It may be slightly higher in children.

Differential Parameter	Conventional Units
Erythrocyte precursors	18–32%
Myeloblasts	0–2%
Promyelocytes	2–6%
Myelocytes	9–17%
Metamyelocytes	7–25%
Bands	10–16%
Neutrophils	18–28%
Eosinophils and precursors	1–5%
Basophils and precursors	0–1%
Monocytes and precursors	1–5%
Lymphocytes	9–19%
Plasma cells	0–1%

DESCRIPTION: This test involves the removal of a small sample of bone marrow by aspiration, needle biopsy, or open surgical biopsy for a complete hematological analysis. The marrow is a suspension of blood, fat, and developing blood cells, which is evaluated for morphology and examined for all stages of maturation; iron stores; and myeloid-to-erythrocyte ratio (M:E). Sudan black B and periodic acid Schiff (PAS) stains can be performed for microscopic examination to differentiate the types of leukemia, although flow cytometry and cytogenetics have become more commonly used techniques for this purpose.

B

INDICATIONS

- Determine marrow differential (proportion of the various types of cells present in the marrow) and M:E
- Evaluate abnormal results of complete blood count or white blood cell count with differential showing increased numbers of leukocyte precursors
- Evaluate hepatomegaly or splenomegaly
- Identify bone marrow hyperplasia or hypoplasia
- Identify infectious organisms present in the bone marrow (histoplasmosis, mycobacteria, cytomegalovirus, parvovirus inclusions)
- Monitor effects of exposure to bone marrow depressants
- Monitor bone marrow response to chemotherapy or radiation therapy

POTENTIAL DIAGNOSIS

Increased Reticulocytes
- Compensated red blood cell (RBC) loss
- Response to vitamin B_{12} therapy

Decreased Reticulocytes
- Aplastic crisis of sickle cell anemia or hereditary spherocytosis

Increased Leukocytes
- *General associations include compensation for infectious process, leukemias, or leukemoid drug reactions*

Decreased Leukocytes
- *General associations include reduction in the marrow space as seen in metastatic neoplasm or myelofibrosis, lack of production of cells, lower production of cells as seen*

in the elderly, or following suppressive therapy such as chemotherapy or radiation

Increased Neutrophils (total)
- Acute myeloblastic leukemia
- Myeloid (chronic) leukemias

Decreased Neutrophils (total)
- Aplastic anemia
- Leukemias (monocytic and lymphoblastic)

Increased Lymphocytes
- Aplastic anemia
- Lymphatic leukemia
- Lymphomas
- Lymphosarcoma
- Mononucleosis
- Viral infections

Increased Plasma Cells
- Cancer
- Cirrhosis of the liver
- Connective tissue disorders
- Hypersensitivity reactions
- Infections
- Macroglobulinemia
- Ulcerative colitis

Increased Megakaryocytes
- Hemorrhage
- Increasing age
- Infections
- Megakaryocytic myelosis
- Myeloid leukemia
- Pneumonia
- Polycythemia vera
- Thrombocytopenia

Decreased Megakaryocytes
- Agranulocytosis
- Cirrhosis of the liver
- Pernicious aplastic anemia
- Radiation therapy
- Thrombocytopenic purpura

Increased M:E
- Bone marrow failure
- Infections
- Leukemoid reactions
- Myeloid leukemia

Decreased M:E
- Anemias
- Hepatic disease
- Polycythemia vera
- Posthemorrhagic hematopoiesis

Increased Normoblasts
- Anemias
- Chronic blood loss
- Polycythemia vera

Decreased Normoblasts
- Aplastic anemia
- Folic acid or vitamin B_{12} deficiency
- Hemolytic anemia

Increased Eosinophils
- Bone marrow cancer
- Lymphadenoma
- Myeloid leukemia

CRITICAL FINDINGS
- Classification or grading of tumor
- Identification of malignancy

It is essential that critical diagnoses be communicated immediately to the requesting health-care provider (HCP). A listing of these diagnoses varies among facilities.

INTERFERING FACTORS
- Recent blood transfusions, iron therapy, or administration of cytotoxic agents may alter test results.
- ❖ This procedure is contraindicated in patients with known bleeding disorders.
- Failure to follow dietary restrictions before the procedure may cause the procedure to be canceled or repeated.

NURSING IMPLICATIONS AND PROCEDURE

PRETEST:
- Positively identify the patient using at least two unique identifiers before providing care, treatment, or services.
- *Patient Teaching:* Inform the patient this procedure can assist in establishing a diagnosis of bone marrow and immune system disease.
- Obtain a history of the patient's complaints, including a list of known allergens, especially allergies or sensitivities to latex or anesthetics.
- Obtain a history of the patient's hematopoietic and immune systems, especially any bleeding disorders and other symptoms, and results of previously performed laboratory tests and diagnostic and surgical procedures.
- Record the date of the last menstrual period and determine the possibility of pregnancy in perimenopausal women.
- Note any recent procedures that can interfere with test results.
- Obtain a list of the patient's current medications, including anticoagulants, aspirin and other salicylates, herbs, nutritional supplements, and nutraceuticals (see Appendix F). Such products should be discontinued by medical direction for the appropriate number of days prior to a surgical procedure.
- Review the procedure with the patient. Inform the patient that it may be necessary to remove hair from the site before the procedure. Address concerns about pain and explain that a sedative and/or analgesia will be administered to promote relaxation and reduce discomfort prior to the percutaneous biopsy; a general anesthesia will be administered prior to the open biopsy. Explain to the patient that no pain will be experienced during the test when general anesthesia is used but that any discomfort with a needle biopsy will be minimized with local anesthetics

and systemic analgesics. Inform the patient that the biopsy is performed under sterile conditions by an HCP specializing in this procedure. The surgical procedure usually takes about 30 min to complete, and sutures may be necessary to close the site. A needle biopsy usually takes about 20 min to complete.

▶ *Sensitivity to social and cultural issues,* as well as concern for modesty, is important in providing psychological support before, during, and after the procedure.

▶ Explain that an IV line may be inserted to allow infusion of IV fluids, anesthetics, or sedatives.

▶ Instruct the patient that nothing should be taken by mouth for at least 4 hr prior to the procedure to reduce the risk of nausea and vomiting. Protocols may vary among facilities.

▶ *Make sure a written and informed consent has been signed prior to the procedure and before administering any medications.*

INTRATEST:

▶ Ensure that the patient has complied with dietary restrictions; ensure that food has been restricted for at least 4 to 8 hr depending on the anesthetic chosen for the procedure.

▶ Ensure that anticoagulant therapy has been withheld for the appropriate number of days prior to the procedure. Number of days to withhold medication is dependent on the type of anticoagulant. Notify the HCP if patient anticoagulant therapy has not been withheld.

▶ Have emergency equipment readily available.

▶ Have the patient void before the procedure.

▶ Observe standard precautions, and follow the general guidelines in Appendix A. Positively identify the patient, and label the appropriate collection containers with the corresponding patient demographics, date and time of collection, and site location.

▶ Assist the patient to the desired position depending on the test site to be used. In young children, the most frequently chosen site is the proximal tibia. Vertebral bodies T10 through L4 are preferred in older children. In adults, the sternum or iliac crests are the preferred sites. Place the patient in the prone, sitting, or side-lying position for the vertebral bodies; the side-lying position for iliac crest or tibial sites; or the supine position for the sternum. Instruct the patient to cooperate fully and to follow directions. Direct the patient to breathe normally and to avoid unnecessary movement during the local anesthetic and the procedure.

▶ Record baseline vital signs, and continue to monitor throughout the procedure. Protocols may vary among facilities.

▶ After the administration of general or local anesthesia, shave and cleanse the site with an antiseptic solution, and drape the area with sterile towels.

Needle Aspiration

▶ The HCP will anesthetize the site with procaine or lidocaine, and then insert a needle with stylet into the marrow. The stylet is removed, a syringe attached, and a 0.5-mL aliquot of marrow withdrawn. The needle is removed, and pressure is applied to the site. The aspirate is applied to slides, and, when dry, a fixative is applied.

Needle Biopsy

▶ Instruct the patient to take slow deep breaths when the local anesthetic is injected. Protect the site with sterile drapes.

▶ Local anesthetic is introduced deeply enough to include periosteum. A cutting biopsy needle is introduced through a small skin incision and bored into the marrow cavity. A core needle is introduced through the cutting needle, and a plug of marrow is removed. The needles are withdrawn, and the specimen is placed in a

B

preservative solution. Pressure is applied to the site for 3 to 5 min, and then a pressure dressing is applied.

General

▶ Monitor the patient for complications related to the procedure (e.g., allergic reaction, anaphylaxis).

▶ Place tissue samples in properly labeled specimen container containing formalin solution, and promptly transport the specimen to the laboratory for processing and analysis.

POST-TEST:

▶ A report of the results will be sent to the requesting HCP, who will discuss the results with the patient.

▶ Instruct the patient to resume preoperative diet, as directed by the HCP.

▶ Monitor vital signs and neurological status every 15 min for 1 hr, then every 2 hr for 4 hr, and then as ordered by the HCP. Monitor temperature every 4 hr for 24 hr. Monitor intake and output at least every 8 hr. Compare with baseline values. Notify the HCP if temperature is elevated. Protocols may vary among facilities.

▶ Observe for delayed allergic reactions, such as rash, urticaria, tachycardia, hyperpnea, hypertension, palpitations, nausea, or vomiting.

▶ Observe/assess the biopsy site for bleeding, inflammation, or hematoma formation.

▶ Instruct the patient in the care and assessment of the site.

▶ Instruct the patient to report any redness, edema, bleeding, or pain at the biopsy site. Instruct the patient to immediately report chills or fever.

▶ Assess for nausea and pain. Administer antiemetic and analgesic medications as needed and as directed by the HCP.

▶ Administer antibiotic therapy if ordered. Remind the patient of the importance of completing the entire course of antibiotic therapy, even if signs and symptoms disappear before completion of therapy.

▶ Recognize anxiety related to test results. Discuss the implications of abnormal test results on the patient's lifestyle. Provide teaching and information regarding the clinical implications of the test results, as appropriate. Educate the patient regarding access to counseling services.

▶ Reinforce information given by the patient's HCP regarding further testing, treatment, or referral to another HCP. Inform the patient of a follow-up appointment for removal of sutures, if indicated. Answer any questions or address any concerns voiced by the patient or family.

▶ Instruct the patient in the use of any ordered medications. Explain the importance of adhering to the therapy regimen. As appropriate, instruct the patient in significant side effects and systemic reactions associated with the prescribed medication. Encourage him or her to review corresponding literature provided by a pharmacist.

▶ Depending on the results of this procedure, additional testing may be performed to evaluate or monitor progression of the disease process and determine the need for a change in therapy. Evaluate test results in relation to the patient's symptoms and other tests performed.

RELATED MONOGRAPHS:

▶ Related tests include biopsy lymph node, CBC, LAP, immunofixation electrophoresis, mediastinoscopy, and vitamin B_{12}.

▶ Refer to the Hematopoietic and Immune systems tables at the end of the book for related tests by body system.

Biopsy, Breast

SYNONYM/ACRONYM: N/A.

COMMON USE: To assist in establishing a diagnosis of breast disease; in the presence of breast cancer, this test is also used to assist in evaluating prognosis and management of response to therapy.

SPECIMEN: Breast tissue or cells.

REFERENCE VALUE: (Method: Macroscopic and microscopic examination of tissue for biopsy; cytochemical or immunohistochemical for estrogen and progesterone receptors, Ki67, PCNA, P53; flow cytometry for DNA ploidy and S-phase fraction; immunohistochemical or FISH for Her-2/neu) Fluorescence in situ hybridization (FISH) is a cytogenic technique that uses fluorescent-labeled DNA probes to detect specific chromosome abnormalities. Favorable findings:

- Biopsy: no abnormal cells or tissue
- DNA ploidy: majority diploid cell population
- SPF: low fraction of replicating cells in total cell population
- Her-2/neu, Ki67, PCNA, and P53: negative to low percentage of stained cells
- Estrogen and progesterone receptors: high percentage of stained cells

DESCRIPTION: Breast cancer is the most common newly diagnosed cancer in American women. It is the second leading cause of cancer-related death. Biopsy is the excision of a sample of tissue that can be analyzed microscopically to determine cell morphology and the presence of tissue abnormalities. Fine-needle and open biopsies of the breast have become more commonly ordered in recent years as increasing emphasis on early detection of breast cancer has become stronger. Breast biopsies are used to assist in the identification and prognosis of breast cancer. A number of tests can be performed on breast tissue to assist in identification and management of breast cancer. *Estrogen and progesterone receptor assays (ER and PR)* are used to identify patients with a type of breast cancer that may be more responsive than other types of tumors to estrogen-deprivation (anti-estrogen) therapy or removal of the ovaries. Patients with these types of tumors generally have a better prognosis. *DNA ploidy* testing by flow cytometry may also be performed on suspicious tissue. Cancer is the unchecked proliferation of tumor cells that contain abnormal amounts of DNA. The higher the grade of tumor cells, the more likely abnormal DNA will be detected. The *ploidy* (number of chromosome sets in the nucleus) is an indication of the speed of cell replication and tumor growth. Cells synthesize DNA in the S phase of mitosis. *S-phase fraction*

B

(SPF) is an indicator of the number of cells undergoing replication. Normal tissue has a higher percentage of resting diploid cells, or cells containing two chromosomes. Aneuploid cells contain multiple chromosomes. Genes on the chromosomes are coded to produce specific proteins. *Ki67 and proliferating cell nuclear antigen (PCNA)* are examples of proteins that can be measured to indicate the degree of cell proliferation in biopsied tissue. Overexpression of a protein called *human epidermal growth factor receptor 2* (HER-2/neu oncoprotein) is helpful in establishing histological evidence of metastatic breast cancer. Metastatic breast cancer patients with high levels of HER-2/neu oncoprotein have a poor prognosis. They have rapid tumor progression, increased rate of recurrence, poor response to standard therapies, and a lower survival rate. Herceptin (trastuzumab) is indicated for treatment of HER-2/neu overexpression. *P53* is a suppressor protein that normally prevents cells with abnormal DNA from multiplying. Mutations in the P53 gene cause the loss of P53 functionality; the checkpoint is lost, and cancerous cells are allowed to proliferate.

INDICATIONS

- Evidence of breast lesion by palpation, mammography, or ultrasound
- Identify patients with breast or other types of cancer that may respond to hormone or antihormone therapy
- Monitor responsiveness to hormone or antihormone therapy

- Observable breast changes such as "peau d'orange" skin, scaly skin of the areola, drainage from the nipple, or ulceration of the skin

POTENTIAL DIAGNOSIS

Positive findings in
- Carcinoma of the breast
- Hormonal therapy (ER and PR)
- Receptor-positive tumors (ER and PR)

CRITICAL FINDINGS

- Assessment of clear margins after tissue excision
- Classification or grading of tumor
- Identification of malignancy

It is essential that critical diagnoses be communicated immediately to the requesting health-care provider (HCP). A listing of these diagnoses varies among facilities.

INTERFERING FACTORS

- ✸ This procedure is contraindicated in patients with bleeding disorders.
- Antiestrogen preparations (e.g., tamoxifen) ingested 2 mo before tissue sampling will affect test results (ER and PR).
- Pretesting preservation of the tissue is method and test dependent. The testing laboratory should be consulted for proper instructions prior to the biopsy procedure.
- Failure to transport specimen to the laboratory immediately can result in degradation of tissue. Prompt and proper specimen processing, storage, and analysis are important to achieve accurate results.
- Massive tumor necrosis or tumors with low cellular composition falsely decrease results.
- Failure to follow dietary restrictions before the procedure may cause the procedure to be canceled or repeated.

NURSING IMPLICATIONS AND PROCEDURE

PRETEST:

▶ Positively identify the patient using at least two unique identifiers before providing care, treatment, or services.

▶ *Patient Teaching:* Inform the patient this procedure can assist in evaluating breast health.

▶ Obtain a history of the patient's complaints, including a list of known allergens, especially allergies or sensitivities to latex or anesthetics.

▶ Obtain a history of the patient's reproductive system, especially any bleeding disorders and other symptoms, and results of previously performed laboratory tests and diagnostic and surgical procedures.

▶ Record the date of the last menstrual period and determine the possibility of pregnancy in perimenopausal women.

▶ Note any recent procedures that can interfere with test results. Ensure that the patient has not received antiestrogen therapy within 2 mo of the test.

▶ Obtain a list of the patient's current medications, including anticoagulants, aspirin and other salicylates, herbs, nutritional supplements, and nutraceuticals (see Appendix F). Such products should be discontinued by medical direction for the appropriate number of days prior to a surgical procedure.

▶ Review the procedure with the patient. Inform the patient that it may be necessary to remove hair from the site before the procedure. Instruct that prophylactic antibiotics may be administered prior to the procedure. Address concerns about pain and explain that a sedative and/or analgesia will be administered to promote relaxation and reduce discomfort prior to the percutaneous biopsy; a general anesthesia will be administered prior to the open biopsy. Explain to the patient that no pain will be experienced during the test when general anesthesia is used but that any discomfort with a needle biopsy will be minimized with local anesthetics and systemic analgesics. Inform the patient that the biopsy is performed under sterile conditions by an HCP specializing in this procedure. The surgical procedure usually takes about 20 to 30 min to complete, and sutures may be necessary to close the site. A needle biopsy usually takes about 15 min to complete.

▶ *Sensitivity to social and cultural issues,* as well as concern for modesty, is important in providing psychological support before, during, and after the procedure.

▶ Explain that an IV line may be inserted to allow infusion of IV fluids, anesthetics, analgesics, or IV sedation.

Open Biopsy

▶ Instruct the patient that nothing should be taken by mouth for 6 to 8 hr prior to a general anesthetic. Protocols may vary among facilities.

Needle Biopsy

▶ Instruct the patient that nothing should be taken by mouth for at least 4 hr prior to the procedure to reduce the risk of nausea and vomiting. Protocols may vary among facilities.

General

▶ Make sure a written and informed consent has been signed prior to the procedure and before administering any medications.

INTRATEST:

▶ Ensure that the patient has complied with dietary restrictions; ensure that food has been restricted for at least 4 to 8 hr depending on the anesthetic chosen for the procedure. Ensure that the patient has not received antiestrogen therapy within 2 mo of the test.

▶ Ensure that anticoagulant therapy has been withheld for the appropriate number of days prior to the procedure. Number of days to withhold medication is dependent on the type of anticoagulant. Notify the HCP if patient anticoagulant therapy has not been withheld.

▶ Have emergency equipment readily available.

▶ Have the patient void before the procedure.

▶ Observe standard precautions, and follow the general guidelines in

Appendix A. Positively identify the patient and label the appropriate collection containers with the corresponding patient demographics, date and time of collection, and site location, especially left or right breast.

▶ Assist the patient to the desired position depending on the test site to be used, and direct the patient to breathe normally during the beginning of the general anesthetic. Instruct the patient to cooperate fully and to follow directions. For the patient undergoing local anesthesia, direct him or her to breathe normally and to avoid unnecessary movement during the procedure.

▶ Record baseline vital signs, and continue to monitor throughout the procedure. Protocols may vary among facilities.

▶ After the administration of general or local anesthesia, shave and cleanse the site with an antiseptic solution, and drape the area with sterile towels.

Open Biopsy

▶ After administration of general anesthesia and surgical preparation are completed, an incision is made, suspicious area(s) are located, and tissue samples are collected.

Needle Biopsy

▶ Direct the patient to take slow deep breaths when the local anesthetic is injected. Protect the site with sterile drapes. Instruct the patient to take a deep breath, exhale forcefully, and hold the breath while the biopsy needle is inserted and rotated to obtain a core of breast tissue. Once the needle is removed, the patient may breathe. Pressure is applied to the site for 3 to 5 min, then a sterile pressure dressing is applied.

General

▶ Monitor the patient for complications related to the procedure (e.g., allergic reaction, anaphylaxis).

▶ Place tissue samples in formalin solution. Label the specimen, indicating site location, and promptly transport the specimen to the laboratory for processing and analysis.

POST-TEST:

▶ A report of the results will be sent to the requesting HCP, who will discuss the results with the patient.

▶ Instruct the patient to resume preoperative diet, as directed by the HCP. Assess the patient's ability to swallow before allowing the patient to attempt liquids or solid foods.

▶ Monitor vital signs and neurological status every 15 min for 1 hr, then every 2 hr for 4 hr, and then as ordered by the HCP. Monitor temperature every 4 hr for 24 hr. Monitor intake and output at least every 8 hr. Compare with baseline values. Notify the HCP if temperature is elevated. Protocols may vary among facilities.

▶ Observe/assess for delayed allergic reactions, such as rash, urticaria, tachycardia, hyperpnea, hypertension, palpitations, nausea, or vomiting.

▶ Observe/assess the biopsy site for bleeding, inflammation, or hematoma formation.

▶ Instruct the patient in the care and assessment of the site.

▶ Instruct the patient to report any redness, edema, bleeding, or pain at the biopsy site. Instruct the patient to immediately report chills or fever.

▶ Assess for nausea and pain. Administer antiemetic and analgesic medications as needed and as directed by the HCP.

▶ Administer antibiotic therapy if ordered. Remind the patient of the importance of completing the entire course of antibiotic therapy, even if signs and symptoms disappear before completion of therapy.

▶ Recognize anxiety related to test results. Discuss the implications of abnormal test results on the patient's lifestyle. Provide teaching and information regarding the clinical implications of the test results, as appropriate. Educate the patient regarding access to counseling services. Provide contact information, if desired, for the American Cancer Society (www.cancer.org).

▶ Reinforce information given by the patient's HCP regarding further testing, treatment, or referral to another HCP. Inform the patient of a follow-up appointment for removal of sutures, if indicated. Decisions regarding the need for and frequency of breast self-examination, mammography, magnetic resonance imaging (MRI) breast, or other cancer screening procedures should be made after consultation between the patient and HCP. The most current guidelines for breast cancer screening of the general population as well as of individuals with increased risk are available from the American Cancer Society (www.cancer.org), the American College of Obstetricians and Gynecologists (ACOG) (www.acog.org), and the American College of Radiology (www.acr.org). Answer any questions or address any concerns voiced by the patient or family.

▶ Instruct the patient in the use of any ordered medications. Explain the importance of adhering to the therapy regimen. As appropriate, instruct the patient in significant side effects and systemic reactions associated with the prescribed medication. Encourage the patient to review corresponding literature provided by a pharmacist.

▶ Depending on the results of this procedure, additional testing may be performed to evaluate or monitor progression of the disease process and determine the need for a change in therapy. Evaluate test results in relation to the patient's symptoms and other tests performed.

RELATED MONOGRAPHS:

▶ Related tests include cancer antigens, ductography, mammogram, MRI breast, stereotactic biopsy breast, and US breast.
▶ Refer to the Reproductive System table at the end of the book for related tests by body system.

Biopsy, Cervical

SYNONYM/ACRONYM: Cone Biopsy, LEEP.

COMMON USE: To assist in diagnosing and staging cervical cancer.

SPECIMEN: Cervical tissue.

REFERENCE VALUE: (Method: Microscopic examination of tissue cells) No abnormal cells or tissue.

DESCRIPTION: Biopsy is the excision of a sample of tissue that can be analyzed microscopically to determine cell morphology and the presence of tissue abnormalities. The cervical biopsy is used to assist in confirmation of cancer when screening tests are positive. Cervical biopsy is obtained using an instrument that punches into the tissue and retrieves a tissue sample. Schiller's test entails applying an iodine solution to the cervix. Normal cells pick up the iodine and stain brown. Abnormal cells do not pick up any color. Punch biopsy results may indicate the need for a cone biopsy of the cervix. Cone biopsy involves removing a wedge of tissue from the cervix by using a surgical knife, a carbon dioxide laser, or a loop electrosurgical excision procedure (LEEP). The LEEP procedure can be performed by placing the patient under a general anesthetic; by a regional anesthesia, such as a spinal or epidural; or by a cervical block whereby a local anesthetic is injected into the cervix. The patient is given oral or IV pain medicine in conjunction with the local anesthetic when this method is used. Following colposcopy or cervical biopsy, LEEP can be used to treat abnormal tissue identified on biopsy.

INDICATIONS

• Follow-up to abnormal Papanicolaou (Pap) smear, Schiller's test, or colposcopy
• Suspected cervical malignancy

POTENTIAL DIAGNOSIS

Positive findings in
• Carcinoma in situ
• Cervical dysplasia
• Cervical polyps

CRITICAL FINDINGS

• Assessment of clear margins after tissue excision
• Classification or grading of tumor
• Identification of malignancy

It is essential that critical diagnoses be communicated immediately to the requesting health-care provider (HCP). A listing of these diagnoses varies among facilities.

INTERFERING FACTORS

• ❖ The test is contraindicated in cases of acute pelvic inflammatory disease or bleeding disorders.
• This test should not be performed while the patient is menstruating.

• Failure to follow dietary restrictions before the procedure may cause the procedure to be canceled or repeated.

NURSING IMPLICATIONS AND PROCEDURE

PRETEST:

▶ Positively identify the patient using at least two unique identifiers before providing care, treatment, or services.
▶ *Patient Teaching:* Inform the patient this procedure can assist in establishing a diagnosis of cervical disease.
▶ Obtain a history of the patient's complaints, including a list of known allergens, especially allergies or sensitivities to latex, iodine, or anesthetics.
▶ Obtain a history of the patient's reproductive system, especially any bleeding disorders and other symptoms, and results of previously performed laboratory tests and diagnostic and surgical procedures.
▶ Record the date of the last menstrual period and determine the possibility of pregnancy in perimenopausal women.
▶ Obtain a list of the patient's current medications, including herbs, nutritional supplements, and nutraceuticals (see Appendix F). Such products should be discontinued by medical direction for the appropriate number of days prior to a surgical procedure.
▶ Review the procedure with the patient. Inform the patient that it may be necessary to remove hair from the site before the procedure. Instruct that prophylactic antibiotics may be administered prior to the procedure. Address concerns about pain and explain that a sedative and/or analgesia will be administered to promote relaxation and reduce discomfort prior to the percutaneous biopsy; general anesthesia will be administered prior to the open biopsy. Explain that no pain will be experienced during the test when general anesthesia is used but that any discomfort with a needle biopsy will be

minimized with local anesthetics and systemic analgesics. Inform the patient the biopsy is performed under sterile conditions by an HCP specializing in this procedure. The surgical procedure usually takes about 20 to 30 min to complete, and sutures may be necessary to close the site.

▶ *Sensitivity to social and cultural issues,* as well as concern for modesty, is important in providing psychological support before, during, and after the procedure.

▶ Explain that an IV line may be inserted to allow infusion of IV fluids, anesthetics, analgesics, or IV sedation.

LEEP as an Outpatient Procedure

▶ Instruct the patient that nothing should be taken by mouth for at least 6 to 8 hr prior to a general anesthetic. Protocols may vary among facilities.

LEEP in HCP's Office

▶ Instruct the patient that nothing should be taken by mouth for at least 4 hr prior to the procedure to reduce the risk of nausea and vomiting. Protocols may vary among facilities.

General

▶ *Make sure a written and informed consent has been signed prior to the procedure and before administering any medications.*

INTRATEST:

▶ Ensure that the patient has complied with dietary restrictions; ensure that food has been restricted for at least 4 to 8 hr depending on the anesthetic chosen for the procedure.

▶ Ensure that anticoagulant therapy has been withheld for the appropriate number of days prior to the procedure. Number of days to withhold medication is dependent on the type of anticoagulant. Notify HCP if patient anticoagulant therapy has not been withheld.

▶ Have emergency equipment readily available.

▶ Have the patient void before the procedure.

▶ Observe standard precautions, and follow the general guidelines in Appendix A. Positively identify the patient and label

the appropriate collection containers with the corresponding patient demographics, date and time of collection, and site location.

▶ Have the patient remove clothes below the waist. Assist the patient into a lithotomy position on a gynecological examination table (with feet in stirrups). Drape the patient's legs. Instruct the patient to cooperate fully and to follow directions. Direct the patient to breathe normally and to avoid unnecessary movement during the local or general anesthetic and the procedure.

Punch Biopsy

▶ A small, round punch is rotated into the skin to the desired depth. The cylinder of skin is pulled upward with forceps and separated at its base with a scalpel or scissors. If needed, sutures are applied. A sterile dressing is applied over the site.

▶ Record baseline vital signs, and continue to monitor throughout the procedure. Protocols may vary among facilities.

▶ After the administration of general or local anesthesia, shave and cleanse the site with an antiseptic solution, and drape the area with sterile towels.

LEEP in the HCP's Office

▶ A speculum is inserted into the vagina and is opened to gently spread apart the vagina for inspection of the cervix.

▶ The diseased tissue is removed along with a small amount of healthy tissue along the margins of the biopsy to ensure that no diseased tissue is left in the cervix after the procedure.

LEEP as an Outpatient Procedure

▶ After administration of general anesthesia and surgical preparation are completed, the procedure is carried out as noted above.

General

▶ Monitor the patient for complications related to the procedure (e.g., allergic reaction, anaphylaxis).

▶ Place tissue samples in properly labeled specimen container containing formalin solution, and promptly transport the specimen to the laboratory for processing and analysis.

B

POST-TEST:

• A report of the results will be sent to the requesting HCP, who will discuss the results with the patient.

• Instruct the patient to resume preoperative diet, as directed by the HCP. Assess the patient's ability to swallow before allowing the patient to attempt liquids or solid foods.

• Monitor vital signs and neurological status every 15 min for 1 hr, then every 2 hr for 4 hr, and then as ordered by the HCP. Monitor temperature every 4 hr for 24 hr. Monitor intake and output at least every 8 hr. Compare with baseline values. Notify the HCP if temperature is elevated. Protocols may vary among facilities.

• Observe/assess for delayed allergic reactions, such as rash, urticaria, tachycardia, hyperpnea, hypertension, palpitations, nausea, or vomiting.

• Advise the patient to expect a gray-green vaginal discharge for several days, that some vaginal bleeding may occur for up to 1 wk but should not be heavier than a normal menses, and that some pelvic pain may occur. Instruct the patient to avoid strenuous activity for 8 to 24 hr; to avoid douching or intercourse for 2 wk or as instructed; and to report excessive bleeding, chills, fever, or any other unusual findings to the HCP.

• Assess for nausea and pain. Administer antiemetic and analgesic medications as needed and as directed by the HCP.

• Administer antibiotic therapy if ordered. Remind the patient of the importance of completing the entire course of antibiotic therapy, even if signs and symptoms disappear before completion of therapy.

• Recognize anxiety related to test results, and offer support. Discuss the implications of abnormal test results on the patient's lifestyle. Provide teaching and information regarding the clinical implications of the test results, as appropriate. Educate the patient regarding access to counseling services.

• Reinforce information given by the patient's HCP regarding further testing, treatment, or referral to another HCP. Decisions regarding the need for and frequency of conventional or liquid-based Pap tests or other cancer screening procedures should be made after consultation between the patient and HCP. The most current guidelines for cervical cancer screening of the general population as well as of individuals with increased risk are available from the American Cancer Society (www.cancer.org) and the American College of Obstetricians and Gynecologists (ACOG) (www.acog.org). Answer any questions or address any concerns voiced by the patient or family.

• Instruct the patient in the use of any ordered medications. Explain the importance of adhering to the therapy regimen. As appropriate, instruct the patient in significant side effects and systemic reactions associated with the prescribed medication. Encourage her to review corresponding literature provided by a pharmacist.

• Depending on the results of this procedure, additional testing may be performed to evaluate or monitor progression of the disease process and determine the need for a change in therapy. Evaluate test results in relation to the patient's symptoms and other tests performed.

RELATED MONOGRAPHS:

• Related tests include *Chlamydia* group antibodies, colposcopy, culture anal/genital, culture viral, Pap smear, and syphilis serology.

• See the Reproductive System table at the end of the book for related tests by body system.

Biopsy, Chorionic Villus

SYNONYM/ACRONYM: N/A.

COMMON USE: To assist in diagnosing genetic fetal abnormalities such as Down syndrome.

SPECIMEN: Chorionic villus tissue.

REFERENCE VALUE: (Method: Tissue culture) Normal karyotype.

DESCRIPTION: This test is used to detect fetal abnormalities caused by numerous genetic disorders. The advantage over amniocentesis is that it can be performed as early as the 8th week of pregnancy, permitting earlier decisions regarding termination of pregnancy. However, unlike amniocentesis, this test will not detect neural tube defects.

INDICATIONS
- Assist in the diagnosis of in utero metabolic disorders such as cystic fibrosis or other errors of lipid, carbohydrate, or amino acid metabolism
- Detect abnormalities in the fetus of women of advanced maternal age
- Determine fetal gender when the mother is a known carrier of a sex-linked abnormal gene that could be transmitted to male offspring, such as hemophilia or Duchenne's muscular dystrophy
- Evaluate fetus in families with a history of genetic disorders, such as Down syndrome, Tay-Sachs disease, chromosome or enzyme anomalies, or inherited hemoglobinopathies

POTENTIAL DIAGNOSIS
Abnormal karyotype: *Numerous genetic disorders. Generally, the laboratory provides detailed interpretive information regarding the specific chromosome abnormality detected.*

CRITICAL FINDINGS
- Identification of abnormalities in chorionic villus tissue
- It is essential that critical diagnoses be communicated immediately to the requesting health-care provider (HCP). A listing of these diagnoses varies among facilities.

INTERFERING FACTORS
- ❖ The test is contraindicated in the patient with a history of or in the presence of incompetent cervix.
- Failure to follow dietary restrictions before the procedure may cause the procedure to be canceled or repeated.

NURSING IMPLICATIONS AND PROCEDURE

PRETEST:
▶ Positively identify the patient using at least two unique identifiers before providing care, treatment, or services.

▸ *Patient Teaching:* Inform the patient this procedure can assist in establishing a diagnosis of in utero genetic disorders.

▸ Obtain a history of the patient's complaints, including a list of known allergens, especially allergies or sensitivities to latex or anesthetics.

▸ Obtain a history of the patient's reproductive system, symptoms, and results of previously performed laboratory tests and diagnostic and surgical procedures. Include any family history of genetic disorders such as cystic fibrosis, Duchenne's muscular dystrophy, hemophilia, sickle cell anemia, Tay-Sachs disease, thalassemia, and trisomy 21. Obtain maternal Rh type. If Rh-negative, check for prior sensitization.

▸ Record the date of the last menstrual period and determine that the pregnancy is in the first trimester between the 10th and 12th weeks.

▸ Obtain a history of intravenous drug use, high-risk sexual activity, or occupational exposure.

▸ Obtain a list of the patient's current medications, including herbs, nutritional supplements, and nutraceuticals (see Appendix F).

▸ Review the procedure with the patient. Warn the patient that normal results do not guarantee a normal fetus. Assure the patient that precautions to avoid injury to the fetus will be taken by locating the fetus with ultrasound. Address concerns about pain related to the procedure. Explain that during the transabdominal procedure, any discomfort with a needle biopsy will be minimized with local anesthetics. Explain that during the transvaginal procedure, some cramping may be experienced as the catheter is guided through the cervix. Encourage relaxation and controlled breathing during the procedure to aid in reducing any mild discomfort. Inform the patient that specimen collection is performed by an HCP specializing in this procedure and usually takes approximately 10 to 15 min to complete.

▸ *Sensitivity to social and cultural issues,* as well as concern for modesty, is important in providing psychological support before, during, and after the procedure.

▸ There are no food, fluid, or medication restrictions unless by medical direction.

▸ Instruct the patient to drink a glass of water about 30 min prior to testing so that the bladder is full. This elevates the uterus higher in the pelvis. The patient should not void before the procedure.

▸ *Make sure a written and informed consent has been signed prior to the procedure and before administering any medications.*

INTRATEST:

▸ Ensure that the patient has a full bladder before the procedure.

▸ Have emergency equipment readily available.

▸ Observe standard precautions, and follow the general guidelines in Appendix A. Positively identify the patient, and label the appropriate collection containers with the corresponding patient demographics, date and time of collection, and site location.

▸ Have the patient remove clothes below the waist. *Transabdominal:* Assist the patient into a supine position on the examination table with abdomen exposed. Drape the patient's legs, leaving abdomen exposed. *Transvaginal:* Assist the patient into a lithotomy position on a gynecologic examination table (with feet in stirrups). Drape the patient's legs. Instruct the patient to cooperate fully and to follow directions. Direct the patient to breathe normally and to avoid unnecessary movement during the local anesthetic and the procedure.

▸ Record maternal and fetal baseline vital signs, and continue to monitor throughout the procedure. Monitor for uterine contractions. Monitor fetal vital signs using ultrasound. Protocols may vary among facilities.

▸ After the administration of local anesthesia, shave and cleanse the site with an antiseptic solution, and drape the area with sterile towels.

Transabdominal Biopsy

- Assess the position of the amniotic fluid, fetus, and placenta using ultrasound.
- A needle is inserted through the abdomen into the uterus, avoiding contact with the fetus. A syringe is connected to the needle, and the specimen of chorionic villus cells is withdrawn from the uteroplacental area. Pressure is applied to the site for 3 to 5 min, and then a sterile pressure dressing is applied.

Transvaginal Biopsy

- Assess the position of the fetus and placenta using ultrasound.
- A speculum is inserted into the vagina and is opened to gently spread apart the vagina for inspection of the cervix. The cervix is cleansed with a swab of antiseptic solution.
- A catheter is inserted through the cervix into the uterus, avoiding contact with the fetus. A syringe is connected to the catheter, and the specimen of chorionic villus cells is withdrawn from the uteroplacental area.

General

- Monitor the patient for complications related to the procedure (e.g., premature labor, allergic reaction, anaphylaxis).
- Place tissue samples in formalin solution. Label the specimen, indicating site location, and promptly transport the specimen to the laboratory for processing and analysis.

POST-TEST:

- A report of the results will be sent to the requesting HCP, who will discuss the results with the patient.
- After the procedure, the patient is placed in the left side-lying position, and both maternal and fetal vital signs are monitored for at least 30 min. Protocols may vary among facilities.
- Observe/assess for delayed allergic reactions, such as rash, urticaria, tachycardia, hyperpnea, hypertension, palpitations, nausea, or vomiting.
- Observe/assess the biopsy site for bleeding, inflammation, or hematoma formation.

- Instruct the patient in the care and assessment of the site.
- Instruct the patient to report any redness, edema, bleeding, or pain at the biopsy site.
- Advise the patient to expect mild cramping, leakage of small amount of amniotic fluid, and vaginal spotting for up to 2 days following the procedure. Instruct the patient to report moderate to severe abdominal pain or cramps, increased or prolonged leaking of amniotic fluid from vagina or abdominal needle site, vaginal bleeding that is heavier than spotting, and either chills or fever.
- Administer $Rh_o(D)$ immune globulin (RhoGAM IM or Rhophylac IM or IV) to maternal Rh-negative patients to prevent maternal Rh sensitization should the fetus be Rh-positive.
- Administer mild analgesic and antibiotic therapy as ordered. Remind the patient of the importance of completing the entire course of antibiotic therapy, even if signs and symptoms disappear before completion of therapy.
- Recognize anxiety related to test results. Discuss the implications of abnormal test results on the patient's lifestyle. Provide teaching and information regarding the clinical implications of the test results, as appropriate. Encourage family to seek counseling if concerned with pregnancy termination or to seek genetic counseling if chromosomal abnormality is determined. Decisions regarding elective abortion should take place in the presence of both parents. Provide a nonjudgmental, nonthreatening atmosphere for a discussion during which risks of delivering a developmentally challenged infant are discussed with options (termination of pregnancy or adoption). It is also important to discuss problems the mother and father may experience (guilt, depression, anger) if fetal abnormalities are detected.
- Reinforce information given by the patient's HCP regarding further testing, treatment, or referral to another HCP. Answer any questions or address any concerns voiced by the patient or family.
- Instruct the patient in the use of any ordered medications. Explain the importance of adhering to the therapy

regimen. As appropriate, instruct the patient in significant side effects and systemic reactions associated with the prescribed medication. Encourage her to review corresponding literature provided by a pharmacist.

▶ Depending on the results of this procedure, additional testing may be performed to evaluate or monitor progression of the disease process and determine the need for a change in therapy. Evaluate test results in relation to the patient's symptoms and other tests performed.

RELATED MONOGRAPHS:

▶ Related tests include amniotic fluid analysis, chromosome analysis, α_1 fetoprotein, HCG, hexosaminidase A and B, L/S ratio, US biophysical profile, and US obstetric.

▶ Refer to the Reproductive System table at the end of the book for related tests by body system.

Biopsy, Intestinal

SYNONYM/ACRONYM: N/A.

COMMON USE: To assist in confirming a diagnosis of intestinal cancer or disease.

SPECIMEN: Intestinal tissue or cells.

REFERENCE VALUE: (Method: Macroscopic and microscopic examination of tissue) No abnormal tissue or cells.

DESCRIPTION: Intestinal biopsy is the excision of a tissue sample from the small intestine for microscopic analysis to determine cell morphology and the presence of tissue abnormalities. This test assists in confirming the diagnosis of cancer or intestinal disorders. Biopsy specimen is usually obtained during endoscopic examination.

INDICATIONS

• Assist in the diagnosis of various intestinal disorders, such as lactose and other enzyme deficiencies, celiac disease, and parasitic infections

• Confirm suspected intestinal malignancy
• Confirm suspicious findings during endoscopic visualization of the intestinal wall

POTENTIAL DIAGNOSIS
Abnormal findings in

• Cancer
• Celiac disease
• Lactose deficiency
• Parasitic infestation
• Tropical sprue

CRITICAL FINDINGS

• Assessment of clear margins after tissue excision
• Classification or grading of tumor
• Identification of malignancy

It is essential that critical diagnoses be communicated immediately to the requesting health-care provider (HCP). A listing of these diagnoses varies among facilities.

INTERFERING FACTORS

- Barium swallow within 48 hr of small intestine biopsy affects results.
- ✦ This procedure is contraindicated in patients with bleeding disorders and aortic arch aneurysm.
- Failure to follow dietary restrictions before the procedure may cause the procedure to be canceled or repeated.

NURSING IMPLICATIONS AND PROCEDURE

PRETEST:

- Positively identify the patient using at least two unique identifiers before providing care, treatment, or services.
- *Patient Teaching:* Inform the patient this procedure can assist in establishing a diagnosis of intestinal disease.
- Obtain a history of the patient's complaints, including a list of known allergens, especially allergies or sensitivities to latex or anesthetics.
- Obtain a history of the patient's gastrointestinal and immune systems, any bleeding disorders, symptoms, and results of previously performed laboratory tests and diagnostic and surgical procedures.
- Record the date of the last menstrual period and determine the possibility of pregnancy in perimenopausal women.
- Note any recent procedures that can interfere with test results.
- Obtain a list of the patient's current medications including anticoagulants, aspirin and other salicylates, herbs, nutritional supplements, and nutraceuticals (see Appendix F). Such products should be discontinued by medical direction for the appropriate number of days prior to a surgical procedure.

- Review the procedure with the patient. Inform the patient that it may be necessary to remove hair from the site before the procedure. Address concerns about pain and explain that a sedative may be administered to promote relaxation during the procedure. Inform the patient that the procedure is performed by an HCP specializing in this procedure and usually takes about 60 min to complete.
- *Sensitivity to social and cultural issues,* as well as concern for modesty, is important in providing psychological support before, during, and after the procedure.
- Explain that an IV line will be inserted to allow infusion of IV fluids, anesthetics, and analgesics.
- Explain that a clear liquid diet is to be consumed 1 day prior to the procedure. Then food and fluids are restricted for 6 to 8 hr before the test. Protocols may vary among facilities.
- Provide the patient with a gown, robe, and foot coverings and instruct him or her to void prior to the procedure.
- Instruct the patient to remove dentures, jewelry (including watches), hairpins, credit cards, and other metallic objects. Inform the HCP if the patient has any crowns or caps on the teeth.
- *Make sure a written and informed consent has been signed prior to the procedure and before administering any medications.*

INTRATEST:

- Ensure that the patient has complied with dietary restrictions; ensure that food has been restricted for at least 6 to 8 hr prior to the procedure if general anesthesia will be used.
- Ensure that anticoagulant therapy has been withheld for the appropriate number of days prior to the procedure. Number of days to withhold medication is dependent on the type of anticoagulant. Notify the HCP if patient anticoagulant therapy has not been withheld.
- Have emergency equipment readily available.
- Observe standard precautions and follow the general guidelines in Appendix A. Positively identify the patient, and label

the appropriate collection containers with the corresponding patient demographics, date and time of collection, and site location.

▶ Assist the patient into a semireclining position. Instruct the patient to cooperate fully and to follow directions. Direct the patient to breathe normally and to avoid unnecessary movement.

▶ Record baseline vital signs, and continue to monitor throughout the procedure. Protocols may vary among facilities.

Esophagogastroduodenoscopy (EGD) Biopsy

▶ A local anesthetic is sprayed into the throat. A protective tooth guard and a bite block may be placed in the mouth.

▶ The flexible endoscope is passed into and through the mouth, and the patient is asked to swallow. Once the endoscope passes into the esophagus, assist the patient into the left lateral position. A suction device is used to drain saliva.

▶ The esophagus, stomach, and duodenum are visually examined as the endoscope passes through each section. A biopsy specimen can be taken from any suspicious sites.

▶ Tissue samples are obtained by inserting a cytology brush or biopsy forceps through the endoscope.

▶ When the examination and tissue removal are complete, the endoscope and suction device are withdrawn and the tooth guard and bite block are removed.

▶ Monitor the patient for complications related to the procedure (e.g., allergic reaction, anaphylaxis).

▶ Place tissue samples in formalin solution. Label the specimen, indicating site location, and promptly transport the specimen to the laboratory for processing and analysis.

POST-TEST:

▶ A report of the results will be sent to the requesting HCP, who will discuss the results with the patient.

▶ Instruct the patient to resume usual diet, as directed by the HCP. Assess

the patient's ability to swallow before allowing the patient to attempt liquids or solid foods.

▶ Monitor vital signs and neurological status every 15 min for 1 hr, then every 2 hr for 4 hr, and then as ordered by the HCP. Monitor temperature every 4 hr for 24 hr. Monitor intake and output at least every 8 hr. Compare with baseline values. Notify the HCP if temperature is elevated. Protocols may vary among facilities.

▶ Observe/assess for delayed allergic reactions, such as rash, urticaria, tachycardia, hyperpnea, hypertension, palpitations, nausea, or vomiting.

▶ Instruct the patient to report any chest pain, upper abdominal pain, pain on swallowing, difficulty breathing, or expectoration of blood. Report these to the HCP immediately.

▶ Administer mild analgesic and antibiotic therapy as ordered. Remind the patient of the importance of completing the entire course of antibiotic therapy, even if signs and symptoms disappear before completion of therapy.

▶ Recognize anxiety related to test results. Discuss the implications of abnormal test results on the patient's lifestyle. Provide teaching and information regarding the clinical implications of the test results, as appropriate. Educate the patient regarding access to counseling services.

▶ Reinforce information given by the patient's HCP regarding further testing, treatment, or referral to another HCP. Answer any questions or address any concerns voiced by the patient or family.

▶ Instruct the patient in the use of any ordered medications. Explain the importance of adhering to the therapy regimen. As appropriate, instruct the patient in significant side effects and systemic reactions associated with the prescribed medication. Encourage him or her to review corresponding literature provided by a pharmacist.

▶ Depending on the results of this procedure, additional testing may be

performed to evaluate or monitor progression of the disease process and determine the need for a change in therapy. Evaluate test results in relation to the patient's symptoms and other tests performed.

RELATED MONOGRAPHS:

▶ Related tests include albumin, antibodies gliadin, calcium, cancer antigens, capsule endoscopy, colonoscopy, D-xylose tolerance, fecal analysis, fecal fat, folic acid, iron/TIBC, LTT, ova and parasite, potassium, PT/INR, sodium, vitamin B_{12}, and vitamin D.

▶ Refer to the Gastrointestinal and Immune systems tables at the end of the book for related tests by body system.

Biopsy, Kidney

SYNONYM/ACRONYM: Renal biopsy.

COMMON USE: To assist in diagnosing cancer and other renal disorders.

SPECIMEN: Kidney tissue or cells.

REFERENCE VALUE: (Method: Macroscopic and microscopic examination of tissue) No abnormal cells or tissue.

DESCRIPTION: Kidney or renal biopsy is the excision of a tissue sample from the kidney for microscopic analysis to determine cell morphology and the presence of tissue abnormalities. This test assists in confirming a diagnosis of cancer found on x-ray or ultrasound or to diagnose certain inflammatory or immunological conditions. Biopsy specimen is usually obtained either percutaneously or after surgical incision.

- Monitor progression of nephrotic syndrome
- Monitor renal function after transplantation

POTENTIAL DIAGNOSIS

Positive findings in
- Acute and chronic poststreptococcal glomerulonephritis
- Amyloidosis infiltration
- Cancer
- Disseminated lupus erythematosus
- Goodpasture's syndrome
- Immunological rejection of transplanted kidney
- Nephrotic syndrome
- Pyelonephritis
- Renal venous thrombosis

CRITICAL FINDINGS
- Assessment of clear margins after tissue excision
- Classification or grading of tumor
- Identification of malignancy

INDICATIONS
- Assist in confirming suspected renal malignancy
- Assist in the diagnosis of the cause of renal disease
- Determine extent of involvement in systemic lupus erythematosus or other immunological disorders

It is essential that critical diagnoses be communicated immediately to the requesting health-care provider (HCP). A listing of these diagnoses varies among facilities.

INTERFERING FACTORS

- ✸ This procedure is contraindicated in bleeding disorders, advanced renal disease, uncontrolled hypertension, or solitary kidney (except transplanted kidney).
- Obesity and severe spinal deformity can make percutaneous biopsy impossible.
- Failure to follow dietary restrictions before the procedure may cause the procedure to be canceled or repeated.

NURSING IMPLICATIONS AND PROCEDURE

PRETEST:

- Positively identify the patient using at least two unique identifiers before providing care, treatment, or services.
- *Patient Teaching:* Inform the patient this procedure can assist in establishing a diagnosis of kidney disease.
- Obtain a history of the patient's complaints, including a list of known allergens, especially allergies or sensitivities to latex or anesthetics.
- Obtain a history of the patient's genitourinary and immune systems, especially any bleeding disorders or other symptoms, and results of previously performed laboratory tests and diagnostic and surgical procedures.
- Record the date of the last menstrual period and determine the possibility of pregnancy in perimenopausal women.
- Note any recent procedures that can interfere with test results.
- Obtain a list of the patient's current medications, including anticoagulants, aspirin and other salicylates, herbs, nutritional supplements, and

nutraceuticals (see Appendix F). Such products should be discontinued by medical direction for the appropriate number of days prior to a surgical procedure.

- Review the procedure with the patient. Inform the patient that it may be necessary to remove hair from the site before the procedure. Instruct that prophylactic antibiotics may be administered prior to the procedure. Address concerns about pain and explain that a sedative and/or analgesia will be administered to promote relaxation and reduce discomfort prior to the percutaneous biopsy; a general anesthesia will be administered prior to the open biopsy. Explain to the patient that no pain will be experienced during the test when general anesthesia is used but that any discomfort with a needle biopsy will be minimized with local anesthetics and systemic analgesics. Inform the patient that the biopsy is performed under sterile conditions by an HCP specializing in this procedure. The surgical procedure usually takes about 60 min to complete, and sutures may be necessary to close the site. A needle biopsy usually takes about 40 min to complete.
- *Sensitivity to social and cultural issues,* as well as concern for modesty, is important in providing psychological support before, during, and after the procedure.
- Explain that an IV line will be inserted to allow infusion of IV fluids, anesthetics, analgesics, or IV sedation.

Open Biopsy

- Instruct the patient that nothing should be taken by mouth for 6 to 8 hr prior to a general anesthetic. Protocols may vary among facilities.

Needle Biopsy

- Instruct the patient that nothing should be taken by mouth for at least 4 hr prior to the procedure to reduce the risk of nausea and vomiting. Protocols may vary among facilities.

General

- *Make sure a written and informed consent has been signed prior to the procedure and before administering any medications.*

INTRATEST:

- Ensure that the patient has complied with dietary restrictions; ensure that food has been restricted for at least 4 to 8 hr depending on the anesthetic chosen for the procedure.
- Ensure that anticoagulant therapy has been withheld for the appropriate number of days prior to the procedure. Number of days to withhold medication is dependent on the type of anticoagulant. Notify the HCP if patient anticoagulant therapy has not been withheld.
- Have emergency equipment readily available.
- Have the patient void before the procedure.
- Observe standard precautions, and follow the general guidelines in Appendix A. Positively identify the patient, and label the appropriate collection containers with the corresponding patient demographics, date and time of collection, and site location, especially left or right kidney.
- Assist the patient to the desired position depending on the test site to be used, and direct the patient to breathe normally during the beginning of the general anesthetic. Instruct the patient to cooperate fully and to follow directions. Direct the patient to avoid unnecessary movement.
- Record baseline vital signs, and continue to monitor throughout the procedure. Protocols may vary among facilities.
- After the administration of general or local anesthesia, shave and cleanse the site with an antiseptic solution, and drape the area with sterile towels.

Open Biopsy

- After administration of general anesthesia and surgical preparation are completed, an incision is made, suspicious area(s) are located, and tissue samples are collected.

Needle Biopsy

- A sandbag may be placed under the abdomen to aid in moving the kidneys to the desired position. Direct the patient to take slow deep breaths when the local anesthetic is injected. Protect the site with sterile drapes. Instruct the patient to take a deep breath, exhale

forcefully, and hold the breath while the biopsy needle is inserted and rotated to obtain a core of renal tissue. Once the needle is removed, the patient may breathe. Pressure is applied to the site for 5 to 20 min, then a sterile pressure dressing is applied.

General

- Monitor the patient for complications related to the procedure (e.g., allergic reaction, anaphylaxis).
- Place tissue samples in formalin solution. Label the specimen, indicating site location, and promptly transport the specimen to the laboratory for processing and analysis.

POST-TEST:

- A report of the results will be sent to the requesting HCP, who will discuss the results with the patient.
- Instruct the patient to resume preoperative diet, as directed by the HCP. Assess the patient's ability to swallow before allowing the patient to attempt liquids or solid foods.
- Monitor vital signs and neurological status every 15 min for 1 hr, then every 2 hr for 4 hr, and then as ordered by the HCP. Monitor temperature every 4 hr for 24 hr. Monitor intake and output at least every 8 hr. Compare with baseline values. Notify the HCP if temperature is elevated. Protocols may vary among facilities.
- Observe/assess for delayed allergic reactions, such as rash, urticaria, tachycardia, hyperpnea, hypertension, palpitations, nausea, or vomiting.
- Instruct the patient to immediately report symptoms such as fast heart rate, difficulty breathing, skin rash, itching, chest pain, persistent right shoulder pain, or abdominal pain. Immediately report symptoms to the appropriate HCP.
- Observe/assess the biopsy site for bleeding, inflammation, or hematoma formation.
- Instruct the patient in the care and assessment of the site.
- Instruct the patient to report any redness, edema, bleeding, or pain at the biopsy site. Instruct the patient to immediately report chills or fever.

Observe/assess the biopsy site for bleeding, inflammation, or hematoma formation.

Inform the patient that blood may be seen in the urine after the first or second postprocedural voiding.

Monitor fluid intake and output for 24 hr. Instruct the patient on intake and output recording and provide appropriate measuring containers.

Instruct the patient to report any changes in urinary pattern or volume or any unusual appearance of the urine. If urinary volume is less than 200 mL in the first 8 hr, encourage the patient to increase fluid intake unless contraindicated by another medical condition.

Assess for nausea and pain. Administer antiemetic and analgesic medications as needed and as directed by the HCP.

Administer antibiotic therapy if ordered. Remind the patient of the importance of completing the entire course of antibiotic therapy, even if signs and symptoms disappear before completion of therapy.

Recognize anxiety related to test results. Discuss the implications of abnormal test results on the patient's lifestyle. Provide teaching and information regarding the clinical implications of the test results, as appropriate. Educate the patient regarding access to counseling services.

Reinforce information given by the patient's HCP regarding further testing, treatment, or referral to another HCP.

Inform the patient of a follow-up appointment for removal of sutures, if indicated. Answer any questions or address any concerns voiced by the patient or family.

Instruct the patient in the use of any ordered medications. Explain the importance of adhering to the therapy regimen. As appropriate, instruct the patient in significant side effects and systemic reactions associated with the prescribed medication. Encourage him or her to review corresponding literature provided by a pharmacist.

Depending on the results of this procedure, additional testing may be performed to evaluate or monitor progression of the disease process and determine the need for a change in therapy. Evaluate test results in relation to the patient's symptoms and other tests performed.

RELATED MONOGRAPHS:

Related tests include albumin, aldosterone, angiography renal, antibodies antiglomerular basement membrane, β_2-microglobulin, BUN, CT renal, creatinine, creatinine clearance, cytology urine, cystoscopy, IVP, KUB studies, osmolality, PTH, potassium, protein, renin, renogram, sodium, US kidney, and UA.

Refer to the Genitourinary and Immune systems tables at the end of the book for related tests by body system.

Biopsy, Liver

SYNONYM/ACRONYM: N/A.

COMMON USE: To assist in diagnosing liver cancer, and other liver disorders such as cirrhosis and hepatitis.

SPECIMEN: Liver tissue or cells.

REFERENCE VALUE: (Method: Macroscopic and microscopic examination of tissue) No abnormal cells or tissue.

DESCRIPTION: Liver biopsy is the excision of a tissue sample from the liver for microscopic analysis to determine cell morphology and the presence of tissue abnormalities. This test is used to assist in confirming a diagnosis of cancer or certain disorders of the hepatic parenchyma. Biopsy specimen is usually obtained either percutaneously or after surgical incision.

It is essential that critical diagnoses be communicated immediately to the requesting health-care provider (HCP). A listing of these diagnoses varies among facilities.

INTERFERING FACTORS

- This procedure is contraindicated in patients with bleeding disorders, suspected vascular tumor of the liver, ascites that may obscure proper insertion site for needle biopsy, subdiaphragmatic or right hemothoracic infection, or biliary tract infection.
- Failure to follow dietary restrictions before the procedure may cause the procedure to be canceled or repeated.

INDICATIONS

- Assist in confirming suspected hepatic malignancy
- Assist in confirming suspected hepatic parenchymal disease
- Assist in diagnosing the cause of persistently elevated liver enzymes, hepatomegaly, or jaundice

POTENTIAL DIAGNOSIS

Positive findings in
- Benign tumor
- Cancer
- Cholesterol ester storage disease
- Cirrhosis
- Galactosemia
- Hemochromatosis
- Hepatic involvement with systemic lupus erythematosus, sarcoidosis, or amyloidosis
- Hepatitis
- Parasitic infestations (e.g., amebiasis, malaria, visceral larva migrans)
- Reye's syndrome
- Wilson's disease

CRITICAL FINDINGS

- Assessment of clear margins after tissue excision
- Classification or grading of tumor
- Identification of malignancy

NURSING IMPLICATIONS AND PROCEDURE

PRETEST:

- Positively identify the patient using at least two unique identifiers before providing care, treatment, or services.
- *Patient Teaching:* Inform the patient this procedure can assist in establishing a diagnosis of liver disease.
- Obtain a history of the patient's complaints, especially fatigue and pain related to inflammation and swelling of the liver. Include a list of known allergens, especially allergies or sensitivities to latex or anesthetics.
- Obtain a history of the patient's hepatobiliary and immune systems, especially any bleeding disorders and other symptoms, and results of previously performed laboratory tests and diagnostic and surgical procedures.
- Record the date of the last menstrual period and determine the possibility of pregnancy in perimenopausal women.
- Note any recent procedures that can interfere with test results.

Obtain a list of the patient's current medications including anticoagulants, aspirin and other salicylates, herbs, nutritional supplements, and nutraceuticals (see Appendix F). Such products should be discontinued by medical direction for the appropriate number of days prior to a surgical procedure.

Review the procedure with the patient. Inform the patient that it may be necessary to remove hair from the site before the procedure. Instruct that prophylactic antibiotics may be administered prior to the procedure. Address concerns about pain and explain that a sedative and/or analgesia will be administered to promote relaxation and reduce discomfort prior to the percutaneous biopsy; a general anesthesia will be administered prior to the open biopsy. Explain to the patient that no pain will be experienced during the test when general anesthesia is used but that any discomfort with a needle biopsy will be minimized with local anesthetics and systemic analgesics. Inform the patient that the biopsy is performed under sterile conditions by an HCP specializing in this procedure. The surgical procedure usually takes about 90 min to complete, and sutures may be necessary to close the site. A needle biopsy usually takes about 15 min to complete.

Sensitivity to social and cultural issues, as well as concern for modesty, is important in providing psychological support before, during, and after the procedure.

Explain that an IV line will be inserted to allow infusion of IV fluids, anesthetics, analgesics, or IV sedation.

Open Biopsy

Instruct the patient that nothing should be taken by mouth for 6 to 8 hr prior to a general anesthetic. Protocols may vary among facilities.

Needle Biopsy

Instruct the patient that nothing should be taken by mouth for at least 4 hr prior to the procedure to reduce the risk of nausea and vomiting. Protocols may vary among facilities.

General

Make sure a written and informed consent has been signed prior to the procedure and before administering any medications.

INTRATEST:

Ensure that the patient has complied with dietary restrictions; ensure that food has been restricted for at least 4 to 8 hr depending on the anesthetic chosen for the procedure.

Ensure that anticoagulant therapy has been withheld for the appropriate number of days prior to the procedure. Number of days to withhold medication is dependent on the type of anticoagulant. Notify the HCP if patient anticoagulant therapy has not been withheld.

Have emergency equipment readily available.

Have the patient void before the procedure.

Observe standard precautions, and follow the general guidelines in Appendix A. Positively identify the patient, and label the appropriate collection containers with the corresponding patient demographics, date and time of collection, and site location.

Assist the patient to the desired position depending on the test site to be used and direct the patient to breathe normally during the beginning of the general anesthetic. Instruct the patient to cooperate fully and to follow directions. For the patient undergoing local anesthesia, direct him or her to breathe normally and to avoid unnecessary movement during the procedure. Instruct the patient to avoid coughing or straining, which may increase intra-abdominal pressure.

Record baseline vital signs, and continue to monitor throughout the procedure. Protocols may vary among facilities.

After the administration of general or local anesthesia, shave and cleanse the site with an antiseptic solution, and drape the area with sterile towels.

Open Biopsy

After administration of general anesthesia and surgical preparation are completed, an incision is made, suspicious area(s) are located, and tissue samples are collected.

Needle Biopsy

Direct the patient to take slow deep breaths when the local anesthetic is injected. Protect the site with sterile drapes. Instruct the patient to take a deep breath, exhale forcefully, and hold the breath while the biopsy needle is inserted and rotated to obtain a core of liver tissue. Once the needle is removed, the patient may breathe. Pressure is applied to the site for 3 to 5 min, then a sterile pressure dressing is applied.

General

◆ Monitor the patient for complications related to the procedure (e.g., allergic reaction, anaphylaxis).
◆ Place tissue samples in formalin solution. Label the specimen, indicating site location, and promptly transport the specimen to the laboratory for processing and analysis.

POST-TEST:

◆ A report of the results will be sent to the requesting HCP, who will discuss the results with the patient.
◆ Instruct the patient to resume preoperative diet, as directed by the HCP. Assess the patient's ability to swallow before allowing the patient to attempt liquids or solid foods.
◆ Monitor vital signs and neurological status every 15 min for 1 hr, then every 2 hr for 4 hr, and then as ordered by the HCP. Monitor temperature every 4 hr for 24 hr. Monitor intake and output at least every 8 hr. Compare with baseline values. Notify the HCP if temperature is elevated. Protocols may vary among facilities.
◆ Observe/assess for delayed allergic reactions, such as rash, urticaria, tachycardia, hyperpnea, hypertension, palpitations, nausea, or vomiting.
◆ Instruct the patient to immediately report symptoms such as fast heart rate, difficulty breathing, skin rash, itching, chest pain, persistent right shoulder pain, or abdominal pain. Immediately report symptoms to the appropriate HCP.
◆ Observe/assess the biopsy site for bleeding, inflammation, or hematoma formation.
◆ Instruct the patient in the care and assessment of the site.
◆ Instruct the patient to report any redness, edema, bleeding, or pain at the biopsy site. Instruct the patient to immediately report chills or fever.

◆ Assess for nausea and pain. Administer antiemetic and analgesic medications as needed and as directed by the HCP.
◆ Administer antibiotic therapy if ordered. Remind the patient of the importance of completing the entire course of antibiotic therapy, even if signs and symptoms disappear before completion of therapy.
◆ Recognize anxiety related to test results. Discuss the implications of abnormal test results on the patient's lifestyle. Provide teaching and information regarding the clinical implications of the test results, as appropriate. Educate the patient regarding access to counseling services.
◆ Reinforce information given by the patient's HCP regarding further testing, treatment, or referral to another HCP. Inform the patient of a follow-up appointment for removal of sutures, if indicated. Answer any questions or address any concerns voiced by the patient or family.
◆ Instruct the patient in the use of any ordered medications. Explain the importance of adhering to the therapy regimen. As appropriate, instruct the patient in significant side effects and systemic reactions associated with the prescribed medication. Encourage him or her to review corresponding literature provided by a pharmacist.
◆ Depending on the results of this procedure, additional testing may be performed to evaluate or monitor progression of the disease process and determine the need for a change in therapy. Evaluate test results in relation to the patient's symptoms and other tests performed.

RELATED MONOGRAPHS:

◆ Related tests include ALT, albumin, ALP, ammonia, amylase, AMA/ASMA, α_1-antitrypsin/phenotyping, AST, bilirubin, cholesterol, coagulation factors, CBC, copper, GGT, hepatitis antigens and antibodies, infectious mononucleosis screen, laparoscopy abdominal, lipase, liver and spleen scan, MRI liver, PT/INR, radiofrequency ablation liver, UA, and US liver.
◆ Refer to the Hepatobiliary and Immune systems tables at the end of the book for related tests by body system.

Biopsy, Lung

SYNONYM/ACRONYM: Transbronchial lung biopsy, open lung biopsy.

COMMON USE: To assist in diagnosing lung cancer and other lung tissue disease.

SPECIMEN: Lung tissue or cells.

REFERENCE VALUE: (Method: Macroscopic and microscopic examination of tissue) No abnormal tissue or cells; no growth in culture.

DESCRIPTION: A biopsy of the lung is performed to obtain lung tissue for examination of pathological features. The specimen can be obtained transbronchially or by open lung biopsy. In a transbronchial biopsy, forceps pass through the bronchoscope to obtain the specimen. In a transbronchial needle aspiration biopsy, a needle passes through a bronchoscope to obtain the specimen. In a transcatheter bronchial brushing, a brush is inserted through the bronchoscope. In an open lung biopsy, the chest is opened and a small thoracic incision is made to remove tissue from the chest wall. Lung biopsies are used to differentiate between infection and other sources of disease indicated by initial radiology studies, computed tomography scans, or sputum analysis. Specimens are cultured to detect pathogenic organisms or directly examined for the presence of malignant cells.

INDICATIONS
• Assist in the diagnosis of lung cancer
• Assist in the diagnosis of fibrosis and degenerative or inflammatory diseases of the lung

• Assist in the diagnosis of sarcoidosis

POTENTIAL DIAGNOSIS

Abnormal findings in
• Amyloidosis
• Cancer
• Granulomas
• Infections caused by *Blastomyces, Histoplasma, Legionella* spp., and *Pneumocystis jiroveci* (formerly *P. carinii*)
• Sarcoidosis
• Systemic lupus erythematosus
• Tuberculosis

CRITICAL FINDINGS
• Any postprocedural decrease in breath sounds noted at the biopsy site should be reported immediately.
• Assessment of clear margins after tissue excision
• Classification or grading of tumor
• Identification of malignancy
• Shortness of breath, cyanosis, or rapid pulse during the procedure must be reported immediately

It is essential that critical diagnoses be communicated immediately to the requesting health-care provider (HCP). A listing of these diagnoses varies among facilities.

INTERFERING FACTORS

- Conditions such as vascular anomalies of the lung, bleeding abnormalities, or pulmonary hypertension may increase the risk of bleeding.
- Conditions such as bullae or cysts and respiratory insufficiency increase the risk of pneumothorax.
- Failure to follow dietary restrictions before the procedure may cause the procedure to be canceled or repeated.

NURSING IMPLICATIONS AND PROCEDURE

PRETEST:

- Positively identify the patient using at least two unique identifiers before providing care, treatment, or services.
- *Patient Teaching:* Inform the patient this procedure can assist in establishing a diagnosis of lung disease.
- Obtain a history of the patient's complaints, including a list of known allergens, especially allergies or sensitivities to latex or anesthetics.
- Obtain a history of the patient's immune and respiratory systems, any bleeding disorders or other symptoms, and results of previously performed laboratory tests and diagnostic and surgical procedures.
- Note any recent procedures that can interfere with test results.
- Record the date of the last menstrual period and determine the possibility of pregnancy in perimenopausal women.
- Obtain a list of the patient's current medications including anticoagulants, aspirin and other salicylates, herbs, nutritional supplements, and nutraceuticals (see Appendix F). Such products should be discontinued by medical direction for the appropriate number of days prior to a surgical procedure.
- Review the procedure with the patient. Inform the patient that it may be necessary to remove hair from the site before the procedure. Instruct that prophylactic antibiotics may be administered prior to the procedure. Address concerns about pain and explain that a sedative and/or analgesia will be administered to promote relaxation and reduce discomfort prior to the transbronchial needle aspiration biopsy; a general anesthesia will be administered prior to the open biopsy. Explain to the patient that no pain will be experienced during the test when general anesthesia is used but that any discomfort with a needle biopsy will be minimized with local anesthetics and systemic analgesics. Atropine is usually given before bronchoscopy examinations to reduce bronchial secretions and prevent vagally induced bradycardia. Meperidine (Demerol) or morphine may be given as a sedative. Lidocaine is sprayed in the patient's throat to reduce discomfort caused by the presence of the tube. Inform the patient that the biopsy is performed under sterile conditions by an HCP specializing in this procedure. The surgical procedure usually takes about 30 min to complete, and sutures may be necessary to close the site. A needle biopsy usually takes about 15 to 30 min to complete.
- *Sensitivity to social and cultural issues,* as well as concern for modesty, is important in providing psychological support before, during, and after the procedure.
- Explain that an IV line will be inserted to allow infusion of IV fluids, antibiotics, anesthetics, and analgesics.
- Instruct the patient that nothing should be taken by mouth for 6 to 8 hr prior to a general anesthetic. Protocols may vary among facilities.
- Have the patient void before the procedure.
- *Make sure a written and informed consent has been signed prior to the procedure and before administering any medications.*

INTRATEST:

▸ Ensure that the patient has complied with dietary restrictions; ensure that food has been restricted for at least 6 to 8 hr prior to the procedure.

▸ Ensure that anticoagulant therapy has been withheld for the appropriate number of days prior to the procedure. Number of days to withhold medication is dependent on the type of anticoagulant. Notify the HCP if patient anticoagulant therapy has not been withheld.

▸ Have emergency equipment readily available. Keep resuscitation equipment on hand in the case of respiratory impairment or laryngospasm after the procedure.

▸ Avoid using morphine sulfate in those with asthma or other pulmonary disease. This drug can further exacerbate bronchospasms and respiratory impairment.

▸ Observe standard precautions, and follow the general guidelines in Appendix A. Positively identify the patient, and label the appropriate collection containers with the corresponding patient demographics, date and time of collection, and site location, especially left or right lung.

▸ Have patient remove dentures, contact lenses, eyeglasses, and jewelry. Notify the HCP if the patient has permanent crowns on teeth. Have the patient remove clothing and change into a gown for the procedure.

▸ Assist the patient to a comfortable position, and direct the patient to breathe normally during the beginning of the general anesthesia. Instruct the patient to cooperate fully and to follow directions. Direct the patient to breathe normally and to avoid unnecessary movement during the local anesthetic and the procedure.

▸ Record baseline vital signs and continue to monitor throughout the procedure. Protocols may vary among facilities.

▸ After the administration of general or local anesthesia, shave and cleanse the site with an antiseptic solution, and drape the area with sterile towels.

Open Biopsy

▸ The patient is prepared for thoracotomy under general anesthesia in the operating room. Tissue specimens are collected from suspicious sites. Place specimen from needle aspiration or brushing on clean glass microscope slides. Place tissue or aspirate specimens in appropriate sterile container for culture or appropriate fixative container for histological studies.

▸ Carefully observe/assess the patient for any signs of respiratory distress during the procedure.

▸ A chest tube is inserted after the procedure.

Needle Biopsy

▸ Instruct the patient to take slow, deep breaths when the local anesthetic is injected. Protect the site with sterile drapes. Assist patient to a sitting position with arms on a pillow over a bed table. Instruct patient to avoid coughing during the procedure. The needle is inserted through the posterior chest wall and into the intercostal space. The needle is rotated to obtain the sample and then withdrawn. Pressure is applied to the site with a petroleum jelly gauze, and a pressure dressing is applied over the petroleum jelly gauze.

Bronchoscopy

▸ Provide mouth care to reduce oral bacterial flora.

▸ After administration of general anesthesia, position the patient in a supine position with the neck hyperextended. If local anesthesia is used, the patient is seated while the tongue and oropharynx are sprayed and swabbed with anesthetic. Provide an emesis basin for the increased saliva and encourage the patient to spit out the saliva because the gag reflex may be impaired. When loss of sensation is adequate, the patient is placed in a supine or side-lying position. The fiberoptic scope can be introduced through the nose, the mouth, an endotracheal tube, a tracheostomy tube, or a rigid bronchoscope. Most common insertion is through the nose. Patients with copious secretions or massive hemoptysis, or in whom airway complications are more likely, may be intubated before the bronchoscopy. Additional local anesthetic is applied through the scope as it approaches the vocal cords and the carina, eliminating reflexes in these sensitive areas. The fiberoptic approach allows visualization of airway segments without having to move the patient's head through various positions.

▸ After visual inspection of the lungs, tissue samples are collected from suspicious sites by bronchial brush or biopsy forceps to be used for cytological and microbiological studies.

▸ After the procedure, the bronchoscope is removed. Patients who had local anesthesia are placed in a semi-Fowler's position to recover.

General

▸ Monitor the patient for complications related to the procedure (e.g., allergic reaction, anaphylaxis).

▸ Place tissue samples in properly labeled specimen containers containing formalin solution, and promptly transport the specimen to the laboratory for processing and analysis.

POST-TEST:

▸ A report of the results will be sent to the requesting HCP, who will discuss the results with the patient.

▸ Instruct the patient to resume preoperative diet, as directed by the HCP. Assess the patient's ability to swallow before allowing the patient to attempt liquids or solid foods.

▸ Inform the patient that he or she may experience some throat soreness and hoarseness. Instruct patient to treat throat discomfort with lozenges and warm gargles when the gag reflex returns.

▸ Monitor vital signs and neurological status every 15 min for 1 hr, then every 2 hr for 4 hr, and then as ordered by the HCP. Monitor temperature every 4 hr for 24 hr. Monitor intake and output at least every 8 hr. Compare with baseline values. Notify the HCP if temperature is elevated. Protocols may vary among facilities.

▸ Emergency resuscitation equipment should be readily available if the vocal cords become spastic after intubation.

▸ Observe/assess for delayed allergic reactions, such as rash, urticaria, tachycardia, hyperpnea, hypertension, palpitations, nausea, or vomiting.

▸ Observe/assess the biopsy site for bleeding, inflammation, or hematoma formation.

▸ Instruct the patient in the care and assessment of the biopsy site.

▸ Instruct the patient to report any redness, edema, bleeding, or pain at the biopsy site.

▸ Observe/assess the patient for hemoptysis, difficulty breathing, cough, air hunger, excessive coughing, pain, or absent breath sounds over the affected area. Monitor chest tube patency and drainage after a thoracotomy.

▸ Evaluate the patient for symptoms indicating the development of pneumothorax, such as dyspnea, tachypnea, anxiety, decreased breathing sounds, or restlessness. A chest x-ray may be ordered to check for the presence of this complication.

▸ Evaluate the patient for symptoms of empyema, such as fever, tachycardia, malaise, or elevated white blood cell count.

▸ Observe/assess the patient's sputum for blood if a biopsy was taken, because large amounts of blood may indicate the development of a problem; a small amount of streaking is expected. Evaluate the patient for signs of bleeding, such as tachycardia, hypotension, or restlessness.

▸ Instruct the patient to remain in a semi-Fowler's position after bronchoscopy or fine-needle aspiration to maximize ventilation. Semi-Fowler's position is a semisitting position with the knees flexed and supported by pillows on the bed or examination table. Instruct the patient to stay in bed lying on the affected side for at least 2 hr with a pillow or rolled towel under the site to prevent bleeding. The patient will also need to remain on bedrest for 24 hr.

◗ Assess for nausea and pain. Administer antiemetic and analgesic medications as needed and as directed by the HCP.

◗ Administer antibiotic therapy if ordered. Remind the patient of the importance of completing the entire course of antibiotic therapy, even if signs and symptoms disappear before completion of therapy.

◗ Recognize anxiety related to test results. Discuss the implications of abnormal test results on the patient's lifestyle. Provide teaching and information regarding the clinical implications of the test results, as appropriate. Educate the patient regarding access to counseling services.

◗ Reinforce information given by the patient's HCP regarding further testing, treatment, or referral to another HCP. Instruct the patient to use lozenges or gargle for throat discomfort. Inform the patient of smoking cessation programs as appropriate. Malnutrition is commonly seen in patients with severe respiratory disease for numerous reasons, including fatigue, lack of appetite, and gastrointestinal distress. Adequate intake of vitamins A and C are also important to prevent pulmonary infection and to decrease the extent of lung tissue damage.

The importance of following the prescribed diet should be stressed to the patient/caregiver. Educate the patient regarding access to counseling services, as appropriate. Answer any questions or address any concerns voiced by the patient or family.

◗ Instruct the patient in the use of any ordered medications. Explain the importance of adhering to the therapy regimen. As appropriate, instruct the patient in significant side effects and systemic reactions associated with the prescribed medication. Encourage him or her to review corresponding literature provided by a pharmacist.

◗ Depending on the results of this procedure, additional testing may be performed to evaluate or monitor progression of the disease process and determine the need for a change in therapy. Evaluate test results in relation to the patient's symptoms and other tests performed.

RELATED MONOGRAPHS:

◗ Related tests include arterial/alveolar oxygen ratio, antibodies antiglomerular basement membrane, blood gases, bronchoscopy, chest x-ray, CBC, CT thoracic, culture sputum, cytology sputum, gallium scan, gram/acid fast stain, lung perfusion scan, lung ventilation scan, MRI chest, mediastinoscopy, pleural fluid analysis, PFT, and TB skin tests.

◗ Refer to the Immune and Respiratory systems tables at the end of the book for related tests by body system.

Biopsy, Lymph Node

SYNONYM/ACRONYM: N/A.

COMMON USE: To assist in diagnosing cancer such as lymphoma and leukemia as well as other systemic disorders.

SPECIMEN: Lymph node tissue or cells.

REFERENCE VALUE: (Method: Macroscopic and microscopic examination of tissue) No abnormal tissue or cells.

DESCRIPTION: Lymph node biopsy is the excision of a tissue sample from one or more lymph nodes for microscopic analysis to determine cell morphology and the presence of tissue abnormalities. This test assists in confirming a diagnosis of cancer, diagnosing disorders causing systemic illness, or determining the stage of metastatic cancer. A biopsy specimen is usually obtained either by needle biopsy or after surgical incision. Biopsies are most commonly performed on the following types of lymph nodes: cervical nodes, which drain the face and scalp; axillary nodes, which drain the arms, breasts, and upper chest; and inguinal nodes, which drain the legs, external genitalia, and lower abdominal wall.

INDICATIONS

- Assist in confirming suspected fungal or parasitic infections of the lymphatics
- Assist in confirming suspected malignant involvement of the lymphatics
- Determine the stage of metastatic cancer

- Differentiate between benign and malignant disorders that may cause lymph node enlargement
- Evaluate persistent enlargement of one or more lymph nodes for unknown reasons

POTENTIAL DIAGNOSIS

Abnormal findings in
- Chancroid
- Fungal infection (e.g., cat scratch disease)
- Immunodeficiency
- Infectious mononucleosis
- Lymph involvement of systemic diseases (e.g., systemic lupus erythematosus, sarcoidosis)
- Lymphangitis
- Lymphogranuloma venereum
- Malignancy (e.g., lymphomas, leukemias)
- Metastatic disease
- Parasitic infestation (e.g., pneumoconiosis)

CRITICAL FINDINGS

- Assessment of clear margins after tissue excision
- Classification or grading of tumor
- Identification of malignancy

It is essential that critical diagnoses be communicated immediately to the requesting health-care provider (HCP).

A listing of these diagnoses varies among facilities.

INTERFERING FACTORS

- ◈ This procedure is contraindicated in patients with bleeding disorders.
- Failure to follow dietary restrictions before the procedure may cause the procedure to be canceled or repeated.

NURSING IMPLICATIONS AND PROCEDURE

PRETEST:

- Positively identify the patient using at least two unique identifiers before providing care, treatment, or services.
- *Patient Teaching:* Inform the patient this procedure can assist in establishing a diagnosis of lymph node disease.
- Obtain a history of the patient's complaints, including a list of known allergens, especially allergies or sensitivities to latex or anesthetics.
- Obtain a history of the patient's immune system, any bleeding disorders or other symptoms, and results of previously performed laboratory tests and diagnostic and surgical procedures.
- Record the date of the last menstrual period and determine the possibility of pregnancy in perimenopausal women.
- Note any recent procedures that can interfere with test results.
- Obtain a list of the patient's current medications including anticoagulants, aspirin and other salicylates, herbs, nutritional supplements, and nutraceuticals (see Appendix F). Such products should be discontinued by medical direction for the appropriate number of days prior to a surgical procedure.
- Review the procedure with the patient. Inform the patient that it may be necessary to remove hair from the site before the procedure. Instruct that prophylactic antibiotics may be administered prior to the procedure. Address concerns about pain and explain that a sedative and/or analgesia will be administered to promote relaxation and reduce discomfort prior to the percutaneous biopsy; a general anesthesia will be administered prior to the open biopsy. Explain to the patient that no pain will be experienced during the test when general anesthesia is used but that any discomfort with a needle biopsy will be minimized with local anesthetics and systemic analgesics. Inform the patient that the biopsy is performed under sterile conditions by an HCP, with support staff, specializing in this procedure. The surgical procedure usually takes about 30 min to complete, and sutures may be necessary to close the site. A needle biopsy usually takes about 15 min to complete.
- *Sensitivity to social and cultural issues,* as well as concern for modesty, is important in providing psychological support before, during, and after the procedure.
- Explain that an IV line will be inserted to allow infusion of IV fluids, anesthetics, analgesics, or IV sedation.

Open Biopsy

- Instruct the patient that nothing should be taken by mouth for 6 to 8 hr prior to a general anesthetic. Protocols may vary among facilities.

Needle Biopsy

- Instruct the patient that nothing should be taken by mouth for at least 4 hr prior to the procedure to reduce the risk of nausea and vomiting. Protocols may vary among facilities.

General

- *Make sure a written and informed consent has been signed prior to the procedure and before administering any medications.*

INTRATEST:

- Ensure that the patient has complied with dietary restrictions; ensure that food has been restricted for at least 4 to 8 hr depending on the anesthetic chosen for the procedure.
- Ensure that anticoagulant therapy has been withheld for the appropriate number of days prior to the procedure. Number of days to withhold medication is dependent on the type of anticoagulant. Notify the HCP if patient

anticoagulant therapy has not been withheld.

♦ Have emergency equipment readily available.

♦ Have the patient void before the procedure.

♦ Observe standard precautions, and follow the general guidelines in Appendix A. Positively identify the patient, and label the appropriate collection containers with the corresponding patient demographics, date and time of collection, and site location.

♦ Assist the patient to the desired position depending on the test site to be used, and direct the patient to breathe normally during the beginning of the general anesthetic. Instruct the patient to cooperate fully and to follow directions. For the patient undergoing local anesthesia, direct him or her to breathe normally and to avoid unnecessary movement during the procedure.

♦ Record baseline vital signs, and continue to monitor throughout the procedure. Protocols may vary among facilities.

♦ After the administration of general or local anesthesia, shave and cleanse the site with an antiseptic solution, and drape the area with sterile towels.

Open Biopsy

♦ After administration of general anesthesia and surgical preparation are completed, an incision is made, suspicious area(s) are located, and tissue samples are collected.

Needle Biopsy

♦ Instruct the patient to take slow, deep breaths when the local anesthetic is injected. Protect the site with sterile drapes. The node is grasped with sterile gloved fingers, and a needle (with attached syringe) is inserted directly into the node. The node is aspirated to collect the specimen. Pressure is applied to the site for 3 to 5 min, then a sterile dressing is applied.

General

♦ Monitor the patient for complications related to the procedure (e.g., allergic reaction, anaphylaxis).

♦ Place tissue samples in formalin solution. Label the specimen, indicating site location, and promptly transport the specimen to the laboratory for processing and analysis.

POST-TEST:

♦ A report of the results will be sent to the requesting HCP, who will discuss the results with the patient.

♦ Instruct the patient to resume preoperative diet, as directed by the HCP. Assess the patient's ability to swallow before allowing the patient to attempt liquids or solid foods.

♦ Monitor vital signs and neurological status every 15 min for 1 hr, then every 2 hr for 4 hr, and then as ordered by the HCP. Monitor temperature every 4 hr for 24 hr. Monitor intake and output at least every 8 hr. Compare with baseline values. Notify the HCP if temperature is elevated. Protocols may vary among facilities.

♦ Observe/assess for delayed allergic reactions, such as rash, urticaria, tachycardia, hyperpnea, hypertension, palpitations, nausea, or vomiting.

♦ Observe/assess the biopsy site for bleeding, inflammation, or hematoma formation.

♦ Instruct the patient in the care and assessment of the site.

♦ Instruct the patient to report any redness, edema, bleeding, or pain at the biopsy site.

♦ Assess for nausea and pain. Administer antiemetic and analgesic medications as needed and as directed by the HCP.

♦ Administer antibiotic therapy if ordered. Remind the patient of the importance of completing the entire course of antibiotic therapy, even if signs and symptoms disappear before completion of therapy.

♦ Recognize anxiety related to test results. Discuss the implications of abnormal test results on the patient's lifestyle. Provide teaching and information regarding the clinical implications of the test results, as appropriate. Educate the patient regarding access to counseling services.

♦ Reinforce information given by the patient's HCP regarding further testing, treatment, or referral to another HCP. Inform the patient of a follow-up

B

appointment for removal of sutures, if indicated. Answer any questions or address any concerns voiced by the patient or family.

▶ Instruct the patient in the use of any ordered medications. Explain the importance of adhering to the therapy regimen. As appropriate, instruct the patient in significant side effects and systemic reactions associated with the prescribed medication. Encourage him or her to review corresponding literature provided by a pharmacist.

▶ Depending on the results of this procedure, additional testing may be performed to evaluate or monitor progression of the disease process and determine the need for a change in therapy. Evaluate test results in relation to the patient's symptoms and other tests performed.

RELATED MONOGRAPHS:

▶ Related tests include biopsy bone marrow, CD4/CD8 enumeration, cerebrospinal fluid analysis, *Chlamydia* serology, CBC, CT pelvis, CT thoracic, culture for bacteria/fungus, CMV, Gram stain, HIV-1/HIV-2 serology, immunofixation electrophoresis, immunoglobulins (A, G, and M), infectious mononucleosis screen, lymphangiography, mammogram, mediastinoscopy, PET pelvis, RF, total protein and fractions, toxoplasmosis serology, and US lymph nodes.

▶ Refer to the Immune System table at the end of the book for related tests by body system.

Biopsy, Muscle

SYNONYM/ACRONYM: N/A.

COMMON USE: To assist in diagnosing muscular disease such as Duchenne's muscular dystrophy as well as other neuropathies and parasitic infections.

SPECIMEN: Muscle tissue or cells.

REFERENCE VALUE: (Method: Macroscopic and microscopic examination of tissue) No abnormal tissue or cells.

DESCRIPTION: Muscle biopsy is the excision of a muscle tissue sample for microscopic analysis to determine cell morphology and the presence of tissue abnormalities. This test is used to confirm a diagnosis of neuropathy or myopathy and to diagnose parasitic infestation. A biopsy specimen is usually obtained from the deltoid or gastrocnemius muscle after a surgical incision.

INDICATIONS

• Assist in confirming suspected fungal infection or parasitic infestation of the muscle
• Assist in diagnosing the cause of neuropathy or myopathy

- Assist in the diagnosis of Duchenne's muscular dystrophy

POTENTIAL DIAGNOSIS

Abnormal findings in
- Alcoholic myopathy
- Amyotrophic lateral sclerosis
- Duchenne's muscular dystrophy
- Fungal infection
- Myasthenia gravis
- Myotonia congenita
- Parasitic infestation
- Polymyalgia rheumatica
- Polymyositis

CRITICAL FINDINGS

- Assessment of clear margins after tissue excision
- Classification or grading of tumor
- Identification of malignancy

It is essential that critical diagnoses be communicated immediately to the requesting health-care provider (HCP). A listing of these diagnoses varies among facilities.

INTERFERING FACTORS

- If electromyography is performed before muscle biopsy, residual inflammation may lead to false-positive biopsy results.
- ❖ This procedure is contraindicated in patients with bleeding disorders.
- Failure to follow dietary restrictions before the procedure may cause the procedure to be canceled or repeated.

NURSING IMPLICATIONS AND PROCEDURE

PRETEST:

- Positively identify the patient using at least two unique identifiers before providing care, treatment, or services.
- *Patient Teaching:* Inform the patient this procedure can assist in

establishing a diagnosis of musculoskeletal disease.
- Obtain a history of the patient's complaints, including a list of known allergens, especially allergies or sensitivities to latex or anesthetics.
- Obtain a history of the patient's immune and musculoskeletal systems, any bleeding disorders or other symptoms, and results of previously performed laboratory tests and diagnostic and surgical procedures.
- Record the date of the last menstrual period and determine the possibility of pregnancy in perimenopausal women.
- Note any recent procedures that can interfere with test results.
- Obtain a list of the patient's current medications including anticoagulants, aspirin and other salicylates, herbs, nutritional supplements, and nutraceuticals (see Appendix F). Such products should be discontinued by medical direction for the appropriate number of days prior to a surgical procedure.
- Review the procedure with the patient. Inform the patient that it may be necessary to remove hair from the site before the procedure. Instruct that prophylactic antibiotics may be administered prior to the procedure. Address concerns about pain and explain that a sedative and/or analgesia will be administered to promote relaxation and reduce discomfort prior to the percutaneous biopsy; a general anesthesia will be administered prior to the open biopsy. Explain that no pain will be experienced during the test when general anesthesia is used but that any discomfort with a needle biopsy will be minimized with local anesthetics and systemic analgesics. Inform the patient that the biopsy is performed under sterile conditions by an HCP specializing in this procedure. The surgical procedure usually takes about 20 min to complete, and sutures may be necessary to close the site. A needle biopsy usually takes about 15 min to complete.
- *Sensitivity to social and cultural issues,* as well as concern for modesty, is important in providing psychological support before, during, and after the procedure.

▶ Explain that an IV line may be inserted to allow infusion of IV fluids, anesthetics, or sedatives.

▶ Instruct the patient that nothing should be taken by mouth for at least 4 hr prior to the procedure to reduce the risk of nausea and vomiting. Protocols may vary among facilities.

▶ *Make sure a written and informed consent has been signed prior to the procedure and before administering any medications.*

INTRATEST:

▶ Ensure that the patient has complied with dietary restrictions; ensure that food has been restricted for at least 4 hr prior to the procedure.

▶ Ensure that anticoagulant therapy has been withheld for the appropriate number of days prior to the procedure. Number of days to withhold medication is dependent on the type of anticoagulant. Notify the HCP if patient anticoagulant therapy has not been withheld.

▶ Have emergency equipment readily available.

▶ Have the patient void before the procedure.

▶ Observe standard precautions, and follow the general guidelines in Appendix A. Positively identify the patient, and label the appropriate collection containers with the corresponding patient demographics, date and time of collection, and site location.

▶ Assist the patient to a comfortable position: a supine position (for deltoid biopsy) or prone position (for gastrocnemius biopsy). Instruct the patient to cooperate fully and to follow directions. Direct the patient to breathe normally and to avoid unnecessary movement during the local anesthetic and the procedure.

▶ Record baseline vital signs, and continue to monitor throughout the procedure. Protocols may vary among facilities.

▶ After the administration of general or local anesthesia, shave and cleanse the site with an antiseptic solution, and drape the area with sterile towels.

Open Biopsy

▶ Assess baseline neurological status. Instruct the patient to take slow deep breaths when the local anesthetic is injected. Protect the site with sterile drapes.

▶ After infiltration of the site with local anesthetic, a small incision is made through the dermis, exposing the muscle. A small area of muscle is excised and removed with forceps. The area is then closed with sutures or similar material, and a sterile dressing is applied.

Needle Biopsy

▶ Instruct the patient to take slow deep breaths when the local anesthetic is injected. Protect the site with sterile drapes.

▶ After infiltration of the site with local anesthetic, a cutting biopsy needle is introduced through a small skin incision and bored into the muscle. A core needle is introduced through the cutting needle, and a plug of muscle is removed. The needles are withdrawn, and the specimen is placed in a preservative solution. Pressure is applied to the site for 3 to 5 min, and then a pressure dressing is applied.

General

▶ Monitor the patient for complications related to the procedure (e.g., allergic reaction, anaphylaxis).

▶ Place tissue samples in properly labeled specimen container containing formalin solution, and promptly transport the specimen to the laboratory for processing and analysis.

POST-TEST:

▶ A report of the results will be sent to the requesting HCP, who will discuss the results with the patient.

▶ Instruct the patient to resume preoperative diet, as directed by the HCP.

▶ Monitor vital signs and neurological status every 15 min for 1 hr, then every 2 hr for 4 hr, and then as ordered by the HCP. Monitor temperature every 4 hr for 24 hr. Compare with baseline values. Notify the HCP if temperature is elevated. Protocols may vary among facilities.

Observe/assess for delayed allergic reactions, such as rash, urticaria, tachycardia, hyperpnea, hypertension, palpitations, nausea, or vomiting.

Observe/assess the biopsy site for bleeding, inflammation, or hematoma formation.

Instruct the patient in the care and assessment of the site.

Instruct the patient to report any redness, edema, bleeding, or pain at the biopsy site.

Assess for nausea and pain. Administer antiemetic and analgesic medications as needed and as directed by the HCP.

Administer antibiotic therapy if ordered. Remind the patient of the importance of completing the entire course of antibiotic therapy, even if signs and symptoms disappear before completion of therapy.

Recognize anxiety related to test results. Discuss the implications of abnormal test results on the patient's lifestyle. Provide teaching and information regarding the clinical implications of the test results, as appropriate. Educate the patient regarding access to counseling services.

Reinforce information given by the patient's HCP regarding further testing, treatment, or referral to another HCP.

Inform the patient of a follow-up appointment for removal of sutures, if indicated. Answer any questions or address any concerns voiced by the patient or family.

Instruct the patient in the use of any ordered medications. Explain the importance of adhering to the therapy regimen. As appropriate, instruct the patient in significant side effects and systemic reactions associated with the prescribed medication. Encourage him or her to review corresponding literature provided by a pharmacist.

Depending on the results of this procedure, additional testing may be performed to evaluate or monitor progression of the disease process and determine the need for a change in therapy. Evaluate test results in relation to the patient's symptoms and other tests performed.

RELATED MONOGRAPHS:

Related tests include AChR, aldolase, ANA, antibody Jo-1, antithyroglobulin antibodies, CK and isoenzymes, EMG, ENG, myoglobin, and RF.

Refer to the Immune and Musculoskeletal systems tables at the end of the book for related tests by body system.

Biopsy, Prostate

SYNONYM/ACRONYM: N/A.

COMMON USE: To assist in diagnosing prostate cancer.

SPECIMEN: Prostate tissue.

REFERENCE VALUE: (Method: Microscopic examination of tissue cells) No abnormal cells or tissue.

DESCRIPTION: Biopsy of the prostate gland is performed to identify cancerous cells, especially if serum prostate-specific antigen (PSA) is increased. New technology makes it possible to combine data such as analysis of molecular biomarkers and cellular structure specific to the individual's biopsy tissue, standard tissue biopsy results, Gleason's score, number of positive tumor cores, tumor stage, presurgical and postsurgical PSA levels, and postsurgical margin status with computerized mathematical programs to create a personalized report that predicts the likelihood of post-prostatectomy disease progression. Serial measurements of PSA in the blood are often performed before and after surgery. Approximately 15% to 40% of patients who have had their prostate removed will encounter an increase in PSA. Patients treated for prostate cancer and who have had a PSA recurrence can still develop a metastasis as much as 8 yr after the postsurgical PSA level increased. The majority of tumors develop slowly and require minimal intervention, but patients with an increase in PSA greater than 2.0 ng/mL in a year are more likely to have an aggressive form of prostate cancer with a greater risk of death. Personalized medicine provides a technology to predict the progression of prostate cancer, likelihood of recurrence, or development of related metastatic disease.

INDICATIONS
- Evaluate prostatic hypertrophy of unknown etiology
- Investigate suspected cancer of the prostate

POTENTIAL DIAGNOSIS
Positive findings in prostate cancer

Gleason Grading	
1	Simple round glands, closely packed rounded masses with well-defined edges. Closely resemble normal prostate tissue.
2	Simple round glands, loosely packed in vague, rounded masses with loosely packed edges. Closely resemble normal prostate tissue.
3	Small, very small, or medium-sized single glands of irregular shape and spacing with poorly defined infiltrating edges.
4	Small, medium, or large glands fused into cords, chains, or ragged infiltrating masses.
5	No glandular differentiation, solid sheets, cords, single cells with central necrosis.

Gleason's score is the sum of two grades assigned by the pathologist during microscopic examination of the biopsy samples. The score ranges from 1 to 10 with 10 being the worst. The first number assigned is the primary grade (1 to 5), which indicates where the cancer is the most prominent. The second number is the secondary grade (1 to 5), which indicates where the cancer is next most prominent. It is important to have the breakdown in grading as well as the total score. For example, Patient A's Gleason's score is $4 + 3 = 7$, and Patient B's Gleason's score is $3 + 4 = 7$. Even though both patients have the same Gleason's score, Patient B has a slightly better prognosis because the primary area is graded a 3.

TNM Classification of Tumors

T refers to the size of the primary tumor
T_0 No evidence of primary tumor
T_{IS} Carcinoma in situ
T_{1-4} Increasing degrees in tumor size and involvement

N refers to lymph node involvement
N_0 No evidence of disease in lymph nodes
N_{1-4} Increasing degrees in lymph node involvement
N_X Regional lymph nodes unable to be assessed clinically

M refers to distant metastases
M_0 No evidence of distant metastases
M_{1-4} Increasing degrees of distant metastatic involvement, including distant nodes

---

CRITICAL FINDINGS

• Assessment of clear margins after tissue excision
• Classification or grading of tumor
• Identification of malignancy

It is essential that critical diagnoses be communicated immediately to the requesting health-care provider (HCP). A listing of these diagnoses varies among facilities.

INTERFERING FACTORS

• ✺ This procedure is contraindicated in patients with bleeding disorders.
• ✺ Failure to follow dietary restrictions before the procedure may cause the procedure to be canceled or repeated.
• The various sampling approaches have individual drawbacks that should be considered: Transurethral sampling does not always ensure that malignant cells will be included in the specimen, whereas transrectal sampling carries the risk of perforating the rectum and creating a channel through which malignant cells can seed normal tissue.

NURSING IMPLICATIONS AND PROCEDURE

PRETEST:

▸ Positively identify the patient using at least two unique identifiers before providing care, treatment, or services.
▸ *Patient Teaching:* Inform the patient this procedure can assist in establishing a diagnosis of prostate disease.
▸ Obtain a history of the patient's complaints, including a list of known allergens, especially allergies or sensitivities to latex or anesthetics.
▸ Obtain a history of the patient's genitourinary system, any bleeding disorders or other symptoms, and results of previously performed laboratory tests and diagnostic and surgical procedures.
▸ Note any recent procedures that can interfere with test results.
▸ Obtain a list of the patient's current medications including anticoagulants, aspirin and other salicylates, herbs, nutritional supplements, and nutraceuticals (see Appendix F). Such products should be discontinued by medical direction for the appropriate number of days prior to a surgical procedure.

B

▸ Review the procedure with the patient. Inform the patient that it may be necessary to remove hair from the site before the procedure. Instruct that prophylactic antibiotics may be administered prior to the procedure. Address concerns about pain and explain that a sedative and/or analgesia will be administered to promote relaxation and reduce discomfort prior to the percutaneous biopsy; a general anesthesia will be administered prior to the open biopsy. Explain to the patient that no pain will be experienced during the test when general anesthesia is used but that any discomfort with a needle biopsy will be minimized with local anesthetics and systemic analgesics. Inform the patient that the biopsy is performed under sterile conditions by an HCP, with support staff, specializing in this procedure. The surgical procedure usually takes about 30 min to complete, and sutures may be necessary to close the site. A needle biopsy usually takes about 20 min to complete. Instructions regarding the appropriate transport container for molecular diagnostic studies should be obtained from the laboratory prior to the procedure.

▸ *Sensitivity to social and cultural issues,* as well as concern for modesty, is important in providing psychological support before, during, and after the procedure.

▸ Explain that an IV line will be inserted to allow infusion of IV fluids, antibiotics, anesthetics, and analgesics.

▸ Ensure that anticoagulant therapy has been withheld for the appropriate number of days prior to the procedure. Number of days to withhold medication is dependent on the type of anticoagulant. Notify the HCP if patient anticoagulant therapy has not been withheld.

▸ Instruct the patient that nothing should be taken by mouth for 6 to 8 hr prior to a general anesthetic. Protocols may vary among facilities.

▸ *Make sure a written and informed consent has been signed prior to the procedure and before administering any medications.*

INTRATEST:

▸ Ensure that the patient has complied with dietary restrictions; ensure that food has been restricted for at least 6 to 8 hr prior to the procedure.

▸ Have emergency equipment readily available.

▸ Have the patient void before the procedure. Administer enemas if ordered.

▸ Observe standard precautions, and follow the general guidelines in Appendix A. Positively identify the patient, and label the appropriate collection containers with the corresponding patient demographics, date and time of collection, and site location.

▸ Assist the patient to a comfortable position, and direct the patient to breathe normally during the beginning of the general anesthesia.

▸ Cleanse the biopsy site with an antiseptic solution, and drape the area with sterile towels.

▸ Record baseline vital signs, and continue to monitor throughout the procedure. Protocols may vary among facilities.

Transurethral Approach

▸ After administration of general anesthesia, position the patient on a urological examination table with the feet in stirrups. The endoscope is inserted into the urethra. The tissue is excised with a cutting loop and is placed in formalin solution.

Transrectal Approach

▸ After administration of general anesthesia, position the patient in the Sims' position. A rectal examination is performed to locate suspicious nodules. A biopsy needle guide is placed at the biopsy site, and the biopsy needle is inserted through the needle guide. The cells are aspirated, the needle is withdrawn, and the sample is placed in formalin solution.

Perineal Approach

▸ After administration of general anesthesia, position the patient in the lithotomy position. Clean the perineum with an antiseptic solution, and protect the biopsy site with sterile drapes. A small incision is made, and the sample is removed by needle biopsy or biopsy punch and placed in formalin solution.

General

- Monitor the patient for complications related to the procedure (e.g., allergic reaction, anaphylaxis).
- Apply digital pressure to the biopsy site. If there is no bleeding after the perineal approach, place a sterile dressing on the biopsy site. Immediately notify the HCP if there is significant bleeding.
- Place tissue samples for standard biopsy examination in properly labeled specimen containers containing formalin solution, place tissue samples for molecular diagnostic studies in properly labeled specimen containers, and promptly transport the specimen to the laboratory for processing and analysis.

POST-TEST:

- A report of the results will be sent to the requesting HCP, who will discuss the results with the patient.
- Instruct the patient to resume preoperative diet, as directed by the HCP. Assess the patient's ability to swallow before allowing the patient to attempt liquids or solid foods.
- *Nutritional Considerations:* There is growing evidence that inflammation and oxidation play key roles in the development of numerous diseases, including prostate cancer. Research also shows that diets containing dried beans, fresh fruits and vegetables, nuts, spices, whole grains, and smaller amounts of red meats can increase the amount of protective antioxidants. Regular exercise, especially in combination with a healthy diet, can bring about changes in the body's metabolism that decrease inflammation and oxidation.
- Monitor vital signs and neurological status every 15 min for 1 hr, then every 2 hr for 4 hr, and then as ordered by the HCP. Monitor temperature every 4 hr for 24 hr. Monitor intake and output at least every 8 hr. Compare with baseline values. Notify the HCP if temperature is elevated. Protocols may vary among facilities.
- Instruct the patient on intake and output recording and provide appropriate measuring containers.

- Encourage fluid intake of 3,000 mL unless contraindicated.
- Observe/assess for delayed allergic reactions, such as rash, urticaria, tachycardia, hyperpnea, hypertension, palpitations, nausea, or vomiting.
- Instruct the patient in the care and assessment of the site.
- Instruct the patient to report any chills, fever, redness, edema, bleeding, or pain at the biopsy site.
- Assess for infection, hemorrhage, or perforation of the urethra or rectum.
- Inform the patient that blood may be seen in the urine after the first or second postprocedural voiding.
- Instruct the patient to report any further changes in urinary pattern, volume, or appearance.
- Assess for nausea, pain, and bladder spasms. Administer antiemetic, analgesic, and antispasmodic medications as needed and as directed by the HCP.
- Administer antibiotic therapy if ordered. Remind the patient of the importance of completing the entire course of antibiotic therapy, even if signs and symptoms disappear before completion of therapy.
- Recognize anxiety related to test results. Discuss the implications of abnormal test results on the patient's lifestyle. Provide teaching and information regarding the clinical implications of the test results, as appropriate. Educate the patient regarding access to counseling services. Provide contact information, if desired, for the National Cancer Institute (www.cancer.gov).
- Reinforce information given by the patient's HCP regarding further testing, treatment, or referral to another HCP. Decisions regarding the need for and frequency of routine PSA testing or other cancer screening procedures should be made after consultation between the patient and HCP. The most current guidelines for prostate cancer screening of the general population as well as of individuals with increased risk are available from the American Cancer Society (www.cancer.org) and the American Urological Association (www.aua.org). Counsel the patient, as appropriate,

that sexual dysfunction related to altered body function, drugs, or radiation may occur. Answer any questions or address any concerns voiced by the patient or family.

▶ Instruct the patient in the use of any ordered medications. Explain the importance of adhering to the therapy regimen. As appropriate, instruct the patient in significant side effects and systemic reactions associated with the prescribed medication. Encourage him to review corresponding literature provided by a pharmacist.

▶ Depending on the results of this procedure, additional testing may be performed to evaluate or monitor progression of the disease process and determine the need for a change in therapy. Evaluate test results in relation to the patient's symptoms and other tests performed.

RELATED MONOGRAPHS:

▶ Related tests include cystoscopy, cystourethrograpy voiding, PAP, PSA, retrograde ureteropyelography, semen analysis, and US prostate.

▶ Refer to the Genitourinary System table at the end of the book for related tests by body system.

Biopsy, Skin

SYNONYM/ACRONYM: N/A.

COMMON USE: To assist in diagnosing skin cancer.

SPECIMEN: Skin tissue or cells.

REFERENCE VALUE: (Method: Macroscopic and microscopic examination of tissue) No abnormal tissue or cells.

DESCRIPTION: Skin biopsy is the excision of a tissue sample from suspicious skin lesions. The microscopic analysis can determine cell morphology and the presence of tissue abnormalities. This test assists in confirming the diagnosis of malignant or benign skin lesions. A skin biopsy can be obtained by any of these four methods: curettage, shaving, excision, or punch. A Tzanck smear may be prepared from vesicles (blisters) present on the skin. Skin cells in the vesicles can be evaluated microscopically to indicate the presence of certain viruses, especially herpes, that cause cells to become enlarged and otherwise abnormal in appearance.

INDICATIONS
• Assist in the diagnosis of keratoses, warts, moles, keloids, fibromas, cysts, or inflamed lesions
• Assist in the diagnosis of inflammatory process of the skin, especially herpes infection
• Assist in the diagnosis of skin cancer
• Evaluate suspicious skin lesions

POTENTIAL DIAGNOSIS

Abnormal findings in
• Basal cell carcinoma
• Cysts
• Dermatitis
• Dermatofibroma
• Keloids
• Malignant melanoma
• Neurofibroma
• Pemphigus
• Pigmented nevi
• Seborrheic keratosis
• Skin involvement in systemic lupus erythematosus, discoid lupus erythematosus, and scleroderma
• Squamous cell carcinoma
• Viral infection (herpes, varicella)
• Warts

CRITICAL FINDINGS

• Assessment of clear margins after tissue excision
• Classification or grading of tumor
• Identification of malignancy

It is essential that critical diagnoses be communicated immediately to the requesting health-care provider (HCP). A listing of these diagnoses varies among facilities.

INTERFERING FACTORS

• ☀ This procedure is contraindicated in patients with bleeding disorders.
• Failure to follow dietary restrictions before the procedure may cause the procedure to be canceled or repeated.

NURSING IMPLICATIONS AND PROCEDURE

PRETEST:

▶ Positively identify the patient using at least two unique identifiers before providing care, treatment, or services.
▶ *Patient Teaching:* Inform the patient this procedure can assist in establishing a diagnosis of skin disease.

▶ Obtain a history of the patient's complaints, including a list of known allergens, especially allergies or sensitivities to latex or anesthetics.
▶ Obtain a history of the patient's immune and musculoskeletal systems, any bleeding disorders or other symptoms, and results of previously performed laboratory tests and diagnostic and surgical procedures.
▶ Record the date of the last menstrual period and determine the possibility of pregnancy in perimenopausal women.
▶ Note any recent procedures that can interfere with test results.
▶ Obtain a list of the patient's current medications including anticoagulants, aspirin and other salicylates, herbs, nutritional supplements, and nutraceuticals (see Appendix F). Such products should be discontinued by medical direction for the appropriate number of days prior to a surgical procedure.
▶ Review the procedure with the patient. Inform the patient that it may be necessary to remove hair from the site before the procedure. Instruct that prophylactic antibiotics may be administered prior to the procedure. Address concerns about pain and explain that a sedative and/or analgesia will be administered to promote relaxation and reduce discomfort prior to the punch biopsy; a general anesthesia will be administered prior to the open biopsy. Explain that no pain will be experienced during the test when general anesthesia is used but that any discomfort with a punch biopsy will be minimized with local anesthetics and systemic analgesics. Inform the patient the biopsy is performed under sterile conditions by an HCP, with support staff, specializing in this procedure. The surgical procedure usually takes about 30 min to complete, and sutures may be necessary to close the site. A punch biopsy usually takes about 20 min to complete.
▶ *Sensitivity to social and cultural issues,* as well as concern for modesty, is important in providing psychological support before, during, and after the procedure.
▶ Explain that an IV line may be inserted to allow infusion of IV fluids, anesthetics, or sedatives, depending on the type of biopsy.

There are no food, fluid, or medication restrictions unless by medical direction.

Make sure a written and informed consent has been signed prior to the procedure and before administering any medications.

B

INTRATEST:

- Ensure that the patient has complied with dietary restrictions if ordered by the HCP.
- Ensure that anticoagulant therapy has been withheld for the appropriate number of days prior to the procedure. Number of days to withhold medication is dependent on the type of anticoagulant. Notify the HCP if patient anticoagulant therapy has not been withheld.
- Have emergency equipment readily available.
- Have the patient void before the procedure.
- Observe standard precautions, and follow the general guidelines in Appendix A. Positively identify the patient, and label the appropriate collection containers with the corresponding patient demographics, date and time of collection, and site location.
- Assist the patient to the desired position depending on the test site to be used, and direct the patient to breathe normally during the local anesthetic and the procedure. Instruct the patient to cooperate fully, follow directions, and avoid unnecessary movement.
- Record baseline vital signs, and continue to monitor throughout the procedure. Protocols may vary among facilities.
- After the administration of general or local anesthesia, shave and cleanse the site with an antiseptic solution, and drape the area with sterile towels.

Curettage
- The skin is scraped with a curette to obtain specimen.

Shaving or Excision
- A scalpel is used to remove a portion of the lesion that protrudes above the epidermis. If the lesion is to be excised, the incision is made as wide and as deep as needed to ensure that the entire lesion is removed. Bleeding is controlled with external pressure to the site. Large wounds are closed with sutures. An adhesive bandage is applied when excision is complete.

Punch Biopsy
- A small, round punch about 4 to 6 mm in diameter is rotated into the skin to the desired depth. The cylinder of skin is pulled upward with forceps and separated at its base with a scalpel or scissors. If needed, sutures are applied. A sterile dressing is applied over the site.
- Monitor the patient for complications related to the procedure (e.g., allergic reaction, anaphylaxis).
- Place tissue samples in properly labeled specimen container containing formalin solution, and promptly transport the specimen to the laboratory for processing and analysis.

POST-TEST:

- A report of the results will be sent to the requesting HCP, who will discuss the results with the patient.
- Instruct the patient to resume preoperative diet, as directed by the HCP. Assess the patient's ability to swallow before allowing the patient to attempt liquids or solid foods.
- Monitor vital signs and neurological status every 15 min for 1 hr, then every 2 hr for 4 hr, and then as ordered by the HCP. Monitor temperature every 4 hr for 24 hr. Compare with baseline values. Notify the HCP if temperature is elevated. Protocols may vary among facilities.
- Observe/assess for delayed allergic reactions, such as rash, urticaria, tachycardia, hyperpnea, hypertension, palpitations, nausea, or vomiting.
- Observe/assess the biopsy site for bleeding, inflammation, or hematoma formation.
- Instruct the patient in the care and assessment of the site.
- Instruct the patient to report any redness, edema, bleeding, or pain at the biopsy site.
- Assess for nausea and pain. Administer antiemetic and analgesic medications as needed and as directed by the HCP.
- Administer antibiotic therapy if ordered. Remind the patient of the importance of completing the entire course of

antibiotic therapy, even if signs and symptoms disappear before completion of therapy.

▸ Recognize anxiety related to test results. Discuss the implications of abnormal test results on the patient's lifestyle. Provide teaching and information regarding the clinical implications of the test results, as appropriate. Educate the patient regarding access to counseling services.

▸ Reinforce information given by the patient's HCP regarding further testing, treatment, or referral to another HCP. Inform the patient of a follow-up appointment for the removal of sutures, if indicated. Answer any questions or address any concerns voiced by the patient or family.

▸ Instruct the patient in the use of any ordered medications. Explain the importance of adhering to the therapy regimen. As appropriate, instruct the patient in significant side effects and systemic reactions associated with the prescribed medication. Encourage him or her to review corresponding literature provided by a pharmacist.

▸ Depending on the results of this procedure, additional testing may be performed to evaluate or monitor progression of the disease process and determine the need for a change in therapy. Evaluate test results in relation to the patient's symptoms and other tests performed.

RELATED MONOGRAPHS:

▸ Related tests include allergen-specific IgE, ANA, culture skin, eosinophil count, ESR, and IgE.

▸ Refer to the Immune and Musculoskeletal systems tables at the end of the book for related tests by body system.

Biopsy, Thyroid

SYNONYM/ACRONYM: N/A.

COMMON USE: To assist in diagnosing thyroid cancer.

SPECIMEN: Thyroid gland tissue or cells.

REFERENCE VALUE: (Method: Macroscopic and microscopic examination of tissue) No abnormal tissue or cells.

DESCRIPTION: Thyroid biopsy is the excision of a tissue sample for microscopic analysis to determine cell morphology and the presence of tissue abnormalities. This test assists in confirming a diagnosis of cancer or determining the cause of persistent thyroid symptoms. A biopsy specimen can be obtained by needle aspiration or by surgical excision.

INDICATIONS

- Assist in the diagnosis of thyroid cancer or benign cysts or tumors
- Determine the cause of inflammatory thyroid disease
- Determine the cause of hyperthyroidism
- Evaluate enlargement of the thyroid gland

POTENTIAL DIAGNOSIS

Positive findings in
- Benign thyroid cyst
- Granulomatous thyroiditis

- Hashimoto's thyroiditis
- Nontoxic nodular goiter
- Thyroid cancer

CRITICAL FINDINGS

- Assessment of clear margins after tissue excision
- Classification or grading of tumor
- Identification of malignancy

It is essential that critical diagnoses be communicated immediately to the requesting health-care provider (HCP). A listing of these diagnoses varies among facilities.

INTERFERING FACTORS

- This procedure is contraindicated in patients with bleeding disorders.
- Failure to follow dietary restrictions before the procedure may cause the procedure to be canceled or repeated.

NURSING IMPLICATIONS AND PROCEDURE

PRETEST:

- Positively identify the patient using at least two unique identifiers before providing care, treatment, or services.
- *Patient Teaching:* Inform the patient this procedure can assist in establishing a diagnosis of thyroid disease.
- Obtain a history of the patient's complaints, including a list of known allergies, especially allergies or sensitivities to latex or anesthetics.
- Obtain a history of the patient's endocrine and immune systems, any bleeding disorders or other symptoms, and results of previously performed laboratory tests and diagnostic and surgical procedures.
- Record the date of the last menstrual period and determine possibility of pregnancy in perimenopausal women.
- Note any recent procedures that can interfere with test results.

- Obtain a list of the patient's current medications including anticoagulants, aspirin and other salicylates, herbs, nutritional supplements, and nutraceuticals (see Appendix F). Such products should be discontinued by medical direction for the appropriate number of days prior to a surgical procedure.
- Review the procedure with the patient. Inform the patient that it may be necessary to remove hair from the site before the procedure. Instruct that prophylactic antibiotics may be administered prior to the procedure. Address concerns about pain and explain that a sedative and/or analgesia will be administered to promote relaxation and reduce discomfort prior to the percutaneous biopsy; general anesthesia will be administered prior to the open biopsy. Explain that no pain will be experienced during the test when general anesthesia is used but that any discomfort with a needle biopsy will be minimized with local anesthetics and systemic analgesics. Inform the patient that the biopsy is performed under sterile conditions by an HCP, with support staff, specializing in this procedure. The surgical procedure usually takes about 30 min to complete, and sutures may be necessary to close the site. A needle biopsy usually takes about 15 min to complete.
- *Sensitivity to social and cultural issues,* as well as concern for modesty, is important in providing psychological support before, during, and after the procedure.
- Explain that an IV line will be inserted to allow infusion of IV fluids, anesthetics, analgesics, or IV sedation.

Open Biopsy

- Instruct the patient that nothing should be taken by mouth for 6 to 8 hr prior to a general anesthetic. Protocols may vary among facilities.

Needle Biopsy

- Instruct the patient that nothing should be taken by mouth for at least 4 hr prior to the procedure to reduce the risk of nausea and vomiting. Protocols may vary among facilities.

▶ Have the patient void before the procedure.

General
▶ *Make sure a written and informed consent has been signed prior to the procedure and before administering any medications.*

INTRATEST:

▶ Ensure that the patient has complied with dietary restrictions; ensure food has been restricted for at least 4 to 8 hr depending on the anesthetic chosen for the procedure.
▶ Ensure that anticoagulant therapy has been withheld for the appropriate number of days prior to the procedure. Number of days to withhold medication is dependent on the type of anticoagulant. Notify HCP if patient anticoagulant therapy has not been withheld.
▶ Have emergency equipment readily available.
▶ Observe standard precautions, and follow the general guidelines in Appendix A. Positively identify the patient and label the appropriate collection containers with the corresponding patient demographics, date and time of collection, and site location.
▶ Assist the patient to the desired position depending on the test site to be used, and direct the patient to breathe normally during the beginning of the general anesthetic. Instruct the patient to cooperate fully and to follow directions. For the patient undergoing local anesthesia, direct him or her to breathe normally and to avoid unnecessary movement during the procedure.
▶ Record baseline vital signs and continue to monitor throughout the procedure. Protocols may vary among facilities.
▶ After the administration of general or local anesthesia, shave and cleanse the site with an antiseptic solution, and drape the area with sterile towels.

Open Biopsy
▶ After administration of general anesthesia and surgical preparation is completed, an incision is made, suspicious area(s) are located, and tissue samples are collected.

Needle Biopsy
▶ Direct the patient to take slow, deep breaths when the local anesthetic is injected. Protect the site with sterile drapes. Instruct the patient to take a deep breath, exhale forcefully, and hold the breath while the biopsy needle is inserted and rotated to obtain a core of thyroid tissue. Once the needle is removed, the patient may breathe. Pressure is applied to the site for 3 to 5 min, then a sterile pressure dressing is applied.

General
▶ Monitor the patient for complications related to the procedure (e.g., allergic reaction, anaphylaxis).
▶ Place tissue samples in properly labeled specimen container containing formalin solution, and promptly transport the specimen to the laboratory for processing and analysis.

POST-TEST:

▶ A report of the results will be sent to the requesting HCP, who will discuss the results with the patient.
▶ Instruct the patient to resume preoperative diet, as directed by the HCP. Assess the patient's ability to swallow before allowing the patient to attempt liquids or solid foods.
▶ Monitor vital signs and neurological status every 15 min for 1 hr, then every 2 hr for 4 hr, and then as ordered by the HCP. Monitor temperature every 4 hr for 24 hr. Monitor intake and output at least every 8 hr. Compare with baseline values. Notify the HCP if temperature is elevated. Protocols may vary among facilities.
▶ Observe/assess for delayed allergic reactions, such as rash, urticaria, tachycardia, hyperpnea, hypertension, palpitations, nausea, or vomiting.

B

B

▸ Observe/assess the biopsy site for bleeding, inflammation, or hematoma formation.

▸ Instruct the patient in the care and assessment of the site.

▸ Instruct the patient to report any redness, edema, bleeding, or pain at the biopsy site.

▸ Assess for nausea and pain. Administer antiemetic and analgesic medications as needed and as directed by the HCP.

▸ Administer antibiotic therapy if ordered. Remind the patient of the importance of completing the entire course of antibiotic therapy, even if signs and symptoms disappear before completion of therapy.

▸ Recognize anxiety related to test. Discuss the implications of the abnormal test results on the patient's lifestyle. Provide teaching and information regarding the clinical implications of the test results, as appropriate. Educate the patient regarding access to counseling services.

▸ Reinforce information given by the patient's HCP regarding further testing, treatment, or referral to another HCP. Inform the patient of a follow-up appointment for removal of sutures, if indicated. Answer any questions or address any concerns voiced by the patient or family.

▸ Instruct the patient in the use of any ordered medications. Explain the importance of adhering to the therapy regimen. As appropriate, instruct the patient in significant side effects and systemic reactions associated with the prescribed medication. Encourage him or her to review corresponding literature provided by a pharmacist.

▸ Depending on the results of this procedure, additional testing may be performed to evaluate or monitor progression of the disease process and determine the need for a change in therapy. Evaluate test results in relation to the patient's symptoms and other tests performed.

RELATED MONOGRAPHS:

▸ Related tests include antibodies, antithyroglobulin, calcitonin and stimulation tests, parathyroid scan, radioactive iodine uptake, thyroid-binding inhibitory immunoglobulin, thyroid scan, TSH, free thyroxine, and US thyroid.

▸ Refer to the Endocrine and Immune systems tables at the end of the book for related tests by body system.

Bladder Cancer Markers, Urine

SYNONYM/ACRONYM: Nuclear matrix protein (NMP) 22, Bard BTA, cytogenic marker for bladder cancer.

COMMON USE: To assist in diagnosing bladder cancer.

SPECIMEN: Urine (5 mL), unpreserved random specimen collected in a clean plastic collection container for NMP22 and Bard BTA; urine (30 mL), first void specimen collected in fixative specific for FISH testing.

REFERENCE VALUE: (Method: Enzyme immunoassay for NMP22, immunochromatographic for Bard BTA, fluorescence in situ hybridization [FISH] for cytogenic marker)

NMP22: Negative: Less than 6 units/mL, borderline: 6 to 10 units/mL, positive: Greater than 10 units/mL

Bard BTA: Negative

Cytogenic Marker: Negative

DESCRIPTION: Cystoscopy is still considered the gold standard for detection of bladder cancer, but other noninvasive tests have been developed, including several urine assays approved by the Food and Drug Administration. Compared to cytological studies, these assays are believed to be more sensitive but less specific for detecting transitional cell carcinoma. FISH is a cytogenic technique that uses fluorescent-labeled DNA probes to detect specific chromosome abnormalities. The FISH bladder cancer assay specifically detects the presence of aneuploidy for chromosomes 3, 7, and 17 and absence of the 9p21 loci, findings associated with transitional cell cancer of the bladder.

NMP22: Nuclear matrix proteins (NMPs) are involved in the regulation and expression of various genes. The NMP identified as NuMA is abundant in bladder tumor cells. The dying tumor cells release the soluble NMP into the urine. This assay is quantitative.

Bladder tumor antigen (BTA): A human complement factor H-related protein (hCFHrp) is thought to be produced by bladder tumor cells as protection from the body's natural immune response. BTA is released from tumor cells into the urine. This assay is qualitative.

INDICATIONS
• Detection of bladder carcinoma
• Management of recurrent bladder cancer

POTENTIAL DIAGNOSIS
Increased in bladder carcinoma.

CRITICAL FINDINGS
• Bladder carcinoma

It is essential that critical diagnoses be communicated immediately to the requesting health-care provider (HCP). A listing of these diagnoses varies among facilities.

INTERFERING FACTORS
• *NMP22:* Any condition that results in inflammation of the bladder or urinary tract may cause falsely elevated values.
• *Bard BTA:* Recent surgery, biopsy, or other trauma to the bladder or urinary tract may cause falsely elevated values. Bacterial overgrowth from active urinary tract infection, renal or bladder calculi, gross contamination from blood, and positive leukocyte dipstick may also cause false-positive results.
• *Cytogenic marker:* Incorrect fixative, gross contamination from blood, bacterial overgrowth from active urinary tract infection, inadequate number of bladder cells in specimen.

B

NURSING IMPLICATIONS AND PROCEDURE

PRETEST:

- Positively identify the patient using at least two unique identifiers before providing care, treatment, or services.
- *Patient Teaching:* Inform the patient this procedure can assist in establishing a diagnosis of bladder disease.
- Obtain a history of the patient's complaints, including a list of known allergens.
- Obtain a history of the patient's genitourinary system, symptoms, and results of previously performed laboratory tests and diagnostic and surgical procedures.
- Note any recent procedures that can interfere with test results.
- Obtain a list of the patient's current medications including herbs, nutritional supplements, and nutraceuticals (see Appendix F).
- Review the procedure with the patient. Address concerns about pain and explain that there should be no discomfort during the procedure. Inform the patient that specimen collection takes approximately 5 min, depending on the cooperation and ability of the patient.
- *Sensitivity to social and cultural issues,* as well as concern for modesty, is important in providing psychological support before, during, and after the procedure.
- There are no food, fluid, or medication restrictions unless by medical direction.

INTRATEST:

- Instruct the patient to cooperate fully and to follow directions.
- Observe standard precautions, and follow the general guidelines in Appendix A. Positively identify the patient, and label the appropriate collection container with the corresponding patient demographics, date, and time of collection.

- Obtain urine specimen in a clean plastic collection container. Promptly transport the specimen to the laboratory for processing and analysis.

POST-TEST:

- A report of the results will be sent to the requesting HCP, who will discuss the results with the patient.
- Recognize anxiety related to test results, and be supportive of fear of shortened life expectancy. Discuss the implications of abnormal test results on the patient's lifestyle. Provide teaching and information regarding the clinical implications of the test results, as appropriate. Educate the patient regarding access to counseling services. Provide contact information, if desired, for the American Cancer Society (www.cancer.org) or the National Cancer Institute (www.cancer.gov).
- Reinforce information given by the patient's HCP regarding further testing, treatment, or referral to another HCP. The greatest risk factor for bladder cancer is smoking. Inform the patient of smoking cessation programs as appropriate. Answer any questions or address any concerns voiced by the patient or family.
- Depending on the results of this procedure, additional testing may be performed to evaluate or monitor progression of the disease process and determine the need for a change in therapy. Evaluate test results in relation to the patient's symptoms and other tests performed.

RELATED MONOGRAPHS:

- Related tests include biopsy bladder, cytology urine, cystoscopy, IVP, and US bladder.
- Refer to the Genitourinary System table at the end of the book for related tests by body system.

Bleeding Time

SYNONYM/ACRONYM: Mielke bleeding time, Simplate bleeding time, template bleeding time, Surgicutt bleeding time, Ivy bleeding time.

COMMON USE: To evaluate platelet function.

SPECIMEN: Whole blood.

REFERENCE VALUE: (Method: Timed observation of incision)
Template: 2.5 to 10 min
Ivy: 2 to 7 min
Slight differences exist in the disposable devices used to make the incision. Although the Mielke or template bleeding time is believed to offer greater standardization to a fairly subjective procedure, both methods are thought to be of equal sensitivity and reproducibility.

POTENTIAL DIAGNOSIS

This test does not predict excessive bleeding during a surgical procedure.

Prolonged In
- Bernard-Soulier syndrome *(evidenced by a rare hereditary condition in which platelet glycoprotein GP1b is deficient and platelet aggregation is decreased)*
- Fibrinogen disorders *(fibrinogen helps platelets link together)*
- Glanzmann's thrombasthenia *(evidenced by a rare hereditary condition in which platelet glycoprotein IIb/IIIa is deficient and platelet aggregation is decreased)*
- Hereditary telangiectasia *(evidenced by fragile blood vessels that do not permit adequate constriction to stop bleeding)*
- Liver disease *(related to decreased production of coagulation proteins that affect bleeding time)*
- Some myeloproliferative disorders *(evidenced by disorders of decreased platelet production)*
- Renal disease *(related to abnormal platelet function)*
- Thrombocytopenia *(evidenced by insufficient platelets to stop bleeding)*
- von Willebrand's disease *(evidenced by deficiency of von Willebrand factor, necessary for normal platelet adhesion)*

Decreased in: N/A

CRITICAL FINDINGS
- Greater than 14 min

Note and immediately report to the health-care provider (HCP) any critically increased values and related symptoms.

Find and print out the full monograph at DavisPlus (http://davisplus.fadavis .com, keyword Van Leeuwen).

Blood Gases

SYNONYM/ACRONYM: Arterial blood gases (ABGs), venous blood gases, capillary blood gases, cord blood gases.

COMMON USE: To assess oxygenation and acid base balance.

SPECIMEN: Whole blood. Specimen volume and collection container may vary with collection method. See Intratest section for specific collection instructions. Specimen should be tightly capped and transported in an ice slurry.

REFERENCE VALUE: (Method: Selective electrodes for pH, Pco_2 and Po_2)

Blood Gas Value (pH)	Birth, Cord, Full Term	Adult/Child
Arterial	7.11–7.36	7.35–7.45
Venous	7.25–7.45	7.32–7.43
Capillary	7.32–7.49	7.35–7.45
Scalp	7.25–7.40	N/A

Note: SI units (conversion factor × 1).

P_{CO_2}	Arterial	SI Units (Conventional Units $\times$ 0.133)	Venous	SI Units (Conventional Units $\times$ 0.133)	Capillary	SI Units (Conventional Units $\times$ 0.133)
Birth, cord, full term	32–66 mm Hg	4.3–8.8 kPa	27–49 mm Hg	3.6–6.5 kPa	—	—
Adult/child	35–45 mm Hg	4.66–5.98 kPa	41–51 mm Hg	5.4–6.8 kPa	26–41 mm Hg	3.5–5.4 kPa

P_{O_2}	Arterial	SI Units (Conventional Units $\times$ 0.133)	Venous	SI Units (Conventional Units $\times$ 0.133)	Capillary	SI Units (Conventional Units $\times$ 0.133)
Birth, cord, full term	8–24 mm Hg	1.1–3.2 kPa	17–41 mm Hg	2.3–5.4 kPa	—	—
Adult/child	80–95 mm Hg	10.6–12.6 kPa	20–49 mm Hg	2.6–6.5 kPa	80–95 mm Hg	10.6–12.6 kPa

HCO_3^-	Arterial SI Units mmol/L (Conventional Units × 1)	Venous SI Units mmol/L (Conventional Units × 1)	Capillary SI Units mmol/L (Conventional Units × 1)
Birth, cord, full term	17–24 mEq/L	17–24 mEq/L	N/A
2 mo to 2 yr	16–23 mEq/L	24–28 mEq/Lq	18–23 mEq/L
Adult	22–26 mEq/L	24–28 mEq/Lq	18–23 mEq/L

O_2 Sat	Arterial	Venous	Capillary
Birth, cord, full term	40–90%	40–70%	–
Adult/child	95–99%	70–75%	95–98%

Tco_2	Arterial Conventional & SI Units	Venous Conventional & SI Units
Birth, cord, full term	13–22 mmol/L	14–22 mmol/L
Adult/child	22–29 mmol/L	25–30 mmol/L

Base Excess Arterial	SI Units mmol/L (Conventional Units × 1)
Birth, cord, full term	(–10) – (–2) mEq/L
Adult/child	(–2) – (+3) mEq/L

DESCRIPTION: Blood gas analysis is used to evaluate respiratory function and provide a measure for determining acid-base balance. Respiratory, renal, and cardiovascular system functions are integrated in order to maintain normal acid-base balance. Therefore, respiratory or metabolic disorders may cause abnormal blood gas findings. The blood gas measurements commonly reported are pH, partial pressure of carbon dioxide in the blood (Pco_2), partial pressure of oxygen in the blood (Po_2), bicarbonate (HCO_3^-), O_2 saturation, and base excess (BE) or base deficit (BD). pH reflects the number of free hydrogen ions (H^+) in the body. A pH less than 7.35 indicates acidosis. A pH greater than 7.45 indicates alkalosis. Changes in the ratio of free H^+ to HCO_3 will result in a compensatory response from the lungs or kidneys to restore proper acid-base balance.

Pco_2 is an important indicator of ventilation. The level of Pco_2 is controlled primarily by the lungs and is referred to as the respiratory component of acid-base balance. The main buffer system in the body is the bicarbonate–carbonic acid system. Bicarbonate is an important alkaline ion that participates along with other anions, such as hemoglobin, proteins, and phosphates, to neutralize acids.

For the body to maintain proper balance, there must be a ratio of 20 parts bicarbonate to one part carbonic acid (20:1). Carbonic acid level is indirectly measured by P_{CO_2}. Bicarbonate level is indirectly measured by the total carbon dioxide content (T_{CO_2}). The carbonic acid level is not measured directly but can be estimated because it is 3% of the P_{CO_2}. Bicarbonate can also be calculated from these numbers once the carbonic acid value has been obtained because of the 20:1 ratio. For example, if the P_{CO_2} were 40, the carbonic acid would be calculated as (3% × 40) or 1.2, and the HCO_3^- would be calculated as (20 × 1.2) or 24. The main acid in the acid-base system is carbonic acid. It is the metabolic or non-respiratory component of the acid-base system and is controlled by the kidney. Bicarbonate levels can either be measured directly or estimated from the T_{CO_2} in the blood. BE/BD reflects the number of anions available in the blood to help buffer changes in pH. A BD (negative BE) indicates metabolic acidosis, whereas a positive BE indicates metabolic alkalosis.

Extremes in acidosis are generally more life threatening than alkalosis. Acidosis can develop either very quickly (e.g., cardiac arrest) or over a longer period of time (e.g., renal failure). Infants can develop acidosis very quickly if they are not kept warm and given enough calories. Children with diabetes tend to go into acidosis more quickly than do adults who have been dealing with the disease over a longer period of time. In many cases, a venous or capillary specimen is satisfactory to obtain the necessary information regarding acid-base balance without subjecting the patient to an arterial puncture with its associated risks.

As seen in the table of reference ranges, P_{O_2} is lower in infants than in children and adults owing to the respective level of maturation of the lungs at birth. P_{O_2} tends to trail off after age 30, decreasing by approximately 3 to 5 mm Hg per decade as the organs age and begin to lose elasticity. The formula used to approximate the relationship between age and P_{O_2} is:

$$P_{O_2} = 104 - (age \times 0.27)$$

Like carbon dioxide, oxygen is carried in the body in a dissolved and combined (oxyhemoglobin) form. Oxygen content is the sum of the dissolved and combined oxygen. The oxygen-carrying capacity of the blood indicates how much oxygen could be carried if all the hemoglobin were saturated with oxygen. Percentage of oxygen saturation is [oxyhemoglobin concentration ÷ (oxyhemoglobin concentration + deoxyhemoglobin concentration)] × 100.

Testing on specimens other than arterial blood is often ordered when oxygen measurements are not needed or when the information regarding oxygen can be obtained by noninvasive techniques such as pulse oximetry. Capillary blood is satisfactory for most purposes for pH and P_{CO_2}; the use of capillary P_{O_2} is limited to the exclusion of hypoxia. Measurements involving oxygen are usually not useful when performed on venous samples; arterial blood is required to accurately measure P_{O_2} and oxygen saturation. Considerable evidence indicates that prolonged exposure to high levels of oxygen can result in injury, such as retinopathy of prematurity in infants or the drying of airways in any patient. Monitoring Po_2 from blood gases is especially appropriate under such circumstances.

INDICATIONS

This group of tests is used to assess conditions such as asthma, chronic obstructive pulmonary disease (COPD), embolism (e.g., fatty or other embolism) during coronary arterial bypass surgery, and hypoxia. It is also used to assist in the diagnosis of respiratory failure, which is defined as a Po_2 less than 50 mm Hg and Pco_2 greater than

50 mm Hg. Blood gases can be valuable in the management of patients on ventilators or being weaned from ventilators. Blood gas values are used to determine acid-base status, the type of imbalance, and the degree of compensation as summarized in the following section. Restoration of pH to near-normal values is referred to as fully compensated balance. When pH values are moving in the same direction (i.e., increasing or decreasing) as the Pco_2 or HCO_3^-, the imbalance is metabolic. When the pH values are moving in the opposite direction from the Pco_2 or HCO_3^-, the imbalance is caused by respiratory disturbances. To remember this concept, the following mnemonic can be useful: MeTRO = **Metabolic Together, Respiratory Opposite.**

Acid-Base Disturbance	pH	Pco_2	Po_2	HCO_3^-
Respiratory Acidosis				
Uncompensated	Decreased	Increased	Normal	Normal
Compensated	Normal	Increased	Increased	Increased
Respiratory Alkalosis				
Uncompensated	Increased	Decreased	Normal	Normal
Compensated	Normal	Decreased	Decreased	Decreased
Uncompensated	Decreased	Normal	Decreased	Decreased
Compensated	Normal	Decreased	Decreased	Decreased
Metabolic (Nonrespiratory) Acidosis				
Uncompensated	Increased	Normal	Increased	Increased
Compensated	Normal	Increased	Increased	Increased

POTENTIAL DIAGNOSIS

Acid-base imbalance is determined by evaluating pH, Pco_2, and HCO_3^- values. pH less than 7.35 reflects an acidic state, whereas pH greater than 7.45 reflects alkalosis. Pco_2 and HCO_3^- determine whether the imbalance is respiratory or nonrespira-

tory (metabolic). Because a patient may have more than one imbalance and may also be in the process of compensating, the interpretation of blood gas values may not always seem straightforward.

Respiratory conditions that interfere with normal breathing *cause CO_2 to be retained in the blood. This results in an increase of circulating carbonic acid and a corresponding decrease in pH (respiratory acidosis). Acute respiratory acidosis can occur in acute pulmonary edema, severe respiratory infections, bronchial obstruction, pneumothorax, hemothorax, open chest wounds, opiate poisoning, respiratory depressant drug therapy, and inhalation of air with a high CO_2 content. Chronic respiratory acidosis can be seen in patients with asthma, pulmonary fibrosis, emphysema, bronchiectasis, and respiratory depressant drug therapy. Respiratory conditions that increase the breathing rate cause CO_2 to be removed from the alveoli more rapidly than it is being produced. This results in an alkaline pH. Acute respiratory alkalosis may be seen in anxiety, hysteria, hyperventilation, and pulmonary embolus and with an increase in artificial ventilation. Chronic respiratory alkalosis may be seen in high fever, administration of drugs (e.g., salicylate and sulfa) that stimulate the respiratory system, hepatic coma, hypoxia of high altitude, and central nervous system (CNS) lesions or injury that result in stimulation of the respiratory center.*

Metabolic (nonrespiratory) conditions that cause the excessive formation or decreased excretion of organic or inorganic acids result in metabolic acidosis. Some of these conditions include ingestion of salicylates, ethylene glycol, and methanol, as well as uncontrolled diabetes, starvation, shock, renal disease, and

biliary or pancreatic fistula. Metabolic alkalosis results from conditions that increase pH, as can be seen in excessive intake of antacids to treat gastritis or peptic ulcer, excessive administration of HCO_3^-, loss of stomach acid caused by protracted vomiting, cystic fibrosis, or potassium and chloride deficiencies.

Respiratory Acidosis

- Decreased pH
- Decreased O_2 saturation
- Increased P_{CO_2}:
  Acute intermittent porphyria
  Anemia (severe)
  Anorexia
  Anoxia
  Asthma
  Atelectasis
  Bronchitis
  Bronchoconstriction
  Carbon monoxide poisoning
  Cardiac disorders
  Congenital heart defects
  Congestive heart failure
  COPD
  Cystic fibrosis
  Depression of respiratory center
  Drugs depressing the respiratory system
  Electrolyte disturbances (severe)
  Emphysema
  Fever
  Head injury
  Hypercapnia
  Hypothyroidism (severe)
  Near drowning
  Pleural effusion
  Pneumonia
  Pneumothorax
  Poisoning
  Poliomyelitis
  Pulmonary edema
  Pulmonary embolism
  Pulmonary tuberculosis
  Respiratory distress syndrome (adult and neonatal)

Respiratory failure
Sarcoidosis
Smoking
Tumor
- A decreased Po_2 that increases Pco_2:
  Decreased alveolar gas exchange: cancer, compression or resection of lung, respiratory distress syndrome (newborns), sarcoidosis
  Decreased ventilation or perfusion: asthma, bronchiectasis, bronchitis, cancer, croup, cystic fibrosis (mucoviscidosis), emphysema, granulomata, pneumonia, pulmonary infarction, shock
  Hypoxemia: anesthesia, carbon monoxide exposure, cardiac disorders, high altitudes, near drowning, presence of abnormal hemoglobins
  Hypoventilation: cerebrovascular incident, drugs depressing the respiratory system, head injury
  Right-to-left shunt: congenital heart disease, intrapulmonary venoarterial shunting

Compensation
- Increased Po_2:
  Hyperbaric oxygenation
  Hyperventilation
- Increased base excess:
  Increased HCO_3^- to bring pH to (near) normal

Respiratory Alkalosis
- Increased pH
- Decreased Pco_2:
  Anxiety
  CNS lesions or injuries that cause stimulation of the respiratory center
  Excessive artificial ventilation
  Fever
  Head injury
  Hyperthermia
  Hyperventilation
  Hysteria
  Salicylate intoxication

Compensation
- Decreased Po_2:
  Rebreather mask

- Decreased base excess:
  Decreased HCO_3^- to bring pH to (near) normal

Metabolic Acidosis
- Decreased pH
- Decreased HCO_3^-
- Decreased base excess
- Decreased Tco_2:
  Decreased excretion of H^+: acquired (e.g., drugs, hypercalcemia), Addison's disease, diabetic ketoacidosis, Fanconi's syndrome, inherited (e.g., cystinosis, Wilson's disease), renal failure, renal tubular acidosis
  Increased acid intake
  Increased formation of acids: diabetic ketoacidosis, high-fat/low-carbohydrate diets
  Increased loss of alkaline body fluids: diarrhea, excess potassium, fistula
  Renal disease

Compensation
- Decreased Pco_2:
  Hyperventilation

Metabolic Alkalosis
- Increased pH
- Increased HCO_3^-
- Increased base excess
- Increased Tco_2:
  Alkali ingestion (excessive)
  Anoxia
  Gastric suctioning
  Hypochloremic states
  Hypokalemic states
  Potassium depletion: Cushing's disease, diarrhea, diuresis, excessive vomiting, excessive ingestion of licorice, inadequate potassium intake, potassium-losing nephropathy, steroid administration
  Salicylate intoxication
  Shock
  Vomiting

Compensation
- Increased Tco_2:
  Hypoventilation

CRITICAL FINDINGS

Arterial Blood Gas Parameter	Less Than	Greater Than
pH	7.20	7.60
HCO_3^-	10 mmol/L	40 mmol/L
Pco_2	20 mm Hg	67 mm Hg
Po_2	45 mm Hg	

Note and immediately report to the health-care provider (HCP) any critically increased or decreased values and related symptoms.

INTERFERING FACTORS

- Drugs that may cause an increase in HCO_3^- include acetylsalicylic acid (initially), antacids, carbenicillin, carbenoxolone, ethacrynic acid, glycyrrhiza (licorice), laxatives, mafenide, and sodium bicarbonate.
- Drugs that may cause a decrease in HCO_3^- include acetazolamide, acetylsalicylic acid (long term or high doses), citrates, dimethadione, ether, ethylene glycol, fluorides, mercury compounds (laxatives), methylenedioxyamphetamine, paraldehyde, and xylitol.
- Drugs that may cause an increase in Pco_2 include acetylsalicylic acid, aldosterone bicarbonate, carbenicillin, carbenoxolone, corticosteroids, dexamethasone, ethacrynic acid, laxatives (chronic abuse), and x-ray contrast agents.
- Drugs that may cause a decrease in Pco_2 include acetazolamide, acetylsalicylic acid, ethamivan, neuromuscular relaxants (secondary to postoperative hyperventilation), NSD 3004 (arterial long-acting carbonic anhydrase inhibitor), theophylline, tromethamine, and xylitol.
- Drugs that may cause an increase in Po_2 include theophylline and urokinase.
- Drugs that may cause a decrease in Po_2 include althesin, barbiturates, granulocyte-macrophage colony-stimulating factor, isoproterenol, and meperidine.

- Samples for blood gases are obtained by arterial puncture, which carries a risk of bleeding, especially in patients who have bleeding disorders or are taking anticoagulants or other blood thinning medications.
- Recent blood transfusion may produce misleading values.
- Specimens with extremely elevated white blood cell counts will undergo misleading decreases in pH resulting from cellular metabolism, if transport to the laboratory is delayed.
- Specimens collected soon after a change in inspired oxygen has occurred will not accurately reflect the patient's oxygenation status.
- Specimens collected within 20 to 30 min of respiratory passage suctioning or other respiratory therapy will not be accurate.
- Excessive differences in actual body temperature relative to normal body temperature will not be reflected in the results. Temperature affects the amount of gas in solution. Blood gas analyzers measure samples at 37°C (98.6°F); therefore, if the patient is hyperthermic or hypothermic, it is important to notify the laboratory of the patient's actual body temperature at the time the specimen was collected. Fever will increase actual Po_2 and Pco_2 values;

therefore, the uncorrected values measured at 37°C will be falsely decreased. Hypothermia decreases actual Po_2 and Pco_2 values; therefore, the uncorrected values measured at 37°C will be falsely increased.

• A falsely increased O_2 saturation may occur because of elevated levels of carbon monoxide in the blood.

• O_2 saturation is a calculated parameter based on an assumption of 100% hemoglobin A. Values may be misleading when hemoglobin variants with different oxygen dissociation curves are present. Hemoglobin S will cause a shift to the right, indicating decreased oxygen binding. Fetal hemoglobin and methemoglobin will cause a shift to the left, indicating increased oxygen binding.

• Excessive amounts of heparin in the sample may falsely decrease pH, Pco_2, and Po_2.

• Citrates should never be used as an anticoagulant in evacuated collection tubes for venous blood gas determinations because citrates will cause a marked analytic decrease in pH.

• Air bubbles or blood clots in the specimen are cause for rejection. Air bubbles in the specimen can falsely elevate or decrease the results depending on the patient's blood gas status. If an evacuated tube is used for venous blood gas specimen collection, the tube must be removed from the needle before the needle is withdrawn from the arm or else the sample will be contaminated with room air.

• Specimens should be placed in ice slurry immediately after collection because blood cells continue to carry out metabolic processes in the specimen after it has been removed from the patient. These

natural life processes can affect pH, Po_2, Pco_2, and the other calculated values in a short period of time. The cold temperature provided by the ice slurry will slow down, but not completely stop, metabolic changes occurring in the sample over time. Iced specimens not analyzed within 60 min of collection should be rejected for analysis.

NURSING IMPLICATIONS AND PROCEDURE

PRETEST:

▶ Positively identify the patient using at least two unique identifiers before providing care, treatment, or services.

▶ *Patient Teaching:* Inform the patient this test can assist in assessing blood oxygen balance and oxygenation level.

▶ Obtain a history of the patient's complaints, including a list of known allergens, especially allergies or sensitivities to latex and anesthetics.

▶ Obtain a history of the patient's cardiovascular, genitourinary, and respiratory systems, any bleeding disorders or other symptoms, and results of previously performed laboratory tests and diagnostic and surgical procedures.

▶ Note any recent procedures that can interfere with test results.

▶ Obtain a list of the patient's current medications, including anticoagulants, aspirin and other salicylates, herbs, nutritional supplements, and nutraceuticals (see Appendix F).

▶ Record the patient's temperature.

▶ Indicate the type of oxygen, mode of oxygen delivery, and delivery rate as part of the test requisition process. Wait 30 min after a change in type or mode of oxygen delivery or rate for specimen collection.

▶ Review the procedure with the patient and advise rest for 30 min before specimen collection. Explain to the patient that an arterial puncture may be painful. The site may be anesthetized with 1% to 2% lidocaine before puncture. Inform the patient that specimen collection and postprocedure care of the puncture site usually take 10 to 15 min. The person collecting the specimen should be notified beforehand if the patient is receiving anticoagulant therapy or taking aspirin or other natural products that may prolong bleeding from the puncture site.

❖ If the sample is to be collected by radial artery puncture, perform an Allen test before puncture to ensure that the patient has adequate collateral circulation to the hand if thrombosis of the radial artery occurs after arterial puncture. The modified Allen test is performed as follows: Extend the patient's wrist over a rolled towel. Ask the patient to make a fist with the hand extended over the towel. Use the second and third fingers to locate the pulses of the ulnar and radial arteries on the palmar surface of the wrist. (The thumb should not be used to locate these arteries because it has a pulse.) Compress both arteries and ask the patient to open and close the fist several times until the palm turns pale. Release pressure on the ulnar artery only. Color should return to the palm within 5 sec if the ulnar artery is functioning. This is a positive Allen test, and blood gases may be drawn from the radial artery site. The Allen test should then be performed on the opposite hand. The hand to which color is restored fastest has better circulation and should be selected for specimen collection.

Sensitivity to social and cultural issues, as well as concern for modesty, is important in providing psychological support before, during, and after the procedure.

There are no food, fluid, or medication restrictions unless by medical direction.

Prepare an ice slurry in a cup or plastic bag to have ready for immediate transport of the specimen to the laboratory.

INTRATEST:

If the patient has a history of allergic reaction to latex, avoid the use of equipment containing latex.

Instruct the patient to cooperate fully and to follow directions. Direct the patient to breathe normally and to avoid unnecessary movement.

Observe standard precautions and follow the general guidelines in Appendix A. Positively identify the patient and label the appropriate tubes with the corresponding patient demographics, date, and time of collection.

Arterial

Perform an arterial puncture and collect the specimen in an air-free heparinized syringe. There is no demonstrable difference in results between samples collected in plastic syringes and samples collected in glass syringes. It is very important that no room air be introduced into the collection container because the gases in the room and in the sample will begin equilibrating immediately. The end of the syringe must be stoppered immediately after the needle is withdrawn and removed. Apply a pressure dressing over the puncture site. Samples should be mixed by gently rolling the syringe to ensure proper mixing of the heparin with the sample, which prevents the formation of small clots leading to rejection of the sample. The tightly capped sample should be placed in an ice slurry immediately after collection. Information on the specimen label should be protected from water in the ice slurry by first placing the specimen in a protective plastic bag. Promptly transport the specimen to the laboratory for processing and analysis.

Venous

Central venous blood is collected in a heparinized syringe.

Venous blood is collected percutaneously by venipuncture in a 5-mL green-top (heparin) tube (for adult patients) or a heparinized Microtainer (for pediatric patients). The vacuum collection tube must be removed from the needle before the needle is removed from the patient's arm. Apply a pressure dressing over the puncture site. Samples should be mixed by gently rolling the syringe to ensure proper mixing of the heparin with the sample, which prevents the formation of small clots leading to rejection of the sample. The tightly capped sample should be placed in an ice slurry immediately after collection. Information on the specimen label should be protected from water in the ice slurry by first placing the specimen in a protective plastic bag. Promptly transport the specimen to the laboratory for processing and analysis.

Capillary
▶ Perform a capillary puncture and collect the specimen in two 250-μL heparinized capillaries (scalp or heel for neonatal patients) or a heparinized Microtainer (for pediatric patients). Observe standard precautions and follow the general guidelines in Appendix A. The capillary tubes should be filled as much as possible and capped on both ends. Some hospitals recommend that metal "fleas" be added to the capillary tube before the ends are capped. During transport, a magnet can be moved up and down the outside of the capillary tube to facilitate mixing and prevent the formation of clots, which would cause rejection of the sample. It is important to inform the laboratory or respiratory therapy staff of the number of fleas used so the fleas can be accounted for and removed before the sample is introduced into the blood gas analyzers. Fleas left in the sample may damage the blood gas equipment if allowed to enter the analyzer. Microtainer samples should be mixed by gently rolling the capillary tube to ensure proper mixing of the heparin with the sample, which prevents the formation of small clots leading to rejection of the sample. Promptly transport the specimen to the laboratory for processing and analysis.

Cord Blood
▶ The sample may be collected directly from the cord, using a syringe. The tightly capped sample should be placed in an ice slurry immediately after collection. Information on the specimen label should be protected from water in the ice slurry by first placing the specimen in a protective plastic bag. Promptly transport the specimen to the laboratory for processing and analysis.

Scalp Sample
▶ Samples for scalp pH may be collected anaerobically before delivery in special

scalp-sample collection capillaries and transported immediately to the laboratory for analysis. Some hospitals recommend that fleas be added to the scalp tube before the ends are capped. See preceding section on capillary collection for discussion of fleas.

POST-TEST:
▶ A report of the results will be sent to the requesting HCP, who will discuss the results with the patient.
▶ Pressure should be applied to the puncture site for at least 5 min in the unanticoagulated patient and for at least 15 min in the case of a patient receiving anticoagulant therapy. Observe/assess puncture site for bleeding or hematoma formation. Apply pressure bandage.
▶ Observe/assess the patient for signs or symptoms of respiratory acidosis, such as dyspnea, headache, tachycardia, pallor, diaphoresis, apprehension, drowsiness, coma, hypertension, or disorientation.
▶ Teach the patient breathing exercises to assist with the appropriate exchange of oxygen and carbon dioxide.
▶ Administer oxygen, if appropriate.
▶ Teach the patient how to properly use the incentive spirometer device or mininebulizer if ordered.
▶ Observe/assess the patient for signs or symptoms of respiratory alkalosis, such as tachypnea, restlessness, agitation, tetany, numbness, seizures, muscle cramps, dizziness, or tingling fingertips.
▶ Instruct the patient to breathe deeply and slowly; performing this type of breathing exercise into a paper bag decreases hyperventilation and quickly helps the patient's breathing return to normal.
▶ Observe/assess the patient for signs or symptoms of metabolic acidosis, such as rapid breathing, flushed skin, nausea, vomiting, dysrhythmias, coma, hypotension, hyperventilation, and restlessness.
▶ Observe/assess the patient for signs or symptoms of metabolic alkalosis, such as shallow breathing, weakness, dysrhythmias, tetany, hypokalemia, hyperactive reflexes, and excessive vomiting.

▶ *Nutritional Considerations:* Abnormal blood gas values may be associated with diseases of the respiratory system. Malnutrition is commonly seen in patients with severe respiratory disease for reasons including fatigue, lack of appetite, and gastrointestinal distress. Research has estimated that the daily caloric intake required for respiration of patients with COPD is 10 times higher than that of normal individuals. Inadequate nutrition can result in hypophosphatemia, especially in the respirator-dependent patient. During periods of starvation, phosphorus leaves the intracellular space and moves outside the tissue, resulting in dangerously decreased phosphorus levels. Adequate intake of vitamins A and C is also important to prevent pulmonary infection and to decrease the extent of lung tissue damage. The importance of following the prescribed diet should be stressed to the patient and/or caregiver.

▶ Water balance needs to be closely monitored in COPD patients. Fluid retention can lead to pulmonary edema.

▶ Reinforce information given by the patient's HCP regarding further testing, treatment, or referral to another HCP. Answer any questions or address any concerns voiced by the patient or family.

▶ Depending on the results of this procedure, additional testing may be performed to evaluate or monitor progression of the disease process and determine the need for a change in therapy. Evaluate test results in relation to the patient's symptoms and other tests performed.

RELATED MONOGRAPHS:

▶ Related tests include α_1-AT, anion gap, arterial/alveolar oxygen ratio, biopsy lung, bronchoscopy, carboxyhemoglobin, chest x-ray, chloride sweat, CBC hemoglobin, CBC WBC and diff, culture and smear for mycobacteria, culture bacterial sputum, culture viral, cytology sputum, electrolytes, gram stain, IgE, lactic acid, lung perfusion scan, lung ventilation scan, osmolality, phosphorus, plethysmography, pleural fluid analysis, pulse oximetry, PFT, and TB skin tests.

▶ Refer to the Cardiovascular, Genitourinary, and Respiratory systems tables at the end of the book for related tests by body system.

Blood Groups and Antibodies

SYNONYM/ACRONYM: ABO group and Rh typing, blood group antibodies, type and screen, type and crossmatch.

COMMON USE: To identify ABO blood group and Rh type, typically for transfusion purposes.

SPECIMEN: Serum (2 mL) collected in a red-top tube or whole blood (2 mL) collected in a lavender-top (EDTA) tube.

REFERENCE VALUE: (Method: FDA-approved reagents with glass slides, glass tubes, gel, or automated systems) Compatibility (no clumping or hemolysis).

Blood Type	Rh Type (With Any ABO)	Other Antibodies That React at 37°C or With Antiglobulin	Other Antibodies That React at Room Temperature or Below
A	Positive	Kell	Lewis
B	Negative	Duffy	P
AB		Kidd	MN
O		S	Cold agglutinins
		s	
		U	

DESCRIPTION: Blood typing is a series of tests that include the ABO and Rh blood-group system performed to detect surface antigens on red blood cells (RBCs) by an agglutination test and compatibility tests to determine antibodies against these antigens. The major antigens in the ABO system are A and B, although AB and O are also common phenotypes. The patient with A antigens has group A blood; the patient with B antigens has group B blood. The patient with both A and B antigens has group AB blood (universal recipient); the patient with neither A nor B antigens has group O blood (universal donor). Blood group and type is genetically determined. After 6 mo of age, individuals develop serum antibodies that react with A or B antigen absent from their own RBCs. These are called *anti-A* and *anti-B antibodies*.

In ABO blood typing, the patient's RBCs mix with anti-A and anti-B sera, a process known as forward grouping. The process then reverses, and the patient's serum mixes with type A and B cells in *reverse grouping*.

Generally, only blood with the same ABO group and Rh type as the recipient is

transfused because the anti-A and anti-B antibodies are strong agglutinins that cause a rapid, complement-mediated destruction of incompatible cells. However, blood donations have decreased nationwide, creating shortages in the available supply. Safe substitutions with blood of a different group and/or Rh type may occur depending on the inventory of available units. Many laboratories require consultation with the requesting health-care provider (HCP) prior to issuing Rh-positive units to an Rh-negative individual.

ABO and Rh testing is also performed as a prenatal screen in pregnant women to identify the risk of hemolytic disease of the newborn. Although most of the anti-A and anti-B activity resides in the immunoglobulin M (IgM) class of immunoglobulins, some activity rests with immunoglobulin G (IgG). Anti-A and anti-B antibodies of the IgG class coat the RBCs without immediately affecting their viability and can readily cross the placenta, resulting in hemolytic disease of the newborn. Individuals with type O blood frequently have more IgG anti-A and anti-B than other people; thus, ABO hemolytic disease of the newborn will affect infants of type O mothers almost exclusively (unless the newborn is also type O).

Major antigens of the Rh system are D (or Rh_o), C, E, c, and e. Individuals whose RBCs possess D antigen are called Rh-positive; those who lack D antigen are called Rh-negative, no matter what other Rh antigens are present. Individuals who are Rh-negative produce anti-D antibodies when exposed to Rh-positive cells by either transfusions or pregnancy. These anti-D antibodies cross the placenta to the fetus and can cause hemolytic disease of the newborn or transfusion reactions if Rh-positive blood is administered.

INDICATIONS

- Determine ABO and Rh compatibility of donor and recipient before transfusion (type and screen or crossmatch).
- Determine anti-D antibody titer of Rh-negative mothers after sensitization by pregnancy with an Rh-positive fetus.
- Determine the need for a micro-dose of immunosuppressive therapy (e.g., with Rhogam) during the first 12 wk of gestation or a standard dose after 12 wk of gestation for complications such as abortion, miscarriage, vaginal hemorrhage, ectopic pregnancy, or abdominal trauma.
- Determine Rh blood type and perform antibody screen of prenatal patients on initial visit to determine maternal Rh type and to indicate whether maternal RBCs have been sensitized by any antibodies known to cause hemolytic disease of the newborn, especially anti-D antibody.

Rh blood type, antibody screen, and antibody titration (if an antibody has been identified) will be rechecked at 28 wk of gestation and prior to injection of prophylactic standard dose of $Rh_o(D)$ immune globulin Rhogam IM or Rhophylac IM or IV for Rh-negative mothers. These tests will also be repeated after delivery of an Rh-positive fetus to an Rh-negative mother and prior to injection of prophylactic standard dose of $Rh_o(D)$ immune globulin (if maternal Rh-negative blood has not been previously sensitized with Rh-positive cells resulting in a positive anti-D antibody titer). A postpartum blood sample must be evaluated for fetal-maternal bleed on all Rh-negative mothers to determine the need for additional doses of Rh immune globulin. One in 300 cases will demonstrate hemorrhage greater than 15 mL of blood and require additional $Rh_o(D)$ immune globulin.

- Identify donor ABO and Rh blood type for stored blood.
- Identify maternal and infant ABO and Rh blood types to predict risk of hemolytic disease of the newborn.
- Identify the patient's ABO and Rh blood type, especially before a procedure in which blood loss is a threat or blood replacement may be needed.
- Identify any unusual transfusion related antibodies in the patient's blood, especially before a procedure in which blood replacement may be needed.

POTENTIAL DIAGNOSIS

- ABO system: A, B, AB, or O specific to person
- Rh system: positive or negative specific to person
- Crossmatching: compatibility between donor and recipient
- Incompatibility indicated by clumping (agglutination) of red blood cells

Group and Type	Incidence (%)	Alternative Transfusion Group and Type of PACKED CELL UNITS in Order of Preference If Patient's Own Group and Type Not Available
O positive	37.4	O negative
O negative	6.6	O positive*
A positive	35.7	A negative, O positive, O negative
A negative	6.3	O negative, A positive,* O positive*
B positive	8.5	B negative, O positive, O negative
B negative	1.5	O negative, B positive,* O positive*
AB positive	3.4	AB negative, A positive, B positive, A negative, B negative, O positive, O negative
AB negative	0.6	A negative, B negative, O negative, AB positive,* A positive,* B positive,* O positive*
Rh Type		
Rh positive	85–90	
Rh negative	10–15	

*If blood units of exact match to the patient's group and type are not available, a switch in ABO blood group is preferable to a change in Rh type. However, in extreme circumstances, Rh-positive blood can be issued to an Rh-negative recipient. It is very likely that the recipient will develop antibodies as the result of receiving Rh-positive red blood cells. Rh antibodies are highly immunogenic, and, once the antibodies are developed, the recipient can only receive Rh-negative blood for subsequent red blood cell transfusion.

CRITICAL FINDINGS

Note and immediately report to the HCP any signs and symptoms associated with a blood transfusion reaction.

Signs and symptoms of blood transfusion reaction range from mildly febrile to anaphylactic and may include chills, dyspnea, fever, headache, nausea, vomiting, palpitations and tachycardia, chest or back pain, apprehension, flushing, hives, angioedema, diarrhea, hypotension, oliguria, hemoglobinuria, renal failure, sepsis, shock, and jaundice. Complications from disseminated intravascular coagulation (DIC) may also occur.

Possible interventions in mildly febrile reactions include slowing the rate of infusion, then verifying and comparing patient identification, transfusion requisition, and blood bag label. The patient should be monitored closely for further development of signs and symptoms. Administration of epinephrine may be ordered.

Possible interventions in a more severe transfusion reaction may include immediate cessation of infusion, notification of the HCP, keeping the IV line open with saline or lactated Ringer's solution, collection of red- and lavender-top tubes for posttransfusion work-up, collection of urine, monitoring vital signs every 5 min, ordering additional testing if DIC is suspected, maintaining patent airway and blood pressure, and administering mannitol. See Appendix D for a more detailed description of transfusion reactions and potential nursing interventions.

INTERFERING FACTORS

• Drugs, including levodopa, methyldopa, methyldopate hydrochloride, and cephalexin, may cause a false-positive result in Rh typing and in antibody screens.
• Recent administration of blood, blood products, dextran, or IV contrast medium causes cellular aggregation resembling agglutination in ABO typing.
• Contrast material such as iodine, barium, and gadolinium may interfere with testing.
• Abnormal proteins, cold agglutinins, and bacteremia may interfere with testing.
• Testing does not detect every antibody and may miss the presence of a weak antibody.
• History of bone marrow transplant, cancer, or leukemia may cause discrepancy in ABO typing.

NURSING IMPLICATIONS AND PROCEDURE

PRETEST:

▶ Positively identify the patient using at least two unique identifiers before providing care, treatment, or services.
▶ *Patient Teaching:* Inform the patient this test can assist in identification of blood type.
▶ Obtain a history of the patient's complaints, including a list of known allergens, especially allergies or sensitivities to latex.
▶ Obtain a history of the patient's immune and hematopoietic systems,

symptoms, and results of previously performed laboratory tests and diagnostic and surgical procedures.
▶ Note any recent or past procedures, especially blood or blood product transfusion or bone marrow transplantation, that could complicate or interfere with test results.
▶ Obtain a list of the patient's current medications including herbs, nutritional supplements, and nutraceuticals (see Appendix F).
▶ Review the procedure with the patient. Inform the patient that specimen collection takes approximately 5 to 10 min. Address concerns about pain and explain that there may be some discomfort during the venipuncture.
▶ *Sensitivity to social and cultural issues,* as well as concern for modesty, is important in providing psychological support before, during, and after the procedure.
▶ There are no food, fluid, or medication restrictions unless by medical direction.
▶ *Make sure a written and informed consent has been signed prior to any transfusion of ABO- and Rh-compatible blood products.*

INTRATEST:

▶ If the patient has a history of allergic reaction to latex, avoid the use of equipment containing latex.
▶ Instruct the patient to cooperate fully and to follow directions. Direct the patient to breathe normally and to avoid unnecessary movement.
▶ Observe standard precautions, and follow the general guidelines in Appendix A. Positively identify the patient, and label the appropriate tubes with the corresponding patient demographics, date, and time of collection. Perform a venipuncture.
▶ Although correct patient identification is important for test specimens, it is crucial when blood is collected for type and crossmatch because clerical error is the most frequent cause of life-threatening ABO

incompatibility. Therefore, additional requirements are necessary, including the verification of two unique identifiers that could include any two unique patient demographics such as name, date of birth, Social Security number, hospital number, date, or blood bank number on requisition and specimen labels; completing and applying a wristband on the arm with the same information; and placing labels with the same information and blood bank number on blood sample tubes.

▶ Remove the needle and apply direct pressure with dry gauze to stop bleeding. Observe/assess venipuncture site for bleeding or hematoma formation and secure gauze with adhesive bandage.

▶ Promptly transport the specimen to the laboratory for processing and analysis.

POST-TEST:

▶ A report of the results will be sent to the requesting HCP, who will discuss the results with the patient.

▶ Inform the patient of ABO blood and Rh type, and advise him or her to record the information on a card or other document routinely carried.

▶ Inform women who are Rh-negative to inform the HCP of their Rh-negative status if they become pregnant or need a transfusion.

▶ Reinforce information given by the patient's HCP regarding further testing, treatment, or referral to another HCP. Answer any questions or address any concerns voiced by the patient or family.

▶ Depending on the results of this procedure, additional testing may be performed to evaluate or monitor progression of the disease process and determine the need for a change in therapy. Evaluate test results in relation to the patient's symptoms and other tests performed.

RELATED MONOGRAPHS:

▶ Related tests include Coomb's antiglobulin, bilirubin, CBC, CBC hematocrit, CBC hemoglobin, CBC platelet count, CBC RBC count, cold agglutinin, FDP, fecal analysis, GI blood loss scan, haptoglobin, Ig A, iron, Kleihauer-Betke, laparoscopy abdominal, Meckel's diverticulum scan, and UA.

▶ Refer to Appendix D, Transfusion Reactions, at the end of the book for further information regarding findings and potential nursing interventions associated with types of transfusion reactions.

▶ Refer to the Immune and Hematopoietic systems tables at the end of the book for related tests by body system.

Blood Pool Imaging

SYNONYM/ACRONYM: Cardiac blood pool scan, ejection fraction study, gated cardiac scan, radionuclide ventriculogram, wall motion study, MUGA.

COMMON USE: To evaluate cardiac function after myocardial infarction.

AREA OF APPLICATION: Heart.

CONTRAST: Intravenous radioactive material.

DESCRIPTION: Multigated blood pool imaging (MUGA; also known as *cardiac blood pool scan*) is used to diagnose cardiac abnormalities involving the left ventricle and myocardial wall abnormalities by imaging the blood within the cardiac chamber rather than the myocardium. The ventricular blood pool can be imaged during the initial transit of a peripherally injected, intravenous bolus of radionuclide (first-pass technique) or when the radionuclide has reached equilibrium concentration. The patient's electrocardiogram (ECG) is synchronized to the gamma camera imager and computer and therefore termed "gated." For multigated studies, technetium-99m (Tc-99m) pertechnetate is injected after an injection of pyrophosphate, allowing the labeling of circulating red blood cells; Tc-99m sulfur colloid is used for first-pass studies. Studies detect abnormalities in heart wall motion at rest or with exercise, ejection fraction, ventricular dilation, stroke volume, and cardiac output. The MUGA procedure, performed with the heart in motion, is used to obtain multiple images of the heart in contraction and relaxation during an R-to-R cardiac cycle. The resulting images can be displayed in a cinematic mode to visualize cardiac function. Repetitive data acquisitions are possible during graded levels of exercise, usually a bicycle ergometer or handgrip, to assess ventricular functional response to exercise.

After the administration of sublingual nitroglycerin, the MUGA scan can evaluate the effectiveness of the drug on ventricular function. Heart shunt imaging is done in conjunction with a resting MUGA scan to obtain ejection fraction and assess regional wall motion.

First-pass cardiac flow study is done to study heart chamber disorders, including left-to-right and right-to-left shunts, determine both right and left ventricular ejection fractions, and assess blood flow through the great vessels. The study uses a jugular or antecubital vein injection of the radionuclide.

INDICATIONS

* Aid in the diagnosis of myocardial infarction
* Aid in the diagnosis of true or false ventricular aneurysms
* Aid in the diagnosis of valvular heart disease and determining the optimal time for valve replacement surgery
* Detect left-to-right shunts and determine pulmonary-to-systemic blood flow ratios, especially in children
* Determine cardiomyopathy
* Determine drug cardiotoxicity to stop therapy before development of congestive heart failure
* Determine ischemic coronary artery disease
* Differentiate between chronic obstructive pulmonary disease and left ventricular failure
* Evaluate ventricular size, function, and wall motion after an acute episode or in chronic heart disease

- Quantitate cardiac output by calculating global or regional ejection fraction

POTENTIAL DIAGNOSIS

Normal findings in

- Normal wall motion, ejection fraction (55% to 65%), coronary blood flow, ventricular size and function, and symmetry in contractions of the left ventricle

Abnormal findings in

- Abnormal wall motion (akinesia or dyskinesia)
- Cardiac hypertrophy
- Cardiac ischemia
- Enlarged left ventricle
- Infarcted areas are akinetic
- Ischemic areas are hypokinetic
- Myocardial infarction

CRITICAL FINDINGS

- Myocardial infarction

It is essential that critical diagnoses be communicated immediately to the appropriate health-care provider (HCP). A listing of these diagnoses varies among facilities. Note and immediately report to the HCP abnormal results and related symptoms.

INTERFERING FACTORS

This procedure is contraindicated for

- Patients who are pregnant or suspected of being pregnant, unless the potential benefits of the procedure far outweigh the risks to the fetus and mother.
- Dipyridamole testing is not performed in patients with anginal pain at rest or in patients with severe atherosclerotic coronary vessels.

- Chemical stress with vasodilators should not be done to patients having asthma; bronchospasm can occur.

Factors that may impair clear imaging

- Inability of the patient to cooperate or remain still during the procedure because of age, significant pain, or mental status.
- Metallic objects within the examination field (e.g., jewelry, body rings), which may inhibit organ visualization and can produce unclear images.

Other considerations

- Conditions such as chest wall trauma, cardiac trauma, angina that is difficult to control, significant cardiac arrhythmias, or a recent cardioversion procedure may affect test results.
- Atrial fibrillation and extrasystoles invalidate the procedure.
- Suboptimal cardiac stress or patient exhaustion, preventing maximum heart rate testing, will affect results when the procedure is done in conjunction with exercise testing.
- Consultation with an HCP should occur before the procedure for radiation safety concerns regarding younger patients or patients who are lactating.
- Risks associated with radiation overexposure can result from frequent x-ray or radionuclide procedures. Personnel working in the examination area should wear badges to record their level of radiation.

NURSING IMPLICATIONS AND PROCEDURE

PRETEST:

- Positively identify the patient using at least two unique identifiers before providing care, treatment, or services.

* *Patient Teaching:* Inform the patient this procedure can assist in assessing the pumping action of the heart.
* Obtain a history of the patient's complaints, including a list of known allergens, especially allergies or sensitivities to latex, iodine, seafood, contrast medium, anesthetics, or dyes.
* Obtain a history of the patient's cardiovascular system, symptoms, and results of previously performed laboratory tests and diagnostic and surgical procedures.
* Note any recent procedures that can interfere with test results, including examinations using iodine-based contrast medium.
* Record the date of the last menstrual period and determine the possibility of pregnancy in perimenopausal women.
* Obtain a list of the patient's current medications including herbs, nutritional supplements, and nutraceuticals (see Appendix F).
* Review the procedure with the patient. Address concerns about pain related to the procedure and explain that some pain may be experienced during the test, or there may be moments of discomfort. Reassure the patient that the radionuclide poses no radioactive hazard and rarely produces side effects. Inform the patient that the procedure is performed in a nuclear medicine department by an HCP specializing in this procedure and takes approximately 60 min.
* *Sensitivity to social and cultural issues,* as well as concern for modesty, is important in providing psychological support before, during, and after the procedure.
* Instruct the patient to wear walking shoes for the treadmill or bicycle exercise. Emphasize to the patient the importance of reporting fatigue, pain, or shortness of breath.
* Instruct the patient to remove external metallic objects from the area to be examined prior to the procedure.
* The patient should fast and restrict fluids for 4 hr prior to the procedure.

Instruct the patient to withhold medications for 24 hr before the test as ordered by the HCP. Protocols may vary among facilities.

* *Make sure a written and informed consent has been signed prior to the procedure and before administering any medications.*

INTRATEST:

* Ensure that the patient has complied with dietary and medication restrictions.
* Ensure that the patient has removed external metallic objects from the area to be examined prior to the procedure.
* If the patient has a history of allergic reactions to any substance or drug, administer ordered prophylactic steroids or antihistamines before the procedure.
* Have emergency equipment readily available.
* Record baseline vital signs and assess neurological status. Protocols may vary among facilities.
* Instruct the patient to cooperate fully and to follow directions. Instruct the patient to remain still throughout the procedure because movement produces unreliable results.
* Observe standard precautions, and follow the general guidelines in Appendix A.
* The patient is placed at rest in the supine position on the scanning table.
* Expose the chest and attach the ECG leads. Record baseline readings.
* IV radionuclide is administered and the heart is scanned with images taken in various positions over the entire cardiac cycle.
* When the scan is to be done under exercise conditions, the patient is assisted onto the treadmill or bicycle ergometer and is exercised to a calculated 80% to 85% of the maximum heart rate as determined by the protocol selected. Images are done at each exercise level and begun immediately after injection of the radionuclide.
* If nitroglycerin is given, an HCP assessing the baseline MUGA scan injects the

medication. Additional scans are repeated until blood pressure reaches the desired level.

- Patients who cannot exercise are given dipyridamole before the radionuclide is injected.
- Monitor the patient for complications related to the procedure (e.g., allergic reaction, anaphylaxis, bronchospasm).
- Remove the needle or catheter and apply a pressure dressing over the puncture site.
- Observe/assess the needle/catheter site for bleeding, hematoma formation, or inflammation.

POST-TEST:

- A report of the results will be sent to the requesting HCP, who will discuss the results with the patient.
- Unless contraindicated, advise patient to drink increased amounts of fluids for 24 to 48 hr to eliminate the radionuclide from the body. Inform the patient that radionuclide is eliminated from the body within 6 to 24 hr.
- No other radionuclide tests should be scheduled for 24 to 48 hr after this procedure.
- Evaluate the patient's vital signs. Monitor vital signs and neurological status every 15 min for 1 hr, then every 2 hr for 4 hr, and then as ordered by HCP. Monitor intake and output at least every 8 hr. Compare with baseline values. Protocols may vary among facilities.
- Instruct the patient to resume usual dietary, medication, and activity, as directed by the HCP.
- Observe for delayed allergic reactions, such as rash, urticaria, tachycardia, hyperpnea, hypertension, palpitations, nausea, or vomiting.
- Instruct the patient to immediately report symptoms such as fast heart rate, difficulty breathing, skin rash, itching, chest pain, persistent right shoulder pain, or abdominal pain. Immediately report symptoms to the appropriate HCP.
- Monitor ECG tracings and compare with baseline readings until stable.

- Observe/assess the needle/catheter site for bleeding, hematoma formation, or inflammation.
- Instruct the patient in the care and assessment of the injection site.
- If a woman who is breastfeeding must have a nuclear scan, she should not breastfeed the infant until the radionuclide has been eliminated. This could take as long as 3 days. She should be instructed to express the milk and discard it during the 3-day period to prevent cessation of milk production.
- Instruct the patient to immediately flush the toilet and to meticulously wash hands with soap and water after each voiding for 24 hr after the procedure.
- Instruct all caregivers to wear gloves when discarding urine for 24 hr after the procedure. Wash gloved hands with soap and water before removing gloves. Then wash hands after the gloves are removed.
- *Nutritional Considerations:* Abnormal findings may be associated with cardiovascular disease. The American Heart Association and National Heart, Lung, and Blood Institute (NHBLI) recommend nutritional therapy for individuals identified to be at high risk for developing coronary artery disease (CAD) or individuals who have specific risk factors and/or existing medical conditions (e.g., elevated low-density lipoprotein LDL cholesterol levels, other lipid disorders, insulin-dependent diabetes, insulin resistance, or metabolic syndrome). If overweight, the patient should be encouraged to achieve a normal weight. The NHLBI's National Cholesterol Education Program (NCEP) revised its dietary guidelines for reducing CAD in 2001. Guidelines for the Therapeutic Lifestyle Changes (TLC) diet are outlined in the Third Report of the Expert Panel on Detection, Evaluation, and Treatment of High Blood Cholesterol in Adults (Adult Treatment Panel III [ATP III]). The TLC diet emphasizes a reduction in foods high in saturated fats and cholesterol. Red meats, eggs, and dairy products are the major sources

of saturated fats and cholesterol. If triglycerides also are elevated, the patient should be advised to eliminate or reduce alcohol and simple carbohydrates from the diet. The TLC approach also includes the use of plant stanols or sterols and increased dissolved fiber as an option for lowering LDL cholesterol levels; nutritional recommendations for daily total caloric intake; recommendations for allowable percentage of calories derived from fat (saturated and unsaturated), carbohydrates, protein, and cholesterol; as well as recommendations for daily expenditure of energy.

Nutritional Considerations: Overweight patients with high blood pressure should be encouraged to achieve a normal weight. Other changeable risk factors warranting patient education include strategies to safely decrease sodium intake, increase physical activity, decrease alcohol consumption, eliminate tobacco use, and decrease cholesterol levels.

Social and Cultural Considerations: Numerous studies point to the prevalence of excess body weight in American children and adolescents. Experts estimate that obesity is present in 25% of the population ages 6 to 11 yr. The medical, social, and emotional consequences of excess body weight are significant. Special attention should be given to instructing the child and caregiver regarding health risks and weight control education.

Recognize anxiety related to test results, and be supportive of fear of shortened life expectancy. Discuss the implications of abnormal test results on the patient's lifestyle. Provide teaching and information regarding the clinical implications of the test results, as appropriate. Educate the patient regarding access to counseling

services. Provide contact information, if desired, for the American Heart Association (www.americanheart.org) or the NHLBI (www.nhlbi.nih.gov).

Recognize anxiety related to test results, and be supportive of perceived loss of independent function. Discuss the implications of abnormal test results on the patient's lifestyle. Provide teaching and information regarding the clinical implications of the test results, as appropriate.

Reinforce information given by the patient's HCP regarding further testing, treatment, or referral to another HCP. Answer any questions or address any concerns voiced by the patient or family.

Depending on the results of this procedure, additional testing may be needed to evaluate and determine the need for a change in therapy or progression of the disease process. Evaluate test results in relation to the patient's symptoms and other tests performed.

RELATED MONOGRAPHS:

Related tests include antiarrhythmic drugs, apolipoprotein A and B, AST, ANP, blood gases, BNP, calcium, ionized calcium, cholesterol (total, HDL, and LDL), CRP, CT cardiac scoring, CK and isoenzymes, culture viral, echocardiography, echocardiography transesophageal, ECG, exercise stress test, glucose, glycated hemoglobin, Holter monitor, homocysteine, ketones, LDH and isoenzymes, lipoprotein electrophoresis, magnesium, MRI chest, MI infarct scan, myocardial perfusion heart scan, myoglobin, pericardial fluid analysis, PET heart scan, potassium, triglycerides, and troponin.

Refer to the Cardiovascular System table at the end of the book for related tests by body system.

Bone Mineral Densitometry

SYNONYM/ACRONYM: DEXA, DXA, SXA, QCT, RA, ultrasound densitometry.

Dual-energy x-ray absorptiometry (DEXA, DXA): Two x-rays of different energy levels measure bone mineral density and predict risk of fracture.

Single-energy x-ray absorptiometry (SXA): A single-energy x-ray measures bone density at peripheral sites.

Quantitative computed tomography (QCT): QCT is used to examine the lumbar vertebrae. It measures trabecular and cortical bone density. Results are compared to a known standard. This test is the most expensive and involves the highest radiation dose of all techniques.

Radiographic absorptiometry (RA): A standard x-ray of the hand. Results are compared to a known standard.

Ultrasound densitometry: Studies bone mineral content in peripheral densitometry sites such as the heel or wrist. It is not as precise as x-ray techniques but is less expensive than other techniques.

COMMON USE: To evaluate bone density related to osteoporosis.

AREA OF APPLICATION: Lumbar spine, heel, hip, wrist, whole body.

CONTRAST: None.

DESCRIPTION: Bone mineral density (BMD) can be measured at any of several body sites, including the spine, hip, wrist, and heel. Machines to measure BMD include computed tomography (CT), radiographic absorptiometry, ultrasound, SXA, and most commonly, DEXA. The radiation exposure from SXA and DEXA machines is approximately one-tenth that of a standard chest x-ray.

The BMD values measured by the various techniques cannot be directly compared. Therefore, they are stated in terms of standard deviation (SD) units. The patient's T-score is the number of SD units above or below the average BMD in young adults. A Z-score is the number of SD units above or below the average value for a person of the same age as the measured patient. For most BMD readings, 1 SD is equivalent to 10% to 12% of the average young-normal BMD value. A T-score of −2.5 is therefore equivalent to a bone mineral loss of 30% when compared to a young adult.

INDICATIONS

Osteoporosis is a condition characterized by low BMD, which results in increased risk of fracture. The National Osteoporosis Foundation estimates that 4 to 6 million postmenopausal women in the United States have osteoporosis, and an additional 13 to 17 million (30% to 50%) have low bone density at the hip. It is estimated that one of every two women will experience a fracture as a result of low bone mineral content in her lifetime. The measurement of BMD gives the best indication of risk for a fracture. The lower the BMD, the greater the risk of fracture. The most common fractures are those of the hip, vertebrae, and distal forearm. Bone mineral loss is a disease of the entire skeleton and not restricted to the areas listed. The effect of the fractures has a wide range, from complete recovery to chronic pain, disability, and possible death.

- Determine the mineral content of bone
- Determine a possible cause of amenorrhea
- Establish a diagnosis of osteoporosis
- Estimate the actual fracture risk compared to young adults
- Evaluate bone demineralization associated with chronic renal failure
- Evaluate bone demineralization associated with immobilization
- Monitor changes in BMD due to medical problems or therapeutic intervention
- Predict future fracture risk

POTENTIAL DIAGNOSIS

Normal findings in
- Normal bone mass with T-score value not less than −1.

Abnormal findings in
- Osteoporosis is defined as T-score value less than −2.5.
- Low bone mass or osteopenia has T-scores from −1 to −2.5.
- Fracture risk increases as BMD declines from young-normal levels (low T-scores).
- Low Z-scores in older adults can be misleading because low BMD is very common.
- Z-scores estimate fracture risk compared to others of the same age (versus young-normal adults).

CRITICAL FINDINGS: N/A

INTERFERING FACTORS (or factors associated with increased risk of osteoporosis)

This procedure is contraindicated for
- Patients who are pregnant or suspected of being pregnant, unless the potential benefits of the procedure far outweigh the risks to the fetus and mother.

Factors that may impair clear imaging
- Inability of the patient to cooperate or remain still during the procedure because of age, significant pain, or mental status.
- Metallic objects within the examination field (e.g., jewelry, earrings, and/or dental amalgams), which may inhibit organ visualization and can produce unclear images.

Other considerations
- The use of anticonvulsant drugs, cytotoxic drugs, tamoxifen, glucocorticoids, lithium, or heparin, as well as increased alcohol intake, increased aluminum levels, excessive thyroxin, renal dialysis, or smoking, may affect the test results by either increasing or decreasing the bone mineral content.
- Consultation with a health-care provider (HCP) should occur before the procedure for radiation safety concerns regarding younger patients or patients who are lactating.
- Risks associated with radiation overexposure can result from frequent x-ray or radionuclide procedures. Personnel in the room with the patient should stand behind a shield, or leave the area while the examination is being done. Personnel working in the examination area

should wear badges to record their radiation exposure level.

Other considerations as a result of altered BMD, not the BMD testing process

• Vertebral fractures may cause complications including back pain, height loss, and kyphosis.
• Limited activity, including difficulty bending and reaching, may result.
• Patient may have poor self-esteem resulting from the cosmetic effects of kyphosis.
• Potential restricted lung function may result from fractures.
• Fractures may alter abdominal anatomy, resulting in constipation, pain, distention, and diminished appetite.
• Potential for a restricted lifestyle may result in depression and other psychological symptoms.
• Possible increased dependency on family for basic care may occur.

NURSING IMPLICATIONS AND PROCEDURE

PRETEST:

▶ Positively identify the patient using at least two unique identifiers before providing care, treatment, or services.
▶ *Patient Teaching:* Inform the patient this procedure can assist in assessing bone density.
▶ Obtain a history of the patient's complaints, including a list of known allergens, especially allergies or sensitivities to latex, iodine, seafood, contrast medium, anesthetics, or dyes.
▶ Obtain a history of the patient's musculoskeletal system, symptoms, and results of previously performed laboratory tests and diagnostic and surgical procedures
▶ Note any recent procedures that can interfere with test results, including examinations using iodine-based contrast medium.

▶ Record the date of the last menstrual period and determine the possibility of pregnancy in perimenopausal women.
▶ Obtain a list of the patient's current medications, including herbs, nutritional supplements, and nutraceuticals (see Appendix F).
▶ Review the procedure with the patient. Address concerns about pain related to the procedure and explain that some pain may be experienced during the test, or there may be moments of discomfort. Inform the patient that the procedure is usually performed in a radiology department by a HCP, and staff, specializing in this procedure and takes approximately 60 min.
▶ Instruct the patient to remove jewelry and other metallic objects from the area to be examined.
▶ There are no food, fluid, or medication restrictions unless by medical direction.
▶ *Sensitivity to social and cultural issues,* as well as concern for modesty, is important in providing psychological support before, during, and after the procedure.

INTRATEST:

▶ Ensure that the patient has removed all external metallic objects from the area to be examined prior to the procedure.
▶ Instruct the patient to void prior to the procedure and to change into the gown, robe, and foot coverings provided. Patient's clothing may not need to be removed unless it contains metal that would interfere with the test.
▶ Instruct the patient to cooperate fully and to follow directions. Instruct the patient to remain still throughout the procedure because movement produces unreliable results.
▶ Observe standard precautions, and follow the general guidelines in Appendix A.
▶ Place the patient in a supine position on a flat table with foam wedges, which help maintain position and immobilization.

POST-TEST:

▶ A report of the results will be sent to the requesting HCP, who will discuss the results with the patient.

Recognize anxiety related to test results, and be supportive of perceived loss of independent function. Discuss the implications of abnormal test results on the patient's lifestyle. Provide teaching and information regarding the clinical implications of the test results, as appropriate.

Reinforce information given by the patient's HCP regarding further testing, treatment, or referral to another HCP. Answer any questions or address any concerns voiced by the patient or family.

Depending on the results of this procedure, additional testing may be needed to evaluate or monitor progression of the disease process and determine the need for a change in therapy. Evaluate test results in relation to the patient's symptoms, previous BMD values, and other tests performed.

RELATED MONOGRAPHS:

Related tests include ALP, antibodies anticyclic citrullinated peptide, ANA, arthrogram, arthroscopy, biopsy bone, bone scan, calcium, CRP, collagen cross-linked telopeptides, CT pelvis, CT spine, ESR, MRI musculoskeletal, MRI pelvis, osteocalcin, PTH, phosphorus, radiography bone, RF, synovial fluid analysis, and vitamin D.

Refer to the Musculoskeletal System table at the end of the book for related tests by body system.

Bone Scan

SYNONYM/ACRONYM: Bone imaging, radionuclide bone scan, bone scintigraphy, whole-body bone scan.

COMMON USE: To assist in diagnosing bone disease such as cancer or other degenerative bone disorders.

AREA OF APPLICATION: Bone/skeleton.

CONTRAST: Intravenous radioactive material (diphosphonate compounds), usually combined with technetium-99m.

DESCRIPTION: This nuclear medicine scan assists in diagnosing and determining the extent of primary and metastatic bone disease and bone trauma and monitors the progression of degenerative disorders. Abnormalities are identified by scanning 1 to 3 hr after the intravenous injection of a radionuclide such as technetium-99m methylene diphosphonate.

Areas of increased uptake and activity on the bone scan represent abnormalities unless they occur in normal areas of increased activity, such as the sternum, sacroiliac, clavicle, and scapular joints in adults, and growth centers and cranial sutures in children. The radionuclide mimics calcium physiologically and therefore localizes in bone with an intensity proportional to the degree of metabolic activity. Gallium, magnetic resonance imaging (MRI), or white blood cell scanning can follow a bone scan to obtain a more sensitive study if acute inflammatory conditions such as osteomyelitis or septic arthritis are suspected. In addition, bone scan can detect fractures in patients who continue to have pain even though x-rays have proved negative. A gamma camera detects the radiation emitted from the injected radioactive material. Whole-body or representative images of the skeletal system can be obtained.

INDICATIONS

- Aid in the diagnosis of benign tumors or cysts
- Aid in the diagnosis of metabolic bone diseases
- Aid in the diagnosis of osteomyelitis
- Aid in the diagnosis of primary malignant bone tumors (e.g., osteogenic sarcoma, chondrosarcoma, Ewing's sarcoma, metastatic malignant tumors)
- Aid in the detection of traumatic or stress fractures
- Assess degenerative joint changes or acute septic arthritis
- Assess suspected child abuse
- Confirm temporomandibular joint derangement
- Detect Legg-Calvé-Perthes disease
- Determine the cause of unexplained bone or joint pain
- Evaluate the healing process following fracture, especially if an underlying bone disease is present
- Evaluate prosthetic joints for infection, loosening, dislocation, or breakage
- Evaluate tumor response to radiation or chemotherapy
- Identify appropriate site for bone biopsy, lesion excision, or débridement

POTENTIAL DIAGNOSIS

Normal findings in
- No abnormalities, as indicated by homogeneous and symmetric distribution of the radionuclide throughout all skeletal structures

Abnormal findings in
- Bone necrosis
- Degenerative arthritis
- Fracture
- Legg-Calvé-Perthes disease
- Metastatic bone neoplasm
- Osteomyelitis
- Paget's disease
- Primary metastatic bone tumors
- Renal osteodystrophy
- Rheumatoid arthritis

CRITICAL FINDINGS: N/A

INTERFERING FACTORS

This procedure is contraindicated for
- Patients who are pregnant or suspected of being pregnant, unless the potential benefits of the procedure far outweigh the risks to the fetus and mother.

Factors that may impair clear imaging
- Inability of the patient to cooperate or remain still during the procedure because of age, significant pain, or mental status.
- Metallic objects within the examination field (e.g., jewelry, earrings, and/or dental amalgams), which may inhibit organ visualization and can produce unclear images.
- Retained barium from a previous radiological procedure may affect the image.

- A distended bladder may obscure pelvic detail.
- Other nuclear scans done within the previous 24 to 48 hr may alter image.

Other considerations
- The existence of multiple myeloma or thyroid cancer can result in a false-negative scan for bone abnormalities.
- Improper injection of the radionuclide may allow the tracer to seep deep into the muscle tissue, producing erroneous hot spots.
- Consultation with a health-care provider (HCP) should occur before the procedure for radiation safety concerns regarding younger patients or patients who are lactating.
- Risks associated with radiation overexposure can result from frequent x-ray or radionuclide procedures. Personnel working in the examination area should wear badges to record their level of radiation exposure.

NURSING IMPLICATIONS AND PROCEDURE

PRETEST:

- Positively identify the patient using at least two unique identifiers before providing care, treatment, or services.
- *Patient Teaching:* Inform the patient this procedure can assist in identification of bone disease before it can be detected with plain x-ray images.
- Obtain a history of the patient's complaints, including a list of known allergens, especially allergies or sensitivities to latex, iodine, seafood, contrast medium, anesthetics, or dyes.
- Obtain a history of results of the patient's musculoskeletal systems, symptoms, and results of previously performed laboratory tests and diagnostic and surgical procedures.
- Note any recent procedures that can interfere with test results, including

examinations using iodine-based contrast medium.
- Record the date of the last menstrual period and determine the possibility of pregnancy in perimenopausal women.
- Obtain a list of the patient's current medications, including herbs, nutritional supplements, and nutraceuticals (see Appendix F).
- Review the procedure with the patient. Address concerns about pain related to the procedure and explain to the patient that some pain may be experienced during the test, or there may be moments of discomfort. Reassure the patient that the radionuclide poses no radioactive hazard and rarely produces side effects. Inform the patient the procedure is performed in a nuclear medicine department by an HCP specializing in this procedure, and takes approximately 30 to 60 min.
- *Sensitivity to social and cultural issues,* as well as concern for modesty, is important in providing psychological support before, during, and after the procedure.
- There are no food, fluid, or medication restrictions unless by medical direction.
- Instruct the patient to remove jewelry and other metallic objects in the area to be examined.
- *Make sure a written and informed consent has been signed prior to the procedure and before administering any medications.*

INTRATEST:

- Ensure that the patient has removed all external metallic objects from the area to be examined prior to the procedure.
- If the patient has a history of allergic reactions to any substance or drug, administer ordered prophylactic steroids or antihistamines before the procedure.
- Have emergency equipment readily available.
- Instruct the patient to void prior to the procedure and to change into the gown, robe, and foot coverings provided.
- Instruct the patient to cooperate fully and to follow directions. Instruct the patient to remain still throughout the

procedure because movement produces unreliable results.

▶ Observe standard precautions, and follow the general guidelines in Appendix A.

▶ Administer sedative to a child or to an uncooperative adult, as ordered.

▶ Place the patient in a supine position on a flat table with foam wedges to help maintain position and immobilization.

▶ IV radionuclide is administered and images are taken immediately to assess blood flow to the bones.

▶ After a delay of 2 to 3 hr to allow the radionuclide to be taken up by the bones, multiple images are obtained over the complete skeleton. Delayed views may be taken up to 24 hr after the injection.

▶ The needle or catheter is removed, and a pressure dressing is applied over the puncture site.

▶ Observe/assess the needle/catheter insertion site for bleeding, inflammation, or hematoma formation.

▶ The patient may be imaged by single-photon emission computed tomography (SPECT) techniques to further clarify areas of suspicious radionuclide localization.

POST-TEST:

▶ A report of the results will be sent to the requesting HCP, who will discuss the results with the patient.

▶ Unless contraindicated, advise patient to drink increased amounts of fluids for 24 to 48 hr to eliminate the radionuclide from the body. Inform the patient that radionuclide is eliminated from the body within 6 to 24 hr.

▶ No other radionuclide tests should be scheduled for 24 to 48 hr after this procedure.

▶ Instruct the patient to resume medication and activity as directed by the HCP.

▶ Observe/assess the needle/catheter insertion site for bleeding, inflammation, or hematoma formation.

▶ Instruct the patient in the care and assessment of the injection site.

▶ If a woman who is breastfeeding must have a nuclear scan, she should not breastfeed the infant until the radionuclide has been eliminated. This could take as long as 3 days. She should be instructed to express the milk and discard it during the 3-day period to prevent cessation of milk production.

▶ Instruct the patient to immediately flush the toilet and to meticulously wash hands with soap and water after each voiding for 24 hr after the procedure.

▶ Instruct all caregivers to wear gloves when discarding urine for 24 hr after the procedure. Wash gloved hands with soap and water before removing gloves. Then wash ungloved hands after the gloves are removed.

▶ Recognize anxiety related to test results, and be supportive of perceived loss of independent function. Discuss the implications of abnormal test results on the patient's lifestyle. Provide teaching and information regarding the clinical implications of the test results, as appropriate.

▶ Reinforce information given by the patient's HCP regarding further testing, treatment, or referral to another HCP. Answer any questions or address any concerns voiced by the patient or family.

▶ Depending on the results of this procedure, additional testing may be needed to evaluate or monitor progression of the disease process and determine the need for a change in therapy. Evaluate test results in relation to the patient's symptoms and other tests performed.

RELATED MONOGRAPHS:

▶ Related tests include antibodies, anti-cyclic citrullinated peptide, ANA, arthroscopy, BMD, calcium, CRP, collagen cross-linked telopeptide, CT pelvis, CT spine, culture blood, ESR, MRI musculoskeletal, MRI pelvis, osteocalcin, radiography bone, RF, synovial fluid analysis, and white blood cell scan.

▶ Refer to the Musculoskeletal System table at the end of the book for related tests by body system.

Bronchoscopy

SYNONYM/ACRONYM: Flexible bronchoscopy.

COMMON USE: To visualize and assess bronchial structure for disease such as cancer and infection.

AREA OF APPLICATION: Bronchial tree, larynx, trachea.

CONTRAST: None.

DESCRIPTION: This procedure provides direct visualization of the larynx, trachea, and bronchial tree by means of either a rigid or a flexible bronchoscope. A fiberoptic bronchoscope with a light incorporated is guided into the tracheobronchial tree. A local anesthetic may be used to allow the scope to be inserted through the mouth or nose into the trachea and into the bronchi. The patient must breathe during insertion and with the scope in place. The purpose of the procedure is both diagnostic and therapeutic.

The rigid bronchoscope allows visualization of the larger airways, including the lobar, segmental, and subsegmental bronchi, while maintaining effective gas exchange. Rigid bronchoscopy is preferred when large volumes of blood or secretions need to be aspirated, foreign bodies are to be removed, large-sized biopsy specimens are to be obtained, and for most bronchoscopies in children.

The flexible fiberoptic bronchoscope has a smaller lumen that is designed to allow for visualization of all segments of the bronchial tree. The accessory lumen of the bronchoscope is used for tissue biopsy, bronchial washings, instillation of anesthetic agents and medications, and to obtain specimens with brushes for cytological examination. In general, fiberoptic bronchoscopy is less traumatic to the surrounding tissues than the larger rigid bronchoscopes. Fiberoptic bronchoscopy is performed under local anesthesia; patient tolerance is better for fiber-optic bronchoscopy than for rigid bronchoscopy.

INDICATIONS
- Detect end-stage bronchogenic cancer
- Detect lung infections and inflammation
- Determine etiology of persistent cough, hemoptysis, hoarseness, unexplained chest x-ray abnormalities, and/or abnormal cytological findings in sputum
- Determine extent of smoke-inhalation or other traumatic injury
- Evaluate airway patency; aspirate deep or retained secretions
- Evaluate endotracheal tube placement or possible adverse sequelae to tube placement
- Evaluate possible airway obstruction in patients with known or suspected sleep apnea
- Evaluate respiratory distress and tachypnea in an infant to rule out

tracheoesophageal fistula or other congenital anomaly
- Identify bleeding sites and remove clots within the tracheobronchial tree
- Identify hemorrhagic and inflammatory changes in Kaposi's sarcoma
- Intubate patients with cervical spine injuries or massive upper airway edema
- Remove foreign body
- Treat lung cancer through instillation of chemotherapeutic agents, implantation of radioisotopes, or laser palliative therapy

POTENTIAL DIAGNOSIS

Normal findings in
- Normal larynx, trachea, bronchi, bronchioles, and alveoli

Abnormal findings in
- Abscess
- Bronchial diverticulum
- Bronchial stenosis
- Bronchogenic cancer
- Coccidioidomycosis, histoplasmosis, blastomycosis, phycomycosis
- Foreign bodies
- Inflammation
- Interstitial pulmonary disease
- Opportunistic lung infections (e.g., pneumocystitis, nocardia, cytomegalovirus)
- Strictures
- Tuberculosis
- Tumors

CRITICAL FINDINGS: N/A

INTERFERING FACTORS

This procedure is contraindicated for
- Patients with bleeding disorders, especially those associated with uremia and cytotoxic chemotherapy.
- Patients with pulmonary hypertension.

- Patients with cardiac conditions or dysrhythmias.
- Patients with disorders that limit extension of the neck.
- Patients with severe obstructive tracheal conditions.
- Patients with or having the potential for respiratory failure; introduction of the bronchoscope alone may cause a 10 to 20 mm Hg drop in Pao_2.

Factors that may impair the results of the examination
- Inability of the patient to cooperate or remain still during the procedure because of age, significant pain, or mental status.
- Metallic objects within the examination field (e.g., jewelry, earrings, and/or dental amalgams), which may inhibit organ visualization and can produce unclear images.

Other considerations
- Hypoxemic or hypercapnic states require continuous oxygen administration.
- Failure to follow dietary restrictions before the procedure may cause the procedure to be canceled or repeated.

NURSING IMPLICATIONS AND PROCEDURE

PRETEST:
- Positively identify the patient using at least two unique identifiers before providing care, treatment, or services.
- *Patient Teaching:* Inform the patient this procedure can assess the lungs and respiratory system.
- Obtain a history of the patient's complaints or symptoms, including a list of known allergens, especially allergies or sensitivities to latex, iodine, seafood, contrast medium, and anesthetics.

- Obtain a history of the patient's immune and respiratory systems, symptoms, and results of previously performed laboratory tests and diagnostic and surgical procedures.
- Note any recent procedures that can interfere with test results. Ensure that this procedure is performed before an upper gastrointestinal study or barium swallow.
- Record the date of the last menstrual period and determine the possibility of pregnancy in perimenopausal women.
- Obtain a list of the patient's current medications including anticoagulants, aspirin and other salicylates, herbs, nutritional supplements, and nutraceuticals (see Appendix F). Such products should be discontinued by medical direction for the appropriate number of days prior to a surgical procedure. Note the last time and dose of medication taken.
- Review the procedure with the patient. Instruct that prophylactic antibiotics may be administered prior to the procedure. Address concerns about pain related to the procedure and explain that some pain may be experienced during the test, and there may be moments of discomfort. Explain that a sedative and/or analgesia may be administered to promote relaxation and reduce discomfort prior to the bronchoscopy. Atropine is usually given before bronchoscopy examinations to reduce bronchial secretions and prevent vagally induced bradycardia. Meperidine (Demerol) or morphine may be given as a sedative. Lidocaine is sprayed in the patient's throat to reduce discomfort caused by the presence of the tube. Inform the patient that the procedure is performed in a gastrointestinal laboratory or radiology department, under sterile conditions, by a health care provider (HCP) specializing in this procedure. The procedure usually takes about 30 to 60 min to complete.
- *Sensitivity to social and cultural issues,* as well as concern for modesty, is important in providing psychological support before, during, and after the procedure.
- Explain that an IV line will be inserted to allow infusion of IV fluids, antibiotics, anesthetics, and analgesics.

- The patient should fast and restrict fluids for 8 hr prior to the procedure. Instruct the patient to avoid taking anticoagulant medication or to reduce dosage as ordered prior to the procedure. Number of days to withhold medication is dependent on the type of anticoagulant. Protocols may vary among facilities.
- *Make sure a written and informed consent has been signed prior to the procedure and before administering any medications.*

INTRATEST:

- Ensure that the patient has complied with food, fluid, and medication restrictions for 8 hr prior to the procedure.
- Ensure that the patient has removed dentures, jewelry, and external metallic objects in the area to be examined prior to the procedure.
- Have emergency equipment readily available.
- Instruct the patient to void prior to the procedure and change into the gown, robe, and foot coverings provided.
- Avoid using morphine sulfate in those with asthma or other pulmonary disease. This drug can further exacerbate bronchospasms and respiratory impairment.
- Observe standard precautions, and follow the general guidelines in Appendix A. Positively identify the patient, and label the appropriate collection containers with the corresponding patient demographics, date and time of collection, and site location, especially left or right lung.
- Assist the patient to a comfortable position, and direct the patient to breathe normally during the beginning of the general anesthesia. Instruct the patient to cooperate fully and to follow directions. Direct the patient to breathe normally and to avoid unnecessary movement during the local anesthetic and the procedure.
- Record baseline vital signs and continue to monitor throughout the procedure. Protocols may vary among facilities.

Rigid Bronchoscopy

- The patient is placed in the supine position and a general anesthetic is administered. The patient's neck is hyperextended, and the lightly lubricated bronchoscope is inserted orally and passed through the glottis. The patient's head is turned or repositioned to aid visualization of various segments.

▶ After inspection, the bronchial brush, suction catheter, biopsy forceps, laser, and electrocautery devices are introduced to obtain specimens for cytological or microbiological study or for therapeutic procedures.

▶ If a bronchial washing is performed, small amounts of solution are instilled into the airways and removed.

▶ After the procedure, the bronchoscope is removed and the patient is placed in a side-lying position with the head slightly elevated to promote recovery.

Fiberoptic Bronchoscopy

▶ Provide mouth care to reduce oral bacterial flora.

▶ The patient is placed in a sitting position while the tongue and oropharynx are sprayed or swabbed with local anesthetic. Provide an emesis basin for the increased saliva and encourage the patient to spit out the saliva because the gag reflex may be impaired. When loss of sensation is adequate, the patient is placed in a supine or side-lying position. The fiberoptic scope can be introduced through the nose, the mouth, an endotracheal tube, a tracheostomy tube, or a rigid bronchoscope. Most common insertion is through the nose. Patients with copious secretions or massive hemoptysis, or in whom airway complications are more likely, may be intubated before the bronchoscopy. Additional local anesthetic is applied through the scope as it approaches the vocal cords and the carina, eliminating reflexes in these sensitive areas. The fiberoptic approach allows visualization of airway segments without having to move the patient's head through various positions.

▶ After visual inspection of the lungs, tissue samples are collected from suspicious sites by bronchial brush or biopsy forceps to be used for cytological and microbiological studies.

▶ After the procedure, the bronchoscope is removed. Patients who had local anesthesia are placed in a semi-Fowler's position to recover.

General

▶ Monitor the patient for complications related to the procedure (e.g., allergic reaction, anaphylaxis).

▶ Place tissue samples in properly labeled specimen containers containing formalin solution, and promptly transport the specimen to the laboratory for processing and analysis.

POST-TEST:

▶ A report of the results will be sent to the requesting HCP, who will discuss the results with the patient.

▶ Instruct the patient to resume preoperative diet, as directed by the HCP. Assess the patient's ability to swallow before allowing the patient to attempt liquids or solid foods.

▶ Inform the patient that he or she may experience some throat soreness and hoarseness. Instruct patient to treat throat discomfort with lozenges and warm gargles when the gag reflex returns.

▶ Monitor vital signs and neurological status every 15 min for 1 hr, then every 2 hr for 4 hr, and then as ordered by the HCP. Monitor temperature every 4 hr for 24 hr. Monitor intake and output at least every 8 hr. Compare with baseline values. Notify the HCP if temperature changes. Protocols may vary among facilities.

▶ Emergency resuscitation equipment should be readily available if the vocal cords become spastic after intubation.

▶ Observe for delayed allergic reactions, such as rash, urticaria, tachycardia, hyperpnea, hypertension, palpitations, nausea, or vomiting.

▶ Observe the patient for hemoptysis, difficulty breathing, cough, air hunger, excessive coughing, pain, or absent breathing sounds over the affected area. Immediately report symptoms to the appropriate HCP.

▶ Evaluate the patient for symptoms indicating the development of pneumothorax, such as dyspnea, tachypnea, anxiety, decreased breathing sounds, or restlessness. A chest x-ray may be ordered to check for the presence of this complication.

- Evaluate the patient for symptoms of empyema, such as fever, tachycardia, malaise, or elevated white blood cell count.
- Observe the patient's sputum for blood if a biopsy was taken, because large amounts of blood may indicate the development of a problem; a small amount of streaking is expected. Evaluate the patient for signs of bleeding such as tachycardia, hypotension, or restlessness.
- Assess for nausea and pain. Administer antiemetic and analgesic medications as needed and as directed by the HCP.
- Administer antibiotic therapy if ordered. Remind the patient of the importance of completing the entire course of antibiotic therapy even if signs and symptoms disappear before completion of therapy.
- Recognize anxiety related to test results. Discuss the implications of abnormal test results on the patient's lifestyle. Provide teaching and information regarding the clinical implications of the test results, as appropriate. Educate the patient regarding access to counseling services.
- Instruct the patient to use lozenges or gargle for throat discomfort. Inform the patient of smoking cessation programs as appropriate. Malnutrition is commonly seen in patients with severe respiratory disease for numerous reasons, including fatigue, lack of appetite,

and gastrointestinal distress. Adequate intake of vitamins A and C is also important to prevent pulmonary infection and to decrease the extent of lung tissue damage. The importance of following the prescribed diet should be stressed to the patient/caregiver. Educate the patient regarding access to counseling services, as appropriate.
- Reinforce information given by the patient's HCP regarding further testing, treatment, or referral to another HCP. Answer any questions or address any concerns voiced by the patient or family.
- Depending on the results of this procedure, additional testing may be needed to evaluate or monitor progression of the disease process and determine the need for a change in therapy. Evaluate test results in relation to the patient's symptoms and other tests performed.

RELATED MONOGRAPHS:

- Related tests include arterial/alveolar oxygen ratio, antibodies, anti–glomerular basement membrane, biopsy lung, blood gases, chest x-ray, complete blood count, CT thorax, culture and smear mycobacteria, culture sputum, culture viral, cytology sputum, Gram stain, lung perfusion scan, lung ventilation scan, MRI chest, mediastinoscopy, and pulse oximetry.
- Refer to the Immune and Respiratory systems tables at the end of the book for related tests by body system.

B-Type Natriuretic Peptide and Pro-B-Type Natriuretic Peptide

SYNONYM/ACRONYM: BNP and proBNP.

COMMON USE: To assist in diagnosing congestive heart failure.

SPECIMEN: Plasma (1 mL) collected in a plastic, lavender-top (EDTA) tube.

REFERENCE VALUE: (Method: Immunochemiluminometric for BNP; immuno-(electro)chemiluminescence for proBNP).

B

	BNP	proBNP (N-Terminal)
Male	Less than 100 pg/mL	Less than or equal to 60 pg/mL
Female	Less than 100 pg/mL	12–150 pg/mL

BNP levels are increased in elderly adults.

New York Heart Association Classification of CHF	Corresponding Range of Median BNP Values Across Different Test Methods	Clinical Symptoms and BNP Values Indicate
Class I: patients with no limitation of activities; they suffer no symptoms from ordinary activities.	100–250 pg/mL	Heart failure is present but no clinical symptoms are evident
Class II: patients with slight, mild limitation of activity; they are comfortable with rest or with mild exertion.	Greater than 300–400 pg/mL	Mild or slight heart failure
Class III: patients with marked limitation of activity; they are comfortable only at rest.	Greater than 400–500 pg/mL	Moderate or marked heart failure
Class IV: patients who should be at complete rest, confined to bed or chair; any physical activity brings on discomfort and symptoms occur at rest.	Greater than 900 pg/mL	Severe heart failure

Note: CHF = congestive heart failure.
Source: New York Heart Association Classification of CHF. Reprinted with permission, www.americanheart.org, © 2010, American Heart Association, Inc.

DESCRIPTION: The peptides B-type natriuretic peptide (BNP) and atrial natriuretic peptide (ANP) assist in the regulation of fluid balance and blood pressure. BNP, proBNP, and ANP are useful markers in the diagnosis of congestive heart failure (CHF). BNP or brain natriuretic peptide, first isolated in the brain of pigs, is a neurohormone synthesized primarily in the ventricles of the human heart in response to increases in ventricular pressure and volume. Circulating levels of BNP and proBNP increase in proportion to the severity of heart failure. A rapid BNP point-of-care immunoassay may be performed, in which a venous blood sample is collected, placed on a strip, and inserted into a device that measures BNP. Results are completed in 10 to 15 min.

INDICATIONS

- Assist in determining the prognosis and therapy of patients with heart failure
- Assist in the diagnosis of heart failure
- Assist in differentiating heart failure from pulmonary disease
- Cost-effective screen for left ventricular dysfunction; positive findings would point to the need for echocardiography and further assessment

POTENTIAL DIAGNOSIS

Increased in

BNP is secreted in response to increased hemodynamic load caused by physiological stimuli, as with ventricular stretch or endocrine stimuli from the aldosterone/renin system.

- Cardiac inflammation (myocarditis, cardiac allograft rejection)
- Cirrhosis
- Cushing's syndrome
- Heart failure
- Kawasaki's disease
- Left ventricular hypertrophy
- Myocardial infarction
- Primary hyperaldosteronism
- Primary pulmonary hypertension
- Renal failure
- Ventricular dysfunction

Decreased in: N/A

CRITICAL FINDINGS: N/A

INTERFERING FACTORS

- Nesiritide (Natrecor) is a recombinant form of BNP that may be given therapeutically by IV to patients in acutely decompensated heart failure; BNP levels may be transiently elevated at the time of administration and must be interpreted with caution.

NURSING IMPLICATIONS AND PROCEDURE

PRETEST:

- Positively identify the patient using at least two unique identifiers before providing care, treatment, or services.
- *Patient Teaching:* Inform the patient this test can assist in diagnosing congestive heart failure.
- Obtain a history of the patient's complaints, including a list of known allergens, especially allergies or sensitivities to latex.
- Obtain a history of the patient's cardiovascular system, symptoms, and results of previously performed laboratory tests and diagnostic and surgical procedures.
- Obtain a list of the patient's current medications, including herbs, nutritional supplements, and nutraceuticals (see Appendix F).
- Review the procedure with the patient. Inform the patient that specimen collection takes approximately 5 to 10 min. Address concerns about pain and explain to the patient that there may be some discomfort during the venipuncture.
- *Sensitivity to social and cultural issues,* as well as concern for modesty, is important in providing psychological support before, during, and after the procedure.
- There are no food, fluid, or medication restrictions unless by medical direction.

INTRATEST:

- If the patient has a history of allergic reaction to latex, avoid the use of equipment containing latex.
- Instruct the patient to cooperate fully and to follow directions. Direct the patient to breathe normally and to avoid unnecessary movement.
- Observe standard precautions, and follow the general guidelines in Appendix A. Positively identify the patient, and label the appropriate tubes with the corresponding patient demographics, date, and time of collection. Perform a venipuncture.

- Remove the needle and apply direct pressure with dry gauze to stop bleeding. Observe/assess venipuncture site for bleeding or hematoma formation and secure gauze with adhesive bandage.
- Promptly transport the specimen to the laboratory for processing and analysis.

POST-TEST:

- A written report of the results will be sent to the requesting health-care provider (HCP), who will discuss the results with the patient.
- *Treatment Considerations for CHF:* Ensure that the patient (if not currently taking) is placed on an angiotensin-converting enzyme inhibitor, β-blocker, and diuretic and is monitored with daily weights.
- *Nutritional Considerations:* Instruct patients to consume a variety of foods within the basic food groups, eat foods high in potassium when taking diuretics, eat a diet high in fiber (25 to 35 g/day), maintain a healthy weight, be physically active, limit salt intake to 2,000 mg/day, limit alcohol intake, and be a nonsmoker.
- *Nutritional Considerations:* Foods high in potassium include citrus fruits such as bananas, strawberries, oranges; cantaloupes; green leafy vegetables such as spinach and broccoli; dried fruits such as dates, prunes, and raisins; legumes such as peas and pinto beans; nuts and whole grains.
- Reinforce information given by the patient's HCP regarding further testing, treatment, or referral to another HCP. Answer any questions or address any concerns voiced by the patient or family.
- Depending on the results of this procedure, additional testing may be performed to evaluate or monitor progression of the disease process and determine the need for a change in therapy. Evaluate test results in relation to the patient's symptoms and other tests performed.

RELATED MONOGRAPHS:

- Related tests include AST, ANF, calcium and ionized calcium, CRP, CK and isoenzymes, CT scoring, echocardiography, glucose, homocysteine, Holter monitor, LDH and isoenzymes, magnesium, MRI chest, MI scan, myocardial perfusion heart scan, myoglobin, PET heart, potassium, and tropinin.
- Refer to the Cardiovascular System table at the end of the book for related tests by body system.

Calcitonin and Calcitonin Stimulation Tests

SYNONYM/ACRONYM: Thyrocalcitonin, hCT.

COMMON USE: To diagnose and monitor the effectiveness of treatment for medullary thyroid cancer.

SPECIMEN: Serum (3 mL) collected in a red- or tiger-top tube.

REFERENCE VALUE: (Method: Immunoassay)

Procedure	Medication Administered	Recommended Collection Times
Calcium and penta-gastrin stimulation	Calcium, 2 mg/kg IV for 1 min, followed by penta-gastrin 0.5 mcg/kg	4 calcitonin levels—baseline immediately before bolus; and 1 min, 2 min, and 5 min postbolus

IV = intravenous.

	Conventional Units	SI Units (Conventional Units × 1)
Calcitonin		
Male	Less than 10 pg/mL	Less than 10 ng/L
Female	Less than 5 pg/mL	Less than 5 ng/L
Maximum Response		
10 min after calcium and pentagastrin stimulation		
Male	Less than 112 pg/mL	Less than 112 ng/L
Female	Less than 23 pg/mL	Less than 23 ng/L

DESCRIPTION: Calcitonin, also called thyrocalcitonin, is secreted by the parafollicular or C cells of the thyroid gland in response to elevated serum calcium levels. Calcitonin antagonizes the effects of parathyroid hormone and vitamin D so that calcium continues to be laid down in bone rather than reabsorbed into the blood. Calcitonin also increases renal clearance of magnesium and inhibits tubular reabsorption of phosphates. The net result is that calcitonin decreases the serum calcium level. The pentagastrin (Peptavlon) provocation test and the calcium pentagastrin provocation test are useful for diagnosing medullary thyroid cancer.

INDICATIONS
- Assist in the diagnosis of hyperparathyroidism
- Assist in the diagnosis of medullary thyroid cancer
- Evaluate altered serum calcium levels
- Monitor response to therapy for medullary thyroid carcinoma
- Predict recurrence of medullary thyroid carcinoma

287

• Screen family members of patients with medullary thyroid carcinoma (20% have a familial pattern)

POTENTIAL DIAGNOSIS

Increased in
• Alcoholic cirrhosis *(related to release of calcium from body stores associated with acute instances of malnutrition)*
• Cancer of the breast, lung, and pancreas *(related to metastasis of calcitonin-producing cells to other organs)*
• Carcinoid syndrome *(related to calcitonin-producing tumor cells)*
• C-cell hyperplasia *(related to increased production due to hyperplasia)*
• Chronic renal failure *(related to increased excretion of calcium and retention of phosphorus resulting in release of calcium from body stores; C cells respond to an increase in serum calcium levels)*
• Ectopic secretion *(especially neuroendocrine origins)*
• Hypercalcemia (any cause) *(related to increased production by C cells in response to increased calcium levels)*
• Medullary thyroid cancer *(related to overproduction by cancerous cells)*
• MEN Type II *(related to calcitonin-producing tumor cells)*
• Pancreatitis *(related to alcoholism or hypercalcemia)*
• Pernicious anemia *(related to hypergastrinemia)*
• Pheochromocytoma *(related to calcitonin-producing tumor cells)*
• Pregnancy (late) *(related to increased maternal loss of circulating calcium to developing fetus; release of calcium from maternal stores stimulates increased release of calcitonin)*
• Pseudohypoparathyroidism *(related to release of calcium from body stores initiates feedback response from C cells)*
• Thyroiditis *(related to calcitonin-producing tumor cells)*
• Zollinger-Ellison syndrome *(related to hypergastrinemia)*

Decreased in: N/A

CRITICAL FINDINGS: N/A

INTERFERING FACTORS
• Drugs that may increase calcitonin levels include calcium, epinephrine, estrogens, glucagon, oral contraceptives, pentagastrin, and sincalide.
• Failure to follow dietary restrictions before the procedure may cause the procedure to be canceled or repeated.

NURSING IMPLICATIONS AND PROCEDURE

PRETEST:
▶ Positively identify the patient using at least two unique identifiers before providing care, treatment, or services.
▶ *Patient Teaching:* Inform the patient this test can assist in assessing the thyroid gland for disease or can monitor effectiveness of therapy.
▶ Obtain a history of the patient's complaints, including a list of known allergens, especially allergies or sensitivities to latex.
▶ Obtain a history of the patient's endocrine system, as well as results of previously performed laboratory tests and diagnostic and surgical procedures.
▶ Note any recent procedures that can interfere with test results.
▶ Obtain a list of the patient's current medications, including herbs, nutritional supplements, and nutraceuticals (see Appendix F).

- Review the procedure with the patient. Inform the patient that specimen collection takes approximately 5 to 10 min; a few extra minutes are required to administer the stimulation tests. Address concerns about pain and explain that there may be some discomfort during the venipuncture.
- *Sensitivity to social and cultural issues,* as well as concern for modesty, is important in providing psychological support before, during, and after the procedure.
- The patient should fast for 10 to 12 hr before specimen collection. Protocols may vary among facilities.
- There are no fluid or medication restrictions unless by medical direction.
- Prepare an ice slurry in a cup or plastic bag to have ready for immediate transport of the specimen to the laboratory. Prechill the collection tube in the ice slurry.

INTRATEST:

- Ensure that the patient has complied with dietary restrictions and pretesting preparations; ensure that food has been restricted for at least 10 to 12 hr prior to the procedure.
- If the patient has a history of allergic reaction to latex, avoid the use of equipment containing latex.
- Instruct the patient to cooperate fully and to follow directions. Direct the patient to breathe normally and to avoid unnecessary movement.
- Observe standard precautions, and follow the general guidelines in Appendix A. Positively identify the patient, and label the appropriate tubes with the corresponding patient demographics, date, and time of collection. Perform a venipuncture; collect the specimen in a prechilled tube.
- Remove the needle and apply direct pressure with dry gauze to stop

bleeding. Observe/assess venipuncture site for bleeding or hematoma formation and secure gauze with adhesive bandage.
- The sample should be placed in an ice slurry immediately after collection. Information on the specimen label should be protected from water in the ice slurry by first placing the specimen in a protective plastic bag. Promptly transport the specimen to the laboratory for processing and analysis.

POST-TEST:

- A report of the results will be sent to the requesting health-care provider (HCP), who will discuss the results with the patient.
- Instruct the patient to resume usual diet as directed by the HCP.
- Reinforce information given by the patient's HCP regarding further testing, treatment, or referral to another HCP. Answer any questions or address any concerns voiced by the patient or family.
- Depending on the results of this procedure, additional testing may be performed to evaluate or monitor progression of the disease process and determine the need for a change in therapy. Evaluate test results in relation to the patient's symptoms and other tests performed.

RELATED MONOGRAPHS:

- Related tests include ACTH, biopsy thyroid, calcium, cancer antigens, catecholamines, CBC, gastrin stimulation test, magnesium, metanephrines, PTH, parathyroid scan, phosphorus, thyroglobulin, thyroid scan, TSH, US thyroid and parathyroid, and vitamin D.
- Refer to the Endocrine System table at the end of the book for related tests by body system.

C

Calcium, Blood

SYNONYM/ACRONYM: Total calcium, Ca.

COMMON USE: To investigate various conditions indicated by abnormally increased or decreased calcium levels.

SPECIMEN: Serum (1 mL) collected in a red- or tiger-top tube. Plasma (1 mL) collected in a green-top (heparin) tube is also acceptable.

REFERENCE VALUE: (Method: Spectrophotometry)

Age	Conventional Units	SI Units (Conventional Units × 0.25)
Cord	8.2–11.2 mg/dL	2.05–2.80 mmol/L
0–10 days	7.6–10.4 mg/dL	1.90–2.60 mmol/L
11 days–2 yr	9.0–11.0 mg/dL	2.25–2.75 mmol/L
3–12 yr	8.8–10.8 mg/dL	2.20–2.70 mmol/L
13–18 yr	8.4–10.2 mg/dL	2.10–2.55 mmol/L
Adult	8.2–10.2 mg/dL	2.05–2.55 mmol/L
Adult older than 90 yr	8.2–9.6 mg/dL	2.05–2.40 mmol/L

DESCRIPTION: Calcium, the most abundant cation in the body, participates in almost all of the vital processes. Calcium concentration is largely regulated by the parathyroid glands and by the action of vitamin D. Of the body's calcium reserves, 98% to 99% is stored in the teeth and skeleton. Calcium values are higher in children because of growth and active bone formation. About 45% of the total amount of blood calcium circulates as free ions that participate in coagulation, neuromuscular conduction, intracellular regulation, glandular secretion, and control of skeletal and cardiac muscle contractility. The remaining calcium is bound to circulating proteins (40% bound mostly to albumin) and anions (15% bound to anions such as bicarbonate, citrate, phosphate, and lactate) and plays no physiological role. Calcium values can be adjusted up or down by 0.8 mg/dL for every 1 g/dL that albumin is greater than or less than 4 g/dL. Calcium and phosphorus levels are inversely proportional.

Fluid and electrolyte imbalances are often seen in patients with serious illness or injury; in these clinical situations, the normal homeostatic balance of the body is altered. During surgery or in the case of a critical illness, bicarbonate, phosphate, and lactate concentrations can change dramatically. Therapeutic treatments may also cause or contribute to electrolyte imbalance. This is why total calcium values can sometimes be misleading. Abnormal calcium levels are used to indicate general malfunctions in various body systems. Ionized calcium is used in more specific conditions (see monograph titled "Calcium, Ionized").

Calcium values should be interpreted in conjunction with results of other tests. Normal calcium with an abnormal phosphorus value indicates impaired calcium absorption (possibly because of altered parathyroid hormone level or activity). Normal calcium with an elevated urea nitrogen value indicates possible hyperparathyroidism (primary or secondary). Normal calcium with decreased albumin value is an indication of hypercalcemia (high calcium levels). The most common cause of hypocalcemia (low calcium levels) is hypoalbuminemia. The most common causes of hypercalcemia are hyperparathyroidism and cancer (with or without bone metastases).

INDICATIONS

- Detect parathyroid gland loss after thyroid or other neck surgery, as indicated by decreased levels
- Evaluate cardiac arrhythmias and coagulation disorders to determine if altered serum calcium level is contributing to the problem
- Evaluate the effects of various disorders on calcium metabolism, especially diseases involving bone
- Monitor the effectiveness of therapy being administered to correct abnormal calcium levels, especially calcium deficiencies
- Monitor the effects of renal failure and various drugs on calcium levels

POTENTIAL DIAGNOSIS

Increased in

- Acidosis *(related to imbalance in electrolytes; longstanding acidosis can result in osteoporosis and release of calcium into circulation)*
- Acromegaly *(related to alteration in vitamin D metabolism, resulting in increased calcium)*
- Addison's disease *(related to adrenal gland dysfunction; decreased blood volume and dehydration occur in the absence of aldosterone)*
- Cancers (bone, Burkitt's lymphoma, Hodgkin's lymphoma, leukemia, myeloma, and metastases from other organs)
- Dehydration *(related to a decrease in the fluid portion of blood, causing an overall increase in the concentration of most plasma constituents)*
- Hyperparathyroidism *(related to increased parathyroid hormone [PTH] and vitamin D levels, which increase circulating calcium levels)*
- Idiopathic hypercalcemia of infancy
- Lung disease (tuberculosis, histoplasmosis, coccidioidomycosis, berylliosis) *(related to activity by macrophages in the epithelium that interfere with vitamin D regulation by converting it to its active form; vitamin D increases circulating calcium levels)*
- Malignant disease without bone involvement *(some cancers [e.g., squamous cell carcinoma of the lung and kidney cancer] produce PTH-related peptide that increases calcium levels)*

- Milk-alkali syndrome (Burnett's syndrome) *(related to excessive intake of calcium-containing milk or antacids, which can increase calcium levels)*
- Paget's disease *(related to calcium released from bone)*
- Pheochromocytoma *(hyperparathyroidism related to multiple endocrine neoplasia type 2A [MEN2A] syndrome associated with some pheochromocytomas; PTH increases calcium levels)*
- Polycythemia vera *(related to dehydration; decreased blood volume due to excessive production of red blood cells)*
- Renal transplant *(related to imbalances in electrolytes; a common post-transplant issue)*
- Sarcoidosis *(related to activity by macrophages in the granulomas that interfere with vitamin D regulation by converting it to its active form; vitamin D increases circulating calcium levels)*
- Thyrotoxicosis *(related to increased bone turnover and release of calcium into the blood)*
- Vitamin D toxicity *(vitamin D increases circulating calcium levels)*

Decreased in
- Acute pancreatitis *(complication of pancreatitis related to hypoalbuminemia and calcium binding by excessive fats)*
- Alcoholism *(related to insufficient nutrition)*
- Alkalosis *(increased blood pH causes intracellular uptake of calcium to increase)*
- Chronic renal failure *(related to decreased synthesis of vitamin D)*
- Cystinosis *(hereditary disorder of the renal tubules that results in excessive calcium loss)*
- Hepatic cirrhosis *(related to impaired metabolism of vitamin D and calcium)*
- Hyperphosphatemia *(phosphorus and calcium have an inverse relationship)*
- Hypoalbuminemia *(related to insufficient levels of albumin, an important carrier protein)*
- Hypomagnesemia *(lack of magnesium inhibits PTH and thereby decreases calcium levels)*
- Hypoparathyroidism (congenital, idiopathic, surgical) *(related to lack of PTH)*
- Inadequate nutrition
- Leprosy *(related to increased bone retention)*
- Long-term anticonvulsant therapy *(these medications block calcium channels and interfere with calcium transport)*
- Malabsorption (celiac disease, tropical sprue, pancreatic insufficiency) *(related to insufficient absorption)*
- Massive blood transfusion *(related to the presence of citrate preservative in blood product that chelates or binds calcium and removes it from circulation)*
- Neonatal prematurity
- Osteomalacia (advanced) *(bone loss is so advanced there is little calcium remaining to be released into circulation)*
- Renal tubular disease *(related to decreased synthesis of vitamin D)*
- Vitamin D deficiency (rickets) *(related to insufficient amounts of vitamin D, resulting in decreased calcium metabolism)*

CRITICAL FINDINGS ◈
- Less than 7 mg/dL
- Greater than 12 mg/dL (some patients can tolerate higher concentrations)

Note and immediately report to the health-care provider (HCP) any critically increased or decreased values and related symptoms.

Observe the patient for symptoms of critically decreased or elevated calcium levels. Hypocalcemia is evidenced by convulsions, arrhythmias, changes in electrocardiogram (ECG) in the form of prolonged ST segment and Q-T interval, facial spasms (positive Chvostek's sign), tetany, muscle cramps, numbness in extremities, tingling, and muscle twitching (positive Trousseau's sign). Possible interventions include seizure precautions, increased frequency of ECG monitoring, and administration of calcium or magnesium.

Severe hypercalcemia is manifested by polyuria, constipation, changes in ECG (shortened ST segment), lethargy, muscle weakness, apathy, anorexia, headache, and nausea and ultimately may result in coma. Possible interventions include the administration of normal saline and diuretics to speed up excretion or administration of calcitonin or steroids to force the circulating calcium into the cells.

INTERFERING FACTORS

- Drugs that may increase calcium levels include anabolic steroids, some antacids, calcitriol, calcium salts, danazol, diuretics (long-term), ergocalciferol, isotretinoin, lithium, oral contraceptives, parathyroid extract, parathyroid hormone, prednisone, progesterone, tamoxifen, vitamin A, and vitamin D.
- Drugs that may decrease calcium levels include albuterol, alprostadil, aminoglycosides, anticonvulsants, calcitonin, diuretics (initially), gastrin, glucagon, glucocorticoids, glucose, insulin, laxatives (excessive use), magnesium salts, methicillin, phosphates, plicamycin, sodium sulfate (given IV), tetracycline (in pregnancy), trazodone, and viomycin.

- Calcium exhibits diurnal variation; serial samples should be collected at the same time of day for comparison.
- Venous hemostasis caused by prolonged use of a tourniquet during venipuncture can falsely elevate calcium levels.
- Patients on ethylenediaminetetraacetic acid (EDTA) therapy (chelation) may show falsely decreased calcium values.
- Hemolysis and icterus cause false-positive results because of interference from biological pigments.
- Specimens should never be collected above an IV line because of the potential for dilution when the specimen and the IV solution combine in the collection container, falsely decreasing the result. There is also the potential of contaminating the sample with the substance of interest if it is present in the IV solution, falsely increasing the result.

NURSING IMPLICATIONS AND PROCEDURE

PRETEST:
- Positively identify the patient using at least two unique identifiers before providing care, treatment, or services.
- *Patient Teaching:* Inform the patient this test can assist as a general indicator in diagnosing health concerns.
- Obtain a history of the patient's complaints, including a list of known allergens, especially allergies or sensitivities to latex.
- Obtain a history of the patient's cardiovascular, gastrointestinal, genitourinary, hematopoietic, hepatobiliary, and musculoskeletal systems, as well as results of previously performed laboratory tests and diagnostic and surgical procedures.
- Note any recent procedures that can interfere with test results.
- Obtain a list of the patient's current medications, including herbs, nutritional supplements, and nutraceuticals (see Appendix F).

- Review the procedure with the patient. Inform the patient that specimen collection takes approximately 5 to 10 min. Address concerns about pain and explain that there may be some discomfort during the venipuncture.
- *Sensitivity to social and cultural issues,* as well as concern for modesty, is important in providing psychological support before, during, and after the procedure.
- There are no food, fluid, or medication restrictions unless by medical direction.

INTRATEST:

- If the patient has a history of allergic reaction to latex, avoid the use of equipment containing latex.
- Instruct the patient to cooperate fully and to follow directions. Direct the patient to breathe normally and to avoid unnecessary movement.
- Observe standard precautions, and follow the general guidelines in Appendix A. Positively identify the patient, and label the appropriate tubes with the corresponding patient demographics, date, and time of collection. Perform a venipuncture.
- Remove the needle and apply direct pressure with dry gauze to stop bleeding. Observe/assess venipuncture site for bleeding or hematoma formation and secure gauze with adhesive bandage.
- Promptly transport the specimen to the laboratory for processing and analysis.

POST-TEST:

- A report of the results will be sent to the requesting HCP, who will discuss the results with the patient.
- *Nutritional Considerations:* Patients with abnormal calcium values should be informed that daily intake of calcium is important even though body stores in the bones can be called on to supplement circulating levels. Dietary calcium can be obtained from animal or plant sources. Milk and milk products, sardines, clams, oysters, salmon, rhubarb, spinach, beet greens, broccoli, kale, tofu, legumes, and fortified orange juice are high in calcium. Milk and milk products also contain vitamin D and lactose, which assist calcium

absorption. Cooked vegetables yield more absorbable calcium than raw vegetables. Patients should be informed of the substances that can inhibit calcium absorption by irreversibly binding to some of the calcium, making it unavailable for absorption, such as oxalates, which naturally occur in some vegetables (e.g., beet greens, collards, leeks, okra, parsley, quinoa, spinach, Swiss chard) and are found in tea; phytic acid, found in some cereals (e.g., wheat bran, wheat germ); phosphoric acid, found in dark cola; and insoluble dietary fiber (in excessive amounts). Excessive protein intake can also negatively affect calcium absorption, especially if it is combined with foods high in phosphorus and in the presence of a reduced dietary calcium intake.

- Reinforce information given by the patient's HCP regarding further testing, treatment, or referral to another HCP. Answer any questions or address any concerns voiced by the patient or family.
- Depending on the results of this procedure, additional testing may be performed to evaluate or monitor progression of the disease process and determine the need for a change in therapy. Evaluate test results in relation to the patient's symptoms and other tests performed.

RELATED MONOGRAPHS:

- Related tests include ACTH, albumin, aldosterone, ALP, biopsy bone marrow, BMD, bone scan, calcitonin, calcium ionized, urine calcium, calculus kidney stone analysis, catecholamines, chloride, collagen cross-linked telopeptides, CBC, CT pelvis, CT spine, cortisol, CK and isoenzymes, DHEA, fecal fat, glucose, HVA, magnesium, metanephrines, osteocalcin, PTH, phosphorus, potassium, protein total, radiography bone, renin, sodium, thyroid scan, thyroxine, US thyroid and parathyroid, UA, and vitamin D.
- Refer to the Cardiovascular, Gastrointestinal, Genitourinary, Hematopoietic, Hepatobiliary, and Musculoskeletal systems tables at the end of the book for related tests by body system.

Calcium, Ionized

SYNONYM/ACRONYM: Free calcium, unbound calcium, Ca^{++}, Ca^{2+}.

COMMON USE: To investigate various conditions associated with altered levels of ionized calcium such as hypocalcemia and hypercalcemia.

SPECIMEN: Serum (1 mL) collected in a red- or tiger-top tube. Specimen should be transported tightly capped and remain unopened until testing. Exposure of serum to room air changes the pH of the specimen due to the release of carbon dioxide and can cause erroneous results.

REFERENCE VALUE: (Method: Ion-selective electrode)

Age	Conventional Units	SI Units (Conventional Units × 0.25)
Whole blood		
1–5 days	4.20–5.84 mg/dL	1.05–1.46 mmol/L
Adult	4.60–5.08 mg/dL	1.12–1.32 mmol/L
Plasma		
Adult	4.12–4.92 mg/dL	1.03–1.23 mmol/L
Serum		
1–18 yr	4.8–5.52 mg/dL	1.2–1.38 mmol/L
Adult	4.64–5.28 mg/dL	1.16–1.32 mmol/L

DESCRIPTION: Calcium is the most abundant cation in the body and participates in almost all vital body processes (see other calcium monographs). Circulating calcium is found in the free or ionized form; bound to organic anions such as lactate, phosphate, or citrate; and bound to proteins such as albumin. Ionized calcium is the physiologically active form of circulating calcium. About half of the total amount of calcium circulates as free ions that participate in blood coagulation, neuromuscular conduction, intracellular regulation, glandular secretion, and control of skeletal and cardiac muscle contractility. Calcium levels are regulated largely by the parathyroid glands and by vitamin D. Compared to total calcium level, ionized calcium is a better measurement of calcium metabolism. Ionized calcium levels are not influenced by protein concentrations, as seen in patients with chronic renal failure, nephrotic syndrome, malabsorption, and multiple myeloma. Levels are also not affected in patients with metabolic acid-base balance disturbances. Elevations in ionized calcium may be seen when the total calcium is normal. Measurement of ionized calcium is useful to monitor patients undergoing cardiothoracic surgery or organ transplantation. It is also useful in the evaluation of patients in cardiac arrest.

INDICATIONS

- Detect ectopic parathyroid hormone (PTH)–producing neoplasms
- Evaluate the effect of protein on calcium levels
- Identify individuals with hypocalcemia
- Identify individuals with toxic levels of vitamin D
- Investigate suspected hyperparathyroidism
- Monitor patients with renal failure or organ transplantation in whom secondary hyperparathyroidism may be a complication
- Monitor patients with sepsis or magnesium deficiency

POTENTIAL DIAGNOSIS

Increased in

- Hyperparathyroidism *(related to increased PTH)*
- PTH-producing neoplasms *(PTH increases calcium levels)*
- Vitamin D toxicity *(related to increased absorption of calcium)*

Decreased in

- Burns, severe *(related to increased amino acid release)*
- Hypoparathyroidism (primary) *(related to decreased PTH)*
- Magnesium deficiency *(inhibits release of PTH)*
- Multiple organ failure
- Pancreatitis *(associated with saponification or binding of calcium to fats in tissue surrounding the pancreas)*
- The postdialysis period *(result of low-calcium dialysate administration)*
- The postsurgical period (i.e., major surgeries) *(related to decreased PTH)*
- The post-transfusion period *(result of the use of citrated blood product preservative [calcium chelator])*
- Premature infants with hypoproteinemia and acidosis *(related to alterations in transport protein levels)*
- Pseudohypoparathyroidism *(related to decreased PTH)*
- Sepsis *(related to decreased PTH)*
- Trauma *(related to decreased PTH)*
- Vitamin D deficiency *(related to decreased absorption of calcium)*

CRITICAL FINDINGS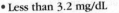

- Less than 3.2 mg/dL
- Greater than 6.2 mg/dL

Note and immediately report to the health-care provider (HCP) any critically increased or decreased values and related symptoms.

Observe the patient for symptoms of critically decreased or elevated calcium levels. Hypocalcemia is evidenced by convulsions, arrhythmias, changes in electrocardiogram (ECG) in the form of prolonged ST segment and Q-T interval, facial spasms (positive Chvostek's sign), tetany, muscle cramps, numbness in extremities, tingling, and muscle twitching (positive Trousseau's sign). Possible interventions include seizure precautions, increased frequency of ECG monitoring, and administration of calcium or magnesium.

Severe hypercalcemia is manifested by polyuria, constipation, changes in ECG (shortened ST segment), lethargy, muscle weakness, apathy, anorexia, headache, and nausea and ultimately may result in coma. Possible interventions include the administration of normal saline and diuretics to speed up excretion or administration of calcitonin or steroids to force the circulating calcium into the cells.

INTERFERING FACTORS

- Drugs that may increase calcium levels include antacids (some), calcitriol, and lithium.
- Drugs that may decrease calcium levels include calcitonin, citrates, foscarnet, and pamidronate (initially).
- Calcium exhibits diurnal variation; serial samples should be collected at the same time of day for comparison.
- Venous hemostasis caused by prolonged use of a tourniquet during venipuncture can falsely elevate calcium levels.
- Patients on ethylenediaminetetraacetic acid (EDTA) therapy (chelation) may show falsely decreased calcium values.
- Specimens should never be collected above an IV line because of the potential for dilution when the specimen and the IV solution combine in the collection container, falsely decreasing the result. There is also the potential of contaminating the sample with the substance of interest if it is present in the IV solution, falsely increasing the result.

NURSING IMPLICATIONS AND PROCEDURE

PRETEST:

- Positively identify the patient using at least two unique identifiers before providing care, treatment, or services.
- *Patient Teaching:* Inform the patient this test can assist in evaluating the level of blood calcium.
- Obtain a history of the patient's complaints, including a list of known allergens, especially allergies or sensitivities to latex.
- Obtain a history of the patient's cardiovascular, gastrointestinal, genitourinary, hematopoietic, hepatobiliary, and musculoskeletal systems, as well as results of previously performed

laboratory tests and diagnostic and surgical procedures.
- Note any recent procedures that could interfere with test results.
- Obtain a list of the patient's current medications, including herbs, nutritional supplements, and nutraceuticals (see Appendix F).
- Review the procedure with the patient. Inform the patient that specimen collection takes approximately 5 to 10 min. Address concerns about pain and explain that there may be some discomfort during the venipuncture.
- *Sensitivity to social and cultural issues,* as well as concern for modesty, is important in providing psychological support before, during, and after the procedure.
- There are no food, fluid, or medication restrictions unless by medical direction.

INTRATEST:

- If the patient has a history of allergic reaction to latex, avoid the use of equipment containing latex.
- Instruct the patient to cooperate fully and to follow directions. Direct the patient to breathe normally and to avoid unnecessary movement.
- Observe standard precautions, and follow the general guidelines in Appendix A. Positively identify the patient, and label the appropriate tubes with the corresponding patient demographics, date, and time of collection. Perform a venipuncture and, without using a tourniquet, collect the specimen.
- Remove the needle and apply direct pressure with dry gauze to stop bleeding. Observe/assess venipuncture site for bleeding or hematoma formation and secure gauze with adhesive bandage.
- The specimen should be stored under anaerobic conditions after collection to prevent the diffusion of gas from the specimen. Falsely decreased values result from unstoppered specimens. Promptly transport the specimen to the laboratory for processing and analysis.

POST-TEST:

- A report of the results will be sent to the requesting HCP, who will discuss the results with the patient.

Nutritional Considerations: Patients with abnormal calcium values should be informed that daily intake of calcium is important even though body stores in the bones can be called on to supplement circulating levels. Dietary calcium can be obtained from animal or plant sources. Milk and milk products, sardines, clams, oysters, salmon, rhubarb, spinach, beet greens, broccoli, kale, tofu, legumes, and fortified orange juice are high in calcium. Milk and milk products also contain vitamin D and lactose, which assist calcium absorption. Cooked vegetables yield more absorbable calcium than raw vegetables. Patients should be informed of the substances that can inhibit calcium absorption by irreversibly binding to some of the calcium, making it unavailable for absorption, such as oxalates, which naturally occur in some vegetables (e.g., beet greens, collards, leeks, okra, parsley, quinoa, spinach, Swiss chard) and are found in tea; phytic acid, found in some cereals (e.g., wheat bran, wheat germ); phosphoric acid, found in dark cola; and insoluble dietary fiber (in excessive amounts). Excessive protein intake can also negatively affect calcium absorption, especially if it is combined with foods high in phosphorus and in the presence of a reduced dietary calcium intake.

- Reinforce information given by the patient's HCP regarding further testing, treatment, or referral to another HCP. Answer any questions or address any concerns voiced by the patient or family.
- Depending on the results of this procedure, additional testing may be performed to evaluate or monitor progression of the disease process and determine the need for a change in therapy. Evaluate test results in relation to the patient's symptoms and other tests performed.

RELATED MONOGRAPHS:

- Related tests include albumin, ALP, calcitonin, calcium, calculus kidney stone panel, gastrin and gastrin stimulation, magnesium, PTH, parathyroid scan, phosphorus, potassium, protein total, sodium, thyroglobulin, US thyroid and parathyroid, UA, and vitamin D.
- Refer to the Cardiovascular, Gastrointestinal, Genitourinary, Hematopoietic, Hepatobiliary, and Musculoskeletal systems tables at the end of the book for related tests by body system.

Calcium, Urine

SYNONYM/ACRONYM: N/A.

COMMON USE: To indicate sufficiency of dietary calcium intake and rate of absorption. Urine calcium levels are also used to assess bone resorption, renal stones, and renal loss of calcium.

SPECIMEN: Urine (5 mL) from an unpreserved random or timed specimen collected in a clean plastic collection container.

REFERENCE VALUE: (Method: Spectrophotometry)

Age	Conventional Units*	SI Units (Conventional Units × 0.25)*
Infant and child	Up to 6 mg/kg per 24 hr	Up to 0.15 mmol/kg per 24 hr
Adult on average diet	100–300 mg/24 hr	2.5–7.5 mmol/24 hr

*Values depend on diet. Average daily intake of calcium: 600–800 mg/24 hr.

DESCRIPTION: Regulating electrolyte balance is a major function of the kidneys. In normally functioning kidneys, urine levels increase when serum levels are high and decrease when serum levels are low to maintain homeostasis. Analyzing urinary electrolyte levels can provide important clues to the functioning of the kidneys and other major organs. Tests for calcium in urine usually involve timed urine collections during a 12- or 24-hr period. Measurement of random specimens may also be requested. Urinary calcium excretion may also be expressed as calcium-to-creatinine ratio: In a healthy individual with constant muscle mass, the ratio is less than 0.14.

INDICATIONS
- Assist in establishing the presence of kidney stones
- Evaluate bone disease
- Evaluate dietary intake and absorption
- Evaluate renal loss
- Monitor patients on calcium replacement

POTENTIAL DIAGNOSIS

Increased in
- Acromegaly *(related to imbalance in vitamin D metabolism)*
- Diabetes *(related to increased loss from damaged kidneys)*
- Fanconi's syndrome *(evidenced by hereditary or acquired disorder of the renal tubules that results in excessive calcium loss)*
- Glucocorticoid excess *(related to action of glucocorticoids, which is to decrease the gastrointestinal absorption of calcium and increase urinary excretion)*
- Hepatolenticular degeneration (Wilson's disease) *(related to excessive electrolyte loss due to renal damage)*
- Hyperparathyroidism *(related to increased levels of PTH which result in increased calcium levels)*
- Hyperthyroidism *(related to increased bone turnover; excess circulating calcium is excreted by the kidneys)*
- Idiopathic hypercalciuria
- Immobilization *(related to disruption in calcium homeostasis and bone loss)*
- Kidney stones *(evidenced by excessive urinary calcium; contributes to the formation of kidney stones)*
- Leukemia and lymphoma (some instances)
- Myeloma *(calcium is released from damaged bone; excess circulating calcium is excreted by the kidneys)*
- Neoplasm of the breast or bladder *(some cancers secrete PTH or PTH-related peptide that increases calcium levels)*
- Osteitis deformans *(calcium is released from damaged bone;*

excess circulating calcium is
excreted by the kidneys)
- Osteolytic bone metastases
  (carcinoma, sarcoma) *(calcium
  is released from damaged
  bone; excess circulating
  calcium is excreted by the
  kidneys)*
- Osteoporosis *(calcium is
  released from damaged bone;
  excess circulating calcium is
  excreted by the kidneys)*
- Paget's disease *(calcium
  is released from damaged
  bone; excess circulating
  calcium is excreted by the
  kidneys)*
- Renal tubular acidosis *(metabolic
  acidosis resulting in loss of
  calcium by the kidneys)*
- Sarcoidosis *(macrophages in
  the granulomas interfere
  with vitamin D regulation by
  converting it to its active
  form; vitamin D increases
  circulating calcium levels,
  and excess is excreted by the
  kidneys)*
- Schistosomiasis
- Thyrotoxicosis *(increased
  bone turnover; excess circulating calcium is excreted by the
  kidneys)*
- Vitamin D intoxication *(increases
  calcium metabolism; excess is
  excreted by the kidneys)*

Decreased in
- Hypocalcemia (other than renal
  disease)
- Hypocalciuric hypercalcemia
  (familial, nonfamilial)
- Hypoparathyroidism *(PTH insti-
  gates release of calcium; if PTH
  levels are low, calcium levels will
  be decreased)*
- Hypothyroidism
- Malabsorption (celiac disease, tropical sprue) *(related to insufficient
  levels of calcium)*
- Malignant bone neoplasm

- Nephrosis and acute nephritis
  *(related to decreased synthesis
  of vitamin D)*
- Osteoblastic metastases
- Osteomalacia *(related to vitamin D
  deficiency)*
- Pre-eclampsia
- Pseudohypoparathyroidism
- Renal osteodystrophy
- Rickets *(related to deficiency in
  vitamin D)*
- Vitamin D deficiency *(deficiency
  in vitamin D results in decreased
  calcium levels)*

CRITICAL FINDINGS: N/A

INTERFERING FACTORS
- Drugs that can increase urine
  calcium levels include acetazolamide, ammonium chloride,
  asparaginase, calcitonin,
  corticosteroids, corticotropin,
  dexamethasone, dihydroxychole-
  calciferol, diuretics (initially),
  ergocalciferol, ethacrynic acid,
  glucocorticoids, mannitol
  (initially), meralluride, mercaptomerin, mersalyl, metolazone, nandrolone, parathyroid extract,
  parathyroid hormone, plicamycin,
  prednisolone, sodium sulfate,
  sulfates, torsemide, triamcinolone,
  triamterene, viomycin, and
  vitamin D.
- Drugs that can decrease urine
  calcium levels include angiotensin,
  bicarbonate, calcitonin, cellulose
  phosphate, citrates, diuretics
  (chronic), lithium, mestranol,
  methyclothiazide, neomycin, oral
  contraceptives, parathyroid
  extract, polythiazide, sodium
  phytate, spironolactone,
  thiazides, trichlormethiazide, and
  vitamin K.
- Failure to collect all the urine and
  store the specimen properly during
  the 24-hr test period invalidates the
  results.

NURSING IMPLICATIONS AND PROCEDURE

PRETEST:

- Positively identify the patient using at least two unique identifiers before providing care, treatment, or services.
- *Patient Teaching:* Inform the patient this test can assist in evaluating the effectiveness of the bodies absorption of calcium.
- Obtain a history of the patient's complaints, including a list of known allergens, especially allergies or sensitivities to latex.
- Obtain a history of the patient's endocrine, genitourinary, and musculo-skeletal systems and results of previously performed laboratory tests and diagnostic and surgical proce-dures.
- Obtain a list of the patient's current medications, including herbs, nutritional supplements, and nutraceuticals (see Appendix F).
- Review the procedure with the patient. Provide a nonmetallic urinal, bedpan, or toilet-mounted collection device. Address concerns about pain and explain that there should be no discomfort during the procedure.
- *Sensitivity to social and cultural issues,* as well as concern for modesty, is important in providing psychological support before, during, and after the procedure.
- Usually a 24-hr time frame for urine collection is ordered. Inform the patient that all urine must be saved during that 24-hr period. Instruct the patient not to void directly into the laboratory collection container. Instruct the patient to avoid defecating in the collection device and to keep toilet tissue out of the collection device to prevent contamination of the specimen. Place a sign in the bathroom to remind the patient to save all urine.
- Instruct the patient to void all urine into the collection device and then to pour the urine into the laboratory collection container. Alternatively, the specimen can be left in the collection device for a health care staff member to add to the laboratory collection container.
- There are no fluid or medication restrictions unless by medical direction.
- Instruct the patient to follow a normal calcium diet for at least 4 days before test. Protocols may vary among facilities.

INTRATEST:

- Ensure that the patient has complied with dietary restrictions; ensure that a normal calcium diet has been followed for at least 4 days prior to the procedure.
- If the patient has a history of allergic reaction to latex, avoid the use of equipment containing latex.
- Instruct the patient to cooperate fully and to follow directions.
- Observe standard precautions, and follow the general guidelines in Appendix A. Positively identify the patient, and label the appropriate collection container with the corresponding patient demographics, date, and time of collection.

Random Specimen (collect in early morning)

- Obtain urine specimen in a properly labeled plastic collection container and immediately transport urine. If an indwelling catheter is in place, it may be necessary to clamp off the catheter for 15 to 30 min before specimen collection. Cleanse specimen port with antiseptic swab, and then aspirate 5 mL of urine with a 21- to 25-gauge needle and syringe. Transfer urine to a plastic container.

Timed Specimen

- Obtain a clean 3-L urine specimen container, toilet-mounted collection device, and plastic bag (for transport of the specimen container). The specimen must be refrigerated or kept on ice through-out the collection period. If an indwelling urinary catheter is in place, the drainage bag must be kept on ice.

C

C

▶ Begin the test between 6 and 8 a.m. if possible. Collect first voiding and discard. Record the time the specimen was discarded as the beginning of the timed collection period. The next morning, ask the patient to void at the same time the collection was started, and add this last voiding to the container. Urinary output should be recorded throughout the collection time.

▶ If an indwelling catheter is in place, replace the tubing and container system at the start of the collection time. Keep the container system on ice during the collection period or empty the urine into a larger container periodically during the collection period; monitor to ensure continued drainage, and conclude the test the next morning at the same hour the collection began.

▶ At the conclusion of the test, compare the quantity of urine with the urinary output record for the collection; if the specimen contains less than the recorded output, some urine may have been discarded, invalidating the test.

▶ Include on the collection container's label the amount of urine collected and test start and stop times. Promptly transport the specimen to the laboratory for processing and analysis.

POST-TEST:

▶ A report of the results will be sent to the requesting health-care provider (HCP), who will discuss the results with the patient.

▶ Instruct the patient to resume usual diet as directed by the HCP.

▶ *Nutritional Considerations:* Increased urine calcium levels may be associated with kidney stones. Educate the patient, if appropriate, as to the importance of drinking a sufficient amount of water when kidney stones are suspected.

▶ Recognize anxiety related to test results. Discuss the implications of abnormal test results on the patient's lifestyle. Provide teaching and information regarding the clinical implications of the test results, as appropriate.

▶ Reinforce information given by the patient's HCP regarding further testing, treatment, or referral to another HCP. Answer any questions or address any concerns voiced by the patient or family.

▶ Depending on the results of this procedure, additional testing may be performed to evaluate or monitor progression of the disease process and determine the need for a change in therapy. Evaluate test results in relation to the patient's symptoms and other tests performed.

RELATED MONOGRAPHS:

▶ Related tests include ACTH, albumin, aldosterone, ALP, biopsy bone marrow, BMD, bone scan, calcitonin, calcium ionized, calculus kidney stone analysis, catecholamines, chloride, collagen cross-linked telopeptides, CBC, CT pelvis, CT spine, cortisol, CK and isoenzymes, DHEA, fecal fat, glucose, HVA, magnesium, metanephrines, osteocalcin, oxalate, PTH, phosphorus, potassium, protein total, radiography bone, renin, sodium, thyroid scan, thyroxine, US thyroid and parathyroid, UA, uric acid, and vitamin D.

▶ Refer to the Endocrine, Genitourinary, and Musculoskeletal systems tables at the end of the book for related tests by body system.

Calculus, Kidney Stone Panel

SYNONYM/ACRONYM: Kidney stone analysis, nephrolithiasis analysis.

COMMON USE: To identify the presence of kidney stones.

SPECIMEN: Kidney stones.

REFERENCE VALUE: (Method: Infrared spectrometry) None detected.

DESCRIPTION: Renal calculi (kidney stones) are formed by the crystallization of calcium oxalate (most common), magnesium ammonium phosphate, calcium phosphate, uric acid, and cystine. Formation of stones may be due to reduced urine flow and excessive amounts of the previously mentioned insoluble substances. The presence of stones is confirmed by diagnostic visualization or passing of the stones in the urine. The chemical nature of the stones is confirmed qualitatively.

INDICATIONS
- Identify substances present in renal calculi

POTENTIAL DIAGNOSIS

Positive findings in
- Presence of renal calculi

Negative findings in: N/A

CRITICAL FINDINGS: N/A

INTERFERING FACTORS
- Drugs and substances that may increase the formation of urine calculi include probenecid and vitamin D.

- Adhesive tape should not be used to attach stones to any transportation or collection container, because the adhesive interferes with infrared spectrometry.

NURSING IMPLICATIONS AND PROCEDURE

PRETEST:
- Positively identify the patient using at least two unique identifiers before providing care, treatment, or services.
- *Patient Teaching:* Inform the patient this test can assist in identification of the presence of kidney stones.
- Obtain a history of the patient's complaints, especially hematuria, recurrent urinary tract infection, and abdominal pain. Also, obtain a list of known allergens.
- Obtain a history of the patient's genitourinary system and results of previously performed laboratory tests and diagnostic and surgical procedures.
- Obtain a list of the patient's current medications, including herbs, nutritional supplements, and nutraceuticals (see Appendix F).
- Review the procedure with the patient. Address concerns about pain and explain that there may be some discomfort during the procedure.
- *Sensitivity to social and cultural issues,* as well as concern for modesty, is important in providing psychological support before, during, and after the procedure.
- There are no food, fluid, or medication restrictions unless by medical direction.

INTRATEST:

- Instruct the patient to cooperate fully and to follow directions.
- Observe standard precautions, and follow the general guidelines in Appendix A. Positively identify the patient, and label the appropriate collection container with the corresponding patient demographics, date, and time of collection.
- The patient presenting with symptoms indicating the presence of kidney stones may be provided with a device to strain the urine. The patient should be informed to transfer any particulate matter remaining in the strainer into the specimen collection container provided. Stones removed by the health-care provider (HCP) should be placed in the appropriate collection container.
- Promptly transport the specimen to the laboratory for processing and analysis.

POST-TEST:

- A report of the results will be sent to the requesting HCP, who will discuss the results with the patient.
- Inform the patient with kidney stones that the likelihood of recurrence is high. Educate the patient regarding risk factors that contribute to the likelihood of kidney stone formation, including family history, osteoporosis, urinary tract infections, gout, magnesium deficiency, Crohn's disease with prior resection, age, gender (males are two to three times more likely than females to develop stones), race (whites are three to four times more likely than African Americans to develop stones), and climate.

Nutritional Considerations: Nutritional therapy is indicated for individuals identified as being at high risk for developing kidney stones. Educate the patient that diets rich in protein, salt, and oxalates increase the risk of stone formation. Adequate fluid intake should be encouraged.

- Recognize anxiety related to test results. Discuss the implications of abnormal test results on the patient's lifestyle. Provide teaching and information regarding the clinical implications of the test results, as appropriate.
- Reinforce information given by the patient's HCP regarding further testing, treatment, or referral to another HCP. Follow-up testing of urine may be requested, but usually not for 1 mo after the stones have passed or been removed. Answer any questions or address any concerns voiced by the patient or family.
- Depending on the results of this procedure, additional testing may be performed to evaluate or monitor progression of the disease process and determine the need for a change in therapy. Evaluate test results in relation to the patient's symptoms and other tests performed.

RELATED MONOGRAPHS:

- Related tests include CT abdomen, calcium, creatinine clearance, culture bacterial urine, cystoscopy, IVP, KUB, magnesium, oxalate, phosphorus, renogram, retrograde ureteropyelography, US kidney, uric acid, and UA.
- Refer to the Genitourinary System table at the end of the book for related tests by body system.

Cancer Antigens: CA 15-3, CA 19-9, CA 125, and Carcinoembryonic

SYNONYM/ACRONYM: Carcinoembryonic antigen (CEA), cancer antigen 125 (CA 125), cancer antigen 15-3 (CA 15-3), cancer antigen 19-9 (CA 19-9), cancer antigen 27.29 (CA 27.29).

COMMON USE: To identify the presence of various cancers, such as breast and ovarian, as well as to evaluate the effectiveness of cancer treatment.

SPECIMEN: Serum (1 mL) collected in a red-top tube. Care must be taken to use the same assay method if serial measurements are to be taken.

REFERENCE VALUE: (Method: Radioactive immunoassay, Immunochemiluminometric assay [ICMA])

Smoking Status	Conventional Units	SI Units (Conventional Units × 1)
CEA		
Smoker	Less than 5.0 ng/mL	Less than 5.0 mcg/L
Nonsmoker	Less than 2.5 ng/mL	Less than 2.5 mcg/L

Conventional Units	SI Units (Conventional Units × 1)
CA 125	
Less than 35 units/mL	Less than 35 kU/L
CA 15-3	
Less than 25 units/mL	Less than 25 kU/L
CA 19-9	
Less than 35 units/mL	Less than 35 kU/L
CA 27.29	
Less than 38.6 units/mL	Less than 38.6 kU/L

DESCRIPTION: Carcinoembryonic antigen (CEA) is a glycoprotein normally produced only during early fetal life and rapid multiplication of epithelial cells, especially those of the digestive system. CEA also appears in the blood of chronic smokers. Although the test is not diagnostic for any specific disease and is not useful as a screening test for cancer, it is very useful for monitoring response to therapy in breast, liver, colon, and gastrointestinal cancer. Serial monitoring is also a useful indicator of recurrence or metastasis in colon or liver carcinoma.

CA 125, a glycoprotein present in normal endometrial tissue, appears in the blood when natural endometrial protective barriers are destroyed, as occurs in cancer or endometriosis. Persistently rising levels indicate a poor prognosis, but absence of the tumor marker does not rule out tumor presence. Levels may also rise in pancreatic, liver, colon, breast, and lung cancers. CA 125 is most useful in monitoring the progression or recurrence of known ovarian cancer. It is not useful as a screening test when used alone.

CA 15-3 monitors patients for recurrence or metastasis of breast carcinoma.

CA 19-9 is a carbohydrate antigen used for post-therapeutic monitoring of patients with gastrointestinal, pancreatic, liver, and colorectal cancer.

CA 27.29 is a glycoprotein product of the muc-1 gene. It is most useful as a serial monitor for response to therapy or recurrence of breast carcinoma.

INDICATIONS

CEA
- Determine stage of colorectal cancer and test for recurrence or metastasis
- Monitor response to treatment of breast and gastrointestinal cancers

CA 125
- Assist in the diagnosis of carcinoma of the cervix and endometrium
- Assist in the diagnosis of ovarian cancer
- Monitor response to treatment of ovarian cancer

CA 15-3 and CA 27.29
- Monitor recurrent carcinoma of the breast

CA 19-9
- Monitor effectiveness of therapy
- Monitor gastrointestinal, head and neck, and gynecological carcinomas
- Predict recurrence of cholangio-carcinoma
- Predict recurrence of stomach, pancreatic, colorectal, gallbladder, liver, and urothelial carcinomas

POTENTIAL DIAGNOSIS

Increased in

CEA
- Benign tumors, including benign breast disease
- Chronic tobacco smoking
- Cirrhosis
- Colorectal, pulmonary, gastric, pancreatic, breast, head and neck, esophageal, ovarian, and prostate cancer

- Inflammatory bowel disease
- Pancreatitis
- Radiation therapy (transient)

CA 125
- Breast, colon, endometrial, liver, lung, ovarian, and pancreatic cancer
- Endometriosis
- First-trimester pregnancy
- Menses
- Ovarian abscess
- Pelvic inflammatory disease
- Peritonitis

CA 15-3 and CA 27.29
- Recurrence of breast carcinoma

CA 19-9
- Gastrointestinal, head and neck, and gynecologic carcinomas
- Recurrence of stomach, pancreatic, colorectal, gallbladder, liver, and urothelial carcinomas
- Recurrence of cholangiocarcinoma

Decreased in
- Effective therapy or removal of the tumor

CRITICAL FINDINGS: N/A

INTERFERING FACTORS
- Recent radioactive scans or radiation within 1 wk before the test can interfere with test results when radioimmunoassay is the test method.

NURSING IMPLICATIONS AND PROCEDURE

PRETEST:
▶ Positively identify the patient using at least two unique identifiers before providing care, treatment, or services.

- *Patient Teaching:* Inform the patient this test can assist in monitoring the progress of various types of disease and evaluate response to therapy.
- Obtain a history of the patient's complaints, including a list of known allergens, especially allergies or sensitivities to latex.
- Obtain a history of the patient's gastrointestinal, immune, and reproductive systems, as well as results of previously performed laboratory tests and diagnostic and surgical procedures.
- Note any recent radiology procedures that can interfere with test results.
- Obtain a list of the patient's current medications, including herbs, nutritional supplements, and nutraceuticals (see Appendix F).
- Determine if the patient smokes, because smokers may have false elevations of CEA.
- Review the procedure with the patient. Inform the patient that specimen collection takes approximately 5 to 10 minutes. Address concerns about pain and explain that there may be some discomfort during the venipuncture.
- *Sensitivity to social and cultural issues,* as well as concern for modesty, is important in providing psychological support before, during, and after the procedure.
- There are no food, fluid, or medication restrictions unless by medical direction.

INTRATEST:

- If the patient has a history of allergic reaction to latex, avoid the use of equipment containing latex.
- Instruct the patient to cooperate fully and to follow directions. Direct the patient to breathe normally and to avoid unnecessary movement.
- Observe standard precautions, and follow the general guidelines in Appendix A. Positively identify the patient, and label the appropriate tubes with the corresponding patient demographics, date, and time of collection. Perform a venipuncture.
- Remove the needle and apply direct pressure with dry gauze to stop bleeding. Observe/assess

venipuncture site for bleeding or hematoma formation and secure gauze with adhesive bandage.
- Promptly transport the specimen to the laboratory for processing and analysis.

POST-TEST:

- A report of the results will be sent to the requesting health-care provider (HCP), who will discuss them with the patient.
- Recognize anxiety related to test results, and be supportive of perceived loss of independence and fear of shortened life expectancy. Discuss the implications of abnormal test results on the patient's lifestyle. Provide teaching and information regarding the clinical implications of the test results, as appropriate. Educate the patient regarding access to counseling services. Provide contact information, if desired, for the American Cancer Association (www.cancer.org).
- Reinforce information given by the patient's HCP regarding further testing, treatment, or referral to another HCP. Decisions regarding the need for and frequency of breast self-examination, mammography, MRI breast, or other cancer screening procedures should be made after consultation between the patient and HCP. The most current guidelines for breast cancer screening of the general population as well as of individuals with increased risk are available from the American Cancer Society (www.cancer.org), the American College of Obstetricians and Gynecologists (ACOG) (www.acog.org), and the American College of Radiology (www.acr.org). Answer any questions or address any concerns voiced by the patient or family.
- Decisions regarding the need for and frequency of occult blood testing, colonoscopy, or other cancer screening procedures should be made after consultation between the patient and HCP. The most current guidelines for colon cancer screening of the general

population as well as of individuals with increased risk are available from the American Cancer Society (www.cancer.org) and the American College of Gastroenterology (www.gi.org).

▶ Depending on the results of this procedure, additional testing may be performed to evaluate or monitor progression of the disease process and determine the need for a change in therapy. Evaluate test results in relation to the patient's symptoms and other tests performed.

RELATED MONOGRAPHS:

▶ Related tests include barium enema, biopsy breast, biopsy cervical, biopsy intestinal, biopsy liver, capsule endoscopy, colonoscopy, colposcopy, fecal analysis, HCG, liver and spleen scan, MRI breast, MRI liver, mammogram, stereotactic breast biopsy, proctosigmoidoscopy, radiofrequency ablation liver, US breast, and US liver.

▶ Refer to the Gastrointestinal, Immune, and Reproductive systems tables at the end of the book for related tests by body system.

Capsule Endoscopy

SYNONYM/ACRONYM: Pill GI endoscopy.

COMMON USE: To assist in visualization of the GI tract to identify disease such as tumor and inflammation.

AREA OF APPLICATION: Esophagus, stomach, upper duodenum, and small bowel.

CONTRAST: None.

DESCRIPTION: This outpatient procedure involves ingesting a small (size of a large vitamin pill) capsule that is wireless and contains a small video camera that will pass naturally through the digestive system while taking pictures of the intestine. The capsule is 11 mm by 30 mm and contains a camera, light source, radio transmitter, and battery. The patient swallows the capsule, and the camera takes and transmits two images per second. The images are transmitted to a recording device, which saves all images for review later by a health-care provider (HCP). This device is approximately the size of a personal compact disk player. The recording device is worn on a belt around the patient's waist, and the video images are transmitted to aerials taped to the body and stored on the device. After 8 hr, the device is removed and returned to the HCP for processing. Thousands of images are downloaded onto a computer for viewing by an HCP specialist. The capsule is disposable and will be excreted naturally in the patient's bowel movements. In the rare case that it is not excreted naturally, it will need to be removed endoscopically or surgically.

INDICATIONS

- Assist in differentiating between benign and neoplastic tumors
- Detect gastric or duodenal ulcers
- Detect gastrointestinal tract (GI) inflammatory disease
- Determine the presence and location of GI bleeding and vascular abnormalities
- Evaluate the extent of esophageal injury after ingestion of chemicals
- Evaluate stomach or duodenum after surgical procedures
- Evaluate suspected gastric obstruction
- Identify Crohn's disease, infectious enteritis, and celiac sprue
- Identify source of chronic diarrhea
- Investigate the cause of abdominal pain, celiac syndrome, and other malabsorption syndromes

POTENTIAL DIAGNOSIS

Normal findings in

- Esophageal mucosa is normally yellow-pink. At about 9 in. from the incisor teeth, a pulsation indicates the location of the aortic arch. The gastric mucosa is orange-red and contains rugae. The proximal duodenum is reddish and contains a few longitudinal folds, whereas the distal duodenum has circular folds lined with villi. No abnormal structures or functions are observed in the esophagus, stomach, or duodenum.

Abnormal findings in

- Achalasia
- Acute and chronic gastric and duodenal ulcers

- Crohn's disease, infectious enteritis, and celiac sprue
- Diverticular disease
- Duodenal cancer, diverticula, and ulcers
- Duodenitis
- Esophageal or pyloric stenosis
- Esophageal varices
- Esophagitis or strictures
- Gastric cancer, tumors, and ulcers
- Gastritis
- Hiatal hernia
- Mallory-Weiss syndrome
- Perforation of the esophagus, stomach, or small bowel
- Polyps
- Small bowel tumors
- Strictures
- Tumors (benign or malignant)

CRITICAL FINDINGS: N/A

INTERFERING FACTORS

This procedure is contraindicated for

- Patients who have had surgery involving the stomach or duodenum, which can make locating the duodenal papilla difficult.
- Patients with a bleeding disorder.
- Patients with unstable cardiopulmonary status, blood coagulation defects, or cholangitis, unless the patient received prophylactic antibiotic therapy before the test (otherwise, the examination must be rescheduled).
- Patients with unstable cardiopulmonary status, blood coagulation defects, known aortic arch aneurysm, large esophageal Zenker's diverticulum, recent GI surgery, esophageal varices, or known esophageal perforation.

Factors that may impair clear imaging

- Gas or feces in the GI tract resulting from inadequate cleansing or failure to restrict food intake before the study.

- Retained barium from a previous radiological procedure.

Other considerations

- The patient should not be near any electromagnetic source, such as magnetic resonance imaging (MRI) or amateur (ham) radio equipment.
- Undergoing an MRI during the procedure may result in serious damage to the patient's intestinal tract or abdomen. The patient should contact his or her HCP for evaluation prior to any other procedure.
- Delayed capsule transit times may be a result of narcotic use, somatostatin use, gastroparesis, or psychiatric illness.

NURSING IMPLICATIONS AND PROCEDURE

PRETEST:

- Positively identify the patient using at least two unique identifiers before providing care, treatment, or services.
- *Patient Teaching:* Inform the patient this procedure can assist in assessing the esophagus, stomach, and upper intestines for disease.
- Obtain a history of the patient's complaints including a list of known allergens, especially allergies or sensitivities to latex, iodine, seafood, contrast medium, anesthetics, and dyes.
- Obtain a history of the patient's gastrointestinal system, symptoms, and results of previously performed laboratory tests and diagnostic and surgical procedures.
- Ensure that this procedure is performed before an upper GI series or barium swallow.
- Record the date of the last menstrual period and determine the possibility of pregnancy in perimenopausal women.

- Obtain a list of the patient's current medications, including anticoagulants, aspirin and other salicylates, herbs, nutritional supplements, and nutraceuticals (see Appendix F). Such products should be discontinued by medical direction for the appropriate number of days prior to a surgical procedure. Note time and date of last dose.
- Review the procedure with the patient. Address concerns about pain and explain that no pain will be experienced during the procedure. Inform the patient that the procedure is begun in a GI laboratory or office, usually by an HCP or support staff, and that it takes approximately 30 to 60 min to begin the procedure.
- *Sensitivity to social and cultural issues,* as well as concern for modesty, is important in providing psychological support before, during, and after the procedure.
- Instruct the patient to stop taking medications that have a coating effect, such as sucralfate and Pepto-Bismol, 3 days before the procedure.
- Instruct the patient to abstain from the use of tobacco products for 24 hr prior to the procedure.
- Instruct the patient to start a liquid diet on the day before the procedure. From 10 p.m. the evening before the procedure, the patient should not eat or drink except for necessary medication with a sip of water. Instruct the patient to take a standard bowel prep the night before the procedure. Protocols may vary from facility to facility.
- Instruct the patient not to take any medication for 2 hr prior to the procedure.
- Inform the patient that there is a chance of intestinal obstruction associated with the procedure.
- Instruct the patient to wear loose, two-piece clothing on the day of the procedure. This assists with the placement of the sensors on the patient's abdomen.
- *Make sure a written and informed consent has been signed prior to the procedure.*

INTRATEST:

- Ensure that the patient has complied with dietary and medication restrictions and pretesting preparations for at least 8 hr prior to the procedure.
- Observe standard precautions, and follow the general guidelines in Appendix A.
- Obtain accurate height, weight, and abdominal girth measurements prior to beginning the examination.
- Instruct the patient to cooperate fully and to follow directions.
- Ask the patient to ingest the capsule with a full glass of water. The water may have simethicone in it to reduce gastric and bile bubbles.
- After ingesting the capsule, the patient should not eat or drink for at least 2 hr. After 4 hr, the patient may have a light snack.
- After ingesting the capsule and until it is excreted, the patient should not be near any source of powerful electromagnetic fields, such as MRI or amateur (ham) radio equipment.
- The procedure lasts approximately 8 hr.
- Instruct the patient not to disconnect the equipment or remove the belt at any time during the test.
- If the data recorder stops functioning, instruct the patient to record the time and the nature of any event such as eating or drinking.
- Instruct the patient to keep a timed diary for the day detailing the food and liquids ingested and symptoms during the recording period.
- Instruct the patient to avoid any strenuous physical activity, bending, or stooping during the test.

POST-TEST:

- Instruct the patient to resume normal activity, medication, and diet after the test is ended, or as tolerated after the examination, as directed by the HCP.
- Instruct the patient to remove the recorder and return it to the HCP.
- Patients are asked to verify the elimination of the capsule but not to retrieve the capsule.

- Inform the patient that the capsule is a single-use device that does not harbor any environmental hazards.
- Emphasize that any abdominal pain, fever, nausea, vomiting, or difficulty breathing must be immediately reported to the HCP.
- A report of the examination will be sent to the requesting HCP, who will discuss the results with the patient.
- Recognize anxiety related to test results. Discuss the implications of abnormal test results on the patient's lifestyle. Provide teaching and information regarding the clinical implications of the test results, as appropriate.
- Reinforce information given by the patient's HCP regarding further testing, treatment, or referral to another HCP. Decisions regarding the need for and frequency of occult blood testing, colonoscopy, or other cancer screening procedures should be made after consultation between the patient and HCP. The most current guidelines for colon cancer screening of the general population as well as individuals with increased risk are available from the American Cancer Society (www.cancer.org) and the American College of Gastroenterology (www.gi.org). Answer any questions or address any concerns voiced by the patient or family. Answer any questions or address any concerns voiced by the patient or family.
- Depending on the results of this procedure, additional testing may be needed to evaluate or monitor progression of the disease process and determine the need for a change in therapy. Evaluate test results in relation to the patient's symptoms and other tests performed.

RELATED MONOGRAPHS:

- Related tests include barium enema, barium swallow, biopsy intestinal, cancer antigens, colonoscopy, CT abdomen, CT colonoscopy, esophageal manometry, esophagogastroduo-denoscopy, fecal analysis, folate, gastric acid emptying scan, gastric acid stimulation test, gastrin, *Helicobacter pylori*, KUB studies, MRI abdomen, PET pelvis, proctosigmoidoscopy,

upper GI and small bowel series, US abdomen, and vitamin B_{12}.
- Refer to the Gastrointestinal System table at the end of the book for related tests by body system.

Carbon Dioxide

SYNONYM/ACRONYM: CO_2 combining power, CO_2, Tco_2.

COMMON USE: To assess the effect of total carbon dioxide levels on respiratory and metabolic acid-base balance.

SPECIMEN: Serum (1 mL) collected in a red- or tiger-top tube, plasma (1 mL) collected in a green-top (lithium or sodium heparin) tube; or whole blood (1 mL) collected in a green-top (lithium or sodium heparin) tube or heparinized syringe.

REFERENCE VALUE: (Method: Colorimetry, enzyme assay, or Pco_2 electrode)

Carbon Dioxide	Conventional & SI Units
Plasma or serum (venous)	
Infant–2 yr	13–29 mmol/L
2 yr–older adult	23–29 mmol/L
Whole blood (venous)	
Infant–2 yr	18–28 mmol/L
2 yr–older adult	22–26 mmol/L

DESCRIPTION: Serum or plasma carbon dioxide (CO_2) measurement is usually done as part of an electrolyte panel. Total CO_2 (Tco_2) is an important component of the body's buffering capability, and measurements are used mainly in the evaluation of acid-base balance. It is important to understand the differences between Tco_2 (CO_2 content) and CO_2 gas (Pco_2). *Total CO_2*

reflects the majority of CO_2 in the body, mainly in the form of bicarbonate (HCO_3^-); is present as a base; and is regulated by the kidneys. CO_2 gas contributes little to the Tco_2 level, is acidic, and is regulated by the lungs (see monograph titled "Blood Gases").

CO_2 provides the basis for the principal buffering system of the extracellular fluid system, which is the bicarbonate–

carbonic acid buffer system. CO_2 circulates in the body either bound to protein or physically dissolved. Constituents in the blood that contribute to Tco_2 levels are bicarbonate, carbamino compounds, and carbonic acid (carbonic acid includes undissociated carbonic acid and dissolved CO_2). Bicarbonate is the second largest group of anions in the extracellular fluid (chloride is the largest). Tco_2 levels closely reflect bicarbonate levels in the blood, because 90% to 95% of CO_2 circulates as HCO_3^-.

INDICATIONS

* Evaluate decreased venous CO_2 in the case of compensated metabolic acidosis
* Evaluate increased venous CO_2 in the case of compensated metabolic alkalosis
* Monitor decreased venous CO_2 as a result of compensated respiratory alkalosis
* Monitor increased venous CO_2 as a result of compensation for respiratory acidosis secondary to significant respiratory system infection or cancer; decreased respiratory rate

POTENTIAL DIAGNOSIS

Increased in

Interpretation requires clinical information and evaluation of other electrolytes

* Acute intermittent porphyria *(related to severe vomiting associated with acute attacks)*
* Airway obstruction *(related to impaired elimination from weak breathing responses)*
* Asthmatic shock *(related to impaired elimination from abnormal breathing responses)*

* Brain tumor *(related to abnormal blood circulation)*
* Bronchitis (chronic) *(related to impaired elimination from weak breathing responses)*
* Cardiac disorders *(related to lack of blood circulation)*
* Depression of respiratory center *(related to impaired elimination from weak breathing responses)*
* Electrolyte disturbance (severe) *(response to maintain acid-base balance)*
* Emphysema *(related to impaired elimination from weak breathing responses)*
* Hypothyroidism *(related to impaired elimination from weak breathing responses)*
* Hypoventilation *(related to impaired elimination from weak breathing responses)*
* Metabolic alkalosis *(various causes; excessive vomiting)*
* Myopathy *(related to impaired ventilation)*
* Pneumonia *(related to impaired elimination from weak breathing responses)*
* Poliomyelitis *(related to impaired elimination from weak breathing responses)*
* Respiratory acidosis *(related to impaired elimination)*
* Tuberculosis (pulmonary) *(related to impaired elimination from weak breathing responses)*

Decreased in

Interpretation requires clinical information and evaluation of other electrolytes

* Acute renal failure *(response to buildup of ketoacids)*
* Anxiety *(related to hyperventilation; too much CO_2 is exhaled)*
* Dehydration *(response to metabolic acidosis that develops)*
* Diabetic ketoacidosis *(response to buildup of ketoacids)*

- Diarrhea (severe) *(acidosis related to loss of base ions like HCO_3^-; most of CO_2 content is in this form)*
- High fever *(response to neutralize acidosis present during fever)*
- Metabolic acidosis *(response to neutralize acidosis)*
- Respiratory alkalosis *(hyperventilation; too much CO_2 is exhaled)*
- Salicylate intoxication *(response to neutralize related metabolic acidosis)*
- Starvation *(CO_2 buffer system used to neutralize buildup of ketoacids)*

CRITICAL FINDINGS

- Less than 15 mmol/L
- Greater than 40 mmol/L

Note and immediately report to the health-care provider (HCP) any critically increased or decreased values and related symptoms.

Observe the patient for signs and symptoms of excessive or insufficient CO_2 levels, and report these findings to the HCP. If the patient has been vomiting for several days and is breathing shallowly, or if the patient has had gastric suctioning and is breathing shallowly, this may indicate elevated CO_2 levels. Decreased CO_2 levels are evidenced by deep, vigorous breathing and flushed skin.

INTERFERING FACTORS

- Drugs that may cause an increase in Tco_2 levels include acetylsalicylic acid, aldosterone, bicarbonate, carbenicillin, carbenoxolone, corticosteroids, dexamethasone, ethacrynic acid, laxatives (chronic abuse), and x-ray contrast agents.

- Drugs that may cause a decrease in Tco_2 levels include acetazolamide, acetylsalicylic acid (initially), amiloride, ammonium chloride, fluorides, metformin, methicillin, nitrofurantoin, NSD 3004 (long-acting carbonic anhydrase inhibitor), paraldehyde, tetracycline, triamterene, and xylitol.
- Prompt and proper specimen processing, storage, and analysis are important to achieve accurate results. The specimen should be stored under anaerobic conditions after collection to prevent the diffusion of CO_2 gas from the specimen. Falsely decreased values result from uncovered specimens. It is estimated that CO_2 diffuses from the sample at the rate of 6 mmol/hr.

NURSING IMPLICATIONS AND PROCEDURE

PRETEST:

- Positively identify the patient using at least two unique identifiers before providing care, treatment, or services.
- *Patient Teaching:* Inform the patient this test can assist in measuring the amount of carbon dioxide in the body.
- Obtain a history of the patient's complaints, including a list of known allergens, especially allergies or sensitivities to latex.
- Obtain a history of the patient's cardiovascular, genitourinary, and respiratory systems, as well as results of previously performed laboratory tests and diagnostic and surgical procedures.
- Note any recent procedures that can interfere with test results.
- Obtain a list of the patient's current medications, including herbs, nutritional supplements, and nutraceuticals (see Appendix F).

- Review the procedure with the patient. Inform the patient that specimen collection takes approximately 5 to 10 min. Address concerns about pain and explain that there may be some discomfort during the venipuncture.
- *Sensitivity to social and cultural issues,* as well as concern for modesty, is important in providing psychological support before, during, and after the procedure.
- There are no food, fluid, or medication restrictions unless by medical direction.

INTRATEST:

- If the patient has a history of allergic reaction to latex, avoid the use of equipment containing latex.
- Instruct the patient to cooperate fully and to follow directions. Direct the patient to breathe normally and to avoid unnecessary movement.
- Observe standard precautions, and follow the general guidelines in Appendix A. Positively identify the patient, and label the appropriate tubes with the corresponding patient demographics, date, and time of collection. Perform a venipuncture.
- Remove the needle and apply direct pressure with dry gauze to stop bleeding. Observe/assess venipuncture site for bleeding or hematoma formation and secure gauze with adhesive bandage.
- Promptly transport the specimen to the laboratory for processing and analysis.

POST-TEST:

- A report of the results will be sent to the requesting HCP, who will discuss the results with the patient.
- *Nutritional Considerations:* Abnormal CO_2 values may be associated with diseases of the respiratory system. Malnutrition is commonly seen in patients with severe respiratory disease for reasons including fatigue, lack of appetite, and gastrointestinal distress. Research has estimated that the daily caloric intake required for respiration of patients with chronic obstructive pulmonary disease is 10 times higher than that of normal individuals. Adequate intake of vitamins A and C is also important to prevent pulmonary infection and to decrease the extent of lung tissue damage. The importance of following the prescribed diet should be stressed to the patient and/or caregiver.
- Reinforce information given by the patient's HCP regarding further testing, treatment, or referral to another HCP. Answer any questions or address any concerns voiced by the patient or family.
- Depending on the results of this procedure, additional testing may be performed to evaluate or monitor progression of the disease process and determine the need for a change in therapy. Evaluate test results in relation to the patient's symptoms and other tests performed.

RELATED MONOGRAPHS:

- Related tests include anion gap, arterial/alveolar oxygen ratio, biopsy lung, blood gases, chest x-ray, chloride, cold agglutinin titer, CBC white blood cell count and differential, culture bacterial blood, culture bacterial sputum, culture mycobacterium, culture viral, cytology sputum, eosinophil count, ESR, gallium scan, Gram stain, IgE, ketones, lung perfusion scan, osmolality, phosphorus, plethysmography, pleural fluid analysis, potassium, PFT, pulse oximetry, and salicylate.
- Refer to the Cardiovascular, Genitourinary, and Respiratory systems tables at the end of the book for related tests by body system.

Carboxyhemoglobin

SYNONYM/ACRONYM: Carbon monoxide, CO, COHb, COH.

COMMON USE: To identify the amount of carbon monoxide in the blood related to poisoning, toxicity from smoke inhalation, or exhaust from cars.

SPECIMEN: Whole blood (1 mL) collected in a green-top (heparin) or lavender-top (EDTA) tube, depending on laboratory requirement. Specimen should be transported tightly capped (anaerobic) and in an ice slurry if blood gases are to be performed simultaneously. Carboxyhemoglobin is stable at room temperature.

REFERENCE VALUE: (Method: Spectrophotometry, co-oximetry)

	% Saturation of Hemoglobin
Newborns	10–12%
Nonsmokers	Up to 2%
Smokers	Up to 10%

DESCRIPTION: Exogenous carbon monoxide (CO) is a colorless, odorless, tasteless by-product of incomplete combustion derived from the exhaust of automobiles, coal and gas burning, and tobacco smoke. Endogenous CO is produced as a result of red blood cell catabolism. CO levels are elevated in newborns as a result of the combined effects of high hemoglobin turnover and the inefficiency of the infant's respiratory system. CO binds tightly to hemoglobin with an affinity 250 times greater than oxygen, competitively and dramatically reducing the oxygen-carrying capacity of hemoglobin. The increased percentage of bound CO reflects the extent to which normal transport of oxygen has been negatively affected. Overexposure causes hypoxia, which results in headache, nausea, vomiting, vertigo, collapse, or convulsions. Toxic exposure causes anoxia, increased levels of lactic acid, and irreversible tissue damage, which can result in coma or death. Acute exposure may be evidenced by a cherry red color to the lips, skin, and nail beds; this observation may not be apparent in cases of chronic exposure. A direct correlation has been implicated between carboxyhemoglobin levels and symptoms of atherosclerotic disease, angina, and myocardial infarction.

INDICATIONS
- Assist in the diagnosis of suspected CO poisoning
- Evaluate the effect of smoking on the patient
- Evaluate exposure to fires and smoke inhalation

POTENTIAL DIAGNOSIS

Increased in
- CO poisoning
- Hemolytic disease *(CO released during red blood cell catabolism)*
- Tobacco smoking

Decreased in: N/A

CRITICAL FINDINGS ✦

Percent of Total Hemoglobin	Symptoms
10%–20%	Asymptomatic
10%–30%	Disturbance of judgment, headache, dizziness
30%–40%	Dizziness, muscle weakness, vision problems, confusion, increased heart rate, increased breathing rate
50%–60%	Loss of consciousness, coma
Greater than 60%	Death

Note and immediately report to the health-care provider (HCP) any critically increased or decreased values and related symptoms.

Women and children may suffer more severe symptoms of carbon monoxide poisoning at lower levels of carbon monoxide than men because women and children usually have lower red blood cell counts.

A possible intervention in moderate CO poisoning is the administration of supplemental oxygen given at atmospheric pressure. In severe CO poisoning, hyperbaric oxygen treatments may be used.

INTERFERING FACTORS

Specimen should be collected before administration of oxygen therapy.

NURSING IMPLICATIONS AND PROCEDURE

PRETEST:

▶ Positively identify the patient using at least two unique identifiers before providing care, treatment, or services.
▶ *Patient Teaching:* Inform the patient this test can assist in evaluating the extent of carbon monoxide poisoning or toxicity.

▶ Obtain a history of the patient's complaints, including a list of known allergens, especially allergies or sensitivities to latex.
▶ Obtain a history of the patient's respiratory system and results of previously performed laboratory tests and diagnostic and surgical procedures.
▶ Note any recent procedures that can interfere with test results.
▶ Obtain a list of the patient's current medications, including herbs, nutritional supplements, and nutraceuticals (see Appendix F).
▶ Review the procedure with the patient. Explain to the patient or family members that the cause of the headache, vomiting, dizziness, convulsions, or coma could be related to CO exposure. Inform the patient that specimen collection takes approximately 5 to 10 min. Address concerns about pain and explain to the patient that there may be some discomfort during the venipuncture.
▶ *Sensitivity to social and cultural issues,* as well as concern for modesty, is important in providing psychological support before, during, and after the procedure.
▶ If carboxyhemoglobin measurement will be performed simultaneously with arterial blood gases, prepare an ice slurry in a cup or plastic bag and have it on hand for immediate transport of the specimen to the laboratory.
▶ There are no food, fluid, or medication restrictions unless by medical direction.

INTRATEST:

- If the patient has a history of allergic reaction to latex, avoid the use of equipment containing latex.
- Instruct the patient to cooperate fully and to follow directions. Direct the patient to breathe normally and to avoid unnecessary movement.
- Observe standard precautions, and follow the general guidelines in Appendix A. Positively identify the patient, and label the appropriate tubes with the corresponding patient demographics, date, and time of collection. Perform a venipuncture. The tightly capped sample should be placed in an ice slurry immediately after collection. Information on the specimen label should be protected from water in the ice slurry by first placing the specimen in a protective plastic bag.
- Remove the needle and apply direct pressure with dry gauze to stop bleeding. Observe/assess venipuncture site for bleeding or hematoma formation and secure gauze with adhesive bandage.
- Promptly transport the specimen to the laboratory for processing and analysis.

POST-TEST:

- A report of the results will be sent to the requesting HCP, who will discuss the results with the patient.
- Recognize anxiety related to test results, and be supportive of impaired activity related to fear of shortened life expectancy. Discuss the implications of abnormal test results on the patient's lifestyle. Provide teaching and information regarding the clinical implications of the test results, as appropriate. Educate the patient regarding access to counseling services. Educate the patient regarding avoiding gas heaters and indoor cooking fires without adequate ventilation and the need to have gas furnaces checked yearly for CO leakage. Inform the patient of smoking cessation programs, as appropriate.
- Reinforce information given by the patient's HCP regarding further testing, treatment, or referral to another HCP. Answer any questions or address any concerns voiced by the patient or family.
- Depending on the results of this procedure, additional testing may be performed to evaluate or monitor progression of the disease process and determine the need for a change in therapy. Evaluate test results in relation to the patient's symptoms and other tests performed.

RELATED MONOGRAPHS:

- Related tests include angiography pulmonary, arterial/alveolar oxygen ratio, blood gases, carbon dioxide, CBC, lung perfusion scan, lung ventilation scan, plethysmography, and PFT.
- Refer to the Respiratory System table at the end of the book for related tests by body system.

Catecholamines, Blood and Urine

SYNONYM/ACRONYM: Epinephrine, norepinephrine, dopamine.

COMMON USE: To assist in diagnosing catecholamine-secreting tumors, such as those found in the adrenal medulla, and in the investigation of hypertension. The urine test is used to assist in diagnosing pheochromocytoma and as a work-up of neuroblastoma.

SPECIMEN: Plasma (2 mL) collected in green-top (heparin) tube. Urine (25 mL) from a timed specimen collected in a clean, plastic, amber collection container with 6N hydrochloric acid as a preservative.

REFERENCE VALUE: (Method: High-performance liquid chromatography)

Blood	Conventional Units	SI Units
		(Conventional Units × 5.46)
Epinephrine		
Supine, 30 min	0–110 pg/mL	0–600 pmol/L
Standing, 30 min	0–140 pg/mL	0–764 pmol/L
		(Conventional Units × 5.91)
Norepinephrine		
Supine, 30 min	70–750 pg/mL	414–4,432 pmol/L
Standing, 30 min	200–1,700 pg/mL	1,182–10,047 pmol/L
		(Conventional Units × 6.53)
Dopamine		
Supine or standing	0–30 pg/mL	0–196 pmol/L

Urine	Conventional Units	SI Units
		(Conventional Units × 5.46)
Epinephrine		
Newborn–9 yr	0–11.0 mcg/24 hr	0–60.1 nmol/24 hr
10–19 yr	0–18.0 mcg/24 hr	0–98.3 nmol/24 hr
20 yr–older adult	0–20 mcg/24 hr	0–109 nmol/24 hr
		(Conventional Units × 5.91)
Norepinephrine		
Newborn–9 yr	0–59 mcg/24 hr	0–349 nmol/24 hr
10–19 yr	0–90 mcg/24 hr	0–532 nmol/24 hr
20 yr–older adult	0–135 mcg/24 hr	0–798 nmol/24 hr
		(Conventional Units × 6.53)
Dopamine		
Newborn–9 yr	0–414 mcg/24 hr	65–1,698 nmol/24 hr
10–19 yr	0–575 mcg/24 hr	0–3,755 nmol/24 hr
20 yr–older adult	0–510 mcg/24 hr	0–3,330 nmol/24 hr

DESCRIPTION: Catecholamines are produced by the chromaffin tissue of the adrenal medulla. They also are found in sympathetic nerve endings and in the brain. The major catecholamines are epinephrine, norepinephrine, and dopamine. They prepare the body for the fight-or-flight stress response, help regulate metabolism, and are excreted from the body by the kidneys. Levels are affected by diurnal variations, fluctuating in response to stress, postural changes, diet, smoking, drugs, and temperature changes. As a result, blood measurement is not as reliable as a 24-hr timed urine test. For test results to be valid, all of the previously mentioned environmental variables must be controlled when the test is performed. Results of blood specimens are most reliable when the specimen is collected during a hypertensive episode. Catecholamines are measured when there is high suspicion of pheochromocytoma but urine results are normal or borderline. Use of a clonidine suppression test with measurement of plasma catecholamines may be requested. Failure to suppress production of catecholamines after administration of clonidine supports the diagnosis of pheochromocytoma. Elevated homovanillic acid levels rule out pheochromocytoma because this tumor primarily secretes epinephrine. Elevated catecholamines without hypertension suggest neuroblastoma or ganglioneuroma. Findings should be compared with metanephrines and vanillylmandelic acid, which are the metabolites of epinephrine and norepinephrine. Findings should also be compared with homovanillic acid, which is the product of dopamine metabolism.

INDICATIONS

- Assist in the diagnosis of neuroblastoma, ganglioneuroma, or dysautonomia
- Assist in the diagnosis of pheochromocytoma
- Evaluate acute hypertensive episode
- Evaluate hypertension of unknown origin
- Screen for pheochromocytoma among family members with an autosomal dominant inheritance pattern for Lindau–von Hippel disease or multiple endocrine neoplasia

POTENTIAL DIAGNOSIS

Increased in

- Diabetic acidosis (epinephrine and norepinephrine) *(related to metabolic stress; are released to initiate glycogenolysis, gluconeogenesis, and lipolysis)*
- Ganglioblastoma (epinephrine, slight increase; norepinephrine, large increase) *(related to production by the tumor)*
- Ganglioneuroma (all are increased; norepinephrine, largest increase) *(related to production by the tumor)*
- Hypothyroidism (epinephrine and norepinephrine) *(possibly related to interactions among the immune, endocrine, and nervous systems)*
- Long-term manic-depressive disorders (epinephrine and norepinephrine) *(some studies indicate a relationship between decreased catecholamine levels and manic depressive illnesses; the pathophysiology is not well understood)*
- Myocardial infarction (epinephrine and norepinephrine) *(related to physical stress)*
- Neuroblastoma (all are increased; norepinephrine and dopamine, largest increase) *(related to production by the tumor)*
- Pheochromocytoma (epinephrine, continuous or intermittent increase; norepinephrine, slight increase) *(related to production by the tumor)*

- Shock (epinephrine and norepinephrine) *(related to physical stress)*
- Strenuous exercise (epinephrine and norepinephrine) *(related to physical stress)*

Decreased in
- Autonomic nervous system dysfunction (norepinephrine)
- Orthostatic hypotension caused by central nervous system disease (norepinephrine) *(related to inability of sympathetic nervous system to activate postganglionic neuron)*
- Parkinson's disease (dopamine) *(some studies indicate a relationship between decreased catecholamine levels and Parkinson's disease; the pathophysiology is not well understood)*

CRITICAL FINDINGS: N/A

INTERFERING FACTORS
- Drugs that may increase plasma catecholamine levels include ajmaline, chlorpromazine, cyclopropane, diazoxide, ether, monoamine oxidase inhibitors, nitroglycerin, pentazocine, perphenazine, phenothiazine, promethazine, and theophylline.
- Drugs that may decrease plasma catecholamine levels include captopril, and reserpine.
- Drugs that may increase urine catecholamine levels include atenolol, isoproterenol, methyldopa, niacin, nitroglycerin, prochlorperazine, rauwolfia, reserpine, syrosingopine, and theophylline.
- Drugs that may decrease urine catecholamine levels include bretylium tosylate, clonidine, decaborane, guanethidine, guanfacine, methyldopa, ouabain, radiographic substances, and reserpine.

- Stress, hypoglycemia, smoking, and drugs can produce elevated catecholamines.
- Secretion of catecholamines exhibits diurnal variation, with the lowest levels occurring at night.
- Secretion of catecholamines varies during the menstrual cycle, with higher levels excreted during the luteal phase and lowest levels during ovulation.
- Diets high in amines (e.g., bananas, avocados, beer, aged cheese, chocolate, cocoa, coffee, fava beans, grains, tea, vanilla, walnuts, Chianti wine) can produce elevated catecholamine levels.
- Failure to collect all urine and store 24-hr specimen properly will yield a falsely low result.
- Failure to follow dietary restrictions before the procedure may cause the procedure to be canceled or repeated.

NURSING IMPLICATIONS AND PROCEDURE

PRETEST:
- Positively identify the patient using at least two unique identifiers before providing care, treatment, or services.
- *Patient Teaching:* Inform the patient this test can assist in investigating the cause of fluctuating hormone levels.
- Obtain a history of the patient's complaints, including a list of known allergens, especially allergies or sensitivities to latex.
- Obtain a history of the patient's endocrine system, as well as results of previously performed laboratory tests and diagnostic and surgical procedures.
- Record the date of the patient's last menstrual period.
- Obtain a list of the patient's current medications, including herbs, nutritional supplements, and nutraceuticals (see Appendix F).
- Review the procedure with the patient.

Blood

▶ Inform the patient that he or she may be asked to keep warm and to rest for 45 to 60 min before the test. Inform the patient that multiple specimens may be required. Inform the patient that specimen collection takes approximately 5 to 10 min. Address concerns about pain and explain that there may be some discomfort during the venipuncture. Inform the patient that a saline lock may be inserted before the test because the stress of repeated venipunctures may increase catecholamine levels.

Urine

▶ Provide a nonmetallic urinal, bedpan, or toilet-mounted collection device. Address concerns about pain related to the procedure. Explain to the patient that there should be no discomfort during the procedure. Usually a 24-hr time frame for urine collection is ordered. Inform the patient that all urine over a 24-hr period must be saved; if a preservative has been added to the container, instruct the patient not to discard the preservative. Instruct the patient not to void directly into the laboratory collection container. Instruct the patient to avoid defecating in the collection device and to keep toilet tissue out of the collection device to prevent contamination of the specimen. Place a sign in the bathroom as a reminder to save all urine. Instruct the patient to void all urine into the collection device, then pour the urine into the laboratory collection container. Alternatively, the specimen can be left in the collection device for a health care staff member to add to the laboratory collection container.

Blood and Urine

▶ Sensitivity to social and cultural issues, as well as concern for modesty, is important in providing psychological support before, during, and after the procedure.

▶ Instruct the patient to follow a normal-sodium diet for 3 days before testing, abstain from smoking tobacco for 24 hr before testing, and avoid consumption of foods high in amines for 48 hr before testing.

▶ Instruct the patient to avoid self-prescribed medications for 2 wk before testing (especially appetite suppressants and cold and allergy medications, such as nose drops, cough suppressants, and bronchodilators).

▶ Instruct the patient to withhold prescribed medication (especially methyldopa, epinephrine, levodopa, and methenamine mandelate) if directed by the health-care provider (HCP).

▶ Instruct the patient to withhold food and fluids for 10 to 12 hr before the test. Protocols may vary from facility to facility.

▶ Instruct the patient collecting a 24-hr urine specimen to avoid excessive stress and exercise during the test collection period.

▶ Prior to blood specimen collection, prepare an ice slurry in a cup or plastic bag to have ready for immediate transport of the specimen to the laboratory. Prechill the collection tube in the ice slurry.

INTRATEST:

▶ Ensure that the patient has complied with dietary, medication, and activity restrictions and with pretesting preparations; ensure that food and fluids have been restricted for at least 10 to 12 hr prior to the procedure, and that excessive exercise and stress have been avoided prior to the procedure. Instruct the patient to continue to avoid excessive exercise and stress during the 24-hr collection of urine.

▶ If the patient has a history of allergic reaction to latex, care should be taken to avoid the use of equipment containing latex.

▶ Instruct the patient to cooperate fully and to follow directions.

▶ Observe standard precautions, and follow the general guidelines in Appendix A. Positively identify the patient, and label the appropriate collection containers with the corresponding patient demographics, date, and time of collection.

Blood

- Perform a venipuncture between 6 and 8 a.m.; collect the specimen in a prechilled tube.
- Remove the needle and apply direct pressure with dry gauze to stop bleeding. Observe/assess venipuncture site for bleeding or hematoma formation and secure gauze with adhesive bandage.
- Ask the patient to stand for 10 min, and then perform a second venipuncture and obtain a sample as previously described.
- Each sample should be placed in an ice slurry immediately after collection. Information on the specimen labels should be protected from water in the ice slurry by first placing the specimens in a protective plastic bag. Promptly transport the specimens to the laboratory for processing and analysis.

Urine

- Obtain a clean 3-L urine specimen container, toilet-mounted collection device, and plastic bag (for transport of the specimen container). The specimen must be refrigerated or kept on ice throughout the collection period. If an indwelling urinary catheter is in place, the drainage bag must be kept on ice.
- Begin the test between 6 and 8 a.m. if possible. Collect first voiding and discard. Record the time the specimen was discarded as the beginning of the timed collection period. The next morning, ask the patient to void at the same time the collection was started and add this last voiding to the container.
- If an indwelling catheter is in place, replace the tubing and container system at the start of the collection time. Keep the container system on ice during the collection period or empty the urine into a larger container periodically during the collection period; monitor to ensure continued drainage, and conclude the test the next morning at the same hour the collection was begun.

- At the conclusion of the test, compare the quantity of urine with the urinary output record for the collection; if the specimen contains less than what was recorded as output, some urine may have been discarded, invalidating the test.

Blood and Urine

- Include on the collection container's label the amount of urine, test start and stop times, and ingestion of any foods or medications that can affect test results.
- Promptly transport the specimen to the laboratory for processing and analysis.

POST-TEST:

- A report of the results will be sent to the requesting HCP, who will discuss the results with the patient.
- Instruct the patient to resume usual diet, fluids, medications, and activity, as directed by the HCP.
- Recognize anxiety related to test results. Discuss the implications of abnormal test results on the patient's lifestyle. Provide teaching and information regarding the clinical implications of the test results, as appropriate.
- Reinforce information given by the patient's HCP regarding further testing, treatment, or referral to another HCP. Answer any questions or address any concerns voiced by the patient or family.
- Depending on the results of this procedure, additional testing may be performed to evaluate or monitor progression of the disease process and determine the need for a change in therapy. Evaluate test results in relation to the patient's symptoms and other tests performed.

RELATED MONOGRAPHS:

- Related tests include angiography adrenal, calcitonin, CT renal, HVA, metanephrines, renin, and VMA.
- Refer to the Endocrine System table at the end of the book for related tests by body system.

CD4/CD8 Enumeration

SYNONYM/ACRONYM: T-cell profile.

COMMON USE: To monitor HIV disease progression and the effectiveness of retroviral therapy.

SPECIMEN: Whole blood (1 mL) collected in a green-top (heparin) tube.

REFERENCE VALUE: (Method: flow cytometry)

Total lymphocytes	1,000–4,800/mm^3 (1.0–4.8 × 10^3)	34%
Mature T cells (CD3)	650–3,036/mm^3	65–92%
Helper T cells (CD4)	310–2,112/mm^3	31–64%
Suppressor T cells (CD8)	80–1,353/mm^3	8–41%
CD4/CD8 ratio	1.0–3.7	

DESCRIPTION: Enumeration of lymphocytes, identification of cell lineage, and identification of cellular stage of development are used to diagnose and classify malignant myeloproliferative diseases and to plan treatment. T-cell enumeration is also useful in the evaluation and management of immunodeficiency and autoimmune disease. A severely depressed CD4 count is an excellent predictor of imminent opportunistic infection. HIV viral load is another important test used to establish a baseline for viral activity when a person is first diagnosed with HIV. Viral load testing is performed on plasma from a whole blood sample. Methods commonly used to perform viral load testing include branched DNA (bDNA) or reverse transcriptase polymerase chain reaction (RT-PCR). Results are not interchangeable from method to method. Therefore, it is important to use the same viral load method for serial testing. Baseline and repeat testing for CD4 count and viral load are usually performed 2 to 4 wk apart. The viral load demonstrates how actively the virus is reproducing and helps determine whether treatment is necessary. CD4 count is a reflection of immune status. Public health guidelines recommend that treatment of asymptomatic patients be considered when CD4 count is greater than 350/mm^3 and viral load is 55,000 copies/mL or greater (bDNA) or 30,000 copies/mL or greater (RT-PCR); treatment is recommended when the patient is symptomatic regardless of test results or when the patient is asymptomatic and CD4 count is less than 350/mm^3 and viral load is detectable. If retroviral therapy is initiated, CD4 counts and viral load studies will be monitored every 3 to 4 mo. Viral mutations occur; increased viral load may indicate resistance to antiviral drugs. Changes in drug therapy may warrant additional viral load studies to verify efficacy of modified therapy.

INDICATIONS

- Assist in the diagnosis of AIDS and plan treatment
- Evaluate malignant myeloproliferative diseases and plan treatment
- Evaluate thymus-dependent or cellular immunocompetence

POTENTIAL DIAGNOSIS

Increased in

- Malignant myeloproliferative diseases (e.g., acute and chronic lymphocytic leukemia, lymphoma)

Decreased in

- AIDS
- Aplastic anemia
- Hodgkin's disease

CRITICAL FINDINGS: N/A

INTERFERING FACTORS

- Drugs that may increase T-cell count include interferon-γ.
- Drugs that may decrease T-cell count include chlorpromazine and prednisone.
- Specimens should be stored at room temperature.
- Recent radioactive scans or radiation can decrease T-cell counts.
- Values may be abnormal in patients with severe recurrent illness or after recent surgery requiring general anesthesia.

NURSING IMPLICATIONS AND PROCEDURE

PRETEST:

▶ Positively identify the patient using at least two unique identifiers before providing care, treatment, or services.

▶ *Patient Teaching:* Inform the patient this test can assist in diagnosing disease and monitoring the effectiveness of disease therapy.

▶ Obtain a history of the patient's complaints, including a list of known allergens, especially allergies or sensitivities to latex.

▶ Obtain a history of the patient's hematopoietic and immune systems and results of previously performed laboratory tests and diagnostic and surgical procedures.

▶ Note any recent procedures that can interfere with test results.

▶ Obtain a list of the patient's current medications, including herbs, nutritional supplements, and nutraceuticals (see Appendix F).

▶ Review the procedure with the patient. Inform the patient that specimen collection takes approximately 5 to 10 min. Address concerns about pain and explain that there may be some discomfort during the venipuncture.

▶ *Sensitivity to social and cultural issues,* as well as concern for modesty, is important in providing psychological support before, during, and after the procedure.

▶ There are no food, fluid, or medication restrictions unless by medical direction.

INTRATEST:

▶ If the patient has a history of allergic reaction to latex, avoid the use of equipment containing latex.

▶ Instruct the patient to cooperate fully and to follow directions. Direct the patient to breathe normally and to avoid unnecessary movement.

▶ Observe standard precautions, and follow the general guidelines in Appendix A. Positively identify the patient, and label the appropriate tubes with the corresponding patient demographics, date, and time of collection. Perform a venipuncture.

▶ Remove the needle and apply direct pressure with dry gauze to stop bleeding. Observe/assess venipuncture site for bleeding or hematoma formation and secure gauze with adhesive bandage.

Promptly transport the specimen to the laboratory for processing and analysis.

POST-TEST:

A report of the results will be sent to the requesting health care provider (HCP), who will discuss the results with the patient.

Nutritional Considerations: As appropriate, stress the importance of good nutrition and suggest that the patient meet with a nutritional specialist. Stress the importance of following the care plan for medications and follow-up visits. Inform the patient that subsequent requests for follow-up blood work at regular intervals should be anticipated.

Recognize anxiety related to test results, and be supportive of impaired activity related to perceived loss of independence and fear of shortened life expectancy. Discuss the implications of abnormal test results on the patient's lifestyle. Provide teaching and information regarding the clinical implications of the test results, as appropriate. Educate the patient as to the risk of infection related to immunosuppressed inflammatory response and fatigue related to decreased energy production. Educate the patient regarding access to counseling services.

Counsel the patient, as appropriate, regarding risk of transmission and proper prophylaxis, and reinforce the importance of strict adherence to the treatment regimen, including consultation with a pharmacist.

Reinforce information given by the patient's HCP regarding further testing, treatment, or referral to another HCP. Provide contact information, if desired, for the Centers for Disease Control and Prevention (www.cdc.org). Answer any questions or address any concerns voiced by the patient or family.

Depending on the results of this procedure, additional testing may be performed to evaluate or monitor progression of the disease process and determine the need for a change in therapy. Evaluate test results in relation to the patient's symptoms and other tests performed.

RELATED MONOGRAPHS:

Related tests include biopsy bone marrow, bronchoscopy, CBC, CBC platelet count, CBC WBC count and differential, culture and smear mycobacteria, culture viral, cytology sputum, gallium scan, HIV-1/HIV-2 antibodies, laparoscopy abdominal, LAP, lymphangiogram, MRI musculoskeletal, mediastinoscopy, and β_2-microglobulin.

Refer to the Hematopoietic and Immune systems tables at the end of the book for related tests by body system.

Cerebrospinal Fluid Analysis

SYNONYM/ACRONYM: CSF analysis.

COMMON USE: To assist in the differential diagnosis of infection or hemorrhage of the brain. Also used in the evaluation of other conditions with significant neuromuscular effects, such as multiple sclerosis.

SPECIMEN: CSF (1 to 3 mL) collected in three or four separate plastic conical tubes. Tube 1 is used for chemistry and serology testing, tube 2 is used for microbiology, tube 3 is used for cell count, and tube 4 is used for miscellaneous testing.

REFERENCE VALUE: (Method: Macroscopic evaluation of appearance; spectrophotometry for glucose, lactic acid, and protein; immunoassay for myelin basic protein; nephelometry for immunoglobulin G [IgG]; electrophoresis for oligoclonal banding; Gram stain, India ink preparation, and culture for microbiology; microscopic examination of fluid for cell count; flocculation for Venereal Disease Research Laboratory [VDRL])

Lumbar Puncture	Conventional Units	SI Units
Color and appearance	Crystal clear	
		(Conventional Units × 10)
Protein		
0–1 mo	Less than 150 mg/dL	Less than 15,000 mg/L
1–6 mo	30–100 mg/dL	3,000–10,000 mg/L
7 mo–adult	15–45 mg/dL	150–450 mg/L
Older adult	15–60 mg/dL	150–600 mg/L
		(Conventional Units × 0.0555)
Glucose		
Infant or child	60–80 mg/dL	3.3–4.4 mmol/L
Adult	40–70 mg/dL	2.2–3.9 mmol/L
		(Conventional Units × 0.111)
Lactic acid		
Neonate	10–60 mg/dL	1.1–6.7 mmol/L
3–10 days	10–40 mg/dL	1.1–4.4 mmol/L
Adult	Less than 25.2 mg/dL	Less than 2.8 mmol/L
		(Conventional Units × 1)
Myelin basic protein	Less than 4.0 ng/mL	Less than 4.0 mcg/L
Oligoclonal bands	Absent	
		(Conventional Units × 10)
IgG	Less than 3.4 mg/dL	Less than 34 mg/L
Gram stain	Negative	
India ink	Negative	
Culture	No growth	
RBC count	0	0
		(Conventional Units × 1)
WBC count		
Neonate–1 mo	0–30/mL	0–30 × 10^6/L
1 mo–1 yr	0–10/mL	0–10 × 10^6/L
1–5 yr	0–8/mL	0–8 × 10^6/L
5 yr–adult	0–5/mL	0–5 × 10^6/L

WBC Differential	Adult	Children
Lymphocytes	40%–80%	5%–13%
Monocytes	15%–45%	50%–90%
Neutrophils	0%–6%	0%–8%

(table continues on page 328)

VDRL	Nonreactive
Cytology	No abnormal cells seen

CSF glucose should be 60%–70% of plasma glucose level.
RBC = red blood cell; VDRL = Venereal Disease Research Laboratory; WBC = white blood cell.
Color should be assessed after sample is centrifuged.

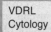

DESCRIPTION: Cerebrospinal fluid (CSF) circulates in the subarachnoid space and has a twofold function: to protect the brain and spinal cord from injury and to transport products of cellular metabolism and neurosecretion. The total volume of CSF is 90 to 150 mL in adults and 60 mL in infants. CSF analysis helps determine the presence and cause of bleeding and assists in diagnosing cancer, infections, and degenerative and autoimmune diseases of the brain and spinal cord. Specimens for analysis are most frequently obtained by lumbar puncture and sometimes by ventricular or cisternal puncture. Lumbar puncture can also have therapeutic uses, including injection of drugs and anesthesia.

INDICATIONS

- Assist in the diagnosis and differentiation of subarachnoid or intracranial hemorrhage
- Assist in the diagnosis and differentiation of viral or bacterial meningitis or encephalitis
- Assist in the diagnosis of diseases such as multiple sclerosis, autoimmune disorders, or degenerative brain disease
- Assist in the diagnosis of neurosyphilis and chronic central nervous system (CNS) infections
- Detect obstruction of CSF circulation due to hemorrhage, tumor, or edema
- Establish the presence of any condition decreasing the flow of oxygen to the brain
- Monitor for metastases of cancer into the CNS
- Monitor severe brain injuries

POTENTIAL DIAGNOSIS

Increased in
- Color and appearance *(xanthochromia is any pink, yellow, or orange color; bloody—hemorrhage; xanthochromic—old hemorrhage, red blood cell [RBC] breakdown, methemoglobin, bilirubin [greater than 6 mg/dL], increased protein [greater than 150 mg/dL], melanin [meningeal melanosarcoma], carotene [systemic carotenemia]; hazy—meningitis; pink to dark yellow—aspiration of epidural fat; turbid—cells, microorganisms, protein, fat, or contrast medium)*
- Protein *(related to alterations in blood-brain barrier that allow permeability to proteins)*: meningitis, encephalitis
- Lactic acid *(related to cerebral hypoxia and correlating anaerobic metabolism)*: bacterial, tubercular, fungal meningitis
- Myelin basic protein *(related to accumulation as a result of nerve sheath demyelination)*: trauma, stroke, tumor, multiple sclerosis, subacute sclerosing panencephalitis
- IgG and oligoclonal banding *(related to autoimmune or*

inflammatory response): multiple sclerosis, CNS syphilis, and subacute sclerosing panencephalitis

- Gram stain: *meningitis due to Escherichia coli, Streptococcus agalactiae, Streptococcus pneumoniae, Haemophilus influenzae, Mycobacterium avium-intracellulare, Mycobacterium leprae, Mycobacterium tuberculosis, Neisseria meningitidis, Cryptococcus neoformans*
- India ink preparation: *meningitis due to C. neoformans*
- Culture: *encephalitis or meningitis due to herpes simplex virus, S. pneumoniae, H. influenzae, N. meningitidis, C. neoformans*
- RBC count: *hemorrhage*
- White blood cell (WBC) count: *General increase—injection of contrast media or anticancer drugs in subarachnoid space; CSF infarct; metastatic tumor in contact with CSF; reaction to repeated lumbar puncture*
  Elevated WBC count with a predominance of neutrophils indicative of bacterial meningitis
  Elevated WBC count with a predominance of lymphocytes indicative of viral, tubercular, parasitic, or fungal meningitis; multiple sclerosis
  Elevated WBC count with a predominance of monocytes indicative of chronic bacterial meningitis, amebic meningitis, multiple sclerosis, toxoplasmosis
  Increased plasma cells indicative of acute viral infections, multiple sclerosis, sarcoidosis, syphilitic meningoencephalitis, subacute sclerosing panencephalitis, tubercular meningitis, parasitic infections, Guillain-Barré syndrome
  Presence of eosinophils indicative of parasitic and fungal infections, acute polyneuritis, idiopathic hypereosinophilic syndrome, reaction to drugs or a shunt in CSF

- VDRL: *syphilis*

Positive findings in
- Cytology: *malignant cells*

Decreased in
- Glucose: *bacterial and tubercular meningitis*

CRITICAL FINDINGS ✧
- Positive Gram stain, India ink preparation, or culture
- Presence of malignant cells or blasts
- Elevated WBC count
- Glucose less than 37 mg/dL

Note and immediately report to the health-care provider (HCP) any positive or critically increased results and related symptoms.

INTERFERING FACTORS

This procedure is contraindicated for
- ✧ This procedure is contraindicated if infection is present at the needle insertion site.
- ✧ It may also be contraindicated in patients with degenerative joint disease or coagulation defects and in patients who are uncooperative during the procedure.
- ✧ Use with extreme caution in patients with increased intracranial pressure because overly rapid removal of CSF can result in herniation.

Other considerations
- Drugs that may decrease CSF protein levels include cefotaxime and dexamethasone.
- Interferon-β may increase myelin basic protein levels.
- Drugs that may increase CSF glucose levels include cefotaxime and dexamethasone.
- RBC count may be falsely elevated with a traumatic spinal tap.

- Delays in analysis may present a false positive appearance of xanthochromia due to RBC lysis that begins within 4 hr of a bloody tap.

NURSING IMPLICATIONS AND PROCEDURE

PRETEST:

- Positively identify the patient using at least two unique identifiers before providing care, treatment, or services.
- *Patient Teaching:* Inform the patient this procedure can assist in evaluating health by providing a sample of fluid from around the spinal cord to be tested for disease and infection.
- Obtain a history of the patient's complaints, including a list of known allergens, especially allergies or sensitivities to latex or anesthetics.
- Obtain a history of the patient's immune and musculoskeletal systems and results of previously performed laboratory tests and diagnostic and surgical procedures.
- Obtain a list of the patient's current medications, including herbs, nutritional supplements, and nutraceuticals (see Appendix F).
- Review the procedure with the patient. Inform the patient that the position required may be awkward but that someone will assist during the procedure. Stress the importance of remaining still and breathing normally throughout the procedure. Inform the patient that specimen collection takes approximately 20 min. Address concerns about pain and explain that a stinging sensation may be felt when the local anesthetic is injected. Instruct the patient to report any pain or other sensations that may require repositioning the spinal needle. Explain that there may be some discomfort during the procedure. Inform the patient the procedure will be performed by a HCP.
- *Sensitivity to social and cultural issues,* as well as concern for modesty, is important in providing psychological support before, during, and after the procedure.

- There are no food, fluid, or medication restrictions unless by medical direction.
- *Make sure a written and informed consent has been signed prior to the procedure and before administering any medications.*

INTRATEST:

- If the patient has a history of allergic reaction to latex, avoid the use of equipment containing latex.
- Ensure that anticoagulant therapy has been withheld for the appropriate number of days prior to the procedure. Number of days to withhold medication is dependent on the type of anticoagulant. Notify HCP if patient anticoagulant therapy has not been withheld.
- Have emergency equipment readily available.
- Instruct the patient to cooperate fully and to follow directions. Direct the patient to breathe normally and to avoid unnecessary movement.
- Observe standard precautions, and follow the general guidelines in Appendix A. Positively identify the patient, and label the appropriate tubes with the corresponding patient demographics, date, and time of collection. Collect the specimen in four plastic conical tubes.
- Record baseline vital signs.
- To perform a lumbar puncture, position the patient in the knee-chest position at the side of the bed. Provide pillows to support the spine or for the patient to grasp. The sitting position is an alternative. In this position, the patient must bend the neck and chest to the knees.
- Prepare the site—usually between L3 and L4, or between L4 and L5—with povidone-iodine and drape the area.
- A local anesthetic is injected. Using sterile technique, the HCP inserts the spinal needle through the spinous processes of the vertebrae and into the subarachnoid space. The stylet is removed. If the needle is properly placed, CSF drips from the needle.
- Attach the stopcock and manometer, and measure initial pressure. Normal pressure for an adult in the lateral

recumbent position is 90 to 180 mm H_2O; normal pressure for a child age 8 years or younger is 10 to 100 mm H_2O. These values depend on the body position and are different in a horizontal or sitting position.

- CSF pressure may be elevated if the patient is anxious, holding his or her breath, or tensing muscles. It may also be elevated if the patient's knees are flexed too firmly against the abdomen. CSF pressure may be significantly elevated in patients with intracranial tumors. If the initial pressure is elevated, the HCP may perform Queckenstedt's test. To perform this test, pressure is applied to the jugular vein for about 10 sec. CSF pressure usually rises rapidly in response to the occlusion and then returns to the pretest level within 10 sec after the pressure is released. Sluggish response may indicate CSF obstruction.
- Obtain four (or five) vials of fluid, according to the HCP's request, in separate tubes (1 to 3 mL in each), and label them numerically (1 to 4 or 5) in the order they were filled.
- A final pressure reading is taken, and the needle is removed. Clean the puncture site with an antiseptic solution and apply direct pressure with dry gauze to stop bleeding or CSF leakage. Observe/assess puncture site for bleeding, CSF leakage, or hematoma formation and secure gauze with adhesive bandage.
- Promptly transport the specimen to the laboratory for processing and analysis.

POST-TEST:

- A report of the results will be sent to the requesting HCP, who will discuss the results with the patient.
- Monitor vital signs and neurological status and for headache every 15 min for 1 hr, then every 2 hr for 4 hr, and then as ordered by the HCP. Monitor temperature every 4 hr for 24 hr. Compare with baseline values. Notify the HCP if temperature is elevated. Protocols may vary among facilities.
- If permitted, administer fluids to replace lost CSF and help prevent or relieve

headache—a side effect of lumbar puncture.
- Position the patient flat in the supine position with head of bed at not more than a 30° elevation, following the HCP's instructions. Maintain position for 8 hr. Changing position is acceptable as long as the body remains horizontal.
- Recognize anxiety related to test results. Discuss the implications of abnormal test results on the patient's lifestyle. Provide teaching and information regarding the clinical implications of the test results, as appropriate.
- Reinforce information given by the patient's HCP regarding further testing, treatment, or referral to another HCP. Provide information regarding vaccine-preventable diseases when indicated (encephalitis, influenza, meningococcal diseases). Answer any questions or address any concerns voiced by the patient or family.
- Instruct the patient in the use of any ordered medications. Explain the importance of adhering to the therapy regimen. As appropriate, instruct the patient in significant side effects and systemic reactions associated with the prescribed medication. Encourage him or her to review corresponding literature provided by a pharmacist.
- Depending on the results of this procedure, additional testing may be performed to evaluate or monitor progression of the disease process and determine the need for a change in therapy. Evaluate test results in relation to the patient's symptoms and other tests performed.

RELATED MONOGRAPHS:

- Related tests include CBC, CT brain, culture for appropriate organisms (blood, fungal, mycobacteria, sputum, throat, viral, wound), EMG, evoked brain potentials, Gram stain, MRI brain, PET brain, and syphilis serology.
- Refer to the Immune and Musculoskeletal systems tables at the end of the book for related tests by body system.

Ceruloplasmin

SYNONYM/ACRONYM: Copper oxidase, Cp.

COMMON USE: To assist in the evaluation of copper intoxication and liver disease, especially Wilson's disease.

SPECIMEN: Serum (1 mL) collected in a red- or tiger-top tube.

REFERENCE VALUE: (Method: Nephelometry)

Age	Conventional Units	SI Units (Conventional Units × 10)
Newborn–3 mo	5–18 mg/dL	50–180 mg/L
6–12 mo	33–43 mg/dL	330–430 mg/L
1–3 yr	26–55 mg/dL	260–550 mg/L
4–5 yr	27–56 mg/dL	270–560 mg/L
6–7 yr	24–48 mg/dL	240–480 mg/L
8 yr–older adult	20–54 mg/dL	200–540 mg/L

DESCRIPTION: Ceruloplasmin is an α_2-globulin produced by the liver that binds copper for transport in the blood after it is absorbed from the gastrointestinal system. Decreased production of this globulin causes copper to be deposited in body tissues such as the brain, liver, corneas, and kidneys.

INDICATIONS
- Assist in the diagnosis of Menkes' (kinky hair) disease
- Assist in the diagnosis of Wilson's disease
- Determine genetic predisposition to Wilson's disease
- Monitor patient response to total parenteral nutrition (hyperalimentation)

POTENTIAL DIAGNOSIS

Increased in
Ceruloplasmin is an acute-phase reactant protein and will be increased in many inflammatory conditions, including cancer
- Acute infections
- Biliary cirrhosis
- Cancer of the bone, lung, stomach
- Copper intoxication
- Hodgkin's disease
- Leukemia
- Pregnancy (last trimester) *(estrogen increases copper levels)*
- Rheumatoid arthritis
- Tissue necrosis

Decreased in
- Menkes' disease *(severe X-linked defect causing failed transport to the liver and tissues)*
- Nutritional deficiency of copper
- Wilson's disease *(genetic defect causing failed transport to the liver and tissues)*

CRITICAL FINDINGS: N/A

INTERFERING FACTORS
- Drugs that may increase ceruloplasmin levels include anticonvulsants,

norethindrone, oral contraceptives, and tamoxifen.

- Drugs that may decrease ceruloplasmin levels include asparaginase and levonorgestrel (Norplant).
- Excessive therapeutic intake of zinc may interfere with intestinal absorption of copper.

NURSING IMPLICATIONS AND PROCEDURE

PRETEST:

- Positively identify the patient using at least two unique identifiers before providing care, treatment, or services.
- *Patient Teaching:* Inform the patient this test can determine copper levels in the blood.
- Obtain a history of the patient's complaints, including a list of known allergens, especially allergies or sensitivities to latex.
- Obtain a history of the patient's hepatobiliary system and results of previously performed laboratory tests and diagnostic and surgical procedures.
- Obtain a list of the patient's current medications, including herbs, nutritional supplements, and nutraceuticals (see Appendix F).
- Review the procedure with the patient. Inform the patient that specimen collection takes approximately 5 to 10 min. Address concerns about pain and explain that there may be some discomfort during the venipuncture.
- *Sensitivity to social and cultural issues,* as well as concern for modesty, is important in providing psychological support before, during, and after the procedure.
- There are no food, fluid, or medication restrictions unless by medical direction.

INTRATEST:

- If the patient has a history of allergic reaction to latex, avoid the use of equipment containing latex.
- Instruct the patient to cooperate fully and to follow directions. Direct the patient to breathe normally and to avoid unnecessary movement.
- Observe standard precautions, and follow the general guidelines in

Appendix A. Positively identify the patient, and label the appropriate tubes with the corresponding patient demographics, date, and time of collection. Perform a venipuncture.
- Remove the needle and apply direct pressure with dry gauze to stop bleeding. Observe/assess venipuncture site for bleeding or hematoma formation and secure gauze with adhesive bandage.
- Promptly transport the specimen to the laboratory for processing and analysis.

POST-TEST:

- A report of the results will be sent to the requesting health-care provider (HCP), who will discuss the results with the patient.
- *Nutritional Considerations:* Instruct the patient with copper deficiency to increase intake of foods rich in copper, as appropriate. Organ meats, shellfish, nuts, and legumes are good sources of dietary copper. High intake of zinc, iron, calcium, and manganese interferes with copper absorption. Copper deficiency does not normally occur in adults; however, patients receiving long-term total parenteral nutrition should be evaluated if signs and symptoms of copper deficiency appear, such as jaundice or eye color changes. Kayser-Fleischer rings (green-gold rings) in the cornea and a liver biopsy specimen showing more than 250 mcg of copper per gram confirms Wilson's disease.
- Reinforce information given by the patient's HCP regarding further testing, treatment, or referral to another HCP. Answer any questions or address any concerns voiced by the patient or family.
- Depending on the results of this procedure, additional testing may be performed to evaluate or monitor progression of the disease process and determine the need for a change in therapy. Evaluate test results in relation to the patient's symptoms and other tests performed.

RELATED MONOGRAPHS:

- Related tests include biopsy liver, copper, and zinc.
- Refer to the Hepatobiliary System table at the end of the book for related tests by body system.

Chest X-Ray

SYNONYM/ACRONYM: Chest radiography, CXR.

COMMON USE: To assist in the evaluation of cardiac, respiratory, and skeletal structure within the lung cavity and diagnose multiple diseases such as pneumonia and congestive heart failure.

AREA OF APPLICATION: Lungs.

CONTRAST: None.

DESCRIPTION: Chest radiography, commonly called chest x-ray, is one of the most frequently performed radiological diagnostic studies. This study yields information about the pulmonary, cardiac, and skeletal systems. The lungs, filled with air, are easily penetrated by x-rays and appear black on chest images. A routine chest x-ray includes a posteroanterior (PA) projection, in which x-rays pass from the posterior to the anterior, and a left lateral projection. Additional projections that may be requested are obliques, lateral decubitus, or lordotic views. Portable x-rays, done in acute or critical situations, can be done at the bedside and usually include only the anteroposterior (AP) projection with additional images taken in a lateral decubitus position if the presence of free pleural fluid or air is in question. Chest images should be taken on full inspiration and erect when possible to minimize heart magnification and demonstrate fluid levels. Expiration images may be added to detect a pneumothorax or locate foreign bodies. Rib detail images may be taken to delineate bone pathology, useful when chest radiographs suggest fractures or metastatic lesions. Fluoroscopic studies of the chest can also be done to evaluate lung and diaphragm movement. In the beginning of the disease process of tuberculosis, asthma, and chronic obstructive pulmonary disease, the results of a chest x-ray may not correlate with the clinical status of the patient and may even be normal.

INDICATIONS
- Aid in the diagnosis of diaphragmatic hernia, lung tumors, intravenous devices, and metastasis
- Evaluate known or suspected pulmonary disorders, chest trauma, cardiovascular disorders, and skeletal disorders
- Evaluate placement and position of an endotracheal tube, tracheostomy tube, nasogastric feeding tube, pacemaker wires, central venous catheters, Swan-Ganz catheters, chest tubes, and intra-aortic balloon pump
- Evaluate positive PPD or Mantoux tests
- Monitor resolution, progression, or maintenance of disease
- Monitor effectiveness of the treatment regimen

POTENTIAL DIAGNOSIS

Normal findings in
• Normal lung fields, cardiac size, mediastinal structures, thoracic spine, ribs, and diaphragm

Abnormal findings in
• Atelectasis
• Bronchitis
• Curvature of the spinal column (scoliosis)
• Enlarged heart
• Enlarged lymph nodes
• Flattened diaphragm
• Foreign bodies lodged in the pulmonary system
• Fractures of the sternum, ribs, and spine
• Lung pathology, including tumors
• Malposition of tubes or wires
• Mediastinal tumor and pathology
• Pericardial effusion
• Pericarditis
• Pleural effusion
• Pneumonia
• Pneumothorax
• Pulmonary bases, fibrosis, infiltrates
• Tuberculosis
• Vascular abnormalities

CRITICAL FINDINGS
• Foreign body
• Malposition of tube, line, or postoperative device (pacemaker)
• Pneumonia
• Pneumoperitoneum
• Pneumothorax
• Spine fracture

It is essential that critical diagnoses be communicated immediately to the appropriate health-care provider (HCP). A listing of these diagnoses varies among facilities. Note and immediately report to the HCP abnormal results and related symptoms.

INTERFERING FACTORS

This procedure is contraindicated for
• Patients who are pregnant or suspected of being pregnant, unless the potential benefits of the procedure far outweigh the risks to the fetus and mother.

Factors that may impair the results of the examination
• Metallic objects within the examination field.
• Improper adjustment of the radiographic equipment to accommodate obese or thin patients, which can cause overexposure or underexposure.
• Incorrect positioning of the patient, which may produce poor visualization of the area to be examined.
• Inability of the patient to cooperate or remain still during the procedure because of age, significant pain, or mental status.

Other considerations
• The procedure may be terminated if chest pain or severe cardiac arrhythmias occur.
• Consultation with a HCP should occur before the procedure for radiation safety concerns regarding younger patients or patients who are lactating.
• Risks associated with radiation overexposure can result from frequent x-ray procedures. Personnel in the examination room with the patient should wear a protective lead apron, stand behind a shield, or leave the area while the examination is being done. Personnel working in the examination area should wear badges to record their level of radiation exposure.

NURSING IMPLICATIONS AND PROCEDURE

PRETEST:
▶ Positively identify the patient using at least two unique identifiers before providing care, treatment, or services.

C

▶ *Patient Teaching:* Inform the patient this procedure can assist in assessing the heart and lungs for disease.

▶ Obtain a history of the patient's complaints, including a list of known allergens.

▶ Obtain a history of the patient's cardiovascular and respiratory systems, symptoms, and results of previously performed laboratory tests and diagnostic and surgical procedures.

▶ Record the date of the last menstrual period and determine the possibility of pregnancy in perimenopausal women.

▶ Obtain a list of the patient's current medications, including herbs, nutritional supplements, and nutraceuticals (see Appendix F).

▶ Review the procedure with the patient. Address concerns about pain and explain that no pain will be experienced during the test. Inform the patient that the procedure is performed in the radiology department or at the bedside by a registered radiological technologist, and takes approximately 5 to 15 min.

▶ *Sensitivity to social and cultural issues,* as well as concern for modesty, is important in providing psychological support before, during, and after the procedure.

▶ Instruct the patient to remove all metallic objects from the area to be examined.

▶ There are no food, fluid, or medication restrictions unless by medical direction.

INTRATEST:

▶ Ensure that the patient has removed all external metallic objects from the area to be examined.

▶ Patients are given a gown, robe, and foot coverings to wear.

▶ Instruct the patient to cooperate fully and to follow directions. Instruct the patient to remain still throughout the procedure because movement produces unreliable results.

▶ Observe standard precautions, and follow the general guidelines in Appendix A.

▶ Place the patient in the standing position facing the cassette or image

detector, with hands on hips, neck extended, and shoulders rolled forward.

▶ Position the chest with the left side against the image holder for a lateral view.

▶ For portable examinations, elevate the head of the bed to the high Fowler's position.

▶ Ask the patient to inhale deeply and hold his or her breath while the x-ray images are taken, and then to exhale after the images are taken.

POST-TEST:

▶ The report will be sent to the requesting HCP, who will discuss the results with the patient.

▶ Recognize anxiety related to test results and be supportive of impaired activity related to respiratory capacity and perceived loss of physical activity. Discuss the implications of abnormal test results on the patient's lifestyle. Provide teaching and information regarding the clinical implications of the test results, as appropriate.

▶ Reinforce information given by the patient's HCP regarding further testing, treatment, or referral to another HCP. Answer any questions or address any concerns voiced by the patient or family.

▶ Depending on the results of this procedure, additional testing may be performed to evaluate and determine the need for a change in therapy or progression of the disease process. Evaluate test results in relation to the patient's symptoms and other tests performed.

RELATED MONOGRAPHS:

▶ Related tests include biopsy lung, blood gases, bronchoscopy, CT thoracic, CBC, culture mycobacteria, culture sputum, culture viral, electrocardiogram, Gram stain, lung perfusion scan, MRI chest, pulmonary function study, pulse oximetry, and TB tests.

▶ Refer to the Cardiovascular and Respiratory systems tables at the end of the book for related tests by body system.

Chlamydia Group Antibody, IgG

SYNONYM/ACRONYM: N/A.

COMMON USE: To diagnose Chlamydia, a common sexually transmitted disease.

SPECIMEN: Serum (1 mL) collected in a red-top tube.

REFERENCE VALUE: (Method: Enzyme immunoassay)

Negative	Index less than 0.91
Equivocal	Index 0.91–1.09
Positive	Index greater than 1.09

DESCRIPTION: Chlamydia, one of the most common sexually transmitted diseases, is caused by *Chlamydia trachomatis*. These gram-negative bacteria are called *obligate cell parasites* because they require living cells for growth. There are three serotypes of *C. trachomatis*. One group causes lymphogranuloma venereum, with symptoms of the first phase of the disease appearing 2 to 6 wk after infection; another causes a genital tract infection different from lymphogranuloma venereum, in which symptoms in men appear 7 to 28 days after intercourse (women are generally asymptomatic); and the third causes the ocular disease trachoma (incubation period, 7 to 10 days). *Chlamydia psittaci* is the cause of psittacosis in birds and humans. It is increasing in prevalence as a pathogen responsible for other significant diseases of the respiratory system. The incubation period for *C. psittaci* infections in humans is 7 to 15 days and is followed by chills, fever, and a persistent nonproductive cough.

Chlamydia is difficult to culture and grow, so antibody testing has become the technology of choice. The antigen used in many screening kits is not species specific and can confirm only the presence of *Chlamydia* spp. Newer technology using DNA probes can identify the species. Assays that detect immunoglobulin G (IgG) antibodies are used to assist in the diagnosis of chlamydial infection. A limitation of IgG antibody screening is that positive results may indicate past rather than current infection. Assays that can specifically identify *C. trachomatis* require special collection and transport kits. They also have specific collection instructions, and the specimens are collected on swabs. The laboratory performing this testing should be consulted before specimen collection.

INDICATIONS
- Establish *Chlamydia* as the cause of atypical pneumonia
- Establish the presence of chlamydial infection

POTENTIAL DIAGNOSIS

Positive findings in
- Chlamydial infection
- Infantile pneumonia *(related to transmission at birth from an infected mother)*
- Infertility *(related to scarring of ovaries or fallopian tubes from untreated chlamydial infection)*
- Lymphogranuloma venereum
- Ophthalmia neonatorum *(related to transmission at birth from an infected mother)*
- Pelvic inflammatory disease
- Urethritis

CRITICAL FINDINGS: N/A

INTERFERING FACTORS
- Hemolysis or lipemia may interfere with analysis.
- Positive results may demonstrate evidence of past infection and not necessarily indicate current infection.

NURSING IMPLICATIONS AND PROCEDURE

PRETEST:

- Positively identify the patient using at least two unique identifiers before providing care, treatment, or services.
- *Patient Teaching:* Inform the patient this test can assist in diagnosing chlamydial infection.
- Obtain a history of the patient's complaints, including a list of known allergens, especially allergies or sensitivities to latex.
- Obtain a history of the patient's immune and reproductive systems, as well as results of previously performed laboratory tests and diagnostic and surgical procedures.
- Obtain a list of the patient's current medications, including herbs, nutritional supplements, and nutraceuticals (see Appendix F).
- Review the procedure with the patient. Inform the patient that specimen collection takes approximately 5 to 10 min. Address concerns about pain and explain that there may be some discomfort during the venipuncture.
- *Sensitivity to social and cultural issues,* as well as concern for modesty, is important in providing psychological support before, during, and after the procedure.
- Inform the patient that several tests may be necessary to confirm diagnosis. Any individual positive result should be repeated in 7 to 10 days to monitor a change in titer.
- There are no food, fluid, or medication restrictions unless by medical direction.

INTRATEST:

- If the patient has a history of allergic reaction to latex, avoid the use of equipment containing latex.
- Instruct the patient to cooperate fully and to follow directions. Direct the patient to breathe normally and to avoid unnecessary movement.
- Observe standard precautions, and follow the general guidelines in Appendix A. Positively identify the patient, and label the appropriate tubes with the corresponding patient demographics, date, and time of collection. Perform a venipuncture.
- Remove the needle and apply direct pressure with dry gauze to stop bleeding. Observe/assess venipuncture site for bleeding or hematoma formation and secure gauze with adhesive bandage.
- Promptly transport the specimen to the laboratory for processing and analysis.

POST-TEST:

- A report of the results will be sent to the requesting health-care provider (HCP), who will discuss the results with the patient.
- Recognize anxiety related to test results, and be supportive. Discuss the implications of abnormal test results on the patient's lifestyle. Provide teaching and information regarding the clinical implications of the test results, as appropriate. Emphasize the need to return to have a convalescent blood sample taken in 7 to 14 days. Educate the patient regarding access to counseling services.

Social and Cultural Considerations: Counsel the patient, as appropriate, as to the risk of sexual transmission and educate the patient regarding proper prophyl-axis. Reinforce the importance of strict adherence to the treatment regimen.

Social and Cultural Considerations: Inform the patient with positive *C. trachomatis* that findings must be reported to a local health department official, who will question the patient regarding his or her sexual partners.

Social and Cultural Considerations: Offer support, as appropriate, to patients who may be the victim of rape or sexual assault. Educate the patient regarding access to counseling services. Provide a nonjudgmental, nonthreatening atmosphere for a discussion during which you explain the risks of sexually transmitted diseases. It is also important to discuss emotions the patient may experience (guilt, depression, anger) as a victim of rape or sexual assault.

Provide emotional support if the patient is pregnant and if results are positive.

Inform the patient that chlamydial infection during pregnancy places the newborn at risk for pneumonia and conjunctivitis.

Reinforce information given by the patient's HCP regarding further testing, treatment, or referral to another HCP. Answer any questions or address any concerns voiced by the patient or family.

Depending on the results of this procedure, additional testing may be performed to evaluate or monitor progression of the disease process and determine the need for a change in therapy. Evaluate test results in relation to the patient's symptoms and other tests performed.

RELATED MONOGRAPHS:

Related tests include culture bacterial (anal, genital), culture viral, Gram stain, Pap smear, and syphilis serology.

Refer to the Immune and Reproductive systems tables at the end of the book for related tests by body system.

Chloride, Blood

SYNONYM/ACRONYM: Cl^-.

COMMON USE: To evaluate electrolytes, acid-base balance, and hydration level.

SPECIMEN: Serum (1 mL) collected in a red- or tiger-top tube. Plasma (1 mL) collected in a green-top (heparin) tube is also acceptable.

REFERENCE VALUE: (Method: Ion-selective electrode)

Age	Conventional Units	SI Units (Conventional Units × 1)
Premature	95–110 mEq/L	95–110 mmol/L
0–1 mo	98–113 mEq/L	98–113 mmol/L
2 mo–older adult	97–107 mEq/L	97–107 mmol/L

DESCRIPTION: Chloride is the most abundant anion in the extracellu-lar fluid. Its most important function is in the maintenance of acid-base balance, in which it competes with bicarbonate for sodium. Chloride levels generally increase and decrease proportionally to sodium levels and inversely proportional to bicarbonate levels. Chloride also participates with sodium in the maintenance of water balance and aids in the regulation of osmotic pressure. Chloride contributes to gastric acid (hydrochloric acid) for digestion and activation of enzymes. The chloride content of venous blood is slightly higher than that of arterial blood because chloride ions enter red blood cells in response to absorption of carbon dioxide into the cell. As carbon dioxide enters the blood cell, bicarbonate leaves and chloride is absorbed in exchange to maintain electrical neutrality within the cell.

Chloride is provided by dietary intake, mostly in the form of sodium chloride. It is absorbed by the gastrointestinal system, filtered out by the glomeruli, and reabsorbed by the renal tubules. Excess chloride is excreted in the urine. Serum values normally remain fairly stable. A slight decrease may be detectable after meals because chloride is used to produce hydrochloric acid as part of the digestive process. Measurement of chloride levels is not as essential as measurement of other electrolytes such as sodium or potassium. Chloride is usually included in standard electrolyte panels to detect the presence of unmeasured anions via calculation of the anion gap. Chloride levels are usually not interpreted apart from sodium, potassium, carbon dioxide, and anion gap.

The patient's clinical picture needs to be considered in the evaluation of electrolytes. Fluid and electrolyte imbalances are often seen in patients with serious illness or injury because in these cases the clinical situation has affected the normal homeostatic balance of the body. It is also possible that therapeutic treatments being administered are causing or contributing to the electrolyte imbalance. Children and adults are at high risk for fluid and electrolyte imbalances when chloride levels are depleted. Children are considered to be at high risk during chloride imbalance because a positive serum chloride balance is important for expansion of the extracellular fluid compartment. Anemia, the result of decreased hemoglobin levels, is a frequent issue for elderly patients. Because hemoglobin participates in a major buffer system in the body, depleted hemoglobin levels affect the efficiency of chloride ion exchange for bicarbonate in red blood cells, which in turn affects acid-base balance. Elderly patients are also at high risk because their renal response to change in pH is slower, resulting in a more rapid development of electrolyte imbalance.

INDICATIONS

- Assist in confirming a diagnosis of disorders associated with abnormal chloride values, as seen in acid-base and fluid imbalances
- Differentiate between types of acidosis (hyperchloremic versus anion gap)
- Monitor effectiveness of drug therapy to increase or decrease serum chloride levels

POTENTIAL DIAGNOSIS

Increased in
- Acute renal failure *(related to decreased renal excretion)*

- Cushing's disease *(related to sodium retention as a result of increased levels of aldosterone; typically, chloride levels follow sodium levels)*
- Dehydration *(related to hemoconcentration)*
- Diabetes insipidus *(hemoconcentration related to excessive urine production)*
- Excessive infusion of normal saline *(related to excessive intake)*
- Head trauma with hypothalamic stimulation or damage
- Hyperparathyroidism (primary) *(high chloride-to-phosphate ratio is used to assist in diagnosis)*
- Metabolic acidosis *(associated with prolonged diarrhea)*
- Renal tubular acidosis *(acidosis related to net retention of chloride ions)*
- Respiratory alkalosis (e.g., hyperventilation) *(related to metabolic exchange of intracellular chloride replaced by bicarbonate; chloride levels increase)*
- Salicylate intoxication *(related to acid-base imbalance resulting in a hyperchloremic acidosis)*

Decreased in
- Addison's disease *(related to insufficient production of aldosterone; potassium is retained while sodium and chloride are lost)*
- Burns *(dilutional effect related to sequestration of extracellular fluid)*
- Congestive heart failure *(related to dilutional effect of fluid buildup)*
- Diabetic ketoacidosis *(related to acid-base imbalance with accumulation of ketone bodies and increased chloride)*
- Excessive sweating *(related to excessive loss of chloride without replacement)*
- Gastrointestinal loss from vomiting (severe), diarrhea, nasogastric suction, or fistula

- Metabolic alkalosis *(related to homeostatic response in which intracellular chloride increases to reduce alkalinity of extracellular fluid)*
- Overhydration *(related to dilutional effect)*
- Respiratory acidosis (chronic)
- Salt-losing nephritis *(related to excessive loss)*
- Syndrome of inappropriate antidiuretic hormone secretion *(related to dilutional effect)*
- Water intoxication *(related to dilutional effect)*

CRITICAL FINDINGS ◈
- Less than 80 mEq/L
- Greater than 115 mEq/L

Note and immediately report to the health-care provider (HCP) any critically increased or decreased values and related symptoms. Observe the patient for symptoms of critically decreased or elevated chloride levels. Proper interpretation of chloride values must be made within the context of other electrolyte values and requires clinical knowledge of the patient.

The following may be seen in hypochloremia: twitching or tremors, which may indicate excitability of the nervous system; slow and shallow breathing; and decreased blood pressure as a result of fluid loss. Possible interventions relate to treatment of the underlying cause.

Signs and symptoms associated with hyperchloremia are weakness; lethargy; and deep, rapid breathing. Proper interventions include treatments that correct the underlying cause.

INTERFERING FACTORS
- Drugs that may cause an increase in chloride levels include acetazolamide, acetylsalicylic acid, ammonium chloride, androgens, bromide,

chlorothiazide, cholestyramine, cyclosporine, estrogens, guanethidine, hydrochlorothiazide, lithium, methyldopa, NSAIDs, oxyphenbutazone, phenylbutazone, and triamterene.

- Drugs that may cause a decrease in chloride levels include aldosterone, bicarbonate, corticosteroids, corticotropin, cortisone, diuretics, ethacrynic acid, furosemide, hydroflumethiazide, laxatives (if chronic abuse occurs), mannitol, meralluride, mersalyl, methyclothiazide, metolazone, and triamterene. Many of these drugs can cause a diuretic action that inhibits the tubular reabsorption of chloride. *Note:* Triamterene has nephrotoxic and azotemic effects, and when organ damage has occurred, increased serum chloride levels result. Potassium chloride (found in salt substitutes) can lower blood chloride levels and raise urine chloride levels.

- Elevated triglyceride or protein levels may cause a volume-displacement error in the specimen, reflecting falsely decreased chloride values when chloride measurement methods employing predilution specimens are used (e.g., indirect ion-selective electrode, flame photometry).

- Specimens should never be collected above an IV line because of the potential for dilution when the specimen and the IV solution combine in the collection container, falsely decreasing the result. There is also the potential of contaminating the sample with the normal saline contained in the IV solution, falsely increasing the result.

NURSING IMPLICATIONS AND PROCEDURE

PRETEST:

- Positively identify the patient using at least two unique identifiers before providing care, treatment, or services.

- *Patient Teaching:* Inform the patient this test can assist in evaluating the amount of chloride in the blood.
- Obtain a history of the patient's complaints, including a list of known allergens, especially allergies or sensitivities to latex.
- Obtain a history of the patient's cardiovascular, endocrine, gastrointestinal, genitourinary, and respiratory systems, as well as results of previously performed laboratory tests and diagnostic and surgical procedures.
- Specimens should not be collected during hemodialysis.
- Obtain a list of the patient's current medications, including herbs, nutritional supplements, and nutraceuticals (see Appendix F).
- Review the procedure with the patient. Inform the patient that specimen collection takes approximately 5 to 10 min. Address concerns about pain and explain that there may be some discomfort during the venipuncture.
- *Sensitivity to social and cultural issues,* as well as concern for modesty, is important in providing psychological support before, during, and after the procedure.
- There are no food, fluid, or medication restrictions unless by medical direction.

INTRATEST:

- If the patient has a history of allergic reaction to latex, avoid the use of equipment containing latex.
- Instruct the patient to cooperate fully and to follow directions. Direct the patient to breathe normally and to avoid unnecessary movement. Instruct the patient not to clench and unclench fist immediately before or during specimen collection.
- Observe standard precautions, and follow the general guidelines in Appendix A. Positively identify the patient, and label the appropriate tubes with the corresponding patient demographics, date, and time of collection. Perform a venipuncture.
- Remove the needle and apply direct pressure with dry gauze to stop bleeding. Observe/assess venipuncture site for bleeding or hematoma formation and secure gauze with adhesive bandage.

▶ Promptly transport the specimen to the laboratory for processing and analysis.

POST-TEST:

▶ A report of the results will be sent to the requesting HCP, who will discuss the results with the patient.

▶ Observe the patient on saline IV fluid replacement therapy for signs of over-hydration, especially in cases in which there is a history of cardiac or renal disease. Signs of overhydration include constant, irritable cough; chest rales; dyspnea; or engorgement of neck and hand veins.

▶ Evaluate the patient for signs and symptoms of dehydration. Check the patient's skin turgor, mucous membrane moisture, and ability to produce tears. Dehydration is a significant and common finding in geriatric and other patients in whom renal function has deteriorated.

▶ Monitor daily weights as well as intake and output to determine whether fluid retention is occurring because of sodium and chloride excess. Patients at risk for or with a history of fluid imbalance are also at risk for electrolyte imbalance.

▶ *Nutritional Considerations:* Careful observation of the patient on IV fluid replacement therapy is important. A patient receiving a continuous 5% dextrose solution (D_5W) may not be taking in an adequate amount of chloride to meet the body's needs. The patient, if allowed, should be encouraged to drink fluids such as broths, tomato juice, or colas and to eat foods such as meats, seafood, or eggs, which contain sodium and chloride. The use of table salt may also be appropriate.

▶ *Nutritional Considerations:* Instruct patients with elevated chloride levels to avoid eating or drinking anything containing sodium chloride salt. The patient or caregiver should also be encouraged to read food labels to determine which products are suitable for a low-sodium diet.

▶ *Nutritional Considerations:* Instruct patients with low chloride levels that a decrease in iron absorption may occur as a result of less chloride available to form gastric acid, which is essential for iron absorption. In prolonged periods of chloride deficit, iron-deficiency anemia could develop.

▶ Reinforce information given by the patient's HCP regarding further testing, treatment, or referral to another HCP. Answer any questions or address any concerns voiced by the patient or family.

▶ Depending on the results of this procedure, additional testing may be performed to evaluate or monitor progression of the disease process and determine the need for a change in therapy. Evaluate test results in relation to the patient's symptoms and other tests performed.

RELATED MONOGRAPHS:

▶ Related tests include ACTH, anion gap, blood gases, carbon dioxide, CBC hematocrit, CBC hemoglobin, osmolality, potassium, protein total and fractions, and sodium.

▶ Refer to the Cardiovascular, Endocrine, Gastrointestinal, Genitourinary, and Respiratory systems tables at the end of the book for related test by body system.

Chloride, Sweat

SYNONYM/ACRONYM: Sweat test, pilocarpine iontophoresis sweat test, sweat chloride.

COMMON USE: To assist in diagnosing cystic fibrosis.

SPECIMEN: Sweat (0.1 mL minimum) collected by pilocarpine iontophoresis.

REFERENCE VALUE: (Method: Ion-specific electrode or titration)

	Conventional Units	SI Units (Conventional Units × 1)
Normal	0–40 mEq/L	0–40 mmol/L
Borderline	41–60 mEq/L	41–60 mmol/L
Consistent with the diagnosis of CF	Greater than 60 mEq/L	Greater than 60 mmol/L

DESCRIPTION: Cystic fibrosis (CF) is a genetic disease that affects normal functioning of the exocrine glands, causing them to excrete large amounts of electrolytes. Patients with CF have sweat electrolyte levels two to five times normal. Sweat test values, with family history and signs and symptoms, are required to establish a diagnosis of CF. CF is transmitted as an autosomal recessive trait and is characterized by abnormal exocrine secretions within the lungs, pancreas, small intestine, bile ducts, and skin. Clinical presentation may include chronic problems of the gastrointestinal and/or respiratory system. CF is more common in Caucasians. Sweat conductivity is a screening method that estimates chloride levels. Sweat conductivity values greater than or equal to 50 mEq/L should be referred for quantitative analysis of sweat chloride. Testing of stool samples for decreased trypsin activity has been used as a screen for CF in infants and children, but this is a much less reliable method than the sweat test. The American College of Obstetricians and Gynecologists (ACOG) suggests that carrier screening be discussed as an option to patients (and couples) who are pregnant or are considering pregnancy. Laboratories generally offer a panel of the current and most common cystic fibrosis mutations recommended by ACOG and the American College of Medical Genetics. Some states include CF in the neonatal screening performed at birth. Genetic testing can also be reliably performed on DNA material harvested from whole blood, amniotic fluid (submitted with maternal blood sample), chorionic villus samples (submitted with maternal blood sample), or buccal swabs to screen for genetic mutations associated with CF and can assist in confirming a diagnosis of CF, but the sweat electrolyte test is still considered the gold standard diagnostic for CF.

The sweat test is a noninvasive study done to assist in the diagnosis of CF when considered with other test results and physical assessments. This test is usually performed on children, although adults may also be tested; it is not usually ordered on adults because results can be highly variable and should be interpreted with caution. Sweat for specimen collection is induced by a small electrical current carrying the drug pilocarpine. The test measures the concentration of chloride produced by the sweat glands of the skin. A high concentration of chloride in the specimen indicates the presence of CF. The sweat test is used less commonly to measure the concentration of sodium ions for the same purpose.

INDICATIONS

• Assist in the diagnosis of CF
• Screen for CF in individuals with a family history of the disease
• Screen for suspected CF in children with recurring respiratory infections
• Screen for suspected CF in infants with failure to thrive and infants who pass meconium late
• Screen for suspected CF in individuals with malabsorption syndrome

POTENTIAL DIAGNOSIS

Increased in
Conditions that affect electrolyte distribution and excretion may produce false-positive sweat test results.
• Addison's disease
• Alcoholic pancreatitis *(dysfunction of CF gene is linked to pancreatic disease susceptibility)*
• CF
• Chronic pulmonary infections *(related to undiagnosed CF)*
• Congenital adrenal hyperplasia
• Diabetes insipidus
• Familial cholestasis
• Familial hypoparathyroidism
• Fucosidosis
• Glucose-6-phosphate dehydrogenase deficiency
• Hypothyroidism
• Mucopolysaccharidosis
• Nephrogenic diabetes insipidus
• Renal failure

Decreased in
Conditions that affect electrolyte distribution and retention may produce false-negative sweat test results.
• Edema
• Hypoaldosteronism
• Hypoproteinemia
• Sodium depletion

CRITICAL FINDINGS ✷

• 20 yr or younger: greater than 60 mEq/L considered diagnostic of CF
• Older than 20 years: greater than 70 mEq/L considered diagnostic of CF

Note and immediately report to the health-care provider (HCP) any critically increased values and related symptoms. Values should be interpreted with consideration of family history and clinical signs and symptoms.

The validity of the test result is affected tremendously by proper specimen collection and handling. Before proceeding with appropriate patient education and counseling, it is important to perform duplicate testing on patients whose results are in the diagnostic or intermediate ranges. A negative test should be repeated if test results do not support the clinical picture.

INTERFERING FACTORS

• An inadequate amount of sweat may produce inaccurate results.
• ✷ This test should not be performed on patients with skin disorders (e.g., rash, erythema, eczema).
• Improper cleaning of the skin or improper application of gauze pad or filter paper for collection affects test results.
• Hot environmental temperatures may reduce the sodium chloride concentration in sweat; cool environmental

temperatures may reduce the amount of sweat collected.

• If the specimen container that stores the gauze or filter paper is handled without gloves, the test results may show a false increase in the final weight of the collection container.

NURSING IMPLICATIONS AND PROCEDURE

PRETEST:

▶ Positively identify the patient using at least two unique identifiers before providing care, treatment, or services.

▶ *Patient Teaching:* Inform the patient this test can assist in diagnosing an inherited disease that affects the lungs.

▶ Obtain a history of the patient's complaints, including a list of known allergens, especially allergies or sensitivities to latex.

▶ Obtain a history of the patient's endocrine and respiratory systems, especially failure to thrive or CF in other family members, as well as results of previously performed laboratory tests and diagnostic and surgical procedures.

▶ Obtain a list of the patient's current medications, including herbs, nutritional supplements, and nutraceuticals (see Appendix F).

▶ Review the procedure with the patient and caregiver. Encourage the caregiver to stay with and support the child during the test. The iontophoresis and specimen collection usually takes approximately 75 to 90 min. Address concerns about pain and explain that there is no pain associated with the test, but a stinging sensation may be experienced when the low electrical current is applied at the site.

▶ *Sensitivity to social and cultural issues,* as well as concern for modesty, is important in providing psychological support before, during, and after the procedure.

▶ There are no food, fluid, or medication restrictions unless by medical direction.

INTRATEST:

▶ Instruct the patient to cooperate fully and to follow directions.

▶ Observe standard precautions, and follow the general guidelines in Appendix A. Positively identify the patient, and label the appropriate collection container with the corresponding patient demographics, date, and time of collection.

▶ ◈ The test should not be performed if the patient is receiving oxygen by means of an open system related to the remote possibility of explosion from an electrical spark. If the patient can temporarily receive oxygen via a facemask or nasal cannula, then sweat testing can be done

▶ ◈ The patient is placed in a position that will allow exposure of the site on the forearm or thigh. To ensure collection of an adequate amount of sweat in a small infant, two sites (right forearm and right thigh) can be used. The patient should be covered to prevent cool environmental temperatures from affecting sweat production. The site selected for iontophoresis should never be the chest or left side because of the risk of cardiac arrest from the electrical current.

▶ The site is washed with distilled water and dried. A positive electrode is attached to the site on the right forearm or right thigh and covered with a pad that is saturated with pilocarpine, a drug that stimulates sweating. A negative electrode is covered with a pad that is saturated with bicarbonate solution. Iontophoresis is achieved by supplying a low (4 to 5 mA) electrical current via the electrode for 12 to 15 min. Battery-powered equipment is preferred over an electrical outlet to supply the current.

▶ The electrodes are removed, revealing a red area at the site, and the site is washed with distilled water and dried to remove any possible contaminants on the skin.

▶ Preweighed disks made of filter paper are placed on the site with a forceps; to prevent evaporation of sweat collected at the site, the disks are covered with paraffin or plastic and sealed at the edges. The disks are left in place for about 1 hr. Distract the child with books or games to allay fears.

▶ After 1 hr, the paraffin covering is removed, and disks are placed in a preweighed container with a forceps. The container is sealed and sent immediately to the laboratory for weighing and analysis of chloride content. At least 100 mg of sweat is required for accurate results.

▶ Terminate the test if the patient complains of burning at the electrode site. Reposition the electrode before the test is resumed.

▶ Promptly transport the specimen to the laboratory for processing and analysis. Do not directly handle the preweighed specimen container or filter paper.

POST-TEST:

▶ A report of the results will be sent to the requesting HCP, who will discuss the results with the patient/caregiver.

▶ Observe/assess the site for unusual color, sensation, or discomfort.

▶ Inform the patient and caregiver that redness at the site fades in 2 to 3 hr.

▶ Instruct the patient to resume usual diet, fluids, medications, and activity, as directed by the HCP.

▶ *Nutritional Considerations:* If appropriate, instruct the patient and caregiver that nutrition may be altered because of impaired digestive processes associated with CF. Increased viscosity of exocrine gland secretion may lead to poor absorption of digestive enzymes and fat-soluble vitamins, necessitating oral intake of digestive enzymes with each meal and calcium and vitamin (A, D, E, and K) supplementation. Malnutrition also is seen commonly in patients with chronic, severe respiratory disease for many reasons, including fatigue, lack of appetite, and gastrointestinal distress. Research has estimated that the daily caloric intake needed for children with CF between 4 and 7 yr may be 2,000 to 2,800 and for teens 3,000 to 5,000. Tube feeding may be necessary to supplement regular high-calorie meals. To prevent pulmonary infection and decrease the extent of lung tissue damage, adequate intake of vitamins A and C is also important. Excessive

loss of sodium chloride through the sweat glands of a patient with CF may necessitate increased salt intake, especially in environments where increased sweating is induced. The importance of following the prescribed diet should be stressed to the patient and caregiver.

▶ If appropriate, instruct the patient and caregiver that ineffective airway clearance related to excessive production of mucus and decreased ciliary action may result. Chest physical therapy and the use of aerosolized antibiotics and mucus-thinning drugs are an important part of the daily treatment regimen.

▶ Recognize anxiety related to test results, and be supportive of impaired activity related to perceived loss of independence and fear of shortened life expectancy. Discuss the implications of abnormal test results on the patient's lifestyle. Provide teaching and information regarding the clinical implications of the test results, as appropriate. Educate the patient regarding access to counseling services. Help the patient and caregiver to cope with long-term implications. Recognize that anticipatory anxiety and grief related to potential lifestyle changes may be expressed when someone is faced with a chronic disorder. Provide information regarding genetic counseling and possible screening of other family members if appropriate. Provide contact information, if desired, for the Cystic Fibrosis Foundation (www.cff.org).

▶ Reinforce information given by the patient's HCP regarding further testing, treatment, or referral to another HCP. Explain that a positive sweat test alone is not diagnostic of CF; repetition of borderline and positive tests is generally recommended. Answer any questions or address any concerns voiced by the patient or family.

▶ Depending on the results of this procedure, additional testing may be performed to evaluate or monitor progression of the disease process and determine the need for a change in therapy. Evaluate test results in relation to the patient's symptoms and other tests performed.

RELATED MONOGRAPHS:

- Related tests include α_1-antitrypsin/ phenotype, amylase, anion gap, biopsy chorionic villus, blood gases, fecal analysis, fecal fat, osmolality, phosphorus, potassium, and sodium.
- Refer to the Endocrine and Respiratory systems tables at the end of the book for related tests by body system.

Cholangiography, Percutaneous Transhepatic

SYNONYM/ACRONYM: Percutaneous cholecystogram, PTC, PTHC.

COMMON USE: To visualize and assess biliary ducts for causes of obstruction and jaundice, such as cancer or stones.

AREA OF APPLICATION: Biliary system.

CONTRAST: Radiopaque iodine-based contrast medium.

DESCRIPTION: Percutaneous transhepatic cholangiography (PTC) is a test used to visualize the biliary system in order to evaluate persistent upper abdominal pain after cholecystectomy and to determine the presence and cause of obstructive jaundice. The liver is punctured with a thin needle under fluoroscopic guidance, and contrast medium is injected as the needle is slowly withdrawn. This test visualizes the biliary ducts without depending on the gallbladder's concentrating ability. The intrahepatic and extrahepatic biliary ducts, and occasionally the gallbladder, can be visualized to determine possible obstruction. In obstruction of the extrahepatic ducts, a catheter can be placed in the duct to allow external drainage of bile. Endoscopic retrograde cholangiopancreatography (ERCP) and PTC are the only methods available to view the biliary tree in the presence of jaundice. ERCP poses less risk and is probably done more often. PTC is an invasive procedure and has potential risks, including bleeding, septicemia, bile peritonitis, and extravasation of the contrast medium.

INDICATIONS

- Aid in the diagnosis of obstruction caused by gallstones, benign strictures, malignant tumors, congenital cysts, and anatomic variations
- Determine the cause, extent, and location of mechanical obstruction
- Determine the cause of upper abdominal pain after cholecystectomy
- Distinguish between obstructive and nonobstructive jaundice

POTENTIAL DIAGNOSIS

Normal findings in

- Biliary ducts are normal in diameter, with no evidence of dilation,

filling defects, duct narrowing, or extravasation.
- Contrast medium fills the ducts and flows freely.
- Gallbladder appears normal in size and shape.

Abnormal findings in
- Anatomic biliary or pancreatic duct variations
- Biliary sclerosis
- Cholangiocarcinoma
- Cirrhosis
- Common bile duct cysts
- Gallbladder carcinoma
- Gallstones
- Hepatitis
- Nonobstructive jaundice
- Pancreatitis
- Sclerosing cholangitis
- Tumors, strictures, inflammation, or gallstones of the common bile duct

CRITICAL FINDINGS: N/A

INTERFERING FACTORS

This procedure is contraindicated for
- ◈ Patients with allergies to shellfish or iodinated dye. The contrast medium used may cause a life-threatening allergic reaction. Patients with a known hypersensitivity to the medium may benefit from premedication with corticosteroids or the use of nonionic contrast medium.
- Patients who are pregnant or suspected of being pregnant, unless the potential benefits of the procedure far outweigh the risks to the fetus and mother.
- ◈ Patients with cholangitis. The injection of the contrast medium can increase biliary pressure, leading to bacteremia, septicemia, and shock.
- Patients with postoperative wound sepsis, hypersensitivity to iodine, or acute renal failure.
- ◈ Patients with bleeding disorders, massive ascites, or acute renal failure.

Factors that may impair clear imaging
- Gas or feces in the gastrointestinal (GI) tract resulting from inadequate cleansing or failure to restrict food intake before the study.
- Retained barium from a previous radiological procedure.
- Metallic objects within the examination field, which may inhibit organ visualization and cause unclear images.
- Inability of the patient to cooperate or remain still during the procedure because of age, significant pain, or mental status.

Other considerations
- The procedure may be terminated if chest pain or severe cardiac arrhythmias occur.
- Failure to follow dietary restrictions and other pretesting preparations may cause the procedure to be canceled or repeated.
- Peritonitis may occur as a result of bile extravasation.
- Consultation with a health-care provider (HCP) should occur before the procedure for radiation safety concerns regarding younger patients or patients who are lactating.
- Risks associated with radiation overexposure can result from frequent x-ray procedures. Personnel in the examination room with the patient should wear a protective lead apron stand behind a shield, or leave the area while the examination is being done. Personnel working in the examination area should wear badges to record their level of radiation exposure.

C

NURSING IMPLICATIONS AND PROCEDURE

PRETEST:

▶ Positively identify the patient using at least two unique identifiers before providing care, treatment, or services.

▶ *Patient Teaching:* Inform the patient this procedure can assist in assessing the bile ducts of the gallbladder and pancreas.

▶ Obtain a history of the patient's complaints, including a list of known allergens, especially allergies or sensitivities to latex, iodine, seafood, contrast medium, anesthetics, and dyes.

▶ Obtain a history of the patient's gastrointestinal and hepatobiliary systems, symptoms, and results of previously performed laboratory tests and diagnostic and surgical procedures.

▶ Ensure that this procedure is performed before an upper GI study or barium swallow.

▶ Record the date of the last menstrual period and determine the possibility of pregnancy in perimenopausal women.

▶ Obtain a list of the patient's current medications, including anticoagulants, aspirin and other salicylates, herbs, nutritional supplements, and nutraceuticals (see Appendix F). Such products should be discontinued by medical direction for the appropriate number of days prior to a surgical procedure. Note time and date of last dose.

▶ If contrast medium is scheduled to be used, patients receiving metformin (glucophage) for non-insulin-dependent (type 2) diabetes should discontinue the drug on the day of the test and continue to withhold it for 48 hr after the test. Failure to do so may result in lactic acidosis.

▶ Review the procedure with the patient. Address concerns about pain and explain that there may be moments of discomfort and some pain experienced during the test. Inform the patient that the procedure is usually performed in the radiology department by an HCP, with support staff, and takes approximately 30 to 60 min.

▶ *Sensitivity to social and cultural issues,* as well as concern for modesty, is important in providing psychological support before, during, and after the procedure.

▶ Explain that an IV line may be inserted to allow infusion of IV fluids, anesthetics, or sedatives.

▶ Type and screen the patient's blood for possible transfusion.

▶ Inform the patient that a laxative and cleansing enema may be needed the day before the procedure, with cleansing enemas on the morning of the procedure depending on the institution's policy.

▶ Instruct the patient to remove all external metallic objects from the area to be examined.

▶ The patient should fast and restrict fluids for 8 hr prior to the procedure. Instruct the patient to avoid taking anticoagulant medication or to reduce dosage as ordered prior to the procedure. Protocols may vary among facilities.

▶ *Make sure a written and informed consent has been signed prior to the procedure and before administering any medications.*

INTRATEST:

▶ Ensure that the patient has complied with dietary, fluid, and medication restrictions for 8 hr prior to the procedure.

▶ Ensure the patient has removed all external metallic objects from the area to be examined.

▶ Assess for completion of bowel preparation according to the institution's procedure.

▶ If the patient has a history of allergic reactions to any relevant substance or drug, administer ordered prophylactic steroids or antihistamines before the procedure. Use nonionic contrast medium for the procedure.

▶ Have emergency equipment readily available.

▶ Instruct the patient to void prior to the procedure and to change into the gown, robe, and foot coverings provided.

▶ Instruct the patient to cooperate fully and to follow directions. Instruct the patient to remain still throughout the procedure because movement produces unreliable results.

- Record baseline vital signs, and continue to monitor throughout the procedure. Protocols may vary among facilities.
- Observe standard precautions, and follow the general guidelines in Appendix A.
- Place the patient in the supine position on an examination table.
- A kidney, ureter, and bladder (KUB) or plain film is taken to ensure that no barium or stool will obscure visualization of the biliary system.
- An area over the abdominal wall is anesthetized, and the needle is inserted and advanced under fluoroscopic guidance. Contrast medium is injected when placement is confirmed by the free flow of bile.
- A specimen of bile may be sent to the laboratory for culture and cytological analysis.
- At the end of the procedure, the contrast medium is aspirated from the biliary ducts, relieving pressure on the dilated ducts.
- If an obstruction is found during the procedure, a catheter is inserted into the bile duct to allow drainage of bile.
- Maintain pressure over the needle insertion site for several hours if bleeding is persistent.
- Observe/assess the needle site for bleeding, inflammation, or hematoma formation.
- Establish a closed and sterile drainage system if a catheter is left in place.

POST-TEST:

- A report of the examination will be sent to the requesting HCP, who will discuss the results with the patient.
- Instruct the patient to resume usual diet, fluids, medications, and activity, as directed by the HCP. Renal function should be assessed before metformin is restarted.
- Monitor vital signs and neurological status every 15 min for 1 hr, then every 2 hr for 4 hr, and as ordered. Take temperature every 4 hr for 24 hr. Monitor intake and output at least every 8 hr. Compare with baseline values. Notify

the HCP if temperature is elevated. Protocols may vary among facilities.
- Monitor for reaction to iodinated contrast medium, including rash, urticaria, tachycardia, hyperpnea, hypertension, palpitations, nausea, or vomiting.
- Observe/assess the puncture site for signs of bleeding, hematoma formation, ecchymosis, or leakage of bile. Notify the HCP if any of these is present.
- Advise the patient to watch for symptoms of infection, such as pain, fever, increased pulse rate, and muscle aches.
- Recognize anxiety related to test results. Discuss the implications of abnormal test results on the patient's lifestyle. Provide teaching and information regarding the clinical implications of the test results, as appropriate.
- Reinforce information given by the patient's HCP regarding further testing, treatment, or referral to another HCP. Answer any questions or address any concerns voiced by the patient or family.
- Depending on the results of this procedure, additional testing may be needed to evaluate or monitor progression of the disease process and determine the need for a change in therapy. Evaluate test results in relation to the patient's symptoms and other tests performed.

RELATED MONOGRAPHS:

- Related tests include ALT, amylase, AMA, AST, biopsy liver, cancer antigens, cholangiography postoperative, cholangiopancreatography endoscopic retrograde, CT abdomen, GGT, hepatitis antigens and antibodies (A, B, C), hepatobiliary scan, KUB studies, laparoscopy abdominal, lipase, MRI abdomen, peritoneal fluid analysis, pleural fluid analysis, and US liver and biliary tract.
- Refer to the Gastrointestinal and Hepatobiliary systems tables at the end of the book for related tests by body system.

C

Cholangiography, Postoperative

SYNONYM/ACRONYM: T-tube cholangiography.

COMMON USE: A postoperative evaluation to provide ongoing assessment of the effectiveness of bile duct surgery.

AREA OF APPLICATION: Gallbladder, bile ducts.

CONTRAST: Iodinated contrast medium.

DESCRIPTION: After cholecystectomy, a self-retaining, T-shaped tube may be inserted into the common bile duct. Postoperative (T-tube) cholangiography is a fluoroscopic and radiographic examination of the biliary tract that involves the injection of a contrast medium through the T-tube inserted during surgery. This test may be performed at the time of surgery and again 7 to 10 days after cholecystectomy to assess the patency of the common bile duct and to detect any remaining calculi. T-tube placement may also be done after a liver transplant because biliary duct obstruction or anastomotic leakage is possible. This test should be performed before any gastrointestinal (GI) studies using barium and after any studies involving the measurement of iodinated compounds.

INDICATIONS
- Determine biliary duct patency before T-tube removal
- Identify the cause, extent, and location of obstruction after surgery

POTENTIAL DIAGNOSIS

Normal findings in
- Biliary ducts are normal in size.
- Contrast medium fills the ductal system and flows freely.

Abnormal findings in
- Appearance of channels of contrast medium outside of the biliary ducts, indicating a fistula
- Filling defects, dilation, or shadows within the biliary ducts, indicating calculi or neoplasm

CRITICAL FINDINGS: N/A

INTERFERING FACTORS

This procedure is contraindicated for
- ❋ Patients with allergies to shellfish or iodinated dye. The contrast medium used may cause a life-threatening allergic reaction. Patients with a known hypersensitivity to the medium may benefit from premedication with corticosteroids or the use of nonionic contrast medium.
- Patients who are pregnant or suspected of being pregnant, unless the potential benefits of the procedure far outweigh the risks to the fetus and mother.
- ❋ Patients with cholangitis. The injection of the contrast medium can increase biliary pressure, leading to bacteremia, septicemia, and shock.
- ❋ Patients with postoperative wound sepsis, hypersensitivity to iodine, or acute renal failure.

Factors that may impair clear imaging
- Gas or feces in the GI tract resulting from inadequate cleansing or

failure to restrict food intake before the study.
- Retained barium from a previous radiological procedure.
- Metallic objects within the examination field, which may inhibit organ visualization and cause unclear images.
- Inability of the patient to cooperate or remain still during the procedure because of age, significant pain, or mental status.

Other considerations
- The procedure may be terminated if chest pain or severe cardiac arrhythmias occur.
- Air bubbles resembling calculi may be seen if there is inadvertent injection of air.
- Peritonitis may occur as a result of bile extravasation.
- Failure to follow dietary restrictions and other pretesting preparations may cause the procedure to be canceled or repeated.
- Consultation with a health-care provider (HCP) should occur before the procedure for radiation safety concerns regarding younger patients or patients who are lactating.
- Risks associated with radiation overexposure can result from frequent x-ray procedures. Personnel in the examination room with the patient should wear a protective lead apron, stand behind a shield, or leave the area while the examination is being done. Personnel working in the examination area should wear badges to record their radiation level.

NURSING IMPLICATIONS AND PROCEDURE

PRETEST:
- Positively identify the patient using at least two unique identifiers before providing care, treatment, or services.

- *Patient Teaching:* Inform the patient this procedure can assist in assessing the bile ducts of the gallbladder and pancreas.
- Obtain a history of the patient's complaints, including a list of known allergens, especially allergies or sensitivities to latex, iodine, seafood, contrast medium, anesthetics and dyes.
- Obtain a history of results of the patient's gastrointestinal and hepatobiliary systems, symptoms, and previously performed laboratory tests and diagnostic and surgical procedures.
- Ensure that this procedure is performed before an upper GI study or barium swallow.
- Record the date of the last menstrual period and determine the possibility of pregnancy in perimenopausal women.
- Obtain a list of the patient's current medications, including herbs, nutritional supplements, and nutraceuticals (see Appendix F).
- If contrast medium is scheduled to be used, patients receiving metformin (glucophage) for non-insulin-dependent (type 2) diabetes should discontinue the drug on the day of the test and continue to withhold it for 48 hr after the test. Failure to do so may result in lactic acidosis.
- Review the procedure with the patient. Address concerns about pain and explain that there may be moments of discomfort and some pain experienced during the test. Inform the patient that the procedure is usually performed in the radiology department by a HCP and takes approximately 30 to 60 min.
- *Sensitivity to social and cultural issues,* as well as concern for modesty, is important in providing psychological support before, during, and after the procedure.
- Instruct the patient to remove jewelry and other metallic objects in the area to be examined.
- Instruct the patient to fast and restrict fluids for 8 hr prior to the procedure. Protocols may vary among facilities.
- *Make sure a written and informed consent has been signed prior to the procedure and before administering any medications.*

INTRATEST:

- Ensure that the patient has complied with dietary, fluid, and medication restrictions for 8 hr prior to the procedure.
- Ensure that the patient has removed all external metallic objects from the area to be examined prior to the procedure.
- If the patient has a history of allergic reactions to any relevant substance or drug, administer ordered prophylactic steroids or antihistamines before the procedure.
- Have emergency equipment readily available.
- Instruct the patient to void prior to the procedure and to change into the gown, robe, and foot coverings provided.
- Observe standard precautions, and follow the general guidelines in Appendix A.
- Instruct the patient to cooperate fully and to follow directions. Instruct the patient to remain still throughout the procedure because movement produces unreliable results.
- Record baseline vital signs, and continue to monitor throughout the procedure. Protocols may vary from facility to facility.
- Clamp the T-tube 24 hr before and during the procedure, if ordered, to help prevent air bubbles from entering the ducts.
- An x-ray of the abdomen is obtained to determine if any residual contrast medium is present from previous studies.
- The patient is placed on an examination table in the supine position.
- The area around the T-tube is draped; the end of the T-tube is cleansed with 70% alcohol. If the T-tube site is inflamed and painful, a local anesthetic (e.g., lidocaine) may be injected around the site. A needle is inserted into the open end of the T-tube, and the clamp is removed.
- Contrast medium is injected, and fluoroscopy is performed to visualize contrast medium moving through the duct system.
- The patient may feel a bloating sensation in the upper right quadrant as the contrast medium is injected. The tube is clamped, and images are taken. A delayed image may be taken 15 min later to visualize passage of the contrast medium into the duodenum.
- For procedures done after surgery, the T-tube is removed if findings are normal; a dry, sterile dressing is applied to the site.
- If retained calculi are identified, the T-tube is left in place for 4 to 6 wk until the tract surrounding the T-tube is healed to perform a percutaneous removal.

POST-TEST:

- A report of the examination will be sent to the requesting HCP, who will discuss the results with the patient.
- Instruct the patient to resume usual diet, fluids, medications, and activity, as directed by the HCP. Renal function should be assessed before metformin is resumed, if contrast was used.
- Monitor vital signs and neurological status every 15 min for 1 hr, then every 2 hr for 4 hr, and as ordered. Take temperature every 4 hr for 24 hr. Monitor intake and output at least every 8 hr. Compare with baseline values. Notify the HCP if temperature is elevated. Protocols may vary among facilities.
- Monitor T-tube site and change sterile dressing, as ordered.
- Instruct the patient on the care of the site and dressing changes.
- Monitor for reaction to iodinated contrast medium, including rash, urticaria, tachycardia, hyperpnea, hypertension, palpitations, nausea, or vomiting.
- Instruct the patient to immediately report symptoms such as fast heart rate, difficulty breathing, skin rash, itching, chest pain, persistent right shoulder pain, or abdominal pain. Immediately report symptoms to the appropriate HCP.
- Carefully monitor the patient for fatigue and fluid and electrolyte imbalance.
- Recognize anxiety related to test results. Discuss the implications of abnormal test results on the patient's lifestyle. Provide teaching and information regarding the clinical implications of the test results, as appropriate.
- Reinforce information given by the patient's HCP regarding further testing, treatment, or referral to another HCP. Answer any questions or

address any concerns voiced by the patient or family.

▶ Depending on the results of this procedure, additional testing may be needed to evaluate or monitor progression of the disease process and determine the need for a change in therapy. Evaluate test results in relation to the patient's symptoms and other tests performed.

RELATED MONOGRAPHS:

▶ Related tests include CT abdomen, hepatobiliary scan, KUB, MRI abdomen, and US liver and biliary system.

▶ Refer to the Gastrointestinal and Hepatobiliary systems tables at the end of the book for tests by related body systems.

Cholangiopancreatography, Endoscopic Retrograde

SYNONYM/ACRONYM: ERCP.

COMMON USE: To visualize and assess the pancreas and common bile ducts for occlusion or stricture.

AREA OF APPLICATION: Gallbladder, bile ducts, pancreatic ducts.

CONTRAST: Iodinated contrast medium.

DESCRIPTION: Endoscopic retrograde cholangiopancreatography (ERCP) allows direct visualization of the pancreatic and biliary ducts with a flexible endoscope and, after injection of contrast material, with x-rays. It allows the physician to view the pancreatic, hepatic, and common bile ducts and the ampulla of Vater. ERCP and percutaneous transhepatic cholangiography (PTC) are the only procedures that allow direct visualization of the biliary and pancreatic ducts. ERCP is less invasive and has less morbidity than PTC. It is useful in the evaluation of patients with jaundice, because the ducts can be visualized even when the patient's bilirubin level is high. (In contrast, oral cholecystography and IV cholangiography cannot

visualize the biliary system when the patient has high bilirubin levels.) By endoscopy, the distal end of the common bile duct can be widened, and gallstones can be removed and stents placed in narrowed bile ducts to allow bile to be drained in jaundiced patients. During endoscopy, specimens of suspicious tissue can be taken for pathological review, and manometry pressure readings can be obtained from the bile and pancreatic ducts. ERCP is used in the diagnosis and follow-up of pancreatic disease.

INDICATIONS

• Assess jaundice of unknown cause to differentiate biliary tract obstruction from liver disease

- Collect specimens for cytology
- Identify obstruction caused by calculi, cysts, ducts, strictures, stenosis, and anatomic abnormalities
- Retrieve calculi from the distal common bile duct and release strictures
- Perform therapeutic procedures, such as sphincterotomy and placement of biliary drains

POTENTIAL DIAGNOSIS

Normal findings in
- Normal appearance of the duodenal papilla
- Patency of the pancreatic and common bile ducts

Abnormal findings in
- Duodenal papilla tumors
- Pancreatic cancer
- Pancreatic fibrosis
- Pancreatitis
- Sclerosing cholangitis

CRITICAL FINDINGS: N/A

INTERFERING FACTORS

This procedure is contraindicated for
- Patients who are pregnant or suspected of being pregnant, unless the potential benefits of the procedure far outweigh the risks to the fetus and mother.
- ◆ Patients with allergies to shellfish or iodinated dye. The contrast medium used may cause a life-threatening allergic reaction. Patients with a known hypersensitivity to the medium may benefit from premedication with corticosteroids or the use of nonionic contrast medium.

Factors that may impair clear imaging
- Gas or feces in the gastrointestinal (GI) tract resulting from inadequate cleansing or failure to restrict food intake before the study.
- Retained barium from a previous radiological procedure.

- Previous surgery involving the stomach or duodenum, which can make locating the duodenal papilla difficult.
- A patient with Zenker's diverticulum involving the esophagus, who may be unable to undergo ERCP.
- A patient with unstable cardiopulmonary status, blood coagulation defects, or cholangitis (test may have to be rescheduled unless the patient received antibiotic therapy before the test).
- A patient with known acute pancreatitis.
- Incorrect positioning of the patient, which may produce poor visualization of the area to be examined.
- Inability of the patient to cooperate or remain still during the procedure because of age, significant pain, or mental status.

Other considerations
- The procedure may be terminated if chest pain or severe cardiac arrhythmias occur.
- Failure to follow dietary restrictions and other pretesting preparations may cause the procedure to be canceled or repeated.
- Consultation with a health-care provider (HCP) should occur before the procedure for radiation safety concerns regarding younger patients or patients who are lactating.
- Risks associated with radiation overexposure can result from frequent x-ray procedures. Personnel in the examination room with the patient should wear a protective lead apron, stand behind a shield, or leave the area while the examination is being done. Personnel working in the examination area should wear badges to record their level of radiation exposure.

NURSING IMPLICATIONS AND PROCEDURE

PRETEST:

- Positively identify the patient using at least two unique identifiers before providing care, treatment, or services.
- *Patient Teaching:* Inform the patient this procedure can assist in assessing the bile ducts of the gallbladder and pancreas.
- Obtain a history of the patient's complaints, including a list of known allergens, especially allergies or sensitivities to latex, iodine, seafood, contrast medium, anesthetics, and dyes.
- Obtain a history of the patient's gastrointestinal and hepatobiliary systems, symptoms, and results of previously performed laboratory tests and diagnostic and surgical procedures.
- Ensure that this procedure is performed before an upper GI study or barium swallow.
- Record the date of the last menstrual period and determine the possibility of pregnancy in perimenopausal women.
- Obtain a list of the patient's current medications including anticoagulants, aspirin and other salicylates, herbs, nutritional supplements, and nutraceuticals (see Appendix F). Note the last time and dose of medication taken.
- If contrast medium is scheduled to be used, patients receiving metformin (glucophage) for non-insulin-dependent (type 2) diabetes should discontinue the drug on the day of the test and continue to withhold it for 48 hr after the test. Failure to do so may result in lactic acidosis.
- Review the procedure with the patient. Address concerns about pain and explain that some pain may be experienced during the test, and there may be moments of discomfort. Inform the patient that the procedure is performed in a GI lab or radiology department, usually by a HCP, with support staff, and takes approximately 30 to 60 min.
- *Sensitivity to social and cultural issues,* as well as concern for modesty, is important in providing psychological support before, during, and after the procedure.

- Explain that an IV line may be inserted to allow infusion of IV fluids, anesthetics, or sedatives.
- Instruct the patient to remove jewelry and other metallic objects from the area to be examined.
- The patient should fast and restrict fluids for 8 hr prior to the procedure. Instruct the patient to avoid taking anticoagulant medication or to reduce dosage as ordered prior to the procedure. Protocols may vary among facilities.
- *Make sure a written and informed consent has been signed prior to the procedure and before administering any medications.*

INTRATEST:

- Ensure the patient has complied with dietary, fluid, and medication restrictions for 8 hr prior to the procedure.
- Ensure the patient has removed all external metallic objects from the area to be examined.
- Assess for completion of bowel preparation according to the institution's procedure.
- If the patient has a history of allergic reactions to any relevant substance or drug, administer ordered prophylactic steroids or antihistamines before the procedure. Use nonionic contrast medium for the procedure.
- Have emergency equipment readily available.
- Instruct the patient to void prior to the procedure and to change into the gown, robe, and foot coverings provided.
- Instruct the patient to cooperate fully and to follow directions. Instruct the patient to remain still throughout the procedure because movement produces unreliable results.
- Record baseline vital signs, and continue to monitor throughout the procedure. Protocols may vary among facilities.
- Observe standard precautions, and follow the general guidelines in Appendix A. Positively identify the patient, and label the appropriate containers with the corresponding patient demographics, date, and time of collection if cytology samples are collected.
- Insert an IV line for administration of drugs, as needed.

- Administer test ordered sedation.
- An x-ray of the abdomen is obtained to determine if any residual contrast medium is present from previous studies.
- The oropharynx is sprayed or swabbed with a topical local anesthetic.
- The patient is placed on an examination table in the left lateral position with the left arm behind the back and right hand at the side with the neck slightly flexed. A protective guard is inserted into the mouth to cover the teeth. A bite block can also be inserted to maintain adequate opening of the mouth.
- The endoscope is passed through the mouth with a dental suction device in place to drain secretions. A side-viewing flexible fiberoptic endoscope is passed into the duodenum, and a small cannula is inserted into the duodenal papilla (ampulla of Vater).
- The patient is placed in the prone position. The duodenal papilla is visualized and cannulated with a catheter. Occasionally the patient can be turned slightly to the right side to aid in visualization of the papilla.
- IV glucagon or anticholinergics can be administered to minimize duodenal spasm and to facilitate visualization of the ampulla of Vater.
- ERCP manometry can be done at this time to measure the pressure in the bile duct, pancreatic duct, and sphincter of Oddi at the papilla area via the catheter as it is placed in the area before the contrast medium is injected.
- When the catheter is in place, contrast medium is injected into the pancreatic and biliary ducts via the catheter, and fluoroscopic images are taken. Biopsy specimens for cytological analysis may be obtained.
- Place specimens in appropriate containers, label them properly, and promptly transport them to the laboratory.

POST-TEST:

- A report of the examination will be sent to the requesting HCP, who will discuss the results with the patient.
- Do not allow the patient to eat or drink until the gag reflex returns, after which the patient is permitted to eat lightly for 12 to 24 hr.

- Instruct the patient to resume usual diet, fluids, medications, and activity after 24 hr, or as directed by the HCP. Renal function should be assessed before metformin is resumed, if contrast was used.
- Monitor vital signs and neurological status every 15 min for 1 hr, then every 2 hr for 4 hr, and as ordered. Take temperature every 4 hr for 24 hr. Monitor intake and output at least every 8 hr. Compare with baseline values. Notify the HCP if temperature is elevated. Protocols may vary among facilities.
- Monitor for reaction to iodinated contrast medium, including rash, urticaria, tachycardia, hyperpnea, hypertension, palpitations, nausea, or vomiting.
- Tell the patient to expect some throat soreness and possible hoarseness. Advise the patient to use warm gargles, lozenges, ice packs to the neck, or cool fluids to alleviate throat discomfort.
- Inform the patient that any belching, bloating, or flatulence is the result of air insufflation.
- Instruct the patient to immediately report symptoms such as fast heart rate, difficulty breathing, skin rash, itching, chest pain, persistent right shoulder pain, or abdominal pain. Immediately report symptoms to the appropriate HCP.
- Recognize anxiety related to test results. Discuss the implications of abnormal test results on the patient's lifestyle. Provide teaching and information regarding the clinical implications of the test results, as appropriate.
- Reinforce information given by the patient's HCP regarding further testing, treatment, or referral to another HCP. Answer any questions or address any concerns voiced by the patient or family.
- Depending on the results of this procedure, additional testing may be needed to evaluate or monitor progression of the disease process and determine the need for a change in therapy. Evaluate test results in relation to the patient's symptoms and other tests performed.

RELATED MONOGRAPHS:

▶ Related tests include amylase, CT abdomen, hepatobiliary scan, KUB studies, lipase, MRI abdomen, peritoneal fluid analysis, pleural

fluid analysis, and US liver and biliary system.
▶ Refer to the Gastrointestinal and Hepatobiliary systems tables at the end of the book for related tests by body system.

Cholesterol, HDL and LDL

SYNONYM/ACRONYM: α_1-Lipoprotein cholesterol, high-density cholesterol, HDLC, and β-lipoprotein cholesterol, low-density cholesterol, LDLC.

COMMON USE: To assess and monitor risk for coronary artery disease.

SPECIMEN: Serum (2 mL) collected in a red- or tiger-top tube.

REFERENCE VALUE: (Method: Spectrophotometry)

HDLC	Conventional Units	SI Units (Conventional Units × 0.0259)
Birth	6–56 mg/dL	0.16–1.45 mmol/L
Children, adults, and older adults		
Desirable	Greater than 60 mg/dL	Greater than 1.56 mmol/L
Acceptable	40–60 mg/dL	0.9–1.56 mmol/L
Low	Less than 40 mg/dL	Less than 0.9 mmol/L

LDLC	Conventional Units	SI Units (Conventional Units × 0.0259)
Optimal	Less than 100 mg/dL	Less than 2.59 mmol/L
Near optimal	100–129 mg/dL	2.59–3.34 mmol/L
Borderline high	130–159 mg/dL	2.67–4.11 mmol/L
High	160–189 mg/dL	4.14–4.90 mmol/L
Very high	Greater than 190 mg/dL	Greater than 4.92 mmol/L

	NMR LDLC Particle Number	NMR LDLC Small Particle Size
High-risk CAD	Less than 1,000 nmol/L	Less than 850 nmol/L
Moderately high-risk CAD	Less than 1,300 nmol/L	Less than 850 nmol/L

CAD, coronary artery disease; NMR = nuclear magnetic resonance.

DESCRIPTION: High-density lipoprotein cholesterol (HDLC) and low-density lipoprotein cholesterol (LDLC) are the major transport proteins for cholesterol in the body. It is believed that HDLC may have protective properties in that its role includes transporting cholesterol from the arteries to the liver. LDLC is the major transport protein for cholesterol to the arteries from the liver. LDLC can be calculated using total cholesterol, total triglycerides, and HDLC levels. Beyond the total cholesterol, HDL and LDL cholesterol values, other important risk factors must be considered. The Framingham algorithm can assist in estimating the risk of developing coronary artery disease (CAD) within a 10-yr period. The National Cholesterol Education Program (NCEP) also provides important guidelines. The latest NCEP guidelines for target lipid levels, major risk factors, and therapeutic interventions are outlined in Adult Treatment Panel III (ATP III) (www.nhlbi.nih.gov/guidelines/cholesterol/index.htm).

Studies have shown that CAD is inversely related to LDLC particle number and size. The nuclear magnetic resonance (NMR) lipid profile uses NMR imaging spectroscopy to determine LDLC particle number and size in addition to measurement of the traditional lipid markers.

HDLC levels less than 40 mg/dL in men and women represent a coronary risk factor. There is an inverse relationship between HDLC and risk of CAD (i.e., lower HDLC levels represent a higher risk of CAD). Levels of LDLC in terms of risk for CAD are directly proportional to risk and vary by age group. The LDLC can be estimated using the Friedewald formula:

$$LDLC = (Total\ Cholesterol) - (HDLC) - (VLDLC)$$

Very-low-density lipoprotein cholesterol (VLDLC) is estimated by dividing the triglycerides (conventional units) by 5. Triglycerides in SI units would be divided by 2.18 to estimate VLDLC. It is important to note that the formula is valid only if the triglycerides are less than 400 mg/dL or 4.52 mmol/L.

INDICATIONS

- Determine the risk of cardiovascular disease
- Evaluate the response to dietary and drug therapy for hypercholesterolemia
- Investigate hypercholesterolemia in light of family history of cardiovascular disease

POTENTIAL DIAGNOSIS

Although the exact pathophysiology is unknown, cholesterol is required for many functions at the cellular and organ levels. Elevations of cholesterol are associated with conditions caused by an inherited defect in lipoprotein metabolism, liver disease, kidney disease, or a disorder of the endocrine system. Decreases in cholesterol levels are associated with conditions caused by enzyme deficiencies, malnutrition, malabsorption, liver disease, and sudden increased utilization.

HDLC increased in
- Alcoholism
- Biliary cirrhosis
- Chronic hepatitis

- Exercise
- Familial hyper-α-lipoproteinemia

HDLC decreased in:
- Abetalipoproteinemia
- Cholestasis
- Chronic renal failure
- Fish-eye disease
- Genetic predisposition or enzyme/cofactor deficiency
- Hepatocellular disorders
- Hypertriglyceridemia
- Nephrotic syndrome
- Obesity
- Premature CAD
- Sedentary lifestyle
- Smoking
- Tangier's disease
- Syndrome X (metabolic syndrome)
- Uncontrolled diabetes

LDLC increased in
- Anorexia nervosa
- Chronic renal failure
- Corneal arcus
- Cushing's syndrome
- Diabetes
- Diet high in cholesterol and saturated fat
- Dysglobulinemias
- Hepatic disease
- Hepatic obstruction
- Hyperlipoproteinemia types IIA and IIB
- Hypothyroidism
- Nephrotic syndrome
- Porphyria
- Pregnancy
- Premature CAD
- Syndrome X (metabolic syndrome)
- Tendon and tuberous xanthomas

LDLC decreased in
- Acute stress (severe burns, illness)
- Chronic anemias
- Chronic pulmonary disease
- Genetic predisposition or enzyme/cofactor deficiency
- Hyperthyroidism
- Hypolipoproteinemia and abetalipoproteinemia

- Inflammatory joint disease
- Myeloma
- Reye's syndrome
- Severe hepatocellular destruction or disease
- Tangier disease

CRITICAL FINDINGS: N/A

INTERFERING FACTORS
- Drugs that may increase HDLC levels include albuterol, anticonvulsants, cholestyramine, cimetidine, clofibrate and other fibric acid derivatives, estrogens, ethanol (moderate use), lovastatin, niacin, oral contraceptives, pindolol, pravastatin, prazosin, and simvastatin.
- Drugs that may decrease HDLC levels include acebutolol, atenolol, danazol, diuretics, etretinate, interferon, isotretinoin, linseed oil, metoprolol, neomycin, nonselective β-adrenergic blocking agents, probucol, progesterone, steroids, and thiazides.
- Drugs that may increase LDLC levels include androgens, catecholamines, chenodiol, cyclosporine, danazol, diuretics, etretinate, glucogenic corticosteroids, and progestins.
- Drugs that may decrease LDLC levels include aminosalicylic acid, cholestyramine, colestipol, estrogens, fibric acid derivatives, interferon, lovastatin, neomycin, niacin, pravastatin, prazosin, probucol, simvastatin, terazosin, and thyroxine.
- Some of the drugs used to lower total cholesterol and LDLC or increase HDLC may cause liver damage.
- Grossly elevated triglyceride levels invalidate the Friedewald formula for mathematical estimation of LDLC; if the triglyceride level is greater than 400 mg/dL, the formula should not be used.

- Fasting before specimen collection is highly recommended. Ideally, the patient should be on a stable diet for 3 wk and fast for 12 hr before specimen collection.
- Failure to follow dietary restrictions before the procedure may cause the procedure to be canceled or repeated.

NURSING IMPLICATIONS AND PROCEDURE

PRETEST:

▶ Positively identify the patient using at least two unique identifiers before providing care, treatment, or services.
▶ *Patient Teaching:* Inform the patient this test can assist with evaluation of cholesterol level.
▶ Obtain a history of the patient's complaints, including a list of known allergens, especially allergies or sensitivities to latex.
▶ Obtain a history of the patient's cardiovascular system and results of previously performed laboratory tests and diagnostic and surgical procedures. The presence of other risk factors, such as family history of heart disease, smoking, obesity, diet, lack of physical activity, hypertension, diabetes, previous myocardial infarction, and previous vascular disease, should be investigated.
▶ Obtain a list of the patient's current medications, including herbs, nutritional supplements, and nutraceuticals (see Appendix F).
▶ Review the procedure with the patient. Inform the patient that specimen collection takes approximately 5 to 10 min. Address concerns about pain and explain that there may be some discomfort during the venipuncture.
▶ *Sensitivity to social and cultural issues,* as well as concern for modesty, is important in providing psychological support before, during, and after the procedure.
▶ Instruct the patient to fast for 12 hr before specimen collection. Protocols may vary among facilities.

▶ Confirm with the requesting health-care provider (HCP) that the patient should withhold medications known to influence test results, and instruct the patient accordingly.
▶ There are no fluid restrictions unless by medical direction.

INTRATEST:

▶ Ensure that the patient has complied with dietary and medication restrictions as well as other pretesting preparations; ensure that food has been restricted for at least 12 hr prior to the procedure.
▶ If the patient has a history of allergic reaction to latex, avoid the use of equipment containing latex.
▶ Instruct the patient to cooperate fully and to follow directions. Direct the patient to breathe normally and to avoid unnecessary movement.
▶ Observe standard precautions, and follow the general guidelines in Appendix A. Positively identify the patient, and label the appropriate tubes with the corresponding patient demographics, date, and time of collection. Perform a venipuncture.
▶ Remove the needle and apply direct pressure with dry gauze to stop bleeding. Observe/assess venipuncture site for bleeding or hematoma formation and secure gauze with adhesive bandage.
▶ Promptly transport the specimen to the laboratory for processing and analysis.

POST-TEST:

▶ A report of the results will be sent to the requesting HCP, who will discuss the results with the patient.
▶ Instruct the patient to resume usual diet, fluids, and medications, as directed by the HCP.
▶ *Nutritional Considerations:* Decreased HDLC level and increased LDLC level may be associated with CAD. Nutritional therapy is recommended for the patient identified to be at high risk for developing CAD. The American Heart Association and National Heart, Lung, and Blood Institute (NHBLI) recommend nutritional therapy for individuals identified to be at high risk for developing CAD or

individuals who have specific risk factors and/or existing medical conditions (e.g., elevated LDL cholesterol levels, other lipid disorders, insulin-dependent diabetes, insulin resistance, or metabolic syndrome). If overweight, the patient should be encouraged to achieve a normal weight. The NHLBI's National Cholesterol Education Program (NCEP) revised its dietary guidelines for reducing CAD in 2001. Guidelines for the Therapeutic Lifestyle Changes (TLC) diet are outlined in the Third Report of the Expert Panel on Detection, Evaluation, and Treatment of High Blood Cholesterol in Adults (Adult Treatment Panel III [ATP III]). The TLC diet emphasizes a reduction in foods high in saturated fats and cholesterol. Red meats, eggs, and dairy products are the major sources of saturated fats and cholesterol. If triglycerides also are elevated, the patient should be advised to eliminate or reduce alcohol and simple carbohydrates from the diet. The TLC approach also includes the use of plant stanols or sterols and increased dissolved fiber as an option for lowering LDL cholesterol levels; nutritional recommendations for daily total caloric intake; recommendations for allowable percentage of calories derived from fat (saturated and unsaturated), carbohydrates, protein, and cholesterol; as well as recommendations for daily expenditure of energy.

▶ *Nutritional Considerations:* Overweight patients with high blood pressure should be encouraged to achieve a normal weight. Other changeable risk factors warranting patient education include strategies to safely decrease sodium intake, increase physical activity, decrease alcohol consumption, eliminate tobacco use, and decrease cholesterol levels.

▶ *Social and Cultural Considerations:* Numerous studies point to the prevalence of excess body weight in American children and adolescents.

Experts estimate that obesity is present in 25% of the population ages 6 to 11 yr. The medical, social, and emotional consequences of excess body weight are significant. Special attention should be given to instructing the child and caregiver regarding health risks and weight-control education.

▶ Recognize anxiety related to test results, and be supportive of fear of shortened life expectancy. Discuss the implications of abnormal test results on the patient's lifestyle. Provide teaching and information regarding the clinical implications of the test results, as appropriate. Educate the patient regarding access to counseling services. Provide contact information, if desired, for the American Heart Association (www.americanheart.org) or the NHLBI (www.nhlbi.nih.gov).

▶ Reinforce information given by the patient's HCP regarding further testing, treatment, or referral to another HCP. Answer any questions or address any concerns voiced by the patient or family.

▶ Depending on the results of this procedure, additional testing may be performed to evaluate or monitor progression of the disease process and determine the need for a change in therapy. Evaluate test results in relation to the patient's symptoms and other tests performed.

RELATED MONOGRAPHS:

▶ Related tests include antiarrhythmic drugs, apolipoprotein A and B, AST, ANP, blood gases, BNP, calcium (total and ionized), cholesterol total, CT cardiac scoring, CRP, CK and isoenzymes, echocardiography, glucose, glycated hemoglobin, Holter monitor, homocysteine, ketones, LDH and isoenzymes, lipoprotein electrophoresis, magnesium, MRI chest, MI scan, myocardial perfusion heart scan, myoglobin, PET heart, potassium, triglycerides, and troponin.

▶ Refer to the Cardiovascular System table at the end of the book for related tests by body system.

Cholesterol, Total

SYNONYM/ACRONYM: N/A.

COMMON USE: To assess and monitor risk for coronary artery disease.

SPECIMEN: Serum (1 mL) collected in a red- or tiger-top tube. Plasma (1 mL) collected in a green-top (heparin) tube is also acceptable. It is important to use the same tube type when serial specimen collections are anticipated for consistency in testing.

REFERENCE VALUE: (Method: Spectrophotometry)

Risk	Conventional Units	SI Units (Conventional Units × 0.0259)
Children and adolescents (less than 20 yr)		
Desirable	Less than 170 mg/dL	Less than 4.4 mmol/L
Borderline	170–199 mg/dL	4.4–5.2 mmol/L
High	Greater than 200 mg/dL	Greater than 5.2 mmol/L
Adults and older adults		
Desirable	Less than 200 mg/dL	Less than 5.18 mmol/L
Borderline	200–239 mg/dL	5.18–6.19 mmol/L
High	Greater than 240 mg/dL	Greater than 6.22 mmol/L

Plasma values may be 10% lower than serum values.

DESCRIPTION: Cholesterol is a lipid needed to form cell membranes and a component of the materials that render the skin waterproof. It also helps form bile salts, adrenal corticosteroids, estrogen, and androgens. Cholesterol is obtained from the diet (exogenous cholesterol) and also synthesized in the body (endogenous cholesterol). Although most body cells can form some cholesterol, it is produced mainly by the liver and intestinal mucosa. Cholesterol is an integral component in cell membrane maintenance and hormone production. Very low cholesterol values, as are sometimes seen in critically ill patients, can be as life-threatening as very high levels.

According to the National Cholesterol Education Program, maintaining cholesterol levels less than 200 mg/dL significantly reduces the risk of coronary heart disease; no age and gender stratification is presented as part of its recommendation. Numerous studies have been done, and there are inconsistencies among the studies as to target "normals" segregated by age and gender. Beyond the total cholesterol and high-density lipoprotein cholesterol (HDLC) values, other important risk factors must be considered. The Framingham algorithm can assist in estimating the risk of developing coronary artery disease (CAD) within a 10-yr period. Many myocardial infarctions occur even in patients whose cholesterol levels are considered to be within acceptable limits or who are in a moderate-risk category. The combination of risk factors and lipid values helps identify individuals at risk so that appropriate interventions can be taken. If the cholesterol level is greater than 200 mg/dL, repeat testing after a 12- to 24-hr fast is recommended.

INDICATIONS

- Assist in determining risk of cardiovascular disease
- Assist in the diagnosis of nephrotic syndrome, hepatic disease, pancreatitis, and thyroid disorders
- Evaluate the response to dietary and drug therapy for hypercholesterolemia
- Investigate hypercholesterolemia in light of family history of cardiovascular disease

POTENTIAL DIAGNOSIS

Increased in

Although the exact pathophysiology is unknown, cholesterol is required for many functions at the cellular and organ level. Elevations of cholesterol are associated with conditions caused by an inherited defect in lipoprotein metabolism, liver disease, kidney disease, or a disorder of the endocrine system.

- Acute intermittent porphyria
- Alcoholism
- Anorexia nervosa
- Cholestasis
- Chronic renal failure
- Diabetes (with poor control)
- Diets high in cholesterol and fats
- Familial hyperlipoproteinemia
- Glomerulonephritis
- Glycogen storage disease (von Gierke's disease)
- Gout
- Hypothyroidism (primary)
- Ischemic heart disease
- Nephrotic syndrome
- Obesity
- Pancreatic and prostatic malignancy
- Pregnancy
- Syndrome X (metabolic syndrome)
- Werner's syndrome

Decreased in

Although the exact pathophysiology is unknown, cholesterol is required for many functions at the cellular and organ level. Decreases in cholesterol levels are associated with conditions caused by malnutrition, malabsorption, liver disease, and sudden increased utilization.

- Burns
- Chronic myelocytic leukemia
- Chronic obstructive pulmonary disease
- Hyperthyroidism
- Liver disease (severe)
- Malabsorption and malnutrition syndromes
- Myeloma
- Pernicious anemia
- Polycythemia vera
- Severe illness
- Sideroblastic anemias
- Tangier disease
- Thalassemia
- Waldenström's macroglobulinemia

CRITICAL FINDINGS: N/A

INTERFERING FACTORS

- Drugs that may increase cholesterol levels include amiodarone, androgens, β-blockers, calcitriol, cortisone, cyclosporine, danazol, diclofenac, disulfiram, fluoxymesterone, glucogenic corticosteroids, ibuprofen, isotretinoin, levodopa, mepazine, methyclothiazide, miconazole (owing to castor oil vehicle, not the drug), nafarelin, nandrolone, some oral contraceptives, oxymetholone, phenobarbital, phenothiazine, prochlorperazine, sotalol, thiabendazole, thiouracil, tretinoin, and trifluoperazine.
- Drugs that may decrease cholesterol levels include acebutolol, amiloride, aminosalicylic acid, androsterone, ascorbic acid, asparaginase, atenolol, atorvastatin, beclobrate, bezafibrate, carbutamide, cerivastatin, cholestyramine, ciprofibrate, clofibrate, clonidine, colestipol, dextrothyroxine, doxazosin, enalapril, estrogens, fenfluramine, fenofibrate, fluvastatin, gemfibrozil, haloperidol, hormone replacement therapy, hydralazine, hydrochlorothiazide, interferon, isoniazid, kanamycin, ketoconazole, lincomycin, lisinopril, lovastatin, metformin, nafenopin, nandrolone, neomycin, niacin, nicotinic acid, nifedipine, oxandrolone, paromomycin, pravastatin, probucol, simvastatin, tamoxifen, terazosin, thyroxine, trazodone, triiodothyronine, ursodiol, valproic acid, and verapamil.
- Ingestion of alcohol 12 to 24 hr before the test can falsely elevate results.
- Ingestion of drugs that alter cholesterol levels within 12 hr of the test may give a false impression of cholesterol levels, unless the test is done to evaluate such effects.
- Positioning can affect results; lower levels are obtained if the specimen is from a patient who has been supine for 20 min.
- Failure to follow dietary restrictions before the procedure may cause the procedure to be canceled or repeated.

NURSING IMPLICATIONS AND PROCEDURE

PRETEST:

- Positively identify the patient using at least two unique identifiers before providing care, treatment, or services.
- *Patient Teaching:* Inform the patient this test can assist with evaluation of cholesterol level.
- Obtain a history of the patient's complaints, including a list of known allergens, especially allergies or sensitivities to latex.
- Obtain a history of the patient's cardiovascular, gastrointestinal, and hepatobiliary systems, as well as results of previously performed laboratory tests and diagnostic and surgical procedures. The presence of other risk factors, such as family history of heart disease, smoking, obesity, diet, lack of physical activity, hypertension, diabetes, previous myocardial infarction, and previous vascular disease, should be investigated.
- Obtain a list of the patient's current medications, including herbs, nutritional supplements, and nutraceuticals (see Appendix F).
- Review the procedure with the patient. Inform the patient that specimen collection takes approximately 5 to 10 min. Address concerns about pain and explain that there may be some discomfort during the venipuncture.
- *Sensitivity to social and cultural issues,* as well as concern for modesty, is important in providing psychological support before, during, and after the procedure.
- Instruct the patient to withhold alcohol and drugs known to alter cholesterol levels for 12 to 24 hr before specimen collection, at the direction of the health-care provider (HCP).

▶ There are no fluid or medication restrictions unless by medical direction.
▶ Fasting 6 to 12 hr before specimen collection is required if triglyceride measurements are included; it is recommended if cholesterol levels alone are measured for screening. Protocols may vary among facilities.

INTRATEST:

▶ Ensure that the patient has complied with dietary restrictions and pretesting preparations; ensure that food has been restricted for at least 6 to 12 hr prior to the procedure if triglycerides are to be measured.
▶ If the patient has a history of allergic reaction to latex, avoid the use of equipment containing latex.
▶ Instruct the patient to cooperate fully and to follow directions. Direct the patient to breathe normally and to avoid unnecessary movement.
▶ Observe standard precautions, and follow the general guidelines in Appendix A. Positively identify the patient, and label the appropriate tubes with the corresponding patient demographics, date, and time of collection. Perform a venipuncture.
▶ Remove the needle and apply direct pressure with dry gauze to stop bleeding. Observe/assess venipuncture site for bleeding or hematoma formation and secure gauze with adhesive bandage.
▶ Promptly transport the specimen to the laboratory for processing and analysis.

POST-TEST:

▶ A report of the results will be sent to the requesting HCP, who will discuss the results with the patient.
▶ Instruct the patient to resume usual diet as directed by the HCP.
▶ Secondary causes for increased cholesterol levels should be ruled out before therapy to decrease levels is initiated by use of drugs.
▶ *Nutritional Considerations:* Increases in total cholesterol levels may be associated with CAD. Nutritional therapy is recommended for patients identified to be at high risk for developing CAD. If overweight, the patient should be encouraged to achieve a normal weight. The American Heart Association and National Heart, Lung, and Blood Institute (NHBLI) recommend nutritional therapy for individuals identified to be at high risk for developing CAD or individuals who have specific risk factors and/or existing medical conditions (e.g., elevated LDL cholesterol levels, other lipid disorders, insulin-dependent diabetes, insulin resistance, or metabolic syndrome). If overweight, the patient should be encouraged to achieve a normal weight. The NHLBI's National Cholesterol Education Program (NCEP) revised its dietary guidelines for reducing CAD in 2001. Guidelines for the Therapeutic Lifestyle Changes (TLC) diet are outlined in the Third Report of the Expert Panel on Detection, Evaluation, and Treatment of High Blood Cholesterol in Adults (Adult Treatment Panel III [ATP III]). The TLC diet emphasizes a reduction in foods high in saturated fats and cholesterol. Red meats, eggs, and dairy products are the major sources of saturated fats and cholesterol. If triglycerides also are elevated, the patient should be advised to eliminate or reduce alcohol and simple carbohydrates from the diet. The TLC approach also includes the use of plant stanols or sterols and increased dissolved fiber as an option for lowering LDL cholesterol levels; nutritional recommendations for daily total caloric intake; recommendations for allowable percentage of calories derived from fat (saturated and unsaturated), carbohydrates, protein, and cholesterol; as well as recommendations for daily expenditure of energy.
▶ *Nutritional Considerations:* Overweight patients with high blood pressure should be encouraged to achieve a normal weight. Other changeable risk factors warranting patient education include strategies to safely decrease sodium intake, increase physical activity, decrease alcohol consumption, eliminate tobacco use, and decrease cholesterol levels.
▶ *Social and Cultural Considerations:* Numerous studies point to the prevalence of excess body weight in American children and adolescents. Experts estimate that obesity is present in 25% of the population ages 6 to 11 yr. The medical, social, and emotional consequences of excess body

weight are significant. Special attention should be given to instructing the child and caregiver regarding health risks and weight-control education.

▸ Recognize anxiety related to test results, and be supportive of fear of shortened life expectancy. Discuss the implications of abnormal test results on the patient's lifestyle. Provide teaching and information regarding the clinical implications of the test results, as appropriate. Educate the patient regarding access to counseling services. Provide contact information, if desired, for the American Heart Association (www.americanheart.org) or the NHLBI (www.nhlbi.nih.gov).

▸ Reinforce information given by the patient's HCP regarding further testing, treatment, or referral to another HCP. Answer any questions or address any concerns voiced by the patient or family.

▸ Depending on the results of this procedure, additional testing may be performed to evaluate or monitor progression of the disease process and determine the need for a change in therapy. Evaluate test results in relation to the patient's symptoms and other tests performed.

RELATED MONOGRAPHS:

▸ Related tests include antiarrhythmic drugs, apolipoprotein A and B, AST, ANP, blood gases, BNP, calcium, cholesterol (HDL and LDL), CT cardiac scoring, CRP, CK and isoenzymes, echocardiography, glucose, glycated hemoglobin, Holter monitor, homocysteine, ketones, LDH and isoenzymes, lipoprotein electrophoresis, MRI chest, magnesium, MI scan, myocardial perfusion heart scan, myoglobin, PET heart, potassium, triglycerides, and troponin.

▸ Refer to the Cardiovascular, Gastrointestinal, and Hepatobiliary systems tables at the end of the book for related tests by body system.

Chromosome Analysis, Blood

SYNONYM/ACRONYM: N/A.

COMMON USE: To test for suspected chromosomal disorders that result in birth defects such as Down's syndrome.

SPECIMEN: Whole blood (2 mL) collected in a green-top (sodium heparin) tube.

REFERENCE VALUE: (Method: Tissue culture and microscopic analysis) No chromosomal abnormalities identified.

DESCRIPTION: Chromosome analysis or karyotyping involves comparison of test samples against normal chromosome patterns of number and structure. A normal karyotype consists of 22 pairs or autosomal chromosomes and one pair sex chromosomes, XX for female and XY for male. Variations in number or structure can be congenital or acquired. Variations can range from a small, single-gene mutation to abnormalities in an entire chromosome or set of chromosomes due to duplication, deletion, substitution, translocation, or other rearrangement. Testing for birth defects as well as mental and physical retardation can be accomplished through the use of several technologies. Chromosome analysis by phytohemagglutination assay is used to detect Down's syndrome and abnormal sexual development. Fluorescence in situ hybridization (FISH) testing is useful in the detection of specific microdeletion syndromes (e.g., Prader-Willi, Angelman, Beckwith-Wiedemann, Smith-Magenis, DiGeorge, Williams, Miller-Dieker) and other acquired chromosomal changes associated with hematological disorders. Amniotic fluid, chorionic villus sampling, and cells from fetal tissue or products of conception can also be evaluated for chromosomal abnormalities.

INDICATIONS

- Evaluate conditions related to cryptorchidism, hypogonadism, primary amenorrhea, and infertility
- Evaluate congenital anomaly, delayed development (physical or mental), mental retardation, and ambiguous sexual organs
- Investigate the carrier status of patients or relatives with known genetic abnormalities
- Investigate the cause of multiple miscarriages
- Provide prenatal care or genetic counseling

POTENTIAL DIAGNOSIS

The following tables list some common genetic defects.

Syndrome	Autosomal Chromosome Defect	Features
Beckwith-Wiedemann	Duplication 11p15	Macroglossia, omphalocele, earlobe creases
Cat's eye	Trisomy 2q11	Anal atresia, coloboma
Cri du chat	Deletion 5p	Catlike cry, microcephaly, hypertelorism, mental retardation, retrognathia
Down	Trisomy 21	Epicanthal folds, simian crease of palm, flat nasal bridge, mental retardation, congenital heart disease
Edwards	Trisomy 18	Micrognathia, clenched third/fourth fingers with the fifth finger overlapping, rockerbottom feet, mental retardation, congenital heart disease
Pallister-Killian	Trisomy 12p	Psychomotor delay, sparse anterior scalp hair, micrognathia, hypotonia
Patau	Trisomy 13	Microcephaly, cleft palate or lip, polydactyly, mental retardation, congenital heart disease

(*table continues on page 370*)

| Warkam | Mosaic trisomy 8 | Malformed ears, bulbous nose, deep palm creases, absent or hypoplastic patellae |
| Wolf-Hirschhorn | Deletion 4p | Microcephaly, growth retardation, mental retardation, carp mouth |

Syndrome	Sex-Chromosome Defect	Features
XYY	47,XYY	Tall, increased risk of behavior problems
Klinefelter	47,XXY	Hypogonadism, infertility, underdeveloped secondary sex characteristics, learning disabilities
Triple X	47,XXX	Increased risk of infertility and learning disabilities
Ullrich-Turner	45,X	Short, gonadal dysgenesis, webbed neck, low posterior hairline, renal and cardiovascular abnormalities

CRITICAL FINDINGS: N/A

INTERFERING FACTORS: N/A

NURSING IMPLICATIONS AND PROCEDURE

PRETEST:

▶ Positively identify the patient using at least two unique identifiers before providing care, treatment, or services.
▶ *Patient Teaching:* Inform the patient this test can assist in identification of potential birth defects.
▶ Obtain a history of the patient's complaints, including a list of known allergens, especially allergies or sensitivities to latex.
▶ Obtain a history of the patient's reproductive system, family history of known or suspected genetic disorders, and results of previously performed laboratory tests and diagnostic and surgical procedures.
▶ Obtain a list of the patient's current medications, including herbs, nutritional

supplements, and nutraceuticals (see Appendix F).
▶ Review the procedure with the patient. Inform the patient that specimen collection takes approximately 5 to 10 min. Address concerns about pain and explain that there may be some discomfort during the venipuncture.
▶ *Sensitivity to social and cultural issues,* as well as concern for modesty, is important in providing psychological support before, during, and after the procedure.
▶ There are no food, fluid, or medication restrictions unless by medical direction.

INTRATEST:

▶ If the patient has a history of allergic reaction to latex, avoid the use of equipment containing latex.
▶ Instruct the patient to cooperate fully and to follow directions. Direct the patient to breathe normally and to avoid unnecessary movement.
▶ Observe standard precautions, and follow the general guidelines in Appendix A. Positively identify the patient, and label the appropriate tubes with the corresponding patient demographics,

date, and time of collection. Perform a venipuncture.

▶ Remove the needle and apply direct pressure with dry gauze to stop bleeding. Observe/assess venipuncture site for bleeding or hematoma formation and secure gauze with adhesive bandage.

▶ Promptly transport the specimen to the laboratory for processing and analysis.

POST-TEST:

▶ A report of the results will be sent to the requesting health-care provider (HCP), who will discuss the results with the patient.

▶ Recognize anxiety related to test results, and be supportive of the sensitive nature of the testing. Discuss the implications of abnormal test results on the patient's lifestyle. Provide teaching and information regarding the clinical implications of the test results, as appropriate. Educate the patient regarding access to counseling services.

▶ *Social and Cultural Considerations:* Encourage the family to seek counseling if they are contemplating pregnancy termination or to seek genetic counseling if a chromosomal abnormality is determined. Decisions regarding elective abortion should occur in the presence of both parents. Provide a nonjudgmental, nonthreatening atmosphere for discussing the risks and difficulties of delivering and raising a developmentally challenged infant, as well as exploring other options (termination of pregnancy or adoption). It is also important to discuss feelings the mother and father may experience (e.g., guilt, depression, anger) if fetal abnormalities are detected. Educate the patient and family regarding access to counseling services, as appropriate.

▶ Reinforce information given by the patient's HCP regarding further testing, treatment, or referral to another HCP. Answer any questions or address any concerns voiced by the patient or family.

▶ Depending on the results of this procedure, additional testing may be performed to evaluate or monitor changes in health status and determine the need for a change in therapy. Evaluate test results in relation to the patient's symptoms and other tests performed.

RELATED MONOGRAPHS:

▶ Related tests include α_1-fetoprotein, amniotic fluid analysis, biopsy chorionic villus, and US biophysical profile obstetric.

▶ Refer to the Reproductive System table at the end of the book for related tests by body system.

Clot Retraction

SYNONYM/ACRONYM: N/A.

COMMON USE: To assist in the diagnosis of bleeding disorders.

SPECIMEN: Whole blood collected in a full 5-mL red-top tube.

REFERENCE VALUE: (Method: Macroscopic observation of sample) A normal clot, gently separated from the side of the test tube and incubated at 37°C, shrinks to about half of its original size within 1 hr. The result is a firm, cylindrical fibrin clot that contains red blood cells and is sharply demarcated from the clear serum. Complete clot retraction can take 6 to 24 hr.

C

DESCRIPTION: The clot retraction test measures the adequacy of platelet function by measuring the speed and extent of clot retraction. Normally, when blood clots in a test tube, it retracts away from the sidewalls of the tube. Platelets play a major role in the clot retraction process. When platelets are decreased or function is impaired, scant serum and a soft, plump, poorly demarcated clot form in the tube. In addition to normal platelets, clot retraction depends on the contractile protein thrombosthenin, magnesium, adenosine triphosphate (ATP), and pyruvate kinase. Clot retraction is also influenced by hematocrit and by fibrinogen structure and concentration.

INDICATIONS
- Evaluate the adequacy of platelet function
- Evaluate thrombocytopenia of unknown origin
- Investigate the possibility of Glanzmann's disease
- Investigate suspected abnormalities of fibrinogen or fibrinolytic activity

POTENTIAL DIAGNOSIS

Increased in
- Anemia (severe) *(related to inadequate numbers of red blood cells (RBCs) that quickly produce a clot)*
- Hypofibrinogenemia, dysfibrinogenemia, disseminated intravascular coagulation (DIC) *(evidenced by rapid formation of a small, loosely formed clot; absence of functional fibrinogen reduces fibrinolysis)*

- Medications like aspirin *(related to effect of acetylsalicylic acid as a potentiator of platelet aggregation)*

Decreased in
- Glanzmann's thrombasthenia *(related to autosomal recessive abnormality of platelet glycoprotein IIb–IIIa required for platelet aggregation)*
- Polycythemia *(related to excessive numbers of RBCs that physically limit the extent to which the clot can retract)*
- Thrombocytopenia *(related to inadequate numbers of platelets to produce a well-formed clot)*
- von Willebrand disease *(related to deficiency of von Willebrand factor required for platelet aggregation)*
- Waldenström's macroglobulinemia *(related to excessive production of paraproteins that physically obstruct platelet aggregation)*

CRITICAL FINDINGS: N/A

INTERFERING FACTORS
- Drugs that may produce a decreased result include apronalide, carbenicillin, and plicamycin.
- Platelet count less than $100 \times 10^3/mm^3$, acetylsalicylic acid therapy, altered fibrinogen/fibrin structure, hypofibrinogenemia, polycythemia or hemoconcentration, and multiple myeloma are conditions in which abnormal clot retraction may occur, limiting the ability to form a valid assessment of platelet function.
- Prompt and proper specimen processing, storage, and analysis are important to achieve accurate results. Specimens received in the laboratory more than 1 hr after collection should be rejected.

NURSING IMPLICATIONS AND PROCEDURE

PRETEST:

▶ Positively identify the patient using at least two unique identifiers before providing care, treatment, or services.

▶ *Patient Teaching:* Inform the patient this test can assist in evaluating the effectiveness of blood clotting.

▶ Obtain a history of the patient's complaints, including a list of known allergens, especially allergies or sensitivities to latex.

▶ Obtain a history of the patient's hematopoietic system and results of previously performed laboratory tests and diagnostic and surgical procedures.

▶ Note any recent procedures that can interfere with test results.

▶ Obtain a list of the patient's current medications, including herbs, nutritional supplements, and nutraceuticals (see Appendix F).

▶ Review the procedure with the patient. Inform the patient that specimen collection takes approximately 5 to 10 min. Address concerns about pain and explain that there may be some discomfort during the venipuncture.

▶ *Sensitivity to social and cultural issues,* as well as concern for modesty, is important in providing psychological support before, during, and after the procedure.

▶ There are no food, fluid, or medication restrictions unless by medical direction.

INTRATEST:

▶ If the patient has a history of allergic reaction to latex, avoid the use of equipment containing latex.

▶ Instruct the patient to cooperate fully and to follow directions. Direct the patient to breathe normally and to avoid unnecessary movement.

▶ Observe standard precautions, and follow the general guidelines in Appendix A. Positively identify the patient, and label the appropriate tubes with the corresponding patient demographics, date, and time of collection. Perform a venipuncture.

▶ Remove the needle and apply direct pressure with dry gauze to stop bleeding. Observe/assess venipuncture site for bleeding or hematoma formation and secure gauze with adhesive bandage.

▶ Promptly transport the specimen to the laboratory within 1 hr of collection for processing and analysis.

POST-TEST:

▶ A report of the results will be sent to the requesting health-care provider (HCP), who will discuss the results with the patient.

▶ Inform the patient with abnormal clot retraction of the importance of taking precautions against bruising and bleeding. These precautions may include the use of a soft bristle toothbrush, use of an electric razor, avoidance of constipation, avoidance of acetylsalicylic acid and similar products, and avoidance of intramuscular injections.

▶ Reinforce information given by the patient's HCP regarding further testing, treatment, or referral to another HCP. Answer any questions or address any concerns voiced by the patient or family.

▶ Depending on the results of this procedure, additional testing may be performed to evaluate or monitor progression of the disease process and determine the need for a change in therapy. Evaluate test results in relation to the patient's symptoms and other tests performed.

RELATED MONOGRAPHS:

▶ Related tests include bleeding time, coagulation factor XIII, CBC, CBC hematocrit, CBC hemoglobin, CBC platelet count, and fibrinogen.

▶ Refer to the Hematopoietic System table at the end of the book for related tests by body system.

C

Coagulation Factors

SYNONYM/ACRONYM: See table.

COMMON USE: To detect factor deficiencies and related coagulopathies such as found in disseminated intravascular coagulation (DIC).

SPECIMEN: Whole blood collected in a completely filled blue-top (3.2% sodium citrate) tube. If the patient's hematocrit exceeds 55%, the volume of citrate in the collection tube must be adjusted.

REFERENCE VALUE: (Method: Photo-optical clot detection) Activity from 50% to 150%.

	Preferred Name	Synonym	Role in Modern Coagulation Cascade Model	Coagulation Test Responses in the Presence of Factor Deficiency
Factor I	Fibrinogen	—	Assists in the formation of the fibrin clot	PT prolonged, aPTT prolonged
Factor II	Prothrombin	Prethrombin	Assists factor Xa in formation of trace thrombin in the initiation phase and assists factors VIIIa, IXa, Xa, and Va to form thrombin in the propagation phase of hemostasis	PT prolonged, aPTT prolonged
Tissue factor (formerly known as factor III)	Tissue factor	Tissue thromboplastin	Assists factor VII and Ca^{2+} in the activation of factors IX and X during the initiation phase of hemostasis	PT prolonged, aPTT prolonged

Calcium (formerly known as factor IV)	Calcium	Ca^{2+}	Essential to the activation of multiple clotting factors	N/A
Factor V	Proaccelerin	Labile factor, accelerator globulin (AcG)	Assists factors VIIIa, IXa, Xa, and II in the formation of thrombin during the amplification and propagation phases of hemostasis	PT prolonged, aPTT prolonged
Factor VII	Proconvertin	Stabile factor, serum prothrombin conversion accelerator, autoprothrombin I	Assists tissue factor and Ca^{2+} in the activation of factors IX and X	PT prolonged, aPTT normal
Factor VIII	Antihemophilic factor (AHF)	Antihemophilic globulin (AHG), antihemophilic factor A, platelet cofactor 1	Activated by trace thrombin during the initiation phase of hemostasis to amplify formation of additional thrombin	aPTT prolonged, PT normal
Factor IX	Plasma thromboplastin component (PTC)	Christmas factor, antihemophilic factor B, platelet cofactor 2	Assists factors Va and VIIIa in the amplification phase and factors VIIIa, Xa, Va, and II to form thrombin in the propagation phase	aPTT prolonged, PT normal
Factor X	Stuart-Prower factor	Autoprothrombin III, thrombokinase	Assists with formation of trace thrombin in the initiation phase and acts with factors VIIIa, IXa, Va, and II to form thrombin in the propagation phase	PT prolonged, aPTT prolonged

(*table continues on page 376*)

C

Factor XI	Plasma thrombo-plastin antecedent (PTA)	Antihemophilic factor C	Activated by thrombin pro-duced in the extrinsic path-way to enhance production of additional thro-mbin inside the fibrin clot via the intrinsic path-way; this factor also participates in slowing down the process of fibrinolysis	aPTT pro-longed, PT normal
Factor XII	Hageman factor	Glass factor, contact factor	Contact activator of the kinin system (e.g., prekallikrein, and high-molec-ular-weight kininogen)	aPTT pro-longed, PT normal
Factor XIII	Fibrin-stabilizing factor (FSF)	Laki-Lorand factor (LLF), fibrinase, plasma transglu-taminase	Activated by thrombin and assists in forma-tion of bonds between fibrin strands to com-plete secondary hemostasis	PT normal, aPTT normal
von Will-ebrand factor	von Willebrand factor	vWF	Assists in platelet adhesion and thrombus formation	Ristocetin cofactor decreased

DESCRIPTION: Hemostasis involves three components: blood vessel walls, platelets, and plasma coagu-lation proteins. The coagulation proteins respond to blood vessel injury in an overlapping chain of events. There is a balance in health between the prothrombot-ic or clot formation process and the antithrombotic or clot disinte-gration process. The prothrombot-ic process, also known as primary hemostasis, includes the forma-tion of a platelet plug. Simultaneously, the coagulation cascade or secondary hemostasis occurs. The contact activation (formerly known as the intrinsic pathway) and tissue factor (for-merly known as the extrinsic pathway) pathways of secondary hemostasis are a series of reac-tions involving the substrate pro-tein fibrinogen, the coagulation factors (also known as *enzyme precursors* or *zymogens*), nonenzymatic cofactors (Ca^{2+}), and phospholipids. The factors were assigned Roman numerals in the order of their discovery, not their place in the coagulation sequence. Factor VI was originally thought to be a separate clotting factor. It was subsequently proved to be the same as a modified form of factor Va, and therefore the number is no longer used.

The antithrombotic process includes tissue factor pathway inhibitor (TFPI), antithrombin, protein C, and fibrinolysis.

The coagulation factors are formed in the liver. They can be divided into three groups based on their common properties:

1. The contact group is activated in vitro by a surface such as glass and is activated in vivo by collagen. The contact group includes factor XI, factor XII, prekallikrein, and high-molecular-weight kininogen.
2. The prothrombin or vitamin K–dependent group includes factors II, VII, IX, and X.
3. The fibrinogen group includes factors I, V, VIII, and XIII. They are the most labile of the factors and are consumed during the coagulation process. The factors listed in the table are the ones most commonly measured.

A more modern concept of the coagulation cascade has replaced the traditional model and is presented on the next page. The modern model includes three overlapping phases in the formation of thrombin: initiation, amplification, and propagation. It is now believed that tissue factor (TF) is the primary initiator of the coagulation cascade either by contact activation or trauma. The cellular theory of coagulation provides evidence that some cells (e.g., endothelial cells, smooth muscle cells, monocytes) can be induced to express TF. Substances such as endotoxins, tumor necrosis factor alpha, and lipoproteins can also stimulate expression of TF. TF, in combination with factor VII and calcium, forms a complex that then activates factors IX and X in the initiation phase. Activated factor X in the presence of factor II (prothrombin) leads to the formation of thrombin. TFPI quickly inactivates this stage of the pathway so that limited or trace amounts of thrombin are produced and which results in the activation of factors VIII and V. Activated factor IX, assisted by activated factors V and VIII, initiate amplification and propagation of thrombin in the cascade. Thrombin activates factor XIII and begins converting fibrinogen into fibrin monomers, which spontaneously polymerize and then become cross-linked into a stable clot by activated factor XIII.

Qualitative and quantitative factor deficiencies can affect the function of the coagulation pathways. Factor V and factor II (prothrombin) mutations are examples of qualitative deficiencies and are the most common inherited predisposing factors for blood clots. Approximately 5% to 7% of Caucasians have the factor V Leiden mutation and 2% to 3% have a prothrombin mutation. Hemophilia A is an inherited deficiency of factor VIII and occurs at a prevalence of about 1 in 5,000 to 10,000 male births. Hemophilia B is an inherited deficiency of factor IX and occurs at a prevalence of about 1 in about 20,000 to 34,000 male births.

The PT/INR measures the function of the extrinsic and common pathways of coagulation and is used to monitor patients receiving warfarin or coumarin-derivative anticoagulant therapy. The aPTT measures

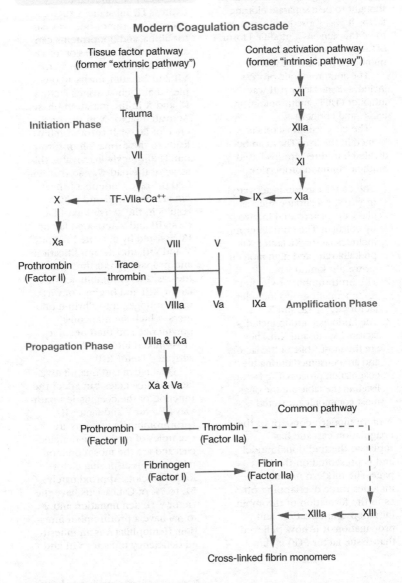

Modern Coagulation Cascade

Tissue factor pathway (former "extrinsic pathway")

Contact activation pathway (former "intrinsic pathway")

XII

Initiation Phase

Trauma

XIIa

VII

XI

X ← TF-VIIa-Ca^{++} → IX ← XIa

Xa

VIII   V

Prothrombin (Factor II) — Trace thrombin

VIIIa   Va   IXa   **Amplification Phase**

Propagation Phase   VIIIa & IXa

Xa & Va

Common pathway

Prothrombin (Factor II) —— Thrombin (Factor IIa) ----

Fibrinogen (Factor I) → Fibrin (Factor IIa)

XIIIa ← XIII

Cross-linked fibrin monomers

the function of the intrinsic and common pathways of coagulation and is used to monitor patients receiving heparin anticoagulant therapy.

INDICATIONS
- Identify the presence of inherited bleeding disorders
- Identify the presence of qualitative or quantitative factor deficiency

POTENTIAL DIAGNOSIS

Increased in: N/A

Decreased in
- Congenital deficiency
- Disseminated intravascular coagulation *(related to consumption of factors as part of the coagulation cascade)*
- Liver disease *(related to inability of damaged liver to synthesize coagulation factors)*

CRITICAL FINDINGS: N/A

INTERFERING FACTORS
- Drugs that may increase factor II levels include fluoxymesterone, methandrostenolone, nandrolone, and oxymetholone.
- Drugs that may decrease factor II levels include warfarin.
- Drugs that may increase factor V, VII, and X levels include anabolic steroids, fluoxymesterone, methandrostenolone, nandrolone, oral contraceptives, and oxymetholone.
- Drugs that may decrease factor V levels include streptokinase.
- Drugs that may decrease factor VII levels include acetylsalicylic acid, asparaginase, cefamandole, ceftriaxone, dextran, dicumarol, gemfibrozil, oral contraceptives, and warfarin.
- Drugs that may increase factor VIII levels include chlormadinone.
- Drugs that may decrease factor VIII levels include asparaginase.
- Drugs that may increase factor IX levels include chlormadinone and oral contraceptives.
- Drugs that may decrease factor IX levels include asparaginase and warfarin.
- Drugs that may decrease factor X levels include chlormadinone, dicumarol, oral contraceptives, and warfarin.
- Drugs that may decrease factor XI levels include asparaginase and captopril.
- Drugs that may decrease factor XII levels include captopril.
- Test results of patients on anticoagulant therapy are unreliable.
- Placement of tourniquet for longer than 1 min can result in venous stasis and changes in the concentration of plasma proteins to be measured. Platelet activation may also occur under these conditions, causing erroneous results.
- Vascular injury during phlebotomy can activate platelets and coagulation factors, causing erroneous results.
- Hemolyzed specimens must be rejected because hemolysis is an indication of platelet and coagulation factor activation.
- Icteric or lipemic specimens interfere with optical testing methods, producing erroneous results.
- Incompletely filled collection tubes, specimens contaminated with heparin, clotted specimens, or unprocessed specimens not delivered to the laboratory within 1 to 2 hr of collection should be rejected.

C

NURSING IMPLICATIONS AND PROCEDURE

PRETEST:

- Positively identify the patient using at least two unique identifiers before providing care, treatment, or services.
- *Patient Teaching:* Inform the patient this test can assist in evaluating the effectiveness of blood clotting.
- Obtain a history of the patient's complaints, including a list of known allergens, especially allergies or sensitivities to latex.
- Obtain a history of the patient's hematopoietic and hepatobiliary systems, any bleeding disorders, and results of previously performed laboratory tests and diagnostic and surgical procedures.
- Obtain a list of the patient's current medications. Include anticoagulants, aspirin and other salicylates, herbs, nutritional supplements, and nutraceuticals (see Appendix F). Such products should be discontinued by medical direction for the appropriate number of days prior to a surgical procedure.
- Review the procedure with the patient. Inform the patient that specimen collection takes approximately 5 to 10 min. Address concerns about pain and explain that there may be some discomfort during the venipuncture.
- *Sensitivity to social and cultural issues,* as well as concern for modesty, is important in providing psychological support before, during, and after the procedure.
- There are no food, fluid, or medication restrictions unless by medical direction.

INTRATEST:

- If the patient has a history of allergic reaction to latex, avoid the use of equipment containing latex.
- Instruct the patient to cooperate fully and to follow directions. Direct the patient to breathe normally and to avoid unnecessary movement.
- Observe standard precautions, and follow the general guidelines in Appendix A. Positively identify the patient, and label the appropriate tubes with the corresponding patient demographics, date,

and time of collection. Perform a venipuncture. When multiple specimens are drawn, the blue-top tube should be collected after sterile (i.e., blood culture) tubes. Otherwise, when using a standard vacutainer system, the blue top is the first tube collected. When a butterfly is used and due to the added tubing, an extra red-top tube should be collected before the blue-top tube to ensure complete filling of the blue top tube.
- Remove the needle and apply direct pressure with dry gauze to stop bleeding. Observe/assess venipuncture site for bleeding or hematoma formation and secure gauze with adhesive bandage.
- Promptly transport the specimen to the laboratory for processing and analysis. The Clinical Laboratory Standards Institute (CLSI) recommendation for processed and unprocessed samples stored in unopened tubes is that testing should be completed within 1 to 4 hr of collection. If the patient has a known hematocrit above 55%, adjust the amount of anticoagulant in the collection tube before drawing the blood according to the CLSI guidelines:

Anticoagulant vol. [x] = (100 − hematocrit)/(595 − hematocrit) × total vol. of anticoagulated blood required

Example:

Patient hematocrit = 60%
= [(100 − 60)/(595 − 60) × 5.0]
= 0.37 mL sodium citrate for a 5-mL standard drawing tube

POST-TEST:

- A report of the results will be sent to the requesting health-care provider (HCP), who will discuss the results with the patient.
- Instruct the patient to report immediately any signs of unusual bleeding or bruising.
- Inform the patient with decreased factor levels of the importance of taking precautions against bruising and bleeding. These precautions may include the use of a soft bristle toothbrush, use of an electric razor, avoidance of

constipation, avoidance of acetylsalicyl-ic acid and similar products, and avoid-ance of intramuscular injections.

- Reinforce information given by the patient's HCP regarding further test-ing, treatment, or referral to another HCP. Answer any questions or address any concerns voiced by the patient or family.
- Depending on the results of this procedure, additional testing may be performed to evaluate or monitor progression of the disease process and determine the need for a change in

therapy. Evaluate test results in relation to the patient's symptoms and other tests performed.

RELATED MONOGRAPHS:

- Related tests include aPTT, ALT, ALP, AT-IIII, AST, clot retraction, CBC platelet count, copper, fibrinogen, FDP, plasmi-nogen, protein C, protein S, PT/INR, and vitamin K.
- Refer to the Hematopoietic and Hepatobiliary systems tables at the end of the book for related tests by body system.

C

Cold Agglutinin Titer

SYNONYM/ACRONYM: Mycoplasma serology.

COMMON USE: To identify and confirm the presence of viral infections such as found in atypical pneumonia.

SPECIMEN: Serum (2 mL) collected in a red-top tube. The tube must be placed in a water bath or heat block at 37°C for 1 hr and allowed to clot before the serum is separated from the red blood cells (RBCs).

REFERENCE VALUE: (Method: Patient serum containing autoantibodies titered against type O RBCs at 2°C to 8°C. Type O cells are used because they have no antigens on the cell membrane surface. Agglutination with patient sera would not occur because of reaction between RBC blood type antigens and patient blood type antibodies.) Negative: Single titer less than 1:32 or less than a four-fold increase in titer over serial samples.

DESCRIPTION: Cold agglutinins are antibodies that cause clumping or agglutination of RBCs at cold tem-peratures in individuals with cer-tain conditions or who are infected by particular organisms. Cold agglu-tinins are associated with *Myco-plasma pneumoniae* infection. *M. pneumoniae* has I antigen speci-ficity to human RBC membranes.

Fetal cells largely contain I antigens, but by 18 mo most cells carry the I antigen. The agglutinins are usually immunoglobulin M (IgM) antibod-ies and cause agglutination of cells at temperatures in the range of 0°C to 10°C. The temperature of circu-lating blood in the extremities may be lower than core temperatures. RBCs of affected individuals may agglutinate and obstruct blood vessels in fingers, toes, and ears, or they may initiate the complement cascade. Affected cells may be lysed immediately within the capillaries and blood vessels as a result of the action of complement on the cell wall, or they may return to the circulatory system and be lysed in the spleen by macrophages.

The titer endpoint is the highest dilution of serum that shows a specific antigen-antibody reaction. Single titers greater than 1:64, or a fourfold increase in titer between specimens collected 5 or more days apart, are clinically significant. Patients affected with primary atypical viral pneumonia exhibit a rise in titer 8 to 10 days after the onset of illness. IgM antibodies peak in 12 to 25 days and begin to diminish 30 days after onset.

INDICATIONS
- Assist in the confirmation of primary atypical pneumonia, influenza, or pulmonary embolus
- Provide additional diagnostic support for cold agglutinin disease associated with viral infections or lymphoreticular cancers

POTENTIAL DIAGNOSIS

Increased in
Mycoplasma infection stimulates production of antibodies against specific RBC antigens in affected individuals
- Cirrhosis
- Gangrene
- Hemolytic anemia
- Infectious diseases (e.g., staphylococcemia, influenza, tuberculosis)
- Infectious mononucleosis
- Malaria

- *M. pneumoniae* (primary atypical pneumonia)
- Multiple myeloma
- Pulmonary embolism
- Raynaud's disease (severe)
- Systemic lupus erythematosus
- Trypanosomiasis

Decreased in: N/A

CRITICAL FINDINGS: N/A

INTERFERING FACTORS
- Antibiotic use may interfere with or decrease antibody production.
- A high antibody titer may interfere with blood typing and crossmatching procedures.
- High titers may appear spontaneously in elderly patients and persist for many years.
- Prompt and proper specimen processing, storage, and analysis are important to achieve accurate results. Specimens should always be transported to the laboratory as quickly as possible after collection. The specimen must clot in a 37°C water bath for 1 hr before separation. Refrigeration of the sample before serum separates from the RBCs may falsely decrease the titer.

NURSING IMPLICATIONS AND PROCEDURE

PRETEST:
- Positively identify the patient using at least two unique identifiers before providing care, treatment, or services.
- *Patient Teaching:* Inform the patient this test can assist in diagnosing viral versus bacterial disease.
- Obtain a history of the patient's complaints, including a list of known allergens, especially allergies or sensitivities to latex.
- Obtain a history of the patient's immune and respiratory systems, as well as results of previously performed

laboratory tests and diagnostic and surgical procedures.

- Obtain a list of the patient's current medications, including herbs, nutritional supplements, and nutraceuticals (see Appendix F).
- Note any recent medications that can interfere with test results.
- Review the procedure with the patient. Inform the patient that multiple specimens may be required. Inform the patient that specimen collection takes approximately 5 to 10 min. Address concerns about pain and explain that there may be some discomfort during the venipuncture.
- *Sensitivity to social and cultural issues,* as well as concern for modesty, is important in providing psychological support before, during, and after the procedure.
- There are no food, fluid, or medication restrictions (except antibiotics) unless by medical direction.

INTRATEST:

- Ensure that the patient has complied with medication restrictions prior to the procedure.
- If the patient has a history of allergic reaction to latex, avoid the use of equipment containing latex.
- Instruct the patient to cooperate fully and to follow directions. Direct the patient to breathe normally and to avoid unnecessary movement.
- Observe standard precautions, and follow the general guidelines in Appendix A. Positively identify the patient, and label the appropriate tubes with the corresponding patient demographics, date, and time of collection. Perform a venipuncture.
- Remove the needle and apply direct pressure with dry gauze to stop bleeding. Observe/assess venipuncture site for bleeding or

hematoma formation and secure gauze with adhesive bandage.
- Promptly transport the specimen to the laboratory for processing and analysis.
- Inform the laboratory if the patient is receiving antibiotics.

POST-TEST:

- A report of the results will be sent to the requesting health-care provider (HCP), who will discuss the results with the patient.
- Instruct the patient to resume antibiotics as directed by the HCP. Instruct the patient in the importance of completing the entire course of antibiotic therapy even if no symptoms are present.
- Reinforce information given by the patient's HCP regarding further testing, treatment, or referral to another HCP. Emphasize the need for the patient to return in 7 to 14 days for a convalescent blood sample. Answer any questions or address any concerns voiced by the patient or family.
- Depending on the results of this procedure, additional testing may be performed to evaluate or monitor progression of the disease process and determine the need for a change in therapy. Evaluate test results in relation to the patient's symptoms and other tests performed.

RELATED MONOGRAPHS:

- Related tests include arterial/alveolar oxygen ratio, blood gases, chest x-ray, CBC, CBC WBC count, Coombs' antiglobulin, culture viral, ESR, gallium scan, infectious mononucleosis screen, lung perfusion scan, plethysmography, and pleural fluid analysis.
- Refer to the Immune and Respiratory systems tables at the end of the book for related tests by body system.

Collagen Cross-Linked N-Telopeptide

SYNONYM/ACRONYM: NT_x.

COMMON USE: To evaluate the effectiveness of treatment for osteoporosis.

SPECIMEN: Urine (2 mL) from a random specimen collected in a clean plastic container.

REFERENCE VALUE: (Method: Immunoassay)

Adult male	Less than 65 mmol bone collagen equivalents/mmol creatinine
Adult female (premenopausal)	Less than 65 mmol bone collagen equivalents/mmol creatinine
Adult female (postmenopausal)	Less than 131 mmol bone collagen equivalents/mmol creatinine

Tanner Stage	Male	Female
I	55–508 (mmol bone collagen equivalents/mmol creatinine)	6–662 (mmol bone collagen equivalents/mmol creatinine)
II	21–423 (mmol bone collagen equivalents/mmol creatinine)	193–514 (mmol bone collagen equivalents/mmol creatinine)
III	27–462 (mmol bone collagen equivalents/mmol creatinine)	13–632 (mmol bone collagen equivalents/mmol creatinine)
IV	Less than 609 (mmol bone collagen equivalents/mmol creatinine)	Less than 389 (mmol bone collagen equivalents/mmol creatinine)
V	Less than 240 (mmol bone collagen equivalents/mmol creatinine)	Less than 132 (mmol bone collagen equivalents/mmol creatinine)

Values are higher in children.

DESCRIPTION: Osteoporosis is the most common bone disease in the West. It is often called the "silent disease" because bone loss occurs without symptoms. The formation and maintenance of bone mass is dependent on a combination of factors that include genetics, nutrition, exercise, and hormone function. Normally, the rate of bone formation is equal to the rate of bone resorption. After midlife, the rate of bone loss begins to increase. Osteoporosis is more commonly identified in women than in men. Other risk factors include thin, small-framed body structure; family history of osteoporosis; diet low in calcium; white or Asian race; excessive use of alcohol; cigarette smoking; sedentary lifestyle; long-term use of corticosteroids, thyroid replacement medications, or antiepileptics; history of bulimia, anorexia nervosa, chronic liver disease, or malabsorption disorders; and postmenopausal state. Osteoporosis is a major consequence of menopause in women owing to the decline of estrogen production. Osteoporosis is rare in premenopausal women. Estrogen replacement therapy (after menopause) is one strategy that has been commonly employed to prevent osteoporosis, although its exact protective mechanism is unknown. Results of some recently published studies indicate that there may be significant adverse side effects to estrogen replacement therapy; more research is needed to understand the long-term effects (positive and negative) of this therapy. Other treatments include raloxifene (selectively modulates estrogen receptors), calcitonin (interacts directly with osteoclasts), and bisphosphates (inhibit osteoclast-mediated bone resorption).

A noninvasive test to detect the presence of collagen cross-linked N-telopeptide (NT_x) is used to follow the progress of patients who have begun treatment for osteoporosis. NT_x is formed when collagenase acts on bone. Small NT_x fragments are excreted in the urine after bone resorption. A desirable response, 2 to 3 mo after therapy is initiated, is a 30% reduction in NT_x and a reduction of 50% below baseline by 12 mo.

INDICATIONS

- Assist in the evaluation of osteoporosis
- Assist in the management and treatment of osteoporosis
- Monitor effects of estrogen replacement therapy

POTENTIAL DIAGNOSIS

Increased in

Conditions that reflect increased bone resorption are associated with increased levels of N-telopeptide in the urine

- Alcoholism *(related to inadequate nutrition)*
- Chronic immobilization
- Chronic treatment with anticonvulsants, corticosteroids, gonadotropin releasing hormone agonists, heparin, or thyroid hormone)
- Conditions that include hypercortisolism, hyperparathyroidism, hyperthyroidism, and hypogonadism.
- Gastrointestinal disease *(related to inadequate dietary intake or absorption of minerals required for bone formation and maintenance)*
- Growth disorders (acromegaly, growth hormone deficiency, osteogenesis imperfecta)
- Hyperparathyroidism *(related to imbalance in calcium and phosphorus that affects the rate of bone resorption)*
- Multiple myeloma and metastatic tumors
- Osteomalacia *(related to defective bone mineralization)*

- Osteoporosis
- Paget's disease
- Postmenopausal women *(related to estrogen deficiency)*
- Recent fracture
- Renal insufficiency *(related to excessive loss through renal dysfunction)*
- Rheumatoid arthritis and other connective tissue diseases *(related to inadequate diet due to loss of appetite)*

Decreased in
- Effective therapy for osteoporosis

CRITICAL FINDINGS: N/A

INTERFERING FACTORS
- NT_x levels are affected by urinary excretion, and values may be influenced by the presence of renal impairment or disease.

NURSING IMPLICATIONS AND PROCEDURE

PRETEST:
- Positively identify the patient using at least two unique identifiers before providing care, treatment, or services.
- *Patient Teaching:* Inform the patient this test can assist in diagnosing osteoporosis and evaluating the effectiveness of therapy.
- Obtain a history of the patient's complaints, including a list of known allergens.
- Obtain a history of the patient's musculoskeletal system and results of previously performed laboratory tests and diagnostic and surgical procedures.
- Obtain a list of the patient's current medications, including herbs, nutritional supplements, and nutraceuticals (see Appendix F).
- Review the procedure with the patient. Inform the patient that specimen collection takes approximately 5 to 10 min. Address concerns about pain and explain that there should be no discomfort during the procedure.

- *Sensitivity to social and cultural issues,* as well as concern for modesty, is important in providing psychological support before, during, and after the procedure.
- There are no food, fluid, or medication restrictions unless by medical direction.

INTRATEST:
- Instruct the patient to cooperate fully and to follow directions.
- Observe standard precautions, and follow the general guidelines in Appendix A. Positively identify the patient, and label the appropriate collection container with the corresponding patient demographics, date, and time of collection.
- Instruct the patient to collect a second-void morning specimen as follows: (1) void and then drink a glass of water; (2) wait 30 min, and then try to void again.
- Promptly transport the specimen to the laboratory for processing and analysis.

POST-TEST:
- A report of the results will be sent to the requesting health-care provider (HCP), who will discuss the results with the patient.
- Instruct the patient to resume usual diet, fluids, medications, and activity, as directed by the HCP.
- *Nutritional Considerations:* Increased NT_x levels may be associated with osteoporosis. Nutritional therapy may be indicated for patients identified as being at high risk for developing osteoporosis. Educate the patient about the National Osteoporosis Foundation's guidelines regarding a regular regimen of weight-bearing exercises, limited alcohol intake, avoidance of tobacco products, and adequate dietary intake of vitamin D (400 to 800 IU/day) and calcium (1,200 to 1,500 mg/day). Dietary calcium can be obtained in animal or plant sources. Milk and milk products, sardines, clams, oysters, salmon, rhubarb, spinach, beet greens, broccoli, kale, tofu, legumes, and fortified orange juice are high in calcium. Milk and milk products also contain vitamin D and lactose to assist in absorption. Cooked vegetables yield more absorbable calcium than raw vegetables. Patients should

also be informed of the substances that can inhibit calcium absorption by irreversibly binding to some of the calcium and making it unavailable for absorption, such as oxalates, which naturally occur in some vegetables; phytic acid, found in some cereals; and excessive intake of insoluble dietary fiber. Excessive protein intake also can affect calcium absorption negatively, especially if it is combined with foods high in phosphorus. Vitamin D is synthesized by the skin and is available in fortified dairy foods and cod liver oil.

▶ Recognize anxiety related to test results, and be supportive of impaired activity related to lack of muscular control, perceived loss of independence, and fear of shortened life expectancy. Discuss the implications of abnormal test results on the patient's lifestyle. Provide teaching and information regarding the clinical implications of the test results, as appropriate. Educate the patient regarding access to counseling services. Provide contact information, if desired, for the National Osteoporosis Foundation (www.nof.org).

▶ Reinforce information given by the patient's HCP regarding further testing, treatment, or referral to another HCP. Answer any questions or address any concerns voiced by the patient or family.

▶ Depending on the results of this procedure, additional testing may be performed to evaluate or monitor progression of the disease process and determine the need for a change in therapy. Evaluate test results in relation to the patient's symptoms and other tests performed.

RELATED MONOGRAPHS:

▶ Related tests include ALP, BMD, calcitonin, calcium, creatinine, creatinine clearance, osteocalcin, PTH, phosphorus, radiography bone, and vitamin D.

▶ Refer to the Musculoskeletal System table at the end of the book for related tests by body system.

Colonoscopy

SYNONYM/ACRONYM: Full colonoscopy, lower endoscopy, lower panendoscopy.

COMMON USE: To visualize and assess the lower colon for tumor, cancer, and infection.

AREA OF APPLICATION: Colon.

CONTRAST: Air.

DESCRIPTION: Colonoscopy allows inspection of the mucosa of the entire colon, ileocecal valve, and terminal ileum using a flexible fiberoptic colonoscope inserted through the anus and advanced to the terminal ileum. The colonoscope is a multichannel instrument that allows viewing of the gastrointestinal (GI) tract lining, insufflation of air, aspiration of fluid, obtaining of tissue biopsy samples, and passage of a laser beam for obliteration of tissue and control of bleeding. Mucosal surfaces of the lower GI tract are examined for ulcerations, polyps, chronic diarrhea, hemorrhagic sites, neoplasms, and strictures.

C

During the procedure, tissue samples may be obtained for cytology, and some therapeutic procedures may be performed, such as excision of small tumors or polyps, coagulation of bleeding sites, and removal of foreign bodies.

INDICATIONS

- Assess GI function in a patient with a personal or family history of colon cancer, polyps, or ulcerative colitis
- Confirm diagnosis of colon cancer and inflammatory bowel disease
- Detect Hirschsprung's disease and determine the areas affected by the disease
- Determine cause of lower GI disorders, especially when barium enema and proctosigmoidoscopy are inconclusive
- Determine source of rectal bleeding and perform hemostasis by coagulation
- Evaluate postsurgical status of colon resection
- Evaluate stools that show a positive occult blood test, lower GI bleeding, or change in bowel habits
- Follow up on previously diagnosed and treated colon cancer
- Investigate iron-deficiency anemia of unknown origin
- Reduce volvulus and intussusception in children
- Remove colon polyps
- Remove foreign bodies and sclerosing strictures by laser

POTENTIAL DIAGNOSIS

Normal findings in
- Normal intestinal mucosa with no abnormalities of structure, function, or mucosal surface in the colon or terminal ileum

Abnormal findings in
- Benign lesions
- Bleeding sites
- Bowel distention
- Bowel infection or inflammation
- Colitis
- Colon cancer
- Crohn's disease
- Diverticula
- Foreign bodies
- Hemorrhoids
- Polyps
- Proctitis
- Tumors
- Vascular abnormalities

CRITICAL FINDINGS: N/A

INTERFERING FACTORS

This procedure is contraindicated for
- Patients with bleeding disorders or cardiac conditions.
- Patients with bowel perforation, acute peritonitis, acute colitis, ischemic bowel necrosis, toxic colitis, recent bowel surgery, advanced pregnancy, severe cardiac or pulmonary disease, recent myocardial infarction, known or suspected pulmonary embolus, and large abdominal aortic or iliac aneurysm.
- Patients who have had a colon anastomosis within the past 14 to 21 days, because an anastomosis may break down with gas insufflation.

Factors that may impair clear imaging
- Gas or feces in the GI tract resulting from inadequate cleansing or failure to restrict food intake before the study.
- Retained barium from a previous radiological procedure.
- Metallic objects (e.g., jewelry, body rings) within the examination field, which may inhibit organ visualization and cause unclear images.

- Patients who are very obese or who may exceed the weight limit for the equipment.
- Inability of the patient to cooperate or remain still during the procedure because of age, significant pain, or mental status.
- Severe lower GI bleeding or the presence of feces, barium, blood, or blood clots, which can interfere with visualization.
- Spasm of the colon, which can mimic the radiographic signs of cancer. (*Note:* The use of IV glucagon minimizes spasm.)
- Inability of the patient to tolerate introduction of or retention of barium, air, or both in the bowel.

Other considerations

- Complications of the procedure may include hemorrhage and cardiac arrhythmias.
- The procedure may be terminated if chest pain or severe cardiac arrhythmias occur.
- Failure to follow dietary restrictions and other pretesting preparations may cause the procedure to be canceled or repeated.
- Bowel preparations that include laxatives or enemas should be avoided in pregnant patients or patients with inflammatory bowel disease unless specifically directed by a health-care provider (HCP).
- Consultation with an HCP should occur before the procedure for radiation safety concerns regarding younger patients or patients who are lactating.
- Risks associated with radiation overexposure can result from frequent x-ray procedures. Personnel in the examination room with the patient should wear a protective lead apron, stand behind a shield, or leave the area while the examination is being done. Personnel working in the examination area should wear badges to record their level of radiation exposure.

NURSING IMPLICATIONS AND PROCEDURE

PRETEST:

▶ Positively identify the patient using at least two unique identifiers before providing care, treatment, or services.

▶ *Patient Teaching:* Inform the patient this procedure can assist in assessing the colon for disease.

▶ Obtain a history of the patient's complaints, including a list of known allergens, especially allergies or sensitivities to latex, iodine, seafood, anesthetics, or contrast medium.

▶ Obtain a history of patient's gastrointestinal system, symptoms, and results of previously performed laboratory tests and diagnostic and surgical procedures.

▶ Note any recent procedures that can interfere with test results, including examinations using barium- or iodine-based contrast medium. Ensure that barium studies were performed more than 4 days before the CT scan.

▶ Ensure that this procedure is performed before an upper GI study or barium swallow.

▶ Record the date of the last menstrual period and determine the possibility of pregnancy in perimenopausal women.

▶ Obtain a list of the patient's current medications including anticoagulants, aspirin and other salicylates, herbs, nutritional supplements, and nutraceuticals (see Appendix F). Such products should be discontinued by medical direction for the appropriate number of days prior to a surgical procedure. Note the last time and dose of medication taken.

▶ Note intake of oral iron preparations within 1 wk before the procedure because these cause black, sticky feces that are difficult to remove with bowel preparation.

▶ Review the procedure with the patient. Address concerns about pain and explain that some pain may be experienced during the test, and there may be

C

moments of discomfort. Inform the patient that the procedure is performed in a GI lab, by an HCP, with support staff, and takes approximately 30 to 60 min.

▸ *Sensitivity to social and cultural issues,* as well as concern for modesty, is important in providing psychological support before, during, and after the procedure.

▸ Inform the patient that it is important that the bowel be cleaned thoroughly so that the physician can visualize the colon. Inform the patient that a laxative and cleansing enema may be needed the day before the procedure, with cleansing enemas on the morning of the procedure, depending on the institution's policy.

▸ Instruct the patient to remove all external metallic objects from the area to be examined.

▸ Instruct the patient to eat a low-residue diet for several days before the procedure and to consume only clear liquids the evening before the test. The patient should fast and restrict fluids for 8 hr prior to the procedure. Protocols may vary among facilities.

▸ *Make sure a written and informed consent has been signed prior to the procedure and before administering any medications.*

INTRATEST:

▸ Ensure that the patient has complied with dietary, fluid and medication restrictions, and pretesting preparations for at least 8 hr prior to the procedure.

▸ Ensure that ordered laxatives were administered late in the afternoon of the day before the procedure.

▸ Assess for completion of bowel preparation according to the institution's procedure.

▸ Instruct the patient to remove all external metallic objects from the area to be examined.

▸ Have emergency equipment readily available.

▸ Instruct the patient to void prior to the procedure and to change into the gown, robe, and foot coverings provided.

▸ Instruct the patient to cooperate fully and to follow directions. Instruct the patient to remain still throughout the procedure because movement produces unreliable results.

▸ Observe standard precautions, and follow the general guidelines in Appendix A. Positively identify the patient, and label the appropriate containers with the corresponding patient demographics, date, and time of collection.

▸ Obtain and record baseline vital signs.

▸ An IV line may be started to allow infusion of a sedative or IV fluids.

▸ Administer medications, as ordered, to reduce discomfort and to promote relaxation and sedation.

▸ Place the patient on an examination table in the left lateral decubitus position and drape with the buttocks exposed.

▸ The HCP performs a visual inspection of the perianal area and a digital rectal examination.

▸ Instruct the patient to bear down as if having a bowel movement as the fiberoptic tube is inserted through the rectum.

▸ The scope is advanced through the sigmoid. The patient's position is changed to supine to facilitate passage into the transverse colon. Air is insufflated through the tube during passage to aid in visualization.

▸ Instruct the patient to take deep breaths to aid in movement of the scope downward through the ascending colon to the cecum and into the terminal portion of the ileum.

▸ Air is insufflated to distend the GI tract, as needed. Biopsies, cultures, or any endoscopic surgery is performed.

▸ Foreign bodies or polyps are removed and placed in appropriate specimen containers, labeled, and sent to the laboratory.

▸ Photographs are obtained for future reference.

▸ At the end of the procedure, excess air and secretions are aspirated through the scope, and the colonoscope is removed.

POST-TEST:

▸ A report of the examination will be sent to the requesting HCP, who will discuss the results with the patient.

▸ Monitor the patient for signs of respiratory depression.

▶ Monitor vital signs and neurological status every 15 min for 1 hr, then every 2 hr for 4 hr, or as ordered. Take temperature every 4 hr for 24 hr. Monitor intake and output at least every 8 hr. Compare with baseline values. Notify the HCP if temperature is elevated. Protocols may vary among facilities.

▶ Observe the patient until the effects of the sedation have worn off.

▶ Instruct the patient to resume usual diet, fluids, medications, and activity, as directed by the HCP.

▶ Monitor for any rectal bleeding. Instruct the patient to expect slight rectal bleeding for 2 days after removal of polyps or biopsy specimens but that an increasing amount of bleeding or sustained bleeding should be reported to the HCP immediately.

▶ Instruct the patient to immediately report symptoms such as fast heart rate, difficulty breathing, skin rash, itching, chest pain, persistent right shoulder pain, or abdominal pain. Immediately report symptoms to the appropriate HCP.

▶ Inform the patient that belching, bloating, or flatulence is the result of air insufflation.

▶ Encourage the patient to drink several glasses of water to help replace fluids lost during the preparation for the test.

▶ Carefully monitor the patient for fatigue and fluid and electrolyte imbalance.

▶ Recognize anxiety related to test results. Discuss the implications of abnormal test results on the patient's lifestyle. Provide teaching and information regarding the clinical implications of the test results, as appropriate.

▶ Reinforce information given by the patient's HCP regarding further testing, treatment, or referral to another HCP. Decisions regarding the need for and frequency of occult blood testing, colonoscopy or other cancer screening procedures should be made after consultation between the patient and HCP. The most current guidelines for colon cancer screening of the general population as well as individuals with increased risk are available from the American Cancer Society (www.cancer.org) and the American College of Gastroenterology (www.gi.org). Answer any questions or address any concerns voiced by the patient or family.

▶ Depending on the results of this procedure, additional testing may be needed to evaluate or monitor progression of the disease process and determine the need for a change in therapy. Evaluate test results in relation to the patient's symptoms and other tests performed.

RELATED MONOGRAPHS:

▶ Related tests include barium enema, biopsy intestinal, capsule endoscopy, carcinoembrionic and cancer antigens, CT abdomen, CT colonoscopy, fecal analysis, KUB, MRI abdomen, and proctosigmoidoscopy.

▶ Refer to the Gastrointestinal System table at the end of the book for related tests by body system.

Color Perception Test

SYNONYM/ACRONYM: Color blindness test, Ishihara color perception test, Ishihara pseudoisochromatic plate test.

COMMON USE: To assist in the diagnosis of color blindness.

AREA OF APPLICATION: Eyes.

CONTRAST: N/A.

DESCRIPTION: Defects in color perception can be hereditary or acquired. The congenital defect for color blindness is carried by the female, who is generally unaffected, and is expressed dominantly in males. Color blindness occurs in 8% of males and 0.4% of females. It may be partial or complete. The partial form is the hereditary form, and in the majority of patients the color deficiency is in the red-green area of the spectrum. Acquired color blindness may occur as a result of diseases of the retina or optic nerve. Color perception tests are performed to determine the acuity of color discrimination. The most common test uses pseudoisochromic plates with numbers or letters buried in a maze of dots. Misreading the numbers or letters indicates a color perception deficiency and may indicate color blindness, a genetic dysfunction, or retinal pathology.

INDICATIONS

- Detect deficiencies in color perception
- Evaluate because of family history of color visual defects
- Investigate suspected retinal pathology affecting the cones

POTENTIAL DIAGNOSIS

Normal findings in
- Normal visual color discrimination; no difficulty in identification of color combinations

Abnormal findings in
- Identification of some but not all colors

CRITICAL FINDINGS: N/A

INTERFERING FACTORS

- Inability of the patient to cooperate or remain still during the procedure because of age, significant pain, or mental status.
- Inability of the patient to read.
- Poor visual acuity or poor lighting.
- Failure of the patient to wear corrective lenses (glasses or contact lenses).
- Damaged or discolored test plates.

NURSING IMPLICATIONS AND PROCEDURE

PRETEST:

- Positively identify the patient using at least two unique identifiers before providing care, treatment, or services.
- *Patient Teaching:* Inform the patient or parent/child this procedure can assist in detection of color vision impairment.
- Obtain a history of the patient's complaints, including a list of known allergens.
- Obtain a history of the patient's known or suspected vision loss; changes in visual acuity, including type and cause; use of glasses or contact lenses; eye conditions with treatment regimens; eye surgery; and other tests and procedures to assess and diagnose visual deficit.
- Obtain a history of symptoms and results of previously performed laboratory tests and diagnostic and surgical procedures.
- Obtain a list of the patient's current medications, including herbs, nutritional supplements, and nutraceuticals (see Appendix F).
- Review the procedure with the patient. Ask the patient if he or she wears corrective lenses; also inquire about the importance of color discrimination in his or her work, as applicable. Address concerns about pain and explain that no discomfort will be experienced during the test. Inform the patient that a health-care provider (HCP) performs the test in a quiet, darkened room, and that to evaluate both eyes, the test can take 5 to 15 or up to 30 min, depending on the complexity of testing required.
- *Sensitivity to social and cultural issues,* as well as concern for modesty, is important in providing psychological support before, during, and after the procedure.

There are no food, fluid, or medication restrictions unless by medical direction.

INTRATEST:

Instruct the patient to cooperate fully and to follow directions.

Seat the patient comfortably. Occlude one eye and hold test booklet 12 to 14 in. in front of the exposed eye.

Ask the patient to identify the numbers or letters buried in the maze of dots or to trace the objects with a handheld pointed object.

Repeat on the other eye.

POST-TEST:

A report of the results will be sent to the requesting HCP, who will discuss the results with the patient.

Recognize anxiety related to test results and be supportive of impaired activity related to color vision loss. Discuss the implications of abnormal test results on the patient's lifestyle. Provide teaching and information regarding the clinical implications of the test results, as appropriate. Provide contact information regarding vision aids for people with impaired color perception, if desired: ABLEDATA (sponsored by the National Institute on Disability and Rehabilitation Research [NIDRR], available at www.abledata.com).

Reinforce information given by the patient's HCP regarding further testing, treatment, or referral to another HCP. Answer any questions or address any concerns voiced by the patient or family.

Depending on the results of this procedure, additional testing may be performed to evaluate or monitor progression of the disease process and determine the need for a change in therapy. Evaluate test results in relation to the patient's symptoms and other tests performed.

RELATED MONOGRAPHS:

Related tests include refraction and slit-lamp biomicroscopy.

Refer to the Ocular System table at the end of the book for related tests by body system.

Colposcopy

SYNONYM/ACRONYM: Cervical biopsy, endometrial biopsy.

COMMON USE: To visualize and assess the cervix and vagina in the case of suspected cancer or other disease.

AREA OF APPLICATION: Vagina and cervix.

CONTRAST: None.

DESCRIPTION: In this procedure, the vagina and cervix are viewed using a colposcope, a special binocular microscope and light system that magnifies the mucosal surfaces. Colposcopy is usually performed after suspicious Papanicolaou (Pap) test results or when suspected lesions cannot be visualized fully by the naked eye. The procedure is useful for identifying areas of cellular dysplasia and diagnosing cervical cancer because it provides the best view of the suspicious lesion, ensuring that the most representative area of the lesion is obtained for cytological analysis to confirm malignant changes. Colposcopy is also valuable for assessing women with a history of exposure to diethylstilbestrol (DES) in utero. The goal is to identify precursor changes in cervical tissue before the changes advance from benign or atypical cells to cervical cancer. Photographs (cervicography) can also be taken of the cervix.

INDICATIONS

- Evaluate the cervix after abnormal Pap smear
- Evaluate vaginal lesions
- Localize the area from which cervical biopsy samples should be obtained because such areas may not be visible to the naked eye
- Monitor conservatively treated cervical intraepithelial neoplasia
- Monitor women whose mothers took DES during pregnancy

POTENTIAL DIAGNOSIS

Normal findings in
- Normal appearance of the vagina and cervix
- No abnormal cells or tissues

Abnormal findings in
- Atrophic changes
- Cervical erosion
- Cervical intraepithelial neoplasia
- Infection
- Inflammation
- Invasive carcinoma
- Leukoplakia
- Papilloma, including condyloma

CRITICAL FINDINGS: N/A

INTERFERING FACTORS

This procedure is contraindicated for
- Patients who are pregnant or suspected of being pregnant, unless the potential benefits of the procedure far outweigh the risks to the fetus and mother.
- Patients with cardiac conditions.
- Patients with bleeding disorders, especially if cervical biopsy specimens are to be obtained.
- Women who are currently menstruating.

Factors that may impair clear imaging
- Inadequate cleansing of the cervix of secretions and medications.
- Scarring of the cervix.
- Inability of the patient to cooperate or remain still during the procedure because of age, significant pain, or mental status.
- Severe bleeding or the presence of feces, blood, or blood clots, which can interfere with visualization.

Other considerations
- Complications of the procedure may include hemorrhage and cardiac arrhythmias.
- The procedure may be terminated if chest pain or severe cardiac arrhythmias occur.

NURSING IMPLICATIONS AND PROCEDURE

PRETEST:
- Positively identify the patient using at least two unique identifiers before providing care, treatment, or services.
- *Patient Teaching:* Inform the patient this procedure can assist in assessing the uterus and cervix for disease.
- Obtain a history of the patient's complaints including a list of known

allergens, especially allergies or sensitivities to latex, iodine, or anesthetics.

▶ Obtain a history of the patient's reproductive system, symptoms, and results of previously performed laboratory tests and diagnostic and surgical procedures.

▶ Record the date of the last menstrual period and determine the possibility of pregnancy in perimenopausal women.

▶ Obtain a list of the patient's current medications, including anticoagulants, aspirin and other salicylates, herbs, nutritional supplements, and nutraceuticals (see Appendix F). Such products should be discontinued by medical direction for the appropriate number of days prior to a surgical procedure. Note the last time and dose of medication taken.

▶ Review the procedure with the patient. Address concerns about pain related to the procedure and explain that some pain may be experienced during the test, and there may be moments of discomfort. Inform the patient that the procedure is performed by a health-care provider (HCP), with support staff, and takes approximately 30 to 60 min.

▶ *Sensitivity to social and cultural issues,* as well as concern for modesty, is important in providing psychological support before, during, and after the procedure.

▶ Explain to the patient that if a biopsy is performed, she may feel menstrual-like cramping during the procedure and experience a minimal amount of bleeding.

▶ There are no food, fluid, or medication restrictions unless by medical direction.

▶ *Make sure a written and informed consent has been signed prior to the procedure and before administering any medications.*

INTRATEST:

▶ Have emergency equipment readily available.

▶ Instruct the patient to void prior to the procedure and to change into the gown, robe, and foot coverings provided.

▶ Observe standard precautions, and follow the general guidelines in Appendix A. Positively identify the patient, and label the appropriate containers with the corresponding patient demographics, date, and time of collection.

▶ Instruct the patient to cooperate fully and to follow directions. Instruct the patient to remain still throughout the procedure because movement produces unreliable results.

▶ Obtain and record baseline vital signs.

▶ An IV line may be started to allow infusion of a sedative or IV fluids.

▶ Administer medications, as ordered, to reduce discomfort and to promote relaxation and sedation.

▶ Place the patient in the lithotomy position on the examining table and drape her. Cleanse the external genitalia with an antiseptic solution.

▶ If a Pap smear is performed, the vaginal speculum is inserted, using water as a lubricant.

▶ The cervix is swabbed with 3% acetic acid to remove mucus or any cream medication and to improve the contrast between tissue types. The scope is positioned at the speculum and is focused on the cervix. The area is examined carefully, using light and magnification. Photographs can be taken for future reference.

▶ Tissues that appear abnormal or atypical undergo biopsy using a forceps inserted through the speculum. Bleeding, which is common after cervical biopsy, may be controlled by cautery, suturing, or application of silver nitrate or ferric subsulfate (Monsel's solution) to the site.

▶ The vagina is rinsed with sterile saline or water to remove the acetic acid and prevent burning after the procedure. If bleeding persists, a tampon may be inserted after removal of the speculum.

▶ Biopsy samples are placed in appropriately labeled containers with special preservative solution, and promptly transported to the laboratory.

POST-TEST:

▶ A report of the results will be sent to the requesting HCP, who will discuss the results with the patient.

▸ Monitor the patient for signs of respiratory depression.

▸ Monitor vital signs and neurological status every 15 min for 1 hr, then every 2 hr for 4 hr, and as ordered. Take temperature every 4 hr for 24 hr. Monitor intake and output at least every 8 hr. Compare with baseline values. Notify the HCP if temperature is elevated. Protocols may vary among facilities.

▸ Observe the patient until the effects of the sedation, if ordered, have worn off.

▸ Instruct the patient to remove the vaginal tampon, if inserted, within 8 to 24 hr; after that time, the patient should wear pads if there is bleeding or drainage.

▸ If a biopsy was performed, inform the patient that a discharge may persist for a few days to a few weeks.

▸ Advise the patient to avoid strenuous exercise 8 to 24 hr after the procedure and to avoid douching and intercourse for about 2 wk or as directed by the HCP.

▸ Monitor for any bleeding.

▸ Instruct the patient to expect slight bleeding for 2 days after removal of biopsy specimens, but emphasize that persistent vaginal bleeding or abnormal vaginal discharge, an increasing amount of bleeding, abdominal pain, and fever must be reported to the HCP immediately.

▸ Instruct the patient to immediately report symptoms such as fast heart rate, difficulty breathing, skin rash, itching, chest pain, persistent right shoulder pain, or abdominal pain. Immediately report symptoms to the appropriate HCP.

▸ Recognize anxiety related to test results. Discuss the implications of abnormal test results on the patient's lifestyle. Provide teaching and information regarding the clinical implications of the test results, as appropriate.

▸ Reinforce information given by the patient's HCP regarding further testing, treatment, or referral to another HCP. Answer any questions or address any concerns voiced by the patient or family.

▸ Depending on the results of this procedure, additional testing may be needed to evaluate or monitor progression of the disease process and determine the need for a change in therapy. Evaluate test results in relation to the patient's symptoms and other tests performed.

RELATED MONOGRAPHS:

▸ Related tests include biopsy cervical, CT abdomen, culture viral, MRI abdomen, Pap smear, and US pelvis.

▸ Refer to the Reproductive System table at the end of the book for related tests by body system.

Complement C3 and Complement C4

SYNONYM/ACRONYM: C3 and C4.

COMMON USE: To assist in the diagnosis of immunological diseases, such as rheumatoid arthritis, and systemic lupus erythematosus (SLE), in which complement is consumed at an increased rate, or to detect inborn deficiency.

SPECIMEN: Serum (1 mL) collected in a red-top tube.

REFERENCE VALUE: (Method: Nephelometry)

C3

Age	Conventional Units	SI Units (Conventional Units × 10)
Newborn	57–116 mg/dL	570–1,160 mg/L
6 mo–adult	74–166 mg/dL	740–1,660 mg/L
Adult	83–177 mg/dL	830–1,770 mg/L

C4

Age	Conventional Units	SI Units (Conventional Units × 10)
Newborn	10–31 mg/dL	100–310 mg/L
6 mo–6 yr	15–52 mg/dL	150–520 mg/L
7–12 yr	19–40 mg/dL	190–400 mg/L
13–15 yr	19–57 mg/dL	190–570 mg/L
16–18 yr	19–42 mg/dL	190–420 mg/L
Adult	12–36 mg/dL	120–360 mg/L

DESCRIPTION: Complement proteins act as enzymes that aid in the immunological and inflammatory response. The complement system is an important mechanism for the destruction and removal of foreign materials. Serum complement levels are used to detect autoimmune diseases. C3 and C4 are the most frequently assayed complement proteins, along with total complement.

Circulating C3 is synthesized in the liver and comprises 70% of the complement system, but cells in other tissues can also produce C3. C3 is an essential activating protein in the classic and alternate complement cascades. It is decreased in patients with immunological diseases, in whom it is consumed at an increased rate. C4 is produced primarily in the liver but can also be produced by monocytes, fibroblasts, and macrophages. C4 participates in the classic complement pathway.

INDICATIONS
- Detect genetic deficiencies
- Evaluate immunological diseases

POTENTIAL DIAGNOSIS

Normal C4 and decreased C3	Acute glomerulonephritis, membranous glomerulonephritis, immune complex diseases, SLE, C3 deficiency
Decreased C4 and normal C3	Immune complex diseases, cryoglobulinemia, C4 deficiency, hereditary angioedema
Decreased C4 and decreased C3	Immune complex diseases

Increased in
Response to sudden increased demand

- C3 and C4
  Acute-phase reactions

- C3
  Amyloidosis
  Cancer
  Diabetes
  Myocardial infarction
  Pneumococcal pneumonia
  Pregnancy
  Rheumatic disease
  Thyroiditis
  Viral hepatitis

- C4
  Certain malignancies

Decreased in
Related to overconsumption during immune response

- C3 and C4
  Hereditary deficiency *(insufficient production)*
  Liver disease *(insufficient production related to damaged liver cells)*
  SLE

- C3
  Chronic infection (bacterial, parasitic, viral)
  Post–membranoproliferative-glomerulonephritis
  Post–streptococcal infection
  Rheumatic arthritis

- C4
  Angioedema *(hereditary and acquired)*
  Autoimmune hemolytic anemia
  Autoimmune thyroiditis
  Cryoglobulinemia
  Glomerulonephritis
  Juvenile dermatomyositis
  Meningitis (bacterial, viral)
  Pneumonia
  Streptococcal or staphylococcal sepsis

CRITICAL FINDINGS: N/A

INTERFERING FACTORS

- Drugs that may increase C3 levels include cimetidine and cyclophosphamide.
- Drugs that may decrease C3 levels include danazol and phenytoin.
- Drugs that may increase C4 levels include cimetidine, cyclophosphamide, and danazol.
- Drugs that may decrease C4 levels include dextran and penicillamine.

NURSING IMPLICATIONS AND PROCEDURE

PRETEST:

- Positively identify the patient using at least two unique identifiers before providing care, treatment, or services.
- *Patient Teaching:* Inform the patient this test can assist in diagnosing diseases of the immune system.
- Obtain a history of the patient's complaints, including a list of known allergens, especially allergies or sensitivities to latex.
- Obtain a history of the patient's immune system and results of previously performed laboratory tests and diagnostic and surgical procedures.
- Obtain a list of the patient's current medications, including herbs, nutritional supplements, and nutraceuticals (see Appendix F).
- Review the procedure with the patient. Inform the patient that specimen collection takes approximately 5 to 10 min. Address concerns about pain and explain that there may be some discomfort during the venipuncture.
- *Sensitivity to social and cultural issues,* as well as concern for modesty, is important in providing psychological support before, during, and after the procedure.
- There are no food, fluid, or medication restrictions unless by medical direction.

INTRATEST:

- If the patient has a history of allergic reaction to latex, avoid the use of equipment containing latex.
- Instruct the patient to cooperate fully and to follow directions. Direct the patient to breathe normally and to avoid unnecessary movement.

▶ Observe standard precautions, and follow the general guidelines in Appendix A. Positively identify the patient, and label the appropriate tubes with the corresponding patient demographics, date, and time of collection. Perform a venipuncture.

▶ Remove the needle and apply direct pressure with dry gauze to stop bleeding. Observe/assess venipuncture site for bleeding or hematoma formation and secure gauze with adhesive bandage.

▶ Promptly transport the specimen to the laboratory for processing and analysis.

POST-TEST:

▶ A report of the results will be sent to the requesting health-care provider (HCP), who will discuss the results with the patient.

▶ Reinforce information given by the patient's HCP regarding further testing, treatment, or referral to another HCP. Answer any questions or address any concerns voiced by the patient or family.

▶ Depending on the results of this procedure, additional testing may be performed to evaluate or monitor progression of the disease process and determine the need for a change in therapy. Evaluate test results in relation to the patient's symptoms and other tests performed.

RELATED MONOGRAPHS:

▶ Related tests include anticardiolipin antibody, ANA, complement total, cryoglobulin, and ESR.

▶ Refer to the Immune System table at the end of the book for related tests by body system.

Complement, Total

SYNONYM/ACRONYM: Total hemolytic complement, CH_{50}, CH_{100}.

COMMON USE: To evaluate immune diseases related to complement activity and follow up on a patient's response to therapy such as treatment for systemic lupus erythematosus (SLE).

SPECIMEN: Serum (1 mL) collected in a red-top tube.

REFERENCE VALUE: (Method: Quantitative hemolysis)

Conventional Units	SI Units (Conventional Units × 1)
25–110 CH_{50} units/mL	25–110 CH_{50} kU/L

DESCRIPTION: The complement system comprises proteins that become activated and interact in a sequential cascade. The complement system is an important part of the body's natural defense against allergic and immune reactions. It is activated by plasmin and is interrelated with the coagulation and fibrinolytic systems. Activation of the complement system results in cell lysis, release of histamine, chemotaxis of white blood cells, increased vascular permeability, and contraction of smooth muscle. The activation of this system can sometimes occur with uncontrolled self-destructive effects on the body. In the serum complement assay, a patient's serum is mixed with sheep red blood cells coated with antibodies. If complement is present in sufficient quantities, 50% of the red blood cells are lysed. Lower amounts of lysed cells are associated with decreased complement levels.

INDICATIONS
- Assist in the diagnosis of hereditary angioedema
- Evaluate complement activity in autoimmune disorders
- Evaluate and monitor therapy for systemic lupus erythematosus (SLE)
- Screen for complement deficiency

POTENTIAL DIAGNOSIS

Increased in
- Acute-phase immune response *(related to sudden response to increased demand)*

Decreased in
- Autoimmune diseases *(related to continuous demand)*
- Autoimmune hemolytic anemia *(related to consumption during hemolytic process)*
- Burns *(related to increased consumption from initiation of complement cascade)*
- Cryoglobulinemia *(related to increased consumption)*
- Hereditary deficiency *(related to insufficient production)*
- Infections *(bacterial, parasitic, viral; related to increased consumption during immune response)*
- Liver disease *(related to decreased production by damaged liver cells)*
- Malignancy *(related to consumption during cellular immune response)*
- Membranous glomerulonephritis *(related to consumption during cellular immune response)*
- Rheumatoid arthritis *(related to consumption during immune response)*
- SLE *(related to consumption during immune response)*
- Trauma *(related to consumption during immune response)*
- Vasculitis *(related to consumption during cellular immune response)*

CRITICAL FINDINGS: N/A

INTERFERING FACTORS
- Drugs that may increase total complement levels include cyclophosphamide and oral contraceptives.
- Specimen should not remain at room temperature longer than 1 hr.

NURSING IMPLICATIONS AND PROCEDURE

PRETEST:
- Positively identify the patient using at least two unique identifiers before providing care, treatment, or services.
- *Patient Teaching:* Inform the patient this test can assist in evaluating response to treatment for infection or disease.
- Obtain a history of the patient's complaints, including a list of known allergies, especially allergies or sensitivities to latex.
- Obtain a history of the patient's immune system and results of previously performed laboratory tests and diagnostic and surgical procedures.
- Obtain a list of the patient's current medications, including herbs, nutritional supplements, and nutraceuticals (see Appendix F).

▶ Review the procedure with the patient. Inform the patient that specimen collection takes approximately 5 to 10 min. Address concerns about pain and explain that there may be some discomfort during the venipuncture.

▶ *Sensitivity to social and cultural issues,* as well as concern for modesty, is important in providing psychological support before, during, and after the procedure.

▶ There are no food, fluid, or medication restrictions unless by medical direction.

INTRATEST:

▶ If the patient has a history of allergic reaction to latex, avoid the use of equipment containing latex.

▶ Instruct the patient to cooperate fully and to follow directions. Direct the patient to breathe normally and to avoid unnecessary movement.

▶ Observe standard precautions, and follow the general guidelines in Appendix A. Positively identify the patient, and label the appropriate tubes with the corresponding patient demographics, date, and time of collection. Perform a venipuncture.

▶ Remove the needle and apply direct pressure with dry gauze to stop bleeding. Observe/assess venipuncture site

for bleeding or hematoma formation and secure gauze with adhesive bandage.

▶ Promptly transport the specimen to the laboratory for processing and analysis.

POST-TEST:

▶ A report of the results will be sent to the requesting health-care provider (HCP), who will discuss the results with the patient.

▶ Reinforce information given by the patient's HCP regarding further testing, treatment, or referral to another HCP. Answer any questions or address any concerns voiced by the patient or family.

▶ Depending on the results of this procedure, additional testing may be performed to evaluate or monitor progression of the disease process and determine the need for a change in therapy. Evaluate test results in relation to the patient's symptoms and other tests performed.

RELATED MONOGRAPHS:

▶ Related tests include antibody anticytoplasmic neutrophilic, ANA, Coomb's antiglobulin, complement C3 and C4, cryoglobulin, ESR, G6PD, Ham's test, osmotic fragility, PK, and RF.

▶ Refer to the Immune System table at the end of the book for related tests by body system.

Complete Blood Count

SYNONYM/ACRONYM: CBC.

COMMON USE: To evaluate numerous conditions involving red blood cells, white blood cells, and platelets. This test is also used to indicate inflammation, infection, and response to chemotherapy.

SPECIMEN: Whole blood from one full lavender-top (EDTA) tube or Microtainer. Whole blood from a green-top (lithium or sodium heparin) tube may be submitted, but the following automated values may not be reported: white blood cell (WBC) count, WBC differential, platelet count, and mean platelet volume.

REFERENCE VALUE: (Method: Automated, computerized multichannel analyzers that sort and size cells on the basis of changes in either electrical impedance or light pulses as the cells pass in front of a laser. Many of these analyzers are capable of determining a five-part WBC differential.) This battery of tests includes hemoglobin, hematocrit, red blood cell (RBC) count, RBC morphology, RBC indices, RBC distribution width index (RDW), platelet count, platelet size, WBC count, and WBC differential. The five-part automated WBC differential identifies and enumerates neutrophils, lymphocytes, monocytes, eosinophils, and basophils.

Hemoglobin

Age	Conventional Units	SI Units (Conventional Units × 10)
Cord blood	13.5–20.7 g/dL	135–207 mmol/L
0–1 wk	15.2–23.6 g/dL	152–236 mmol/L
2–3 wk	12.7–18.7 g/dL	127–187 mmol/L
1–2 mo	9.7–17.3 g/dL	97–173 mmol/L
3–11 mo	9.3–13.3 g/dL	93–133 mmol/L
1–5 yr	10.4–13.6 g/dL	104–136 mmol/L
6–8 yr	10.9–14.5 g/dL	109–145 mmol/L
9–14 yr	11.5–15.5 g/dL	115–155 mmol/L
15 yr–adult		
Male	13.2–17.3 g/dL	132–173 mmol/L
Female	11.7–15.5 g/dL	117–155 mmol/L
Older adult		
Male	12.6–17.4 g/dL	126–174 mmol/L
Female	11.7–16.1 g/dL	117–161 mmol/L

Note: See "Complete Blood Count, Hemoglobin" monograph for more detailed information.

Hematocrit

Age	Conventional Units (%)	SI Units (Conventional Units × 0.01)
Cord blood	42–62	0.42–0.62
0–1 wk	46–68	0.46–0.68
2–3 wk	40–56	0.40–0.56
1–2 mo	32–54	0.32–0.54
3–11 mo	32–44	0.32–0.44
1–5 yr	31–44	0.31–0.44
6–8 yr	33–41	0.33–0.41
9–14 yr	33–45	0.33–0.45
15 yr–adult		
Male	37–49	0.37–0.49
Female	33–45	0.33–0.45
Older adult		
Male	36–52	0.36–0.52
Female	34–46	0.34–0.46

Note: See "Complete Blood Count, Hematocrit" monograph for more detailed information.

White Blood Cell Count and Differential

Age	Conventional Units WBC × 10³/mm³*	Total Neutrophils (Absolute) and %	Neutrophils Bands (Absolute) and %	Neutrophils Segments (Absolute) and %	Lymphocytes (Absolute) and %	Monocytes (Absolute) and %	Eosinophils (Absolute) and %	Basophils (Absolute) and %
Birth	9.0–30.0	(5.5–18.3) 61%	(0.8–2.7) 9.1%	(4.7–15.6) 52%	(2.8–9.3) 31%	(0.5–1.7) 5.8%	(0.02–0.7) 2.2%	(0.1–0.2) 0.6%
1–23 mo	6.0–17.5	(1.9–5.4) 31%	(0.2–0.5) 3.1%	(1.7–4.9) 28%	(3.7–10.7) 61%	(0.3–0.8) 4.8%	(0.2–0.5) 2.6%	(0–0.1) 0.5%
2–10 yr	4.5–13.5	(2.4–7.3) 54%	(0.1–0.4) 3.0%	(2.3–6.9) 51%	(1.7–5.1) 38%	(0.2–0.6) 4.3%	(0.1–0.3) 2.4%	(0–0.1) 0.5%
11 yr–older adult	4.5–11.0	(2.7–6.5) 59%	(0.1–0.3) 3.0%	(2.5–6.2) 56%	(1.5–3.7) 34%	(0.2–0.4) 4.0%	(0.05–0.5) 2.7%	(0–0.1) 0.5%

*SI Units (Conventional Units × 1 × 10⁹/L or WBC × 1,000/mm³).
Note: See "White Blood Cell Count and Cell Differential" monograph for more detailed information.

Red Blood Cell Count

Age	Conventional Units $(10^6$ cells/mm^3)	SI Units $(10^{12}$ cells/L) (Conventional Units $\times$ 1)
Cord blood	3.60–5.80	3.60–5.80
0–1 wk	4.50–7.00	4.50–7.00
2–3 wk	3.70–6.10	3.70–6.10
1–2 mo	3.10–5.10	3.10–5.10
3–11 mo	3.00–5.00	3.00–5.00
1–5 yr	3.80–5.00	3.80–5.00
6–8 yr	3.90–5.10	3.90–5.10
9–14 yr	3.90–5.60	3.90–5.60
15 yr–adult		
Male	5.20–5.80	5.20–5.80
Female	3.90–5.10	3.90–5.10
Older adult		
Male	3.80–5.80	3.80–5.80
Female	3.70–5.30	3.70–5.30

Note: See "Complete Blood Count, Red Blood Cell Count" monograph for more detailed information.

Red Blood Cell Indices

Age	MCV (fl)	MCH (pg/cell)	MCHC (g/dL)	RDW
Cord blood	107–119	35–39	31–35	14.9–18.7
0–1 wk	104–116	29–45	24–36	14.9–18.7
2–3 wk	95–117	26–38	26–34	14.9–18.7
1–2 mo	81–125	25–37	26–34	14.9–18.7
3–11 mo	78–110	22–34	26–34	14.9–18.7
1–5 yr	74–94	24–32	30–34	11.6–14.8
6–8 yr	73–93	24–32	32–36	11.6–14.8
9–14 yr	74–94	25–33	32–36	11.6–14.8
15 yr–adult				
Male	77–97	26–34	32–36	11.6–14.8
Female	78–98	26–34	32–36	11.6–14.8
Older adult				
Male	79–103	27–35	32–36	11.6–14.8
Female	78–102	27–35	32–36	11.6–14.8

MCH = mean corpuscular hemoglobin; MCHC = mean corpuscular hemoglobin concentration; MCV = mean corpuscular volume; RDW = RBC distribution width index.
Note: See "Complete Blood Count, Red Blood Cell Indices" monograph for more detailed information.

Red Blood Cell Morphology

Morphology	Within Normal Limits	1+	2+	3+	4+
Size					
Anisocytosis	0–5+	5–10	10–20	20–50	Greater than 50
Macrocytes	0–5+	5–10	10–20	20–50	Greater than 50
Microcytes	0–5+	5–10	10–20	20–50	Greater than 50
Shape					
Poikilocytes	0–2+	3–10	10–20	20–50	Greater than 50
Burr cells	0–2+	3–10	10–20	20–50	Greater than 50
Acanthocytes	Less than 1+	2–5	5–10	10–20	Greater than 20
Schistocytes	Less than 1+	2–5	5–10	10–20	Greater than 20
Dacryocytes (teardrop cells)	0–2+	2–5	5–10	10–20	Greater than 20
Codocytes (target cells)	0–2+	2–10	10–20	20–50	Greater than 50
Spherocytes	0–2+	2–10	10–20	20–50	Greater than 50
Ovalocytes	0–2+	2–10	10–20	20–50	Greater than 50
Stomatocytes	0–2+	2–10	10–20	20–50	Greater than 50
Drepanocytes (sickle cells)	Absent	Reported as present or absent			
Helmet cells	Absent	Reported as present or absent			
Agglutination	Absent	Reported as present or absent			
Rouleaux	Absent	Reported as present or absent			
Hemoglobin Content					
Hypochromia	0–2+	3–10	10–50	50–75	Greater than 75
Polychromasia					
Adult	Less than 1+	2–5	5–10	10–20	Greater than 20
Newborn	1–6+	7–15	15–20	20–50	Greater than 50

Note: See "Complete Blood Count, Red Blood Cell Morphology and Inclusions" monograph for more detailed information.

Red Blood Cell Inclusions

Inclusions	Within Normal Limits	1+	2+	3+	4+
Cabot's rings	Absent	Reported as present or absent			
Basophilic stippling	0–1+	1–5	5–10	10–20	Greater than 20
Howell-Jolly bodies	Absent	1–2	3–5	5–10	Greater than 10
Heinz bodies	Absent	Reported as present or absent			
Hemoglobin C crystals	Absent	Reported as present or absent			
Pappenheimer bodies	Absent	Reported as present or absent			
Intracellular parasites (e.g., *Plasmodium*, *Babesia*, trypanosomes)	Absent	Reported as present or absent			

Note: See "Complete Blood Count, Red Blood Cell Morphology and Inclusions" monograph for more detailed information.

Platelet Count

Age	Conventional Units	SI Units (Conventional Units × 1)	MPV (fl)
Newborn–11 mo	150,000–350,000/mm^3	150–350 × 10^9/L	7.0–10.2
1–5 yr	217,000–497,000/mm^3	217–497 × 10^9/L	7.2–10.0
Adult	150,000–450,000/mm^3	150–450 × 10^9/L	7.0–10.2

Note: See "Complete Blood Count, Platelet Count" monograph for more detailed information. Platelet counts may decrease slightly with age.

DESCRIPTION: A complete blood count (CBC) is a group of tests used for basic screening purposes. It is probably the most widely ordered laboratory test. Results provide the enumeration of the cellular elements of the blood, measurement of red blood cell (RBC) indices, and determination of cell morphology by automation and evaluation of stained smears. The results can provide valuable diagnostic information regarding the overall health of the patient and the patient's response to disease and treatment. Detailed information is found in monographs titled

"Complete Blood Count, Hemoglobin"; "Complete Blood Count, Hematocrit"; "Complete Blood Count, Red Blood Cell Indices"; "Complete Blood Count, Red Blood Cell Morphology and Inclusions"; "Complete Blood Count, Red Blood Cell Count"; "Complete Blood Count, Platelet Count"; and "Complete Blood Count, White Blood Cell Count and Cell Differential."

Count, RBC Indices"; "Complete Blood Count, RBC Morphology and Inclusions"; "Complete Blood Count, RBC Count"; "Complete Blood Count, Platelet Count"; and "Complete Blood Count, WBC Count and Differential."

Increased in
See above-listed monographs.

Decreased in
See above-listed monographs.

CRITICAL FINDINGS

INDICATIONS
- Detect hematological disorder, neoplasm, leukemia, or immunological abnormality
- Determine the presence of hereditary hematological abnormality
- Evaluate known or suspected anemia and related treatment
- Monitor blood loss and response to blood replacement
- Monitor the effects of physical or emotional stress
- Monitor fluid imbalances or treatment for fluid imbalances
- Monitor hematological status during pregnancy
- Monitor progression of nonhematological disorders, such as chronic obstructive pulmonary disease, malabsorption syndromes, cancer, and renal disease
- Monitor response to chemotherapy and evaluate undesired reactions to drugs that may cause blood dyscrasias
- Provide screening as part of a general physical examination, especially on admission to a health-care facility or before surgery

POTENTIAL DIAGNOSIS
- See monographs titled "Complete Blood Count, Hemoglobin"; "Complete Blood Count, Hematocrit"; "Complete Blood

Hemoglobin
- Less than 6 g/dL
- Greater than 18 g/dL

Hematocrit
- Less than 18%
- Greater than 54%

WBC Count (on Admission)
- Less than 2,500/mm^3
- Greater than 30,000/mm^3

Platelet Count
- Less than 50,000/mm^3
- Greater than 1,000,000/mm^3

Note and immediately report to the health-care provider (HCP) any critically increased or decreased values and related symptoms.

The presence of abnormal cells, other morphological characteristics, or cellular inclusions may signify a potentially life-threatening or serious health condition and should be investigated. Examples are the presence of sickle cells, moderate numbers of spherocytes, marked schistocytosis, oval macrocytes, basophilic stippling, eosinophil count greater than 10%, monocytosis greater than 15%, nucleated RBCs (if patient is not an infant), malarial organisms, hypersegmented neutrophils, agranular neutrophils, blasts or other immature cells, Auer rods, Döhle bodies, marked toxic granulation, or plasma cells.

INTERFERING FACTORS

- Failure to fill the tube sufficiently (less than three-fourths full) may yield inadequate sample volume for automated analyzers and may be a reason for specimen rejection.
- Hemolyzed or clotted specimens should be rejected for analysis.
- Elevated serum glucose or sodium levels may produce elevated mean corpuscular volume values because of swelling of erythrocytes.
- Recent transfusion history should be considered when evaluating the CBC.

NURSING IMPLICATIONS AND PROCEDURE

PRETEST:

- Positively identify the patient using at least two unique identifiers before providing care, treatment, or services.
- *Patient Teaching:* Inform the patient this test can assist in evaluating the body's response to illness.
- Obtain a history of the patient's complaints, including a list of known allergens, especially allergies or sensitivities to latex.
- Obtain a history of the patient's gastrointestinal, hematopoietic, immune, and respiratory systems as well as results of previously performed laboratory tests and diagnostic and surgical procedures.
- Obtain a list of the patient's current medications, including herbs, nutritional supplements, and nutraceuticals (see Appendix F).
- Review the procedure with the patient. Inform the patient that specimen collection takes approximately 5 to 10 min. Address concerns about pain and explain that there may be some discomfort during the venipuncture.
- *Sensitivity to social and cultural issues,* as well as concern for modesty, is

important in providing psychological support before, during, and after the procedure.
- There are no food, fluid, or medication restrictions unless by medical direction.

INTRATEST:

- If the patient has a history of allergic reaction to latex, avoid the use of equipment containing latex.
- Instruct the patient to cooperate fully and to follow directions. Direct the patient to breathe normally and to avoid unnecessary movement.
- Observe standard precautions, and follow the general guidelines in Appendix A. Positively identify the patient, and label the appropriate tubes with the corresponding patient demographics, date, and time of collection. Perform a venipuncture. An EDTA Microtainer sample may be obtained from infants, children, and adults for whom venipuncture may not be feasible. The specimen should be analyzed within 24 hr when stored at room temperature or within 48 hr if stored at refrigerated temperature. If it is anticipated the specimen will not be analyzed within 24 hr, two blood smears should be made immediately after the venipuncture and submitted with the blood sample. Smears made from specimens older than 24 hr may contain an unacceptable number of misleading artifactual abnormalities of the RBCs, such as echinocytes and spherocytes, as well as necrobiotic white blood cells.
- Remove the needle and apply direct pressure with dry gauze to stop bleeding. Observe/assess venipuncture site for bleeding or hematoma formation and secure gauze with adhesive bandage.
- Promptly transport the specimen to the laboratory for processing and analysis.

POST-TEST:

- A report of the results will be sent to the requesting HCP, who will discuss the results with the patient.
- *Nutritional Considerations:* Instruct patients to consume a variety of foods within the basic food groups, maintain a healthy weight, be physically active, limit salt intake, limit alcohol intake, and avoid use of tobacco.

▸ Reinforce information given by the patient's HCP regarding further testing, treatment, or referral to another HCP. Answer any questions or address any concerns voiced by the patient or family.

▸ Depending on the results of this procedure, additional testing may be performed to evaluate or monitor progression of the disease process and determine the need for a change in therapy. Evaluate test results in relation to the patient's symptoms and other tests performed.

RELATED MONOGRAPHS:

▸ Related tests include alveolar arterial ratio, biopsy bone marrow, blood gases, blood groups and antibodies, erythropoietin, ferritin, CBC hematocrit, CBC hemoglobin, CBC platelet count, CBC RBC count, CBC RBC indices, CBC RBC morphology, CBC WBC count and cell differential, iron/TIBC, lead, pulse oximetry, and reticulocyte count.

▸ Refer to the Gastrointestinal, Hematopoietic, Immune, and Respiratory systems tables at the end of the book for related tests by body system.

Complete Blood Count, Hematocrit

SYNONYM/ACRONYM: Packed cell volume (PCV), Hct.

COMMON USE: To evaluate anemia, polycythemia, and hydration status and to monitor therapy.

SPECIMEN: Whole blood from one full lavender-top (EDTA) tube, Microtainer, or capillary. Whole blood from a green-top (lithium or sodium heparin) tube may also be submitted.

REFERENCE VALUE: (Method: Automated, computerized, multichannel analyzers)

Age	Conventional Units (%)	SI Units (Conventional Units × 0.01)
Cord blood	42–62	0.42–0.62
0–1 wk	46–68	0.46–0.68
2–3 wk	40–56	0.40–0.56
1–2 mo	32–54	0.32–0.54
3–11 mo	31–43	0.31–0.43
1–5 yr	31–43	0.31–0.43
6–8 yr	33–41	0.33–0.41
9–14 yr	33–45	0.33–0.45
15 yr–adult		
Male	38–51	0.38–0.51
Female	33–45	0.33–0.45
Older adult		
Male	36–52	0.36–0.52
Female	34–46	0.34–0.46

DESCRIPTION: Blood consists of a fluid portion (plasma) and a solid portion that includes red blood cells (RBCs), white blood cells, and platelets. The hematocrit, or packed cell volume, is the percentage of RBCs in a volume of whole blood. For example, a hematocrit (Hct) of 45% means that a 100-mL sample of blood contains 45 mL of packed RBCs. Although the Hct depends primarily on the number of RBCs, the average size of the RBCs plays a role. Conditions that cause the RBCs to swell, such as when the serum sodium concentration is elevated, may increase the Hct level.

Hct level is included in the complete blood count (CBC) and is generally tested together with hemoglobin (Hgb). These levels parallel each other and are the best determinant of the degree of anemia or polycythemia. *Polycythemia* is a term used in conjunction with conditions resulting from an abnormal increase in Hgb, Hct, and RBC counts. *Anemia* is a term associated with conditions resulting from an abnormal decrease in Hgb, Hct, and RBC counts. Results of the Hgb, Hct, and RBC counts should be evaluated simultaneously because the same underlying conditions affect this triad of tests similarly. The RBC count multiplied by 3 should approximate the Hgb concentration. The Hct should be within 3 times the Hgb if the RBC population is normal in size and shape. The Hct plus 6 should approximate the first two figures of the RBC count within 3 (e.g., Hct is 40%; therefore 40 + 6 = 46, and the RBC count should be 4.6 or in the range of 4.3 to 4.9). There are some cultural variations in Hgb and Hct (H&H) values. After the first decade of life, the mean Hgb in African Americans is 0.5 to 1.0 g lower than in whites. Mexican Americans and Asian Americans have higher H&H values than whites.

INDICATIONS

- Detect hematological disorder, neoplasm, or immunological abnormality
- Determine the presence of hereditary hematological abnormality
- Evaluate known or suspected anemia and related treatment, in combination with Hgb
- Monitor blood loss and response to blood replacement, in combination with Hgb
- Monitor the effects of physical or emotional stress on the patient
- Monitor fluid imbalances or their treatment
- Monitor hematological status during pregnancy, in combination with Hgb
- Monitor the progression of nonhematological disorders such as chronic obstructive pulmonary disease, malabsorption syndromes, cancer, and renal disease
- Monitor response to drugs or chemotherapy, and evaluate undesired reactions to drugs that may cause blood dyscrasias
- Provide screening as part of a CBC in a general physical examination, especially upon admission to a health-care facility or before surgery

POTENTIAL DIAGNOSIS

Increased in
- Burns *(related to dehydration; total blood volume is decreased, but RBC count remains the same)*
- Congestive heart failure *(when the underlying cause is anemia, the*

body responds by increasing production of RBCs with a corresponding increase in Hct)
- Chronic obstructive pulmonary disease (related to chronic hypoxia that stimulates production of RBC and a corresponding increase in Hct)
- Dehydration (total blood volume is decreased, but RBC count remains the same)
- Erythrocytosis (total blood volume remains the same, but RBC count is increased)
- Hemoconcentration (same effect as seen in dehydration)
- High altitudes (related to hypoxia that stimulates production of RBC and therefore increases Hct)
- Polycythemia (abnormal bone marrow response resulting in overproduction of RBC)
- Shock

Decreased in
- Anemia (overall decrease in RBC and corresponding decrease in Hct)
- Blood loss (acute and chronic) (overall decrease in RBC and corresponding decrease in Hct)
- Bone marrow hyperplasia (bone marrow failure that results in decreased RBC production)
- Carcinoma (anemia is often associated with chronic disease)
- Cirrhosis (related to accumulation of fluid)
- Chronic disease (anemia is often associated with chronic disease)
- Fluid retention (dilutional effect of increased blood volume while RBC count remains stable)
- Hemoglobinopathies (reduced RBC survival with corresponding decrease in Hgb)
- Hemolytic disorders (e.g., hemolytic anemias, prosthetic valves) (reduced RBC survival with corresponding decrease in Hct)

- Hemorrhage (acute and chronic) (related to loss of RBC that exceeds rate of production)
- Hodgkin's disease (bone marrow failure that results in decreased RBC production)
- Incompatible blood transfusion (reduced RBC survival with corresponding decrease in Hgb)
- Intravenous overload (dilutional effect)
- Fluid retention (dilutional effect of increased blood volume while RBC count remains stable)
- Leukemia (bone marrow failure that results in decreased RBC production)
- Lymphomas (bone marrow failure that results in decreased RBC production)
- Nutritional deficit (anemia related to dietary deficiency in iron, vitamins, folate needed to produce sufficient RBC; decreased RBC count with corresponding decrease in Hct)
- Pregnancy (related to anemia)
- Renal disease (related to decreased levels of erythropoietin, which stimulates production of RBCs)
- Splenomegaly (total blood volume remains the same, but spleen retains RBCs and Hct reflects decreased RBC count)

CRITICAL FINDINGS
- Less than 18%
- Greater than 54%

Note and immediately report to the health-care provider (HCP) any critically increased or decreased values and related symptoms.

Low Hct leads to anemia. Anemia can be caused by blood loss, decreased blood cell production, increased blood cell destruction, and hemodilution. Causes of blood loss include menstrual excess or frequency, gastrointestinal bleeding, inflammatory bowel disease, and hematuria. Decreased blood cell production can be caused by folic acid deficiency, vitamin B_{12} deficiency, iron deficiency, and chronic disease. Increased blood cell destruction can be caused by a hemolytic reaction, chemical reaction, medication reaction, and sickle cell disease. Hemodilution can be caused by congestive heart failure, renal failure, polydipsia, and overhydration. Symptoms of anemia (due to these causes) include anxiety, dyspnea, edema, hypertension, hypotension, hypoxia, jugular venous distention, fatigue, pallor, rales, restlessness, and weakness. Treatment of anemia depends on the cause.

High Hct leads to polycythemia. Polycythemia can be caused by dehydration, decreased oxygen levels in the body, and an overproduction of RBCs by the bone marrow. Dehydration from diuretic use, vomiting, diarrhea, excessive sweating, severe burns, or decreased fluid intake decreases the plasma component of whole blood, thereby increasing the ratio of RBCs to plasma, and leads to a higher than normal Hct. Causes of decreased oxygen include smoking, exposure to carbon monoxide, high altitude, and chronic lung disease, which leads to a mild hemoconcentration of blood in the body to carry more oxygen to the body's tissues. An overproduction of RBCs by the bone marrow leads to polycythemia vera, which is a rare chronic myeloproliferative disorder that leads to a severe hemoconcentration of blood. Severe hemoconcentration can lead to thrombosis (spontaneous blood clotting). Symptoms of hemoconcentration include decreased pulse pressure and volume, loss of skin turgor, dry mucous membranes,

headaches, hepatomegaly, low central venous pressure, orthostatic hypotension, pruritus (especially after a hot bath), splenomegaly, tachycardia, thirst, tinnitus, vertigo, and weakness. Treatment of polycythemia depends on the cause. Possible interventions for hemoconcentration due to dehydration include intravenous fluids and discontinuance of diuretics if they are believed to be contributing to critically elevated Hct. Polycythemia due to decreased oxygen states can be treated by removal of the offending substance, such as smoke or carbon monoxide. Treatment includes oxygen therapy in cases of smoke inhalation, carbon monoxide poisoning, and desaturating chronic lung disease. Symptoms of polycythemic overload crisis include signs of thrombosis, pain and redness in the extremities, facial flushing, and irritability. Possible interventions for hemoconcentration due to polycythemia include therapeutic phlebotomy and intravenous fluids.

INTERFERING FACTORS

- Drugs and substances that may cause a decrease in Hct include those that induce hemolysis due to drug sensitivity or enzyme deficiency and those that result in anemia (see monograph titled "Complete Blood Count, RBC Count").
- Some drugs may also affect Hct values by increasing the RBC count (see monograph titled "Complete Blood Count, RBC Count").
- The results of RBC counts may vary depending on the patient's position: Hct can decrease when the patient is recumbent as a result of hemodilution and can increase when the patient rises as a result of hemoconcentration.

- Leaving the tourniquet in place for longer than 60 sec can falsely increase Hct levels by 2% to 5%.
- Traumatic venipuncture and hemolysis may result in falsely decreased Hct values.
- Failure to fill the tube sufficiently (i.e., tube less than three-quarters full) may yield inadequate sample volume for automated analyzers and may be a reason for specimen rejection.
- Clotted or hemolyzed specimens must be rejected for analysis.
- Care should be taken in evaluating the Hct during the first few hours after transfusion or acute blood loss because the value may appear to be normal and may not be a reliable indicator of anemia.
- Abnormalities in the RBC size (macrocytes, microcytes) or shape (spherocytes, sickle cells) may alter Hct values, as in diseases and conditions including sickle cell anemia, hereditary spherocytosis, and iron deficiency.
- Elevated blood glucose or serum sodium levels may produce elevated Hct levels because of swelling of the erythrocytes.

NURSING IMPLICATIONS AND PROCEDURE

PRETEST:

- Positively identify the patient using at least two unique identifiers before providing care, treatment, or services.
- *Patient Teaching:* Inform the patient this test can assist in evaluating the body's blood status.
- Obtain a history of the patient's complaints, including a list of known allergens, especially allergies or sensitivities to latex.
- Obtain a history of the patient's cardiovascular, gastrointestinal, hematopoietic, hepatobiliary, immune, and respiratory systems; symptoms; and results of previously performed laboratory tests and diagnostic and surgical procedures.
- Note any recent procedures that can interfere with test results.
- Obtain a list of the patient s current medications, including herbs, nutritional supplements, and nutraceuticals (see Appendix F).
- Review the procedure with the patient. Inform the patient that specimen collection takes approximately 5 to 10 min. Address concerns about pain and explain that there may be some discomfort during the venipuncture.
- *Sensitivity to social and cultural issues,* as well as concern for modesty, is important in providing psychological support before, during, and after the procedure.
- There are no food, fluid, or medication restrictions unless by medical direction.

INTRATEST:

- If the patient has a history of allergic reaction to latex, avoid the use of equipment containing latex.
- Instruct the patient to cooperate fully and to follow directions. Direct the patient to breathe normally and to avoid unnecessary movement.
- Observe standard precautions, and follow the general guidelines in Appendix A. Positively identify the patient, and label the appropriate tubes with the corresponding patient demographics, date, and time of collection. Perform a venipuncture; collect the specimen in a 5-mL lavender-top (EDTA) tube. An EDTA Microtainer sample may be obtained from infants, children, and adults for whom venipuncture may not be feasible. The specimen should be mixed gently by inverting the tube 10 times. The specimen should be analyzed within 24 hr when stored at room temperature or within 48 hr if stored at refrigerated temperature. If it is anticipated the specimen will not be analyzed within 24 hr, two blood smears should be made immediately

after the venipuncture and submitted with the blood sample. Smears made from specimens older than 24 hr may contain an unacceptable number of misleading artifactual abnormalities of the RBCs, such as echinocytes and spherocytes, as well as necrobiotic white blood cells.

- Remove the needle and apply direct pressure with dry gauze to stop bleeding. Observe/assess venipuncture site for bleeding or hematoma formation and secure gauze with adhesive bandage.

- Promptly transport the specimen to the laboratory for processing and analysis.

POST-TEST:

- A report of the results will be sent to the requesting HCP, who will discuss the results with the patient.

- *Nutritional Considerations:* Nutritional therapy may be indicated for patients with decreased Hct. Iron deficiency is the most common nutrient deficiency in the United States. Patients at risk (e.g., children, pregnant women and women of childbearing age, low-income populations) should be instructed to include foods that are high in iron in their diet, such as meats (especially liver), eggs, grains, green leafy vegetables, and multivitamins with iron. Iron absorption is affected by numerous factors (see monograph titled "Iron").

- Reinforce information given by the patient's HCP regarding further testing, treatment, or referral to another HCP. Answer any questions or address any concerns voiced by the patient or family.

- Depending on the results of this procedure, additional testing may be performed to evaluate or monitor progression of the disease process and determine the need for a change in therapy. Evaluate test results in relation to the patient's symptoms and other tests performed.

RELATED MONOGRAPHS:

- Related tests include biopsy bone marrow, CBC, CBC hemoglobin, CBC RBC indices, CBC RBC morphology, erythropoietin, ferritin, iron/TIBC, and reticulocyte count.

- Refer to the Cardiovascular, Gastrointestinal, Hematopoietic, Hepatobiliary, Immune, and Respiratory systems tables at the end of the book for related tests by body system.

Complete Blood Count, Hemoglobin

SYNONYM/ACRONYM: Hgb.

COMMON USE: To evaluate anemia, polycythemia, hydration status, and monitor therapy such as transfusion.

SPECIMEN: Whole blood from one full lavender-top (EDTA) tube, Microtainer, or capillary. Whole blood from a green-top (lithium or sodium heparin) tube may also be submitted.

REFERENCE VALUE: (Method: Spectrophotometry)

Age	Conventional Units	SI Units (Conventional Units × 10)
Cord blood	13.5–20.7 g/dL	135–207 mmol/L
0–1 wk	15.2–23.6 g/dL	152–236 mmol/L
2–3 wk	12.7–18.7 g/dL	127–187 mmol/L
1–2 mo	9.7–17.3 g/dL	97–173 mmol/L
3–11 mo	9.3–13.3 g/dL	93–133 mmol/L
1–5 yr	10.4–13.6 g/dL	104–136 mmol/L
6–8 yr	10.9–14.5 g/dL	109–145 mmol/L
9–14 yr	11.5–15.5 g/dL	115–155 mmol/L
15 yr–adult		
Male	13.2–17.3 g/dL	132–173 mmol/L
Female	11.7–15.5 g/dL	117–155 mmol/L
Older adult		
Male	12.6–17.4 g/dL	126–174 mmol/L
Female	11.7–16.1 g/dL	117–161 mmol/L

DESCRIPTION: Hemoglobin (Hgb) is the main intracellular protein of erythrocytes. It carries oxygen (O_2) to and removes carbon dioxide (CO_2) from red blood cells (RBCs). It also serves as a buffer to maintain acid-base balance in the extracellular fluid. Each Hgb molecule consists of heme and globulin. Copper is a cofactor necessary for the enzymatic incorporation of iron molecules into heme. Heme contains iron and porphyrin molecules that have a high affinity for O_2. The affinity of Hgb molecules for O_2 is influenced by 2,3-diphosphoglycerate (2,3-DPG), a substance produced by anaerobic glycolysis to generate energy for the RBCs. When Hgb binds with 2,3-DPG, O_2 affinity decreases. The ability of Hgb to bind and release O_2 can be graphically represented by an oxyhemoglobin dissociation curve. The term *shift to the left* describes an increase in the affinity of Hgb for O_2. Conditions that can cause this leftward shift include decreased body temperature, decreased 2,3-DPG, decreased CO_2 concentration, and increased pH. Conversely, a *shift to the right* represents a decrease in the affinity of Hgb for O_2. Conditions that can cause a rightward shift include increased body temperature, increased 2,3-DPG levels, increased CO_2 concentration, and decreased pH.

Hgb levels are a direct reflection of the O_2-combining capacity of the blood. It is the combination of heme and O_2 that gives blood its characteristic red color. RBC counts parallel the O_2-combining capacity of Hgb, but because some RBCs contain more Hgb than others, the relationship is not directly proportional. As CO_2 diffuses into RBCs, an enzyme called carbonic anhydrase converts the CO_2 into bicarbonate and hydrogen ions. Hgb that is not bound to O_2 combines with the free hydrogen ions, increasing pH. As this binding is occurring, bicarbonate is leaving the RBC in exchange for chloride ions. (For additional information about the relationship between the respiratory and renal components of this buffer system, see monograph titled "Blood Gases.")

Hgb is included in the complete blood count (CBC) and generally performed with a hematocrit (Hct). These levels parallel each other and are frequently used to evaluate anemia. *Polycythemia* is a condition resulting from an abnormal increase in Hgb, Hct, and RBC count. *Anemia* is a condition resulting from an abnormal decrease in Hgb, Hct, and RBC count. Results of the Hgb, Hct, and RBC count should be evaluated simultaneously because the same underlying conditions affect this triad of tests similarly. The RBC count multiplied by 3 should approximate the Hgb concentration. The Hct should be within three times the Hgb if the RBC population is normal in size and shape. The Hct plus 6 should approximate the first two figures of the RBC count within 3 (e.g., Hct is 40%; therefore 40 + 6 = 46, and the RBC count should be 4.6 or in the range of 4.3 to 4.9). There are some cultural variations in Hgb and Hct (H&H) values. After the first decade of life, the mean Hgb in African Americans is 0.5 to 1.0 g lower than in whites. Mexican Americans and Asian Americans have higher Hgb and H&H values than whites.

INDICATIONS

- Detect hematological disorder, neoplasm, or immunological abnormality
- Determine the presence of hereditary hematological abnormality
- Evaluate known or suspected anemia and related treatment, in combination with Hct
- Monitor blood loss and response to blood replacement, in combination with Hct
- Monitor the effects of physical or emotional stress on the patient
- Monitor fluid imbalances or their treatment
- Monitor hematological status during pregnancy, in combination with Hct
- Monitor the progression of nonhematological disorders, such as chronic obstructive pulmonary disease (COPD), malabsorption syndromes, cancer, and renal disease
- Monitor response to drugs or chemotherapy and evaluate undesired reactions to drugs that may cause blood dyscrasias
- Provide screening as part of a CBC in a general physical examination, especially upon admission to a health care facility or before surgery

POTENTIAL DIAGNOSIS

Increased in
- Burns *(related to dehydration; total blood volume is decreased, but RBC count remains the same)*
- Congestive heart failure *(when the underlying cause is anemia, the body will respond by increasing production of RBCs; with a responding increase in Hct)*
- COPD *(related to chronic hypoxia that stimulates production of RBCs and a corresponding increase in Hgb)*

- Dehydration *(total blood volume is decreased, but RBC count remains the same)*
- Erythrocytosis *(total blood volume remains the same, but RBC count is increased)*
- Hemoconcentration *(same effect as seen in dehydration)*
- High altitudes *(related to hypoxia that stimulates production of RBCs and therefore increases Hgb)*
- Polycythemia vera *(abnormal bone marrow response resulting in overproduction of RBCs)*
- Shock

Decreased in
- Anemias *(overall decrease in RBCs and corresponding decrease in Hgb)*
- Blood loss (acute and chronic) *(overall decrease in RBC and corresponding decrease in Hct)*
- Bone marrow hyperplasia *(bone marrow failure that results in decreased RBC production)*
- Carcinoma *(anemia is often associated with chronic disease)*
- Cirrhosis *(related to accumulation of fluid)*
- Chronic disease *(anemia is often associated with chronic disease)*
- Fluid retention *(dilutional effect of increased blood volume while RBC count remains stable)*
- Hemoglobinopathies *(reduced RBC survival with corresponding decrease in Hgb)*
- Hemolytic disorders (e.g. hemolytic anemias, prosthetic valves) *(reduced RBC survival with corresponding decrease in Hct)*
- Hemorrhage (acute and chronic) *(overall decrease in RBCs and corresponding decrease in Hgb)*

- Hodgkin's disease *(bone marrow failure that results in decreased RBC production)*
- Incompatible blood transfusion *(reduced RBC survival with corresponding decrease in Hgb)*
- Intravenous overload *(dilutional effect)*
- Leukemia *(bone marrow failure that results in decreased RBC production)*
- Lymphomas *(bone marrow failure that results in decreased RBC production)*
- Nutritional deficit *(anemia related to dietary deficiency in iron, vitamins, folate needed to produce sufficient RBCs; decreased RBC count with corresponding decrease in Hgb)*
- Pregnancy *(related to anemia)*
- Renal disease *(related to decreased levels of erythropoietin, which stimulates production of RBCs)*
- Splenomegaly *(total blood volume remains the same, but spleen retains RBCs and Hgb reflects decreased RBC count)*

CRITICAL FINDINGS
- Less than 6.0 g/dL
- Greater than 18.0 g/dL

Note and immediately report to the health-care provider (HCP) any critically increased or decreased values and related symptoms.

Low Hgb leads to anemia. Anemia can be caused by blood loss, decreased blood cell production, increased blood cell destruction, and hemodilution. Causes of blood loss include menstrual excess or frequency, gastrointestinal bleeding, inflammatory bowel disease, and hematuria. Decreased blood cell production can be caused by folic acid deficiency, vitamin B_{12} deficiency, iron deficiency, and chronic disease. Increased blood cell destruction can be caused by a hemolytic reaction, chemical reaction, medication reaction, and sickle cell disease. Hemodilution can be caused by congestive heart failure, renal failure, polydipsia, and overhydration. Symptoms of anemia (due to these causes) include anxiety, dyspnea, edema, fatigue, hypertension, hypotension, hypoxia, jugular venous distention, pallor, rales, restlessness, and weakness. Treatment of anemia depends on the cause.

High Hgb leads to polycythemia. Polycythemia can be caused by dehydration, decreased oxygen levels in the body, and an overproduction of RBCs by the bone marrow. Dehydration from diuretic use, vomiting, diarrhea, excessive sweating, severe burns, or decreased fluid intake decreases the plasma component of whole blood, thereby increasing the ratio of RBCs to plasma, and leads to a higher than normal Hgb. Causes of decreased oxygen include smoking, exposure to carbon monoxide, high altitude, and chronic lung disease, which leads to a mild hemoconcentration of blood in the body to carry more oxygen to the body's tissues. An overproduction of RBCs by the bone marrow leads to polycythemia vera, which is a rare chronic myeloproliferative disorder that leads to a severe hemoconcentration of blood. Severe hemoconcentration can lead to thrombosis (spontaneous blood clotting). Symptoms of hemoconcentration include decreased pulse pressure and volume, loss of skin turgor, dry mucous membranes, headaches, hepatomegaly, low central venous pressure, orthostatic hypotension, pruritis (especially after a hot bath), splenomegaly, tachycardia, thirst, tinnitus, vertigo, and weakness. Treatment of polycythemia depends on the cause. Possible interventions for hemoconcentration due to dehydration include intravenous fluids and discontinuance of diuretics if they are believed to be contributing to critically elevated Hgb. Polycythemia due to decreased oxygen states can be treated by removal of the offending substance, such as smoke or carbon monoxide. Treatment includes oxygen therapy in cases of smoke inhalation, carbon monoxide poisoning, and desaturating chronic lung disease. Symptoms of polycythemic overload crisis include signs of thrombosis, pain and redness in extremities, facial flushing, and irritability. Possible interventions for hemoconcentration due to polycythemia include therapeutic phlebotomy and intravenous fluids.

INTERFERING FACTORS

- Drugs and substances that may cause a decrease in Hgb include those that induce hemolysis due to drug sensitivity or enzyme deficiency and those that result in anemia (see monograph titled "Complete Blood Count, RBC Count").
- Some drugs may also affect Hgb values by increasing the RBC count (see monograph titled "Complete Blood Count, RBC Count").
- The results of RBC counts may vary depending on the patient's position: Hgb can decrease when the patient is recumbent as a result of hemodilution and can increase when the patient rises as a result of hemoconcentration.

- Use of the nutraceutical liver extract is strongly contraindicated in iron-storage disorders, such as hemochromatosis, because it is rich in heme (the iron-containing pigment in Hgb).
- A severe copper deficiency may result in decreased Hgb levels.
- Cold agglutinins may falsely increase the mean corpuscular Hgb concentration (MCHC) and decrease the RBC count, affecting Hgb values. This can be corrected by warming the blood or replacing the plasma with warmed saline and repeating the analysis.
- Leaving the tourniquet in place for longer than 60 sec can falsely increase Hgb levels by 2% to 5%.
- Failure to fill the tube sufficiently (i.e., tube less than three-quarters full) may yield inadequate sample volume for automated analyzers and may be a reason for specimen rejection.
- Clotted or hemolyzed specimens must be rejected for analysis.
- Care should be taken in evaluating the Hgb during the first few hours after transfusion or acute blood loss because the value may appear to be normal.
- Abnormalities in the RBC size (macrocytes, microcytes) or shape (spherocytes, sickle cells) may alter Hgb values, as in diseases and conditions including sickle cell anemia, hereditary spherocytosis, and iron deficiency.
- Lipemia will falsely increase the Hgb measurement, also affecting the mean corpuscular volume (MCV) and MCHC. This can be corrected by replacing the plasma with saline, repeating the measurement, and manually correcting the Hgb, MCH, and MCHC using specific mathematical formulas.

NURSING IMPLICATIONS AND PROCEDURE

PRETEST:

▶ Positively identify the patient using at least two unique identifiers before providing care, treatment, or services.

▶ *Patient Teaching:* Inform the patient this test can assist in evaluating the amount of hemoglobin in the blood to assist in diagnosis and monitor therapy.

▶ Obtain a history of the patient's complaints, including a list of known allergens, especially allergies or sensitivities to latex.

▶ Obtain a history of the patient's cardiovascular, gastrointestinal, hematopoietic, hepatobiliary, immune, and respiratory systems; symptoms; and results of previously performed laboratory tests and diagnostic and surgical procedures.

▶ Note any recent procedures that can interfere with test results.

▶ Obtain a list of the patient's current medications, including herbs, nutritional supplements, and nutraceuticals (see Appendix F).

▶ Review the procedure with the patient. Inform the patient that specimen collection takes approximately 5 to 10 min. Address concerns about pain and explain that there may be some discomfort during the venipuncture.

▶ *Sensitivity to social and cultural issues,* as well as concern for modesty, is important in providing psychological support before, during, and after the procedure.

▶ There are no food, fluid, or medication restrictions unless by medical direction.

INTRATEST:

▶ If the patient has a history of allergic reaction to latex, avoid the use of equipment containing latex.

▶ Instruct the patient to cooperate fully and to follow directions. Direct the patient to breathe normally and to avoid unnecessary movement.

Observe standard precautions, and follow the general guidelines in Appendix A. Positively identify the patient, and label the appropriate tubes with the corresponding patient demographics, date, and time of collection. Perform a venipuncture; collect the specimen in a 5-mL lavender-top (EDTA) tube. An EDTA Microtainer sample may be obtained from infants, children, and adults for whom venipuncture may not be feasible. The specimen should be mixed gently by inverting the tube 10 times. The specimen should be analyzed within 24 hr when stored at room temperature or within 48 hr if stored at refrigerated temperature. If it is anticipated the specimen will not be analyzed within 24 hr, two blood smears should be made immediately after the venipuncture and submitted with the blood sample. Smears made from specimens older than 24 hr may contain an unacceptable number of misleading artifactual abnormalities of the RBCs, such as echinocytes and spherocytes, as well as necrobiotic white blood cells.

Remove the needle and apply direct pressure with dry gauze to stop bleeding. Observe/assess venipuncture site for bleeding or hematoma formation and secure gauze with adhesive bandage.

Promptly transport the specimen to the laboratory for processing and analysis.

POST-TEST:

A report of the results will be sent to the requesting HCP, who will discuss the results with the patient.

Nutritional Considerations: Nutritional therapy may be indicated for patients with decreased Hgb. Iron deficiency is the most common nutrient deficiency in the United States. Patients at risk (e.g., children, pregnant women and women of childbearing age, low-income populations) should be instructed to include in their diet foods that are high in iron, such as meats (especially liver), eggs, grains, green leafy vegetables, and multivitamins with iron. Iron absorption is affected by numerous factors (see monograph titled "Iron").

Reinforce information given by the patient's HCP regarding further testing, treatment, or referral to another HCP. Answer any questions or address any concerns voiced by the patient or family.

Depending on the results of this procedure, additional testing may be performed to evaluate or monitor progression of the disease process and determine the need for a change in therapy. Evaluate test results in relation to the patient's symptoms and other tests performed.

RELATED MONOGRAPHS:

Related tests include biopsy bone marrow, biopsy lymph node, biopsy kidney, blood groups and antibodies, CBC, CBC hematocrit, Coomb's antiglobulin, CT thoracic, erythropoietin, fecal analysis (occult blood), ferritin, gallium scan, haptoglobin, hemoglobin electrophoresis, iron/TIBC, lymphangiogram, Meckel's diverticulum scan, reticulocyte count, and sickle cell screen.

Refer to the Cardiovascular, Gastrointestinal, Hematopoietic, Hepatobiliary, Immune, and Respiratory systems tables at the end of the book for related tests by body system.

Complete Blood Count, Platelet Count

SYNONYM/ACRONYM: Thrombocytes.

COMMON USE: To assist in diagnosing and evaluating treatment for blood disorders such as thrombocytosis and thrombocytopenia and to evaluate preprocedure or preoperative coagulation status.

SPECIMEN: Whole blood from one full lavender-top (EDTA) tube.

REFERENCE VALUE: (Method: Automated, computerized multichannel analyzers that sort and size cells on the basis of changes in either electrical impedance or light pulses as the cells pass in front of a laser)

Age	Platelet Count*	SI Units (Conventional Units × 10⁶)	MPV (fL)
Newborn–11 mo	150–350 × 10³/mm³ or 150,000–350,000/mm³	150–350 × 10⁹/L	7.0–10.2
1–5 yr	217–497 × 10³/mm³ or 217,000–497,000/mm³	217–497 × 10⁹/L	7.2–10.0
Adult and older adult	150–450 × 10³/mm³ or 150,000–450,000/mm³	150–450 × 10⁹/L	7.0–10.2

Note: Platelet counts may decrease slightly with age.
*Conventional units.
MPV = mean platelet volume.

DESCRIPTION: *Platelets* are non-nucleated, cytoplasmic, round or oval disks formed by budding off of large, multinucleated cells (megakaryocytes). Platelets have an essential function in coagulation, hemostasis, and blood thrombus formation. *Thrombocytosis* is an increase in platelet count. In reactive thrombocytosis, the increase is transient and short-lived, and it usually does not pose a health risk. One exception may be reactive thrombocytosis occurring after coronary bypass surgery. This circumstance has been identified as an important risk factor for postoperative infarction and thrombosis. The term *thrombocythemia* describes platelet increases associated with chronic myeloproliferative disorders; *thrombocytopenia* describes platelet counts of less than 140 × 10³/mm³. Decreased platelet counts occur whenever the body's need for platelets exceeds the rate of platelet production; this circumstance will arise if production rate decreases or platelet loss increases. The severity of bleeding is related to platelet count as well as platelet function. Platelet counts can be within normal limits, but the patient may exhibit signs of internal bleeding; this circumstance usually indicates an anomaly in platelet function. Abnormal findings by automated cell counters may indicate the need to review a smear of peripheral blood for platelet estimate. Abnormally large or giant platelets may result in underestimation of automated counts by 30% to 50%. A large discrepancy between the automated count and the estimate requires that a manual count be performed. Platelet clumping may result in the underestimation of the platelet count. Clumping may be detected by the automated cell counter or upon microscopic review of a blood smear. A citrated platelet count, performed on a specimen collected in a blue-top tube, can be performed to obtain an accurate platelet count from patients who demonstrate platelet clumping in EDTA-preserved samples.

The significance of platelet sizing is becoming more widely known, as modern cell counters are capable of reporting platelet indexes that are analogous to red blood cell (RBC) indices. Platelet size, reflected by mean platelet volume (MPV), and cellular age are inversely related; that is, younger platelets tend to be larger. An increase in MPV indicates an increase in platelet turnover. Therefore, in a healthy patient, the platelet count and MPV have an inverse relationship. Abnormal platelet size may also indicate the presence of a disorder. MPV and platelet distribution width (PDW) are both increased in idiopathic thrombocytopenic purpura. MPV is also increased in May-Hegglin

anomaly, Bernard-Soulier syndrome, myeloproliferative disorders, hyperthyroidism, and pre-eclampsia. MPV is decreased in Wiskott-Aldrich syndrome, septic thrombocytopenia, and hypersplenism.

Medications like clopidogrel (Plavix) and aspirin have antiplatelet effects and are prescribed to prevent heart attack, stroke, and blockage of coronary stents. Studies have confirmed that up to 30% of patients receiving these medications may be nonresponsive. Tests to assess platelet function can provide information that confirms platelet response. Platelet response testing helps ensure alternative or additional platelet therapy is instituted, if necessary. The test results can also be used preoperatively to determine whether antiplatelet medications have been sufficiently cleared from the patient's circulation such that surgery can safely be performed without risk of excessive bleeding.

INDICATIONS

- Confirm an elevated platelet count (thrombocytosis), which can cause increased clotting
- Confirm a low platelet count (thrombocytopenia), which can be associated with bleeding
- Identify the possible cause of abnormal bleeding, such as epistaxis, hematoma, gingival bleeding, hematuria, and menorrhagia
- Provide screening as part of a complete blood count (CBC) in a general physical examination, especially upon admission to a healthcare facility or before surgery

POTENTIAL DIAGNOSIS

Increased in

Conditions that involve inflammation activate and increase the number of circulating platelets:

- Acute infections
- After exercise (transient)
- Anemias (posthemorrhagic, hemolytic, iron-deficiency) *(bone marrow response to anemia; platelet formation is unaffected by iron deficiency)*
- Chronic heart disease
- Cirrhosis
- Essential thrombocythemia
- Leukemias (chronic)
- Malignancies (carcinoma, Hodgkin's, lymphomas)
- Pancreatitis (chronic)
- Polycythemia vera *(hyperplastic bone marrow response in all cell lines)*
- Rebound recovery from thrombocytopenia *(initial response)*
- Rheumatic fever (acute)
- Rheumatoid arthritis
- Splenectomy (2 mo postprocedure) *(normal function of the spleen is to cull aging cells from the blood; without the spleen, the count increases)*
- Surgery (2 wk postprocedure)
- Trauma
- Tuberculosis
- Ulcerative colitis

Decreased in

Decreased in (as a result of megakaryocytic hypoproliferation)
- Alcohol toxicity
- Aplastic anemia
- Congenital states (Fanconi's syndrome, May-Hegglin anomaly, Bernard-Soulier syndrome, Wiskott-Aldrich syndrome, Gaucher's disease, Chédiak-Higashi syndrome)
- Drug toxicity
- Prolonged hypoxia

Decreased in (as a result of ineffective thrombopoiesis)
- Ethanol abuse without malnutrition
- Iron-deficiency anemia
- Megaloblastic anemia (B_{12}/folate deficiency)
- Paroxysmal nocturnal hemoglobinuria
- Thrombopoietin deficiency
- Viral infection

Decreased in (as a result of bone marrow replacement)
- Lymphoma
- Granulomatous infections
- Metastatic carcinoma
- Myelofibrosis

Increased in

Increased destruction in (as a result of increased loss/consumption)
- Contact with foreign surfaces (dialysis membranes, artificial organs, grafts, prosthetic devices)
- Disseminated intravascular coagulation
- Extensive transfusion
- Severe hemorrhage
- Thrombotic thrombocytopenic purpura
- Uremia

Increased destruction in (as a result of immune reaction)
- Antibody/human leukocyte antigen reactions
- Hemolytic disease of the newborn *(target is platelets instead of RBCs)*
- Idiopathic thrombocytopenic purpura
- Refractory reaction to platelet transfusion

Increased destruction in (as a result of immune reaction secondary to infection)
- Bacterial infections
- Burns

- Congenital infections (cytomegalovirus, herpes, syphilis, toxoplasmosis)
- Histoplasmosis
- Malaria
- Rocky Mountain spotted fever

Increased destruction in (as a result of other causes)
- Radiation
- Splenomegaly caused by liver disease

CRITICAL FINDINGS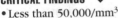
- Less than 50,000/mm³
- Greater than 1,000,000/mm³

Note and immediately report to the health-care provider (HCP) any critically increased or decreased values and related symptoms. Possible interventions for decreased platelet count may include transfusion of platelets.

INTERFERING FACTORS
- Drugs that may decrease platelet counts include acetohexamide, acetophenazine, amphotericin B, antazoline, anticonvulsants, antimony compounds, apronalide, arsenicals, azathioprine, barbiturates, benzene, busulfan, butaperazine, chlordane, chlorophenothane, chlortetracycline, dactinomycin, dextromethorphan, diethylstilbestrol, ethinamate, ethoxzolamide, floxuridine, hexachlorobenzene, hydantoin derivatives, hydroflumethiazide, hydroxychloroquine, iproniazid, mechlorethamine, mefenamic acid, mepazine, miconazole, mitomycin, nitrofurantoin, novobiocin, nystatin, phenolphthalein, phenothiazine, pipamazine, plicamycin, procarbazine, pyrazolones, streptomycin, sulfonamides, tetracycline, thiabendazole, thiouracil, tolazamide, tolazoline, tolbutamide, trifluoperazine, and urethane.

- Drugs that may increase platelet counts include glucocorticoids.
- X-ray therapy may also decrease platelet counts.
- The results of blood counts may vary depending on the patient's position. Platelet counts can decrease when the patient is recumbent, as a result of hemodilution, and can increase when the patient rises, as a result of hemoconcentration.
- Platelet counts normally increase under a variety of stressors, such as high altitudes or strenuous exercise.
- Platelet counts are normally decreased before menstruation and during pregnancy.
- Leaving the tourniquet in place for longer than 60 sec can affect the results.
- Traumatic venipunctures may lead to erroneous results as a result of activation of the coagulation sequence.
- Failure to fill the tube sufficiently (i.e., tube less than three-quarters full) may yield inadequate sample volume for automated analyzers and may be a reason for specimen rejection.
- Hemolysis or clotted specimens are reasons for rejection.
- CBC should be carefully evaluated after transfusion or acute blood loss because the value may appear to be normal.
- A white blood cell count greater than 100 × 10³/mm³, severe RBC fragmentation, and extraneous particles in the fluid used to dilute the sample can alter test results.

NURSING IMPLICATIONS AND PROCEDURE

PRETEST:
▶ Positively identify the patient using at least two unique identifiers

before providing care, treatment, or services.

- *Patient Teaching:* Inform the patient this test can assist in diagnosing, evaluating, and monitoring bleeding disorders.
- Obtain a history of the patient's complaints, including a list of known allergens, especially allergies or sensitivities to latex.
- Obtain a history of the patient's hematopoietic and immune systems, especially any bleeding disorders and other symptoms, as well as results of previously performed laboratory tests and diagnostic and surgical procedures.
- Note any recent procedures that can interfere with test results.
- Obtain a list of the patient's current medications, including anticoagulants, aspirin and other salicylates, herbs, nutritional supplements, and nutraceuticals (see Appendix F).
- Review the procedure with the patient. Inform the patient that specimen collection takes approximately 5 to 10 min. Address concerns about pain and explain that there may be some discomfort during the venipuncture.
- *Sensitivity to social and cultural issues,* as well as concern for modesty, is important in providing psychological support before, during, and after the procedure.
- There are no food, fluid, or medication restrictions unless by medical direction.

INTRATEST:

- If the patient has a history of allergic reaction to latex, avoid the use of equipment containing latex.
- Instruct the patient to cooperate fully and to follow directions. Direct the patient to breathe normally and to avoid unnecessary movement.
- Observe standard precautions, and follow the general guidelines in Appendix A. Positively identify the patient, and label the appropriate tubes with the corresponding patient demographics, date, and time of collection. Perform a venipuncture. The specimen should be mixed gently by inverting the tube 10 times. The specimen should be analyzed within 24 hr when stored at room temperature or within 48 hr if stored at refrigerated temperature. If it is anticipated the specimen will not be analyzed within 24 hr, two blood smears should be made immediately after the venipuncture and submitted with the blood sample.
- Remove the needle and apply direct pressure with dry gauze to stop bleeding. Observe/assess venipuncture site for bleeding or hematoma formation and secure gauze with adhesive bandage.
- Promptly transport the specimen to the laboratory for processing and analysis.

POST-TEST:

- A report of the results will be sent to the requesting HCP, who will discuss the results with the patient.
- Instruct the patient to report bleeding from any areas of the skin or mucous membranes.
- Inform the patient with a decreased platelet count of the importance of taking precautions against bruising and bleeding, including the use of a soft bristle toothbrush, use of an electric razor, avoidance of constipation, avoidance of acetylsalicylic acid and similar products, and avoidance of intramuscular injections.
- Inform the patient of the importance of periodic laboratory testing if he or she is taking an anticoagulant.
- *Nutritional Considerations:* Instruct patients to consume a variety of foods within the basic food groups, maintain a healthy weight, be physically active, limit salt intake, limit alcohol intake, and avoid the use of tobacco.
- Recognize anxiety related to test results. Discuss the implications of abnormal test results on the patient's lifestyle. Provide teaching and information regarding the clinical implications of the test results, as appropriate.

▶ Reinforce information given by the patient's HCP regarding further testing, treatment, or referral to another HCP. Answer any questions or address any concerns voiced by the patient or family.

▶ Depending on the results of this procedure, additional testing may be performed to evaluate or monitor progression of the disease process and determine the need for a change in therapy. Evaluate test results in relation to the patient's symptoms and other tests performed.

RELATED MONOGRAPHS:

▶ Related tests include antiarrhythmic drugs (quinidine), biopsy bone marrow, bleeding time, blood groups and antibodies, clot retraction, coagulation factors, CBC, CBC RBC morphology and inclusions, CBC WBC count and differential, CT angiography, CT brain, FDP, fibrinogen, PTT, platelet antibodies, PT/INR, and US pelvis.

▶ Refer to the Hematopoietic and Immune systems tables at the end of the book for related tests by body system.

Complete Blood Count, RBC Count

SYNONYM/ACRONYM: RBC.

COMMON USE: To evaluate the number of circulating red cells in the blood to assist in diagnosing disease and monitor therapeutic treatment. Variations in the number of cells is most often seen in anemias, cancer, and hemorrhage.

SPECIMEN: Whole blood (1 mL) collected in a lavender-top (EDTA) tube.

REFERENCE VALUE: (Method: Automated, computerized, multichannel analyzers that sort and size cells on the basis of changes in either electrical impedance or light pulses as the cells pass in front of a laser)

Age	Conventional Units (10^6 cells/mm^3)	SI Units (10^{12} cells/L) (Conventional Units × 1)
Cord blood	3.60–5.80	3.60–5.80
0–1 wk	4.50–7.00	4.50–7.00
2–3 wk	3.70–6.10	3.70–6.10
1–2 mo	3.10–5.10	3.10–5.10
3–11 mo	3.00–5.00	3.00–5.00
1–5 yr	3.80–5.00	3.80–5.00
6–8 yr	3.90–5.10	3.90–5.10
9–14 yr	3.90–5.60	3.90–5.60
15 yr–adult		
Male	5.20–5.80	5.20–5.80
Female	3.90–5.10	3.90–5.10

Age	Conventional Units (10^6 cells/mm^3)	SI Units (10^{12} cells/L) (Conventional Units × 1)
Older adult		
Male	3.80–5.80	3.80–5.80
Female	3.70–5.30	3.70–5.30

DESCRIPTION: A component of the complete blood count (CBC), the red blood cell (RBC) count determines the number of RBCs per cubic millimeters (expressed as the number of RBCs per liter of blood according to the international system of units [SI]). Because RBCs contain hemoglobin (Hgb), which is responsible for the transport and exchange of oxygen, the number of circulating RBCs is important. Although the life span of the normal RBC is 120 days, other factors besides cell age and decreased production can cause decreased values; examples are abnormal destruction due to intravascular trauma caused by atherosclerosis or due to an enlarged spleen caused by leukemia. The main sites of RBC production in healthy adults include the bone marrow of the vertebrae, pelvis, ribs, sternum, skull, and proximal ends of the femur and humerus. The main sites of RBC destruction are the spleen and liver. Erythropoietin, a hormone produced by the kidneys, regulates RBC production. Normal RBC development and function are also dependent on adequate levels of vitamin B$_{12}$, folic acid, and iron. A deficiency in vitamin E (a-tocopherol), which is needed to protect the RBC membrane from oxidizers, can result in increased cellular destruction. *Polycythemia* is a condition resulting from an abnormal increase in Hgb, hematocrit (Hct), and RBC count. *Anemia* is a condition resulting from an abnormal decrease in Hgb, Hct, and RBC count. Results of the Hgb, Hct, and RBC count should be evaluated simultaneously because the same underlying conditions affect this triad of tests similarly. The RBC count multiplied by 3 should approximate the Hgb concentration. The Hct should be within three times the Hgb if the RBC population is normal in size and shape. The Hct plus 6 should approximate the first two figures of the RBC count within 3 (e.g., Hct is 40%; therefore 40 + 6 = 46, and the RBC count should be 4.6 or in the range 4.3 to 4.9). (See monographs titled "CBC Hematocrit," "CBC Hemoglobin," and "CBC RBC Indices.")

INDICATIONS

- Detect a hematological disorder involving RBC destruction (e.g., hemolytic anemia)
- Determine the presence of hereditary hematological abnormality
- Monitor the effects of acute or chronic blood loss
- Monitor the effects of physical or emotional stress on the patient
- Monitor patients with disorders associated with elevated erythrocyte counts (e.g., polycythemia vera, chronic obstructive pulmonary disease [COPD])
- Monitor the progression of non-hematological disorders associated with elevated erythrocyte counts,

such as COPD, liver disease, hypothyroidism, adrenal dysfunction, bone marrow failure, malabsorption syndromes, cancer, and renal disease

• Monitor the response to drugs or chemotherapy and evaluate undesired reactions to drugs that may cause blood dyscrasias

• Provide screening as part of a CBC in a general physical examination, especially upon admission to a health care facility or before surgery

POTENTIAL DIAGNOSIS

Increased in

• Anxiety or stress *(related to physiological response)*

• Bone marrow failure *(initial response is stimulation of RBC production)*

• COPD with hypoxia and secondary polycythemia *(related to chronic hypoxia that stimulates production of RBCs and a corresponding increase in RBCs)*

• Dehydration with hemoconcentration *(related to decrease in total blood volume relative to unchanged RBC count)*

• Erythremic erythrocytosis *(related to unchanged total blood volume relative to increase in RBC count)*

• High altitude *(related to hypoxia that stimulates production of RBCs)*

• Polycythemia vera *(related to abnormal bone marrow response resulting in overproduction of RBCs)*

Decreased in

• Chemotherapy *(related to reduced RBC survival)*

• Chronic inflammatory diseases *(related to anemia of chronic disease)*

• Hemoglobinopathy *(related to reduced RBC survival)*

• Hemolytic anemia *(related to reduced RBC survival)*

• Hemorrhage *(related to overall decrease in RBC count)*

• Hodgkin's disease *(evidenced by bone marrow failure that results in decreased RBC production)*

• Leukemia *(evidenced by bone marrow failure that results in decreased RBC production)*

• Multiple myeloma *(evidenced by bone marrow failure that results in decreased RBC production)*

• Nutritional deficit *(related to deficiency of iron or vitamins required for RBC production and/or maturation)*

• Overhydration *(related to increase in blood volume relative to unchanged RBC count)*

• Pregnancy *(related to anemia; normal dilutional effect)*

• Renal disease *(related to decreased production of erythropoietin)*

• Subacute endocarditis

CRITICAL FINDINGS ◈

The presence of abnormal cells, other morphological characteristics, or cellular inclusions may signify a potentially life-threatening or serious health condition and should be investigated. Examples are the presence of sickle cells, moderate numbers of spherocytes, marked schistocytosis, oval macrocytes, basophilic stippling, nucleated RBCs (if the patient is not an infant), or malarial organisms.

Note and immediately report to the health-care provider (HCP) any critically increased or decreased values and related symptoms.

Low RBC count leads to anemia. Anemia can be caused by blood loss, decreased blood cell production, increased blood cell destruction, or hemodilution. Causes of blood loss include menstrual excess or frequency, gastrointestinal bleeding, inflammatory bowel disease, or hematuria. Decreased blood cell production can be caused by folic acid deficiency, vitamin B_{12} deficiency, iron deficiency, or chronic disease. Increased blood cell destruction can be caused by a hemolytic reaction, chemical reaction, medication reaction, or sickle cell disease. Hemodilution can be caused by congestive heart failure, renal failure, polydipsia, or overhydration. Symptoms of anemia (due to these causes) include anxiety, dyspnea, edema, hypertension, hypotension, hypoxia, jugular venous distention, fatigue, pallor, rales, restlessness, and weakness. Treatment of anemia depends on the cause.

High RBC count leads to polycythemia. Polycythemia can be caused by dehydration, decreased oxygen levels in the body, and an overproduction of RBCs by the bone marrow. Dehydration by diuretic use, vomiting, diarrhea, excessive sweating, severe burns, or decreased fluid intake decreases the plasma component of whole blood, thereby increasing the ratio of RBCs to plasma, and leads to a higher than normal Hct. Causes of decreased oxygen include smoking, exposure to carbon monoxide, high altitude, and chronic lung disease, which leads to a mild hemoconcentration of blood in the body to carry more oxygen to the body's tissues. An overproduction of RBCs by the bone marrow leads to polycythemia vera, which is a rare chronic myeloproliferative disorder that leads to a severe hemoconcentration of blood. Severe hemoconcentration can lead to thrombosis (spontaneous blood clotting).

Symptoms of hemoconcentration include decreased pulse pressure and volume, loss of skin turgor, dry mucous membranes, headaches, hepatomegaly, low central venous pressure, orthostatic hypotension, pruritis (especially after a hot bath), splenomegaly, tachycardia, thirst, tinnitus, vertigo, and weakness. Treatment of polycythemia depends on the cause. Possible interventions for hemoconcentration due to dehydration include intravenous fluids and discontinuance of diuretics if they are believed to be contributing to critically elevated Hct. Polycythemia due to decreased oxygen states can be treated by removal of the offending substance, such as smoke or carbon monoxide. Treatment includes oxygen therapy in cases of smoke inhalation, carbon monoxide poisoning, and desaturating chronic lung disease. Symptoms of polycythemic overload crisis include signs of thrombosis, pain and redness in extremities, facial flushing, and irritability. Possible interventions for hemoconcentration due to polycythemia include therapeutic phlebotomy and intravenous fluids.

INTERFERING FACTORS

- Drugs and substances that may decrease RBC count by causing hemolysis resulting from drug sensitivity or enzyme deficiency include acetaminophen, aminopyrine, aminosalicylic acid, amphetamine, anticonvulsants, antipyrine, arsenicals, benzene, busulfan, carbenicillin, cephalothin, chemotherapy drugs, chlorate, chloroquine, chlorothiazide, chlorpromazine, colchicine, diphenhydramine, dipyrone, glucosulfone, gold, hydroflumethiazide, indomethacin, mephenytoin, nalidixic acid, neomycin, nitrofurantoin, penicillin, phenacemide, phenazopyridine, and phenothiazine.

- Drugs that may decrease RBC count by causing anemia include miconazole, penicillamine, phenylhydrazine, primaquine, probenecid, pyrazolones, pyrimethamine, quinines, streptomycin, sulfamethizole, sulfamethoxypyridazine, sulfisoxazole, suramin, thioridazine, tolbutamide, trimethadione, and tripelennamine.
- Drugs that may decrease RBC count by causing bone marrow suppression include ammphotericin B, floxuridine, and phenylbutazone.
- Drugs and vitamins that may increase the RBC count include glucocorticosteroids, pilocarpine, and vitamin B_{12}.
- Use of the nutraceutical liver extract is strongly contraindicated in patients with iron-storage disorders such as hemochromatosis because it is rich in heme (the iron-containing pigment in Hgb).
- Hemodilution (e.g., excessive administration of intravenous fluids, normal pregnancy) in the presence of a normal number of RBCs may lead to false decreases in RBC count.
- Cold agglutinins may falsely increase the mean corpuscular volume (MCV) and decrease the RBC count. This can be corrected by warming the blood or diluting the sample with warmed saline and repeating the analysis.
- Excessive exercise, anxiety, pain, and dehydration may cause false elevations in RBC count.
- A grossly elevated white blood cell (WBC) count (greater than $500 \times 10^3/mm^3$) will cause a falsely elevated RBC count. This can be corrected by diluting the sample with saline to obtain an accurate WBC count and then correcting the RBC mathematically.

- Care should be taken in evaluating the CBC after transfusion.
- RBC counts can vary depending on the patient's position, decreasing when the patient is recumbent as a result of hemodilution and increasing when the patient rises as a result of hemoconcentration.
- Venous stasis can falsely elevate RBC counts; therefore, the tourniquet should not be left on the arm for longer than 60 sec.
- Failure to fill the tube sufficiently (i.e., tube less than three-quarters full) may yield inadequate sample volume for automated analyzers and may be a reason for specimen rejection.
- Hemolyzed or clotted specimens must be rejected for analysis.

NURSING IMPLICATIONS AND PROCEDURE

PRETEST:

▶ Positively identify the patient using at least two unique identifiers before providing care, treatment, or services.

▶ *Patient Teaching:* Inform the patient this test can assist in assessing for anemia and disorders affecting the number of circulating RBCs.

▶ Obtain a history of the patient's complaints, including a list of known allergens, especially allergies or sensitivities to latex.

▶ Obtain a history of the patient's cardiovascular, gastrointestinal, genitourinary, hematopoietic, hepatobiliary, immune, and respiratory systems; symptoms; and results of previously performed laboratory tests and diagnostic and surgical procedures.

▶ Note any recent procedures that can interfere with test results.

▶ Obtain a list of the patient's current medications, including herbs, nutritional supplements, and nutraceuticals (see Appendix F).

▶ Review the procedure with the patient. Inform the patient that specimen collection takes approximately 5 to 10 min. Address concerns about pain and explain that there may be some discomfort during the venipuncture.

▶ *Sensitivity to social and cultural issues,* as well as concern for modesty, is important in providing psychological support before, during, and after the procedure.

▶ There are no food, fluid, or medication restrictions unless by medical direction.

INTRATEST:

▶ If the patient has a history of allergic reaction to latex, avoid the use of equipment containing latex.

▶ Instruct the patient to cooperate fully and to follow directions. Direct the patient to breathe normally and to avoid unnecessary movement.

▶ Observe standard precautions, and follow the general guidelines in Appendix A. Positively identify the patient, and label the appropriate tubes with the corresponding patient demographics, date, and time of collection. Perform a venipuncture. An EDTA Microtainer sample may be obtained from infants, children, and adults for whom venipuncture may not be feasible. The specimen should be mixed gently by inverting the tube 10 times. The specimen should be analyzed within 24 hr when stored at room temperature or within 48 hr if stored at refrigerated temperature. If it is anticipated the specimen will not be analyzed within 24 hr, two blood smears should be made immediately after the venipuncture and submitted with the blood sample. Smears made from specimens older than 24 hr will contain an unacceptable number of misleading artifactual abnormalities of the RBCs, such as echinocytes and spherocytes, as well as necrobiotic WBCs.

▶ Remove the needle and apply direct pressure with dry gauze to stop bleeding. Observe/assess venipuncture site for bleeding or hematoma formation and secure gauze with adhesive bandage.

▶ Promptly transport the specimen to the laboratory for processing and analysis.

POST-TEST:

▶ A report of the results will be sent to the requesting HCP, who will discuss the results with the patient.

▶ *Nutritional Considerations:* Nutritional therapy may be indicated for patients with decreased RBC count. Iron deficiency is the most common nutrient deficiency in the United States. Patients at risk (e.g., children, pregnant women and women of childbearing age, low-income populations) should be instructed to include foods that are high in iron in their diet, such as meats (especially liver), eggs, grains, green leafy vegetables, and multivitamins with iron. Iron absorption is affected by numerous factors (see monograph titled "Iron").

▶ *Nutritional Considerations:* Patients at risk for vitamin B_{12} or folate deficiency include those with the following conditions: malnourishment (inadequate intake), pregnancy (increased need), infancy, malabsorption syndromes (inadequate absorption/increased metabolic rate), infections, cancer, hyperthyroidism, serious burns, excessive blood loss, and gastrointestinal damage. These patients should be instructed, as appropriate, to ingest food sources rich in vitamin B_{12}, such as meats, milk, cheese, eggs, and fortified soy milk products. Sources of folate are meats (especially liver), kidney beans, beets, vegetables in the cabbage family, oranges, cantaloupe, and green leafy vegetables such as spinach, asparagus, and broccoli.

▶ *Nutritional Considerations:* A diet deficient in vitamin E puts the patient at risk for increased RBC destruction, which could lead to anemia. Nutritional therapy may be indicated for these patients. Vitamin E is found in many of the previously mentioned foods, as well as in vegetable oils and wheat germ. Supplemental vitamin E may also be taken, but the danger of toxicity should be explained to the patient. Very large supplemental doses, in excess of

600 mg of vitamin E over a period of 1 yr, may result in excess bleeding. Vitamin E is heat stable but is very negatively affected by light.
▸ Reinforce information given by the patient's HCP regarding further testing, treatment, or referral to another HCP. Answer any questions or address any concerns voiced by the patient or family.
▸ Depending on the results of this procedure, additional testing may be performed to evaluate or monitor progression of the disease process and determine the need for a change in therapy. Evaluate test results in relation to the patient's symptoms and other tests performed.

RELATED MONOGRAPHS:
▸ Related tests include biopsy bone marrow, biopsy kidney, blood groups and antibodies, CBC, CBC hematocrit, CBC hemoglobin, CBC RBC morphology and inclusions, Coomb's antiglobulin, erythropoietin, fecal analysis, ferritin, folate, gallium scan, haptoglobin, iron/TIBC, lymphangiogram, Meckel's diverticulum scan, reticulocyte count, and vitamin B_{12}.
▸ Refer to the Cardiovascular, Gastrointestinal, Genitourinary, Hematopoietic, Hepatobiliary, Immune, and Respiratory systems tables at the end of the book for related tests by body system.

Complete Blood Count, RBC Indices

SYNONYM/ACRONYM: Mean corpuscular hemoglobin (MCH), mean corpuscular volume (MCV), mean corpuscular hemoglobin concentration (MCHC), red blood cell distribution width (RDW).

COMMON USE: To evaluate cell size, shape, weight, and hemoglobin concentration. Used to diagnose and monitor therapy for diagnoses such as iron-deficiency anemia.

SPECIMEN: Whole blood (1 mL) collected in a lavender-top (EDTA) tube.

REFERENCE VALUE: (Method: Automated, computerized, multichannel analyzers that sort and size cells on the basis of changes in either electrical impedance or light pulses as the cells pass in front of a laser)

Age	MCV(fL)	MCH (pg/cell)	MCHC (g/dL)	RDW
Cord blood	107–119	35–39	31–35	14.9–18.7
0–1 wk	104–116	29–45	24–36	14.9–18.7
2–3 wk	95–117	26–38	26–34	14.9–18.7
1–2 mo	81–125	25–37	26–34	14.9–18.7
3–11 mo	78–110	22–34	26–34	14.9–18.7
1–5 yr	74–94	24–32	30–34	11.6–14.8
6–8 yr	73–93	24–32	32–36	11.6–14.8
9–14 yr	74–94	25–33	32–36	11.6–14.8

Age	MCV(fL)	MCH (pg/cell)	MCHC (g/dL)	RDW
15 yr–adult				
Male	77–97	26–34	32–36	11.6–14.8
Female	78–98	26–34	32–36	11.6–14.8
Older adult				
Male	79–103	27–35	32–36	11.6–14.8
Female	78–102	27–35	32–36	11.6–14.8

MCV = mean corpuscular volume; MCH = mean corpuscular hemoglobin; MCHC = mean corpuscular hemoglobin concentration; RDW = red blood cell distribution width.

DESCRIPTION: Red blood cell (RBC) indices provide information about the mean corpuscular volume (MCV), mean corpuscular hemoglobin (MCH), mean corpuscular hemoglobin concentration (MCHC), and RBC distribution width (RDW). The hematocrit, RBC count, and total hemoglobin tests are used to determine the RBC indices. MCV is determined by dividing the hematocrit by the total RBC count and is helpful in classifying anemias. MCH is determined by dividing the total hemoglobin concentration by the RBC count. MCHC is determined by dividing total hemoglobin by hematocrit. Hemoglobin content is indicated as normochromic, hypochromic, and hyperchromic. The RDW is a measurement of cell size distribution over the entire RBC population measured. It can indicate anisocytosis, or excessive variations in cell size. Cell size is indicated as normocytic, microcytic, and macrocytic. (See monographs titled "Complete Blood Count Hemoglobin," "Complete Blood Count Hematocrit," "Complete Blood Count RBC Count," and "Complete Blood Count Red Blood Cell Morphology and Inclusions.")

INDICATIONS

* Assist in the diagnosis of anemia
* Detect a hematological disorder, neoplasm, or immunological abnormality
* Determine the presence of a hereditary hematological abnormality
* Monitor the effects of physical or emotional stress
* Monitor the progression of nonhematological disorders such as chronic obstructive pulmonary disease, malabsorption syndromes, cancer, and renal disease
* Monitor the response to drugs or chemotherapy, and evaluate undesired reactions to drugs that may cause blood dyscrasias
* Provide screening as part of a complete blood count (CBC) in a general physical examination, especially upon admission to a health care facility or before surgery

POTENTIAL DIAGNOSIS

Increased in

MCV

* Alcoholism *(vitamin deficiency related to malnutrition)*
* Antimetabolite therapy *(the therapy inhibits vitamin B_{12} and folate)*
* Liver disease *(complex effect on RBCs that includes malnutrition, alterations in RBC shape and size, effects of chronic disease)*
* Pernicious anemia (vitamin B_{12}/folate anemia)

C

MCH

• Macrocytic anemias *(related to increased hemoglobin or cell size)*

MCHC

• Spherocytosis *(artifact in measurement caused by abnormal cell shape)*

RDW

• Anemias with heterogeneous cell size as a result of hemoglobinopathy, hemolytic anemia, anemia following acute blood loss, iron-deficiency anemia, vitamin- and folate-deficiency anemia *(related to a mixture of cell sizes as the bone marrow responds to the anemia and/or to a mixture of cell shapes due to cell fragmentation as a result of the disease)*

Decreased in

MCV

• Iron-deficiency anemia *(related to low hemoglobin)*
• Thalassemias *(related to low hemoglobin)*

MCH

• Hypochromic anemias *(related to low hemoglobin)*
• Microcytic anemias *(related to low hemoglobin)*

MCHC

• Iron-deficiency anemia *(the amount of hemoglobin in the RBC is small relative to RBC size)*

RDW: N/A

CRITICAL FINDINGS: N/A

INTERFERING FACTORS

• Drugs and substances that may decrease the MCHC include styrene (occupational exposure).
• Drugs that may decrease the MCV include nitrofurantoin.

• Drugs that may increase the MCV include colchicine, pentamidine, pyrimethamine, and triamterene.
• Drugs that may increase the MCH and MCHC include oral contraceptives (long-term use).
• Diseases that cause agglutination of RBCs will alter test results.
• Cold agglutinins may falsely increase the MCV and decrease the RBC count. This can be corrected by warming the blood or diluting the sample with warmed saline and then correcting the RBC count mathematically.
• RBC counts can vary depending on the patient's position, decreasing when the patient is recumbent as a result of hemodilution and increasing when the patient rises as a result of hemoconcentration.
• Care should be taken in evaluating the CBC after transfusion.
• Venous stasis can falsely elevate RBC counts; therefore, the tourniquet should not be left on the arm for longer than 60 sec.
• Failure to fill the tube sufficiently (i.e., tube less than three-quarters full) may yield inadequate sample volume for automated analyzers and may be a reason for specimen rejection.
• Hemolyzed or clotted specimens should be rejected.
• Lipemia and elevated white blood cell (WBC) count (greater than $50 \text{ WBC} \times 10^3/\text{mm}^3$, or $50,000/\text{mm}^3$) will falsely increase the hemoglobin measurement, also affecting the MCV and MCH.

NURSING IMPLICATIONS AND PROCEDURE

PRETEST:

▶ Positively identify the patient using at least two unique identifiers before providing care, treatment, or services.

Patient Teaching: Inform the patient this test can assist in assessing RBC shape and size.

◆ Obtain a history of the patient's complaints, including a list of known allergens especially allergies or sensitivities to latex.

◆ Obtain a history of the patient's gastrointestinal, hematopoietic, immune, and respiratory systems; symptoms; and results of previously performed laboratory tests and diagnostic and surgical procedures.

◆ Note any recent procedures that can interfere with test results.

◆ Obtain a list of the patient's current medications including herbs, nutritional supplements, and nutraceuticals (see Appendix F).

◆ Review the procedure with the patient. Inform the patient that specimen collection takes approximately 5 to 10 min. Address concerns about pain and explain that there may be some discomfort during the venipuncture.

◆ *Sensitivity to social and cultural issues,* as well as concern for modesty, is important in providing psychological support before, during, and after the procedure.

◆ There are no food, fluid, or medication restrictions unless by medical direction.

INTRATEST:

◆ If the patient has a history of allergic reaction to latex, avoid the use of equipment containing latex.

◆ Instruct the patient to cooperate fully and to follow directions. Direct the patient to breathe normally and to avoid unnecessary movement.

◆ Observe standard precautions, and follow the general guidelines in Appendix A. Positively identify the patient, and label the appropriate tubes with the corresponding patient demographics, date, and time of collection. Perform a venipuncture. An EDTA Microtainer sample may be obtained from infants, children, and adults for whom venipuncture may not be feasible. The specimen should be mixed gently by inverting the tube 10 times. The specimen should be analyzed within 24 hr when stored at room

temperature or within 48 hr if stored at refrigerated temperature. If it is anticipated the specimen will not be analyzed within 24 hr, two blood smears should be made immediately after the venipuncture and submitted with the blood sample. Smears made from specimens older than 24 hr may contain an unacceptable number of misleading artifactual abnormalities of the RBCs, such as echinocytes and spherocytes, as well as necrobiotic white blood cells.

◆ Remove the needle and apply direct pressure with dry gauze to stop bleeding. Observe/assess venipuncture site for bleeding or hematoma formation and secure gauze with adhesive bandage.

◆ Promptly transport the specimen to the laboratory for processing and analysis.

POST-TEST:

◆ A report of the results will be sent to the requesting health-care provider (HCP), who will discuss the results with the patient.

◆ Reinforce information given by the patient's HCP regarding further testing, treatment, or referral to another HCP. Answer any questions or address any concerns voiced by the patient or family.

◆ Depending on the results of this procedure, additional testing may be performed to evaluate or monitor progression of the disease process and determine the need for a change in therapy. Evaluate test results in relation to the patient's symptoms and other tests performed.

RELATED MONOGRAPHS:

◆ Related tests include biopsy bone marrow, CBC, CBC hematocrit, CBC hemoglobin, CBC RBC count, CBC RBC morphology and inclusions, CBC WBC count and differential, erythropoietin, ferritin, folate, Hgb electrophoresis, iron/TIBC, lead, reticulocyte count, sickle cell screen, and vitamin B_{12}.

◆ Refer to the Gastrointestinal, Hematopoietic, Immune, and Respiratory systems tables at the end of the book for related tests by body system.

Complete Blood Count, RBC Morphology and Inclusions

SYNONYM/ACRONYM: N/A.

COMMON USE: To make a visual evaluation of the red cell shape and/or size as a confirmation in assisting to diagnose and monitor disease progression.

SPECIMEN: Whole blood from one full lavender-top (EDTA) tube or Wright's-stained, thin-film peripheral blood smear. The laboratory should be consulted as to the necessity of thick-film smears for the evaluation of malarial inclusions.

REFERENCE VALUE: (Method: Microscopic, manual review of stained blood smear)

Red Blood Cell Morphology	Within Normal Limits	1+	2+	3+	4+
Size					
Anisocytosis	0–5+	5–10	10–20	20–50	Greater than 50
Macrocytes	0–5+	5–10	10–20	20–50	Greater than 50
Microcytes	0–5+	5–10	10–20	20–50	Greater than 50
Shape					
Poikilocytes	0–2+	3–10	10–20	20–50	Greater than 50
Burr cells	0–2+	3–10	10–20	20–50	Greater than 50
Acanthocytes	Less than 1+	2–5	5–10	10–20	Greater than 20
Schistocytes	Less than 1+	2–5	5–10	10–20	Greater than 20
Dacryocytes (teardrop cells)	0–2+	2–5	5–10	20–50	Greater than 20
Codocytes (target cells)	0–2+	2–10	10–20	20–50	Greater than 50
Spherocytes	0–2+	2–10	10–20	20–50	Greater than 50
Ovalocytes	0–2+	2–10	10–20	20–50	Greater than 50
Stomatocytes	0–2+	2–10	10–20	20–50	Greater than 50
Drepanocytes (sickle cells)	Absent	Reported as present or absent			
Helmet cells	Absent	Reported as present or absent			

Red Blood Cell Morphology	Within Normal Limits	1+	2+	3+	4+
Agglutination	Absent	Reported as present or absent			
Rouleaux	Absent	Reported as present or absent			
Hemoglobin (Hgb) Content					
Hypochromia	0–2+	3–10	10–50	50–75	Greater than 75
Polychromasia					
Adult	Less than 1+	2–5	5–10	10–20	Greater than 20
Newborn	1–6+	7–15	15–20	20–50	Greater than 50
Inclusions					
Cabot rings	Absent	Reported as present or absent			
Basophilic stippling	0–1+	1–5	5–10	10–20	Greater than 20
Howell-Jolly bodies	Absent	1–2	3–5	5–10	Greater than 10
Heinz bodies	Absent	Reported as present or absent			
Hgb C crystals	Absent	Reported as present or absent			
Pappenheimer bodies	Absent	Reported as present or absent			
Intracellular parasites (e.g., *Plasmodium, Babesia, Trypanosoma*)	Absent	Reported as present or absent			

DESCRIPTION: The decision to manually review a peripheral blood smear for abnormalities in red blood cell (RBC) shape or size is made on the basis of criteria established by the reporting laboratory. Cues in the results of the complete blood count (CBC) will point to specific abnormalities that can be confirmed visually by microscopic review of the sample on a stained blood smear.

INDICATIONS

• Assist in the diagnosis of anemia
• Detect a hematological disorder, neoplasm, or immunological abnormality

- Determine the presence of a hereditary hematological abnormality
- Monitor the effects of physical or emotional stress on the patient
- Monitor the progression of nonhematological disorders, such as chronic obstructive pulmonary disease, malabsorption syndromes, cancer, and renal disease
- Monitor the response to drugs or chemotherapy, and evaluate undesired reactions to drugs that may cause blood dyscrasias
- Provide screening as part of a CBC in a general physical examination, especially upon admission to a health-care facility or before surgery

POTENTIAL DIAGNOSIS

Red Blood Cell Size

Increased in

Cell Size
- Alcoholism
- Aplastic anemia
- Chemotherapy
- Chronic hemolytic anemia
- Grossly elevated glucose (hyperosmotic)
- Hemolytic disease of the newborn
- Hypothyroidism
- Leukemia
- Lymphoma
- Metastatic carcinoma
- Myelofibrosis
- Myeloma
- Refractory anemia
- Sideroblastic anemia
- Vitamin B_{12}/folate deficiency

Decreased in

Cell Size
- Hemoglobin C disease
- Hemolytic anemias

- Hereditary spherocytosis
- Inflammation
- Iron-deficiency anemia
- Thalassemias

Red Blood Cell Shape

Variations in cell shape are the result of hereditary conditions such as elliptocytosis, sickle cell anemia, spherocytosis, thalassemias, or hemoglobinopathies (e.g., hemoglobin C disease). Irregularities in cell shape can also result from acquired conditions, such as physical/mechanical cellular trauma, exposure to chemicals, or reactions to medications.

- Acquired spherocytosis can result from Heinz body hemolytic anemia, microangiopathic hemolytic anemia, secondary isoimmunohemolytic anemia, and transfusion of old banked blood.
- Acanthocytes are associated with acquired conditions such as alcoholic cirrhosis with hemolytic anemia, disorders of lipid metabolism, hepatitis of newborns, malabsorptive diseases, metastatic liver disease, the postsplenectomy period, and pyruvate kinase deficiency.
- Burr cells are commonly seen in acquired renal insufficiency, burns, cardiac valve disease, disseminated intravascular coagulation (DIC), hypertension, intravenous fibrin deposition, metastatic malignancy, normal neonatal period, and uremia.
- Codocytes are seen in hemoglobinopathies, iron-deficiency anemia, obstructive liver disease, and the postsplenectomy period.
- Dacryocytes are most commonly associated with metastases to the bone marrow, myelofibrosis, myeloid metaplasia, pernicious anemia, and tuberculosis.
- Schistocytes are seen in burns, cardiac valve disease, DIC,

glomerulonephritis, hemolytic anemia, microangiopathic hemolytic anemia, renal graft rejection, thrombotic thrombocytopenic purpura, uremia, and vasculitis.

Red Blood Cell Hemoglobin Content

- RBCs with a normal hemoglobin (Hgb) level have a clear central pallor and are referred to as *normochromic*.
- Cells with low Hgb and lacking in central pallor are referred to as *hypochromic*. Hypochromia is associated with iron-deficiency anemia, thalassemias, and sideroblastic anemia.
- Cells with excessive Hgb levels are referred to as *hyperchromic* even though they technically lack a central pallor. Hyperchromia is usually associated with an elevated mean corpuscular Hgb concentration as well as hemolytic anemias.
- Cells referred to as *polychromic* are young erythrocytes that still contain ribonucleic acid (RNA). The RNA is picked up by the Wright's stain. Polychromasia is indicative of premature release of RBCs from bone marrow secondary to increased erythropoietin stimulation.

Red Blood Cell Inclusions

RBC inclusions can result from certain types of anemia, abnormal Hgb precipitation, or parasitic infection.

- Cabot rings may be seen in megaloblastic and other anemias, lead poisoning, and conditions in which RBCs are destroyed before they are released from bone marrow.
- Basophilic stippling is seen whenever there is altered Hgb synthesis, as in thalassemias, megaloblastic

anemias, alcoholism, and lead or arsenic intoxication.

- Howell-Jolly bodies are seen in sickle cell anemia, other hemolytic anemias, megaloblastic anemia, congenital absence of the spleen, and the postsplenectomy period.
- Pappenheimer bodies may be seen in cases of sideroblastic anemia, thalassemias, refractory anemia, dyserythropoietic anemias, hemosiderosis, and hemochromatosis.
- Heinz bodies are most often seen in the blood of patients who have ingested drugs known to induce the formation of these inclusion bodies. They are also seen in patients with hereditary glucose-6-phosphate dehydrogenase (G6PD) deficiency.
- Hgb C crystals can often be identified in stained peripheral smears of patients with hereditary hemoglobin C disease.
- Parasites such as *Plasmodium* (transmitted by mosquitoes and causing malaria) and *Babesia* (transmitted by ticks), known to invade human RBCs, can be visualized with Wright's stain and other special stains of the peripheral blood.

CRITICAL FINDINGS ◈

Note and immediately report to the health-care provider (HCP) any critically increased or decreased values and related symptoms.

The presence of sickle cells or parasitic inclusions should be brought to the immediate attention of the requesting HCP.

INTERFERING FACTORS

- Drugs and substances that may increase Heinz body formation as an initial precursor to significant hemolysis include acetanilid, acetylsalicylic acid, aminopyrine, antimalarials, antipyretics, furadaltone, furazolidone, methylene blue, naphthalene, and nitrofurans.

• Care should be taken in evaluating the CBC after transfusion.

• Leaving the tourniquet in place for longer than 60 sec can falsely affect the results.

• Morphology can be evaluated to some extent via indices; therefore, failure to fill the tube sufficiently (i.e., tube less than three-quarters full) may yield inadequate sample volume for automated analyzers and may be a reason for specimen rejection.

• Hemolyzed or clotted specimens should be rejected.

NURSING IMPLICATIONS AND PROCEDURE

PRETEST:

▶ Positively identify the patient using at least two unique identifiers before providing care, treatment, or services.

▶ *Patient Teaching:* Inform the patient this test can assist in assessing red cell appearance.

▶ Obtain a history of the patient's complaints, including a list of known allergens, especially allergies or sensitivities to latex.

▶ Obtain a history of the patient's gastrointestinal, hematopoietic, hepatobiliary, immune, and respiratory systems; symptoms; and results of previously performed laboratory tests and diagnostic and surgical procedures.

▶ Note any recent procedures that can interfere with test results.

▶ Obtain a list of the patient's current medications, including herbs, nutritional supplements, and nutraceuticals (see Appendix F).

▶ Review the procedure with the patient. Inform the patient that specimen collection takes approximately 5 to 10 min. Address concerns about pain and explain that there may be some discomfort during the venipuncture.

▶ *Sensitivity to social and cultural issues,* as well as concern for modesty, is important in providing psychological support before, during, and after the procedure.

▶ There are no food, fluid, or medication restrictions unless by medical direction.

INTRATEST:

▶ If the patient has a history of allergic reaction to latex, avoid the use of equipment containing latex.

▶ Instruct the patient to cooperate fully and to follow directions. Direct the patient to breathe normally and to avoid unnecessary movement.

▶ Observe standard precautions, and follow the general guidelines in Appendix A. Positively identify the patient, and label the appropriate tubes with the corresponding patient demographics, date, and time of collection. Perform a venipuncture. An EDTA Microtainer sample may be obtained from infants, children, and adults for whom venipuncture may not be feasible. The specimen should be mixed gently by inverting the tube 10 times. The specimen should be analyzed within 6 hr when stored at room temperature or within 24 hr if stored at refrigerated temperature. If it is anticipated the specimen will not be analyzed within 4 to 6 hr, two blood smears should be made immediately after the venipuncture and submitted with the blood sample. Smears made from specimens older than 6 hr will contain an unacceptable number of misleading artifactual abnormalities of the RBCs, such as echinocytes and spherocytes, as well as necrobiotic white blood cells.

▶ Remove the needle and apply direct pressure with dry gauze to stop bleeding.

Observe/assess venipuncture site for bleeding or hematoma formation and secure gauze with adhesive bandage.

Promptly transport the specimen to the laboratory for processing and analysis.

POST-TEST:

A report of the results will be sent to the requesting HCP, who will discuss the results with the patient.

Nutritional Considerations: Instruct patients to consume a variety of foods within the basic food groups, maintain a healthy weight, be physically active, limit salt intake, limit alcohol intake, and avoid the use of tobacco.

Reinforce information given by the patient's HCP regarding further testing, treatment, or referral to another HCP. Answer any questions or address any concerns voiced by the patient or family.

Depending on the results of this procedure, additional testing may be performed to evaluate or monitor progression of the disease process and determine the need for a change in therapy. Evaluate test results in relation to the patient's symptoms and other tests performed.

RELATED MONOGRAPHS:

Related tests include biopsy bone marrow, CBC, CBC hematocrit, CBC hemoglobin, CBC platelet count, CBC RBC count, CBC RBC indices, CBC WBC count with differential, δ-aminolevulinic acid, erythropoietin, ferritin, G6PD, hemoglobin electrophoresis, iron/TIBC, lead, and reticulocyte count.

Refer to the Gastrointestinal, Hematopoietic, Hepatobiliary, Immune, and Respiratory systems tables at the end of the book for related tests by body system.

Complete Blood Count, WBC Count and Differential

SYNONYM/ACRONYM: WBC with diff, leukocyte count, white cell count.

COMMON USE: To evaluate viral and bacterial infections and to assist in diagnosing and monitoring leukemic disorders.

SPECIMEN: Whole blood from one full lavender-top (EDTA) tube.

REFERENCE VALUE: (Method: Automated, computerized, multichannel analyzers that sort and size cells on the basis of changes in either electrical impedance or light pulses as the cells pass in front of a laser.) Many analyzers can determine a five-part WBC differential. The WBC count and differential enumerates and identifies granulocytes, lymphocytes, monocytes, eosinophils, and basophils. (See "White Blood Cell Count and Cell Differential" monograph for more detailed information.)

White Blood Cell Count and Differential

Age	Conventional Units WBC × 10³/mm³*	Neutrophils			Lymphocytes	Monocytes	Eosinophils	Basophils
		Total Neutrophils (Absolute) and %	Bands (Absolute) and %	Segments (Absolute) and %	(Absolute) and %	(Absolute) and %	(Absolute) and %	(Absolute) and %
Birth	9.0–30.0	(5.5–18.3) 61%	(0.8–2.7) 9.1%	(4.7–15.6) 52%	(2.8–9.3) 31%	(0.5–1.7) 5.8%	(0.02–0.7) 2.2%	(0.1–0.2) 0.6%
1–23 mo	6.0–17.5	(1.9–5.4) 31%	(0.2–0.5) 3.1%	(1.7–4.9) 28%	(3.7–10.7) 61%	(0.3–0.8) 4.8%	(0.2–0.5) 2.6%	(0–0.1) 0.5%
2–10 yr	4.5–13.5	(2.4–7.3) 54%	(0.1–0.4) 3.0%	(2.3–6.9) 51%	(1.7–5.1) 38%	(0.2–0.6) 4.3%	(0.1–0.3) 2.4%	(0–0.1) 0.5%
11 yr–older adult	4.5–11.0	(2.7–6.5) 59%	(0.1–0.3) 3.0%	(2.5–6.2) 56%	(1.5–3.7) 34%	(0.2–0.4) 4.0%	(0.05–0.5) 2.7%	(0–0.1) 0.5%

*SI Units (Conventional Units × 1 × 10⁹/L or WBC × 1,000/mm³).

DESCRIPTION: White blood cells (WBCs) constitute the body's primary defense system against foreign organisms, tissues, and other substances. The life span of a normal WBC is 13 to 20 days. Old WBCs are destroyed by the lymphatic system and excreted in the feces. Reference values for WBC counts vary significantly with age. WBC counts vary diurnally, with counts being lowest in the morning and highest in the late afternoon. Other variables such as stress and high levels of activity or physical exercise can trigger transient increases of 2,000 to 5,000 mm^3. The main WBC types are neutrophils (band and segmented neutrophils), eosinophils, basophils, monocytes, and lymphocytes. WBCs are produced in the bone marrow. B-cell lymphocytes remain in the bone marrow to mature. T-cell lymphocytes migrate to and mature in the thymus. The WBC count can be performed alone with the differential cell count or as part of the complete blood count (CBC). The WBC differential can be performed by an automated instrument or manually on a slide prepared from a stained peripheral blood sample. Automated instruments provide excellent, reliable information, but the accuracy of the WBC count can be affected by the presence of circulating nucleated red blood cells (RBCs), clumped platelets, fibrin strands, cold agglutinins, cryoglubulins, intracellular parasitic organisms, or other significant blood cell inclusions and may not be identified in the interpretation of an automated blood count. The decision to report a manual or automated differential is based on specific criteria established by the laboratory. The criteria are designed to identify findings that warrant further investigation or confirmation by manual review. An increased WBC count is termed *leukocytosis,* and a decreased WBC count is termed *leukopenia.* A total WBC count indicates the degree of response to a pathological process, but a more complete evaluation for specific diagnoses for any one disorder is provided by the differential count. The WBCs in the count and differential are reported as an *absolute value* and as a percentage. The relative percentages of cell types are arrived at by basing the enumeration of each cell type on a 100-cell count. The absolute value is obtained by multiplying the relative percentage value of each cell type by the total WBC count. For example, on a CBC report, with a total WBC of 9×10^9 and WBC differential with 92% segmented neutrophils, 1% band neutrophils, 5% lymphocytes, and 1% monocytes the absolute values are calculated as follows: $92/100 \times 9 = 8.3$ segs, $1/100 \times 9 = 0.1$ bands, $5/100 \times 9 = 0.45$ lymphs, $1/100 \times 9 = 0.1$ monos for a total of 9.0 WBC count.

Acute leukocytosis is initially accompanied by changes in the WBC count population, followed by changes within the individual WBCs. Leukocytosis usually occurs by way of increase in a single WBC family rather than a proportional increase in all cell types. Toxic granulation and vacuolation are commonly seen in leukocytosis accompanied by a *shift to the left,* or increase in the percentage of immature band neutrophils to mature segmented neutrophils. *Bandemia* is defined by the presence of greater than 6% band neutrophils in the total neutrophil cell population. These changes in the white cell population are most commonly associated with an infectious process, usually bacterial, but they can occur in healthy individuals who are under stress (in response to epinephrine production), such as women in childbirth and very young infants. The WBC count and differential of a woman in labor or of an actively crying infant may show an overall increase in WBCs with a shift to the left. Before initiating any kind of intervention, it is important to determine whether an increased WBC count is the result of a normal condition involving physiological stress or a pathological process. The use of multiple specimen types may confuse the interpretation of results in infants. Multiple samples from the same collection site (i.e., capillary versus venous) may be necessary to obtain an accurate assessment of the WBC picture in these young patients.

Neutrophils are normally found as the predominant WBC type in the circulating blood. Also called *polymorphonuclear cells,* they are the body's first line of defense through the process of phagocytosis. They also contain enzymes and pyogens, which combat foreign invaders.

Lymphocytes are agranular, mononuclear blood cells that are smaller than granulocytes. They are found in the next highest percentage in normal circulation. Lymphocytes are classified as B cells and T cells. Both types are formed in the bone marrow, but B cells mature in the bone marrow and T cells mature in the thymus. Lymphocytes play a major role in the body's natural defense system. B cells differentiate into immunoglobulin-synthesizing plasma cells. T cells function as cellular mediators of immunity and comprise helper/inducer (CD4) lymphocytes, delayed hypersensitivity lymphocytes, cytotoxic (CD8 or CD4) lymphocytes, and suppressor (CD8) lymphocytes.

Monocytes are mononuclear cells similar to lymphocytes, but they are related more closely to granulocytes in terms of their function. They are formed in the bone marrow from the same cells as those that produce neutrophils. The major function of monocytes is phagocytosis. Monocytes stay in the peripheral blood for about 70 hr, after which they migrate into the tissues and become macrophages.

The function of eosinophils is phagocytosis of antigen-antibody complexes. They become active in the later stages of inflammation. Eosinophils respond to allergic and parasitic diseases: They have granules that contain histamine used to kill foreign cells in the body and proteolytic enzymes that damage parasitic worms (see monograph titled "Eosinophil Count").

Basophils are found in small numbers in the circulating blood. They have a phagocytic function and, similar to eosinophils, contain numerous specific granules. Basophilic granules contain heparin, histamines, and serotonin. Basophils may also be found in tissue and as such are classified as mast cells. Basophilia is noted in conditions such as leukemia, Hodgkin's disease, polycythemia vera, ulcerative colitis, nephrosis, and chronic hypersensitivity states.

INDICATIONS

- Assist in confirming suspected bone marrow depression
- Assist in determining the cause of an elevated WBC count (e.g., infection, inflammatory process)
- Detect hematological disorder, neoplasm, or immunological abnormality
- Determine the presence of a hereditary hematological abnormality
- Monitor the effects of physical or emotional stress
- Monitor the progression of nonhematological disorders, such as chronic obstructive pulmonary disease, malabsorption syndromes, cancer, and renal disease
- Monitor the response to drugs or chemotherapy and evaluate undesired reactions to drugs that may cause blood dyscrasias
- Provide screening as part of a CBC in a general physical examination, especially on admission to a healthcare facility or before surgery

POTENTIAL DIAGNOSIS

Increased in

Leukocytosis
- Normal physiological and environmental conditions:
  Early infancy (*increases are believed to be related to the physiological stress of birth and metabolic demands of rapid development*)
  Emotional stress (*related to secretion of epinephrine*)
  Exposure to extreme heat or cold (*related to physiological stress*)

Pregnancy and labor (*WBC counts may be modestly elevated due to increased neutrophils into the third trimester and during labor, returning to normal within a week postpartum*)
Strenuous exercise (*related to epinephrine secretion; increases are short in duration, minutes to hours*)
Ultraviolet light (*related to physiological stress and possible inflammatory response*)
- Pathological conditions:
  Acute hemolysis, especially due to splenectomy or transfusion reactions (*related to leukocyte response to remove lysed RBC fragments*)
  All types of infections (*related to an inflammatory or infectious response*)
  Anemias (*bone marrow disorders affecting RBC production may result in elevated WBC count*)
  Appendicitis (*related to an inflammatory or infectious response*)
  Collagen disorders (*related to an inflammatory response*)
  Cushing's disease (*related to overproduction of cortisol, a corticosteroid, which stimulates WBC production*)
  Inflammatory disorders (*related to an inflammatory or infectious response*)
  Leukemias and other malignancies (*related to bone marrow disorders that result in abnormal WBC production*)
  Parasitic infestations (*related to an inflammatory or infectious response*)
  Polycythemia vera (*myeloproliferative bone marrow disorder causing an increase in all cell lines*)

Decreased in

Leukopenia
- Normal physiological conditions
  Diurnal rhythms (lowest in the morning)
- Pathological conditions
  Alcoholism (*related to WBC changes associated with nutritional deficiencies of vitamin B_{12} or folate*)
  Anemias (*related to WBC changes associated with nutritional deficiencies of*

vitamin B_{12} or folate, especially in megaloblastic anemias)

Bone marrow depression *(related to decreased production)*

Malaria *(related to hypersplenism)*

Malnutrition *(related to WBC changes associated with nutritional deficiencies of vitamin B_{12} or folate)*

Radiation *(related to physical cell destruction due to toxic effects of radiation)*

Rheumatoid arthritis *(related to side effect of medications used to treat the condition)*

Systemic lupus erythematosus (SLE) and other autoimmune disorders *(related to side effect of medications used to treat the condition)*

Toxic and antineoplastic drugs *(related to bone marrow suppression)*

Very low birth weight neonates *(related to bone marrow activity being diverted to develop RBCs in response to hypoxia)*

Viral infections *(leukopenia, lymphocytopenia, and abnormal lymphocytes may be present in the early stages of viral infections)*

Neutrophils Increased (neutrophilia)

- Acute hemolysis
- Acute hemorrhage
- Extremes in temperature
- Infectious diseases
- Inflammatory conditions (rheumatic fever, gout, rheumatoid arthritis, vasculitis, myositis)
- Malignancies
- Metabolic disorders (uremia, eclampsia, diabetic ketoacidosis, thyroid storm, Cushing's syndrome)
- Myelocytic leukemia
- Physiological stress (e.g., allergies, asthma, exercise, childbirth, surgery)
- Tissue necrosis (burns, crushing injuries, abscesses, myocardial infarction)
- Tissue poisoning with toxins and venoms

Neutrophils Decreased (neutropenia)

- Acromegaly
- Addison's disease
- Anaphylaxis
- Anorexia nervosa, starvation, malnutrition
- Bone marrow depression (viruses, toxic chemicals, overwhelming infection, radiation, Gaucher's disease)
- Disseminated SLE
- Thyrotoxicosis
- Viral infection (mononucleosis, hepatitis, influenza)
- Vitamin B_{12} or folate deficiency

Lymphocytes Increased (lymphocytosis)

- Addison's disease
- Felty's syndrome
- Infections
- Lymphocytic leukemia
- Lymphomas
- Lymphosarcoma
- Myeloma
- Rickets
- Thyrotoxicosis
- Ulcerative colitis
- Waldenström's macroglobulinemia

Lymphocytes Decreased (lymphopenia)

- Antineoplastic drugs
- Aplastic anemia
- Bone marrow failure
- Burns
- Gaucher's disease
- Hemolytic disease of the newborn
- High doses of adrenocorticosteroids
- Hodgkin's disease
- Hypersplenism
- Immunodeficiency diseases
- Malnutrition
- Pernicious anemia
- Pneumonia
- Radiation
- Rheumatic fever
- Septicemia

- Thrombocytopenic purpura
- Toxic chemical exposure
- Transfusion reaction

Monocytes Increased (monocytosis)
- Carcinomas
- Cirrhosis
- Collagen diseases
- Gaucher's disease
- Hemolytic anemias
- Hodgkin's disease
- Infections
- Lymphomas
- Monocytic leukemia
- Polycythemia vera
- Radiation
- Sarcoidosis
- SLE
- Thrombocytopenic purpura
- Ulcerative colitis

CRITICAL FINDINGS
- Less than $2.5 \times 10^3/mm^3$ or $2,500/mm^3$
- Greater than $30.0 \times 10^3/mm^3$ or $30,000/mm^3$

Note and immediately report to the requesting health-care provider (HCP) any critically increased or decreased values and related symptoms.

The presence of abnormal cells, other morphological characteristics, or cellular inclusions may signify a potentially life-threatening or serious health condition and should be investigated. Examples are hypersegmented neutrophils, agranular neutrophils, blasts or other immature cells, Auer rods, Döhle bodies, marked toxic granulation, or plasma cells.

INTERFERING FACTORS
- Drugs that may decrease the overall WBC count include acetyldigitoxin, acetylsalicylic acid, aminoglutethimide, aminopyrine, aminosalicylic acid, ampicillin, amsacrine, antazoline, anticonvulsants, antineoplastic agents (therapeutic intent), antipyrine, barbiturates, busulfan, carbutamide, carmustine, chlorambucil, chloramphenicol, chlordane, chlorophenothane, chlortetracycline, chlorthalidone, cisplatin, colchicine, colistimethate, cycloheximide, cyclophosphamide, cytarabine, dacarbazine, dactinomycin, diaprim, diazepam, diethylpropion, digitalis, dipyridamole, dipyrone, fumagillin, glaucarubin, glucosulfone, hexachlorobenzene, hydroflumethiazide, hydroxychloroquine, iothiouracil, iproniazid, lincomycin, local anesthetics, mefenamic acid, mepazine, meprobamate, mercaptopurine, methotrexate, methylpromazine, mitomycin, paramethadione, parathion, penicillin, phenacemide, phenindione, phenothiazine, pipamazine, prednisone (by Coulter S method), primaquine, procainamide, procarbazine, prochlorperazine, promazine, promethazine, pyrazolones, quinacrine, quinines, radioactive compounds, razoxane, ristocetin, sulfa drugs, tamoxifen, tetracycline, thenalidine, thioridazine, tolazamide, tolazoline, tolbutamide, trimethadione, and urethane.
- A significant decrease in basophil count occurs rapidly after intravenous injection of propanidid and thiopental.
- A significant decrease in lymphocyte count occurs rapidly after administration of corticotropin, mechlorethamine, methysergide, and x-ray therapy; and after megadoses of niacin, pyridoxine, and thiamine.
- Drugs that may increase the overall WBC count include amphetamine, amphotericin B, chloramphenicol, chloroform (normal response to anesthesia), colchicine (leukocytosis follows leukopenia), corticotropin, erythromycin, ether (normal response to anesthesia), fluroxene

(normal response to anesthesia), isoflurane (normal response to anesthesia), niacinamide, phenylbutazone, prednisone, and quinine.

- Drug allergies may have a significant effect on eosinophil count and may affect the overall WBC count. Refer to the monograph titled "Eosinophil Count" for a detailed listing of interfering drugs.
- The WBC count may vary depending on the patient's position, decreasing when the patient is recumbent owing to hemodilution and increasing when the patient rises owing to hemoconcentration.
- Venous stasis can falsely elevate results; the tourniquet should not be left on the arm for longer than 60 sec.
- Failure to fill the tube sufficiently (i.e., tube less than three-quarters full) may yield inadequate sample volume for automated analyzers and may be reason for specimen rejection.
- Hemolyzed or clotted specimens should be rejected for analysis.
- The presence of nucleated red blood cells or giant or clumped platelets affects the automated WBC, requiring a manual correction of the WBC count.
- Care should be taken in evaluating the CBC during the first few hours after transfusion.
- Patients with cold agglutinins or monoclonal gammopathies may have a falsely decreased WBC count as a result of cell clumping.

NURSING IMPLICATIONS AND PROCEDURE

PRETEST:

- Positively identify the patient using at least two unique identifiers before providing care, treatment, or services.

- *Patient Teaching:* Inform the patient this test can assist in assessing for infection or monitoring leukemia.
- Obtain a history of the patient's complaints, including a list of known allergens, especially allergies or sensitivities to latex.
- Obtain a history of the patient's hematopoietic, immune, and respiratory systems; symptoms; and results of previously performed laboratory tests and diagnostic and surgical procedures.
- Note any recent procedures that can interfere with test results.
- Obtain a list of the patient's current medications, including herbs, nutritional supplements, and nutraceuticals (see Appendix F).
- Review the procedure with the patient. Inform the patient that specimen collection takes approximately 5 to 10 min. Address concerns about pain and explain that there may be some discomfort during the venipuncture.
- *Sensitivity to social and cultural issues,* as well as concern for modesty, is important in providing psychological support before, during, and after the procedure.
- There are no food, fluid, or medication restrictions unless by medical direction.

INTRATEST:

- If the patient has a history of allergic reaction to latex, avoid the use of equipment containing latex.
- Instruct the patient to cooperate fully and to follow directions. Direct the patient to breathe normally and to avoid unnecessary movement.
- Observe standard precautions, and follow the general guidelines in Appendix A. Positively identify the patient, and label the appropriate tubes with the corresponding patient demographics, date, and time of collection. Perform a venipuncture. The specimen should be mixed gently by inverting the tube 10 times. The specimen should be analyzed within 24 hr when stored at room temperature or within 48 hr if stored at refrigerated temperature. If it is anticipated the specimen will not be analyzed within 24 hr, two blood smears should be made immediately

after the venipuncture and submitted with the blood sample. Smears made from specimens older than 24 hr may contain an unacceptable number of misleading artifactual abnormalities of the RBCs, such as echinocytes and spherocytes, as well as necrobiotic white blood cells.

- Remove the needle and apply direct pressure with dry gauze to stop bleeding. Observe/assess venipuncture site for bleeding or hematoma formation and secure gauze with adhesive bandage.
- Promptly transport the specimen to the laboratory for processing and analysis.

POST-TEST:

- A report of the results will be sent to the requesting HCP, who will discuss the results with the patient.
- *Nutritional Considerations:* Infection, fever, sepsis, and trauma can result in an impaired nutritional status. Malnutrition can occur for many reasons, including fatigue, lack of appetite, and gastrointestinal distress.
- *Nutritional Considerations:* Adequate intake of vitamins A and C are also important for regenerating body stores depleted by the effort exerted in fighting infections. Educate the patient or caregiver regarding the importance of following the prescribed diet.
- Recognize anxiety related to test results, and be supportive of fear of shortened life expectancy. Discuss the implications of abnormal test results

on the patient's lifestyle. Provide teaching and information regarding the clinical implications of the test results, as appropriate. Educate the patient regarding access to counseling services. Provide contact information, if desired, for the National Cancer Institute (www.nci.nih.org).

- Reinforce information given by the patient's HCP regarding further testing, treatment, or referral to another HCP. Answer any questions or address any concerns voiced by the patient or family.
- Depending on the results of this procedure, additional testing may be performed to evaluate or monitor progression of the disease process and determine the need for a change in therapy. Evaluate test results in relation to the patient's symptoms and other tests performed.

RELATED MONOGRAPHS:

- Related tests include albumin, antibody, anti–neutrophilic cytoplasmic biopsy bone marrow, biopsy lymph node, CBC, CBC RBC count, CBC RBC indices, CBC RBC morphology, culture bacterial (see individually listed culture monographs), culture fungal, culture viral, eosinophil count, ESR, fecal analysis, Gram stain, infectious mononucleosis, LAP, UA, and WBC scan.
- Refer to the Hematopoietic, Immune, and Respiratory systems tables at the end of the book for related tests by body system.

Computed Tomography, Abdomen

SYNONYM/ACRONYM: Computed axial tomography (CAT), computed transaxial tomography (CTT), abdominal CT, helical/spiral CT.

COMMON USE: To visualize and assess abdominal structures and to assist in diagnosing tumors, bleeding, and abscess. Used as an evaluation tool for surgical, radiation, and medical therapeutic interventions.

AREA OF APPLICATION: Abdomen.

CONTRAST: With or without oral or IV iodinated contrast medium.

DESCRIPTION: Abdominal computed tomography (CT) is a noninvasive procedure used to enhance certain anatomic views of the abdominal structures. It becomes invasive when contrast medium is used. During the procedure, the patient lies on a table and is moved in and out of a doughnut-like device called a *gantry*, which houses the x-ray tube and associated electronics. The scanner uses multiple x-ray beams and a series of detectors that rotate around the patient to produce cross-sectional views in a three-dimensional fashion. Differences in tissue density are detected and recorded and are viewable as computerized digital images. Slices or thin sections of certain anatomic views of the liver, biliary tract, pancreas, kidneys, spleen, intestines, and vascular system are reviewed to allow differentiations of solid, cystic, inflammatory, or vascular lesions, as well as identification of suspected hematomas and aneurysms. The procedure is repeated after intravenous injection of iodinated contrast medium for vascular evaluation or after oral ingestion of contrast medium for evaluation of bowel and adjacent structures. Images can be recorded on photographic or x-ray film or stored in digital format as digitized computer data. Cine scanning is used to produce a series of moving images of the area scanned. The CT scan can be used to guide biopsy needles into areas of abdominal tumors to obtain tissue for laboratory analysis and to guide placement of catheters for drainage of intra-abdominal abscesses. Tumors, before and after therapy, may be monitored with CT scanning.

INDICATIONS

- Assist in differentiating between benign and malignant tumors
- Detect aortic aneurysms
- Detect tumor extension of masses and metastasis into the abdominal area
- Differentiate aortic aneurysms from tumors near the aorta
- Differentiate between infectious and inflammatory processes
- Evaluate cysts, masses, abscesses, renal calculi, gastrointestinal (GI) bleeding and obstruction, and trauma
- Evaluate retroperitoneal lymph nodes
- Monitor and evaluate the effectiveness of medical, radiation, or surgical therapies

POTENTIAL DIAGNOSIS

Normal findings in
- Normal size, position, and shape of abdominal organs and vascular system

Abnormal findings in
- Abdominal abscess
- Abdominal aortic aneurysm
- Adrenal tumor or hyperplasia
- Appendicitis
- Bowel obstruction
- Bowel perforation
- Dilation of the common hepatic duct, common bile duct, or gallbladder
- GI bleeding
- Hematomas, diverticulitis, gallstones
- Hemoperitoneum
- Hepatic cysts or abscesses
- Pancreatic pseudocyst
- Primary and metastatic neoplasms
- Renal calculi
- Splenic laceration, tumor, infiltration, and trauma

CRITICAL FINDINGS

- Abscess
- Acute GI bleed
- Aortic aneurysm
- Appendicitis
- Aortic dissection

- Bowel perforation
- Bowel obstruction
- Mesenteric torsion
- Tumor with significant mass effect
- Visceral injury; significant solid organ laceration

It is essential that critical diagnoses be communicated immediately to the appropriate health-care provider (HCP). A listing of these diagnoses varies among facilities. Note and immediately report to the HCP abnormal results and related symptoms.

INTERFERING FACTORS

This procedure is contraindicated for

- ✺ Patients with allergies to shellfish or iodinated dye. The contrast medium used may cause a life-threatening allergic reaction. Patients with a known hypersensitivity to the medium may benefit from premedication with corticosteroids or the use of nonionic contrast medium.
- Patients who are claustrophobic.
- Patients who are pregnant or suspected of being pregnant, unless the potential benefits of the procedure far outweigh the risks to the fetus and mother.
- ✺ Elderly and other patients who are chronically dehydrated before the test, because of their risk of contrast-induced renal failure.
- ✺ Patients who are in renal failure.
- Young patients (17 yr and younger), unless the benefits of the x-ray diagnosis outweigh the risks of exposure to high levels of radiation.

Factors that may impair clear imaging

- Gas or feces in the GI tract resulting from inadequate cleansing or failure to restrict food intake before the study.
- Retained barium from a previous radiological procedure.

- Metallic objects within the examination field (e.g., jewelry, body rings), which may inhibit organ visualization and cause unclear images.
- Patients with extreme claustrophobia unless sedation is given before the study.
- Inability of the patient to cooperate or remain still during the procedure because of age, significant pain, or mental status.

Other considerations

- Complications of the procedure may include hemorrhage, infection at the IV needle insertion site, and cardiac arrhythmias.
- The procedure may be terminated if chest pain or severe cardiac arrhythmias occur.
- Failure to follow dietary restrictions and other pretesting preparations may cause the procedure to be canceled or repeated.
- Consultation with an HCP should occur before the procedure for radiation safety concerns regarding younger patients or patients who are lactating.
- Risks associated with radiation overexposure can result from frequent x-ray procedures. Personnel in the room with the patient should wear a protective lead apron, stand behind a shield, or leave the area while the examination is being done. Personnel working in the examination area should wear badges to record their level of radiation exposure.

NURSING IMPLICATIONS AND PROCEDURE

PRETEST:

▷ Positively identify the patient using at least two unique identifiers before providing care, treatment, or services.
▷ *Patient Teaching:* Inform the patient this procedure can assist in assessing the abdominal organs.

- Obtain a history of the patient's complaints, including a list of known allergens, especially allergies or sensitivities to latex, iodine, seafood, anesthetics, or contrast medium.
- Obtain a history of the patient's gastrointestinal and hepatobiliary systems, symptoms, and results of previously performed laboratory tests and diagnostic and surgical procedures.
- Ensure results of coagulation testing are obtained and recorded prior to the procedure; BUN and creatinine results are also needed if contrast medium is to be used.
- Note any recent procedures that can interfere with test results, including examinations using barium- or iodine-based contrast medium. Ensure that barium studies were performed more than 4 days before the CT scan.
- Record the date of the last menstrual period and determine the possibility of pregnancy in perimenopausal women.
- Obtain a list of the patient's current medications including anticoagulants, aspirin and other salicylates, herbs, nutritional supplements, and nutraceuticals (see Appendix F). Note the last time and dose of medication taken.
- If contrast medium is scheduled to be used, patients receiving metformin (Glucophage) for non-insulin-dependent (type 2) diabetes should discontinue the drug on the day of the test and continue to withhold it for 48 hr after the test. Failure to do so may result in lactic acidosis.
- Review the procedure with the patient. Explain the purpose of the test and how the procedure is performed. Address concerns about pain and explain that there may be moments of discomfort and some pain experienced during the test. Inform the patient that the procedure is performed in a radiology suite usually by an HCP and takes approximately 30 to 60 min.
- *Sensitivity to social and cultural issues,* as well as concern for modesty, is important in providing psychological support before, during, and after the procedure.
- Explain that an IV line may be inserted to allow infusion of IV fluids, anesthetics, or sedatives.

- Inform the patient that he or she may experience nausea, a feeling of warmth, a salty or metallic taste, or a transient headache after injection of contrast medium, if given.
- The patient may be requested to drink approximately 450 mL of a dilute barium solution (approximately 1% barium) beginning 1 hr before the examination. This is administered to distinguish GI organs from the other abdominal organs.
- Instruct the patient to remove jewelry and other metallic objects from the area to be examined.
- The patient should fast and restrict fluids for 8 hr prior to the procedure. Instruct the patient to avoid taking anticoagulant medication or to reduce dosage as ordered prior to the procedure. Protocols may vary among facilities.
- *Make sure a written and informed consent has been signed prior to the procedure and before administering any medications.*

INTRATEST:

- Ensure the patient has complied with dietary, fluids, and medication restrictions for 8 hr prior to the procedure.
- Ensure the patient has removed all external metallic objects from the area to be examined.
- If the patient has a history of allergic reactions to any substance or drug, administer ordered prophylactic steroids or antihistamines before the procedure. Use nonionic contrast medium for the procedure.
- Have emergency equipment readily available.
- Instruct the patient to void prior to the procedure and to change into the gown, robe, and foot coverings provided.
- Instruct the patient to cooperate fully and to follow directions. Instruct the patient to remain still throughout the procedure because movement produces unreliable results.
- Record baseline vital signs, and continue to monitor throughout the procedure. Protocols may vary among facilities.
- Observe standard precautions, and follow the general guidelines in Appendix A.
- Establish an IV fluid line for the injection of contrast, emergency drugs, and sedatives.

- Administer an antianxiety agent, as ordered, if the patient has claustrophobia. Administer a sedative to a child or to an uncooperative adult, as ordered.
- Place the patient in the supine position on an examination table.
- If IV contrast media is used, during and after injection a rapid series of images is taken.
- Instruct the patient to inhale deeply and hold his or her breathe while the x-ray images are taken, and then to exhale after the images are taken.
- Instruct the patient to take slow, deep breaths if nausea occurs during the procedure.
- Monitor the patient for complications related to the procedure (e.g., allergic reaction, anaphylaxis, bronchospasm) if contrast is used.
- The needle is removed, and a pressure dressing is applied over the puncture site.
- Observe/assess the needle site for bleeding, inflammation, or hematoma formation.

POST-TEST:

- A report of the examination will be sent to the requesting HCP, who will discuss the results with the patient.
- Instruct the patient to resume usual diet, fluids, medications, and activity, as directed by the HCP. Renal function should be assessed before metformin is resumed, if contrast was used.
- Monitor vital signs and neurological status every 15 min for 1 hr, then every 2 hr for 4 hr, and then as ordered by the HCP. Monitor temperature every 4 hr for 24 hr. Monitor intake and output at least every 8 hr. Compare with baseline values. Notify the HCP if temperature is elevated. Protocols may vary from facility to facility.
- If contrast was used, observe for delayed allergic reactions, such as rash, urticaria, tachycardia, hyperpnea, hypertension, palpitations, nausea, or vomiting.
- Instruct the patient to immediately report symptoms such as fast heart rate, difficulty breathing, skin rash,

itching, chest pain, persistent right shoulder pain, or abdominal pain. Immediately report symptoms to the appropriate HCP.
- Observe/assess the needle insertion site for bleeding, inflammation, or hematoma formation.
- Instruct the patient in the care and assessment of the site.
- Instruct the patient to apply cold compresses to the insertion site as needed, to reduce discomfort or edema.
- Instruct the patient to increase fluid intake to help eliminate the contrast medium, if used.
- Inform the patient that diarrhea may occur after ingestion of oral contrast medium.
- Recognize anxiety related to test results. Discuss the implications of abnormal test results on the patient's lifestyle. Provide teaching and information regarding the clinical implications of the test results, as appropriate.
- Reinforce information given by the patient's HCP regarding further testing, treatment, or referral to another HCP. Answer any questions or address any concerns voiced by the patient or family.
- Depending on the results of this procedure, additional testing may be needed to evaluate or monitor progression of the disease process and determine the need for a change in therapy. Evaluate test results in relation to the patien's symptoms and other tests performed.

RELATED MONOGRAPHS:

- Related tests include ACTH and challenge tests, amylase, angiography abdomen, biopsy intestinal, BUN, calculus kidney stone panel, CBC, CBC hematocrit, CBC hemoglobin, cortisol and challenge tests, creatinine, cystoscopy, hepatobiliary scan, IVP, KUB studies, MRI abdomen, peritoneal fluid analysis, PT/INR, renogram, and US pelvis.
- Refer to the Gastrointestinal and Hepatobiliary systems tables at the end of the book for related tests by body system.

Computed Tomography, Angiography

SYNONYM/ACRONYM: Computed axial tomography (CAT) angiography, CTA.

COMMON USE: To visualize and assess the vascular structure to assist in the diagnosis of aneurysm, embolism, or stenosis.

AREA OF APPLICATION: Vessels.

CONTRAST: IV iodinated contrast medium.

DESCRIPTION: Computed tomography angiography (CTA) is a noninvasive procedure that enhances certain anatomic views of vascular structures. This procedure complements traditional angiography and allows reconstruction of the images in different planes and removal of surrounding structures, leaving only the vessels to be studied. While lying on a table, the patient is moved in and out of a doughnut-like device called a *gantry*, which houses the x-ray tube and associated electronics. The scanner uses multiple x-ray beams and a series of detectors that rotate around the patient to produce cross-sectional views in a three-dimensional fashion by detecting and recording differences in tissue density after having an x-ray beam passed through the tissues. CTA uses spiral CT technology and collects large amounts of data with each scan. Retrospectively, the data can be manipulated to produce the desired image without exposure to additional radiation or contrast medium. Multiplanar reconstruction images are reviewed by the health-care provider (HCP) at a computerized workstation. These

images are helpful when there are heavily calcified vessels. The axial images give the most precise information regarding the true extent of stenosis, and they can also evaluate intracerebral aneurysms. Small ulcerations and plaque irregularity are readily seen with CTA; the degree of stenosis can be estimated better with CTA because of the increased number of imaging planes. Density measurements are sent to a computer that produces a digital image of the anatomy, enabling the HCP to look at slices or thin sections of certain anatomic views of the vessels. Iodinated contrast medium is given IV for vascular evaluation. Images can be recorded on photographic or x-ray film or stored in digital format as digitized computer data.

INDICATIONS
- Detect aneurysms
- Detect embolism or other occlusions
- Detect fistula
- Detect stenosis
- Detect vascular disease
- Differentiate aortic aneurysms from tumors near the aorta

- Differentiate between vascular and nonvascular tumors
- Evaluate atherosclerosis
- Evaluate hemorrhage or trauma
- Monitor and evaluate the effectiveness of medical or surgical therapies

POTENTIAL DIAGNOSIS

Normal findings in
- Normal size, position, and shape of vascular structures

Abnormal findings in
- Aortic aneurysm
- Cysts or abscesses
- Emboli
- Hemorrhage
- Neoplasm
- Occlusion
- Shunting
- Stenosis

CRITICAL FINDINGS
- Brain or spinal cord ischemia
- Emboli
- Hemorrhage
- Leaking aortic aneurysm
- Occlusion
- Tumor with significant mass effect

It is essential that critical diagnoses be communicated immediately to the appropriate HCP. A listing of these diagnoses varies among facilities. Note and immediately report to the HCP abnormal results and related symptoms.

INTERFERING FACTORS

This procedure is contraindicated for
- ❖ Patients with allergies to shellfish or iodinated dye. The contrast medium used may cause a life-threatening allergic reaction. Patients with a known hypersensitivity to the medium may benefit from premedication with corticosteroids or the use of nonionic contrast medium.
- Patients who are claustrophobic.
- Patients who are pregnant or suspected of being pregnant, unless the potential benefits of the procedure far outweigh the risks to the fetus and mother.
- ❖ Elderly and other patients who are chronically dehydrated before the test, because of their risk of contrast-induced renal failure.
- ❖ Patients who are in renal failure.
- Young patients (17 yr and younger), unless the benefits of the x-ray diagnosis outweigh the risks of exposure to high levels of radiation.

Factors that may impair clear imaging
- Gas or feces in the gastrointestinal tract resulting from inadequate cleansing or failure to restrict food intake before the study.
- Retained barium from a previous radiological procedure.
- Metallic objects within the examination field (e.g., jewelry, body rings), which may inhibit organ visualization and cause unclear images.
- Patients who are very obese or who may exceed the weight limit for the equipment.
- Patients with extreme claustrophobia unless sedation is given before the study.
- Inability of the patient to cooperate or remain still during the procedure because of age, significant pain, or mental status.

Other considerations
- Complications of the procedure include hemorrhage, infection at the IV needle insertion site, and cardiac arrhythmias.
- The procedure may be terminated if chest pain or severe cardiac arrhythmias occur.

- Failure to follow dietary restrictions and other pretesting preparations may cause the procedure to be canceled or repeated.
- Consultation with the HCP should occur before the procedure for radiation safety concerns regarding younger patients or patients who are lactating.
- Risks associated with radiation overexposure can result from frequent x-ray procedures. Personnel in the room with the patient should wear a protective lead apron, stand behind a shield, or leave the area while the examination is being done. Personnel working in the examination area should wear badges to record their level of radiation exposure.

NURSING IMPLICATIONS AND PROCEDURE

PRETEST:

▶ Positively identify the patient using at least two unique identifiers before providing care, treatment, or services.
▶ *Patient Teaching:* Inform the patient this procedure can assist in assessing the cardiovascular system.
▶ Obtain a history of the patient's complaints or clinical symptoms, including a list of known allergens, especially allergies or sensitivities to latex, iodine, seafood, anesthetics, or contrast mediums.
▶ Obtain a history of patient's cardiovascular system, symptoms, and results of previously performed laboratory tests and diagnostic and surgical procedures.
▶ Ensure results of coagulation testing are obtained and recorded prior to the procedure; BUN and creatinine results are also needed if contrast medium is to be used.
▶ Note any recent procedures that can interfere with test results, including

examinations using barium- or iodine-based contrast medium. Ensure that barium studies were performed more than 4 days before the CT scan.
▶ Record the date of the last menstrual period and determine the possibility of pregnancy in perimenopausal women.
▶ Obtain a list of the patient's current medications, including anticoagulants, aspirin and other salicylates, herbs, nutritional supplements, and nutraceuticals (see Appendix F). Such products should be discontinued by medical direction for the appropriate number of days prior to a surgical procedure. Note the last time and dose of medication taken.
▶ If contrast medium is scheduled to be used, patients receiving metformin (Glucophage) for non-insulin-dependent (type 2) diabetes should discontinue the drug on the day of the test and continue to withhold it for 48 hr after the test. Failure to do so may result in lactic acidosis.
▶ Review the procedure with the patient. Address concerns about pain and explain that there may be moments of discomfort and some pain experienced during the test. Inform the patient that the procedure is usually performed in a radiology suite by an HCP specializing in this procedure, with support staff, and takes approximately 30 to 60 min.
▶ *Sensitivity to social and cultural issues,* as well as concern for modesty, is important in providing psychological support before, during, and after the procedure.
▶ Explain that an IV line may be inserted to allow infusion of IV fluids, anesthetics, or sedatives.
▶ Inform the patient that a burning and flushing sensation may be felt throughout the body during injection of the contrast medium. After injection of the contrast medium, the patient may experience an urge to cough, flushing, nausea, or a salty or metallic taste.
▶ Instruct the patient to remove all external metallic objects from the area to be examined.
▶ The patient should fast and restrict fluids for 8 hr prior to the procedure.

Instruct the patient to avoid taking anticoagulant medication or to reduce dosage as ordered prior to the procedure. Protocols may vary among facilities.

Make sure a written and informed consent has been signed prior to the procedure and before administering any medications.

INTRATEST:

▶ Ensure that the patient has complied with dietary, fluid, and medication restrictions for 8 hr prior to the procedure.

▶ Ensure that the patient has removed all external metallic objects from the area to be examined.

▶ If the patient has a history of allergic reactions to any substance or drug, administer ordered prophylactic steroids or antihistamines before the procedure. Use nonionic contrast medium for the procedure.

▶ Have emergency equipment readily available.

▶ Instruct the patient to void prior to the procedure and to change into the gown, robe, and foot coverings provided.

▶ Instruct the patient to cooperate fully and to follow directions. Instruct the patient to remain still throughout the procedure because movement produces unreliable results.

▶ Observe standard precautions, and follow the general guidelines in Appendix A.

▶ Establish an IV fluid line for the injection of contrast, emergency drugs, and sedatives.

▶ Administer an antianxiety agent, as ordered, if the patient has claustrophobia. Administer a sedative to a child or to an uncooperative adult, as ordered.

▶ Place the patient in the supine position on an examination table.

▶ The contrast medium is injected, and a rapid series of images is taken during and after the filling of the vessels to be examined. Delayed images may be taken to examine the vessels after a time and to monitor the venous phase of the procedure.

▶ Ask the patient to inhale deeply and hold his or her breath while the x-ray images are taken, and then to exhale after the images are taken.

▶ Instruct the patient to take slow, deep breaths if nausea occurs during the procedure. Monitor and administer an antiemetic agent if ordered. Ready an emesis basin for use.

▶ Monitor the patient for complications related to the procedure (e.g., allergic reaction, anaphylaxis, bronchospasm).

▶ The needle is removed and a pressure dressing is applied over the puncture site.

▶ Observe/assess the needle site for bleeding, inflammation, or hematoma formation.

POST-TEST:

▶ A report of the examination will be sent to the requesting HCP, who will discuss the results with the patient.

▶ Instruct the patient to resume pretesting diet, as directed by the HCP. Assess the patient's ability to swallow before allowing the patient to attempt liquids or solid foods. Renal function should be assessed before metformin is resumed.

▶ Monitor vital signs and neurological status every 15 min for 1 hr, then every 2 hr for 4 hr, and then as ordered by the HCP. Monitor temperature every 4 hr for 24 hr. Monitor intake and output at least every 8 hr. Compare with baseline values. Notify the HCP if temperature is elevated. Protocols may vary among facilities.

▶ If contrast was used, observe for delayed allergic reactions, such as rash, urticaria, tachycardia, hyperpnea, hypertension, palpitations, nausea, or vomiting.

▶ Instruct the patient to immediately report symptoms such as fast heart rate, difficulty breathing, skin rash, itching, chest pain, persistent right shoulder pain, or abdominal pain. Immediately report symptoms to the appropriate HCP.

▶ Assess extremities for signs of ischemia or absence of distal pulse caused by a catheter-induced thrombus.

▶ Observe/assess the needle insertion site for bleeding, inflammation, or hematoma formation.

C

▶ Instruct the patient to apply cold compresses to the insertion site as needed, to reduce discomfort or edema.

▶ Instruct the patient to increase fluid intake to help eliminate the contrast medium, if used.

▶ Inform the patient that diarrhea may occur after ingestion of oral contrast medium.

▶ Instruct the patient to maintain bed rest for 4 to 6 hr after the procedure.

▶ *Nutritional Considerations:* Abnormal findings may be associated with cardiovascular disease. The American Heart Association and National Heart, Lung, and Blood Institute (NHBLI) recommend nutritional therapy for individuals identified to be at high risk for developing coronary artery disease (CAD) or individuals who have specific risk factors and/or existing medical conditions (e.g., elevated LDL cholesterol levels, other lipid disorders, insulin-dependent diabetes, insulin resistance, or metabolic syndrome). If overweight, the patient should be encouraged to achieve a normal weight. The NHLBI's National Cholesterol Education Program (NCEP) revised its dietary guidelines for reducing CAD in 2001. Guidelines for the Therapeutic Lifestyle Changes (TLC) diet are outlined in the Third Report of the Expert Panel on Detection, Evaluation, and Treatment of High Blood Cholesterol in Adults (Adult Treatment Panel III [ATP III]). The TLC diet emphasizes a reduction in foods high in saturated fats and cholesterol. Red meats, eggs, and dairy products are the major sources of saturated fats and cholesterol. If triglycerides also are elevated, the patient should be advised to eliminate or reduce alcohol and simple carbohydrates from the diet. The TLC approach also includes the use of plant stanols or sterols and increased dissolved fiber as an option for lowering LDL cholesterol levels; nutritional recommendations for daily total caloric intake; recommendations for allowable percentage of calories derived from fat (saturated and unsaturated), carbohydrates, protein, and cholesterol; as well as recommendations for daily expenditure of energy.

▶ *Nutritional Considerations:* Overweight patients with high blood pressure should be encouraged to achieve a normal weight. Other changeable risk factors warranting patient education include strategies to safely decrease sodium intake, increase physical activity, decrease alcohol consumption, eliminate tobacco use, and decrease cholesterol levels.

▶ *Social and Cultural Considerations:* Numerous studies point to the prevalence of excess body weight in American children and adolescents. Experts estimate that obesity is present in 25% of the population ages 6 to 11 yr. The medical, social, and emotional consequences of excess body weight are significant. Special attention should be given to instructing the child and caregiver regarding health risks and weight control education.

▶ Recognize anxiety related to test results, and be supportive of fear of shortened life expectancy. Discuss the implications of abnormal test results on the patient's lifestyle. Provide teaching and information regarding the clinical implications of the test results, as appropriate. Educate the patient regarding access to counseling services. Provide contact information, if desired, for the American Heart Association (www.americanheart.org) or the NHLBI (www.nhlbi.nih.gov).

▶ Inform the patient that diarrhea may occur after ingestion of oral contrast medium.

▶ Recognize anxiety related to test results. Discuss the implications of abnormal test results on the patient's lifestyle. Provide teaching and information regarding the clinical implications of the test results, as appropriate.

▶ Reinforce information given by the patient's HCP regarding further testing, treatment, or referral to another HCP. Answer any questions or address any concerns voiced by the patient or family.

▶ Instruct the patient in the use of any ordered medications. Explain the importance of adhering to the therapy regimen. As appropriate, instruct the patient in significant side effects and systemic reactions associated with the prescribed medication. Encourage him or her to review corresponding literature provided by a pharmacist.

▶ Depending on the results of this procedure, additional testing may be needed to evaluate or monitor progression of the disease process and determine the need for a change in therapy. Evaluate test results in relation to the patient's symptoms and other tests performed.

RELATED MONOGRAPHS:

▶ Related tests include angiography of the specific area (abdomen, adrenal, carotid, coronary, pulmonary, renal), blood pool imaging, BUN, chest x-ray, colonoscopy, CBC, CBC hematocrit, CBC hemoglobin, CT of the specific area (abdomen, biliary/liver, brain, pituitary, renal, spine, spleen, thoracic), creatinine echocardiography, echocardiography transesophageal, fluorescein angiography, fundus photography, MRA, MRI of the specific area (abdomen, brain, chest, pituitary), MI scan, plethysmography, PET (brain, heart), proctosigmoidoscopy, PT/INR, US carotid, and US venous Doppler extremity.

▶ Refer to the Cardiovascular System table at the end of the book for related tests by body system.

Computed Tomography, Biliary Tract and Liver

SYNONYM/ACRONYM: Computed axial tomography (CAT), computed transaxial tomography (CTT), abdominal CT, helical/spiral CT.

COMMON USE: To visualize and assess the structure of the liver and biliary tract to assist in the diagnosis of tumor, obstruction, bleeding, and infection. Used as an evaluation tool for surgical, radiation, and medical therapeutic interventions.

AREA OF APPLICATION: Liver, biliary tract, and adjacent structures.

CONTRAST: With or without IV iodinated contrast medium.

DESCRIPTION: Computed tomography (CT) of the liver and biliary tract is a noninvasive procedure that enhances certain anatomic views of these structures. It becomes invasive with the use of contrast medium. During the procedure, the patient lies on a table and is moved in and out of a doughnut-like device called a *gantry*, which houses the x-ray tube and associated electronics.

The scanner uses multiple x-ray beams and a series of detectors that rotate around the patient to produce cross-sectional views in a three-dimensional fashion. Differences in tissue density are detected and recorded and are viewable as computerized digital images. Slices or thin sections of certain anatomic views of the kidneys and associated vascular system are reviewed to allow differentiation of solid, cystic, inflammatory, or vascular lesions, as well as identification of suspected hematomas and aneurysms. The procedure is repeated after IV injection of iodinated contrast medium for vascular evaluation or after oral ingestion of contrast medium for evaluation of bowel and adjacent structures. Images can be recorded on photographic or x-ray film or stored in digital format as digitized computer data. Cine scanning produces a series of moving images of the scanned area. The CT scan can be used to guide biopsy needles into areas of liver and biliary tract masses to obtain tissue for laboratory analysis and for placement of needles to aspirate cysts or abscesses. CT scanning can monitor mass, cyst, or tumor growth and post-therapy response.

INDICATIONS

- Assist in differentiating between benign and malignant tumors
- Detect dilation or obstruction of the biliary ducts with or without calcification or gallstone
- Detect liver abnormalities, such as cirrhosis with ascites and fatty liver
- Detect tumor extension of masses and metastasis into the hepatic area
- Differentiate aortic aneurysms from tumors near the aorta
- Differentiate between obstructive and nonobstructive jaundice
- Differentiate infectious from inflammatory processes
- Evaluate hepatic cysts, masses, abscesses, and hematomas, or hepatic trauma
- Monitor and evaluate effectiveness of medical, radiation, or surgical therapies

POTENTIAL DIAGNOSIS

Normal findings in
- Normal size, position, and contour of the liver and biliary ducts

Abnormal findings in
- Dilation of the common hepatic duct, common bile duct, or gallbladder
- Gallstones
- Hematomas
- Hepatic cysts or abscesses
- Jaundice (obstructive or nonobstructive)
- Primary and metastatic neoplasms

CRITICAL FINDINGS: N/A

INTERFERING FACTORS

This procedure is contraindicated for

- ❖ Patients with allergies to shellfish or iodinated dye. The contrast medium used may cause a life-threatening allergic reaction. Patients with a known hypersensitivity to the medium may benefit from premedication with corticosteroids or the use of nonionic contrast medium.
- Patients who are claustrophobic.
- Patients who are pregnant or suspected of being pregnant, unless the potential benefits of the procedure far outweigh the risks to the fetus and mother.
- ❖ Elderly and other patients who are chronically dehydrated before the test, because of their risk of contrast-induced renal failure.
- ❖ Patients who are in renal failure.
- Young patients (17 yr and younger), unless the benefits of the x-ray diagnosis outweigh the risks of exposure to high levels of radiation.

Factors that may impair clear imaging

- Gas or feces in the gastrointestinal (GI) tract resulting from inadequate cleansing or failure to restrict food intake before the study.
- Retained barium from a previous radiological procedure.
- Metallic objects (e.g., jewelry, body rings) within the examination field, which may inhibit organ visualization and cause unclear images.
- Patients who are very obese or who may exceed the weight limit for the equipment.
- Patients with extreme claustrophobia unless sedation is given before the study.
- Inability of the patient to cooperate or remain still during the procedure because of age, significant pain, or mental status.

Other considerations

- Complications of the procedure include hemorrhage, infection at the IV needle insertion site, and cardiac arrhythmias.
- The procedure may be terminated if chest pain or severe cardiac arrhythmias occur.
- Failure to follow dietary restrictions and other pretesting preparations may cause the procedure to be canceled or repeated.
- Consultation with a health-care provider (HCP) should occur before the procedure for radiation safety concerns regarding younger patients or patients who are lactating.
- Risks associated with radiation overexposure can result from frequent x-ray procedures. Personnel in the room with the patient should wear a protective lead apron, stand behind a shield, or leave the area while the examination is being done. Personnel working in the examination area should wear badges to record their level of radiation exposure.

NURSING IMPLICATIONS AND PROCEDURE

PRETEST:

- Positively identify the patient using at least two unique identifiers before providing care, treatment, or services.
- *Patient Teaching:* Inform the patient this procedure can assist in assessing the liver, biliary tract, and surrounding structures.
- Obtain a history of the patient's complaints or clinical symptoms, including a list of known allergens, especially allergies or sensitivities to latex, iodine, seafood, anesthetics, or contrast medium.
- Obtain a history of the patient's hepatobiliary system, symptoms, and results of previously performed laboratory tests and diagnostic and surgical procedures.
- Ensure results of coagulation testing are obtained and recorded prior to the procedure; BUN and creatinine results are also needed if contrast medium is to be used.
- Note any recent procedures that can interfere with test results, including examinations using barium- or iodine-based contrast medium. Ensure that barium studies were performed more than 4 days before the CT scan.
- Record the date of the last menstrual period and determine the possibility of pregnancy in perimenopausal women.
- Obtain a list of the patient's current medications, including anticoagulants, aspirin and other salicylates, herbs, nutritional supplements, and nutraceuticals (see Appendix F). Note the last time and dose of medication taken.
- If contrast medium is scheduled to be used, patients receiving metformin (Glucophage) for non-insulin-dependent (type 2) diabetes should discontinue the drug on the day of the test and continue to withhold it for 48 hr after the test. Failure to do so may result in lactic acidosis.

▶ Review the procedure with the patient. Address concerns about pain and explain that there may be moments of discomfort and some pain experienced during the test. Inform the patient the procedure is usually performed in a radiology suite by an HCP specializing in this procedure, with support staff, and takes approximately 30 to 60 min.

▶ *Sensitivity to social and cultural issues,* as well as concern for modesty, is important in providing psychological support before, during, and after the procedure.

▶ Explain that an IV line may be inserted to allow infusion of IV fluids, anesthetics, or sedatives.

▶ Inform the patient that he or she may experience nausea, a feeling of warmth, a salty or metallic taste, or a transient headache after injection of contrast medium, if given.

▶ The patient may be requested to drink approximately 450 mL of a dilute barium solution (approximately 1% barium) beginning 1 hr before the examination. This is administered to distinguish GI organs from the other abdominal organs.

▶ Instruct the patient to remove all external metallic objects from the area to be examined.

▶ The patient should fast and restrict fluids for 8 hr prior to the procedure. Instruct the patient to avoid taking anticoagulant medication or to reduce dosage as ordered prior to the procedure. Protocols may vary among facilities.

▶ *Make sure a written and informed consent has been signed prior to the procedure and before administering any medications.*

INTRATEST:

▶ Ensure the patient has complied with dietary, fluids, and medication restrictions and pretesting preparations for 8 hr prior to the procedure.

▶ Ensure the patient has removed all external metallic objects from the area to be examined.

▶ If the patient has a history of allergic reactions to any substance or drug, administer ordered prophylactic steroids or antihistamines before the procedure. Use nonionic contrast medium for the procedure.

▶ Have emergency equipment readily available.

▶ Instruct the patient to void prior to the procedure and to change into the gown, robe, and foot coverings provided.

▶ Instruct the patient to cooperate fully and to follow directions. Instruct the patient to remain still throughout the procedure because movement produces unreliable results.

▶ Record baseline vital signs, and continue to monitor throughout the procedure. Protocols may vary from facility to facility.

▶ Observe standard precautions, and follow the general guidelines in Appendix A.

▶ Establish an IV fluid line for the injection of contrast medium, emergency drugs, and sedatives.

▶ Administer an antianxiety agent, as ordered, if the patient has claustrophobia. Administer a sedative to a child or to an uncooperative adult, as ordered.

▶ Place the patient in the supine position on an examination table.

▶ If IV contrast medium is used, a rapid series of images is taken during and after injection.

▶ Instruct the patient to inhale deeply and hold his or her breath while the x-ray images are taken, and then to exhale after the images are taken.

▶ Instruct the patient to take slow, deep breaths if nausea occurs during the procedure.

▶ Monitor the patient for complications related to the procedure (e.g., allergic reaction, anaphylaxis, bronchospasm) if contrast is used.

▶ The needle is removed, and a pressure dressing is applied over the puncture site.

▶ Observe/assess the needle site for bleeding, inflammation, or hematoma formation.

POST-TEST:

▶ A report of the examination will be sent to the requesting HCP, who will discuss the results with the patient.

▶ Instruct the patient to resume usual diet, fluids, medications, and activity, as directed by the HCP. Renal function should be assessed before metformin is resumed, if contrast was used.

- Monitor vital signs and neurological status every 15 min for 1 hr, then every 2 hr for 4 hr, and then as ordered by the HCP. Monitor temperature every 4 hr for 24 hr. Monitor intake and output at least every 8 hr. Compare with baseline values. Notify the HCP if temperature is elevated. Protocols may vary among facilities.
- If contrast was used, observe for delayed allergic reactions, such as rash, urticaria, tachycardia, hyperpnea, hypertension, palpitations, nausea, or vomiting.
- Instruct the patient to immediately report symptoms such as fast heart rate, difficulty breathing, skin rash, itching, chest pain, persistent right shoulder pain, or abdominal pain. Immediately report symptoms to the appropriate HCP.
- Observe/assess the needle insertion site for bleeding, inflammation, or hematoma formation.
- Instruct the patient in the care and assessment of the site.
- Instruct the patient to apply cold compresses to the insertion site as needed, to reduce discomfort or edema.
- Instruct the patient to increase fluid intake to help eliminate the contrast medium, if used.
- Inform the patient that diarrhea may occur after ingestion of oral contrast media.
- Recognize anxiety related to test results. Discuss the implications of abnormal test results on the patient's lifestyle. Provide teaching and information regarding the clinical implications of the test results, as appropriate.
- Reinforce information given by the patient's HCP regarding further testing, treatment, or referral to another HCP. Answer any questions or address any concerns voiced by the patient or family.
- Depending on the results of this procedure, additional testing may be needed to evaluate or monitor progression of the disease process and determine the need for a change in therapy. Evaluate test results in relation to the patient's symptoms and other tests performed.

RELATED MONOGRAPHS:

- Related tests include ALT, AST, bilirubin, biopsy liver, BUN, CBC, CBC hematocrit, CBC hemoglobin, creatinine, GGT, hepatobiliary scan, KUB, liver and spleen scan, MRI abdomen, PT/INR, and US liver.
- Refer to the Hepatobiliary System table at the end of the book for related tests by body system.

Computed Tomography, Brain

SYNONYM/ACRONYM: Computed axial tomography (CAT) of the head, computed transaxial tomography (CTT) of the head, brain CT, helical/spiral CT.

COMMON USE: To visualize and assess the brain to assist in diagnosing tumor, bleeding, infarct, infection, structural changes, and edema. Also valuable in evaluation of medical, radiation, and surgical interventions.

AREA OF APPLICATION: Brain.

CONTRAST: With or without IV iodinated contrast medium.

DESCRIPTION: Computed tomography (CT) of the brain is a non-invasive procedure used to assist in diagnosing abnormalities of the head, brain tissue, cerebrospinal fluid, and blood circulation. It becomes invasive if contrast medium is used. The patient lies on a table and is moved in and out of a doughnut-like device called a *gantry*, which houses the x-ray tube and associated electronics. The scanner uses multiple x-ray beams and a series of detectors that rotate around the patient to produce cross-sectional views in a three-dimensional fashion. Differences in tissue density are detected and recorded and are viewable as computerized digital images for the healthcare provider (HCP) to look at. Slices or thin sections of certain anatomic views of the brain and associated vascular system are viewed to allow differentiations of solid, cystic, inflammatory, or vascular lesions, as well as identification of suspected hematomas or aneurysms. The procedure is repeated after intravenous injection of iodinated contrast medium for vascular evaluation. Images can be recorded on photographic or x-ray film or stored in digital format as digitized computer data. Cine scanning is used to produce a series of moving images of the area scanned. Tumor progression, before and after therapy, and effectiveness of medical interventions may be monitored by CT scanning.

INDICATIONS
- Detect brain infection, abscess, or necrosis, as evidenced by decreased density on the image
- Detect ventricular enlargement or displacement by increased cerebrospinal fluid
- Determine benign and cancerous intracranial tumors and cyst formation, as evidenced by changes in tissue densities
- Determine cause of increased intracranial pressure
- Determine presence and type of hemorrhage in infants and children experiencing signs and symptoms of intracranial trauma or congenital conditions such as hydrocephalus and arteriovenous malformations (AVMs)
- Determine presence of multiple sclerosis, as evidenced by sclerotic plaques
- Determine lesion size and location causing infarct or hemorrhage
- Differentiate hematoma location after trauma (e.g., subdural, epidural, cerebral) and determine extent of edema, as evidenced by higher blood densities
- Differentiate between cerebral infarction and hemorrhage
- Evaluate abnormalities of the middle ear ossicles, auditory nerve, and optic nerve
- Monitor and evaluate the effectiveness of medical, radiation, or surgical therapies

POTENTIAL DIAGNOSIS

Normal findings in
- Normal size, position, and shape of intracranial structures and vascular system

Abnormal findings in
- Abscess
- Aneurysm
- AVMs
- Cerebral atrophy
- Cerebral edema
- Cerebral infarction
- Congenital abnormalities
- Craniopharyngioma

- Cysts
- Hematomas (e.g., epidural, subdural, intracerebral)
- Hemorrhage
- Hydrocephaly
- Increased intracranial pressure or trauma
- Infection
- Sclerotic plaques suggesting multiple sclerosis
- Tumor
- Ventricular or tissue displacement or enlargement

CRITICAL FINDINGS

- Abscess
- Acute hemorrhage
- Aneurysm
- Infarction
- Infection
- Tumor with significant mass effect

It is essential that critical diagnoses be communicated immediately to the appropriate HCP. A listing of these diagnoses varies among facilities. Note and immediately report to the HCP abnormal results and related symptoms.

INTERFERING FACTORS

This procedure is contraindicated for

- ❋ Patients with allergies to shellfish or iodinated dye. The contrast medium used may cause a life-threatening allergic reaction. Patients with a known hypersensitivity to the medium may benefit from premedication with corticosteroids or the use of nonionic contrast medium.
- Patients who are claustrophobic.
- Patients who are pregnant or suspected of being pregnant, unless the potential benefits of the procedure far outweigh the risks to the fetus and mother.
- ❋ Elderly and other patients who are chronically

dehydrated before the test, because of their risk of contrast-induced renal failure.
- ❋ Patients who are in renal failure.
- Young patients (17 yr and younger), unless the benefits of the x-ray diagnosis outweigh the risks of exposure to high levels of radiation.

Factors that may impair clear imaging

- Metallic objects (e.g., jewelry, dentures, body rings) within the examination field, which may inhibit organ visualization and cause unclear images.
- Patients who are very obese or who may exceed the weight limit for the equipment.
- Patients with extreme claustrophobia unless sedation is given before the study.
- Inability of the patient to cooperate or remain still during the procedure because of age, significant pain, or mental status.

Other considerations

- Complications of the procedure may include hemorrhage, infection at the IV needle insertion site, and cardiac arrhythmias.
- The procedure may be terminated if chest pain or severe cardiac arrhythmias occur.
- Failure to follow dietary restrictions and other pretesting preparations may cause the procedure to be canceled or repeated.
- Consultation with the HCP should occur before the procedure for radiation safety concerns regarding younger patients or patients who are lactating.
- Risks associated with radiation overexposure can result from frequent x-ray procedures. Personnel in the room with the patient should wear a protective lead apron, stand behind a shield, or leave the area

while the examination is being done. Personnel working in the examination area should wear badges to record their level of radiation exposure.

NURSING IMPLICATIONS AND PROCEDURE

PRETEST:

▶ Positively identify the patient using at least two unique identifiers before providing care, treatment, or services.

▶ *Patient Teaching:* Inform the patient this procedure can assist in assessing the brain.

▶ Obtain a history of the patient's complaints or clinical symptoms, including a list of known allergens, especially allergies or sensitivities to latex, iodine, seafood, anesthetics, or contrast medium.

▶ Obtain a history of the patient's musculoskeletal system, symptoms, and results of previously performed laboratory tests and diagnostic and surgical procedures.

▶ Ensure results of coagulation testing are obtained and recorded prior to the procedure; BUN and creatinine results are also needed if contrast medium is to be used.

▶ Note any recent procedures that can interfere with test results, including examinations using barium- or iodine-based contrast medium. Ensure that barium studies were performed more than 4 days before the CT scan.

▶ Record the date of the last menstrual period and determine the possibility of pregnancy in perimenopausal women.

▶ Obtain a list of the patient's current medications including anticoagulants, aspirin and other salicylates, herbs, nutritional supplements, and nutraceuticals (see Appendix F). Note the last time and dose of medication taken.

▶ If contrast media is scheduled to be used, patients receiving metformin (Glucophage) for non-insulin-dependent (type 2) diabetes should discontinue the drug on the day of the test and continue to withhold it for 48 hr after the test. Failure to do so may result in lactic acidosis.

▶ Review the procedure with the patient. Address concerns about pain and explain that there may be moments of discomfort and some pain experienced during the test. Inform the patient the procedure is usually performed in a radiology suite by an HCP specializing in this procedure, with support staff, and takes approximately 15 to 30 min.

▶ *Sensitivity to social and cultural issues,* as well as concern for modesty, is important in providing psychological support before, during, and after the procedure.

▶ Explain that an IV line may be inserted to allow infusion of IV fluids, contrast medium, dye, or sedatives. Usually contrast medium and normal saline are infused.

▶ Inform the patient that he or she may experience nausea, a feeling of warmth, a salty or metallic taste, or a transient headache after injection of contrast medium.

▶ Instruct the patient to remove dentures and jewelry and other metallic objects from the area to be examined.

▶ There are no food or fluid restrictions unless by medical direction. Instruct the patient to avoid taking anticoagulant medication or to reduce dosage as ordered prior to the procedure. Protocols may vary among facilities.

▶ *Make sure a written and informed consent has been signed prior to the procedure and before administering any medications.*

INTRATEST:

▶ Ensure the patient has complied with medication restrictions and pretesting preparations.

▶ Ensure the patient has removed dentures and all external metallic objects from the area to be examined prior to the procedure.

▶ If the patient has a history of allergic reactions to any substance or drug, administer ordered prophylactic steroids or antihistamines before the procedure. Use nonionic contrast medium for the procedure.

▶ Have emergency equipment readily available.

▶ Instruct the patient to cooperate fully and to follow directions. Instruct the patient to remain still throughout the procedure because movement produces unreliable results.

- Observe standard precautions, and follow the general guidelines in Appendix A.
- Establish an IV fluid line for the injection of contrast medium, emergency drugs, and sedatives.
- Administer an antianxiety agent, as ordered, if the patient has claustrophobia. Administer a sedative to a child or to an uncooperative adult, as ordered.
- Place the patient in the supine position on an examination table.
- If contrast media is used, a rapid series of images is taken during and after injection.
- Instruct the patient to take slow, deep breaths if nausea occurs during the procedure.
- Monitor the patient for complications related to the procedure (e.g., allergic reaction, anaphylaxis, bronchospasm) if contrast is used.
- The needle is removed, and a pressure dressing is applied over the puncture site.
- Observe/assess the needle insertion site for bleeding, inflammation, or hematoma formation.

POST-TEST:

- A report of the examination will be sent to the requesting HCP, who will discuss the results with the patient.
- Instruct the patient to resume medications and activity, as directed by the HCP. Renal function should be assessed before metformin is resumed, if contrast was used.
- Monitor vital signs and neurological status every 15 min for 1 hr, then every 2 hr for 4 hr, and then as ordered by the HCP. Monitor temperature every 4 hr for 24 hr. Monitor intake and output at least every 8 hr. Compare with baseline values. Notify the HCP if temperature is elevated. Protocols may vary from facility to facility.
- If contrast was used, observe for delayed allergic reactions, such as rash, urticaria, tachycardia, hyperpnea, hypertension, palpitations, nausea, or vomiting.

- Instruct the patient to immediately report symptoms such as fast heart rate, difficulty breathing, skin rash, itching, chest pain, persistent right shoulder pain, or abdominal pain. Immediately report symptoms to the appropriate HCP.
- Observe/assess the needle insertion site for bleeding, inflammation, or hematoma formation.
- Instruct the patient in the care and assessment of the site.
- Instruct the patient to apply cold compresses to the puncture site as needed, to reduce discomfort or edema.
- Instruct the patient to increase fluid intake to help eliminate the contrast medium, if used.
- Inform the patient that diarrhea may occur after ingestion of oral contrast medium.
- Recognize anxiety related to test results. Discuss the implications of abnormal test results on the patient's lifestyle. Provide teaching and information regarding the clinical implications of the test results, as appropriate.
- Reinforce information given by the patient's HCP regarding further testing, treatment, or referral to another HCP. Answer any questions or address any concerns voiced by the patient or family.
- Depending on the results of this procedure, additional testing may be needed to evaluate or monitor progression of the disease process and determine the need for a change in therapy. Evaluate test results in relation to the patient's symptoms and other tests performed.

RELATED MONOGRAPHS:

- Related tests include angiography carotid, audiometry hearing loss, BUN, CSF analysis, CBC, CBC hematocrit, CBC hemoglobin, CT angiography, creatinine, EEG, EMG, evoked brain potentials, MR angiography, MRI brain, nerve fiber analysis, otoscopy, PET brain, PT/INR, spondee speech reception threshold, and tuning fork tests.
- Refer to the Musculoskeletal System table at the end of the book for related tests by body system.

C

Computed Tomography, Cardiac Scoring

SYNONYM/ACRONYM: Computed axial tomography (CAT), computed transaxial tomography (CTT), heart vessel calcium CT, helical/spiral CT, cardiac plaque CT.

COMMON USE: To visualize and assess coronary artery status related to plaque buildup, associated with coronary artery disease, and heart failure. Used as an evaluation tool for surgical, radiation, and medical therapeutic interventions.

AREA OF APPLICATION: Heart.

CONTRAST: None.

DESCRIPTION: Cardiac scoring is a noninvasive test for quantifying coronary artery calcium content. Coronary artery disease (CAD) occurs when the arteries that carry blood and oxygen to the heart muscle become clogged or built up with plaque. Plaque buildup slows the flow of blood to the heart muscle, causing ischemia and increasing the risk of heart failure. The procedure begins with a computed tomography (CT) scan of the heart. The patient lies on a table and is moved in and out of a doughnut-like device called a *gantry*, which houses the x-ray tube and associated electronics. The scanner uses multiple x-ray beams and a series of detectors that rotate around the patient to produce cross-sectional views in a three-dimensional fashion by detecting and recording differences in plaque density after having an x-ray beam passed through the tissues. The scanner takes an image of the beating heart while the patient holds his or her breath for approximately 20 sec. The procedure requires no contrast medium injections. These density measurements are sent to a computer that produces a digital analysis of the anatomy, enabling the health-care provider (HCP) to look at the quantified amount of calcium (cardiac plaque score) in the coronary arteries. The data can be recorded on photographic or x-ray film or stored in digital format as digitized computer data.

INDICATIONS

- Detect and quantify coronary artery calcium content
  CAD is the leading cause of death in most industrialized nations.
  Cardiac scoring is a more powerful predictor of CAD than cholesterol screening.
  Of all myocardial infarctions (MIs), 45% occur in people younger than age 65.
  Of women who have had MIs, 44% will die within 1 yr after the attack.
  Women are more likely to die of heart disease than of breast cancer.
- Family history of heart disease
- Screening for coronary artery calcium in patients with:
  Diabetes
  High blood pressure
  High cholesterol

High-stress lifestyle
Overweight by 20% or more
Personal history of smoking
Sedentary lifestyle
- Screening for coronary artery plaque in patients with chest pain of unknown cause

POTENTIAL DIAGNOSIS

Normal findings in
- If the score is 100 or less, the probability of having significant CAD is minimal or is unlikely to be causing a narrowing at the time of the examination.

Abnormal findings in
- If the score is between 101 and 400, a significant amount of calcified plaque was found in the coronary arteries. There is an increased risk of a future MI, and a medical assessment of cardiac risk factors needs to be done. Additional testing may be needed.
- If the score is greater than 400, the procedure has detected extensive calcified plaque in the coronary arteries, which may have caused a critical narrowing of the vessels. A full medical assessment is needed as soon as possible. Further testing may be needed, and treatment may be needed to reduce the risk of MI.

CRITICAL FINDINGS: N/A

INTERFERING FACTORS

This procedure is contraindicated for
- Patients who are claustrophobic.
- Patients who are pregnant or suspected of being pregnant, unless the potential benefits of the procedure far outweigh the risks to the fetus and mother.

- Young patients (17 yr and younger), unless the benefits of the x-ray diagnosis outweigh the risks of exposure to high levels of radiation.

Factors that may impair clear imaging
- Retained barium or radiological contrast from a previous radiological procedure.
- Metallic objects (e.g., jewelry, body rings) within the examination field, which may inhibit organ visualization and cause unclear images.
- Improper adjustment of the radiographic equipment to accommodate obese or thin patients, which can cause overexposure or underexposure and a poor-quality study.
- Patients with extreme claustrophobia unless sedation is given before the study.
- Inability of the patient to cooperate or remain still during the procedure because of age, significant pain, or mental status.

Other considerations
- The procedure may be terminated if chest pain or severe cardiac arrhythmias occur.
- Consultation with the HCP should occur before the procedure for radiation safety concerns regarding younger patients or patients who are lactating.
- Risks associated with radiation overexposure can result from frequent x-ray procedures. Personnel in the room with the patient should wear a protective lead apron, stand behind a shield, or leave the area while the examination is being done. Personnel working in the examination area should wear badges to record their level of radiation exposure.

C

NURSING IMPLICATIONS AND PROCEDURE

PRETEST:

- Positively identify the patient using at least two unique identifiers before providing care, treatment, or services.
- *Patient Teaching:* Inform the patient this procedure can assist in assessing the coronary arteries.
- Obtain a history of the patient's complaints or clinical symptoms, including a list of known allergens, especially allergies or sensitivities to latex, iodine, seafood, anesthetics, or contrast medium.
- Obtain a history of patient's cardiovascular system, symptoms, and results of previously performed laboratory tests and diagnostic and surgical procedures.
- Ensure results of coagulation testing are obtained and recorded prior to the procedure; BUN and creatinine results are also needed if contrast medium is to be used.
- Note any recent procedures that can interfere with test results, including examinations using barium- or iodine-based contrast medium. Ensure that barium studies were performed more than 4 days before the CT scan.
- Record the date of the last menstrual period and determine the possibility of pregnancy in perimenopausal women.
- Obtain a list of the patient's current medications, including anticoagulants, aspirin and other salicylates, herbs, nutritional supplements, and nutraceuticals (see Appendix F). Note the last time and dose of medication taken.
- If contrast medium is scheduled to be used, patients receiving metformin (Glucophage) for non-insulin-dependent (type 2) diabetes should discontinue the drug on the day of the test and continue to withhold it for 48 hr after the test. Failure to do so may result in lactic acidosis.
- Review the procedure with the patient. Address concerns about pain and explain that there may be moments of discomfort and some pain experienced during the test. Inform the patient the procedure is usually performed in a radiology suite by an HCP specializing in this procedure, with support staff, and takes approximately 30 to 60 min.
- *Sensitivity to social and cultural issues,* as well as concern for modesty, is important in providing psychological support before, during, and after the procedure.
- Explain that an IV line may be inserted to allow infusion of IV fluids, anesthetics, or sedatives.
- Inform the patient that he or she may experience nausea, a feeling of warmth, a salty or metallic taste, or a transient headache after injection of contrast medium, if given.
- The patient should not fast or restrict fluids prior to the procedure. Protocols may vary among facilities.
- Instruct the patient to remove all external metallic objects from the area to be examined.

INTRATEST:

- Ensure the patient has complied with pretesting preparations.
- Ensure that the patient has removed all external metallic objects from the area to be examined.
- If the patient has a history of allergic reactions to any substance or drug, administer ordered prophylactic steroids or antihistamines before the procedure. Use nonionic contrast medium for the procedure.
- Have emergency equipment readily available.
- Instruct the patient to void prior to the procedure and to change into the gown, robe, and foot coverings provided.
- Instruct the patient to cooperate fully and to follow directions. Instruct the patient to remain still throughout the procedure because movement produces unreliable results.
- Record baseline vital signs, and continue to monitor throughout the procedure. Protocols may vary among facilities.

- Observe standard precautions, and follow the general guidelines in Appendix A.
- Establish an IV fluid line for the injection of contrast medium, emergency drugs, and sedatives.
- Administer an antianxiety agent, as ordered, if the patient has claustrophobia. Administer a sedative to a child or to an uncooperative adult, as ordered.
- Place the patient in the supine position on an examination table.
- A rapid series of images is taken of the vessels to be examined.
- Instruct the patient to inhale deeply and hold his or her breath while the x-ray images are taken, and then to exhale after the images are taken.
- Instruct the patient to take slow, deep breaths if nausea occurs during the procedure.
- Monitor the patient for complications related to the procedure (e.g., allergic reaction, anaphylaxis, bronchospasm) if contrast is used.
- The needle is removed, and a pressure dressing is applied over the puncture site.
- Observe/assess the needle site for bleeding, inflammation, or hematoma formation.

POST-TEST:

- A report of the examination will be sent to the requesting HCP who will discuss the results with the patient.
- Instruct the patient to resume usual diet, fluids, medications, and activity, as directed by the HCP. Renal function should be assessed before metformin is resumed, if contrast was used.
- Monitor vital signs and neurological status every 15 min for 1 hr, then every 2 hr for 4 hr, and then as ordered by the HCP. Monitor temperature every 4 hr for 24 hr. Monitor intake and output at least every 8 hr. Compare with baseline values. Notify the HCP if temperature is elevated. Protocols may vary among facilities.
- If contrast was used, observe for delayed allergic reactions, such as

rash, urticaria, tachycardia, hyperpnea, hypertension, palpitations, nausea, or vomiting.
- Instruct the patient to immediately report symptoms such as fast heart rate, difficulty breathing, skin rash, itching, chest pain, persistent right shoulder pain, or abdominal pain. Immediately report symptoms to the appropriate HCP.
- Observe/assess the needle insertion site for bleeding, inflammation, or hematoma formation.
- Instruct the patient in the care and assessment of the site.
- Instruct the patient to apply cold compresses to the insertion site as needed, to reduce discomfort or edema.
- Instruct the patient to increase fluid intake to help eliminate the contrast medium, if used.
- Inform the patient that diarrhea may occur after ingestion of oral contrast media.
- Recognize anxiety related to test results. Discuss the implications of abnormal test results on the patient's lifestyle. Provide teaching and information regarding the clinical implications of the test results, as appropriate.
- *Nutritional Considerations:* Abnormal findings may be associated with cardiovascular disease. The American Heart Association and National Heart, Lung, and Blood Institute (NHBLI) recommend nutritional therapy for individuals identified to be at high risk for developing CAD or individuals who have specific risk factors and/or existing medical conditions (e.g., elevated LDL cholesterol levels, other lipid disorders, insulin-dependent diabetes, insulin resistance, or metabolic syndrome). If overweight, the patient should be encouraged to achieve a normal weight. The NHLBI's National Cholesterol Education Program (NCEP) revised its dietary guidelines for reducing CAD in 2001. Guidelines for the Therapeutic Lifestyle Changes (TLC) diet are outlined in the Third Report of the Expert Panel on Detection, Evaluation,

and Treatment of High Blood Cholesterol in Adults (Adult Treatment Panel III [ATP III]). The TLC diet emphasizes a reduction in foods high in saturated fats and cholesterol. Red meats, eggs, and dairy products are the major sources of saturated fats and cholesterol. If triglycerides also are elevated, the patient should be advised to eliminate or reduce alcohol and simple carbohydrates from the diet. The TLC approach also includes the use of plant stanols or sterols and increased dissolved fiber as an option for lowering LDL cholesterol levels; nutritional recommendations for daily total caloric intake; recommendations for allowable percentage of calories derived from fat (saturated and unsaturated), carbohydrates, protein, and cholesterol; as well as recommendations for daily expenditure of energy.

‣ *Nutritional Considerations:* Overweight patients with high blood pressure should be encouraged to achieve a normal weight. Other changeable risk factors warranting patient education include strategies to safely decrease sodium intake, increase physical activity, decrease alcohol consumption, eliminate tobacco use, and decrease cholesterol levels.

‣ *Social and Cultural Considerations:* Numerous studies point to the prevalence of excess body weight in American children and adolescents. Experts estimate that obesity is present in 25% of the population ages 6 to 11 yr. The medical, social, and emotional consequences of excess body weight are significant. Special attention should be given to instructing the child and caregiver regarding health risks and weight control education.

‣ Recognize anxiety related to test results, and be supportive of fear of shortened life expectancy. Discuss the implications of abnormal test results on the patient's lifestyle. Provide teaching and information regarding the clinical implications of the test results, as appropriate. Educate the patient regarding access to counseling services. Provide contact information, if desired, for the American Heart Association (www.americanheart.org) or the NHLBI (www.nhlbi.nih.gov).

‣ Reinforce information given by the patient's HCP regarding further testing, treatment, or referral to another HCP. Answer any questions or address any concerns voiced by the patient or family.

‣ Depending on the results of this procedure, additional testing may be needed to evaluate or monitor progression of the disease process and determine the need for a change in therapy. Evaluate test results in relation to the patient's symptoms and other tests performed.

RELATED MONOGRAPHS:

‣ Related tests include antiarrhythmic drugs, apolipoprotein A and B, AST, atrial natriuretic peptide, BNP, BUN, calcium, chest x-ray, cholesterol (total, HDL, LDL), CRP, CBC, CBC hematocrit, CBC hemoglobin, coronary angiography, CT thorax, CK and isoenzymes, creatinine echocardiography, echocardiography transesophageal ECG, glucose, glycated hemoglobin, Holter monitor, homocysteine, ketones, LDH and isoenzymes, lipoprotein electrophoresis, lung scan, magnesium, MRI chest, MI scan, myocardial perfusion heart scan, myoglobin, PET heart, potassium, PT/INR, triglycerides, and troponin.

‣ Refer to the Cardiovascular System table at the end of the book for related tests by body system.

Computed Tomography, Colonoscopy

SYNONYM/ACRONYM: Computed axial tomography (CAT), computed transaxial tomography (CTT), CT colonography, CT virtual colonoscopy.

COMMON USE: To visualize and assess the rectum and colon related to identification and evaluation of large polyps, lesions, and tumors. Also used to assess the effectiveness of therapeutic interventions such as surgery. Primarily used for patients who cannot tolerate conventional colonoscopy.

AREA OF APPLICATION: Colon.

CONTRAST: Screening examinations are done without IV iodinated contrast medium. Examinations done to clarify questionable or abnormal areas may require IV iodinated contrast medium.

DESCRIPTION: Computed tomography (CT) colonoscopy is a noninvasive technique that involves examining the colon by taking multiple CT scans of the patient's colon and rectum and using computer software to create three-dimensional images. The procedure is used to detect polyps, which are growths of tissue in the colon or rectum. Some types of polyps increase the risk of colon cancer, especially if they are large or if a patient has several polyps. Compared to conventional colonoscopy, CT colonoscopy is less effective in detecting polyps smaller than 5 mm, more effective when the polyps are between 5 and 9.9 mm, and most effective when the polyps are 10 mm or larger. This test may be valuable for patients who have diseases rendering them unable to undergo conventional colonoscopy (e.g., bleeding disorders, lung or heart disease) and for patients who are unable to undergo the sedation required for traditional colonoscopy. The procedure is less invasive than conventional colonoscopy, with little risk of complications and no recovery time. CT colonoscopy can be done as an outpatient procedure, and the patient may return to work or usual activities the same day.

CT colonoscopy and conventional colonoscopy require the bowel to be cleansed before the examination. The patient lies on a table and is moved in and out of a doughnut-like device called a *gantry,* which houses the x-ray tube and associated electronics. The scanner uses multiple x-ray beams and a series of detectors that rotate around the patient to produce cross-sectional views in a three-dimensional fashion by detecting and recording differences in densities in the colon after having an x-ray beam passed through it. The screening procedure requires no contrast medium injections, but if a suspicious area or abnormality is detected, a repeat series of images may be completed after IV contrast medium is given. These density measurements are sent to a computer that produces a digital analysis of the anatomy, enabling a health care provider (HCP) to look at slices or thin sections of certain anatomic views of the colon and vascular system. The data can be recorded on photographic or x-ray film or stored in digital format as digitized computer data. A drawback of CT colonoscopy is that polyp removal and biopsies of tissue in the colon must be done using conventional colonoscopy. Therefore, if polyps are discovered during CT colonoscopy and biopsy becomes necessary, the patient must undergo bowel preparation a second time.

INDICATIONS

- Detect polyps in the colon
- Evaluate the colon for metachronous lesions
- Evaluate the colon in patients with obstructing rectosigmoid disease
- Evaluate polyposis syndromes
- Evaluate the site of resection for local recurrence of lesions
- Examine the colon in patients with heart or lung disease, patients unable to be sedated, and patients unable to undergo colonoscopy
- Failure to visualize the entire colon during conventional colonoscopy
- Identify metastases
- Investigate cause of positive occult blood test
- Investigate further after an abnormal barium enema
- Investigate further when flexible sigmoidoscopy is positive for polyps

POTENTIAL DIAGNOSIS

Normal findings in

- Normal colon and rectum, with no evidence of polyps or growths

Abnormal findings in

- Abnormal endoluminal wall of the colon
- Extraluminal extension of primary cancer
- Mesenteric and retroperitoneal lymphadenopathy
- Metachronous lesions
- Metastases of cancer
- Polyps or growths in colon or rectum
- Tumor recurrence after surgery

CRITICAL FINDINGS: N/A

INTERFERING FACTORS

This procedure is contraindicated for

- ◆ Patients with allergies to shellfish or iodinated dye. The contrast medium used may cause a life-threatening allergic reaction. Patients with a known hypersensitivity to the medium may benefit from premedication with corticosteroids or the use of nonionic contrast medium, if contrast is used.
- Patients who are claustrophobic.
- Patients who are pregnant or suspected of being pregnant, unless the potential benefits of the procedure far outweigh the risks to the fetus and mother.
- ◆ Elderly and other patients who are chronically dehydrated before the test, because of their risk of contrast-induced renal failure, if contrast is used.
- ◆ Patients who are in renal failure, if contrast is used.
- Young patients (17 yr and younger), unless the benefits of the x-ray diagnosis outweigh the risks of exposure to high levels of radiation.

Factors that may impair clear imaging

- Gas or feces in the gastrointestinal tract resulting from inadequate cleansing or failure to restrict food intake before the study.
- Retained barium from a previous radiological procedure.
- Metallic objects (e.g., jewelry, body rings) within the examination field, which may inhibit organ visualization and cause unclear images.
- Patients who are very obese or who may exceed the weight limit for the equipment.
- Patients with extreme claustrophobia unless sedation is given before the study.
- Inability of the patient to cooperate or remain still during the procedure because of age, significant pain, or mental status.

Other considerations

- Complications of the procedure may include hemorrhage, infection at the IV needle insertion site, and cardiac arrhythmias.
- The procedure may be terminated if chest pain or severe cardiac arrhythmias occur.
- Failure to follow dietary restrictions and other pretesting preparations may cause the procedure to be canceled or repeated.
- Consultation with the HCP should occur before the procedure for radiation safety concerns regarding younger patients or patients who are lactating.
- Risks associated with radiation overexposure can result from frequent x-ray procedures. Personnel in the room with the patient should wear a protective lead apron, stand behind a shield, or leave the area while the examination is being done. Personnel working in the examination area should wear badges to record their level of radiation exposure.

NURSING IMPLICATIONS AND PROCEDURE

PRETEST:

- Positively identify the patient using at least two unique identifiers before providing care, treatment, or services.
- *Patient Teaching:* Inform the patient this procedure can assist in assessing the colon.
- Obtain a history of the patient's complaints or clinical symptoms, including a list of known allergens, especially allergies or sensitivities to latex, iodine, seafood, anesthetics, or contrast mediums.
- Obtain a history of the patient's gastrointestinal system, symptoms, and results of previously performed laboratory tests and diagnostic and surgical procedures.
- Ensure results of coagulation testing are obtained and recorded prior to the procedure; BUN and creatinine results are also needed if contrast medium is to be used.
- Note any recent procedures that can interfere with test results, including examinations using barium- or iodine-based contrast medium. Ensure that barium studies were performed more than 4 days before the CT scan.
- Record the date of the last menstrual period and determine the possibility of pregnancy in perimenopausal women.
- Obtain a list of the patient's current medications, including anticoagulants, aspirin and other salicylates, herbs, nutritional supplements, and nutraceuticals (see Appendix F). Note the last time and dose of medication taken.
- If contrast is scheduled to be used, patients receiving metformin (Glucophage) for non-insulin-dependent (type 2) diabetes should discontinue the drug on the day of the test and continue to withhold it for 48 hr after the test. Failure to do so may result in lactic acidosis.
- Review the procedure with the patient. Address concerns about pain and explain that some pain may be experienced during the test, and there may

be moments of discomfort. Inform the patient that the procedure is performed in a radiology department, usually by an HCP specializing in this procedure, with support staff, and takes approximately 30 to 60 min.

▶ *Sensitivity to social and cultural issues,* as well as concern for modesty, is important in providing psychological support before, during, and after the procedure.

▶ Explain that an IV line may be inserted to allow infusion of IV fluids, contrast medium, dye, or sedatives.

▶ Inform the patient that he or she may experience nausea, a feeling of warmth, a salty or metallic taste, or a transient headache after injection of contrast medium.

▶ Instruct the patient to remove jewelry and other metallic objects from the area to be examined.

▶ The patient should fast and restrict fluids for 6 to 8 hr prior to the procedure. Instruct the patient to avoid taking anticoagulant medication or to reduce dosage as ordered prior to the procedure. Protocols may vary among facilities.

▶ *Make sure a written and informed consent has been signed prior to the procedure and before administering any medications.*

INTRATEST:

▶ Ensure that the patient has complied with dietary, fluids, and medication restrictions and pretesting preparations; ensure that food and fluids have been restricted for at least 6 hr prior to the procedure.

▶ Ensure that the patient has removed all external metallic objects from the area to be examined prior to the procedure.

▶ If the patient has a history of allergic reactions to any substance or drug, administer ordered prophylactic steroids or antihistamines before the procedure. Use nonionic contrast medium for the procedure.

▶ Have emergency equipment readily available.

▶ Instruct the patient to void prior to the procedure and to change into the

gown, robe, and foot coverings provided.

▶ Instruct the patient to cooperate fully and to follow directions. Instruct the patient to remain still throughout the procedure because movement produces unreliable results.

▶ Record baseline vital signs, and continue to monitor throughout the procedure. Protocols may vary among facilities.

▶ Observe standard precautions, and follow the general guidelines in Appendix A.

▶ Establish an IV fluid line for the injection of contrast (if used), emergency drugs, and sedatives.

▶ Administer an antianxiety agent, as ordered, if the patient has claustrophobia. Administer a sedative to a child or to an uncooperative adult, as ordered.

▶ Place the patient in the supine position on an examination table.

▶ The colon is distended with room air or carbon dioxide by means of a rectal tube and balloon retention device. Maximal colonic distention is guided by patient tolerance.

▶ If IV contrast is used, a rapid series of images is taken during and after injection.

▶ Instruct the patient to inhale deeply and hold his or her breath while the x-ray images are taken, and then to exhale after the images are taken.

▶ The sequence of images is repeated in the prone position.

▶ Instruct the patient to take slow, deep breaths if nausea occurs during the procedure.

▶ Monitor the patient for complications related to the procedure (e.g., allergic reaction, anaphylaxis, bronchospasm) if contrast is used.

▶ The needle is removed, and a pressure dressing is applied over the puncture site.

▶ Observe/assess the needle site for bleeding, inflammation, or hematoma formation.

POST-TEST:

▶ A report of the examination will be sent to the requesting HCP, who will discuss the results with the patient.

- Instruct the patient to resume usual diet, fluids, medications, and activity, as directed by the HCP. Renal function should be assessed before metformin is resumed, if contrast was used.
- Monitor vital signs and neurological status every 15 min for 1 hr, then every 2 hr for 4 hr, and then as ordered by the HCP. Monitor temperature every 4 hr for 24 hr. Monitor intake and output at least every 8 hr. Compare with baseline values. Notify the HCP if temperature is elevated. Protocols may vary among facilities.
- If contrast was used, observe for delayed allergic reactions, such as rash, urticaria, tachycardia, hyperpnea, hypertension, palpitations, nausea, or vomiting.
- Instruct the patient to immediately report symptoms such as fast heart rate, difficulty breathing, skin rash, itching, chest pain, persistent right shoulder pain, or abdominal pain. Immediately report symptoms to the appropriate HCP.
- Observe/assess the needle/catheter insertion site for bleeding, inflammation, or hematoma formation.
- Instruct the patient in the care and assessment of the site.
- Instruct the patient to apply cold compresses to the puncture site as needed, to reduce discomfort or edema.
- Instruct the patient to increase fluid intake to help eliminate the contrast medium, if used.
- Inform the patient that diarrhea may occur after ingestion of oral contrast media.
- Recognize anxiety related to test results. Discuss the implications of abnormal test results on the patient's lifestyle. Provide teaching and information regarding the clinical implications of the test results, as appropriate.
- Reinforce information given by the patient's HCP regarding further testing, treatment, or referral to another HCP. Decisions regarding the need for and frequency of occult blood testing, colonoscopy, or other cancer screening procedures should be made after consultation between the patient and HCP. The most current guidelines for colon cancer screening of the general population as well as individuals with increased risk are available from the American Cancer Society (www.cancer.org) and the American College of Gastroenterology (www.gi.org). Answer any questions or address any concerns voiced by the patient or family.
- Depending on the results of this procedure, additional testing may be needed to evaluate or monitor progression of the disease process and determine the need for a change in therapy. Evaluate test results in relation to the patient's symptoms and other tests performed.

RELATED MONOGRAPHS:

- Related tests include barium enema, BUN, cancer antigens, capsule endoscopy, colonoscopy, CBC, CBC hematocrit, CBC hemoglobin, CT abdomen, creatinine, fecal analysis, KUB studies, MRI abdomen, PET pelvis, proctosigmoidoscopy, PT/INR, and US pelvis.
- Refer to the Gastrointestinal System table at the end of the book for related tests by body system.

C

Computed Tomography, Pancreas

SYNONYM/ACRONYM: Computed axial tomography (CAT), computed transaxial tomography (CTT, abdominal CT, helical/spiral CT).

COMMON USE: To visualize and assess the pancreas to assist in diagnosing tumors, masses, cancer, bleeding, infection, and abscess. Used as an evaluation tool for surgical, radiation, and medical therapeutic interventions.

AREA OF APPLICATION: Pancreas.

CONTRAST: With or without oral or IV iodinated contrast medium.

DESCRIPTION: Computed tomography (CT) is a noninvasive procedure used to enhance certain anatomic views of the abdominal structures. It becomes an invasive procedure when contrast medium is used. CT of the pancreas aids in the diagnosis or evaluation of pancreatic cysts, pseudocysts, inflammation, tumors, masses, metastases, abscesses, and trauma. In all but the thinnest or most emaciated patients, the pancreas is surrounded by fat that clearly defines its margins. During the procedure, the patient lies on a table and is moved in and out of a doughnut-like device called a *gantry*, which houses the x-ray tube and associated electronics. The scanner uses multiple x-ray beams and a series of detectors that rotate around the patient to produce cross-sectional views in a three-dimensional fashion. Differences in tissue density are detected and recorded and are viewable as computerized digital images. Slices or thin sections of certain anatomic views of the kidneys and associated vascular system are reviewed to allow differentiation of solid, cystic, inflammatory, or vascular lesions, as well as identification of suspected hematomas and aneurysms. The procedure is repeated after intravenous injection of iodinated contrast medium for vascular evaluation or after oral ingestion of contrast medium for evaluation of bowel and adjacent structures. Images can be recorded on photographic or x-ray film or stored in digital format as digitized computer data. Cine scanning produces a series of moving images of the scanned area. The CT scan can be used to guide biopsy needles into areas of pancreatic masses to obtain tissue for laboratory analysis and for placement of needles to aspirate cysts or abscesses. CT scanning can monitor mass, cyst, or tumor growth and post-therapy response.

INDICATIONS

- Detect dilation or obstruction of the pancreatic ducts
- Differentiate between pancreatic disorders and disorders of the retroperitoneum

- Evaluate benign or cancerous tumors or metastasis to the pancreas
- Evaluate pancreatic abnormalities (e.g., bleeding, pancreatitis, pseudocyst, abscesses)
- Evaluate unexplained weight loss, jaundice, and epigastric pain
- Monitor and evaluate effectiveness of medical or surgical therapies

POTENTIAL DIAGNOSIS

Normal findings in
- Normal size, position, and contour of the pancreas, which lies obliquely in the upper abdomen

Abnormal findings in
- Acute or chronic pancreatitis
- Obstruction of the pancreatic ducts
- Pancreatic abscesses
- Pancreatic carcinoma
- Pancreatic pseudocyst
- Pancreatic tumor

CRITICAL FINDINGS: N/A

INTERFERING FACTORS

This procedure is contraindicated for
- ❖ Patients with allergies to shellfish or iodinated dye. The contrast medium used may cause a life-threatening allergic reaction. Patients with a known hypersensitivity to the medium may benefit from premedication with corticosteroids or the use of nonionic contrast medium.
- Patients who are claustrophobic.
- Patients who are pregnant or suspected of being pregnant, unless the potential benefits of the procedure far outweigh the risks to the fetus and mother.
- ❖ Elderly and other patients who are chronically dehydrated before the test, because of their risk of contrast-induced renal failure.
- ❖ Patients who are in renal failure.

- Young patients (17 yr and younger), unless the benefits of the x-ray diagnosis outweigh the risks of exposure to high levels of radiation.

Factors that may impair clear imaging
- Gas or feces in the gastrointestinal (GI) tract resulting from inadequate cleansing or failure to restrict food intake before the study.
- Retained barium from a previous radiological procedure.
- Metallic objects (e.g., jewelry, body rings) within the examination field, which may inhibit organ visualization and cause unclear images.
- Patients who are very obese or who may exceed the weight limit for the equipment.
- Patients with extreme claustrophobia unless sedation is given before the study.
- Inability of the patient to cooperate or remain still during the procedure because of age, significant pain, or mental status.

Other considerations
- Complications of the procedure include hemorrhage, infection at the IV needle insertion site, and cardiac arrhythmias.
- The procedure may be terminated if chest pain or severe cardiac arrhythmias occur.
- Failure to follow dietary restrictions and other pretesting preparations may cause the procedure to be canceled or repeated.
- Consultation with a health-care provider (HCP) should occur before the procedure for radiation safety concerns regarding younger patients or patients who are lactating.
- Risks associated with radiation overexposure can result from frequent x-ray procedures. Personnel in the room with the patient should wear a protective

lead apron, stand behind a shield, or leave the area while the examination is being done. Personnel working in the examination area should wear badges to record their level of radiation exposure.

NURSING IMPLICATIONS AND PROCEDURE

PRETEST:

▶ Positively identify the patient using at least two unique identifiers before providing care, treatment, or services.

▶ *Patient Teaching:* Inform the patient this procedure can assist in assessing the abdomen and pancreatic area.

▶ Obtain a history of the patient's complaints, including a list of known allergens, especially allergies or sensitivities to latex, iodine, seafood, anesthetics, or other contrast medium.

▶ Obtain a history of the patient's gastrointestinal and hepatobiliary system, symptoms, and results of previously performed laboratory tests and diagnostic and surgical procedures.

▶ Ensure results of coagulation testing are obtained and recorded prior to the procedure; BUN and creatinine results are also needed if contrast medium is to be used.

▶ Note any recent procedures that can interfere with test results, including examinations using barium- or iodine-based contrast medium. Ensure that barium studies were performed more than 4 days before the CT scan.

▶ Record the date of the last menstrual period and determine the possibility of pregnancy in perimenopausal women.

▶ Obtain a list of the patient's current medications, including anticoagulants, aspirin and other salicylates, herbs, nutritional supplements, and nutraceuticals (see Appendix F). Note the last time and dose of medication taken.

▶ If contrast medium is scheduled to be used, patients receiving metformin (Glucophage) for non-insulin-dependent (type 2) diabetes should discontinue the drug on the day of the test and continue to withhold it for 48 hr after the test. Failure to do so may result in lactic acidosis.

▶ Review the procedure with the patient. Address concerns about pain and explain that there may be moments of discomfort and some pain experienced during the test. Inform the patient the procedure is usually performed in a radiology suite by an HCP specializing in this procedure, with support staff, and takes approximately 30 to 60 min.

▶ *Sensitivity to social and cultural issues,* as well as concern for modesty, is important in providing psychological support before, during, and after the procedure.

▶ Explain that an IV line may be inserted to allow infusion of IV fluids, contrast medium, dye, or sedatives. Usually contrast medium and normal saline are infused.

▶ Inform the patient that he or she may experience nausea, a feeling of warmth, a salty or metallic taste, or a transient headache after injection of contrast medium.

▶ The patient should fast and restrict fluids for 2 to 4 hr prior to the procedure. Instruct the patient to avoid taking anticoagulant medication or to reduce dosage as ordered prior to the procedure. Protocols may vary among facilities.

▶ The patient may be requested to drink approximately 450 mL of a dilute barium solution (approximately 1% barium) beginning 1 hr before the examination. This is administered to distinguish GI organs from the other abdominal organs.

▶ Instruct the patient to remove jewelry and other metallic objects from the area to be examined.

▶ *Make sure a written and informed consent has been signed prior to the procedure and before administering any medications.*

INTRATEST:

▶ Ensure the patient has complied with dietary, fluids, and medication restrictions and pretesting preparations; ensure that food and fluids have been restricted for at least 2 to 4 hr prior to the procedure.

▶ Ensure that the patient has removed all external metallic objects from the area to be examined prior to the procedure.

▶ If the patient has a history of allergic reactions to any substance or drug, administer ordered prophylactic steroids or antihistamines before the procedure. Use nonionic contrast medium for the procedure.

▶ Have emergency equipment readily available.

▶ Instruct the patient to void prior to the procedure and to change into the gown, robe, and foot coverings provided.

▶ Instruct the patient to cooperate fully and to follow directions. Instruct the patient to remain still throughout the procedure because movement produces unreliable results.

▶ Observe standard precautions, and follow the general guidelines in Appendix A.

▶ Establish an IV fluid line for the injection of contrast medium, emergency drugs, and sedatives.

▶ Administer an antianxiety agent, as ordered, if the patient has claustrophobia. Administer a sedative to a child or to an uncooperative adult, as ordered.

▶ Place the patient in the supine position on an examination table.

▶ If IV contrast medium is used, a rapid series of images is taken during and after injection.

▶ Instruct the patient to inhale deeply and hold his or her breath while the x-ray images are taken, and then to exhale after the images are taken.

▶ Instruct the patient to take slow, deep breaths if nausea occurs during the procedure.

▶ Monitor the patient for complications related to the procedure (e.g., allergic reaction, anaphylaxis, bronchospasm) if contrast is used.

▶ The needle is removed, and a pressure dressing is applied over the puncture site.

▶ Observe/assess the needle site for bleeding, inflammation, or hematoma formation.

POST-TEST:

▶ A report of the examination will be sent to the requesting HCP, who will discuss the results with the patient.

▶ Instruct the patient to resume usual diet, fluids, medications, and activity, as directed by the HCP. Renal function should be assessed before metformin is resumed, if contrast was used.

▶ Monitor vital signs and neurological status every 15 min for 1 hr, then every 2 hr for 4 hr, and then as ordered by the HCP. Monitor temperature every 4 hr for 24 hr. Monitor intake and output at least every 8 hr. Compare with baseline values. Notify the HCP if temperature is elevated. Protocols may vary among facilities.

▶ If contrast was used, observe for delayed allergic reactions, such as rash, urticaria, tachycardia, hyperpnea, hypertension, palpitations, nausea, or vomiting.

▶ Instruct the patient to immediately report symptoms such as fast heart rate, difficulty breathing, skin rash, itching, chest pain, persistent right shoulder pain, or abdominal pain. Immediately report symptoms to the appropriate HCP.

▶ Observe/assess the needle site for bleeding, inflammation, or hematoma formation.

▶ Instruct the patient in the care and assessment of the site.

▶ Instruct the patient to apply cold compresses to the puncture site as needed, to reduce discomfort or edema.

▶ Instruct the patient to increase fluid intake to help eliminate the contrast medium, if used.

▶ Inform the patient that diarrhea may occur after ingestion of oral contrast medium.

▶ Recognize anxiety related to test results. Discuss the implications of abnormal test results on the patient's lifestyle. Provide teaching and information regarding the clinical implications of the test results, as appropriate.

▶ Reinforce information given by the patient's HCP regarding further testing, treatment, or referral to another HCP. Answer any questions or address any concerns voiced by the patient or family.

▶ Depending on the results of this procedure, additional testing may be needed to evaluate or monitor progression of the disease process and determine the need for a change in therapy. Evaluate test results in relation to the patient's symptoms and other tests performed.

RELATED MONOGRAPHS:

▶ Related tests include amylase, angiography of the abdomen, biopsy intestinal, BUN, cancer antigens, CBC hemoglobin, creatinine, ERCP, lipase, MRI abdomen, PT/INR, and US pancreas.

▶ Refer to the Gastrointestinal and Hepatobiliary systems tables at the end of the book for related tests by body system.

C

Computed Tomography, Pelvis

SYNONYM/ACRONYM: Computed axial tomography (CAT), computed transaxial tomography (CTT), pelvis CT, helical/spiral CT.

COMMON USE: To visualize and assess pelvic structures and vascularities related to assisting in diagnosing bleeding, infection, masses, and cyst aspiration (needle-guided biopsy). Used to monitor the effectiveness of medical, radiation, and surgical therapeutic interventions.

AREA OF APPLICATION: Pelvis.

CONTRAST: With or without oral or IV iodinated contrast medium.

DESCRIPTION: Computed tomography (CT) of the pelvis is a noninvasive procedure used to enhance certain anatomic views of the pelvic structures. It becomes an invasive procedure when intravenous contrast medium is used. During the procedure, the patient lies on a table and is moved in and out of a doughnut-like device called a *gantry,* which houses the x-ray tube and associated electronics. The scanner uses multiple x-ray beams and a series of detectors that rotate around the patient to produce cross-sectional views in a three-dimensional fashion. Differences in tissue density are detected and recorded and are viewable as computerized digital images. Slices or thin sections of certain anatomic views of the pelvic strucures and associated vascular system are reviewed to allow differentiation of solid, cystic, inflammatory, or vascular lesions, as well as identification of suspected hematomas and aneurysms. The procedure is repeated after intravenous injection of iodinated contrast medium for vascular evaluation or after oral ingestion of contrast medium for evaluation of bowel and adjacent structures. Images can be recorded on photographic or x-ray film or stored in digital format as digitized computer data. Cine scanning produces a series of moving images of the scanned area. The CT scan can be used to guide biopsy needles into areas of pelvic masses to obtain tissue for laboratory analysis and for placement of needles to aspirate cysts or abscesses. CT scanning can monitor mass, cyst, or tumor growth and post-therapy response.

INDICATIONS

- Assist in differentiating between benign and malignant tumors
- Detect tumor extension of masses and metastasis into the pelvic area
- Differentiate infectious from inflammatory processes
- Evaluate pelvic lymph nodes
- Evaluate cysts, masses, abscesses, ureteral and bladder calculi, gastrointestinal (GI) bleeding and obstruction, and trauma
- Monitor and evaluate effectiveness of medical, radiation, or surgical therapies

POTENTIAL DIAGNOSIS

Normal findings in

- Normal size, position, and shape of pelvic organs and vascular system

Abnormal findings in

- Bladder calculi
- Ectopic pregnancy
- Fibroid tumors
- Hydrosalpinx
- Ovarian cyst or abscess
- Primary and metastatic neoplasms

CRITICAL FINDINGS

- Ectopic pregnancy
- Tumor with significant mass effect

It is essential that critical diagnoses be communicated immediately to the appropriate health-care provider (HCP). A listing of these diagnoses varies among facilities. Note and immediately report to the HCP abnormal results and related symptoms.

INTERFERING FACTORS

This procedure is contraindicated for

- ❖ Patients with allergies to shellfish or iodinated dye. The contrast medium used may cause a life-threatening allergic reaction. Patients with a known hypersensitivity to the medium may benefit from premedication with corticosteroids or the use of nonionic contrast medium.
- Patients who are claustrophobic.
- Patients who are pregnant or suspected of being pregnant, unless the potential benefits of the procedure far outweigh the risks to the fetus and mother.
- ❖ Elderly and other patients who are chronically dehydrated before the test, because of their risk of contrast-induced renal failure.
- ❖ Patients who are in renal failure.
- Young patients (17 yr and younger), unless the benefits of the x-ray diagnosis outweigh the risks of exposure to high levels of radiation.

Factors that may impair clear imaging

- Gas or feces in the GI tract resulting from inadequate cleansing or failure to restrict food intake before the study.
- Retained barium from a previous radiological procedure.
- Metallic objects (e.g., jewelry, body rings) within the examination field, which may inhibit organ visualization and can produce unclear images.
- Patients who are very obese or who may exceed the weight limit for the equipment.

- Patients with extreme claustrophobia unless sedation is given before the study.
- Inability of the patient to cooperate or remain still during the procedure because of age, significant pain, or mental status.

Other considerations

- Complications of the procedure include hemorrhage, infection at the IV needle insertion site, and cardiac arrhythmias.
- The procedure may be terminated if chest pain or severe cardiac arrhythmias occur.
- Failure to follow dietary restrictions and other pretesting preparations may cause the procedure to be canceled or repeated.
- Consultation with an HCP should occur before the procedure for radiation safety concerns regarding younger patients or patients who are lactating.
- Risks associated with radiation overexposure can result from frequent x-ray procedures. Personnel in the room with the patient should wear a protective lead apron, stand behind a shield, or leave the area while the examination is being done. Personnel working in the examination area should wear badges to record their level of radiation exposure.

NURSING IMPLICATIONS AND PROCEDURE

PRETEST:

- Positively identify the patient using at least two unique identifiers before providing care, treatment, or services.
- *Patient Teaching:* Inform the patient this procedure can assist in assessing the pelvis and pelvic organs.
- Obtain a history of the patient's complaints or clinical symptoms, including a list of known allergens, especially allergies or sensitivities to latex, iodine, seafood, anesthetics, or contrast medium.
- Obtain a history of the patient's gastrointestinal, genitourinary, and reproductive systems; symptoms; and results of previously performed laboratory tests and diagnostic and surgical procedures.
- Ensure results of coagulation testing are obtained and recorded prior to the procedure; BUN and creatinine results are also needed if contrast medium is to be used.
- Note any recent procedures that can interfere with test results, including examinations using barium- or iodine-based contrast medium. Ensure that barium studies were performed more than 4 days before the CT scan.
- Record the date of the last menstrual period and determine the possibility of pregnancy in perimenopausal women.
- Obtain a list of the patient's current medications including anticoagulants, aspirin and other salicylates, herbs, nutritional supplements, and nutraceuticals (see Appendix F). Note the last time and dose of medication taken.
- If contrast medium is scheduled to be used, patients receiving metformin (Glucophage) for non-insulin-dependent (type 2) diabetes should discontinue the drug on the day of the test and continue to withhold it for 48 hr after the test. Failure to do so may result in lactic acidosis.
- Review the procedure with the patient. Address concerns about pain and explain that there may be moments of discomfort and some pain experienced during the test. Inform the patient the procedure is usually performed in a radiology suite by an HCP specializing in this procedure, with support staff, and takes approximately 30 to 60 min.
- *Sensitivity to social and cultural issues,* as well as concern for modesty, is important in providing psychological support before, during, and after the procedure.

- Explain that an IV line may be inserted to allow infusion of IV fluids, contrast medium, dye, or sedatives. Usually contrast medium and normal saline are infused.
- Inform the patient that he or she may experience nausea, a feeling of warmth, a salty or metallic taste, or a transient headache after injection of contrast medium.
- The patient should fast and restrict fluids for 2 to 4 hr prior to the procedure. Instruct the patient to avoid taking anticoagulant medication or to reduce dosage as ordered prior to the procedure. Protocols may vary among facilities.
- The patient may be requested to drink approximately 450 mL of a dilute barium solution (approximately 1% barium) beginning 1 hr before the examination. This is administered to distinguish GI organs from the other abdominal organs.
- Instruct the patient to remove jewelry and other metallic objects from the area to be examined.
- *Make sure a written and informed consent has been signed prior to the procedure and before administering any medications.*

INTRATEST:

- Ensure the patient has complied with dietary, fluids, and medication restrictions and pretesting preparations; ensure that food and fluids have been restricted for at least 2 to 4 hr prior to the procedure.
- Ensure the patient has removed all external metallic objects from the area to be examined prior to the procedure.
- If the patient has a history of allergic reactions to any substance or drug, administer ordered prophylactic steroids or antihistamines before the procedure. Use nonionic contrast medium for the procedure.
- Have emergency equipment readily available.
- Instruct the patient to void prior to the procedure and to change into the gown, robe, and foot coverings provided.

- Instruct the patient to cooperate fully and to follow directions. Instruct the patient to remain still throughout the procedure because movement produces unreliable results.
- Observe standard precautions, and follow the general guidelines in Appendix A.
- Establish an IV fluid line for the injection of contrast, emergency drugs, and sedatives.
- Administer an antianxiety agent, as ordered, if the patient has claustrophobia. Administer a sedative to a child or to an uncooperative adult, as ordered.
- Place the patient in the supine position on an examination table.
- If IV contrast medium is used, a rapid series of images is taken during and after injection.
- Instruct the patient to inhale deeply and hold his or her breath while the x-ray images are taken, and then to exhale after the images are taken.
- Instruct the patient to take slow, deep breaths if nausea occurs during the procedure.
- Monitor the patient for complications related to the procedure (e.g., allergic reaction, anaphylaxis, bronchospasm) if contrast is used.
- The needle is removed, and a pressure dressing is applied over the puncture site.
- Observe/assess the needle site for bleeding, inflammation, or hematoma formation.

POST-TEST:

- A report of the examination will be sent to the requesting HCP, who will discuss the results with the patient.
- Instruct the patient to resume usual diet, fluids, medications, and activity, as directed by the HCP. Renal function should be assessed before metformin is resumed, if contrast was used.
- Monitor vital signs and neurological status every 15 min for 1 hr, then every 2 hr for 4 hr, and then as ordered by the HCP. Monitor temperature every 4 hr for 24 hr. Monitor intake and

output at least every 8 hr. Compare with baseline values. Notify the HCP if temperature is elevated. Protocols may vary among facilities.

▸ If contrast was used, observe for delayed allergic reactions, such as rash, urticaria, tachycardia, hyperpnea, hypertension, palpitations, nausea, or vomiting.

▸ Instruct the patient to immediately report symptoms such as fast heart rate, difficulty breathing, skin rash, itching, chest pain, persistent right shoulder pain, or abdominal pain. Immediately report symptoms to the appropriate HCP.

▸ Observe/assess the needle insertion site for bleeding, inflammation, or hematoma formation.

▸ Instruct the patient in the care and assessment of the site.

▸ Instruct the patient to apply cold compresses to the insertion site as needed, to reduce discomfort or edema.

▸ Instruct the patient to increase fluid intake to help eliminate the contrast medium, if used.

▸ Inform the patient that diarrhea may occur after ingestion of oral contrast medium.

▸ Recognize anxiety related to test results. Discuss the implications of abnormal test results on the patient's lifestyle. Provide teaching and information regarding the clinical implications of the test results, as appropriate.

▸ Reinforce information given by the patient's HCP regarding further testing, treatment, or referral to another HCP. Answer any questions or address any concerns voiced by the patient or family.

▸ Depending on the results of this procedure, additional testing may be needed to evaluate or monitor progression of the disease process and determine the need for a change in therapy. Evaluate test results in relation to the patient's symptoms and other tests performed.

RELATED MONOGRAPHS:

▸ Related tests include angiography pelvis, barium enema, BUN, calculus kidney stone panel, cancer antigens, CBC, CBC hematocrit, CBC hemoglobin, creatinine, HCG, IVP, KUB film, MRI abdomen, proctosigmoidoscopy, PT/INR, US pelvis, and UA.

▸ Refer to the Gastrointestinal, Genitourinary, and Reproductive systems tables at the end of the book for related tests by body system.

Computed Tomography, Pituitary

SYNONYM/ACRONYM: Computed axial tomography (CAT), computed transaxial tomography (CTT), pituitary CT, helical/spiral CT.

COMMON USE: To visualize and assess portions of the brain and pituitary gland for cancer, tumor, and bleeding. Used as an evaluation tool for surgical, radiation, and medical therapeutic interventions.

AREA OF APPLICATION: Pituitary/brain.

CONTRAST: With or without IV iodinated contrast medium.

DESCRIPTION: Computed tomography (CT) of the pituitary is a noninvasive procedure that enhances certain anatomic views of the pituitary gland and perisellar region. It becomes invasive when a contrast medium is used. This procedure aids in the evaluation of pituitary adenoma, craniopharyngioma, meningioma, aneurysm, metastatic disease, exophthalmos, and cysts. Visualization of bony septa in the sphenoid sinus and evaluation for nonpneumatization of the sphenoid sinus are best performed with this procedure. During the procedure, the patient lies on a table and moves in and out of a doughnut-like device called a *gantry,* which houses the x-ray tube and associated electronics. The scanner uses multiple x-ray beams and a series of detectors that rotate around the patient to produce cross-sectional views in a three-dimensional fashion. Differences in tissue density are detected and recorded and are viewable as computerized digital images. Slices or thin sections of certain anatomic views of the pituitary and associated vascular system are reviewed to allow differentiations of solid, cystic, inflammatory, or vascular lesions, as well as identification of suspected hematomas and aneurysms. The procedure may be repeated after iodinated contrast medium is given IV for blood vessel and vascular evaluation. Images can be recorded on photographic or x-ray film or stored in digital format as digitized computer data. Cine scanning produces a series of moving images of the scanned area. Tumors, before and after therapy, may be monitored by CT scanning.

INDICATIONS
- Assist in differentiating between benign and malignant tumors
- Detect aneurysms and vascular abnormalities
- Detect congenital anomalies, such as partially empty sella
- Detect tumor extension of masses and metastasis
- Determine pituitary size and location in relation to surrounding structures
- Evaluate cysts, masses, abscesses, and trauma
- Monitor and evaluate effectiveness of medical, radiation, or surgical therapies

POTENTIAL DIAGNOSIS

Normal findings in
- Normal size, position, and shape of the pituitary fossa, cavernous sinuses, and vascular system

Abnormal findings in
- Abscess
- Adenoma
- Aneurysm
- Chordoma
- Craniopharyngioma
- Cyst
- Meningioma
- Metastasis
- Pituitary hemorrhage

CRITICAL FINDINGS: N/A

INTERFERING FACTORS

This procedure is contraindicated for
- ✷ Patients with allergies to shellfish or iodinated dye. The

contrast medium used may cause a life-threatening allergic reaction. Patients with a known hypersensitivity to the medium may benefit from premedication with corticosteroids or the use of nonionic contrast medium.

• Patients who are claustrophobic.

• Patients who are pregnant or suspected of being pregnant, unless the potential benefits of the procedure far outweigh the risks to the fetus and mother.

• ❖ Elderly and other patients who are chronically dehydrated before the test, because of their risk of contrast-induced renal failure.

• ❖ Patients who are in renal failure.

• Young patients (17 yr and younger), unless the benefits of the x-ray diagnosis outweigh the risks of exposure to high levels of radiation.

Factors that may impair clear imaging

• Retained contrast from a previous radiological procedure.

• Metallic objects (e.g., jewelry, dentures, body rings) within the examination field, which may inhibit organ visualization and cause unclear images.

• Patients who are very obese or who may exceed the weight limit for the equipment.

• Patients with extreme claustrophobia unless sedation is given before the study.

• Inability of the patient to cooperate or remain still during the procedure because of age, significant pain, or mental status.

Other considerations

• Complications of the procedure may include hemorrhage, infection at the IV needle insertion site, and cardiac arrhythmias.

• The procedure may be terminated if chest pain or severe cardiac arrhythmias occur.

• Failure to follow pretesting preparations may cause the procedure to be canceled or repeated.

• Consultation with a health-care provider (HCP) should occur before the procedure for radiation safety concerns regarding younger patients or patients who are lactating.

• Risks associated with radiation overexposure can result from frequent x-ray procedures. Personnel in the room with the patient should wear a protective lead apron, stand behind a shield, or leave the area while the examination is being done. Personnel working in the examination area should wear badges to record their level of radiation exposure.

NURSING IMPLICATIONS AND PROCEDURE

PRETEST:

▸ Positively identify the patient using at least two unique identifiers before providing care, treatment, or services.

▸ *Patient Teaching:* Inform the patient this procedure can assist in assessing the brain and pituitary gland.

▸ Obtain a history of the patient's complaints or clinical symptoms, including a list of known allergens, especially allergies or sensitivities to latex, iodine, seafood, anesthetics, or contrast medium.

▸ Obtain a history of the patient's endocrine system, symptoms, and results of previously performed laboratory tests and diagnostic and surgical procedures.

▸ Ensure results of coagulation testing are obtained and recorded prior to the procedure; BUN and creatinine results are also needed if contrast medium is to be used.

• Note any recent procedures that can interfere with test results, including examinations using barium- or iodine-based contrast medium. Ensure that barium studies were performed more than 4 days before the CT scan.

• Record the date of the last menstrual period and determine the possibility of pregnancy in perimenopausal women.

• Obtain a list of the patient's current medications, including anticoagulants, aspirin and other salicylates, herbs, nutritional supplements, and nutraceuticals (see Appendix F). Note the last time and dose of medication taken.

• If contrast medium is scheduled to be used, patients receiving metformin (Glucophage) for non-insulin-dependent (type 2) diabetes should discontinue the drug on the day of the test and continue to withhold it for 48 hr after the test. Failure to do so may result in lactic acidosis.

• Review the procedure with the patient. Address concerns about pain and explain that there may be moments of discomfort and some pain experienced during the test. Inform the patient the procedure is usually performed in a radiology suite by an HCP specializing in this procedure, with support staff, and takes approximately 30 to 60 min.

• *Sensitivity to social and cultural issues,* as well as concern for modesty, is important in providing psychological support before, during and after the procedure.

• Explain that an IV line may be inserted to allow infusion of IV fluids, contrast medium, dye, or sedatives. Usually contrast medium and normal saline are infused.

• Inform the patient that he or she may experience nausea, a feeling of warmth, a salty or metallic taste, or a transient headache after injection of contrast medium.

• Instruct the patient to remove dentures and other metallic objects from the area to be examined.

• There are no food or fluid restrictions unless by medical direction. Instruct the patient to avoid taking anticoagulant medication or to reduce dosage as ordered prior to the procedure. Protocols may vary among facilities.

• *Make sure a written and informed consent has been signed prior to the procedure and before administering any medications.*

INTRATEST:

• Ensure the patient has complied with medication restrictions and pretesting preparations.

• Ensure the patient has removed dentures and all external metallic objects from the area to be examined prior to the procedure.

• If the patient has a history of allergic reactions to any substance or drug, administer ordered prophylactic steroids or antihistamines before the procedure. Use nonionic contrast medium for the procedure.

• Have emergency equipment readily available.

• Instruct the patient to cooperate fully and to follow directions. Instruct the patient to remain still throughout the procedure because movement produces unreliable results.

• Observe standard precautions, and follow the general guidelines in Appendix A.

• Establish an IV fluid line for the injection of contrast medium, emergency drugs, and sedatives.

• Administer an antianxiety agent, as ordered, if the patient has claustrophobia. Administer a sedative to a child or to an uncooperative adult, as ordered.

• Place the patient in the supine position on an examination table.

• If IV contrast medium is used, a rapid series of images is taken during and after injection.

• Instruct the patient to take slow, deep breaths if nausea occurs during the procedure.
• Monitor the patient for complications related to the procedure (e.g., allergic reaction, anaphylaxis, bronchospasm) if contrast medium is used.
• The needle is removed, and a pressure dressing is applied over the puncture site.
• Observe/assess the needle site for bleeding, inflammation, or hematoma formation.

POST-TEST:

• A report of the examination will be sent to the requesting HCP, who will discuss the results with the patient.
• Instruct the patient to resume usual medications and activity, as directed by the HCP. Renal function should be assessed before metformin is resumed, if contrast was used.
• Monitor vital signs and neurological status every 15 min for 1 hr, then every 2 hr for 4 hr, and then as ordered by the HCP. Monitor temperature every 4 hr for 24 hr. Monitor intake and output at least every 8 hr. Compare with baseline values. Notify the HCP if temperature is elevated. Protocols may vary among facilities.
• If contrast was used, observe for delayed allergic reactions, such as rash, urticaria, tachycardia, hyperpnea, hypertension, palpitations, nausea, or vomiting.
• Instruct the patient to immediately report symptoms such as fast heart rate, difficulty breathing, skin rash, itching, chest pain, persistent right shoulder pain, or abdominal pain. Immediately report symptoms to the appropriate HCP.

• Observe/assess the needle insertion site for bleeding, inflammation, or hematoma formation.
• Instruct the patient in the care and assessment of the site.
• Instruct the patient to apply cold compresses to the insertion site as needed, to reduce discomfort or edema.
• Instruct the patient to increase fluid intake to help eliminate the contrast medium, if used.
• Inform the patient that diarrhea may occur after ingestion of oral contrast medium.
• Recognize anxiety related to test results. Discuss the implications of abnormal test results on the patient's lifestyle. Provide teaching and information regarding the clinical implications of the test results, as appropriate.
• Reinforce information given by the patient's HCP regarding further testing, treatment, or referral to another HCP. Answer any questions or address any concerns voiced by the patient or family.
• Depending on the results of this procedure, additional testing may be needed to evaluate or monitor progression of the disease process and determine the need for a change in therapy. Evaluate test results in relation to the patient's symptoms and other tests performed.

RELATED MONOGRAPHS:

• Related tests include ACTH and challenge tests, BUN, CT angiography, CBC, CBC hematocrit, CBC hemoglobin, CT brain, cortisol and challenge tests, creatinine, MRA, MRI brain, PET brain, and PT/INR.
• Refer to the Endocrine System table at the end of the book for related tests by body system.

Computed Tomography, Renal

SYNONYM/ACRONYM: Computed axial tomography (CAT), computed transaxial tomography (CTT), kidney CT, helical/spiral CT.

COMMON USE: To visualize and assess the kidney and surrounding structures to assist in diagnosing cancer, tumor, infection, and congenital anomalies. Used to evaluate the success of therapeutic medical, surgical, and radiation interventions.

AREA OF APPLICATION: Kidney.

CONTRAST: With or without oral or IV iodinated contrast medium.

DESCRIPTION: Renal computed tomography (CT) is a noninvasive procedure used to enhance certain anatomic views of the renal structures. It becomes an invasive procedure when contrast medium is used. CT scanning is a safe, rapid method for renal evaluation that is independent of renal function. It provides unique cross-sectional anatomic information and is unsurpassed in evaluating lesions containing fat or calcium. During the procedure, the patient lies on a table and is moved in and out of a doughnut-like device called a *gantry,* which houses the x-ray tube and associated electronics. The scanner uses multiple x-ray beams and a series of detectors that rotate around the patient to produce cross-sectional views in a three-dimensional fashion. Differences in tissue density are detected and recorded and are viewable as computerized digital images. Slices or thin sections of certain anatomic views of the kidneys and associated vascular system are reviewed to allow differentiation of solid, cystic, inflammatory, or vascular lesions, as well as identification of

suspected hematomas and aneurysms. The procedure is repeated after IV injection of iodinated contrast medium for vascular evaluation or after oral ingestion of contrast medium for evaluation of bowel and adjacent structures. Images can be recorded on photographic or x-ray film or stored in digital format as digitized computer data. Cine scanning produces a series of moving images of the area scanned. The CT scan can be used to guide biopsy needles into areas of suspected tumors to obtain tissue for laboratory analysis and to guide placement of catheters for drainage of renal abscesses. Tumors, before and after therapy, may be monitored with CT scanning.

INDICATIONS

- Aid in the diagnosis of congenital anomalies, such as polycystic kidney disease, horseshoe kidney, absence of one kidney, or kidney displacement
- Aid in the diagnosis of perirenal hematomas and abscesses and assist in localizing for drainage

- Assist in differentiating between benign and malignant tumors
- Assist in differentiating between an infectious and an inflammatory process
- Detect aneurysms and vascular abnormalities
- Detect bleeding or hyperplasia of the adrenal glands
- Detect tumor extension of masses and metastasis into the renal area
- Determine kidney size and location in relation to the bladder in post-transplant patients
- Determine presence and type of adrenal tumor, such as benign adenoma, cancer, or pheochromocytoma
- Evaluate abnormal fluid accumulation around the kidney
- Evaluate cysts, masses, abscesses, renal calculi, obstruction, and trauma
- Evaluate spread of a tumor or invasion of nearby retroperitoneal organs
- Monitor and evaluate effectiveness of medical, radiation, or surgical therapies

POTENTIAL DIAGNOSIS

Normal findings in
- Normal size, position, and shape of kidneys and vascular system

Abnormal findings in
- Adrenal tumor or hyperplasia
- Congenital anomalies, such as polycystic kidney disease, horseshoe kidney, absence of one kidney, or kidney displacement
- Dilation of the common hepatic duct, common bile duct, or gallbladder
- Renal artery aneurysm
- Renal calculi and ureteral obstruction
- Renal cell carcinoma
- Renal cysts or abscesses
- Renal laceration, fracture, tumor, and trauma

- Perirenal abscesses and hematomas
- Primary and metastatic neoplasms

CRITICAL FINDINGS: N/A

INTERFERING FACTORS

This procedure is contraindicated for
- ❖ Patients with allergies to shellfish or iodinated dye. The contrast medium used may cause a life-threatening allergic reaction. Patients with a known hypersensitivity to the medium may benefit from premedication with corticosteroids or the use of nonionic contrast medium.
- Patients who are claustrophobic.
- Patients who are pregnant or suspected of being pregnant, unless the potential benefits of the procedure far outweigh the risks to the fetus and mother.
- ❖ Elderly and other patients who are chronically dehydrated before the test, because of their risk of contrast-induced renal failure.
- ❖ Patients who are in renal failure.
- Young patients (17 yr and younger), unless the benefits of the x-ray diagnosis outweigh the risks of exposure to high levels of radiation.

Factors that may impair clear imaging
- Gas or feces in the gastrointestinal (GI) tract resulting from inadequate cleansing or failure to restrict food intake before the study.
- Retained barium from a previous radiological procedure.
- Metallic objects (e.g., jewelry, body rings) within the examination field, which may inhibit organ visualization and cause unclear images.
- Patients who are very obese or who may exceed the weight limit for the equipment.

- Patients with extreme claustrophobia unless sedation is given before the study.
- Inability of the patient to cooperate or remain still during the procedure because of age, significant pain, or mental status.

Other considerations
- Complications of the procedure include hemorrhage, infection at the IV needle insertion site, and cardiac arrhythmias.
- The procedure may be terminated if chest pain or severe cardiac arrhythmias occur.
- Failure to follow dietary restrictions and other pretesting preparations may cause the procedure to be canceled or repeated.
- Consultation with a health-care provider (HCP) should occur before the procedure for radiation safety concerns regarding younger patients or patients who are lactating.
- Risks associated with radiation overexposure can result from frequent x-ray procedures. Personnel in the room with the patient should wear a protective lead apron, stand behind a shield, or leave the area while the examination is being done. Personnel working in the examination area should wear badges to record their level of radiation exposure.

NURSING IMPLICATIONS AND PROCEDURE

PRETEST:

▶ Positively identify the patient using at least two unique identifiers before providing care, treatment, or services.
▶ *Patient Teaching:* Inform the patient this procedure can assist in assessing the kidney.
▶ Obtain a history of the patient's complaints or clinical symptoms, including a list of known allergens, especially allergies or sensitivities to latex, iodine, seafood, anesthetics, or contrast mediums.
▶ Obtain a history of the patient's genitourinary system, symptoms, and results of previously performed laboratory tests and diagnostic and surgical procedures.
▶ Ensure results of coagulation testing are obtained and recorded prior to the procedure; BUN and creatinine results are also needed if contrast medium is to be used.
▶ Note any recent procedures that can interfere with test results, including examinations using barium- or iodine-based contrast medium. Ensure that barium studies were performed more than 4 days before the CT scan.
▶ Record the date of the last menstrual period and determine the possibility of pregnancy in perimenopausal women.
▶ Obtain a list of the patient's current medications including anticoagulants, aspirin and other salicylates, herbs, nutritional supplements, and nutraceuticals (see Appendix F). Note the last time and dose of medication taken.
▶ If contrast medium is scheduled to be used, patients receiving metformin (Glucophage) for non-insulin-dependent (type 2) diabetes should discontinue the drug on the day of the test and continue to withhold it for 48 hr after the test. Failure to do so may result in lactic acidosis.
▶ Review the procedure with the patient. Address concerns about pain and explain that there may be moments of discomfort and some pain experienced during the test. Inform the patient the procedure is usually performed in a radiology suite by an HCP specializing in this procedure, with support staff, and takes approximately 30 to 60 min.
▶ Explain that an IV line may be inserted to allow infusion of IV fluids, contrast medium, dye, or sedatives. Usually contrast medium and normal saline are infused.
▶ *Sensitivity to social and cultural issues,* as well as concern for modesty, is important in providing psychological support before, during, and after the procedure.

▶ The patient may be requested to drink approximately 450 mL of a dilute barium solution (approximately 1% barium) beginning 1 hr before the examination. This is administered to distinguish GI organs from the other abdominal organs.

▶ Inform the patient that he or she may experience nausea, a feeling of warmth, a salty or metallic taste, or a transient headache after injection of contrast medium.

▶ Instruct the patient to remove jewelry and other metallic objects from the area to be examined.

▶ The patient should fast and restrict fluids for 2 to 4 hr prior to the procedure. Instruct the patient to avoid taking anticoagulant medication or to reduce dosage as ordered prior to the procedure. Protocols may vary among facilities.

▶ *Make sure a written and informed consent has been signed prior to the procedure and before administering any medications.*

INTRATEST:

▶ Ensure the patient has complied with dietary, fluids, and medication restrictions for 2 to 4 hr prior to the procedure.

▶ Ensure the patient has removed all external metallic objects from the area to be examined prior to the procedure.

▶ If the patient has a history of allergic reactions to any substance or drug, administer ordered prophylactic steroids or antihistamines before the procedure. Use nonionic contrast medium for the procedure.

▶ Have emergency equipment readily available.

▶ Instruct the patient to void prior to the procedure and to change into the gown, robe, and foot coverings provided.

▶ Instruct the patient to cooperate fully and to follow directions. Instruct the patient to remain still throughout the procedure because movement produces unreliable results.

▶ Observe standard precautions, and follow the general guidelines in Appendix A.

▶ Establish an IV fluid line for the injection of contrast, emergency drugs, and sedatives.

▶ Administer an antianxiety agent, as ordered, if the patient has claustrophobia. Administer a sedative to a child or to an uncooperative adult, as ordered.

▶ Place the patient in the supine position on an examination table.

▶ If IV contrast is used, a rapid series of images is taken during and after injection.

▶ Instruct the patient to inhale deeply and hold his or her breath while the x-ray images are taken, and then to exhale after the images are taken.

▶ Instruct the patient to take slow, deep breaths if nausea occurs during the procedure.

▶ Monitor the patient for complications related to the procedure (e.g., allergic reaction, anaphylaxis, bronchospasm) if contrast is used.

▶ The needle is removed, and a pressure dressing is applied over the puncture site.

▶ Observe/assess the needle site for bleeding, inflammation, or hematoma formation.

POST-TEST:

▶ A report of the examination will be sent to the requesting HCP, who will discuss the results with the patient.

▶ Instruct the patient to resume usual diet, fluids, medications, and activity, as directed by the HCP. Renal function should be assessed before metformin is resumed, if contrast was used.

▶ Monitor vital signs and neurological status every 15 min for 1 hr, then every 2 hr for 4 hr, and then as ordered by the HCP. Monitor temperature every 4 hr for 24 hr. Monitor intake and output at least every 8 hr. Compare with baseline values. Notify the HCP if temperature is elevated. Protocols may vary among facilities.

▶ If contrast was used, observe for delayed allergic reactions, such as rash, urticaria, tachycardia, hyperpnea, hypertension, palpitations, nausea, or vomiting.

▶ Instruct the patient to immediately report symptoms such as fast heart rate, difficulty breathing, skin rash, itching, chest pain, persistent right shoulder pain, or abdominal pain.

Immediately report symptoms to the appropriate HCP.

- Observe/assess the needle insertion site for bleeding, inflammation, or hematoma formation.
- Instruct the patient in the care and assessment of the site.
- Instruct the patient to apply cold compresses to the insertion site as needed, to reduce discomfort or edema.
- Instruct the patient to increase fluid intake to help eliminate the contrast medium, if used.
- Inform the patient that diarrhea may occur after ingestion of oral contrast medium.
- Recognize anxiety related to test results. Discuss the implications of abnormal test results on the patient's lifestyle. Provide teaching and information regarding the clinical implications of the test results, as appropriate.
- Reinforce information given by the patient's HCP regarding further testing, treatment, or referral to another HCP. Answer any questions or address any concerns voiced by the patient or family.
- Depending on the results of this procedure, additional testing may be needed to evaluate or monitor progression of the disease process and determine the need for a change in therapy. Evaluate test results in relation to the patient's symptoms and other tests performed.

RELATED MONOGRAPHS:

- Related tests include ACTH, angiography adrenal, renal biopsy, BUN, calculus/kidney stone panel, catecholamines, CBC, CBC hematocrit, CBC hemoglobin, creatinine, CT abdomen, homovanillic acid, IVP, KUB, MRI abdomen, PT/INR, US renal, and VMA.
- Refer to the Genitourinary System table at the end of the book for related tests by body system.

Computed Tomography, Spine

SYNONYM/ACRONYM: Computed axial tomography (CAT), computed transaxial tomography (CTT), spine CT, CT myelogram.

COMMON USE: To visualize and assess spinal structure related to tumor, injury, bleeding, and infection. Used as an evaluation tool for surgical, radiation, and medical therapeutic interventions.

AREA OF APPLICATION: Spine.

CONTRAST: With or without oral or IV iodinated contrast medium.

DESCRIPTION: Computed tomography (CT) of the spine is a noninvasive procedure that enhances certain anatomic views of the spinal structures. CT scanning is more versatile than conventional radiography and can easily detect and identify tumors and their types. During the procedure, the patient lies on a table and is moved in and out of a doughnut-like device called a *gantry*, which houses the x-ray tube and associated electronics. The scanner uses multiple x-ray beams and a series of detectors that rotate around the patient to produce cross-sectional views in a three-dimensional fashion. Differences in tissue density are detected and recorded and are viewable as computerized digital images. Slices or thin sections of certain anatomic views of the spine and associated vascular system are reviewed to allow differentiations of solid, cystic, inflammatory, or vascular lesions, as well as identification of suspected hematomas and aneurysms. The procedure may be repeated after intravenous injection of iodinated contrast medium for vascular evaluation. Images can be recorded on photographic or x-ray film or stored in digital format as digitized computer data. Cine scanning produces a series of moving images of the scanned area. CT scanning can be used to guide biopsy needles into areas of suspected tumor to obtain tissue for laboratory analysis and to guide placement of catheters for drainage of abscesses. Tumor size, progression, and pre- and post-therapy changes may be monitored with CT scanning.

INDICATIONS

- Assist in differentiating between benign and malignant tumors
- Detect congenital spinal anomalies, such as spina bifida, meningocele, and myelocele
- Detect herniated intervertebral disks
- Detect paraspinal cysts
- Detect vascular malformations
- Monitor and evaluate effectiveness of medical, radiation, or surgical therapies

POTENTIAL DIAGNOSIS

Normal findings in

- Normal density, size, position, and shape of spinal structures

Abnormal findings in

- Congenital spinal malformations, such as meningocele, myelocele, or spina bifida
- Herniated intervertebral disks
- Paraspinal cysts
- Spinal tumors
- Spondylosis (cervical or lumbar)
- Vascular malformations

CRITICAL FINDINGS

- Cord compression
- Fracture
- Tumor with significant mass effect

It is essential that critical diagnoses be communicated immediately to the appropriate health-care provider (HCP). A listing of these diagnoses varies among facilities. Note and immediately report to the HCP abnormal results and related symptoms.

INTERFERING FACTORS

This procedure is contraindicated for

- Patients with allergies to shellfish or iodinated dye. The contrast medium used may cause a life-threatening allergic reaction. Patients with a known hypersensitivity to the medium may benefit from premedication with corticosteroids or the use of nonionic contrast medium.
- Patients who are claustrophobic.
- Patients who are pregnant or suspected of being pregnant, unless the potential benefits of the procedure far outweigh the risks to the fetus and mother.
- Elderly and other patients who are chronically dehydrated before the test, because of their risk of contrast-induced renal failure.
- Patients who are in renal failure.
- Young patients (17 yr and younger), unless the benefits of the x-ray diagnosis outweigh the risks of exposure to high levels of radiation.

Factors that may impair clear imaging

- Gas or feces in the gastrointestinal tract resulting from inadequate cleansing or failure to restrict food intake before the study.
- Retained barium from a previous radiological procedure.
- Metallic objects (e.g., jewelry, body rings) within the examination field, which may inhibit organ visualization and cause unclear images.
- Patients who are very obese or who may exceed the weight limit for the equipment.
- Patients with extreme claustrophobia unless sedation is given before the study.
- Inability of the patient to cooperate or remain still during the procedure because of age, significant pain, or mental status.

Other considerations

- Complications of the procedure may include hemorrhage, infection at the IV needle insertion site, and cardiac arrhythmias.
- The procedure may be terminated if chest pain or severe cardiac arrhythmias occur.
- Failure to follow pretesting preparations may cause the procedure to be canceled or repeated.
- Consultation with an HCP should occur before the procedure for radiation safety concerns regarding younger patients or patients who are lactating.
- Risks associated with radiation overexposure can result from frequent x-ray procedures. Personnel in the room with the patient should wear a protective lead apron, stand behind a shield, or leave the area while the examination is being done. Personnel working in the examination area should wear badges to record their level of radiation exposure.

NURSING IMPLICATIONS AND PROCEDURE

PRETEST:

- Positively identify the patient using at least two unique identifiers before providing care, treatment, or services.
- *Patient Teaching:* Inform the patient this procedure can assist in assessing the spine.
- Obtain a history of the patient's complaints or clinical symptoms, including a list of known allergens, especially allergies or sensitivities to latex, iodine, seafood, anesthetics, or contrast medium.
- Obtain a history of the patient's musculoskeletal system, symptoms, and results of previously performed laboratory tests and diagnostic and surgical procedures.
- Ensure results of coagulation testing are obtained and recorded prior to the procedure; BUN and creatinine results are also needed if contrast medium is to be used.
- Note any recent procedures that can interfere with test results, including examinations using barium- or iodine-based contrast medium. Ensure that barium studies were performed more than 4 days before the CT scan.
- Record the date of the last menstrual period and determine the possibility of pregnancy in perimenopausal women.
- Obtain a list of the patient's current medications including anticoagulants, aspirin and other salicylates, herbs and nutritional supplements, and nutraceuticals (see Appendix F). Note the last time and dose of medication taken.
- If contrast medium is scheduled to be used, patients receiving metformin (Glucophage) for non-insulin-dependent (type 2) diabetes should discontinue the drug on the day of the test and continue to withhold it for 48 hr after the test. Failure to do so may result in lactic acidosis.
- Review the procedure with the patient. Address concerns about pain and explain that there may be moments of discomfort and some pain experienced during the test. Inform the patient the procedure is usually performed in a

radiology suite by an HCP specializing in this procedure, with support staff, and takes approximately 30 to 60 min.

▶ *Sensitivity to social and cultural issues,* as well as concern for modesty, is important in providing psychological support before, during, and after the procedure.

▶ Explain that an IV line may be inserted to allow infusion of IV fluids, contrast medium, dye, or sedatives. Usually contrast medium and normal saline are infused.

▶ Inform the patient that he or she may experience nausea, a feeling of warmth, a salty or metallic taste, or a transient headache after injection of contrast medium.

▶ Instruct the patient to remove jewelry and other metallic objects from the area to be examined.

▶ There are no food or fluid restrictions unless by medical direction. Instruct the patient to avoid taking anticoagulant medication or to reduce dosage as ordered prior to the procedure. Protocols may vary among facilities.

▶ *Make sure a written and informed consent has been signed prior to the procedure and before administering any medications.*

INTRATEST:

▶ Ensure that the patient has complied with medication restrictions and pretesting preparations.

▶ Ensure that the patient has removed all external metallic objects from the area to be examined prior to the procedure.

▶ If the patient has a history of allergic reactions to any substance or drug, administer ordered prophylactic steroids or antihistamines before the procedure. Use nonionic contrast medium for the procedure.

▶ Have emergency equipment readily available.

▶ Instruct the patient to void prior to the procedure and to change into the gown, robe, and foot coverings provided.

▶ Instruct the patient to cooperate fully and to follow directions. Instruct the patient to remain still throughout the procedure because movement produces unreliable results.

▶ Observe standard precautions, and follow the general guidelines in Appendix A.

▶ If ordered, establish an IV fluid line for the injection of contrast medium, emergency drugs, and sedatives.

▶ Administer an antianxiety agent, as ordered, if the patient has claustrophobia. Administer a sedative to a child or to an uncooperative adult, as ordered.

▶ Place the patient in the supine position on an examination table.

▶ If IV contrast medium is used, a rapid series of images is taken during and after injection.

▶ Instruct the patient to inhale deeply and hold his or her breath while the x-ray images are taken, and then to exhale after the images are taken.

▶ Instruct the patient to take slow, deep breaths if nausea occurs during the procedure.

▶ Monitor the patient for complications related to the procedure (e.g., allergic reaction, anaphylaxis, bronchospasm) if contrast is used.

▶ The needle is removed, and a pressure dressing is applied over the puncture site.

▶ Observe/assess the needle insertion site for bleeding, inflammation, or hematoma formation.

POST-TEST:

▶ A report of the examination will be sent to the requesting HCP, who will discuss the results with the patient.

▶ Instruct the patient to resume usual medications and activity, as directed by the HCP. Renal function should be assessed before metformin is resumed, if contrast was used.

▶ Monitor vital signs and neurological status every 15 min for 1 hr, then every 2 hr for 4 hr, and then as ordered by the HCP. Monitor temperature every 4 hr for 24 hr. Monitor intake and output at least every 8 hr. Compare with baseline values. Notify the HCP if temperature is elevated. Protocols may vary among facilities.

▶ If contrast was used, observe for delayed allergic reactions, such as rash, urticaria, tachycardia, hyperpnea, hypertension, palpitations, nausea, or vomiting.

▶ Instruct the patient to immediately report symptoms such as fast heart rate, difficulty breathing, skin rash, itching, chest pain, persistent right shoulder pain, or abdominal pain. Immediately report symptoms to the appropriate HCP.

▶ Observe/assess the needle insertion site for bleeding, inflammation, or hematoma formation.

▶ Instruct the patient in the care and assessment of the site.

▶ Instruct the patient to apply cold compresses to the insertion site as needed, to reduce discomfort or edema.

▶ Instruct the patient to increase fluid intake to help eliminate the contrast medium, if used.

▶ Recognize anxiety related to test results. Discuss the implications of abnormal test results on the patient's lifestyle. Provide teaching and information

regarding the clinical implications of the test results, as appropriate.

▶ Reinforce information given by the patient's HCP regarding further testing, treatment, or referral to another HCP. Answer any questions or address any concerns voiced by the patient or family.

▶ Depending on the results of this procedure, additional testing may be needed to evaluate or monitor progression of the disease process and determine the need for a change in therapy. Evaluate test results in relation to the patient's symptoms and other tests performed.

RELATED MONOGRAPHS:

▶ Related tests include ALP, BUN, bone scan, CBC, CBC hematocrit, CBC hemoglobin, creatinine, MRI bone, PT/INR, and radiography of the bones.

▶ Refer to the Musculoskeletal System table at the end of the book for related tests by body system.

Computed Tomography, Spleen

SYNONYM/ACRONYM: Computed axial tomography (CAT), computed transaxial tomography (CTT), helical/spiral CT, splenic CT.

COMMON USE: To visualize and assess the spleen and surrounding structure for tumor, bleeding, infection, and trauma. Used to monitor the effectiveness of medical, surgical, and radiation therapeutic interventions.

AREA OF APPLICATION: Abdomen/spleen.

CONTRAST: With or without oral or IV iodinated contrast medium.

DESCRIPTION: Computed tomography (CT) of the spleen is a noninvasive procedure that enhances certain anatomic views of the splenic structures. It becomes an invasive procedure with the use

of contrast medium. The spleen is not often the organ of interest when abdominal CT scans are obtained. However, a wide variety of splenic variations and abnormalities may be detected on abdominal scans designed to evaluate the liver, pancreas, or retroperitoneum. During the procedure, the patient lies on a table and is moved in and out of a doughnut-like device called a *gantry*, which houses the x-ray tube and associated electronics. The scanner uses multiple x-ray beams and a series of detectors that rotate around the patient to produce cross-sectional views in a three-dimensional fashion. Differences in tissue density are detected and recorded and are viewable as computerized digital images. Slices or thin sections of certain anatomic views of the spleen and associated vascular system are reviewed to allow differentiation of solid, cystic, inflammatory, or vascular lesions, as well as identification of suspected hematomas and aneurysms. The procedure is repeated after IV injection of iodinated contrast medium for vascular evaluation or after oral ingestion of contrast medium for evaluation of bowel and adjacent structures. Images can be recorded on photographic or x-ray film or stored in digital format as digitized computer data. Cine scanning produces a series of moving images of the scanned area. The CT scan can be used to guide biopsy needles into areas of splenic masses to obtain tissue for laboratory analysis and for placement of needles to aspirate cysts or abscesses. CT scanning can monitor mass, cyst, or tumor growth and post-therapy response.

INDICATIONS

- Assist in differentiating between benign and malignant tumors
- Detect tumor extension of masses and metastasis
- Differentiate infectious from inflammatory processes
- Evaluate cysts, masses, abscesses, and trauma
- Evaluate the presence of an accessory spleen, polysplenia, or asplenia
- Evaluate splenic vein thrombosis
- Monitor and evaluate effectiveness of medical, radiation, or surgical therapies

POTENTIAL DIAGNOSIS

Normal findings in
- Normal size, position, and shape of the spleen and associated vascular system

Abnormal findings in
- Abdominal aortic aneurysm
- Hematomas
- Hemoperitoneum
- Primary and metastatic neoplasms
- Splenic cysts or abscesses
- Splenic laceration, tumor, infiltration, and trauma

CRITICAL FINDINGS
- Abscess
- Hemorrhage
- Laceration

It is essential that critical diagnoses be communicated immediately to the appropriate health-care provider (HCP). A listing of these diagnoses varies among facilities. Note and immediately report to the HCP abnormal results and related symptoms.

INTERFERING FACTORS

This procedure is contraindicated for
- Patients with allergies to shellfish or iodinated dye. The contrast medium used may cause a life-threatening allergic reaction. Patients with a known

hypersensitivity to the medium may benefit from premedication with corticosteroids or the use of nonionic contrast medium.

- Patients who are claustrophobic.
- Patients who are pregnant or suspected of being pregnant, unless the potential benefits of the procedure far outweigh the risks to the fetus and mother.
- ❖ Elderly and other patients who are chronically dehydrated before the test, because of their risk of contrast-induced renal failure.
- ❖ Patients who are in renal failure.
- Young patients (17 yr and younger), unless the benefits of the x-ray diagnosis outweigh the risks of exposure to high levels of radiation.

Factors that may impair clear imaging

- Gas or feces in the gastrointestinal (GI) tract resulting from inadequate cleansing or failure to restrict food intake before the study.
- Retained barium from a previous radiological procedure.
- Metallic objects (e.g., jewelry, body rings) within the examination field, which may inhibit organ visualization and cause unclear images.
- Patients who are very obese or who may exceed the weight limit for the equipment.
- Patients with extreme claustrophobia unless sedation is given before the study.
- Inability of the patient to cooperate or remain still during the procedure because of age, significant pain, or mental status.

Other considerations

- Complications of the procedure include hemorrhage, infection at the IV needle insertion site, and cardiac arrhythmias.

- The procedure may be terminated if chest pain or severe cardiac arrhythmias occur.
- Failure to follow dietary restrictions and other pretesting preparations may cause the procedure to be canceled or repeated.
- Consultation with an HCP should occur before the procedure for radiation safety concerns regarding younger patients or patients who are lactating.
- Risks associated with radiation overexposure can result from frequent x-ray procedures. Personnel in the room with the patient should wear a protective lead apron, stand behind a shield, or leave the area while the examination is being done. Personnel working in the examination area should wear badges to record their level of radiation exposure.

NURSING IMPLICATIONS AND PROCEDURE

PRETEST:

- Positively identify the patient using at least two unique identifiers before providing care, treatment, or services.
- *Patient Teaching:* Inform the patient this procedure can assist in assessing the abdomen and spleen.
- Obtain a history of the patient's complaints, including a list of known allergens, especially allergies or sensitivities to latex, iodine, seafood, anesthetics, or contrast medium.
- Obtain a history of the patient's hematopoietic system, symptoms, and results of previously performed laboratory tests and diagnostic and surgical procedures.
- Ensure results of coagulation testing are obtained and recorded prior to the procedure; BUN and creatinine results are also needed if contrast medium is to be used.
- Note any recent procedures that can interfere with test results, including

examinations using barium- or iodine-based contrast medium. Ensure that barium studies were performed more than 4 days before the CT scan.

- Record the date of the last menstrual period and determine the possibility of pregnancy in perimenopausal women.
- Obtain a list of the patient's current medications including anticoagulants, aspirin and other salicylates, herbs, nutritional supplements, and nutraceuticals (see Appendix F). Note the last time and dose of medication taken.
- If contrast medium is scheduled to be used, patients receiving metformin (Glucophage) for non-insulin-dependent (type 2) diabetes should discontinue the drug on the day of the test and continue to withhold it for 48 hr after the test. Failure to do so may result in lactic acidosis.
- Review the procedure with the patient. Address concerns about pain and explain that there may be moments of discomfort and some pain experienced during the test. Inform the patient the procedure is usually performed in a radiology suite by an HCP specializing in this procedure, with support staff, and takes approximately 30 to 60 min.
- Explain that an IV line may be inserted to allow infusion of IV fluids, contrast medium, dye, or sedatives. Usually contrast medium and normal saline are infused.
- *Sensitivity to social and cultural issues,* as well as concern for modesty, is important in providing psychological support before, during, and after the procedure.
- The patient may be requested to drink approximately 450 mL of a dilute barium solution (approximately 1% barium) beginning 1 hr before the examination. This is administered to distinguish GI organs from the other abdominal organs.
- Inform the patient that he or she may experience nausea, a feeling of warmth, a salty or metallic taste, or a transient headache after injection of contrast medium.

- Instruct the patient to remove jewelry and other metallic objects from the area to be examined.
- The patient should fast and restrict fluids for 2 to 4 hr prior to the procedure. Instruct the patient to avoid taking anticoagulant medication or to reduce dosage as ordered prior to the procedure. Protocols may vary among facilities.
- *Make sure a written and informed consent has been signed prior to the procedure and before administering any medications.*

INTRATEST:

- Ensure the patient has complied with dietary, fluids, and medication restrictions for 2 to 4 hr prior to the procedure.
- Ensure the patient has removed all external metallic objects from the area to be examined prior to the procedure.
- If the patient has a history of allergic reactions to any substance or drug, administer ordered prophylactic steroids or antihistamines before the procedure. Use nonionic contrast medium for the procedure.
- Have emergency equipment readily available.
- Instruct the patient to void prior to the procedure and to change into the gown, robe, and foot coverings provided.
- Instruct the patient to cooperate fully and to follow directions. Instruct the patient to remain still throughout the procedure because movement produces unreliable results.
- Observe standard precautions, and follow the general guidelines in Appendix A.
- Establish an IV fluid line for the injection of contrast medium, emergency drugs, and sedatives.
- Administer an antianxiety agent, as ordered, if the patient has claustrophobia. Administer a sedative to a child or to an uncooperative adult, as ordered.
- Place the patient in the supine position on an examination table.
- If IV contrast medium is used, a rapid series of images is taken during and after injection.

- Instruct the patient to inhale deeply and hold his or her breath while the x-ray images are taken, and then to exhale after the images are taken.
- Instruct the patient to take slow, deep breaths if nausea occurs during the procedure.
- Monitor the patient for complications related to the procedure (e.g., allergic reaction, anaphylaxis, bronchospasm) if contrast medium is used.
- The needle is removed, and a pressure dressing is applied over the puncture site.
- Observe/assess the needle site for bleeding, inflammation, or hematoma formation.

POST-TEST:

- A report of the examination will be sent to the requesting HCP, who will discuss the results with the patient.
- Instruct the patient to resume usual diet, fluids, medications, and activity, as directed by the HCP. Renal function should be assessed before metformin is resumed, if contrast was used.
- Monitor vital signs and neurological status every 15 min for 1 hr, then every 2 hr for 4 hr, and then as ordered by the HCP. Monitor temperature every 4 hr for 24 hr. Monitor intake and output at least every 8 hr. Compare with baseline values. Notify the HCP if temperature is elevated. Protocols may vary among facilities.
- If contrast was used, observe for delayed allergic reactions, such as rash, urticaria, tachycardia, hyperpnea, hypertension, palpitations, nausea, or vomiting.
- Instruct the patient to immediately report symptoms such as fast heart rate, difficulty breathing, skin rash, itching, chest pain, persistent right shoulder pain, or abdominal pain.

- Immediately report symptoms to the appropriate HCP.
- Observe/assess the needle site for bleeding, inflammation, or hematoma formation.
- Instruct the patient in the care and assessment of the site.
- Instruct the patient to apply cold compresses to the puncture site as needed, to reduce discomfort or edema.
- Instruct the patient to increase fluid intake to help eliminate the contrast medium, if used.
- Inform the patient that diarrhea may occur after ingestion of oral contrast medium.
- Recognize anxiety related to test results. Discuss the implications of abnormal test results on the patient's lifestyle. Provide teaching and information regarding the clinical implications of the test results, as appropriate.
- Reinforce information given by the patient's HCP regarding further testing, treatment, or referral to another HCP. Answer any questions or address any concerns voiced by the patient or family.
- Depending on the results of this procedure, additional testing may be needed to evaluate or monitor progression of the disease process and determine the need for a change in therapy. Evaluate test results in relation to the patient's symptoms and other tests performed.

RELATED MONOGRAPHS:

- Related tests include angiography abdomen, BUN, CBC, CBC hematocrit, CBC hemoglobin, creatinine, KUB film, MRI abdomen, PT/INR, and US liver.
- Refer to the Hematopoietic System table at the end of the book for related tests by body system.

Computed Tomography, Thoracic

SYNONYM/ACRONYM: Chest CT, computed axial tomography (CAT), computed transaxial tomography (CTT), helical/spiral CT.

COMMON USE: To visualize and assess structures within the thoracic cavity such as the heart, lungs, and mediastinal structures to evaluate for aneurysm, cancer, tumor, and infection. Used as an evaluation tool for surgical, radiation, and medical therapeutic interventions.

AREA OF APPLICATION: Thorax.

CONTRAST: With or without oral or IV iodinated contrast medium.

DESCRIPTION: Computed tomography (CT) of the thorax is more detailed than a chest x-ray. It is a noninvasive procedure used to enhance certain anatomic views of the lungs, heart, and mediastinal structures. It becomes invasive when a contrast medium is used. During the procedure, the patient lies on a table and is moved in and out of a doughnut-like device called a *gantry*, which houses the x-ray tube and associated electronics. The scanner uses multiple x-ray beams and a series of detectors that rotate around the patient to produce cross-sectional views in a three-dimensional fashion. Differences in tissue density are detected and recorded and are viewable as computerized digital images. Slices or thin sections of certain anatomic views of the spine, spinal cord, and lung areas are reviewed to allow differentiations of solid, cystic, inflammatory, or vascular lesions. Images can be recorded on photographic or x-ray film or stored in digital format as digitized computer data. Cine scanning is used to produce moving images of the heart.

INDICATIONS
- Detect aortic aneurysms
- Detect bronchial abnormalities, such as stenosis, dilation, or tumor
- Detect lymphomas, especially Hodgkin's disease
- Detect mediastinal and hilar lymphadenopathy
- Detect primary and metastatic pulmonary, esophageal, or mediastinal tumors
- Detect tumor extension of neck mass to thoracic area
- Determine blood, fluid, or fat accumulation in tissues, pleuritic space, or vessels
- Differentiate aortic aneurysms from tumors near the aorta
- Differentiate between benign and malignant tumors
- Differentiate infectious from inflammatory processes
- Differentiate tumor from tuberculosis
- Evaluate cardiac chambers and pulmonary vessels
- Evaluate the presence of plaque in cardiac vessels
- Monitor and evaluate effectiveness of medical or surgical therapeutic regimen

POTENTIAL DIAGNOSIS

Normal findings in
• Normal size, position, and shape of thoracic organs, tissues, and structures

Abnormal findings in
• Aortic aneurysm
• Chest, mediastinal, spine, or rib lesions
• Cysts or abscesses
• Enlarged lymph nodes
• Esophageal pathology, including tumors
• Hodgkin's disease
• Pleural effusion
• Pneumonitis
• Pneumothorax
• Pulmonary embolism

CRITICAL FINDINGS

• Aortic aneurysm
• Aortic dissection
• Pneumothorax
• Pulmonary embolism

It is essential that critical diagnoses be communicated immediately to the appropriate health-care provider (HCP). A listing of these diagnoses varies among facilities. Note and immediately report to the HCP abnormal results and related symptoms.

INTERFERING FACTORS

This procedure is contraindicated for
• ❖ Patients with allergies to shellfish or iodinated dye. The contrast medium used may cause a life-threatening allergic reaction. Patients with a known hypersensitivity to the medium may benefit from premedication with corticosteroids or the use of nonionic contrast medium.
• Patients who are claustrophobic.
• Patients who are pregnant or suspected of being pregnant, unless the potential benefits of

the procedure far outweigh the risks to the fetus and mother.
• ❖ Elderly and other patients who are chronically dehydrated before the test, because of their risk of contrast-induced renal failure.
• ❖ Patients who are in renal failure.
• Young patients (17 yr and younger), unless the benefits of the x-ray diagnosis outweigh the risks of exposure to high levels of radiation.

Factors that may impair clear imaging
• Metallic objects (e.g., jewelry, body rings) within the examination field, which may inhibit organ visualization and cause unclear images.
• Patients who are very obese or who may exceed the weight limit for the equipment.
• Patients with extreme claustrophobia unless sedation is given before the study.
• Inability of the patient to cooperate or remain still during the procedure because of age, significant pain, or mental status.

Other considerations
• Complications of the procedure may include hemorrhage, infection at the IV needle insertion site, and cardiac arrhythmias.
• The procedure may be terminated if chest pain or severe cardiac arrhythmias occur.
• Failure to follow dietary restrictions and other pretesting preparations may cause the procedure to be canceled or repeated.
• Consultation with an HCP should occur before the procedure for radiation safety concerns regarding younger patients or patients who are lactating.
• Risks associated with radiation overexposure can result from

frequent x-ray procedures. Personnel in the room with the patient should wear a protective lead apron, stand behind a shield, or leave the area while the examination is being done. Personnel working in the examination area should wear badges to record their level of radiation exposure.

NURSING IMPLICATIONS AND PROCEDURE

PRETEST:

▶ Positively identify the patient using at least two unique identifiers before providing care, treatment, or services.

▶ *Patient Teaching:* Inform the patient this procedure can assist in assessing the chest.

▶ Obtain a history of the patient's complaints or clinical symptoms, including a list of known allergens, especially allergies or sensitivities to latex, iodine, seafood, anesthetics, or contrast medium.

▶ Obtain a history of the patient's respiratory system, symptoms, and results of previously performed laboratory tests and diagnostic and surgical procedures.

▶ Ensure results of coagulation testing are obtained and recorded prior to the procedure; BUN and creatinine results are also needed if contrast medium is to be used.

▶ Note any recent procedures that can interfere with test results, including examinations using barium- or iodine-based contrast medium. Ensure that barium studies were performed more than 4 days before the CT scan.

▶ Record the date of the last menstrual period and determine the possibility of pregnancy in perimenopausal women.

▶ Obtain a list of the patient's current medications, including anticoagulants, aspirin and other salicylates, herbs, nutritional supplements, and nutraceuticals (see Appendix F). Note the last time and dose of medication taken.

▶ If contrast medium is scheduled to be used, patients receiving metformin (Glucophage) for non-insulin-dependent (type 2) diabetes should discontinue the drug on the day of the test and continue to withhold it for 48 hr after the test. Failure to do so may result in lactic acidosis.

▶ Review the procedure with the patient. Address concerns about pain and explain that there may be moments of discomfort and some pain experienced during the test. Inform the patient the procedure is usually performed in a radiology suite by an HCP specializing in this procedure, with support staff, and takes approximately 30 to 60 min.

▶ Explain that an IV line may be inserted to allow infusion of IV fluids, contrast medium, dye, or sedatives. Usually contrast medium and normal saline are infused.

▶ *Sensitivity to social and cultural issues,* as well as concern for modesty, is important in providing psychological support before, during, and after the procedure.

▶ Inform the patient that he or she may experience nausea, a feeling of warmth, a salty or metallic taste, or a transient headache after injection of contrast medium.

▶ Instruct the patient to remove jewelry and other metallic objects from the area to be examined.

▶ The patient should fast and restrict fluids for 2 to 4 hr prior to the procedure. Instruct the patient to avoid taking anticoagulant medication or to reduce dosage as ordered prior to the procedure. Protocols may vary among facilities.

▶ *Make sure a written and informed consent has been signed prior to the procedure and before administering any medications.*

INTRATEST:

▶ Ensure the patient has complied with dietary, fluid, and medication restrictions for 2 to 4 hr prior to the procedure.

- Ensure the patient has removed all external metallic objects from the area to be examined prior to the procedure.
- If the patient has a history of allergic reactions to any substance or drug, administer ordered prophylactic steroids or antihistamines before the procedure. Use nonionic contrast medium for the procedure.
- Have emergency equipment readily available.
- Instruct the patient to void prior to the procedure and to change into the gown, robe, and foot coverings provided.
- Instruct the patient to cooperate fully and to follow directions. Instruct the patient to remain still throughout the procedure because movement produces unreliable results.
- Observe standard precautions, and follow the general guidelines in Appendix A.
- Establish an IV fluid line for the injection of contrast medium, emergency drugs, and sedatives.
- Administer an antianxiety agent, as ordered, if the patient has claustro- phobia. Administer a sedative to a child or to an uncooperative adult, as ordered.
- Place the patient in the supine position on an examination table.
- If IV contrast medium is used, a rapid series of images is taken during and after injection.
- Ask the patient to inhale deeply and hold his or her breath while the x-ray images are taken, and then to exhale after the images are taken.
- Instruct the patient to take slow, deep breaths if nausea occurs during the procedure. Monitor and administer an antiemetic agent if ordered. Ready an emesis basin for use.
- Monitor the patient for complications related to the procedure (e.g., allergic reaction, anaphylaxis, bronchospasm) if contrast is used.
- The needle is removed, and a pressure dressing is applied over the puncture site.
- Observe/assess the needle insertion site for bleeding, inflammation, or hematoma formation.

POST-TEST:

- A report of the examination will be sent to the requesting HCP, who will discuss the results with the patient.
- Instruct the patient to resume usual medications and activity, as directed by the HCP. Renal function should be assessed before metformin is resumed, if contrast was used.
- Monitor vital signs and neurological status every 15 min for 1 hr, then every 2 hr for 4 hr, and then as ordered by the HCP. Monitor temperature every 4 hr for 24 hr. Monitor intake and output at least every 8 hr. Compare with baseline values. Notify the HCP if temperature is elevated. Protocols may vary among facilities.
- If contrast was used, observe for delayed allergic reactions, such as rash, urticaria, tachycardia, hyperpnea, hypertension, palpitations, nausea, or vomiting.
- Instruct the patient to immediately report symptoms such as fast heart rate, difficulty breathing, skin rash, itching, chest pain, persistent right shoulder pain, or abdominal pain. Immediately report symptoms to the appropriate HCP.
- Observe/assess the needle site for bleeding, inflammation, or hematoma formation.
- Instruct the patient in the care and assessment of the site.
- Instruct the patient to apply cold compresses to the insertion site as needed, to reduce discomfort or edema.
- Instruct the patient to increase fluid intake to help eliminate the contrast medium, if used.
- Inform the patient that diarrhea may occur after ingestion of oral contrast medium.
- Recognize anxiety related to test results. Discuss the implications of abnormal test results on the patient's lifestyle. Provide teaching and informa- tion regarding the clinical implications of the test results, as appropriate.
- Reinforce information given by the patient's HCP regarding further testing, treatment, or referral to another HCP. Answer any questions or

address any concerns voiced by the patient or family.

‣ Depending on the results of this procedure, additional testing may be needed to evaluate or monitor progression of the disease process and determine the need for a change in therapy. Evaluate test results in relation to the patient's symptoms and other tests performed.

RELATED MONOGRAPHS:

‣ Related tests include biopsy bone marrow, BUN, chest x-ray, CBC, CBC hematocrit, CBC hemoglobin, creatinine, echocardiogram, gallium scan, lung scan, MRI chest, mediastinoscopy, pleural fluid analysis, and PT/INR.
‣ Refer to the Respiratory System table at the end of the book for related tests by body system.

Coombs' Antiglobulin, Direct

SYNONYM/ACRONYM: Direct antiglobulin testing (DAT).

COMMON USE: To detect associated conditions or drug therapies that can result in cell hemolysis, such as found in hemolytic disease of newborns, and hemolytic transfusion reactions.

SPECIMEN: Serum (1 mL) collected in a red-top tube and whole blood (1 mL) collected in a lavender-top (EDTA) tube.

REFERENCE VALUE: (Method: Agglutination) Negative (no agglutination).

DESCRIPTION: Direct antiglobulin testing (DAT) detects in vivo antibody sensitization of red blood cells (RBCs). Immunoglobulin G (IgG) produced in certain disease states or in response to certain drugs can coat the surface of RBCs, resulting in cellular damage and hemolysis. When DAT is performed, RBCs are taken from the patient's blood sample, washed with saline to remove residual globulins, and mixed with anti–human globulin reagent. If the anti–human globulin reagent causes agglutination of the patient's RBCs, specific antiglobulin reagents can be used to determine whether the patient's RBCs are coated with IgG, complement, or both.

(See monograph titled "Blood Groups and Antibodies" and Appendix D for more information regarding transfusion reactions.)

INDICATIONS
• Detect autoimmune hemolytic anemia or hemolytic disease of the newborn
• Evaluate suspected drug-induced hemolytic anemia
• Evaluate transfusion reaction

POTENTIAL DIAGNOSIS

Positive findings in

Antibodies formed during these circumstances or conditions attach to the patient's RBCs, and hemolysis occurs.

- Anemia **(autoimmune hemolytic, drug-induced)**
- Hemolytic disease of the newborn
- Infectious mononucleosis
- Lymphomas
- Mycoplasma pneumonia
- Paroxysmal cold hemoglobinuria **(idiopathic or disease-related)**
- Passively acquired antibodies from plasma products
- Post–cardiac vascular surgery
- Systemic lupus erythematosus and other connective tissue immune disorders
- Transfusion reactions **(related to blood incompatibility)**

Negative findings in
- Samples in which sensitization of erythrocytes has not occurred

CRITICAL FINDINGS: N/A

INTERFERING FACTORS
- Drugs and substances that may cause a positive DAT include acetaminophen, aminopyrine, aminosalicylic acid, ampicillin, antihistamines, aztreonam, cephalosporins, chlorinated hydrocarbon insecticides, chlorpromazine, chlorpropamide, cisplatin, clonidine, dipyrone, ethosuximide, fenfluramine, hydralazine, hydrochlorothiazide, ibuprofen, insulin, isoniazid, levodopa, mefenamic acid, melphalan, methadone, methicillin, methyldopa, moxalactam, penicillin, phenytoin, probenecid, procainamide, quinidine, quinine, rifampin, stibophen, streptomycin, sulfonamides, and tetracycline.
- Wharton's jelly may cause a false-positive DAT.
- Cold agglutinins and large amounts of paraproteins in the specimen may cause false-positive results.
- Newborns' cells may give negative results in ABO hemolytic disease.

NURSING IMPLICATIONS AND PROCEDURE

PRETEST:
- Positively identify the patient using at least two unique identifiers before providing care, treatment, or services.
- *Patient Teaching:* Inform the patient/parent this test can assist in assessing for disorders that break down red blood cells.
- Obtain a history of the patient's complaints, including a list of known allergens, especially allergies or sensitivities to latex.
- Obtain a history of the patient's hematopoietic system as well as results of previously performed laboratory tests and diagnostic and surgical procedures.
- Obtain a list of the patient's current medications, including herbs, nutritional supplements, and nutraceuticals (see Appendix F).
- Review the procedure with the patient. Inform the patient that specimen collection takes approximately 5 to 10 min. Address concerns about pain and explain that there may be some discomfort during the venipuncture. If a cord sample is to be taken from a newborn, inform parents that the sample will be obtained at the time of delivery and will not result in blood loss to the infant.
- *Sensitivity to social and cultural issues,* as well as concern for modesty, is important in providing psychological support before, during, and after the procedure.
- There are no food, fluid, or medication restrictions unless by medical direction.

INTRATEST:
- If the patient has a history of allergic reaction to latex, avoid the use of equipment containing latex.
- Instruct the patient to cooperate fully and to follow directions. Direct the patient to breathe normally and to avoid unnecessary movement.
- Observe standard precautions, and follow the general guidelines in Appendix A. Positively identify the patient, and label the appropriate tubes with the

corresponding patient demographics, date, and time of collection. Perform a venipuncture. Cord specimens are obtained by inserting a needle attached to a syringe into the umbilical vein. The specimen is drawn into the syringe and gently expressed into the appropriate collection container.

▸ Remove the needle and apply direct pressure with dry gauze to stop bleeding. Observe/assess venipuncture site for bleeding or hematoma formation and secure gauze with adhesive bandage.

▸ Promptly transport the specimen to the laboratory for processing and analysis.

POST-TEST:

▸ A report of the results will be sent to the requesting health-care provider (HCP), who will discuss the results with the patient.

▸ Note positive test results in cord blood of neonate; also assess newborn's bilirubin and hematocrit levels. Results may indicate the need for immediate exchange transfusion of fresh whole blood that has been typed and cross-matched with the mother's serum.

▸ Inform the postpartum patient of the implications of positive test results in cord blood. Prepare the newborn for exchange transfusion, on medical direction.

▸ Reinforce information given by the patient's HCP regarding further testing, treatment, or referral to another HCP. Answer any questions or address any concerns voiced by the patient or family.

▸ Depending on the results of this procedure, additional testing may be performed to evaluate or monitor progression of the disease process and determine the need for a change in therapy. Evaluate test results in relation to the patient's symptoms and other tests performed.

RELATED MONOGRAPHS:

▸ Related tests include bilirubin, blood groups and antibodies, CBC hematocrit, CBC hemoglobin, Coombs' indirect antiglobulin (IAT), Ham's test, and haptoglobin.

▸ Refer to the Hematopoietic System table at the end of the book for related tests by body system.

Coombs' Antiglobulin, Indirect

SYNONYM/ACRONYM: Indirect antiglobulin test (IAT), antibody screen.

COMMON USE: To check donor and recipient blood cells for antibodies prior to blood transfusion.

SPECIMEN: Serum (1 mL) collected in a red-top tube.

REFERENCE VALUE: (Method: Agglutination) Negative (no agglutination).

DESCRIPTION: The indirect antiglobulin test (IAT) detects and identifies unexpected circulating complement molecules or antibodies in the patient's serum. The first use of this test was for the detection and identification of anti-D using an indirect method. The test is now commonly used to screen a patient's serum for the presence of antibodies that may react against transfused red blood cells (RBCs). During testing, the patient's serum is allowed to incubate with reagent RBCs. The reagent RBCs used are from group O donors and have most of the clinically significant antigens present (D, C, E c, e, K, M, N, S, s, Fy^a, Fy^b, Jk^a, and Jk^b). Antibodies present in the patient's serum coat antigenic sites on the RBC membrane. The reagent cells are washed with saline to remove any unbound antibody. Antihuman globulin is added in the final step of the test. If the patient's serum contains antibodies, the antihuman globulin will cause the antibody-coated RBCs to stick together or agglutinate. (See monograph titled "Blood Groups and Antibodies" and Appendix D for more information regarding transfusion reactions.)

INDICATIONS

- Detect other antibodies in maternal blood that can be potentially harmful to the fetus
- Determine antibody titers in Rh-negative women sensitized by an Rh-positive fetus
- Screen for antibodies before blood transfusions
- Test for the weak Rh-variant antigen D^u.

POTENTIAL DIAGNOSIS

Positive findings in

Circulating antibodies or medications attach to the patient's RBCs, and hemolysis occurs.

- Hemolytic anemia *(drug-induced or autoimmune)*
- Hemolytic disease of the newborn
- Incompatible crossmatch
- Maternal-fetal Rh incompatibility

Negative findings in

- Samples in which the patient's antibodies exhibit dosage effects (i.e., stronger reaction with homozygous than with heterozygous expression of an antigen) and reagent erythrocyte antigens contain single-dose expressions of the corresponding antigen (heterozygous)
- Samples in which reagent erythrocyte antigens are unable to detect low-prevalence antibodies
- Samples in which sensitization of erythrocytes has not occurred (complete absence of antibodies)

CRITICAL FINDINGS: N/A

INTERFERING FACTORS

- Drugs that may cause a positive IAT include meropenem, methyldopa, penicillin, phenacetin, quinidine, and rifampin.
- Recent administration of dextran, whole blood or fractions, or IV contrast media can result in a false-positive reaction.

NURSING IMPLICATIONS AND PROCEDURE

PRETEST:

- Positively identify the patient using at least two unique identifiers before providing care, treatment, or services.
- *Patient Teaching:* Inform the patient this test can assist in assessing for blood compatibility prior to transfusion.

- Obtain a history of the patient's complaints, including a list of known allergens, especially allergies or sensitivities to latex.
- Obtain a history of the patient's hematopoietic system as well as results of previously performed laboratory tests and diagnostic and surgical procedures.
- Note any recent procedures that can interfere with test results.
- Obtain a list of the patient's current medications, including herbs, nutritional supplements, and nutraceuticals (see Appendix F).
- Review the procedure with the patient. Inform the patient that specimen collection takes approximately 5 to 10 min. Address concerns about pain and explain that there may be some discomfort during the venipuncture.
- *Sensitivity to social and cultural issues,* as well as concern for modesty, is important in providing psychological support before, during, and after the procedure.
- There are no food, fluid, or medication restrictions unless by medical direction.

INTRATEST:

- If the patient has a history of allergic reaction to latex, avoid the use of equipment containing latex.
- Instruct the patient to cooperate fully and to follow directions. Direct the patient to breathe normally and to avoid unnecessary movement.
- Observe standard precautions, and follow the general guidelines in Appendix A. Positively identify the patient, and label the appropriate tubes with the corresponding patient demographics, date, and time of collection. Perform a venipuncture.

- Remove the needle and apply direct pressure with dry gauze to stop bleeding. Observe/assess venipuncture site for bleeding or hematoma formation and secure gauze with adhesive bandage.
- Promptly transport the specimen to the laboratory for processing and analysis.

POST-TEST:

- A report of the results will be sent to the requesting health-care provider (HCP), who will discuss the results with the patient.
- Inform pregnant women that negative tests during the first 12 wk of gestation should be repeated at 28 wk to rule out the presence of an antibody.
- Positive test results in pregnant women after 28 wk of gestation indicate the need for antibody identification testing.
- Reinforce information given by the patient's HCP regarding further testing, treatment, or referral to another HCP. Answer any questions or address any concerns voiced by the patient or family.
- Depending on the results of this procedure, additional testing may be performed to evaluate or monitor progression of the disease process and determine the need for a change in therapy. Evaluate test results in relation to the patient's symptoms and other tests performed.

RELATED MONOGRAPHS:

- Related tests include bilirubin, blood groups and antibodies, CBC hematocrit, CBC hemoglobin, Coombs' direct antiglobulin (DAT), and haptoglobin.
- Refer to the Hematopoietic System table at the end of the book for related tests by body system.

Copper

SYNONYM/ACRONYM: Cu.

COMMON USE: To evaluate and monitor exposure to copper and to assist in diagnosing Wilson's disease.

SPECIMEN: Serum (1 mL) collected in a royal blue-top, trace element–free tube.

REFERENCE VALUE: (Method: Inductively coupled plasma-mass spectrometry)

Age	Conventional Units	SI Units (Conventional Units × 0.157)
Newborn–5 days	9–46 mcg/dL	1.4–7.2 micromol/L
1–5 yr	80–150 mcg/dL	12.6–23.6 micromol/L
6–9 yr	84–136 mcg/dL	13.2–21.4 micromol/L
10–14 yr	80–121 mcg/dL	12.6–19.0 micromol/L
15–19 yr	80–171 mcg/dL	10.1–18.4 micromol/L
Adult		
Male	70–140 mcg/dL	11.0–22.0 micromol/L
Female	80–155 mcg/dL	12.6–24.3 micromol/L
Pregnant female	118–302 mcg/dL	18.5–47.4 micromol/L

Values for African Americans are 8% to 12% higher.

DESCRIPTION: Copper is an important cofactor for the enzymes that participate in the formation of hemoglobin and collagen. Copper is also a component of coagulation factor V and assists in the oxidation of glucose. It is required for melanin pigment formation and maintenance of myelin sheaths and is used to synthesize ceruloplasmin. Copper levels vary with intake. Levels vary diurnally and peak during morning hours. This mineral is absorbed in the stomach and duodenum, stored in the liver, and excreted in urine and in feces with bile salts. Copper deficiency results in neutropenia and a hypochromic, microcytic anemia that is not responsive to iron therapy. Other signs and symptoms of copper deficiency include osteoporosis, depigmentation of skin and hair, impaired immune system response, and possible neurological and cardiac abnormalities.

INDICATIONS

- Assist in establishing a diagnosis of Menkes' disease
- Assist in establishing a diagnosis of Wilson's disease
- Monitor patients receiving long-term parenteral nutrition therapy

POTENTIAL DIAGNOSIS

Increased in

Ceruloplasmin is an acute-phase reactant protein and the main protein binder of copper; therefore, copper levels will be increased in many inflammatory conditions, including cancer. Estrogens increase levels of binding protein; therefore, copper is elevated in pregnancy and estrogen therapy.

- Anemias *(related to increased RBC production)*
- Ankylosing rheumatoid spondylitis
- Biliary cirrhosis *(related to release from damaged liver tissue)*
- Collagen diseases
- Complications of renal dialysis *(trace element disturbances related to contamination from dialysate fluid and the disease process itself can be significant and can compound over time)*
- Hodgkin's disease
- Infections
- Inflammation
- Leukemia
- Malignant neoplasms
- Myocardial infarction (MI) *(a correlation exists among copper levels, CK, and LDH in MI; the pathophysiology is unclear but some studies indicate a relationship between trace metal levels and risk of AMI)*
- Pellagra *(related to niacin deficiency; niacin is an essential cofactor in reactions involving copper)*
- Poisoning from copper-contaminated solutions or insecticides *(related to excessive accumulation due to environmental exposure)*
- Pregnancy
- Pulmonary tuberculosis
- Rheumatic fever
- Rheumatoid arthritis
- Systemic lupus erythematosus
- Thalassemias *(related to zinc deficiency of thalassemia and increased rate of release from hemolyzed RBCs; copper and zinc compete for the same binding sites so that a deficiency in one results in an increase of the other)*
- Thyroid disease (hypothyroid or hyperthyroid) *(related to stimulation of thyroid hormone production by copper)*
- Trauma
- Typhoid fever
- Use of copper intrauterine device *(related to copper leaching from the device)*

Decreased in

- Burns *(related to loss of stores in tissue and possibly to competitive inhibition of zinc-containing medications or vitamins administered as part of burn therapy)*
- Cystic fibrosis *(related to inadequate intake and absorption)*
- Dysproteinemia *(related to decreased transport to and from stores)*
- Infants *(related to inadequate intake of milk or consumption of milk deficient in copper; especially premature infants)*
- Iron-deficiency anemias (some) *(related to decreased absorption of iron from the intestines and transfer from tissues to plasma; it is essential to hemoglobin formation)*
- Long-term total parenteral nutrition *(related to inadequate intake)*
- Malabsorption disorders (celiac disease, tropical sprue) *(related to inadequate absorption)*
- Malnutrition *(related to inadequate intake)*
- Menkes' disease *(evidenced by a severe genetic X-linked defect causing failed transport to the liver and tissues)*

- Nephrotic syndrome *(related to loss of transport proteins)*
- Occipital horn syndrome (OHS) *(evidenced by an inherited disorder of copper metabolism; similar to Menkes' disease)*
- Wilson's disease *(evidenced by a genetic defect causing failed transport to the liver and tissues)*

CRITICAL FINDINGS: N/A

INTERFERING FACTORS

- Drugs that may increase copper levels include anticonvulsants and oral contraceptives.
- Drugs that may decrease copper levels include citrates, penicillamine, and valproic acid.
- Excessive therapeutic intake of zinc may interfere with intestinal absorption of copper.

NURSING IMPLICATIONS AND PROCEDURE

PRETEST:

▶ Positively identify the patient using at least two unique identifiers before providing care, treatment, or services.
▶ *Patient Teaching:* Inform the patient this test can assist in monitoring the amount of copper in the body.
▶ Obtain a history of the patient's complaints, including a list of known allergens, especially allergies or sensitivities to latex.
▶ Obtain a history of the patient's hematopoietic, hepatobiliary, and immune systems, as well as results of previously performed laboratory tests and diagnostic and surgical procedures.
▶ Obtain a list of the patient's current medications, including herbs, nutritional supplements, and nutraceuticals (see Appendix F).
▶ Review the procedure with the patient. Inform the patient that specimen collection takes approximately 5 to 10 min. Address concerns about pain

and explain that there may be some discomfort during the venipuncture.
▶ *Sensitivity to social and cultural issues,* as well as concern for modesty, is important in providing psychological support before, during, and after the procedure.
▶ There are no food, fluid, or medication restrictions unless by medical direction.

INTRATEST:

▶ If the patient has a history of allergic reaction to latex, avoid the use of equipment containing latex.
▶ Instruct the patient to cooperate fully and to follow directions. Direct the patient to breathe normally and to avoid unnecessary movement.
▶ Observe standard precautions, and follow the general guidelines in Appendix A. Positively identify the patient, and label the appropriate tubes with the corresponding patient demographics, date, and time of collection. Perform a venipuncture.
▶ Remove the needle and apply direct pressure with dry gauze to stop bleeding. Observe/assess venipuncture site for bleeding or hematoma formation and secure gauze with adhesive bandage.
▶ Promptly transport the specimen to the laboratory for processing and analysis.

POST-TEST:

▶ A report of the results will be sent to the requesting health-care provider (HCP), who will discuss the results with the patient.
▶ *Nutritional Considerations:* Instruct the patient with increased copper levels to avoid foods rich in copper and to increase intake of elements (zinc, iron, calcium, and manganese) that interfere with copper absorption, as appropriate. Copper deficiency does not normally occur in adults, but patients receiving long-term total parenteral nutrition should be evaluated if signs and symptoms of copper deficiency appear. These patients should be informed that organ meats, shellfish, nuts, and legumes are good sources of dietary copper.
▶ Reinforce information given by the patient's HCP regarding further testing, treatment, or referral to another HCP. Answer any questions or address any concerns voiced by the patient or family.

▶ Depending on the results of this procedure, additional testing may be performed to evaluate or monitor progression of the disease process and determine the need for a change in therapy. Evaluate test results in relation to the patient's symptoms and other tests performed.

C

RELATED MONOGRAPHS:
▶ Related tests include biopsy liver, ceruloplasmin, CBC, and zinc.
▶ Refer to the Hematopoietic, Hepatobiliary, and Immune systems tables at the end of the book for related tests by body system.

Cortisol and Challenge Tests

SYNONYM/ACRONYM: Hydrocortisone, compound F.

COMMON USE: To assist in diagnosing adrenocortical insufficiency such as in Cushing's syndrome and Addison's disease.

SPECIMEN: Serum (1 mL) collected in a red- or tiger-top tube. Plasma (1 mL) collected in a green-top (heparin) tube is also acceptable. Care must be taken to use the same type of collection container if serial measurements are to be taken.

Procedure	Medication Administered	Recommended Collection Times
ACTH stimulation, rapid test	1 mcg (low-dose protocol) cosyntropin IM	3 cortisol levels: baseline immediately before bolus, 30 min after bolus, and 60 min after bolus
CRH stimulation	IV dose of 1 mg/kg ovine or human CRH	8 cortisol and 8 ACTH levels: baseline collected 15 min before injection, 0 min before injection, and then 5, 15, 30, 60, 120, and 180 min after injection
Dexamethasone suppression (overnight)	Oral dose of 1 mg dexamethasone (Decadron) at 11 p.m.	Collect cortisol at 8 a.m. on the morning after the dexamethasone dose
Metyrapone stimulation (overnight)	Oral dose of 30 mg/kg metyrapone with snack at midnight	Collect cortisol and ACTH at 8 a.m. on the morning after the metyrapone dose

ACTH = adrenocorticotropic hormone; CRH = corticotropin-releasing hormone; IM = intramuscular; IV = intravenous.

REFERENCE VALUE: (Method: Immunochemiluminescent assay)

Cortisol

Time	Conventional Units	SI Units (Conventional Units × 27.6)
8 a.m.	5–25 mcg/dL	138–690 nmol/L
4 p.m.	3–16 mcg/dL	83–442 nmol/L

ACTH Challenge Tests

ACTH (Cosyntropin) Stimulated, Rapid Test	Conventional Units	SI Units (Conventional Units × 27.6)
Baseline 30- or 60-min response	Cortisol greater than 5 mg/dL Cortisol 18–20 mcg/dL or incremental increase of 7 mcg/dL over baseline value	Greater than 138 nmol/L 496–552 nmol/L

Corticotropin-Releasing Hormone Stimulated	Conventional Units	SI Units (Conventional Units × 27.6)
	Cortisol peaks at greater than 20 mcg/dL within 30–60 min	Greater than 552 nmol/L
		SI Units (Conventional Units × 0.22)
	ACTH increases two to fourfold within 30–60 min	Twofold to fourfold increase within 30–60 min

Dexamethasone Suppressed Overnight Test	Conventional Units	SI Units (Conventional Units × 27.6)
	Cortisol less than 1.8 mcg/dL next day	Less than 49.7 nmol/L

Metyrapone Stimulated Overnight Test	Conventional Units	SI Units (Conventional Units × 27.6)
	Cortisol less than 3 mcg/dL next day	Less than 83 nmol/L
		SI Units (Conventional Units × 0.22)
	ACTH greater than 75 pg/mL	Greater than 16.5 pmol/L
		SI Units (Conventional Units × 30)
	11-deoxycortisol greater than 70 ng/mL	Greater than 210 pmol/L

DESCRIPTION: Cortisol (hydrocortisone) is the predominant glucocorticoid secreted in response to stimulation by the hypothalamus and pituitary adrenocorticotropic hormone (ACTH). Cortisol stimulates gluconeogenesis, mobilizes fats and proteins, antagonizes insulin, and suppresses inflammation. Measuring levels of cortisol in blood is the best indicator of adrenal function. Cortisol secretion varies diurnally, with highest levels occurring on awakening and lowest levels occurring late in the day. Bursts of cortisol excretion can occur at night. Cortisol and ACTH test results are evaluated together because they each control the other's concentrations (i.e., any change in one causes a change in the other). ACTH levels exhibit a diurnal variation, peaking between 6 and 8 a.m. and reaching the lowest point between 6 and 11 p.m. Evening levels are generally one-half to two-thirds lower than morning levels. (See monograph titled "Adrenocorticotropic Hormone [and Challenge Tests].")

INDICATIONS

• Detect adrenal hyperfunction (Cushing's syndrome)

• Detect adrenal hypofunction (Addison's disease)

POTENTIAL DIAGNOSIS

The dexamethasone suppression test is useful in differentiating the causes for increased cortisol levels. Dexamethasone is a synthetic steroid that suppresses secretion of ACTH. With this test, a baseline morning cortisol level is collected, and the patient is given a 1-mg dose of dexamethasone at bedtime. A second specimen is collected the following morning. If cortisol levels have not been suppressed, adrenal adenoma may be suspected. The dexamethasone suppression test also produces abnormal results in patients with psychiatric illnesses.

The corticotropin-releasing hormone (CRH) stimulation test works as well as the dexamethasone suppression test in distinguishing Cushing's disease from conditions in which ACTH is secreted ectopically. In this test, cortisol levels are measured after an injection of CRH. A fourfold increase in cortisol levels above baseline is seen in Cushing's disease. No increase in cortisol is seen if ectopic ACTH secretion is the cause.

C

The ACTH (cosyntropin) stimulated rapid test is used when adrenal insufficiency is suspected. Cosyntropin is a synthetic form of ACTH. A baseline cortisol level is collected before the injection of cosyntropin. Specimens are subsequently collected at 30- and 60-min intervals. If the adrenal glands are functioning normally, cortisol levels rise significantly after administration of cosyntropin.

The metyrapone stimulation test is used to distinguish corticotropin-dependent (pituitary Cushing's disease and ectopic Cushing's disease) from corticotropin-independent (carcinoma of the lung or thyroid) causes of increased cortisol levels. Metyrapone inhibits the conversion of 11-deoxycortisol to cortisol. Cortisol levels should decrease to less than 3 mcg/dL if normal pituitary stimulation by ACTH occurs after an oral dose of metyrapone. Specimen collection and administration of the medication are performed as with the overnight dexamethasone test.

Increased in

Conditions that result in excessive production of cortisol.
- Adrenal adenoma
- Cushing's syndrome
- Ectopic ACTH production
- Hyperglycemia
- Pregnancy
- Stress

Decreased in

Conditions that result in adrenal hypofunction and corresponding low levels of cortisol.
- Addison's disease
- Adrenogenital syndrome
- Hypopituitarism

CRITICAL FINDINGS: N/A

INTERFERING FACTORS

- Drugs and substances that may increase cortisol levels include anticonvulsants, clomipramine, corticotropin, cortisone, CRH, ether, fenfluramine, gemfibrozil, hydrocortisone, insulin, lithium, methadone, metoclopramide, mifepristone, naloxone, opiates, oral contraceptives, ranitidine, tetracosactrin, and vasopressin.
- Drugs and substances that may decrease cortisol levels include barbiturates, beclomethasone, betamethasone, clonidine, desoximetasone, dexamethasone, ephedrine, etomidate, fluocinolone, ketoconazole, levodopa, lithium, methylprednisolone, metyrapone, midazolam, morphine, nitrous oxide, oxazepam, phenytoin, ranitidine, and trimipramine.
- Test results are affected by the time this test is done because cortisol levels vary diurnally.
- Stress and excessive physical activity can produce elevated levels.
- Normal values can be obtained in the presence of partial pituitary deficiency.
- Recent radioactive scans within 1 wk of the test can interfere with test results.
- ❖ The metyrapone stimulation test is contraindicated in patients with suspected adrenal insufficiency.
- ❖ Metyrapone may cause gastrointestinal distress and/or confusion. Administer oral dose of metyrapone with milk and snack.

NURSING IMPLICATIONS AND PROCEDURE

PRETEST:

▶ Positively identify the patient using at least two unique identifiers before providing care, treatment, or services.
▶ *Patient Teaching:* Inform the patient this test can assist in assessing for the amount of cortisol in the blood.

- Obtain a history of the patient's complaints, including a list of known allergens, especially allergies or sensitivities to latex.
- Obtain a history of the patient's endocrine system, as well as results of previously performed laboratory tests and diagnostic and surgical procedures.
- Obtain a list of the patient's current medications, including herbs, nutritional supplements, and nutraceuticals (see Appendix F).
- Review the procedure with the patient. Inform the patient that multiple specimens may be required. Inform the patient that specimen collection takes approximately 5 to 10 min. Address concerns about pain and explain that there may be some discomfort during the venipuncture.
- *Sensitivity to social and cultural issues,* as well as concern for modesty, is important in providing psychological support before, during, and after the procedure.
- There are no food, fluid, or medication restrictions unless by medical direction.
- Drugs that enhance steroid metabolism may be withheld by medical direction prior to metyrapone stimulation testing.
- Instruct the patient to minimize stress to avoid raising cortisol levels.

INTRATEST:

- Have emergency equipment readily available.
- If the patient has a history of allergic reaction to latex, avoid the use of equipment containing latex.
- Instruct the patient to cooperate fully and to follow directions. Direct the patient to breathe normally and to avoid unnecessary movement.
- Observe standard precautions, and follow the general guidelines in Appendix A. Positively identify the patient, and label the appropriate tubes with the corresponding patient demographics, date, and time of collection. Collect specimen between 6 and 8 a.m., when cortisol levels are highest. Perform a venipuncture.
- Adverse reactions to metyrapone include nausea and vomiting (N/V), abdominal pain, headache, dizziness, sedation, allergic rash, decreased white blood cell count, or bone marrow

depression. Signs and symptoms of overdose or acute adrenocortical insufficiency include cardiac arrhythmias, hypotension, dehydration, anxiety, confusion, weakness, impairment of consciousness, N/V, epigastric pain, diarrhea, hyponatremia, and hyperkalemia.
- Remove the needle and apply direct pressure with dry gauze to stop bleeding. Observe/assess venipuncture site for bleeding or hematoma formation and secure gauze with adhesive bandage.
- Promptly transport the specimen to the laboratory for processing and analysis.

POST-TEST:

- A report of the results will be sent to the requesting health-care provider (HCP), who will discuss the results with the patient.
- Instruct the patient to resume usual medications, as directed by the HCP.
- Recognize anxiety related to test results. Discuss the implications of abnormal test results on the patient's lifestyle. Provide teaching and information regarding the clinical implications of the test results, as appropriate. Educate the patient regarding access to counseling services. Provide contact information, if desired, for the Cushing's Support and Research Foundation (www.csrf.net).
- Reinforce information given by the patient's HCP regarding further testing, treatment, or referral to another HCP. Answer any questions or address any concerns voiced by the patient or family.
- Depending on the results of this procedure, additional testing may be performed to evaluate or monitor progression of the disease process and determine the need for a change in therapy. Evaluate test results in relation to the patient's symptoms and other tests performed.

RELATED MONOGRAPHS:

- Related tests include ACTH and challenge tests, angiography adrenal, chloride, CT abdomen, CT pituitary, DHEA, glucagon, glucose, glucose tolerance test, growth hormone, insulin, MRI abdomen, MRI pituitary, renin, sodium, and testosterone.
- Refer to the Endocrine System table at the end of the book for related tests by body system.

C-Peptide

SYNONYM/ACRONYM: Connecting peptide insulin, insulin C-peptide, proinsulin C-peptide.

COMMON USE: To evaluate hypoglycemia, assess beta cell function, and distinguish between type 1 and type 2 diabetes.

SPECIMEN: Serum (1 mL) collected in a red-top tube.

REFERENCE VALUE: (Method: Immunochemiluminometric assay, ICMA)

Age	Conventional Units	SI Units (Conventional Units × 0.333)
9 yr	0.0–3.3 ng/mL	0.0–1.1 nmol/L
10–16 yr	0.4–3.3 ng/mL	0.1–1.1 nmol/L
Greater than 16 yr	1.1–5.0 ng/mL	3.3–1.7 nmol/L

DESCRIPTION: C-peptide is a biologically inactive peptide formed when beta cells of the pancreas convert proinsulin to insulin. Most of C-peptide is secreted by the kidneys. C-peptide levels usually correlate with insulin levels and provide a reliable indication of how well the beta cells secrete insulin. Release of C-peptide is not affected by exogenous insulin administration. C-peptide values double after stimulation with glucose or glucagon, and measurement of C-peptide levels are very useful in the evaluation of hypoglycemia. An insulin/C-peptide ratio less than 1.0 indicates endogenous insulin secretion, whereas a ratio greater than 1.0 indicates an excess of exogenous insulin. An elevated C-peptide level in the presence of plasma glucose less than 40 mg/dL supports a diagnosis of pancreatic islet cell tumor.

INDICATIONS

- Assist in the diagnosis of insulinoma: serum levels of insulin and C-peptide are elevated.
- Detect suspected factitious cause of hypoglycemia (excessive insulin administration): an increase in blood insulin from injection does not increase C-peptide levels.
- Determine beta cell function when insulin antibodies preclude accurate measurement of serum insulin production.
- Distinguish between insulin-dependent (type 1) and non-insulin-dependent (type 2) diabetes (with C-peptide–stimulating test): Patients with diabetes whose C-peptide stimulation level is greater than 18 ng/mL can be managed without insulin treatment.
- Evaluate hypoglycemia.
- Evaluate viability of pancreatic transplant.

POTENTIAL DIAGNOSIS

Increased in

- Islet cell tumor *(related to excessive endogenous insulin production)*
- Non-insulin-dependent (type 2) diabetes *(related to increased insulin production)*
- Pancreas or beta cell transplants *(related to increased insulin production)*
- Renal failure *(increase in circulating levels of C-peptide related to decreased renal excretion)*

Decreased in

- Factitious hypoglycemia *(related to decrease in blood glucose levels in response to insulin injection)*
- Insulin-dependent (type 1) diabetes *(evidenced by insufficient production of insulin by the pancreas)*
- Pancreatectomy *(evidenced by absence of the pancreas)*

CRITICAL FINDINGS: N/A

INTERFERING FACTORS

- Drugs that may increase C-peptide levels include betamethasone, chloroquine, danazol, deferoxamine, ethinyl estradiol, glibenclamide, glimepiride, indapamide, oral contraceptives, piretanide, prednisone, and rifampin.
- Drugs that may decrease C-peptide levels include atenolol and calcitonin.
- C-peptide and endogenous insulin levels do not always correlate in obese patients.
- Failure to follow dietary restrictions before the procedure may cause the procedure to be canceled or repeated.

NURSING IMPLICATIONS AND PROCEDURE

PRETEST:

- Positively identify the patient using at least two unique identifiers before providing care, treatment, or services.
- *Patient Teaching:* Inform the patient this test can assist in assessing for low blood sugar.
- Obtain a history of the patient's complaints, including a list of known allergens, especially allergies or sensitivities to latex.
- Obtain a history of the patient's endocrine system, symptoms, and results of previously performed laboratory tests and diagnostic and surgical procedures.
- Obtain a list of the patient's current medications, including herbs, nutritional supplements, and nutraceuticals (see Appendix F).
- Review the procedure with the patient. Inform the patient that specimen collection takes approximately 5 to 10 min. Address concerns about pain and explain that there may be some discomfort during the venipuncture.
- *Sensitivity to social and cultural issues,* as well as concern for modesty, is important in providing psychological support before, during, and after the procedure.
- The patient should fast for at least 10 hr before specimen collection. Protocols may vary among facilities.
- There are no fluid or medication restrictions unless by medical direction.

INTRATEST:

- Ensure that the patient has complied with dietary restrictions and pretesting preparations; assure that food has been restricted for at least 10 hr prior to the procedure.
- If the patient has a history of allergic reaction to latex, avoid the use of equipment containing latex.
- Instruct the patient to cooperate fully and to follow directions. Direct the patient to breathe normally and to avoid unnecessary movement.
- Observe standard precautions, and follow the general guidelines in

Appendix A. Positively identify the patient, and label the appropriate tubes with the corresponding patient demographics, date, and time of collection. Perform a venipuncture.

- Remove the needle and apply direct pressure with dry gauze to stop bleeding. Observe/assess venipuncture site for bleeding or hematoma formation and secure gauze with adhesive bandage.
- Promptly transport the specimen to the laboratory for processing and analysis.

POST-TEST:

- A report of the results will be sent to the requesting health-care provider (HCP), who will discuss the results with the patient.
- Instruct the patient to resume usual diet as directed by the HCP.
- *Nutritional Considerations:* Abnormal C-peptide levels may be associated with diabetes. There is no "diabetic diet"; however, many meal-planning approaches with nutritional goals are endorsed by the American Dietetic Association. Patients who adhere to dietary recommendations report a better general feeling of health, better weight management, greater control of glucose and lipid values, and improved use of insulin. Instruct the patient, as appropriate, in nutritional management of diabetes. In June 2006, the American Heart Association developed a Therapeutic Lifestyle Changes (TLC) diet with goals directed at people with specific risk factors and/or existing medical conditions (e.g., elevated low-density lipoprotein [LDL] cholesterol levels, other lipid disorders, coronary artery disease [CAD], insulin-dependent diabetes, insulin resistance, or metabolic syndrome). The dietary therapy includes nutritional recommendations for daily total caloric intake and recommendations for allowable percentage of calories derived from fat (saturated and unsaturated), carbohydrates, protein, and cholesterol, as well as recommendations for daily expenditure of energy. The nutritional needs of each diabetic patient need to be determined individually (especially during pregnancy) with the appropriate health care professionals, particularly professionals trained in nutrition.

- Instruct the patient and caregiver to report signs and symptoms of hypoglycemia (weakness, confusion, diaphoresis, rapid pulse) or hyperglycemia (thirst, polyuria, hunger, lethargy). Emphasize, as appropriate, that good control of glucose levels delays the onset and slows the progression of diabetic retinopathy, nephropathy, and neuropathy.
- Recognize anxiety related to test results, and be supportive of perceived loss of independence and fear of shortened life expectancy. Discuss the implications of abnormal test results on the patient's lifestyle. Provide teaching and information regarding the clinical implications of the test results, as appropriate. Emphasize, if indicated, that good glycemic control delays the onset and slows the progression of diabetic retinopathy, nephropathy, and neuropathy. Educate the patient regarding access to counseling services, as appropriate. Provide contact information, if desired, for the American Diabetes Association (www.diabetes.org) or the American Heart Association (www.americanheart.org).
- Reinforce information given by the patient's HCP regarding further testing, treatment, or referral to another HCP. Answer any questions or address any concerns voiced by the patient or family.
- Depending on the results of this procedure, additional testing may be performed to evaluate or monitor progression of the disease process and determine the need for a change in therapy. Evaluate test results in relation to the patient's symptoms and other tests performed.

RELATED MONOGRAPHS:

- Related tests include CT cardiac scoring, cortisol, creatinine, creatinine clearance, EMG, ENG, fluorescein angiography, fructose, fundus photography, glucagon, glucose, glucose tolerance tests, glycated hemoglobin, insulin, insulin antibodies, microalbumin, plethysmography, and visual fields test.
- Refer to the Endocrine System table at the end of the book for related tests by body system.

C-Reactive Protein

SYNONYM/ACRONYM: CRP.

COMMON USE: To indicate nonspecific inflammatory response; this highly sensitive test is used to assess risk for cardiovascular and peripheral vascular disease.

SPECIMEN: Serum (1 mL) collected in a red- or tiger-top tube.

REFERENCE VALUE: (Method: High-sensitivity immunoassay, nephelometry)

High-sensitivity immunoassay (cardiac applications)	1.0–3.0 mg/L

Nephelometry	Conventional Units
Adult	0–4.9 mg/L

DESCRIPTION: C-reactive protein (CRP) is a glycoprotein produced by the liver in response to acute inflammation. The CRP assay is a nonspecific test that determines the presence (not the cause) of inflammation; it is often ordered in conjunction with erythrocyte sedimentation rate (ESR). CRP assay is a more sensitive and rapid indicator of the presence of an inflammatory process than ESR. CRP disappears from the serum rapidly when inflammation has subsided. The inflammatory process and its association with atherosclerosis make the presence of CRP, as detected by highly sensitive CRP assays, a potential marker for coronary artery disease. It is believed that the inflammatory process may instigate the conversion of a stable plaque to a weaker one that can rupture and occlude an artery.

INDICATIONS

- Assist in the differential diagnosis of appendicitis and acute pelvic inflammatory disease
- Assist in the differential diagnosis of Crohn's disease and ulcerative colitis
- Assist in the differential diagnosis of rheumatoid arthritis and uncomplicated systemic lupus erythematosus (SLE)
- Assist in the evaluation of coronary artery disease
- Detect the presence or exacerbation of inflammatory processes
- Monitor response to therapy for autoimmune disorders such as rheumatoid arthritis

POTENTIAL DIAGNOSIS

Increased in
Conditions associated with an inflammatory response stimulate production of CRP.
- Acute bacterial infections
- Crohn's disease
- Inflammatory bowel disease
- Myocardial infarction *(inflammation of the coronary vessels is associated with increased CRP levels and increased risk for*

coronary vessel injury, which may result in distal vessel plaque occlusions)
- Pregnancy (second half)
- Rheumatic fever
- Rheumatoid arthritis
- SLE
- Syndrome X (metabolic syndrome) *(inflammation of the coronary vessels is associated with increased CRP levels and increased risk for coronary vessel injury, which may result in distal vessel plaque occlusions)*

Decreased in: N/A

CRITICAL FINDINGS: N/A

INTERFERING FACTORS
- Drugs that may increase CRP levels include chemotherapy, interleukin-2, oral contraceptives, and pamidronate.
- Drugs that may decrease CRP levels include aurothiomalate, dexamethasone, gemfibrozil, leflunomide, methotrexate, NSAIDs, oral contraceptives (progestogen effect), penicillamine, pentopril, prednisolone, prinomide, and sulfasalazine.
- NSAIDs, salicylates, and steroids may cause false-negative results because of suppression of inflammation.
- Falsely elevated levels may occur with the presence of an intrauterine device.
- Lipemic samples that are turbid in appearance may be rejected for analysis when nephelometry is the test method.

NURSING IMPLICATIONS AND PROCEDURE

PRETEST:
- Positively identify the patient using at least two unique identifiers before providing care, treatment, or services.

- *Patient Teaching:* Inform the patient this test can assist in assessing for inflammation.
- Obtain a history of the patient's complaints, including a list of known allergens, especially allergies or sensitivities to latex. The patient may complain of pain related to the inflammatory process in connective or other tissues.
- Obtain a history of the patient's cardiovascular and immune systems, symptoms, and results of previously performed laboratory tests and diagnostic and surgical procedures.
- Obtain a list of the patient's current medications, including herbs, nutritional supplements, and nutraceuticals (see Appendix F).
- Review the procedure with the patient. Inform the patient that specimen collection takes approximately 5 to 10 min. Address concerns about pain and explain that there may be some discomfort during the venipuncture.
- *Sensitivity to social and cultural issues,* as well as concern for modesty, is important in providing psychological support before, during, and after the procedure.
- There are no food, fluid, or medication restrictions unless by medical direction.

INTRATEST:
- If the patient has a history of allergic reaction to latex, avoid the use of equipment containing latex.
- Instruct the patient to cooperate fully and to follow directions. Direct the patient to breathe normally and to avoid unnecessary movement.
- Observe standard precautions, and follow the general guidelines in Appendix A. Positively identify the patient, and label the appropriate tubes with the corresponding patient demographics, date, and time of collection. Perform a venipuncture.
- Remove the needle and apply direct pressure with dry gauze to stop bleeding. Observe/assess venipuncture site for bleeding or hematoma formation and secure gauze with adhesive bandage.

C

▶ Promptly transport the specimen to the laboratory for processing and analysis.

POST-TEST:

▶ A report of the results will be sent to the requesting health-care provider (HCP), who will discuss the results with the patient.

▶ Reinforce information given by the patient's HCP regarding further testing, treatment, or referral to another HCP. Answer any questions or address any concerns voiced by the patient or family.

▶ Depending on the results of this procedure, additional testing may be performed to evaluate or monitor progression of the disease process and determine the need for a change in therapy. Evaluate test results in relation to the patient's symptoms and other tests performed.

RELATED MONOGRAPHS:

▶ Related tests include antiarrhythmic drugs, antibodies anticyclic citrullinated peptide, ANA, apolipoprotein A and B, AST, arthroscopy, ANP, blood gases, BMD, bone scan, BNP, calcium (blood and ionized), cholesterol (total, HDL, and LDL), CBC, CBC WBC count and differential, CRP, CT, cardiac scoring, CK and isoenzymes, echocardiography, ESR, glucose, glycated hemoglobin, Holter monitor, homocysteine, ketones, LDH and isoenzymes, MRI chest, MRI musculoskeletal, MI scan, myocardial perfusion scan, myoglobin, PET heart, potassium, radiography bone, RF, synovial fluid analysis, triglycerides, and troponin.

▶ Refer to the Cardiovascular and Immune systems tables at the end of the book for related tests by body system.

Creatine Kinase and Isoenzymes

SYNONYM/ACRONYM: CK and isoenzymes.

COMMON USE: To monitor myocardial infarction and some disorders of the musculoskeletal system such as Duchenne's muscular dystrophy.

SPECIMEN: Serum (1 mL) collected in a red- or tiger-top tube. Serial specimens are highly recommended. Care must be taken to use the same type of collection container if serial measurements are to be taken.

REFERENCE VALUE: (Method: Enzymatic for CK, electrophoresis for isoenzymes; enzyme immunoassay techniques are in common use for CK-MB)

	Conventional & SI Units
Total CK	
Newborn–1 yr	2 × adult values
Male (children and adults)	50–204 units/L
Female (children and adults)	36–160 units/L

	Conventional & SI Units
CK Isoenzymes by Electrophoresis	
CK-BB	Absent
CK-MB	Less than 4–6%
CK-MM	94–96%
CK-MB by Immunoassay	0–3 ng/mL
CK-MB Index	0–2.5

CK = creatine kinase; CK-BB = CK isoenzyme in brain; CK-MB = CK isoenzyme in heart; CK-MM = CK isoenzyme in skeletal muscle. The CK-MB index is the CK-MB (by immunoassay) divided by the total CK and then multiplied by 100. For example, a CK-MB by immunoassay of 25 ng/mL with a total CK of 250 units/L would have a CK-MB index of 10. Elevations in total CK occur after exercise. Values in older adults may decline slightly related to loss of muscle mass.

DESCRIPTION: Creatine kinase (CK) is an enzyme that exists almost exclusively in skeletal muscle, heart muscle, and, in smaller amounts, in the brain and lungs. This enzyme is important in intracellular storage and energy release. Three isoenzymes, based on primary location, have been identified by electrophoresis: brain and lungs CK-BB, cardiac CK-MB, and skeletal muscle CK-MM. When injury to these tissues occurs, the enzymes are released into the bloodstream. Levels increase and decrease in a predictable time frame. Measuring the serum levels can help determine the extent and timing of the damage. Noting the presence of the specific isoenzyme helps determine the location of the tissue damage. Atypical forms of CK can be identified. Macro-CK, an immunoglobulin complex of normal CK isoenzymes, has no clinical significance. Mitochondrial-CK is sometimes identified in the sera of seriously ill patients, especially those with metastatic carcinoma.

Acute myocardial infarction (MI) releases CK into the serum within the first 48 hr; values return to normal in about 3 days. The isoenzyme CK-MB appears in the first 4 to 6 hr, peaks in 24 hr, and usually returns to normal in 72 hr. Recurrent elevation of CK suggests reinfarction or extension of ischemic damage. Significant elevations of CK are expected in early phases of muscular dystrophy, even before the clinical signs and symptoms appear. CK elevation diminishes as the disease progresses and muscle mass decreases. Differences in total CK with age and gender relate to the fact that the predominant isoenzyme is muscular in origin. Body builders have higher values, whereas older individuals have lower values because of deterioration of muscle mass.

Serial use of the mass assay for CK-MB with serial cardiac troponin I, myoglobin, and serial electrocardiograms in the assessment of MI has largely replaced the use of CK isoenzyme assay by electrophoresis. CK-MB mass assays are more sensitive and rapid than electrophoresis. Studies have demonstrated a high positive predictive value for acute MI when the CK-MB (by immunoassay) is greater than 10 ng/mL with a relative CK-MB index greater than 3.0.

Timing for Appearance and Resolution of Serum/Plasma Cardiac Markers in Acute MI

Cardiac Marker	Appearance (hr)	Peak (hr)	Resolution (days)
AST	6–8	24–48	3–4
CK (total)	4–6	24	2–3
CK-MB	4–6	15–20	2–3
LDH	12	24–48	10–14
Myoglobin	1–3	4–12	1
Troponin I	2–6	15–20	5–7

INDICATIONS

- Assist in the diagnosis of acute MI and evaluate cardiac ischemia (CK-MB)
- Detect musculoskeletal disorders that do not have a neurological basis, such as dermatomyositis or Duchenne's muscular dystrophy (CK-MM)
- Determine the success of coronary artery reperfusion after streptokinase infusion or percutaneous transluminal angioplasty, as evidenced by a decrease in CK-MB

POTENTIAL DIAGNOSIS

Increased in

CK is released from any damaged cell in which it is stored, so conditions that affect the brain, heart, or skeletal muscle and cause cellular destruction demonstrate elevated CK levels and correlating isoenzyme source CK-BB, CK-MB, CK-MM.

- Alcoholism *(CK-MM)*
- Brain infarction (extensive) *(CK-BB)*
- Congestive heart failure *(CK-MB)*
- Delirium tremens *(CK-MM)*
- Dermatomyositis *(CK-MM)*
- Head injury *(CK-BB)*
- Hypothyroidism *(CK-MM related to metabolic effect on and damage to skeletal muscle tissue)*

- Hypoxic shock *(CK-MM related to muscle damage from lack of oxygen)*
- Gastrointestinal (GI) tract infarction *(CK-MM)*
- Loss of blood supply to any muscle *(CK-MM)*
- Malignant hyperthermia *(CK-MM related to skeletal muscle injury)*
- MI *(CK-MB)*
- Muscular dystrophies *(CK-MM)*
- Myocarditis *(CK-MB)*
- Neoplasms of the prostate, bladder, and GI tract *(CK-MM)*
- Polymyositis *(CK-MM)*
- Pregnancy; during labor *(CK-MM)*
- Prolonged hypothermia *(CK-MM)*
- Pulmonary edema *(CK-MM)*
- Pulmonary embolism *(CK-MM)*
- Reye's syndrome *(CK-BB)*
- Rhabdomyolysis *(CK-MM)*
- Surgery *(CK-MM)*
- Tachycardia *(CK-MB)*
- Tetanus *(CK-MM related to muscle injury from injection)*
- Trauma *(CK-MM)*

Decreased in
- Small stature *(related to lower muscle mass than average stature)*
- Sedentary lifestyle *(related to decreased muscle mass)*

CRITICAL FINDINGS: N/A

INTERFERING FACTORS

- Drugs that may increase total CK levels include any intramuscularly injected preparations because of tissue trauma caused by injection.
- Drugs that may decrease total CK levels include dantrolene and statins.

NURSING IMPLICATIONS AND PROCEDURE

PRETEST:

▶ Positively identify the patient using at least two unique identifiers before providing care, treatment, or services.

▶ *Patient Teaching:* Inform the patient this test can assist in assessing for heart muscle cell damage.

▶ Obtain a history of the patient's complaints, including a list of known allergens, especially allergies or sensitivities to latex.

▶ Obtain a history of the patient's cardiovascular and musculoskeletal systems, symptoms, and results of previously performed laboratory tests and diagnostic and surgical procedures.

▶ Obtain a list of the patient's current medications, including herbs, nutritional supplements, and nutraceuticals (see Appendix F).

▶ Review the procedure with the patient. Inform the patient that a series of samples will be required. (Samples at time of admission and 2 to 4 hr, 6 to 8 hr, and 12 hr after admission are the minimal recommendations. Protocols may vary among facilities. Additional samples may be requested.) Inform the patient that specimen collection takes approximately 5 to 10 min. Address concerns about pain and explain that there may be some discomfort during the venipuncture.

▶ There are no food, fluid, or medication restrictions unless by medical direction.

INTRATEST:

▶ If the patient has a history of allergic reaction to latex, avoid the use of equipment containing latex.

▶ Instruct the patient to cooperate fully and to follow directions. Direct the patient to breathe normally and to avoid unnecessary movement.

▶ Observe standard precautions, and follow the general guidelines in Appendix A. Positively identify the patient, and label the appropriate tubes with the corresponding patient demographics, date, and time of collection. Perform a venipuncture.

▶ Remove the needle and apply direct pressure with dry gauze to stop bleeding. Observe/assess venipuncture site for bleeding or hematoma formation and secure gauze with adhesive bandage.

▶ Promptly transport the specimen to the laboratory for processing and analysis.

POST-TEST:

▶ A report of the results will be sent to the requesting health-care provider (HCP), who will discuss the results with the patient.

▶ *Nutritional Considerations:* Increased CK levels may be associated with coronary artery disease (CAD). The American Heart Association and National Heart, Lung, and Blood Institute (NHBLI) recommend nutritional therapy for individuals identified to be at high risk for developing CAD or individuals who have specific risk factors and/or existing medical conditions (e.g., elevated ILDL cholesterol levels, other lipid disorders, insulin-dependent diabetes, insulin resistance, or metabolic syndrome). If overweight, the patient should be encouraged to achieve a normal weight. The NHLBI's National Cholesterol Education Program (NCEP) revised its dietary guidelines for reducing CAD in 2001. Guidelines for the Therapeutic Lifestyle Changes (TLC) diet are outlined in the Third

Report of the Expert Panel on Detection, Evaluation, and Treatment of High Blood Cholesterol in Adults (Adult Treatment Panel III [ATP III]). The TLC diet emphasizes a reduction in foods high in saturated fats and cholesterol. Red meats, eggs, and dairy products are the major sources of saturated fats and cholesterol. If triglycerides also are elevated, the patient should be advised to eliminate or reduce alcohol and simple carbohydrates from the diet. The TLC approach also includes the use of plant stanols or sterols and increased dissolved fiber as an option for lowering LDL cholesterol levels; nutritional recommendations for daily total caloric intake; recommendations for allowable percentage of calories derived from fat (saturated and unsaturated), carbohydrates, protein, and cholesterol; as well as recommendations for daily expenditure of energy.

▶ *Nutritional Considerations:* Overweight patients with high blood pressure should be encouraged to achieve a normal weight. Other changeable risk factors warranting patient education include strategies to safely decrease sodium intake, increase physical activity, decrease alcohol consumption, eliminate tobacco use, and decrease cholesterol levels.

▶ *Social and Cultural Considerations:* Numerous studies point to the prevalence of excess body weight in American children and adolescents. Experts estimate that obesity is present in 25% of the population ages 6 to 11 yr. The medical, social, and emotional consequences of excess body weight are significant. Special attention should be given to instructing the child and caregiver regarding health risks and weight-control education.

▶ Recognize anxiety related to test results, and be supportive of fear of shortened life expectancy. Discuss the implications of abnormal test results on the patient's lifestyle. Provide teaching and information regarding the clinical implications of the test results, as appropriate. Educate the patient regarding access to counseling services. Provide contact information, if desired, for the American Heart Association (www.americanheart.org), or the NHLBI (www.nhlbi.nih.gov).

▶ Reinforce information given by the patient's HCP regarding further testing, treatment, or referral to another HCP. Answer any questions or address any concerns voiced by the patient or family.

▶ Depending on the results of this procedure, additional testing may be performed to evaluate or monitor progression of the disease process and determine the need for a change in therapy. Evaluate test results in relation to the patient's symptoms and other tests performed.

RELATED MONOGRAPHS:

▶ Related tests include antiarrhythmic drugs, apolipoprotein A and B, AST, ANP, blood gases, BNP, calcium (blood and ionized), cholesterol (total, HDL and LDL), CRP, CT cardiac scoring, echocardiography, glucose, glycated hemoglobin, Holter monitor, homocysteine, ketones, LDH and isoenzymes, lipoprotein electrophoresis, magnesium, MRI chest, MI scan, myocardial perfusion scan, myoglobin, pericardial fluid, PET heart, potassium, triglycerides, and troponin.

▶ Refer to the Cardiovascular and Musculoskeletal systems tables at the end of the book for related tests by body system.

Creatinine, Blood

SYNONYM/ACRONYM: N/A.

COMMON USE: To assess kidney function found in acute and chronic renal failure, related to drug reaction and disease such as diabetes.

SPECIMEN: Serum (1 mL) collected in a red- or tiger-top tube. Plasma (1 mL) collected in a green-top (heparin) tube is also acceptable.

REFERENCE VALUE: (Method: Spectrophotometry)

Age	Conventional Units	SI Units (Conventional Units × 88.4)
Newborn	0.3–1.2 mg/dL	27–106 micromol/L
Infant	0.2–0.4 mg/dL	18–35 micromol/L
1–5 yr	0.3–0.5 mg/dL	27–44 micromol/L
6–10 yr	0.5–0.8 mg/dL	44–71 micromol/L
Adult male	0.6–1.2 mg/dL	53–106 micromol/L
Adult female	0.5–1.1 mg/dL	44–97 micromol/L

Values in older adults may decline slightly related to loss of muscle mass. National Kidney Foundation recommends the use of two decimal places in reporting serum creatinine for use in calculating estimated glomerular filtration rate.

DESCRIPTION: Creatinine is the end product of creatine metabolism. Creatine resides almost exclusively in skeletal muscle, where it participates in energy-requiring metabolic reactions. In these processes, a small amount of creatine is irreversibly converted to creatinine, which then circulates to the kidneys and is excreted. The amount of creatinine generated in an individual is proportional to the mass of skeletal muscle present and remains fairly constant unless there is massive muscle damage resulting from crushing injury or degenerative muscle disease. Creatinine values also decrease with age owing to diminishing muscle mass. Blood urea nitrogen (BUN) is often ordered with creatinine for comparison. The BUN/creatinine ratio is also a useful indicator of disease. The ratio should be between 10:1 and 20:1. Creatinine is the ideal substance for determining renal clearance because a fairly constant quantity is produced within the body. The creatinine clearance test measures a blood sample and a urine sample to determine the rate at which the kidneys are clearing creatinine from the blood; this reflects the glomerular filtration rate, or GFR (see monograph titled "Creatinine, Urine, and Creatinine Clearance, Urine").

Chronic kidney disease (CKD) is a significant health concern worldwide. An international effort to standardize methods to identify and monitor CKD has been undertaken by the National

Kidney Disease Education Program (NKDEP), the International Confederation of Clinical Chemistry and Laboratory Medicine, and the European Communities Confederation of Clinical Chemistry. International efforts have resulted in development of an isotope dilution mass spectrometry (IDMS) reference method for standardized measurement of creatinine. The National Kidney Foundation (NKF) has recommended use of an equation to estimate glomerular filtration rate (eGFR). The equation is based on factors identified in the NKF Modification of Diet in Renal Disease (MDRD) study. The equation includes four factors: serum or plasma creatinine value, age (in years), gender, and race. The equation is valid only for patients between the ages of 18 and 70. A correction factor is incorporated in the equation if the patient is African American because CKD is more prevalent in African Americans; results are approximately 20% higher. It is very important to know whether the creatinine has been measured using an IDMS traceable test method because the values will differ; results are lower. The equations have not been validated for pregnant women (GFR is significantly increased in pregnancy); patients younger than 18 or older than 70; patients with serious comorbidities; or patients with extremes in body size, muscle mass, or nutritional status. eGFR calculators can be found at the National Kidney Disease Education Program (www.nkdep.nih.gov/professionals/gfr_calculators/index.htm).

The equation used for creatinine methods that are *not* traceable to IDMS reference method is:

- **If creatinine is reported in mg/L:**

$$[eGFR \text{ (mL/min/1.73 m}^2) = 186 \times (\text{creat})^{-1.154} \times (\text{Age})^{-0.203} \times (0.742 \text{ if female}) \times (1.210 \text{ if African American})]$$

- **If creatinine is reported in (SI) micromol/L:**

$$[eGFR \text{ (mL/min/1.73 m}^2) = 186 \times (\text{creat}/88.4)^{-1.154} \times (\text{Age})^{-0.203} \times (0.742 \text{ if female}) \times (1.210 \text{ if African American})]$$

The equation used for creatinine methods that *are* traceable to IDMS reference method is:

- **If creatinine is reported in mg/dL:**

$$[eGFR \text{ (mL/min/1.73 m}^2) = 175 \times (\text{creat})^{-1.154} \times (\text{Age})^{-0.203} \times (0.742 \text{ if female}) \times (1.210 \text{ if African American})]$$

- **If creatinine is reported in (SI) micromol/L:**

$$[eGFR \text{ (mL/min/1.73 m}^2) = 175 \times (\text{creat}/88.4)^{-1.154} \times (\text{Age})^{-0.203} \times (0.742 \text{ if female}) \times (1.210 \text{ if African American})]$$

- **Creatinine clearance can be estimated from a blood creatinine level:**

Creatinine clearance = $[1.2 \times (140 - \text{age in years}) \times (\text{weight in kg})]/\text{blood creatinine level}$.

The result is multiplied by 0.85 if the patient is female; the result is multiplied by 1.18 if the patient is African American.

INDICATIONS
- Assess a known or suspected disorder involving muscles in the absence of renal disease
- Evaluate known or suspected impairment of renal function

POTENTIAL DIAGNOSIS

Increased in
- Acromegaly *(related to increased muscle mass)*
- Congestive heart failure *(related to decreased renal blood flow)*
- Dehydration *(related to hemoconcentration)*
- Gigantism *(related to increased muscle mass)*
- Poliomyelitis *(related to increased release from damaged muscle)*
- Renal calculi *(related to decreased renal excretion due to obstruction)*
- Renal disease, acute and chronic renal failure *(related to decreased urinary excretion)*
- Rhabdomyolysis *(related to increased release from damaged muscle)*
- Shock *(related to increased release from damaged muscle)*

Decreased in
- Decreased muscle mass *(related to debilitating disease or increasing age)*
- Hyperthyroidism *(related to increased GFR)*
- Inadequate protein intake *(related to decreased muscle mass)*
- Liver disease (severe) *(related to fluid retention)*
- Muscular dystrophy *(related to decreased muscle mass)*

- Pregnancy *(related to increased GFR and renal clearance)*
- Small stature *(related to decreased muscle mass)*

CRITICAL FINDINGS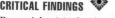
Potential critical value is greater than 7.4 mg/dL (nondialysis patient).

Note and immediately report to the health-care provider (HCP) any critically increased values and related symptoms.

Chronic renal insufficiency is identified by creatinine levels between 1.5 and 3.0 mg/dL; chronic renal failure is present at levels greater than 3.0 mg/dL.

Possible interventions may include renal or peritoneal dialysis and organ transplant, but early discovery of the cause of elevated creatinine levels might avoid such drastic interventions.

INTERFERING FACTORS
- Drugs and substances that may increase creatinine levels include acebutolol, acetaminophen (overdose), acetylsalicylic acid, aldatense, amikacin, amiodarone, amphotericin B, arginine, arsenicals, ascorbic acid, asparaginase, barbiturates, capreomycin, captopril, carbutamide, carvedilol, cephalothin, chlorthalidone, cimetidine, cisplatin, clofibrate, colistin, corn oil (Lipomul), cyclosporine, dextran, doxycycline, enalapril, ethylene glycol, gentamicin, indomethacin, ipodate, kanamycin, levodopa, mannitol, methicillin, methoxyflurane, mitomycin, neomycin, netilmicin, nitrofurantoin, NSAIDs, oxyphenbutazone, paromomycin, penicillin, pentamidine, phosphorus, plicamycin, radiographic agents, semustine, streptokinase, streptozocin, tetracycline, thiazides, tobramycin, triamterene, vancomycin, vasopressin, viomycin, and vitamin D.

C

- Drugs that may decrease creatinine levels include citrates, dopamine, ibuprofen, and lisinopril.
- High blood levels of bilirubin and glucose can cause false decreases in creatinine.
- A diet high in meat can cause increased creatinine levels.
- Ketosis can cause a significant increase in creatinine.
- Hemolyzed specimens are unsuitable for analysis.

NURSING IMPLICATIONS AND PROCEDURE

PRETEST:

- Positively identify the patient using at least two unique identifiers before providing care, treatment, or services.
- *Patient Teaching:* Inform the patient this test can assist in assessing kidney function.
- Obtain a history of the patient's complaints, including a list of known allergens, especially allergies or sensitivities to latex.
- Obtain a history of the patient's genitourinary and musculoskeletal systems, symptoms, and results of previously performed laboratory tests and diagnostic and surgical procedures.
- Obtain a list of the patient's current medications, including herbs, nutritional supplements, and nutraceuticals (see Appendix F).
- Review the procedure with the patient. Inform the patient that specimen collection takes approximately 5 to 10 min. Address concerns about pain and explain that there may be some discomfort during the venipuncture.
- *Sensitivity to social and cultural issues,* as well as concern for modesty, is important in providing psychological support before, during, and after the procedure.
- There are no food, fluid, or medication restrictions unless by medical direction.
- Instruct the patient to refrain from excessive exercise for 8 hr before the test.

INTRATEST:

- Ensure that the patient has complied with activity restrictions; assure that

activity has been restricted for at least 8 hr prior to the procedure.
- If the patient has a history of allergic reaction to latex, avoid the use of equipment containing latex.
- Instruct the patient to cooperate fully and to follow directions. Direct the patient to breathe normally and to avoid unnecessary movement.
- Observe standard precautions, and follow the general guidelines in Appendix A. Positively identify the patient, and label the appropriate tubes with the corresponding patient demographics, date, and time of collection. Perform a venipuncture.
- Remove the needle and apply direct pressure with dry gauze to stop bleeding. Observe/assess venipuncture site for bleeding or hematoma formation and secure gauze with adhesive bandage.
- Promptly transport the specimen to the laboratory for processing and analysis.

POST-TEST:

- A report of the results will be sent to the requesting HCP, who will discuss the results with the patient.
- Instruct the patient to resume usual activity as directed by the HCP.
- *Nutritional Considerations:* Increased creatinine levels may be associated with kidney disease. The nutritional needs of patients with kidney disease vary widely and are in constant flux. Anorexia, nausea, and vomiting commonly occur, prompting the need for continuous nutritional monitoring for malnutrition, especially among patients receiving long-term hemodialysis therapy.
- Recognize anxiety related to test results and be supportive of impaired activity related to fear of shortened life expectancy. Discuss the implications of abnormal test results on the patient's lifestyle. Provide teaching and information regarding the clinical implications of the test results, as appropriate. Educate the patient regarding access to counseling services. Help the patient to cope with long-term implications. Recognize that anticipatory anxiety and grief related to potential lifestyle changes may be expressed when someone is faced with a chronic disorder.

Provide contact information, if desired, for the National Kidney Foundation (www.kidney.org) or the National Kidney Disease Education Program (www.nkdep.nih.gov).
▶ Reinforce information given by the patient's HCP regarding further testing, treatment, or referral to another HCP. Answer any questions or address any concerns voiced by the patient or family.
▶ Depending on the results of this procedure, additional testing may be performed to evaluate or monitor progression of the disease process and determine the need for a change in therapy. Evaluate test results in relation to the patient's symptoms and other tests performed.

RELATED MONOGRAPHS:

▶ Related tests include anion gap, antibiotic drugs, ANF, BNP, biopsy muscle, blood gases, BUN, calcium, calculus kidney stone panel, CT abdomen, CT renal, CK and isoenzymes, creatinine clearance, cystoscopy, echocardiography, echocardiography transesophageal, electrolytes, EMG, ENG, glucagon, glucose, glycolated hemoglobin, insulin, IVP, KUB studies, lung perfusion scan, microalbumin, osmolality, phosphorus, renogram, retrograde ureteropyelography, TSH, thyroxine, uric acid, and UA.
▶ Refer to the Genitourinary and Musculoskeletal systems tables at the end of the book for related tests by body system.

Creatinine, Urine, and Creatinine Clearance, Urine

SYNONYM/ACRONYM: N/A.

COMMON USE: To assess and monitor kidney function related to acute or chronic nephritis.

SPECIMEN: Urine (5 mL) from an unpreserved random or timed specimen collected in a clean plastic collection container.

REFERENCE VALUE: (Method: Spectrophotometry)

Age	Conventional Units	SI Units
		Urine Creatinine (Conventional Units × 8.84)
2–3 yr	6–22 mg/kg/24 hr	53–194 micromol/kg/24 hr
4–18 yr	12–30 mg/kg/24 hr	106–265 micromol/kg/24 hr
Adult male	14–26 mg/kg/24 hr	124–230 micromol/kg/24 hr
Adult female	11–20 mg/kg/24 hr	97–177 micromol/kg/24 hr
		Creatinine Clearance (Conventional Units × 0.0167)
Children	70–140 mL/min/1.73 m^2	1.17–2.33 mL/s/1.73 m^2
Adult male	85–125 mL/min/1.73 m^2	1.42–2.08 mL/s/1.73 m^2
Adult female	75–115 mL/min/1.73 m^2	1.25–1.92 mL/s/1.73 m^2
For each decade after 40 yr	Decrease of 6–7 mL/min/1.73 m^2	Decrease of 0.06–0.07 mL/s/1.73 m^2

DESCRIPTION: Creatinine is the end product of creatine metabolism. Creatine resides almost exclusively in skeletal muscle, where it participates in energy-requiring metabolic reactions. In these processes, a small amount of creatine is irreversibly converted to creatinine, which then circulates to the kidneys and is excreted. The amount of creatinine generated in an individual is proportional to the mass of skeletal muscle present and remains fairly constant, unless there is massive muscle damage resulting from crushing injury or degenerative muscle disease. Creatinine values decrease with advancing age owing to diminishing muscle mass. Although the measurement of urine creatinine is an effective indicator of renal function, the creatinine clearance test is more precise. The creatinine clearance test measures a blood sample and a urine sample to determine the rate at which the kidneys are clearing creatinine from the blood; this reflects the glomerular filtration rate (GFR) and is based on an estimate of body surface.

Chronic kidney disease (CKD) is a significant health concern worldwide. An international effort to standardize methods to identify and monitor CKD has been undertaken by the National Kidney Disease Education Program (NKDEP), the International Confederation of Clinical Chemistry and Laboratory Medicine, and the European Communities Confederation of Clinical Chemistry. International efforts have resulted in development of an isotope dilution mass spectrometry (IDMS) reference method for standardized measurement of creatinine. The National Kidney Foundation (NKF) has recommended use of an equation to estimate glomerular filtration rate (eGFR). The equation is based on factors identified in the NKF Modification of Diet in Renal Disease (MDRD) study. The equation includes four factors: serum or plasma creatinine value, age in years, gender, and race. The equation is valid only for patients between the ages of 18 and 70. A correction factor is incorporated in the equation if the patient is African American because CKD is more prevalent in African Americans; results are approximately 20% higher. It is very important to know whether the creatinine has been measured using an IDMS traceable test method because the values will differ; results are lower. The equations have not been validated for pregnant women (GFR is significantly increased in pregnancy); patients younger than 18 or older than 70; patients with serious comorbidities; or patients with extremes in body size, muscle mass, or nutritional status. eGFR calculators can be found at the NKDEP (www.nkdep.nih.gov/professionals/gfr_calculators/index.htm).

The equation used for creatinine methods that are *not* traceable to IDMS reference method is:

- **If creatinine is reported in mg/dL:**

$$\text{eGFR (mL/min/1.73 m}^2) = 186 \times (\text{creat})^{-1.154} \times (\text{Age})^{-0.203} \times (0.742 \text{ if female}) \times (1.210 \text{ if African American})$$

- **If creatinine is reported in (SI) micromol/L:**

$$[eGFR\ (mL/min/1.73\ m^2) = 186 \times (creat/88.4)^{-1.154} \times (Age)^{-0.203} \times (0.742\ \text{if female}) \times (1.210\ \text{if African American})]$$

The equation used for creatinine methods that *are* traceable to IDMS reference method is:

- **If creatinine is reported in mg/dL:**

$$[eGFR\ (mL/min/1.73\ m^2) = 175 \times (creat)^{-1.154} \times (Age)^{-0.203} \times (0.742\ \text{if female}) \times (1.210\ \text{if African American})]$$

- **If creatinine is reported in (SI) micromol/L:**

$$[eGFR\ (mL/min/1.73\ m^2) = 175 \times (creat/88.4)^{-1.154} \times (Age)^{-0.203} \times (0.742\ \text{if female}) \times (1.210\ \text{if African American})]$$

- **Creatinine clearance can be estimated from a blood creatinine level:**

$$\text{Creatinine clearance} = [1.2 \times (140 - \text{age in years}) \times (\text{weight in kg})]/\text{blood creatinine level.}$$

The result is multiplied by 0.85 if the patient is female; the result is multiplied by 1.18 if the patient is African American.

INDICATIONS

- Determine the extent of nephron damage in known renal disease (at least 50% of functioning nephrons must be lost before values are decreased)
- Determine renal function before administering nephrotoxic drugs
- Evaluate accuracy of a 24-hr urine collection based on the constant level of creatinine excretion
- Evaluate glomerular function
- Monitor effectiveness of treatment in renal disease

POTENTIAL DIAGNOSIS

Increased in
- Acromegaly *(related to increased muscle mass)*
- Carnivorous diets *(related to increased intake of creatine, which is metabolized to creatinine and excreted by the kidneys)*
- Exercise *(related to muscle damage; increased renal blood flow)*
- Gigantism *(related to increased muscle mass)*

Decreased in
Conditions that decrease GFR, impair kidney function, or reduce renal blood flow will decrease renal excretion of creatinine
- Acute or chronic glomerulonephritis
- Chronic bilateral pyelonephritis
- Leukemia
- Muscle wasting diseases *(related to abnormal creatinine production; decreased production reflected in decreased excretion)*
- Paralysis *(related to abnormal creatinine production; decreased production reflected in decreased excretion)*
- Polycystic kidney disease
- Shock
- Urinary tract obstruction (e.g., from calculi)
- Vegetarian diets *(evidenced by diets that exclude intake of animal muscle, the creatine source metabolized to creatinine and excreted by the kidneys)*

CRITICAL FINDINGS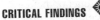

- Degree of impairment:
  Borderline: 62.5–80 mL/min/1.73 m^2
  Slight: 52–62.5 mL/min/1.73 m^2
  Mild: 42–52 mL/min/1.73 m^2
  Moderate: 28–42 mL/min/1.73 m^2
  Marked: Less than 28 mL/min/1.73 m^2

Note and immediately report to the health-care provider (HCP) any critically increased values and related symptoms.

INTERFERING FACTORS

- Drugs that may increase urine creatinine levels include ascorbic acid, cefoxitin, cephalothin, corticosteroids, fluoxymesterone, levodopa, methandrostenolone, methotrexate, methyldopa, nitrofurans (including nitrofurazone), oxymetholone, phenolphthalein, and prednisone.
- Drugs that may increase urine creatinine clearance include enalapril, oral contraceptives, prednisone, and ramipril.
- Drugs that may decrease urine creatinine levels include anabolic steroids, androgens, captopril, and thiazides.
- Drugs that may decrease the urine creatinine clearance include acetylsalicylic acid, amphotericin B, carbenoxolone, chlorthalidone, cimetidine, cisplatin, cyclosporine, guancidine, ibuprofen, indomethacin, mitomycin, oxyphenbutazone, probenecid (coadministered with digoxin), puromycin, and thiazides.
- Excessive ketones in urine may cause falsely decreased values.
- Failure to follow proper technique in collecting 24-hr specimen may invalidate test results.
- Failure to refrigerate specimen throughout urine collection period allows decomposition of creatinine, causing falsely decreased values.
- Consumption of large amounts of meat, excessive exercise, and stress should be avoided for 24 hr before the test. Protocols may vary among facilities.
- Failure to follow dietary restrictions before the procedure may cause the procedure to be canceled or repeated.

NURSING IMPLICATIONS AND PROCEDURE

PRETEST:

- Positively identify the patient using at least two unique identifiers before providing care, treatment, or services.
- *Patient Teaching:* Inform the patient this test can assist in assessing kidney function.
- Obtain a history of the patient's complaints, including a list of known allergens, especially allergies or sensitivities to latex.
- Obtain a history of the patient's genitourinary system, symptoms, and results of previously performed laboratory tests and diagnostic and surgical procedures.
- Obtain a list of the patient's current medications, including herbs, nutritional supplements, and nutraceuticals (see Appendix F).
- Review the procedure with the patient. Provide a nonmetallic urinal, bedpan, or toilet-mounted collection device. Address concerns about pain and explain to the patient that there should be no discomfort during the urine collection procedure. Inform the patient that a blood sample for creatinine will be required on the day urine collection begins or at some point during the 24 hr collection period (see monograph titled "Creatinine, Blood" for additional information).
- *Sensitivity to social and cultural issues,* as well as concern for modesty, is important in providing psychological support before, during, and after the procedure.
- Usually a 24-hr time frame for urine collection is ordered. Inform the patient that all urine must be saved during that 24-hr period. Instruct the patient not to void directly into the laboratory

collection container. Instruct the patient to avoid defecating in the collection device and to keep toilet tissue out of the collection device to prevent contamination of the specimen. Place a sign in the bathroom to remind the patient to save all urine.

▶ Instruct the patient to void all urine into the collection device and then to pour the urine into the laboratory collection container. Alternatively, the specimen can be left in the collection device for a health-care staff member to add to the laboratory collection container.

▶ There are no fluid or medication restrictions unless by medical direction.

▶ Instruct the patient to refrain from eating meat during the test. Protocols may vary among facilities.

INTRATEST:

▶ Ensure that the patient has complied with dietary and activity restrictions for 24 hr prior to the procedure; assure that ingestion of meat has been restricted during the test.

▶ If the patient has a history of allergic reaction to latex, avoid the use of equipment containing latex.

▶ Instruct the patient to cooperate fully and to follow directions.

▶ Observe standard precautions, and follow the general guidelines in Appendix A. Positively identify the patient, and label the appropriate collection container with the corresponding patient demographics, date, and time of collection.

Random Specimen (collect in early morning) Clean-Catch Specimen

▶ Instruct the male patient to (1) thoroughly wash his hands, (2) cleanse the meatus, (3) void a small amount into the toilet, and (4) void directly into the specimen container.

▶ Instruct the female patient to (1) thoroughly wash her hands; (2) cleanse the labia from front to back; (3) while keeping the labia separated, void a small amount into the toilet; and (4) without interrupting the urine stream, void directly into the specimen container.

Pediatric Urine Collector

▶ Put on gloves. Appropriately cleanse the genital area and allow the area to dry. Remove the covering over the adhesive strips on the collector bag and apply over the genital area. Diaper the child. When specimen is obtained, place the entire collection bag in a sterile urine container.

Indwelling Catheter

▶ Put on gloves. Empty drainage tube of urine. It may be necessary to clamp off the catheter for 15 to 30 min before specimen collection. Cleanse specimen port with antiseptic swab, and then aspirate 5 mL of urine with a 21- to 25-gauge needle and syringe. Transfer urine to a sterile container.

Urinary Catheterization

▶ Place female patient in lithotomy position or male patient in supine position. Using sterile technique, open the straight urinary catheterization kit and perform urinary catheterization. Place the retained urine in a sterile specimen container.

Suprapubic Aspiration

▶ Place the patient in a supine position. Cleanse the area with antiseptic and drape with sterile drapes. A needle is inserted through the skin into the bladder. A syringe attached to the needle is used to aspirate the urine sample. The needle is then removed and a sterile dressing is applied to the site. Place the sterile sample in a sterile specimen container.

▶ Do not collect urine from the pouch from the patient with a urinary diversion (e.g., ileal conduit). Instead, perform catheterization through the stoma.

Timed Specimen

▶ Obtain a clean 3-L urine specimen container, toilet-mounted collection device, and plastic bag (for transport of the specimen container). The specimen must be refrigerated or kept on ice throughout the entire collection period. If an indwelling urinary catheter is in place, the drainage bag must be kept on ice.

▶ Begin the test between 6 and 8 a.m. if possible. Collect first voiding and

C

discard. Record the time the specimen was discarded as the beginning of the timed collection period. The next morning, ask the patient to void at the same time the collection was started and add this last voiding to the container. Urinary output should be recorded throughout the collection time.

▶ If an indwelling catheter is in place, replace the tubing and container system at the start of the collection time. Keep the container system on ice during the collection period, or empty the urine into a larger container periodically during the collection period; monitor to ensure continued drainage, and conclude the test the next morning at the same time the collection was begun.

▶ At the conclusion of the test, compare the quantity of urine with the urinary output record for the collection; if the specimen contains less than what was recorded as output, some urine may have been discarded, invalidating the test.

▶ Include on the collection container's label the amount of urine, test start and stop times, and any foods or medications that can affect test results.

▶ Promptly transport the specimen to the laboratory for processing and analysis.

POST-TEST:

▶ A report of the results will be sent to the requesting HCP, who will discuss the results with the patient.

▶ Instruct the patient to resume usual diet, medications, and activity, as directed by the HCP.

▶ Recognize anxiety related to test results and be supportive of impaired activity related to fear of shortened life expectancy. Discuss the implications of abnormal test results on the patient's lifestyle. Provide teaching

and information regarding the clinical implications of the test results, as appropriate. Educate the patient regarding access to counseling services. Help the patient to cope with long-term implications. Recognize that anticipatory anxiety and grief related to potential lifestyle changes may be expressed when someone is faced with a chronic disorder. Provide contact information, if desired, for the NKF (www.kidney.org) or the NKDEP (www.nkdep.nih.gov).

▶ Reinforce information given by the patient's HCP regarding further testing, treatment, or referral to another HCP. Answer any questions or address any concerns voiced by the patient or family.

▶ Depending on the results of this procedure, additional testing may be performed to evaluate or monitor progression of the disease process and determine the need for a change in therapy. Evaluate test results in relation to the patient's symptoms and other tests performed.

RELATED MONOGRAPHS:

▶ Related tests include anion gap, antibiotic drugs, antibodies antiglomerular basement membrane, ANF, biopsy kidney, biopsy muscle, blood gases, BNP, BUN, calcium, calculus kidney stone analysis, C4, CT abdomen, CT renal, CK and isoenzymes, creatinine, culture urine, cytology urine, cystoscopy, echocardiography, echocardiography transesophageal, electrolytes, EMG, ENG, EPO, gallium scan, glucagon, glucose, haptoglobin, insulin, IVP, KUB studies, lung perfusion scan, microalbumin, osmolality, phosphorus, renogram, retrograde ureteropyelography, TSH, thyroxine, US kidney, uric acid, and UA.

▶ Refer to the Genitourinary System table at the end of the book for related tests by body system.

Cryoglobulin

SYNONYM/ACRONYM: Cryo.

COMMON USE: To assist in identification of the presence of certain immunological disorders such as Reynaud's phenomenon.

SPECIMEN: Serum (1 mL) collected in a red-top tube.

REFERENCE VALUE: (Method: Visual observation for changes in appearance) Negative.

DESCRIPTION: Cryoglobulins are abnormal serum proteins that cannot be detected by protein electrophoresis. Cryoglobulins cause vascular problems because they can precipitate in the blood vessels of the fingers when exposed to cold, causing Raynaud's phenomenon. They are usually associated with immunological disease. The laboratory procedure to detect cryoglobulins is a two-step process. The serum sample is observed for cold precipitation after 72 hr of storage at 4°C. True cryoglobulins disappear on warming to room temperature, so in the second step of the procedure, the sample is rewarmed to confirm reversibility of the reaction.

- Type I cryoglobulin (monoclonal)
  Chronic lymphocytic leukemia
  Lymphoma
  Multiple myeloma

- Type II cryoglobulin (mixtures of monoclonal immunoglobulin [Ig] M and polyclonal IgG)
  Autoimmune hepatitis
  Rheumatoid arthritis
  Sjögren's syndrome
  Waldenström's macroglobulinemia

- Type III cryoglobulin (mixtures of polyclonal IgM and IgG)
  Acute poststreptococcal glomerulonephritis
  Chronic infection (especially hepatitis C)
  Cirrhosis
  Endocarditis
  Infectious mononucleosis
  Polymyalgia rheumatica
  Rheumatoid arthritis
  Sarcoidosis
  Systemic lupus erythematosus

Decreased in: N/A

CRITICAL FINDINGS: N/A

INDICATIONS

- Assist in diagnosis of neoplastic diseases, acute and chronic infections, and collagen diseases
- Detect cryoglobulinemia in patients with symptoms indicating or mimicking Raynaud's disease
- Monitor course of collagen and rheumatic disorders

POTENTIAL DIAGNOSIS

Increased in
Cryoglobulins are present in varying degrees in associated conditions.

INTERFERING FACTORS

- Testing the sample prematurely (before total precipitation) may yield incorrect results.
- Failure to maintain sample at normal body temperature before centrifugation can affect results.

Access additional resources at davisplus.fadavis.com

• A recent fatty meal can increase turbidity of the blood, decreasing visibility.

NURSING IMPLICATIONS AND PROCEDURE

PRETEST:

▶ Positively identify the patient using at least two unique identifiers before providing care, treatment, or services.

▶ *Patient Teaching:* Inform the patient this test can assist in assessing for immune system disorders.

▶ Obtain a history of the patient's complaints, including a list of known allergens, especially allergies or sensitivities to latex.

▶ Obtain a history of the patient's immune system as well as results of previously performed laboratory tests and diagnostic and surgical procedures.

▶ Obtain a list of the patient's current medications, including herbs, nutritional supplements, and nutraceuticals (see Appendix F).

▶ Review the procedure with the patient. Inform the patient that specimen collection takes approximately 5 to 10 min. Address concerns about pain and explain that there may be some discomfort during the venipuncture.

▶ *Sensitivity to social and cultural issues,* as well as concern for modesty, is important in providing psychological support before, during, and after the procedure.

▶ There are no food, fluid, or medication restrictions unless by medical direction.

INTRATEST:

▶ If the patient has a history of allergic reaction to latex, avoid the use of equipment containing latex.

▶ Instruct the patient to cooperate fully and to follow directions. Direct the patient to breathe normally and to avoid unnecessary movement.

▶ Observe standard precautions, and follow the general guidelines in Appendix A. Positively identify the patient, and label the appropriate tubes with the corresponding patient demographics, date, and time of collection. Perform a venipuncture.

▶ Remove the needle and apply direct pressure with dry gauze to stop bleeding. Observe/assess venipuncture site for bleeding or hematoma formation and secure gauze with adhesive bandage.

▶ Promptly transport the specimen to the laboratory for processing and analysis.

POST-TEST:

▶ A report of the results will be sent to the requesting health-care provider (HCP), who will discuss the results with the patient.

▶ Reinforce information given by the patient's HCP regarding further testing, treatment, or referral to another HCP. Answer any questions or address any concerns voiced by the patient or family.

▶ Depending on the results of this procedure, additional testing may be performed to evaluate or monitor progression of the disease process and determine the need for a change in therapy. Evaluate test results in relation to the patient's symptoms and other tests performed.

RELATED MONOGRAPHS:

▶ Related tests include ALT, ANA, arthroscopy, AST, bilirubin, biopsy liver, bone scan, ceruloplasmin, copper, CRP, ESR, GGT, infectious mono screen, hepatitis C antibody, IgA, IgG, IgM, IFE, liver and spleen scan, protein, protein electrophoresis, RF, synovial fluid analysis, and US liver.

▶ Refer to the Immune System table at the end of the book for related tests by body system.

Culture and Smear, Mycobacteria

SYNONYM/ACRONYM: Acid-fast bacilli (AFB) culture and smear, tuberculosis (TB) culture and smear, *Mycobacterium* culture and smear.

COMMON USE: To assist in the diagnosis of tuberculosis.

C

SPECIMEN: Sputum (5 to 10 mL), bronchopulmonary lavage, tissue, material from fine-needle aspiration, bone marrow, cerebrospinal fluid (CSF), gastric aspiration, urine, and stool.

REFERENCE VALUE: (Method: Culture on selected media, microscopic examination of sputum by acid-fast or auramine-rhodamine fluorochrome stain) Rapid methods include: chemiluminescent-labeled DNA probes that target ribosomal RNA of the *Mycobacterium* radiometric carbon dioxide detection from ^{14}C-labeled media, polymerase chain reaction/amplification techniques.

> *Culture*: No growth
> *Smear*: Negative for AFB

DESCRIPTION: A culture and smear test is used primarily to detect *Mycobacterium tuberculosis*, which is a tubercular bacillus. The cell wall of this mycobacterium contains complex lipids and waxes that do not take up ordinary stains. Cells that resist decolorization by acid alcohol are termed *acid-fast*. There are only a few groups of acid-fast bacilli (AFB); this characteristic is helpful in rapid identification so that therapy can be initiated in a timely manner. Smears may be negative 50% of the time even though the culture develops positive growth 3 to 8 wk later. AFB cultures are used to confirm positive and negative AFB smears. *M. tuberculosis* grows in culture slowly. Automated liquid culture systems, such as the Bactec and MGIT (Becton Dickinson and Company, 1 Becton Drive,

Franklin Lakes, NJ, 07417), have a turnaround time of approximately 10 days. Results of tests by polymerase chain reaction culture methods are available in 24 to 72 hr.

M. tuberculosis is transmitted via the airborne route to the lungs. It causes areas of granulomatous inflammation, cough, fever, and hemoptysis. It can remain dormant in the lungs for long periods. The incidence of tuberculosis has increased since the late 1980s in depressed inner-city areas, among prison populations, and among HIV-positive patients. Of great concern is the increase in antibiotic-resistant strains. HIV-positive patients often become ill from concomitant infections caused by *M. tuberculosis* and *Mycobacterium avium intracellulare*. *M. avium intracellulare* is acquired via the gastrointestinal tract through ingestion of contaminated food or water. The organism's waxy cell wall protects it from acids in the human digestive tract. Isolation of mycobacteria in the stool does not mean the patient has tuberculosis of the intestines because mycobacteria in stool are zmost often present in sputum that has been swallowed.

INDICATIONS
- Assist in the diagnosis of mycobacteriosis
- Assist in the diagnosis of suspected pulmonary tuberculosis secondary to AIDS
- Assist in the differentiation of tuberculosis from carcinoma or bronchiectasis
- Investigate suspected pulmonary tuberculosis
- Monitor the response to treatment for pulmonary tuberculosis

POTENTIAL DIAGNOSIS

Identified Organism	Primary Specimen Source	Condition
Mycobacterium avium intracellulare	CSF, lymph nodes, semen, sputum, urine	Opportunistic pulmonary infection
M. fortuitum	Bone, body fluid, sputum, surgical wound, tissue	Opportunistic infection (usually pulmonary)
M. leprae	CSF, skin scrapings, lymph nodes	Hanson's disease (leprosy)
M. kansasii	Joint, lymph nodes, skin, sputum	Pulmonary tuberculosis
M. marinum	Joint	Granulomatous skin lesions
M. tuberculosis	CSF, gastric washing, sputum, urine	Pulmonary tuberculosis
M. xenopi	Sputum	Pulmonary tuberculosis

CRITICAL FINDINGS
- *Smear:* Positive for AFB
- *Culture:* Growth of pathogenic bacteria

Note and immediately report to the health-care provider (HCP) positive results and related symptoms. Lists of specific organisms may vary among facilities; specific organisms are required to be reported to local, state, and national departments of health.

INTERFERING FACTORS
- Specimen collection after initiation of treatment with antituberculosis drug therapy may result in inhibited or no growth of organisms.
- Contamination of the sterile container with organisms from an exogenous source may produce misleading results.
- Specimens received on a dry swab should be rejected: A dry swab indicates that the sample is unlikely to have been collected properly

or unlikely to contain a representative quantity of significant organisms for proper evaluation.
- Inadequate or improper (e.g., saliva) samples should be rejected.
- Failure to follow dietary restrictions before the procedure may cause the procedure to be canceled or repeated.

NURSING IMPLICATIONS AND PROCEDURE

PRETEST:

▸ Positively identify the patient using at least two unique identifiers before providing care, treatment, or services.
▸ *Patient Teaching:* Inform the patient this test can assist in diagnosing respiratory disease.
▸ Obtain a history of the patient's complaints, including a list of known allergens, especially allergies or sensitivities to latex. Obtain a history of the patient's exposure to tuberculosis.
▸ Obtain a history of the patient's immune and respiratory systems, symptoms, and results of previously performed laboratory tests and diagnostic and surgical procedures.
▸ Obtain a list of the patient's current medications, including herbs, nutritional supplements, and nutraceuticals (see Appendix F).
▸ Note any recent procedures that can interfere with test results.
▸ Review the procedure with the patient. Reassure the patient that he or she will be able to breathe during the procedure if sputum specimen is collected via suction method. Ensure that oxygen has been administered 20 to 30 min before the procedure if the specimen is to be obtained by tracheal suction. Address concerns about pain related to the procedure. Atropine is usually given before bronchoscopy examinations to reduce bronchial secretions and prevent vagally induced bradycardia. Meperidine (Demerol) or morphine may be given as a sedative. Lidocaine is sprayed in the patient's throat to reduce discomfort caused by the presence of the tube.
▸ Explain to the patient that the time it takes to collect a proper specimen varies according to the level of cooperation of the patient and the specimen collection site. Emphasize that sputum and saliva are not the same. Inform the patient that multiple specimens may be required at timed intervals. Inform the patient that the culture results will not be reported for 3 to 8 wk.
▸ *Sensitivity to social and cultural issues,* as well as concern for modesty, is important in providing psychological support before, during, and after the procedure.

Bronchoscopy

▸ *Make sure a written and informed consent has been signed prior to the procedure and before administering any medications.*
▸ Other than antimicrobial drugs, there are no medication restrictions unless by medical direction.
▸ The patient should fast and refrain from drinking liquids beginning at midnight the night before the procedure. Protocols may vary among facilities.

Expectorated Specimen

▸ Additional liquids the night before may assist in liquefying secretions during expectoration the following morning.
▸ Assist the patient with oral cleaning before sample collection to reduce the amount of sample contamination by organisms that normally inhabit the mouth.
▸ Instruct the patient not to touch the edge or inside of the container with the hands or mouth.
▸ Other than antimicrobial drugs, there are no medication restrictions unless by medical direction.
▸ There are no food or fluid restrictions unless by medical direction.

Tracheal Suctioning

▸ Assist in providing extra fluids, unless contraindicated, and proper humidification to decrease tenacious secretions. Inform the patient that increasing fluid intake before retiring on the night before the test aids in liquefying secretions and may make it easier to expectorate in the morning. Also explain that humidifying inspired air also helps liquefy secretions.

▶ Other than antimicrobial drugs, there are no medication restrictions unless by medical direction.

▶ There are no food or fluid restrictions unless by medical direction.

INTRATEST:

▶ Ensure that the patient has complied with dietary and medication restrictions; assure that food and fluids have been restricted for at least 8 hr prior to the bronchoscopy procedure.

▶ Have patient remove dentures, contact lenses, eyeglasses, and jewelry. Notify the HCP if the patient has permanent crowns on teeth. Have the patient remove clothing and change into a gown for the procedure.

▶ Have emergency equipment readily available. Keep resuscitation equipment on hand in case of respiratory impairment or laryngospasm after the procedure.

▶ Avoid using morphine sulfate in patients with asthma or other pulmonary disease. This drug can further exacerbate bronchospasms and respiratory impairment.

▶ If the patient has a history of allergic reaction to latex, avoid the use of equipment containing latex.

▶ Assist the patient to a comfortable position, and direct the patient to breathe normally during the beginning of the local anesthesia. Instruct the patient to cooperate fully and to follow directions. Direct the patient to breathe normally and to avoid unnecessary movement during the local anesthetic and the procedure.

▶ Observe standard precautions, and follow the general guidelines in Appendix A. Positively identify the patient, and label the appropriate collection container with the corresponding patient demographics, date and time of collection, and any medication the patient is taking that may interfere with test results (e.g., antibiotics).

Bronchoscopy

▶ Record baseline vital signs.

▶ The patient is positioned in relation to the type of anesthesia being used. If local anesthesia is used, the patient is seated and the tongue and oropharynx are sprayed and swabbed with anesthetic before the bronchoscope is inserted. For general anesthesia, the patient is placed in a supine position with the neck hyperextended. After anesthesia, the patient is kept in supine or shifted to a side-lying position and the bronchoscope is inserted. After inspection, the samples are collected from suspicious sites by bronchial brush or biopsy forceps.

Expectorated Specimen

▶ Ask the patient to sit upright, with assistance and support (e.g., with an overbed table) as needed.

▶ Ask the patient to take two or three deep breaths and cough deeply. Any sputum raised should be expectorated directly into a sterile sputum collection container.

▶ If the patient is unable to produce the desired amount of sputum, several strategies may be attempted. One approach is to have the patient drink two glasses of water, and then assume the position for postural drainage of the upper and middle lung segments. Effective coughing may be assisted by placing either the hands or a pillow over the diaphragmatic area and applying slight pressure.

▶ Another approach is to place a vaporizer or other humidifying device at the bedside. After sufficient exposure to adequate humidification, postural drainage of the upper and middle lung segments may be repeated before attempting to obtain the specimen.

▶ Other methods may include obtaining an order for an expectorant to be administered with additional water approximately 2 hr before attempting to obtain the specimen. Chest percussion and postural drainage of all lung segments may also be employed. If the patient is still unable to raise sputum, the use of an ultrasonic nebulizer ("induced sputum") may be necessary; this is usually done by a respiratory therapist.

Tracheal Suctioning

- Obtain the necessary equipment, including a suction device, suction kit, and Lukens tube or in-line trap.
- Position the patient with head elevated as high as tolerated.
- Put on sterile gloves. Maintain the dominant hand as sterile and the non-dominant hand as clean.
- Using the sterile hand, attach the suction catheter to the rubber tubing of the Lukens tube or in-line trap. Then attach the suction tubing to the male adapter of the trap with the clean hand. Lubricate the suction catheter with sterile saline.
- Tell nonintubated patients to protrude the tongue and to take a deep breath as the suction catheter is passed through the nostril. When the catheter enters the trachea, a reflex cough is stimulated; immediately advance the catheter into the trachea and apply suction. Maintain suction for approximately 10 sec, but never longer than 15 sec. Withdraw the catheter without applying suction. Separate the suction catheter and suction tubing from the trap, and place the rubber tubing over the male adapter to seal the unit.
- For intubated patients or patients with a tracheostomy, the previous procedure is followed except that the suction catheter is passed through the existing endotracheal or tracheostomy tube rather than through the nostril. The patient should be hyperoxygenated before and after the procedure in accordance with standard protocols for suctioning these patients.
- Generally, a series of three to five early morning sputum samples are collected in sterile containers. If leprosy is suspected, obtain a smear from nasal scrapings or a biopsy specimen from lesions in a sterile container.

General

- Monitor the patient for complications related to the procedure (e.g., allergic reaction, anaphylaxis, bronchospasm).
- Promptly transport the specimen to the laboratory for processing and analysis.

POST-TEST:

- A report of the results will be sent to the requesting HCP, who will discuss the results with the patient.
- Instruct the patient to resume preoperative diet, as directed by the HCP. Assess the patient's ability to swallow before allowing the patient to attempt liquids or solid foods.
- Inform the patient that he or she may experience some throat soreness and hoarseness. Instruct patient to treat throat discomfort with lozenges and warm gargles when the gag reflex returns.
- Monitor vital signs and compare with baseline values every 15 min for 1 hr, then every 2 hr for 4 hr, and then as ordered by the HCP. Monitor temperature every 4 hr for 24 hr. Notify the HCP if temperature is elevated. Protocols may vary among facilities.
- Emergency resuscitation equipment should be readily available if the vocal cords become spastic after intubation.
- Observe for delayed allergic reactions, such as rash, urticaria, tachycardia, hyperpnea, hypertension, palpitations, nausea, or vomiting.
- Observe the patient for hemoptysis, difficulty breathing, cough, air hunger, excessive coughing, pain, or absent breathing sounds over the affected area. Report any symptoms to the HCP.
- Evaluate the patient for symptoms indicating the development of pneumothorax, such as dyspnea, tachypnea, anxiety, decreased breathing sounds, or restlessness. A chest x-ray may be ordered to check for the presence of this complication.
- Evaluate the patient for symptoms of empyema, such as fever, tachycardia, malaise, or elevated white blood cell count.
- Administer antibiotic therapy if ordered. Remind the patient of the importance of completing the entire course of antibiotic therapy, even if signs and symptoms disappear before completion of therapy.
- **Nutritional Considerations:** Malnutrition is commonly seen in patients with severe respiratory disease for numerous

reasons, including fatigue, lack of appetite, and gastrointestinal distress. Adequate intake of vitamins A and C are also important to prevent pulmonary infection and to decrease the extent of lung tissue damage.

- Recognize anxiety related to test results. Discuss the implications of abnormal test results on the patient's lifestyle. Provide teaching and information regarding the clinical implications of the test results, as appropriate.
- Reinforce information given by the patient's HCP regarding further testing, treatment, or referral to another HCP. Instruct the patient to use lozenges or gargle for throat discomfort. Inform the patient of smoking cessation programs as appropriate. The importance of following the prescribed diet should be stressed to the patient/caregiver. Educate the patient regarding access to counseling services, as appropriate. Answer any questions or address any concerns voiced by the patient or family.
- Instruct the patient in the use of any ordered medications. Explain the importance of adhering to the therapy regimen. As appropriate, instruct the patient in significant side effects and systemic reactions associated with the prescribed medication. Encourage him or her to review corresponding literature provided by a pharmacist.
- Depending on the results of this procedure, additional testing may be needed to evaluate or monitor progression of the disease process and determine the need for a change in therapy. Evaluate test results in relation to the patient's symptoms and other tests performed.

RELATED MONOGRAPHS:

- Related tests include antibodies, anti-glomerular basement membrane, arterial/alveolar oxygen ratio, blood gases, bronchoscopy, chest x-ray, complete blood count, CT thoracic, cultures (fungal, sputum, throat, viral), cytology sputum, gallium scan, Gram stain, lung perfusion scan, lung ventilation scan, MRI chest, mediastinoscopy, pleural fluid analysis, pulmonary function tests, and TB tests.
- Refer to the Immune and Respiratory systems tables at the end of the book for related tests by body system.

Culture, Bacterial, Anal/Genital, Ear, Eye, Skin, and Wound

SYNONYM/ACRONYM: N/A.

COMMON USE: To identify pathogenic bacterial organisms as an indicator for appropriate therapeutic interventions for multiple sites of infection.

SPECIMEN: Sterile fluid or swab from affected area placed in transport media tube provided by laboratory.

REFERENCE VALUE: (Method: Culture aerobic and/or anaerobic on selected media; nucleic acid amplification and DNA probe assays [e.g., Gen-Probe] are available for identification of *Neisseria gonorrhoeae* and *Chlamydia trachomatis*.) Negative: no growth of pathogens.

DESCRIPTION: When indicated by patient history, anal and genital cultures may be performed to isolate the organism responsible for sexually transmitted disease. Group B streptococcus (GBS) is a significant and serious neonatal infection. The Centers for Disease Control and Prevention (CDC) recommends universal GBS screening for all pregnant women at 35 to 37 wk gestation. Rapid GBS test kits can provide results within minutes on vaginal or rectal fluid swab specimens submitted in a sterile red-top tube.

Ear and eye cultures are performed to isolate the organism responsible for chronic or acute infectious disease of the ear and eye.

Skin and soft tissue samples from infected sites must be collected carefully to avoid contamination from the surrounding normal skin flora. Skin and tissue infections may be caused by both aerobic and anaerobic organisms. Therefore, a portion of the sample should be placed in aerobic and a portion in anaerobic transport media. Care must be taken to use transport media that are approved by the laboratory performing the testing.

Sterile fluids can be collected from the affected site. Refer to related body fluid monographs (i.e., amniotic fluid, cerebrospinal fluid, pericardial fluid, peritoneal fluid, pleural fluid, synovial fluid) for specimen collection.

A wound culture involves collecting a specimen of exudates, drainage, or tissue so that the causative organism can be isolated and pathogens identified. Specimens can be obtained from superficial and deep wounds.

Optimally, specimens should be obtained before antibiotic use. The method used to culture and grow the organism depends on the suspected infectious organism. There are transport media specifically for bacterial agents. The laboratory will select the appropriate media for suspect organisms and will initiate antibiotic sensitivity testing if indicated by test results. Sensitivity testing identifies the antibiotics to which organisms are susceptible to ensure an effective treatment plan.

INDICATIONS

Anal/Genital
- Assist in the diagnosis of sexually transmitted diseases
- Determine the cause of genital itching or purulent drainage
- Determine effective antimicrobial therapy specific to the identified pathogen
- Routine prenatal screening for vaginal and rectal GBS colonization

Ear
- Isolate and identify organisms responsible for ear pain, drainage, or changes in hearing
- Isolate and identify organisms responsible for outer-, middle-, or inner-ear infection
- Determine effective antimicrobial therapy specific to the identified pathogen

Eye
- Isolate and identify pathogenic microorganisms responsible for infection of the eye
- Determine effective antimicrobial therapy specific to identified pathogen

Skin
- Isolate and identify organisms responsible for skin eruptions,

drainage, or other evidence of infection
• Determine effective antimicrobial therapy specific to the identified pathogen

Sterile Fluids
• Isolate and identify organisms before surrounding tissue becomes infected
• Determine effective antimicrobial therapy specific to the identified pathogen

Wound
• Detect abscess or deep-wound infectious process
• Determine if an infectious agent is the cause of wound redness, warmth, or edema with drainage at a site
• Determine presence of infectious agents in a stage 3 and stage 4 decubitus ulcer
• Isolate and identify organisms responsible for the presence of pus or other exudate in an open wound
• Determine effective antimicrobial therapy specific to the identified pathogen

POTENTIAL DIAGNOSIS

Positive findings in

Anal/Endocervical/Genital
Infections or carrier states are caused by the following organisms: *C. trachomatis*, *Gardnerella vaginalis*, *N. gonorrhoeae*, toxin-producing strains of *Staphylococcus aureus*, group B streptococcus, and *Treponema pallidum*.

Ear
Commonly identified organisms include *Escherichia coli*, *Proteus* spp., *Pseudomonas aeruginosa*, *S. aureus*, and β-hemolytic streptococci.

Eye
Commonly identified organisms include *C. trachomatis* (transmitted to newborns from infected mothers), *Haemophilus influenzae* (transmitted to newborns from infected mothers), *H. aegyptius*, *N. gonorrhoeae* (transmitted to newborns from infected mothers), *P. aeruginosa*, *S. aureus*, and *Streptococcus pneumoniae*.

Skin
Commonly identified organisms include *Bacteroides*, *Clostridium*, *Corynebacterium*, *Pseudomonas*, staphylococci, and group A streptococci.

Sterile Fluids
Commonly identified pathogens include *Bacteroides*, *Enterococcus* spp., *E. coli*, *P. aeruginosa*, and *Peptostreptococcus* spp.

Wound
Aerobic and anaerobic microorganisms can be identified in wound culture specimens. Commonly identified organisms include *Clostridium perfringens*, *Klebsiella*, *Proteus*, *Pseudomonas*, *S. aureus*, and group A streptococci.

CRITICAL FINDINGS
• *Listeria* in genital cultures
• Methicillin-resistant *S. aureus* (MRSA) in skin or wound cultures

Note and immediately report to the health-care provider (HCP) positive results and related symptoms. Lists of specific organisms may vary from facility to facility; specific organisms are required to be reported to local, state, and national departments of health.

INTERFERING FACTORS

- Failure to collect adequate specimen, improper collection or storage technique, and failure to transport specimen in a timely fashion are causes for specimen rejection.
- Pretest antimicrobial therapy will delay or inhibit the growth of pathogens.
- Testing specimens more than 1 hr after collection may result in decreased growth or no growth of organisms.

NURSING IMPLICATIONS AND PROCEDURE

PRETEST:

- Positively identify the patient using at least two unique identifiers before providing care, treatment, or services.
- *Patient Teaching:* Inform the patient that test can assist in identification of the organism causing infection.
- Obtain a history of the patient's complaints, including a list of known allergens.
- Obtain a history of the patient's immune system, symptoms, and results of previously performed laboratory tests and diagnostic and surgical procedures. Obtain, as appropriate, a history of sexual activity.
- Obtain a list of the patient's current medications, including herbs, nutritional supplements, and nutraceuticals (see Appendix F).
- Note any recent medications that can interfere with test results.
- Review the procedure with the patient. Inform the patient that specimen collection takes approximately 5 min. Address concerns about pain and explain that there may be some discomfort during the specimen collection. Instruct female patients not to douche for 24 hr before a cervical or vaginal specimen is to be obtained.
- *Sensitivity to social and cultural issues,* as well as concern for modesty, is important in providing psychological support before, during, and after the procedure.
- There are no food or fluid restrictions, unless by medical direction.

INTRATEST:

- Ensure that the patient has complied with medication restrictions prior to the procedure.
- Instruct the patient to cooperate fully and to follow directions. Direct the patient to breathe normally and to avoid unnecessary movement.
- Observe standard precautions, and follow the general guidelines in Appendix A. Positively identify the patient, and label the appropriate specimen containers with the corresponding patient demographics, specimen source (left or right as appropriate), patient age and gender, date and time of collection, and any medication the patient is taking that may interfere with the test results (e.g., antibiotics). Do not freeze the specimen or allow it to dry.

Anal

- Place the patient in a lithotomy or side-lying position and drape for privacy. Insert the swab 1 in. into the anal canal and rotate, moving it from side to side to allow it to come into contact with the microorganisms. Remove the swab. Place the swab in the Culturette tube, and squeeze the bottom of the tube to release the transport medium. Ensure that the end of the swab is immersed in the medium. Repeat with a clean swab if the swab is pushed into feces.

Genital

Female Patient

- Position the patient on the gynecological examination table with the feet up in stirrups. Drape the patient's legs to provide privacy and reduce chilling.
- Cleanse the external genitalia and perineum from front to back with towelettes provided in culture kit. Using a Culturette swab, obtain a sample of the lesion or discharge from the urethra or

vulva. Place the swab in the Culturette tube, and squeeze the bottom of the tube to release the transport medium. Ensure that the end of the swab is immersed in the medium.

▶ To obtain a vaginal and endocervical culture, insert a water-lubricated vaginal speculum. Insert the swab into the cervical orifice and rotate the swab to collect the secretions containing the microorganisms. Remove and place in the appropriate culture medium or Gen-Probe transport tube. Material from the vagina can be collected by moving a swab along the sides of the vaginal mucosa. The swab is removed and then placed in a tube of saline medium.

Male Patient

▶ To obtain a urethral culture, cleanse the penis (retracting the foreskin), have the patient milk the penis to express discharge from the urethra. Insert a swab into the urethral orifice and rotate the swab to obtain a sample of the discharge. Place the swab in the Culturette or Gen-Probe transport tube, and squeeze the bottom of the tube to release the transport medium. Ensure that the end of the swab is immersed in the medium.

Ear

▶ Cleanse the area surrounding the site with a swab containing cleaning solution to remove any contaminating material or flora that have collected in the ear canal. If needed, assist the appropriate health-care provider (HCP) in removing any cerumen that has collected.

▶ Insert a Culturette swab approximately 1/4 in. into the external ear canal. Rotate the swab in the area containing the exudate. Carefully remove the swab, ensuring that it does not touch the side or opening of the ear canal.

▶ Place the swab in the Culturette tube, and squeeze the bottom of the tube to release the transport medium. Ensure that the end of the swab is immersed in the medium.

Eye

▶ Pass a moistened swab over the appropriate site, avoiding eyelid and

eyelashes unless those areas are selected for study. Collect any visible pus or other exudate. Place the swab in the Culturette or Gen-Probe transport tube, and squeeze the bottom of the tube to release the transport medium. Ensure that the end of the swab is immersed in the medium.

▶ An appropriate HCP should perform procedures requiring eye scrapings.

Skin

▶ Assist the appropriate HCP in obtaining a skin sample from several areas of the affected site. If indicated, the dark, moist areas of the folds of the skin and outer growing edges of the infection where microorganisms are most likely to flourish should be selected. Place the scrapings in a collection container or spread on a slide. Aspirate any fluid from a pustule or vesicle using a sterile needle and tuberculin syringe. The exudate will be flushed into a sterile collection tube. If the lesion is not fluid filled, open the lesion with a scalpel and swab the area with a sterile cotton-tipped swab. Place the swab in the Culturette tube, and squeeze the bottom of the tube to release the transport medium. Ensure that the end of the swab is immersed in the medium.

Sterile Fluid

▶ Refer to related body fluid monographs (i.e., amniotic fluid, cerebrospinal fluid, pericardial fluid, peritoneal fluid, pleural fluid, synovial fluid) for specimen collection.

Wound

▶ Place the patient in a comfortable position, and drape the site to be cultured. Cleanse the area around the wound to remove flora indigenous to the skin.

▶ Place a Culturette swab in a superficial wound where the exudate is the most excessive without touching the wound edges. Place the swab in the Culturette tube, and squeeze the bottom of the tube to release the transport medium. Ensure that the end of the swab is immersed in the medium. Use more than one swab and Culturette tube to obtain specimens from other areas of the wound.

▶ To obtain a deep wound specimen, insert a sterile syringe and needle into the wound and aspirate the drainage. Following aspiration, inject the material into a tube containing an anaerobic culture medium.

General

▶ Promptly transport the specimen to the laboratory for processing and analysis.

POST-TEST:

▶ Instruct the patient to resume usual medication as directed by the HCP.
▶ Instruct the patient to report symptoms such as pain related to tissue inflammation or irritation.
▶ Instruct the patient to begin antibiotic therapy, as prescribed. Instruct the patient in the importance of completing the entire course of antibiotic therapy even if no symptoms are present.
▶ Inform the patient that a repeat culture may be needed in 1 wk after completion of the antimicrobial regimen.
▶ Advise the patient that final test results may take 24 to 72 hr depending on the organism suspected but that antibiotic therapy may be started immediately.

Anal/Endocervical/Genital

▶ Inform the patient that final results may take from 24 hr to 4 wk, depending on the test performed.
▶ Advise the patient to avoid sexual contact until test results are available.
▶ Instruct the patient in vaginal suppository and medicated cream installation and administration of topical medication to treat specific conditions, as indicated.
▶ Inform infected patients that all sexual partners must be tested for the microorganism.
▶ Inform the patient that positive culture findings for certain organisms must be reported to a local health department official, who will question him or her regarding sexual partners.
▶ **Social and Cultural Considerations:** Offer support, as appropriate, to patients who may be the victims of rape or sexual assault. Educate the patient regarding access to counseling services. Provide a

nonjudgmental, nonthreatening atmosphere for discussing the risks of sexually transmitted diseases. It is also important to address problems the patient may experience (e.g., guilt, depression, anger).

Wound

▶ Instruct the patient in wound care and nutritional requirements (e.g., protein, vitamin C) to promote wound healing.

General

▶ A written report of the examination will be sent to the requesting HCP, who will discuss the results with the patient.
▶ Recognize anxiety related to test results. Discuss the implications of abnormal test results on the patient's lifestyle. Provide teaching and information regarding the clinical implications of the test results, as appropriate.
▶ Reinforce information given by the patient's HCP regarding further testing, treatment, or referral to another HCP. Emphasize the importance of reporting continued signs and symptoms of the infection. Provide information regarding vaccine-preventable diseases where indicated (e.g., hepatitis A and B, human papillomavirus). Answer any questions or address any concerns voiced by the patient or family.
▶ Instruct the patient in the use of any ordered medications (oral, topical, drops). Instruct the patient in the proper use of sterile technique for cleansing the affected site and application of dressings, as directed. Explain the importance of adhering to the therapy regimen. As appropriate, instruct the patient in significant side effects and systemic reactions associated with the prescribed medication. Encourage him or her to review corresponding literature provided by a pharmacist.
▶ Depending on the results of this procedure, additional testing may be performed to evaluate or monitor progression of the disease process and determine the need for a change in therapy. Evaluate test results in relation to the patient's symptoms and other tests performed.

▶ Related tests include relevant amniotic fluid analysis, audiometry hearing loss, biopsy site, CSF analysis, culture viral, Gram stain, otoscopy, pericardial fluid analysis, Pap smear, peritoneal fluid analysis, pleural fluid analysis, spondee speech reception threshold, synovial fluid analysis, syphilis serology, tuning fork tests, vitamin C, and zinc.

▶ Refer to the Immune System table at the end of the book for related tests by body system.

C

Culture, Bacterial, Blood

SYNONYM/ACRONYM: N/A.

COMMON USE: To identify pathogenic bacterial organisms in the blood as an indicator for appropriate therapeutic interventions for sepsis.

SPECIMEN: Whole blood collected in bottles containing standard aerobic and anaerobic culture media; 10 to 20 mL for adult patients or 1 to 5 mL for pediatric patients.

REFERENCE VALUE: (Method: Growth of organisms in standard culture media identified by radiometric or infrared automation, or by manual reading of subculture.) Negative: no growth of pathogens.

DESCRIPTION: Blood cultures are collected whenever bacteremia or septicemia is suspected. Although mild bacteremia is found in many infectious diseases, a persistent, continuous, or recurrent bacteremia indicates a more serious condition that may require immediate treatment. Early detection of pathogens in the blood may aid in making clinical and etiological diagnoses.

Blood culture involves the introduction of a specimen of blood into artificial aerobic and anaerobic growth culture medium. The culture is incubated for a specific length of time, at a specific temperature, and under other conditions suitable for the growth of pathogenic microorganisms. Pathogens enter the bloodstream from soft-tissue infection sites, contaminated IV lines, or invasive procedures (e.g., surgery, tooth extraction, cystoscopy). A blood culture may also be done with an antimicrobial removal device (ARD). This involves transferring some of the blood sample into a special vial containing absorbent resins that remove antibiotics from the sample before the culture is performed. The laboratory will initiate antibiotic sensitivity testing if indicated by test results. Sensitivity testing identifies the antibiotics to which the organisms are susceptible to ensure an effective treatment plan.

INDICATIONS

- Determine sepsis in the newborn as a result of prolonged labor, early rupture of membranes, maternal infection, or neonatal aspiration
- Evaluate chills and fever in patients with infected burns, urinary tract infections, rapidly progressing tissue infection, postoperative wound sepsis, and indwelling venous or arterial catheter
- Evaluate intermittent or continuous temperature elevation of unknown origin
- Evaluate persistent, intermittent fever associated with a heart murmur
- Evaluate a sudden change in pulse and temperature with or without chills and diaphoresis
- Evaluate suspected bacteremia after invasive procedures
- Identify the cause of shock in the postoperative period

POTENTIAL DIAGNOSIS

Positive findings in
- Bacteremia or septicemia: *Aerobacter, Bacteroides, Brucella, Clostridium perfringens, Enterococci, Escherichia coli*, and other coliform bacilli, *Haemophilus influenzae, Klebsiella, Listeria monocytogenes, Pseudomonas aeruginosa, Salmonella, Staphylococcus aureus, Staphylococcus epidermidis*, and β-hemolytic streptococci.
- Plague
- Malaria (by special request, a stained capillary smear would be examined)
- Typhoid fever

Note: *Candida albicans* is a yeast that can cause disease and can be isolated by blood culture.

CRITICAL FINDINGS ❖

- Positive findings in any sterile body fluid such as blood

Note and immediately report to the health-care provider (HCP) positive results and related symptoms. Lists of specific organisms may vary among facilities; specific organisms are required to be reported to local, state, and national departments of health.

INTERFERING FACTORS

- Pretest antimicrobial therapy will delay or inhibit growth of pathogens.
- Contamination of the specimen by the skin's resident flora may invalidate interpretation of test results.
- An inadequate amount of blood or number of blood specimens drawn for examination may invalidate interpretation of results.
- Testing specimens more than 1 hr after collection may result in decreased growth or no growth of organisms. Delay in transport of specimen to the laboratory may result in specimen rejection. Verify submission requirements with the laboratory prior to specimen collection.
- Collection of the specimen in an expired media tube will result in specimen rejection.
- Negative findings do not ensure the absence of infection.

NURSING IMPLICATIONS AND PROCEDURE

PRETEST:
- Positively identify the patient using at least two unique identifiers before providing care, treatment, or services.
- *Patient Teaching:* Inform the patient this test can assist in identification of the organism causing infection.
- Obtain a history of the patient's complaints, including a list of known

allergens, especially allergies or sensitivities to iodine.

- Obtain a history of the patient's immune system, symptoms, and results of previously performed laboratory tests and diagnostic and surgical procedures.
- Obtain a list of the patient's current medications, including herbs, nutritional supplements, and nutraceuticals (see Appendix F).
- Note any recent medications that can interfere with test results.
- Review the procedure with the patient. Inform the patient that specimen collection takes approximately 5 min. Inform the patient that multiple specimens may be required at timed intervals. Address concerns about pain and explain to the patient that there may be some discomfort during the venipuncture.
- *Sensitivity to social and cultural issues,* as well as concern for modesty, is important in providing psychological support before, during, and after the procedure.
- There are no food or fluid restrictions unless by medical direction.

INTRATEST:

- Ensure that the patient has complied with medication restrictions prior to the procedure.
- If the patient has a history of severe allergic reaction to iodine, care should be taken to avoid the use of iodine.
- Instruct the patient to cooperate fully and to follow directions. Direct the patient to breathe normally and to avoid unnecessary movement.
- Observe standard precautions, and follow the general guidelines in Appendix A. Positively identify the patient, and label the appropriate specimen containers with the corresponding patient demographics, date and time of collection, and any medication the patient is taking that may interfere with test results (e.g., antibiotics). Perform a venipuncture; collect the specimen in the appropriate blood culture collection container.
- The high risk for infecting a patient by venipuncture can be decreased by

using an aseptic technique during specimen collection.

- The contamination of blood cultures by skin and other flora can also be dramatically reduced by careful preparation of the puncture site and collection containers before specimen collection. Cleanse the rubber stoppers of the collection containers with the appropriate disinfectant as recommended by the laboratory, allow to air-dry, and cleanse with 70% alcohol. Once the vein has been located by palpation, cleanse the site with 70% alcohol followed by swabbing with an iodine solution. The iodine should be swabbed in a circular, concentric motion, moving outward or away from the puncture site. The iodine should be allowed to completely dry before the sample is collected. If the patient is sensitive to iodine, a double alcohol scrub or green soap may be substituted.
- If collection is performed by directly drawing the sample into a culture tube, fill the aerobic culture tube first.
- If collection is performed using a syringe, transfer the blood sample directly into each culture bottle.
- Remove the needle, and apply direct pressure with a dry gauze to stop bleeding. Observe/assess venipuncture site for bleeding and secure gauze with adhesive bandage.
- Promptly transport the specimen to the laboratory for processing and analysis.
- More than three sets of cultures per day do not significantly add to the likelihood of pathogen capture. Capture rates are more likely affected by obtaining a sufficient volume of blood per culture.
- The use of ARDs or resin bottles is costly and controversial with respect to their effectiveness versus standard culture techniques. They may be useful in selected cases, such as when septicemia or bacteremia is suspected after antimicrobial therapy has been initiated.

Disease Suspected	Recommended Collection
Bacterial pneumonia, fever of unknown origin, meningitis, osteomyelitis, sepsis	Two sets of cultures, each collected from a separate site, 30 min apart
Acute or subacute endocarditis	Three sets of cultures, each collected from a separate site, 30–40 min apart. If cultures are negative after 24 to 48 hr, repeat collections
Septicemia, fungal or mycobacterial infection in immunocompromised patient	Two sets of cultures, each collected from a separate site, 30 to 60 min apart (laboratory may use a lysis concentration technique to enhance recovery)
Septicemia, bacteremia after therapy has been initiated, or request to monitor effectiveness of antimicrobial therapy	Two sets of cultures, each collected from a separate site, 30 to 60 min apart (consider use of ARD to enhance recovery)

POST-TEST:

▶ A report of the results will be sent to the requesting HCP, who will discuss the results with the patient.

▶ Instruct the patient to resume usual medication as directed by the HCP.

▶ Cleanse the iodine from the collection site.

▶ Instruct the patient to report symptoms such as pain related to tissue inflammation or irritation.

▶ Instruct the patient to report fever, chills, and other signs and symptoms of acute infection to the HCP.

▶ Instruct the patient to begin antibiotic therapy, as prescribed. Instruct the patient in the importance of completing the entire course of antibiotic therapy even if no symptoms are present.

▶ Inform the patient that preliminary results should be available in 24 to 72 hr, but final results are not available for 5 to 7 days.

▶ Recognize anxiety related to test results. Discuss the implications of abnormal test results on the patient's lifestyle. Provide teaching and information regarding the clinical implications of the test results, as appropriate.

▶ Reinforce information given by the patient's HCP regarding further testing, treatment, or referral to another HCP. Emphasize the importance of reporting continued signs and symptoms of the infection. Provide information regarding vaccine-preventable diseases where indicated (e.g., influenza, meningococcal, pneumococcal). Answer any questions or address any concerns voiced by the patient or family.

▶ Depending on the results of this procedure, additional testing may be performed to evaluate or monitor progression of the disease process and determine the need for a change in therapy. Evaluate test results in relation to the patient's symptoms and other tests performed.

RELATED MONOGRAPHS:

▶ Related tests include bone scan, bronchoscopy, CBC, cultures (fungal, mycobacteria, throat, sputum, viral), CSF analysis, ESR, gallium scan, Gram stain, HIV-1/2 antibodies, MRI musculoskeletal, PFT, radiography bone, and TB tests.

▶ Refer to the Immune System table at the end of the book for related tests by body system.

C

Culture, Bacterial, Sputum

SYNONYM/ACRONYM: Routine culture of sputum.

COMMON USE: To identify pathogenic bacterial organisms in the sputum as an indicator for appropriate therapeutic interventions for respiratory infections.

SPECIMEN: Sputum (10 to 15 mL).

REFERENCE VALUE: (Method: Aerobic culture on selective and enriched media; microscopic examination of sputum by Gram stain.) The presence of normal upper respiratory tract flora should be expected. Tracheal aspirates and bronchoscopy samples can be contaminated with normal flora, but transtracheal aspiration specimens should show no growth. Normal respiratory flora include *Neisseria catarrhalis*, *Candida albicans*, diphtheroids, α-hemolytic streptococci, and some staphylococci. The presence of normal flora does not rule out infection. A normal Gram stain of sputum contains polymorphonuclear leukocytes, alveolar macrophages, and a few squamous epithelial cells.

DESCRIPTION: This test involves collecting a sputum specimen so the pathogen can be isolated and identified. The test results will reflect the type and number of organisms present in the specimen as well as the antibiotics to which the identified pathogenic organisms are susceptible. Sputum collected by expectoration or suctioning with catheters and by bronchoscopy cannot be cultured for anaerobic organisms; instead, transtracheal aspiration or lung biopsy must be used. The laboratory will initiate antibiotic sensitivity testing if indicated by test results. Sensitivity testing identifies antibiotics to which the organisms are susceptible to ensure an effective treatment plan.

INDICATIONS

Culture
• Assist in the diagnosis of respiratory infections, as indicated by the presence or absence of organisms in culture

Gram Stain
• Assist in the differentiation of gram-positive from gram-negative bacteria in respiratory infection
• Assist in the differentiation of sputum from upper respiratory tract secretions, the latter being indicated by excessive squamous cells or absence of polymorphonuclear leukocytes

POTENTIAL DIAGNOSIS
• The major difficulty in evaluating results is in distinguishing organisms infecting the lower respiratory tract from organisms that have colonized but not infected the lower respiratory tract. Review of the Gram stain assists in this process. The presence of greater than 25 squamous epithelial cells per low-power field (lpf) indicates oral contamination, and the specimen should

be rejected. The presence of many polymorphonuclear neutrophils and few squamous epithelial cells indicates that the specimen was collected from an area of infection and is satisfactory for further analysis.

- Bacterial pneumonia can be caused by *Streptococcus pneumoniae*, *Haemophilus influenzae*, staphylococci, and some gram-negative bacteria. Other pathogens that can be identified by culture are *Corynebacterium diphtheriae*, *Klebsiella pneumoniae*, and *Pseudomonas aeruginosa*. Some infectious agents, such as *C. diphtheriae*, are more fastidious in their growth requirements and cannot be cultured and identified without special treatment. Suspicion of infection by less commonly identified and/or fastidious organisms must be communicated to the laboratory to ensure selection of the proper procedure required for identification.

CRITICAL FINDINGS

- *C. diphtheriae*
- *Legionella*

Note and immediately report to the health-care provider (HCP) positive results and related symptoms. Lists of specific organisms may vary among facilities; specific organisms are required to be reported to local, state, and national departments of health.

INTERFERING FACTORS

- Contamination with oral flora may invalidate results.
- Specimen collection after antibiotic therapy has been initiated may result in inhibited or no growth of organisms.

NURSING IMPLICATIONS AND PROCEDURE

PRETEST:

- Positively identify the patient using at least two unique identifiers before providing care, treatment, or services.
- *Patient Teaching:* Inform the patient this test can assist in identification of the organism causing infection.
- Obtain a history of the patient's complaints, including a list of known allergens, especially allergies or sensitivities to latex.
- Obtain a history of the patient's immune and respiratory systems, symptoms, and results of previously performed laboratory tests and diagnostic and surgical procedures.
- Obtain a list of the patient's current medications, including herbs, nutritional supplements, and nutraceuticals (see Appendix F).
- Note any recent medications that can interfere with test results.
- Review the procedure with the patient. Reassure the patient that he or she will be able to breathe during the procedure if specimen collection is accomplished via suction method. Ensure that oxygen has been administered 20 to 30 min before the procedure if the specimen is to be obtained by tracheal suctioning. Address concerns about pain related to the procedure. Atropine is usually given before bronchoscopy examinations to reduce bronchial secretions and prevent vagally induced bradycardia. Meperidine (Demerol) or morphine may be given as a sedative. Lidocaine is sprayed in the patient's throat to reduce discomfort caused by the presence of the tube.
- Explain to the patient that the time it takes to collect a proper specimen varies according to the level of cooperation of the patient and the specimen collection site. Emphasize that sputum and saliva are not the same. Inform the patient that multiple specimens may be required at timed intervals.
- *Sensitivity to social and cultural issues,* as well as concern for modesty, is important in providing psychological support before, during, and after the procedure.

Bronchoscopy

▶ *Make sure a written and informed consent has been signed prior to the bronchoscopy/biopsy procedure and before administering any medications.*

▶ Other than antimicrobial drugs, there are no medication restrictions, unless by medical direction.

▶ The patient should fast and refrain from drinking liquids beginning at midnight the night before the procedure. Protocols may vary among facilities.

Expectorated Specimen

▶ Additional liquids the night before may assist in liquefying secretions during expectoration the following morning.

▶ Assist the patient with oral cleaning before sample collection to reduce the amount of sample contamination by organisms that normally inhabit the mouth.

▶ Instruct the patient not to touch the edge or inside of the container with the hands or mouth.

▶ Other than antimicrobial drugs, there are no medication restrictions, unless by medical direction.

▶ There are no food or fluid restrictions, unless by medical direction.

Tracheal Suctioning

▶ Assist in providing extra fluids, unless contraindicated, and proper humidification to decrease tenacious secretions. Inform the patient that increasing fluid intake before retiring on the night before the test aids in liquefying secretions and may make it easier to expectorate in the morning. Also explain that humidifying inspired air also helps liquefy secretions.

▶ Other than antimicrobial drugs, there are no medication restrictions, unless by medical direction.

▶ There are no food or fluid restrictions, unless by medical direction.

▶ If the specimen is collected by expectoration or tracheal suctioning, there are no food, fluid, or medication restrictions (except antibiotics), unless by medical direction.

INTRATEST:

▶ Ensure that the patient has complied with dietary and medication restrictions;

ensure that food and fluids have been restricted for at least 8 hr prior to the bronchoscopy procedure.

▶ Have patient remove dentures, contact lenses, eyeglasses, and jewelry. Notify the health-care provider (HCP) if the patient has permanent crowns on teeth. Have the patient remove clothing and change into a gown for the procedure.

▶ Have emergency equipment readily available. Keep resuscitation equipment on hand in case of respiratory impairment or laryngospasm after the procedure.

▶ Avoid using morphine sulfate in patients with asthma or other pulmonary disease. This drug can further exacerbate bronchospasms and respiratory impairment.

▶ If the patient has a history of allergic reaction to latex, avoid the use of equipment containing latex.

▶ Assist the patient to a comfortable position and direct the patient to breathe normally during the beginning of the general anesthesia. Instruct the patient to cooperate fully and to follow directions. Direct the patient to breathe normally and to avoid unnecessary movement during the local anesthetic and the procedure.

▶ Observe standard precautions and follow the general guidelines in Appendix A. Positively identify the patient, and label the appropriate tubes with the corresponding patient demographics, date and time of collection, and any medication the patient is taking that may interfere with test results (e.g., antibiotics). Collect the specimen in the appropriate sterile collection container.

Bronchoscopy

▶ Record baseline vital signs.

▶ The patient is positioned in relation to the type of anesthesia being used. If local anesthesia is used, the patient is seated and the tongue and oropharynx are sprayed and swabbed with anesthetic before the bronchoscope is inserted. For general anesthesia, the patient is placed in a supine position with the neck hyperextended. After anesthesia, the patient is kept in supine or shifted to a side-lying position and the bronchoscope is inserted. After inspection, the samples are collected from suspicious sites by bronchial brush or biopsy forceps.

Expectorated Specimen

▸ Ask the patient to sit upright, with assistance and support (e.g., with an overbed table) as needed.

▸ Ask the patient to take two or three deep breaths and cough deeply. Any sputum raised should be expectorated directly into a sterile sputum collection container.

▸ If the patient is unable to produce the desired amount of sputum, several strategies may be attempted. One approach is to have the patient drink two glasses of water, and then assume the position for postural drainage of the upper and middle lung segments. Effective coughing may be assisted by placing either the hands or a pillow over the diaphragmatic area and applying slight pressure.

▸ Another approach is to place a vaporizer or other humidifying device at the bedside. After sufficient exposure to adequate humidification, postural drainage of the upper and middle lung segments may be repeated before attempting to obtain the specimen.

▸ Other methods may include obtaining an order for an expectorant to be administered with additional water approximately 2 hr before attempting to obtain the specimen. Chest percussion and postural drainage of all lung segments may also be employed. If the patient is still unable to raise sputum, the use of an ultrasonic nebulizer ("induced sputum") may be necessary; this is usually done by a respiratory therapist.

Tracheal Suctioning

▸ Obtain the necessary equipment, including a suction device, suction kit, and Lukens tube or in-line trap.

▸ Position the patient with head elevated as high as tolerated.

▸ Put on sterile gloves. Maintain the dominant hand as sterile and the nondominant hand as clean.

▸ Using the sterile hand, attach the suction catheter to the rubber tubing of the Lukens tube or in-line trap. Then attach the suction tubing to the male adapter

of the trap with the clean hand. Lubricate the suction catheter with sterile saline.

▸ Tell nonintubated patients to protrude the tongue and to take a deep breath as the suction catheter is passed through the nostril. When the catheter enters the trachea, a reflex cough is stimulated; immediately advance the catheter into the trachea and apply suction. Maintain suction for approximately 10 sec, but never longer than 15 sec. Withdraw the catheter without applying suction. Separate the suction catheter and suction tubing from the trap, and place the rubber tubing over the male adapter to seal the unit.

▸ For intubated patients or patients with a tracheostomy, the previous procedure is followed except that the suction catheter is passed through the existing endotracheal or tracheostomy tube rather than through the nostril. The patient should be hyperoxygenated before and after the procedure in accordance with standard protocols for suctioning these patients.

▸ Generally, a series of three to five early morning sputum samples are collected in sterile containers.

General

▸ Monitor the patient for complications related to the procedure (e.g., allergic reaction, anaphylaxis, bronchospasm).

▸ Promptly transport the specimen to the laboratory for processing and analysis.

POST-TEST:

▸ A report of the results will be sent to the requesting HCP, who will discuss the results with the patient.

▸ Instruct the patient to resume preoperative diet, as directed by the HCP. Assess the patient's ability to swallow before allowing the patient to attempt liquids or solid foods.

▸ Inform the patient that he or she may experience some throat soreness and hoarseness. Instruct patient to treat throat discomfort with lozenges and warm gargles when the gag reflex returns.

▸ Monitor vital signs and compare with baseline values every 15 min for 1 hr, then every 2 hr for 4 hr, and then as ordered by the HCP. Monitor temperature every 4 hr for 24 hr. Notify the HCP if temperature is elevated. Protocols may vary among facilities.

‣ Emergency resuscitation equipment should be readily available if the vocal cords become spastic after intubation.

‣ Observe for delayed allergic reactions, such as rash, urticaria, tachycardia, hyperpnea, hypertension, palpitations, nausea, or vomiting.

‣ Observe the patient for hemoptysis, difficulty breathing, cough, air hunger, excessive coughing, pain, or absent breathing sounds over the affected area. Report any symptoms to the HCP.

‣ Evaluate the patient for symptoms indicating the development of pneumothorax, such as dyspnea, tachypnea, anxiety, decreased breathing sounds, or restlessness. A chest x-ray may be ordered to check for the presence of this complication.

‣ Evaluate the patient for symptoms of empyema, such as fever, tachycardia, malaise, or elevated white blood cell count.

‣ Administer antibiotic therapy if ordered. Remind the patient of the importance of completing the entire course of antibiotic therapy, even if signs and symptoms disappear before completion of therapy.

‣ *Nutritional Considerations:* Malnutrition is commonly seen in patients with severe respiratory disease for numerous reasons including fatigue, lack of appetite, and gastrointestinal distress. Adequate intake of vitamins A and C are also important to prevent pulmonary infection and to decrease the extent of lung tissue damage.

‣ Recognize anxiety related to test results. Discuss the implications of abnormal test results on the patient's lifestyle. Provide teaching and information regarding the clinical implications of the test results, as appropriate.

Educate the patient regarding access to counseling services.

‣ Reinforce information given by the patient's HCP regarding further testing, treatment, or referral to another HCP. Instruct the patient to use lozenges or gargle for throat discomfort. Inform the patient of smoking cessation programs as appropriate. The importance of following the prescribed diet should be stressed to the patient/caregiver. Educate the patient regarding access to counseling services, as appropriate. Provide information regarding vaccine preventable diseases where indicated (e.g., diphtheria, influenza, measles, mumps, pertussis, rubella, smallpox, varicella). Answer any questions or address any concerns voiced by the patient or family.

‣ Instruct the patient in the use of any ordered medications. Explain the importance of adhering to the therapy regimen. As appropriate, instruct the patient in significant side effects and systemic reactions associated with the prescribed medication. Encourage him or her to review corresponding literature provided by a pharmacist.

‣ Depending on the results of this procedure, additional testing may be needed to evaluate or monitor progression of the disease process and determine the need for a change in therapy. Evaluate test results in relation to the patient's symptoms and other tests performed.

RELATED MONOGRAPHS:

‣ Related tests include antibodies, anti–glomerular basement membrane, arterial/alveolar oxygen ratio, biopsy lung, blood gases, bronchoscopy, chest x-ray, CBC, CT thoracic, culture (fungal, mycobacterium, throat, viral), cytology sputum, gallium scan, Gram stain/acid-fast stain, HIV-1/2 antibodies, lung perfusion scan, lung ventilation scan, MRI chest, mediastinoscopy, pleural fluid analysis, PFT, and TB tests.

‣ Refer to the Immune and Respiratory systems tables at the end of the book for related tests by body system.

Culture, Bacterial, Stool

SYNONYM/ACRONYM: N/A.

COMMON USE: To identify pathogenic bacterial organisms in the stool as an indicator for appropriate therapeutic interventions to treat organisms such as *Clostridium difficile* and *Escherichia coli*.

C

SPECIMEN: Fresh, random stool collected in a clean plastic container.

REFERENCE VALUE: (Method: Culture on selective media for identification of pathogens usually to include *Salmonella, Shigella, Escherichia coli,* O157:H7, *Yersinia enterocolitica,* and *Campylobacter;* latex agglutination or enzyme immunoassay for *Clostridium* A and B toxins) Negative: No growth of pathogens. Normal fecal flora is 96% to 99% anaerobes and 1% to 4% aerobes. Normal flora present may include *Bacteroides, Candida albicans, Clostridium, Enterococcus, E. coli, Proteus, Pseudomonas,* and *Staphylococcus aureus*.

DESCRIPTION: Stool culture involves collecting a sample of feces so that organisms present can be isolated and identified. Certain bacteria are normally found in feces. However, when overgrowth of these organisms occurs or pathological organisms are present, diarrhea or other signs and symptoms of systemic infection occur. These symptoms are the result of damage to the intestinal tissue by the pathogenic organisms. Routine stool culture normally screens for a small number of common pathogens, such as *Campylobacter, Salmonella,* and *Shigella.* Identification of other bacteria is initiated by special request or upon consultation with a microbiologist when there is knowledge of special circumstances. The laboratory will initiate antibiotic sensitivity testing if indicated by test results. Sensitivity testing identifies the antibiotics to which organisms are susceptible to ensure an effective treatment plan. Life-threatening *Clostridium*

difficile infection of the bowel may occur in patients who are immunocompromised or are receiving broad-spectrum antibiotic therapy (e.g., clindamycin, ampicillin, cephalosporins). The bacteria release a toxin that causes necrosis of the colon tissue. The toxin can be more rapidly identified from a stool sample using an immunochemical method than from a routine culture. Appropriate interventions can be quickly initiated and might include IV replacement of fluid and electrolytes, cessation of broad-spectrum antibiotic administration, and institution of vancomycin or metronidazole antibiotic therapy.

INDICATIONS
- Assist in establishing a diagnosis for diarrhea of unknown etiology
- Identify pathogenic organisms causing gastrointestinal disease and carrier states

POTENTIAL DIAGNOSIS

Positive findings in
- Bacterial infection: *Aeromonas* spp., *Bacillus cereus, Campylobacter, Clostridium difficile, E. coli, including serotype O157:H7, Plesiomonas shigelloides, Salmonella, Shigella, Yersinia*, and *Vibrio*. Isolation of *Staphylococcus aureus* may indicate infection or a carrier state
- Botulism: *Clostridium botulinum* (the bacteria must also be isolated from the food or the presence of toxin confirmed in the stool specimen)
- Parasitic enterocolitis

CRITICAL FINDINGS

- Bacterial pathogens *Campylobacter, Clostridium difficile, E. coli,* 0157:H7, *Listeria,* Rotavirus, *Salmonella, Shigella, Vibrio, Yersinia,* or parasites *Acanthamoeba, Ascaris* (hookworm), *Cyclospora, Cryptosporidium, Entamoeba histolytica,* Giardia, *Strongyloides* (tapeworm), parasitic ova, proglottid, and larvae.

Note and immediately report to the health-care provider (HCP) positive results for bacterial pathogens or parasites. Lists of specific organisms may vary among facilities; specific organisms are required to be reported to local, state, and national departments of health.

INTERFERING FACTORS

- A rectal swab does not provide an adequate amount of specimen for evaluating the carrier state and should be avoided in favor of a standard stool specimen.
- A rectal swab should never be submitted for *Clostridium* toxin studies. Specimens for *Clostridium* toxins should be refrigerated if they are not immediately transported to the laboratory because toxins degrade rapidly.
- A rectal swab should never be submitted for *Campylobacter* culture. Excessive exposure of the sample to air or room temperature may damage this bacterium so that it will not grow in the culture.
- Therapy with antibiotics before specimen collection may decrease the type and the amount of bacteria.
- Failure to transport the culture within 1 hr of collection or urine contamination of the sample may affect results.
- Barium and laxatives used less than 1 wk before the test may reduce bacterial growth.

NURSING IMPLICATIONS AND PROCEDURE

PRETEST:
- Positively identify the patient using at least two unique identifiers before providing care, treatment, or services.
- *Patient Teaching:* Inform the patient this test can assist in identification of the organism causing infection.
- Obtain a history of the patient's complaints, including a list of known allergens.
- Obtain a history of the patient's gastrointestinal and immune systems, symptoms, and results of previously performed laboratory tests and diagnostic and surgical procedures.
- Obtain a history of the patient's travel to foreign countries.
- Obtain a list of the patient's current medications, including herbs, nutritional supplements, and nutraceuticals (see Appendix F).
- Note any recent medications that can interfere with test results.
- Review the procedure with the patient. Address concerns about pain and explain that there may be some

discomfort during the specimen collection. Inform the patient that specimen collection takes approximately 5 min.

▸ *Sensitivity to social and cultural issues,* as well as concern for modesty, is important in providing psychological support before, during, and after the procedure.

▸ There are no food or fluid restrictions unless by medical direction.

INTRATEST:

▸ Ensure that the patient has complied with medication restrictions prior to the procedure.

▸ Instruct the patient to cooperate fully and to follow directions. Direct the patient to breathe normally and to avoid unnecessary movement.

▸ Observe standard precautions, and follow the general guidelines in Appendix A. Positively identify the patient, and label the appropriate collection containers with the corresponding patient demographics, date and time of collection, and any medication the patient is taking that may interfere with test results (e.g., antibiotics).

▸ Collect a stool specimen directly into a clean container. If the patient requires a bedpan, make sure it is clean and dry, and use a tongue blade to transfer the specimen to the container. Make sure representative portions of the stool are sent for analysis. Note specimen appearance on collection container label.

▸ Promptly transport the specimen to the laboratory for processing and analysis.

POST-TEST:

▸ A report of the results will be sent to the requesting HCP, who will discuss the results with the patient.

▸ Instruct the patient to resume usual medication as directed by the HCP.

▸ Instruct the patient to report symptoms such as pain related to tissue inflammation or irritation.

▸ Advise the patient that final test results may take up to 72 hr but that antibiotic therapy may be started immediately. Instruct the patient about the importance of completing the entire course of antibiotic therapy even if no symptoms are present. Note: Antibiotic therapy is frequently contraindicated for *Salmonella* infection unless the infection has progressed to a systemic state.

▸ Recognize anxiety related to test results. Discuss the implications of abnormal test results on the patient's lifestyle. Provide teaching and information regarding the clinical implications of the test results, as appropriate.

▸ Reinforce information given by the patient's HCP regarding further testing, treatment, or referral to another HCP. Emphasize the importance of reporting continued signs and symptoms of the infection. Provide information regarding vaccine-preventable diseases where indicated (e.g., cholera, hepatitis A and B, human papillomavirus, typhoid, yellow fever). Answer any questions or address any concerns voiced by the patient or family.

▸ Depending on the results of this procedure, additional testing may be performed to evaluate or monitor progression of the disease process and determine the need for a change in therapy. Evaluate test results in relation to the patient's symptoms and other tests performed.

RELATED MONOGRAPHS:

▸ Related tests include capsule endoscopy, colonoscopy, fecal analysis, ova and parasites, and proctosigmoidoscopy.

▸ Refer to the Gastrointestinal and Immune systems tables at the end of the book for related tests by body system.

C

Culture, Bacterial, Throat or Nasopharyngeal

SYNONYM/ACRONYM: Routine throat culture.

COMMON USE: To identify pathogenic bacterial organisms in the throat and nares as an indicator for appropriate therapeutic interventions. Treat infections such as pharyngitis, thrush, strep throat, and screen for methicillin-resistant *Staphylococcus aureus* (MRSA).

SPECIMEN: Throat or nasopharyngeal swab.

REFERENCE VALUE: (Method: Aerobic culture) No growth.

DESCRIPTION: The routine throat culture is a commonly ordered test to screen for the presence of group A β-hemolytic streptococci. *Streptococcus pyogenes* is the organism that most commonly causes acute pharyngitis. The more dangerous sequelae of scarlet fever, rheumatic heart disease, and glomerulonephritis are less frequently seen because of the early treatment of infection at the pharyngitis stage. There are a number of other bacterial agents responsible for pharyngitis. Specific cultures can be set up to detect other pathogens such as *Bordetella, Corynebacteria, Haemophilus,* or *Neisseria* if they are suspected or by special request from the health-care provider (HCP). *Corynebacterium diphtheriae* is the causative agent of diphtheria. *Neisseria gonorrhoeae* is a sexually transmitted pathogen. In children, a positive throat culture for *Neisseria* usually indicates sexual abuse. The laboratory will initiate antibiotic sensitivity

testing if indicated by test results. Sensitivity testing identifies the antibiotics to which the organisms are susceptible to ensure an effective treatment plan.

INDICATIONS
- Assist in the diagnosis of bacterial infections such as tonsillitis, diphtheria, gonorrhea, or pertussis
- Assist in the diagnosis of upper respiratory infections resulting in bronchitis, pharyngitis, croup, and influenza
- Isolate and identify group A β-hemolytic streptococci as the cause of strep throat, acute glomerulonephritis, scarlet fever, or rheumatic fever

POTENTIAL DIAGNOSIS
Reports on cultures that are positive for group A β-hemolytic streptococci are generally available within 24 to 48 hr. Cultures that report on normal respiratory flora are issued after 48 hr. Culture results of no growth for *Corynebacterium* require 72 hr to

report; 48 hr are required to report negative *Neisseria* cultures.

CRITICAL FINDINGS
- Culture: Growth of *Corynebacterium* or MRSA

Note and immediately report to the HCP positive results and related symptoms. Lists of specific organisms may vary among facilities; specific organisms are required to be reported to local, state, and national departments of health.

INTERFERING FACTORS
- Contamination with oral flora may invalidate results.
- Specimen collection after antibiotic therapy has been initiated may result in inhibited or no growth of organisms.

NURSING IMPLICATIONS AND PROCEDURE

PRETEST:
- Positively identify the patient using at least two unique identifiers before providing care, treatment, or services.
- *Patient Teaching:* Inform the patient this test can assist in identification of the organism causing infection.
- Obtain a history of the patient's complaints, including a list of known allergens, especially allergies or sensitivities to latex.
- Obtain a history of the patient's immune and respiratory systems, symptoms, and results of previously performed laboratory tests and diagnostic and surgical procedures.
- Obtain a list of the patient's current medications, including herbs, nutritional supplements, and nutraceuticals (see Appendix F).
- Note any recent medications that can interfere with test results.

- Review the procedure with the patient. In cases of acute epiglottitis, do not swab the throat. This can cause a laryngospasm resulting in a loss of airway. A patient with epiglottitis will be sitting up and leaning forward in the tripod position with the head and jaw thrust forward to breathe. Address concerns about pain and explain that there may be some discomfort during the specimen collection. The time it takes to collect a proper specimen varies according to the level of cooperation of the patient. Inform the patient that specimen collection takes approximately 5 min.
- There are no food or fluid restrictions unless by medical direction.
- *Sensitivity to social and cultural issues,* as well as concern for modesty, is important in providing psychological support before, during, and after the procedure.

INTRATEST:
- Ensure that the patient has complied with medication restrictions prior to the procedure.
- Have emergency equipment readily available. Keep resuscitation equipment on hand in case of respiratory impairment or laryngospasm after the procedure.
- Instruct the patient to cooperate fully and to follow directions. Direct the patient to breathe normally and to avoid unnecessary movement.
- Observe standard precautions, and follow the general guidelines in Appendix A. Positively identify the patient, and label the appropriate collection containers with the corresponding patient demographics, date and time of collection, and any medication the patient is taking that may interfere with test results (e.g., antibiotics).
- To collect the throat culture, tilt the patient's head back. Swab both tonsillar pillars and oropharynx with the sterile Culturette. A tongue depressor can be used to ensure that contact with the tongue and uvula is avoided.

C

- A nasopharyngeal specimen is collected through the use of a flexible probe inserted through the nose and directed toward the back of the throat.
- Place the swab in the Culturette tube and squeeze the bottom of the Culturette tube to release the liquid transport medium. Ensure that the end of the swab is immersed in the liquid transport medium.
- Promptly transport the specimen to the laboratory for processing and analysis.

POST-TEST:

- A report of the results will be sent to the requesting HCP, who will discuss the results with the patient.
- Instruct the patient to resume usual medication as directed by the HCP.
- Instruct the patient to notify the HCP immediately if difficulty in breathing or swallowing occurs or if bleeding occurs.
- Instruct the patient to perform mouth care after the specimen has been obtained.
- Provide comfort measures and treatment such as antiseptic gargles; inhalants; and warm, moist applications as needed. A cool beverage may aid in relieving throat irritation caused by coughing or suctioning.
- Administer antibiotic therapy if ordered. Remind the patient of the importance of completing the entire course of antibiotic therapy, even if signs and symptoms disappear before completion of therapy.
- *Nutritional Considerations:* Dehydration can been seen in patients with a bacterial throat infection due to pain with swallowing. Pain medications

reduce patient's dysphagia and allow for adequate intake of fluids and foods.

- Recognize anxiety related to test results. Discuss the implications of abnormal test results on the patient's lifestyle. Provide teaching and information regarding the clinical implications of the test results, as appropriate.
- Reinforce information given by the patient's HCP regarding further testing, treatment, or referral to another HCP. Instruct the patient to use lozenges or gargle for throat discomfort. Inform the patient of smoking cessation programs as appropriate. Emphasize the importance of reporting continued signs and symptoms of the infection. Provide information regarding vaccine-preventable diseases where indicated (e.g., diphtheria, hepatitis B, HPV, influenza, measles, mumps, pertussis, pneumococcal, rubella). Answer any questions or address any concerns voiced by the patient or family.
- Depending on the results of this procedure, additional testing may be performed to evaluate or monitor progression of the disease process and determine the need for a change in therapy. Evaluate test results in relation to the patient's symptoms and other tests performed.

RELATED MONOGRAPHS:

- Related tests include CBC and group A streptococcal (rapid) screen.
- Refer to the Immune and Respiratory systems tables at the end of the book for related tests by body system.

Culture, Bacterial, Urine

SYNONYM/ACRONYM: Routine urine culture.

COMMON USE: To identify the pathogenic bacterial organisms in the urine as an indicator for appropriate therapeutic interventions to treat urinary tract infections.

SPECIMEN: Urine (5 mL) collected in a sterile plastic collection container. Transport tubes containing a preservative are highly recommended if testing will not occur within 2 hr of collection.

REFERENCE VALUE: (Method: Culture on selective and enriched media) Negative: no growth.

DESCRIPTION: A urine culture involves collecting a urine specimen so that the organism causing disease can be isolated and identified. Urine can be collected by clean catch, urinary catheterization, or suprapubic aspiration. The severity of the infection or contamination of the specimen can be determined by knowing the type and number of organisms (colonies) present in the specimen. The laboratory will initiate sensitivity testing if indicated by test results. Sensitivity testing identifies the antibiotics to which the organisms are susceptible to ensure an effective treatment plan.

Commonly detected organisms are those normally found in the genitourinary tract, including *Enterococci*, *Escherichia coli*, *Klebsiella*, *Proteus*, and *Pseudomonas*. A culture showing multiple organisms indicates a contaminated specimen.

Colony counts of 100,000/mL or more indicate urinary tract infection (UTI).

Colony counts of 1,000/mL or less suggest contamination resulting from poor collection technique.

Colony counts between 1,000 and 10,000/mL may be significant depending on a variety of factors, including patient's age, gender, number of types of organisms present, method of specimen collection, and presence of antibiotics.

INDICATIONS
- Assist in the diagnosis of suspected UTI
- Determine the sensitivity of significant organisms to antibiotics
- Monitor the response to UTI treatment

POTENTIAL DIAGNOSIS

Positive findings in
- UTIs

Negative findings in: N/A

CRITICAL FINDINGS
- Extended spectrum beta lactamases (ESBL) *E. coli* or *Klebsiella*
- *Legionella*
- Vancomycin-resistant *Enterococci* (VRE)

Note and immediately report to the health-care provider (HCP) positive results and related symptoms. Lists of specific organisms may vary among facilities; specific organisms are required to be reported to local, state, and national departments of health.

INTERFERING FACTORS

• Antibiotic therapy initiated before specimen collection may produce false-negative results.

• Improper collection techniques may result in specimen contamination.

• Specimen storage for longer than 2 hr at room temperature or 24 hr at refrigerated temperature may result in overgrowth of bacteria and false-positive results. Such specimens may be rejected for analysis.

• Results of urine culture are often interpreted along with routine urinalysis findings.

• Discrepancies between culture and urinalysis may be reason to re-collect the specimen.

• Specimens submitted in expired urine transport tubes will be rejected for analysis.

NURSING IMPLICATIONS AND PROCEDURE

PRETEST:

▶ Positively identify the patient using at least two unique identifiers before providing care, treatment, or services.

▶ *Patient Teaching:* Inform the patient this test can assist in identification of the organism causing infection.

▶ Obtain a history of the patient's complaints, including a list of known allergens.

▶ Obtain a history of the patient's genitourinary and immune systems, symptoms, and results of previously performed laboratory tests and diagnostic and surgical procedures.

▶ Obtain a list of the patient's current medications, including herbs, nutritional supplements, and nutraceuticals (see Appendix F).

▶ Note any recent medications that can interfere with test results.

▶ Review the procedure with the patient. Address concerns about pain and explain that there should be no discomfort during the specimen collection. Inform the patient that specimen collection depends on patient cooperation and usually takes approximately 5 to 10 min.

▶ *Sensitivity to social and cultural issues,* as well as concern for modesty, is important in providing psychological support before, during, and after the procedure.

▶ There are no food or fluid restrictions, unless by medical direction.

▶ Instruct the patient on clean-catch procedure and provide necessary supplies.

INTRATEST:

▶ Ensure that the patient has complied with medication restrictions prior to the procedure.

▶ Instruct the patient to cooperate fully and to follow directions. Direct the patient to breathe normally and to avoid unnecessary movement.

▶ Observe standard precautions, and follow the general guidelines in Appendix A. Positively identify the patient, and label the appropriate collection containers with the corresponding patient demographics, date and time of collection, method of specimen collection, and any medications the patient has taken that may interfere with test results (e.g., antibiotics).

Clean-Catch Specimen

▶ Instruct the male patient to (1) thoroughly wash his hands, (2) cleanse the meatus, (3) void a small amount into the toilet, and (4) void directly into the specimen container.

▶ Instruct the female patient to (1) thoroughly wash her hands; (2) cleanse the labia from front to back; (3) while keeping the labia separated, void a small amount into the toilet; and (4) without interrupting the urine stream, void directly into the specimen container.

Pediatric Urine Collector

Put on gloves. Appropriately cleanse the genital area, and allow the area to dry. Remove the covering over the adhesive strips on the collector bag and apply over the genital area. Diaper the child. When specimen is obtained, place the entire collection bag in a sterile urine container.

Indwelling Catheter

Put on gloves. Empty drainage tube of urine. It may be necessary to clamp off the catheter for 15 to 30 min before specimen collection. Cleanse specimen port with antiseptic swab, and then aspirate 5 mL of urine with a 21- to 25-gauge needle and syringe. Transfer urine to a sterile container.

Urinary Catheterization

Place female patient in lithotomy position or male patient in supine position. Using sterile technique, open the straight urinary catheterization kit and perform urinary catheterization. Place the retained urine in a sterile specimen container.

Suprapubic Aspiration

Place the patient in supine position. Cleanse the area with antiseptic, and drape with sterile drapes. A needle is inserted through the skin into the bladder. A syringe attached to the needle is used to aspirate the urine sample. The needle is then removed and a sterile dressing is applied to the site. Place the sterile sample in a sterile specimen container.

Do not collect urine from the pouch from a patient with a urinary diversion (e.g., ileal conduit). Instead, perform catheterization through the stoma.

General

Promptly transport the specimen to the laboratory for processing and analysis. If a delay in transport is expected, an aliquot of the specimen into a special tube containing a preservative is recommended. Urine transport tubes can be requested from the laboratory.

POST-TEST:

A report of the results will be sent to the requesting HCP, who will discuss the results with the patient.

Instruct the patient to resume usual medication as directed by the HCP.

Instruct the patient to report symptoms such as pain related to tissue inflammation, pain or irritation during void, bladder spasms, or alterations in urinary elimination.

Observe for signs of inflammation if the specimen is obtained by suprapubic aspiration.

Administer antibiotic therapy as ordered. Remind the patient of the importance of completing the entire course of antibiotic therapy, even if signs and symptoms disappear before completion of therapy.

Nutritional Considerations: Instruct the patient to increase water consumption by drinking 8 to 12 glasses of water to assist in flushing the urinary tract. Instruct the patient to avoid alcohol, caffeine, and carbonated beverages, which can cause bladder irritation.

Prevention of UTIs includes increasing daily water consumption, urinating when urge occurs, wiping the perineal area from front to back after urination/defecation, and urinating immediately after intercourse. Prevention also includes maintaining the normal flora of the body. Patients should avoid using spermicidal creams with diaphragms or condoms (when recommended by an HCP), becoming constipated, douching, taking bubble baths, wearing tight-fitting garments, and using deodorizing feminine hygiene products that alter the body's normal flora and increase susceptibility to UTIs.

Recognize anxiety related to test results. Discuss the implications of abnormal test results on the patient's lifestyle. Provide teaching and information regarding the clinical implications of the test results, as appropriate.

Reinforce information given by the patient's HCP regarding further testing, treatment, or referral to another HCP. Emphasize the importance of reporting continued signs and symptoms of the infection. Instruct patient on the proper technique for wiping the perineal area (front to back) after a bowel movement. Answer any questions or address any concerns voiced by the patient or family.

▶ Depending on the results of this procedure, additional testing may be performed to evaluate or monitor progression of the disease process and determine the need for a change in therapy. Evaluate test results in relation to the patient's symptoms and other tests performed.

RELATED MONOGRAPHS:

▶ Related tests include CBC, CBC WBC count and differential, cystometry, cystoscopy, cystourethrography voiding, cytology urine, Gram stain, renogram, and UA.

▶ Refer to the Genitourinary and Immune systems tables at the end of the book for related tests by body system.

Culture, Fungal

SYNONYM/ACRONYM: N/A.

COMMON USE: To identify the pathogenic fungal organisms causing infection.

SPECIMEN: Hair, skin, nail, pus, sterile fluids, blood, bone marrow, stool, bronchial washings, sputum, or tissue samples collected in a sterile plastic, tightly capped container.

REFERENCE VALUE: (Method: Culture on selective media; macroscopic and microscopic examination) No presence of fungi.

DESCRIPTION: Fungi, organisms that normally live in soil, can be introduced into humans through the accidental inhalation of spores or inoculation of spores into tissue through trauma. Individuals most susceptible to fungal infection usually are debilitated by chronic disease, are receiving prolonged antibiotic therapy, or have impaired immune systems. Fungal diseases may be classified according to the involved tissue type: dermatophytoses involve superficial and cutaneous tissue; there are also subcutaneous and systemic mycoses.

INDICATIONS

- Determine antimicrobial sensitivity of the organism
- Isolate and identify organisms responsible for nail infections or abnormalities
- Isolate and identify organisms responsible for skin eruptions, drainage, or other evidence of infection

POTENTIAL DIAGNOSIS

Positive findings in
- Blood
  Candida albicans
  Histoplasma capsulatum

- Cerebrospinal fluid
  Coccidioides immitis

Cryptococcus neoformans
Members of the order Mucorales
Paracoccidioides brasiliensis
Sporothrix schenckii

- Hair
  Epidermophyton
  Microsporum
  Trichophyton

- Nails
  C. albicans
  Cephalosporium
  Epidermophyton
  Trichophyton

- Skin
  Actinomyces israelii
  C. albicans
  C. immitis
  Epidermophyton
  Microsporum
  Trichophyton

- Tissue
  A. israelii
  Aspergillus
  C. albicans
  Nocardia
  P. brasiliensis

CRITICAL FINDINGS ✦

- Positive findings in any sterile body fluid such as blood or cerebrospinal fluid

Note and immediately report to the health-care provider (HCP) positive results and related symptoms. Lists of specific organisms may vary among facilities; specific organisms are required to be reported to local, state, and national departments of health.

INTERFERING FACTORS

Prompt and proper specimen processing, storage, and analysis are important to achieve accurate results.

NURSING IMPLICATIONS AND PROCEDURE

PRETEST:

- Positively identify the patient using at least two unique identifiers before providing care, treatment, or services.
- *Patient Teaching:* Inform the patient this test can assist in identification of the organism causing infection.
- Obtain a history of the patient's complaints, including a list of known allergens.
- Obtain a history of the patient's immune system, symptoms, and results of previously performed laboratory tests and diagnostic and surgical procedures.
- Obtain a list of the patient's current medications, including herbs, nutritional supplements, and nutraceuticals (see Appendix F).
- Note any recent medications that can interfere with test results.
- Review the procedure with the patient. Inform the patient that specimen collection takes approximately 5 min. Address concerns about pain and explain that there may be some discomfort during the specimen collection.
- *Sensitivity to social and cultural issues,* as well as concern for modesty, is important in providing psychological support before, during, and after the procedure.
- There are no food or fluid restrictions unless by medical direction.

INTRATEST:

- Instruct the patient to cooperate fully and to follow directions. Direct the patient to breathe normally and to avoid unnecessary movement.
- Observe standard precautions, and follow the general guidelines in Appendix A. Instructions regarding the appropriate transport materials for blood, bone marrow, bronchial washings, sputum, sterile fluids, stool, and tissue samples should be obtained from the laboratory. Positively identify the patient, and label the appropriate collection containers with the

corresponding patient demographics, date, and time of collection.

▶ Promptly transport the specimen to the laboratory for processing and analysis.

Skin

▶ Clean the collection site with 70% alcohol. Scrape the peripheral margin of the collection site with a sterile scalpel or wooden spatula. Place the scrapings in a sterile collection container.

Hair

▶ Fungi usually grow at the base of the hair shaft. Infected hairs can be identified by using a Wood's lamp in a darkened room. A Wood's lamp provides rays of ultraviolet light at a wavelength of 366 nm, or 3,660 Å. Infected hairs fluoresce a bright yellow-green when exposed to light from the Wood's lamp. Using tweezers, pluck hair from skin.

Nails

▶ Ideally, softened material from the nailbed is sampled from beneath the nail plate. Alternatively, shavings from the deeper portions of the nail itself can be collected.

▶ The potassium hydroxide (KOH) test is used to indicate the presence of mycelium, mycelial fragments, spores, or budding yeast cells. A portion of the specimen is mixed with 15% KOH on a glass slide, and then the slide is covered and gently heated briefly. The slide is examined under a microscope for the presence of fungal elements.

POST-TEST:

▶ A report of the results will be sent to the requesting HCP, who will discuss the results with the patient.

▶ Instruct patient to begin antifungal therapy, as prescribed. Instruct the patient in the importance of completing the entire course of antifungal therapy even if no symptoms are present.

▶ Recognize anxiety related to test results. Discuss the implications of abnormal test results on the patient's lifestyle. Provide teaching and information regarding the clinical implications of the test results, as appropriate.

▶ Reinforce information given by the patient's HCP regarding further testing, treatment, or referral to another HCP. Emphasize the importance of reporting continued signs and symptoms of the infection. Answer any questions or address any concerns voiced by the patient or family.

▶ Depending on the results of this procedure, additional testing may be performed to evaluate or monitor progression of the disease process and determine the need for a change in therapy. Evaluate test results in relation to the patient's symptoms and other tests performed.

RELATED MONOGRAPHS:

▶ Related tests include relevant biopsies (lung, lymph node, skin), bronchoscopy, cultures (blood, mycobacteria, throat, sputum, viral), CSF analysis, gallium scan, HIV-1/2 antibodies, pulmonary function tests, and TB tests.

▶ Refer to the Immune System table at the end of the book for related tests by body system.

Culture, Viral

SYNONYM/ACRONYM: N/A.

COMMON USE: To identify infection caused by pathogenic viral organisms as evidenced by ocular, genitourinary, intestinal, or respiratory symptoms. Common diagnoses are HIV, respiratory syncytial virus (RSV), Epstein-Barr virus, cytomegalovirus (CMV), meningitis, herpes simplex, varicella zoster, and shingles.

SPECIMEN: Urine, semen, blood, body fluid, stool, tissue, or swabs from the affected site.

REFERENCE VALUE: (Method: Culture in special media, enzyme-linked immunoassays, direct fluorescent antibody techniques, latex agglutination, immunoperoxidase techniques) No virus isolated.

DESCRIPTION: Viruses, the most common cause of human infection, are submicroscopic organisms that invade living cells. They can be classified as either RNA- or DNA-type viruses. Viral titers are highest in the early stages of disease before the host has begun to manufacture significant antibodies against the invader. Specimens need to be collected as early as possible in the disease process.

INDICATIONS

Assist in the identification of viral infection

POTENTIAL DIAGNOSIS

Positive findings in

- AIDS
  HIV

- Acute respiratory failure
  Hantavirus

- Anorectal infections
  Herpes simplex virus (HSV)
  Human papillomavirus (HPV)

- Bronchitis
  Parainfluenza virus
  Respiratory syncytial virus (RSV)

- Cervical cancer
  Human papillomavirus

- Condylomata
  Human papillomavirus

- Conjunctivitis/keratitis
  Adenovirus
  Epstein-Barr virus
  HSV
  Measles virus

  Parvovirus
  Rubella virus
  Varicella zoster virus

- Croup
  Parainfluenza virus
  RSV

- Cutaneous infection with rash
  Enteroviruses
  HSV
  Varicella zoster virus

- Encephalitis
  Enteroviruses
  Flaviviruses
  HSV
  HIV
  Measles virus
  Rabies virus
  Togaviruses
  West Nile virus (mosquito-borne arbovirus)

- Febrile illness with rash
  Coxsackieviruses
  Echovirus

- Gastroenteritis
  Norwalk virus
  Rotavirus

- Genital herpes
  HSV-1
  HSV-2

- Genital warts
  HPV

- Hemorrhagic cystitis
  Adenovirus

- Hemorrhagic fever
  Ebola virus
  Hantavirus
  Lassa virus
  Marburg virus

- Herpangina
  Coxsackievirus (group A)

- Infectious mononucleosis
  Cytomegalovirus
  Epstein-Barr virus

- Meningitis
  Coxsackieviruses
  Echovirus
  HSV-2
  Lymphocytic choriomeningitis virus

- Myocarditis/pericarditis
  Coxsackievirus
  Echovirus

- Parotitis
  Mumps virus
  Parainfluenza virus

- Pharyngitis
  Adenovirus
  Coxsackievirus (group A)
  Epstein-Barr virus
  HSV
  H1N1 influenza virus (swine flu)
  Influenza virus
  Parainfluenza virus
  Rhinovirus

- Pleurodynia
  Coxsackievirus (group B)

- Pneumonia
  Adenovirus
  H1N1 influenza virus (swine flu)
  Influenza virus
  Parainfluenza virus
  RSV

- Upper respiratory tract infection
  Adenovirus
  Coronavirus
  H1N1 influenza virus (swine flu)
  Influenza virus
  Parainfluenza virus
  RSV
  Rhinovirus

CRITICAL FINDINGS

Positive RSV, influenza, and varicella zoster cultures should be reported immediately to the requesting health-care provider (HCP).

Note and immediately report to the HCP positive results and related

symptoms. Lists of specific organisms may vary among facilities; specific organisms are required to be reported to local, state, and national departments of health.

INTERFERING FACTORS

Viral specimens are unstable. Prompt and proper specimen processing, storage, and analysis are important to achieve accurate results.

NURSING IMPLICATIONS AND PROCEDURE

PRETEST:

- Positively identify the patient using at least two unique identifiers before providing care, treatment, or services.
- *Patient Teaching:* Inform the patient this test can assist in identification of the organism causing infection.
- Obtain a history of the patient's complaints, including a list of known allergens, especially allergies or sensitivities to latex.
- Obtain a history of the patient's gastro-intestinal, genitourinary, immune, reproductive, and respiratory systems; symptoms; and results of previously performed laboratory tests and diagnostic and surgical procedures.
- Obtain a list of the patient's current medications, including herbs, nutritional supplements, and nutraceuticals (see Appendix F).
- Note any recent medications that can interfere with test results.
- Review the procedure with the patient. Inform the patient that specimen collection takes approximately 5 min. Address concerns about pain and explain that there may be some discomfort during the specimen collection.
- There are no food, fluid, or medication restrictions unless by medical direction.
- *Sensitivity to social and cultural issues*, as well as concern for modesty, is important in providing psychological support before, during, and after the procedure.

C

INTRATEST:

▶ Instruct the patient to cooperate fully and to follow directions. Direct the patient to breathe normally and to avoid unnecessary movement.

▶ Observe standard precautions, and follow the general guidelines in Appendix A. Positively identify the patient, and label the appropriate collection containers with the corresponding patient demographics, date and time of collection, exact site, contact person for notification of results, and other pertinent information (e.g., patient immunocompromised owing to organ transplant, radiation, or chemotherapy).

▶ Instructions regarding the appropriate transport materials for blood, bronchial washings, sputum, sterile fluids, stool, and tissue samples should be obtained from the laboratory. The type of applicator used to obtain swabs should be verified by consultation with the testing laboratory personnel.

▶ The appropriate viral transport material should be obtained from the laboratory. Nasopharyngeal washings or swabs for RSV testing should be immediately placed in cold viral transport media.

▶ Promptly transport the specimen to the laboratory for processing and analysis.

POST-TEST:

▶ A report of the results will be sent to the requesting HCP, who will discuss the results with the patient.

▶ *Nutritional Considerations:* Dehydration can been seen in patients with viral infections due to loss of fluids through fever, diarrhea, and/or vomiting. Antipyretic medication includes acetaminophen to decrease fever and allow for adequate intake of fluids and foods. Do not give acetylsalicylic acid to pediatric patients with a viral illness because it increases the risk of Reye's syndrome.

▶ *Sensitivity to social and cultural issues:* Offer support, as appropriate, to patients who may be the victims of rape or sexual assault. Educate the patient regarding access to counseling services. Provide a nonjudgmental, nonthreatening atmosphere for discussing the risks of sexually transmitted diseases. It is also important to address problems the patient may experience (e.g., guilt, depression, anger).

▶ Recognize anxiety related to test results. Discuss the implications of abnormal test results on the patient's lifestyle. Provide teaching and information regarding the clinical implications of the test results, as appropriate.

▶ Reinforce information given by the patient's HCP regarding further testing, treatment, or referral to another HCP. Provide information regarding vaccine-preventable diseases where indicated (e.g., encephalitis, hepatitis A and B, HPV, influenza, measles, mumps, polio, rubella, smallpox, varicella, yellow fever). Answer any questions or address any concerns voiced by the patient or family.

▶ Depending on the results of this procedure, additional testing may be performed to evaluate or monitor progression of the disease process and determine the need for a change in therapy. Evaluate test results in relation to the patient's symptoms and other tests performed.

RELATED MONOGRAPHS:

▶ Related tests include alveolar/arterial gradient, β-2-microglobulin, barium enema, biopsy (cervical, intestinal, kidney, liver, lung, lymph node, muscle, skin), blood gases, bronchoscopy, CD4/CD8 ratio, CSF analysis, *Chlamydia* group antibody, chest x-ray, cultures (anal, blood, ear, eye, fungal, genital, mycobacteria, skin, sputum, stool, throat, urine, wound), CBC, cytology (sputum, urine), gallium scan, gastric emptying scan, lung perfusion scan, lung ventilation scan, Pap smear, pericardial fluid analysis, plethysmography, pulse oximetry, PFT, slit-lamp biomicroscopy, syphilis serology, TB tests, and viral serology tests (hepatitis, HIV, HTLV, infectious mononucleosis, mumps, rubella, rubeola, varicella).

▶ Refer to the Gastrointestinal, Genitourinary, Immune, Reproductive, and Respiratory systems tables at the end of the book for related tests by body system.

Cystometry

SYNONYM/ACRONYM: CMG, urodynamic testing of bladder function.

COMMON USE: To assess bladder function related to obstruction, neurogenic pathology, and infection including evaluation of surgical, and medical management.

AREA OF APPLICATION: Bladder, urethra.

CONTRAST: None.

DESCRIPTION: Cystometry evaluates the motor and sensory function of the bladder when incontinence is present or neurological bladder dysfunction is suspected and monitors the effects of treatment for the abnormalities. This noninvasive manometric study measures the bladder pressure and volume characteristics in milliliters of water (cm H_2O) during the filling and emptying phases. The test provides information about bladder structure and function that can lead to uninhibited bladder contractions, sensations of bladder fullness and need to void, and ability to inhibit voiding. These abnormalities cause incontinence and other impaired patterns of micturition. Cystometry can be performed with cystoscopy and sphincter electromyography.

INDICATIONS
- Detect congenital urinary abnormalities
- Determine cause of bladder dysfunction and pathology
- Determine cause of recurrent urinary tract infections (UTIs)
- Determine cause of urinary retention

- Determine type of incontinence: *functional* (involuntary and unpredictable), *reflex* (involuntary when a specific volume is reached), *stress* (weak pelvic muscles), *total* (continuous and unpredictable), *urge* (involuntary when urgency is sensed), and *psychological* (e.g., dementia, confusion affecting awareness)
- Determine type of neurogenic bladder (motor or sensory)
- Evaluate the management of neurological bladder before surgical intervention
- Evaluate postprostatectomy incontinence
- Evaluate signs and symptoms of urinary elimination pattern dysfunction
- Evaluate urinary obstruction in male patients experiencing urinary retention
- Evaluate the usefulness of drug therapy on detrusor muscle function and tonicity and on internal and external sphincter function
- Evaluate voiding disorders associated with spinal cord injury

POTENTIAL DIAGNOSIS

Normal findings in
- Absence of residual urine (0 mL)
- Normal sensory perception of bladder fullness, desire to void,

and ability to inhibit urination; appropriate response to temperature (hot and cold)
- Normal bladder capacity: 350 to 750 mL for men and 250 to 550 mL for women
- Normal functioning bladder pressure: 8 to 15 cm H_2O
- Normal sensation of fullness: 40 to 100 cm H_2O or 300 to 500 mL
- Normal bladder pressure during voiding: 30 to 40 cm H_2O
- Normal detrusor pressure: less than 10 cm H_2O
- Normal urge to void: 150 to 450 mL
- Normal filling pattern
- Urethral pressure that is higher than bladder pressure, ensuring continence

Abnormal findings in
- Flaccid bladder that fills without contracting
- Inability to perceive bladder fullness
- Inability to initiate or maintain urination without applying external pressure
- Sensory or motor paralysis of bladder
- Total loss of conscious sensation and vesical control or uncontrollable micturition (incontinence)

CRITICAL FINDINGS: N/A

INTERFERING FACTORS

This procedure is contraindicated for
- Patients with acute UTIs because the study can cause infection to spread to the kidneys.
- Patients who are pregnant or suspected of being pregnant, unless the potential benefits of the procedure far outweigh the risks to the fetus and mother.
- Patients with urethral obstruction.

- Patients with cervical cord lesions because they may exhibit autonomic dysreflexia, as seen by bradycardia, flushing, hypertension, diaphoresis, and headache.
- Inability to catheterize the patient.

Factors that may impair the results of the examination
- Inability of the patient to cooperate or remain still during the procedure because of age, significant pain, or mental status.
- Inability of the patient to void in a supine position or straining to void during the study.
- A high level of patient anxiety or embarrassment, which may interfere with the study, making it difficult to distinguish whether the results are due to stress or organic pathology.
- Administration of drugs that affect bladder function, such as muscle relaxants or antihistamines.

NURSING IMPLICATIONS AND PROCEDURE

PRETEST:
- Positively identify the patient using at least two unique identifiers before providing care, treatment, or services.
- *Patient Teaching:* Inform the patient this procedure can assist in assessing bladder function.
- Obtain a history of the patient's complaints including a list of known allergens, especially allergies or sensitivities to latex, iodine, seafood, contrast medium, anesthetics, and dyes.
- Obtain a history of the patient's genitourinary system, symptoms, and results of previously performed laboratory tests and diagnostic and surgical procedures.
- Ensure results of coagulation and urinalysis testing are obtained and recorded prior to the procedure.
- Record the date of the last menstrual period and determine the possibility of pregnancy in perimenopausal women.

C

▶ Obtain a list of the patient's current medications, including anticoagulants, aspirin and other salicylates, herbs, nutritional supplements, and nutraceuticals (see Appendix F). Note the last time and dose of medication taken.

▶ Review the procedure with the patient. Address concerns about pain and explain that there may be moments of discomfort and some pain experienced during the test. Inform the patient that the procedure is performed in a special urology room or in a clinic setting by the health-care provider (HCP), with support staff, and takes approximately 30 to 45 min.

▶ *Sensitivity to social and cultural issues,* as well as concern for modesty, is important in providing psychological support before, during, and after the procedure.

▶ Instruct the patient to report pain, sweating, nausea, headache, and the urge to void during the study.

▶ Instruct the patient to remove jewelry and other metallic objects in the area to be examined.

▶ There are no food, fluid, or medication restrictions unless by medical direction.

▶ *Make sure a written and informed consent has been signed prior to the procedure and before administering any medications.*

INTRATEST:

▶ Ensure that the patient has removed all external metallic objects from the area to be examined prior to the procedure.

▶ Instruct the patient to change into the gown, robe, and foot coverings provided, but not to void.

▶ Position the patient in a supine or lithotomy position on the examination table. If spinal cord injury is present, the patient can remain on a stretcher in a supine position and be draped appropriately.

▶ Ask the patient to void. During voiding, note characteristics such as start time; force and continuity of the stream; volume voided; presence of dribbling, straining, or hesitancy; and stop time.

▶ Instruct the patient to cooperate fully and to follow directions. Instruct the patient to remain still during the procedure.

▶ Observe standard precautions, and follow the general guidelines in Appendix A.

▶ A urinary catheter is inserted into the bladder under sterile conditions, and residual urine is measured and recorded. A test for sensory response to temperature is done by instilling 30 mL of room-temperature sterile water followed by 30 mL of warm sterile water. Sensations are assessed and recorded.

▶ Fluid is removed from the bladder, and the catheter is connected to a custometer that measures the pressure. Sterile normal saline, distilled water, or carbon dioxide gas is instilled in controlled amounts into the bladder. When the client indicates the urge to void, the bladder is considered full. The patient is instructed to void, and urination amounts as well as start and stop times are then recorded.

▶ Pressure and volume readings are recorded and graphed for response to heat, full bladder, urge to void, and ability to inhibit voiding. The patient is requested to void without straining, and pressures are taken and recorded during this activity.

▶ After completion of voiding, the bladder is emptied of any other fluid, and the catheter is withdrawn, unless further testing is planned.

▶ Further testing may be done to determine if abnormal bladder function is being caused by muscle incompetence or interruption in innervation; anticholinergic medication (e.g., atropine) or cholinergic medication (e.g., bethanechol [Urecholine]) can be injected and the study repeated in 20 or 30 min.

POST-TEST:

▶ A report of the examination will be sent to the requesting HCP, who will discuss the results with the patient.

▶ Monitor fluid intake and urinary output for 24 hr after the procedure.

▶ Monitor vital signs after the procedure every 15 min for 2 hr or as directed. Monitor intake and output at least every 8 hr. Elevated temperature may indicate infection. Notify the HCP if temperature is elevated. Protocols may vary among facilities.

- Instruct the patient to immediately report symptoms such as fast heart rate, difficulty breathing, skin rash, itching, chest pain, persistent right shoulder pain, or abdominal pain. Immediately report symptoms to the appropriate HCP.
- Inform the patient that he or she may experience burning or discomfort on urination for a few voidings after the procedure.
- Persistent flank or suprapubic pain, fever, chills, blood in the urine, difficulty urinating, or change in urinary pattern must be reported immediately to the HCP.
- Recognize anxiety related to test results. Discuss the implications of abnormal test results on the patient's lifestyle. Provide teaching and information regarding the clinical implications of the test results, as appropriate.

- Reinforce information given by the patient's HCP regarding further testing, treatment, or referral to another HCP. Answer any questions or address any concerns voiced by the patient or family.
- Depending on the results of this procedure, additional testing may be needed to evaluate or monitor progression of the disease process and determine the need for a change in therapy. Evaluate test results in relation to the patient's symptoms and other tests performed.

RELATED MONOGRAPHS:

- Related tests include bladder cancer markers, calculus kidney stone panel, *Chlamydia* group antibody, CBC, CBC hematocrit, CBC hemoglobin, CT pelvis, culture urine, cytology urine, IVP, MRI pelvis, PT/INR, US pelvis, and UA.
- Refer to the Genitourinary System table at the end of the book for related tests by body system.

Cystoscopy

SYNONYM/ACRONYM: Cystoureterography, prostatography.

COMMON USE: To assess the urinary tract for bleeding, cancer, tumor, and prostate health.

AREA OF APPLICATION: Bladder, urethra, ureteral orifices.

CONTRAST: None.

DESCRIPTION: Cystoscopy provides direct visualization of the urethra, urinary bladder, and ureteral orifices—areas not usually visible with x-ray procedures. This procedure is also used to obtain specimens and treat pathology associated with the aforementioned structures. Cystoscopy is accomplished by transurethral insertion of a cystoscope into the bladder. Rigid cystoscopes contain an obturator and a telescope with a lens and light system; there are also flexible cystoscopes, which use fiberoptic technology. The procedure may be performed during or after ultrasonography or radiography, or during urethroscopy or retrograde pyelography.

C

INDICATIONS
- Coagulate bleeding areas
- Determine the possible source of persistent urinary tract infections
- Determine the source of hematuria of unknown cause
- Differentiate, through tissue biopsy, between benign and cancerous lesions involving the bladder
- Dilate the urethra and ureters
- Evacuate blood clots and perform fulguration of bleeding sites within the lower urinary tract
- Evaluate changes in urinary elimination patterns
- Evaluate the extent of prostatic hyperplasia and degree of obstruction
- Evaluate the function of each kidney by obtaining urine samples via ureteral catheters
- Evaluate urinary tract abnormalities such as dysuria, frequency, retention, inadequate stream, urgency, and incontinence
- Identify and remove polyps and small tumors (including by fulguration) from the bladder
- Identify congenital anomalies, such as duplicate ureters, ureteroceles, urethral or ureteral strictures, diverticula, and areas of inflammation or ulceration
- Implant radioactive seeds
- Place ureteral catheters to drain urine from the renal pelvis or for retrograde pyelography
- Place ureteral stents and resect prostate gland tissue (transurethral resection of the prostate)
- Remove renal calculi from the bladder or ureters
- Resect small tumors

POTENTIAL DIAGNOSIS

Normal findings in
- Normal ureter, bladder, and urethral structure

Abnormal findings in
- Diverticulum of the bladder, fistula, stones, and strictures
- Inflammation or infection
- Obstruction
- Polyps
- Prostatic hypertrophy or hyperplasia
- Renal calculi
- Tumors
- Ureteral or urethral stricture
- Urinary tract malformation and congenital anomalies

CRITICAL FINDINGS: N/A

INTERFERING FACTORS

This procedure is contraindicated for
- Patients who are pregnant or suspected of being pregnant, unless the potential benefits of the procedure far outweigh the risks to the fetus and mother.
- Patients with bleeding disorders because instrumentation may lead to excessive bleeding from the lower urinary tract.
- Patients with acute cystitis or urethritis because instrumentation could allow bacteria to enter the bloodstream, resulting in septicemia.

Factors that may impair the results of the examination
- Inability of the patient to cooperate or remain still during the procedure because of age, significant pain, or mental status.

Other considerations
- Failure to follow dietary restrictions before the procedure may cause the procedure to be canceled or repeated.

NURSING IMPLICATIONS AND PROCEDURE

PRETEST:

▶ Positively identify the patient using at least two unique identifiers before providing care, treatment, or services.

▶ *Patient Teaching:* Inform the patient this procedure can assist in assessing the urinary tract.

▶ Obtain a history of the patient's complaints, including a list of known allergens, especially allergies or sensitivities to latex, iodine, seafood, contrast medium, anesthetics, and dyes.

▶ Obtain a history of results of the patient's genitourinary system, symptoms, and previously performed laboratory tests and diagnostic and surgical procedures.

▶ Record the date of the last menstrual period and determine the possibility of pregnancy in perimenopausal women.

▶ Obtain a list of the patient's current medications, including anticoagulants, aspirin and other salicylates, herbs, nutritional supplements, and nutraceuticals (see Appendix F). Such products should be discontinued by medical direction for the appropriate number of days prior to a surgical procedure. Note the last time and dose of medication taken.

▶ Review the procedure with the patient. Address concerns about pain and explain that there may be moments of discomfort and some pain experienced during the test. Inform the patient that the procedure is usually performed in a special cystoscopy suite near or in the surgery department by a health-care provider (HCP), with support staff, and takes approximately 30 to 60 min.

▶ *Sensitivity to social and cultural issues,* as well as concern for modesty, is important in providing psychological support before, during, and after the procedure.

▶ Restrict food and fluids for 8 hr if the patient is having general or spinal anesthesia. For local anesthesia, allow only clear liquids 8 hr before the procedure. Protocols may vary among facilities.

▶ Obtain and record the patient's vital signs.

▶ *Make sure a written and informed consent has been signed prior to the procedure and before administering any medications.*

INTRATEST:

▶ Ensure that the patient has complied with dietary restrictions; ensure that food has been restricted for at least 8 hr depending on the anesthetic chosen for the procedure.

▶ Administer ordered preoperative sedation.

▶ Instruct the patient to void prior to the procedure and to change into the gown, robe, and foot coverings provided.

▶ Observe standard precautions, and follow the general guidelines in Appendix A. Positively identify the patient, and label the appropriate collection container with the corresponding patient demographics, date, and time of collection.

▶ Position patient on the examination table, draped and with legs in stirrups. If general or spinal anesthesia is to be used, it is administered before positioning the patient on the table.

▶ Cleanse external genitalia with antiseptic solution. If local anesthetic is used, it is instilled into the urethra and retained for 5 to 10 min. A penile clamp may be used for male patients to aid in retention of anesthetic.

▶ The HCP inserts a cystoscope or a urethroscope to examine the urethra before cystoscopy. The urethroscope has a sheath that may be left in place, and the cystoscope is inserted through it, avoiding multiple instrumentations.

▶ After insertion of the cystoscope, a sample of residual urine may be obtained for culture or other analysis.

▶ The bladder is irrigated via an irrigation system attached to the scope. The irrigation fluid aids in bladder visualization.

▶ If a prostatic tumor is found, a biopsy specimen may be obtained by means of a cytology brush or biopsy forceps inserted through the scope. If the tumor is small and localized, it can be excised and fulgurated. This procedure is termed transurethral resection of the bladder. Polyps can also be identified and excised.

▶ Ulcers or bleeding sites can be fulgurated using electrocautery.

▶ Renal calculi can be crushed and removed from the ureters and bladder.

▶ Ureteral catheters can be inserted via the scope to obtain urine samples from each kidney for comparative analysis and radiographic studies.

▶ Ureteral and urethral strictures can also be dilated during this procedure.

▶ Upon completion of the examination and related procedures, the cystoscope is withdrawn.

▶ Place obtained specimens in proper containers, label them properly, and immediately transport them to the laboratory.

POST-TEST:

▶ A report of the examination will be sent to the requesting HCP, who will discuss the results with the patient.

▶ Instruct the patient to resume his or her usual diet and medications, as directed by the HCP.

▶ Encourage the patient to drink increased amounts of fluids (125 mL/hr for 24 hr) after the procedure.

▶ Monitor vital signs and neurological status every 15 min for 1 hr, then every 2 hr for 4 hr, and then as ordered by the HCP. Take the temperature every 4 hr for 24 hr. Monitor intake and output at least every 8 hr. Compare with baseline values. Notify the HCP if temperature is elevated. Protocols may vary among facilities.

▶ Instruct the patient to immediately report symptoms such as fast heart rate, difficulty breathing, skin rash, itching, chest pain, persistent right shoulder pain, or abdominal pain. Immediately report symptoms to the appropriate HCP.

▶ Inform the patient that burning or discomfort on urination can be experienced for a few voidings after the procedure and that the urine may be blood-tinged for the first and second voidings after the procedure.

▶ Persistent flank or suprapubic pain, fever, chills, blood in the urine, difficulty urinating, or change in urinary pattern must be reported immediately to the HCP.

▶ Recognize anxiety related to test results. Discuss the implications of abnormal test results on the patient's lifestyle. Provide teaching and information regarding the clinical implications of the test results, as appropriate.

▶ Reinforce information given by the patient's HCP regarding further testing, treatment, or referral to another HCP. Answer any questions or address any concerns voiced by the patient or family.

▶ Depending on the results of this procedure, additional testing may be needed to evaluate or monitor progression of the disease process and determine the need for a change in therapy. Evaluate test results in relation to the patient's symptoms and other tests performed.

RELATED MONOGRAPHS:

▶ Related tests include biopsy kidney, biopsy prostate, calculus kidney stone panel, *Chlamydia* group antibody, CT pelvis, culture urine, cytology urine, IVP, MRI pelvis, PSA, US pelvis, and UA.

▶ Refer to the Genitourinary System table at the end of the book for related tests by body system.

Cystourethrography, Voiding

SYNONYM/ACRONYM: Voiding cystography (VCU).

COMMON USE: To visualize and assess the bladder during voiding for evaluation of chronic urinary tract infections.

AREA OF APPLICATION: Bladder, urethra.

CONTRAST: Radiopaque iodine-based contrast medium.

DESCRIPTION: Voiding cystourethrography involves visualization of the bladder filled with contrast medium instilled through a catheter by use of a syringe or gravity, and, after the catheter is removed, the excretion of the contrast medium. Excretion or micturition is recorded electronically or on videotape for confirmation or exclusion of ureteral reflux and evaluation of the urethra. Fluoroscopic or plain images may also be taken to record bladder filling and emptying. This procedure is often used to evaluate chronic urinary tract infections (UTIs).

INDICATIONS

- Assess the degree of compromise of a stenotic prostatic urethra
- Assess hypertrophy of the prostate lobes
- Assess ureteral stricture
- Confirm the diagnosis of congenital lower urinary tract anomaly
- Evaluate abnormal bladder emptying and incontinence
- Evaluate the effects of bladder trauma
- Evaluate possible cause of frequent UTIs

- Evaluate the presence and extent of ureteral reflux
- Evaluate the urethra for obstruction and strictures

POTENTIAL DIAGNOSIS

Normal findings in
- Normal bladder and urethra structure and function

Abnormal findings in
- Bladder trauma
- Bladder tumors
- Hematomas
- Neurogenic bladder
- Pelvic tumors
- Prostatic enlargement
- Ureteral stricture
- Ureterocele
- Urethral diverticula
- Vesicoureteral reflux

CRITICAL FINDINGS: N/A

INTERFERING FACTORS

This procedure is contraindicated for

- Patients with allergies to shellfish or iodinated dye. The contrast medium used may cause a life-threatening allergic reaction. Patients with a known hypersensitivity to the contrast medium may benefit from premedication with corticosteroids or the use of nonionic contrast medium.

- Patients with bleeding disorders.
- Patients who are pregnant or suspected of being pregnant, unless the potential benefits of the procedure far outweigh the risks to the fetus and mother.
- Patients with UTI, obstruction, or injury.
- ◈ Elderly and other patients who are chronically dehydrated before the test, because of their risk of contrast-induced renal failure.
- ◈ Patients who are in renal failure.

Factors that may impair clear imaging

- Metallic objects within the examination field, which may inhibit organ visualization and cause unclear images.
- Inability of the patient to cooperate or remain still during the procedure because of age, significant pain, or mental status.
- Gas or feces in the gastrointestinal tract resulting from inadequate cleansing or failure to restrict food intake before the study.
- Retained barium from a previous radiological procedure.

Other considerations

- Consultation with a health-care provider (HCP) should occur before the procedure for radiation safety concerns regarding younger patients or patients who are lactating.
- Risks associated with radiation overexposure can result from frequent x-ray procedures. Personnel in the room with the patient should wear a protective lead apron, stand behind a shield, or leave the area while the examination is being done. Personnel working in the examination area should wear badges to record their level of radiation exposure.

NURSING IMPLICATIONS AND PROCEDURE

PRETEST:

▸ Positively identify the patient using at least two unique identifiers before providing care, treatment, or services.

▸ *Patient Teaching:* Inform the patient this procedure can assist in assessing the urinary tract.

▸ Obtain a history of the patient's complaints, including a list of known allergens, especially allergies or sensitivities to latex, iodine, seafood, contrast medium, anesthetics, and dyes.

▸ Obtain a history of results of the patient's genitourinary system, symptoms, and previously performed laboratory tests and diagnostic and surgical procedures. Ensure that the results of blood tests are obtained and recorded before the procedure, especially coagulation tests, BUN, and creatinine if contrast medium is to be used.

▸ Ensure that this procedure is performed before an upper gastrointestinal study or barium swallow.

▸ Record the date of the last menstrual period and determine the possibility of pregnancy in perimenopausal women.

▸ Obtain a list of the patient's current medications, including anticoagulants, aspirin and other salicylates, herbs, nutritional supplements, and nutraceuticals (see Appendix F). Note the last time and dose of medication taken.

▸ Review the procedure with the patient. Address concerns about pain and explain that there may be moments of discomfort and some pain experienced during the test. Inform the patient that the procedure is usually performed in the radiology department by an HCP, with support staff, and takes approximately 30 to 60 min.

▸ *Sensitivity to social and cultural issues,* as well as concern for modesty, is important in providing psychological support before, during, and after the procedure.

▶ Inform the patient that he or she may receive a laxative the night before the test or an enema or a cathartic the morning of the test, as ordered.

▶ Instruct the patient to increase fluid intake the day before the test and to have only clear fluids 8 hr before the test.

Make sure a written and informed consent has been signed prior to the procedure and before administering any medications.

INTRATEST:

▶ Ensure that the patient has complied with dietary restrictions. Assess for completion of bowel preparation if ordered.

▶ Ensure that the patient has removed all external metallic objects from the area to be examined prior to the procedure.

▶ If the patient has a history of allergic reactions to any substance or drug, administer ordered prophylactic steroids or antihistamines before the procedure.

▶ Have emergency equipment readily available.

▶ Instruct the patient to void prior to the procedure and to change into the gown, robe, and foot coverings provided.

▶ Observe standard precautions, and follow the general guidelines in Appendix A. Instruct the patient to cooperate fully and to follow directions.

▶ Insert a Foley catheter before the procedure, if ordered. Inform the patient that he or she may feel some pressure when the catheter is inserted and when the contrast medium is instilled through the catheter.

▶ Place the patient on the table in a supine or lithotomy position.

▶ A kidney, ureter, and bladder film or plain radiograph is taken to ensure that no barium or stool obscures visualization of the urinary system.

▶ A catheter is filled with contrast medium to eliminate air pockets and is inserted until the balloon reaches the meatus if not previously inserted in the patient.

▶ When three-fourths of the contrast medium has been injected, a radiographic exposure is made while the remainder of the contrast medium is injected.

▶ When the patient is able to void, the catheter is removed and the patient is asked to urinate while images of the bladder and urethra are recorded.

▶ Monitor the patient for complications related to the procedure (e.g., allergic reaction, anaphylaxis, bronchospasm).

POST-TEST:

▶ A report of the examination will be sent to the requesting HCP, who will discuss the results with the patient.

▶ Instruct the patient to resume usual diet and medications, as directed by the HCP.

▶ Monitor vital signs and neurological status every 15 min for 1 hr, then every 2 hr for 4 hr, and then as ordered by the HCP. Take the temperature every 4 hr for 24 hr. Monitor intake and output at least every 8 hr. Compare with baseline values. Notify the HCP if temperature is elevated. Protocols may vary from among facilities.

▶ Monitor for reaction to iodinated contrast medium, including rash, urticaria, tachycardia, hyperpnea, hypertension, palpitations, nausea, or vomiting.

▶ Instruct the patient to immediately report symptoms such as fast heart rate, difficulty breathing, skin rash, itching, chest pain, persistent right shoulder pain, or abdominal pain. Immediately report symptoms to the appropriate HCP.

▶ Maintain the patient on adequate hydration after the procedure. Encourage the patient to drink increased amounts of fluids (125 mL/hr for 24 hr) after the procedure to prevent stasis and bacterial buildup.

▶ Recognize anxiety related to test results. Discuss the implications of abnormal test results on the patient's lifestyle. Provide teaching and information regarding the clinical implications of the test results, as appropriate.

▶ Reinforce information given by the patient's HCP regarding further testing, treatment, or referral to another HCP. Answer any questions or

address any concerns voiced by the patient or family.

- Depending on the results of this procedure, additional testing may be needed to evaluate or monitor progression of the disease process and determine the need for a change in therapy. Evaluate test results in relation to the patient's symptoms and other tests performed.

RELATED MONOGRAPHS:

- Related tests include biopsy prostate, bladder cancer markers, BUN, CT pelvis, creatinine cytology urine, IVP, MRI pelvis, PSA, PT/INR, and US pelvis.
- Refer to the Genitourinary System table at the end of the book for related tests by body system.

Cytology, Sputum

SYNONYM/ACRONYM: N/A.

COMMON USE: To identify cellular changes associated with neoplasms or organisms that result in respiratory tract infections, such as *Pneumocystis jiroveci* (formerly *P. carinii*).

SPECIMEN: Sputum (10 to 15 mL) collected on three to five consecutive first-morning, deep-cough expectorations.

REFERENCE VALUE: (Method: Macroscopic and microscopic examination) Negative for abnormal cells, fungi, ova, and parasites.

DESCRIPTION: Cytology is the study of the origin, structure, function, and pathology of cells. In clinical practice, cytological examinations are generally performed to detect cell changes resulting from neoplastic or inflammatory conditions. Sputum specimens for cytological examinations may be collected by expectoration alone, by suctioning, by lung biopsy, during bronchoscopy, or by expectoration after bronchoscopy. A description of the method of specimen collection by bronchoscopy and biopsy is found in the monograph titled "Biopsy, Lung."

INDICATIONS

- Assist in the diagnosis of lung cancer

- Assist in the identification of *Pneumocystis jiroveci* (formerly *P. carinii*) in persons with AIDS
- Detect known or suspected fungal or parasitic infection involving the lung
- Detect known or suspected viral disease involving the lung
- Screen cigarette smokers for neoplastic (nonmalignant) cellular changes
- Screen patients with history of acute or chronic inflammatory or infectious lung disorders, which may lead to benign atypical or metaplastic changes

POTENTIAL DIAGNOSIS

(Method: Microscopic examination) The method of reporting results of cytology examinations varies according to the laboratory performing the test.

Terms used to report results may include *negative* (no abnormal cells seen), *inflammatory, benign atypical, suspect for neoplasm, and positive for neoplasm*.

Positive findings in
• Infections caused by fungi, ova, or parasites
• Lipoid or aspiration pneumonia, as seen by lipid droplets contained in macrophages
• Neoplasms
• Viral infections and lung disease

CRITICAL FINDINGS
• Identification of malignancy

It is essential that critical diagnoses be communicated immediately to the requesting health-care provider (HCP). A listing of these diagnoses varies among facilities.

If the patient becomes hypoxic or cyanotic, remove catheter immediately and administer oxygen.

If patient has asthma or chronic bronchitis, watch for aggravated bronchospasms with use of normal saline or acetylcysteine in an aerosol.

INTERFERING FACTORS
• Improper specimen fixation may be cause for specimen rejection.
• Improper technique used to obtain bronchial washing may be cause for specimen rejection.
• Failure to follow dietary restrictions before the procedure may cause the procedure to be canceled or repeated.

NURSING IMPLICATIONS AND PROCEDURE

PRETEST:
▶ Positively identify the patient using at least two unique identifiers before providing care, treatment, or services.

▶ *Patient Teaching:* Inform the patient this test can assist in identification of the organism causing infection.
▶ Obtain a history of the patient's complaints, including a list of known allergens, especially allergies or sensitivities to latex.
▶ Obtain a history of the patient's immune and respiratory systems, symptoms, and results of previously performed laboratory tests and diagnostic and surgical procedures.
▶ Obtain a list of the patient's current medications, including herbs, nutritional supplements, and nutraceuticals (see Appendix F).
▶ Note any recent procedures that can interfere with test results.
▶ Review the procedure with the patient. If the laboratory has provided a container with fixative, instruct the patient that the fixative contents of the specimen collection container should not be ingested or otherwise removed. Instruct the patient not to touch the edge or inside of the specimen container with the hands or mouth. Inform the patient that three samples may be required, on three separate mornings, either by passing a small tube (tracheal catheter) and adding suction or by expectoration. The time it takes to collect a proper specimen varies according to the level of cooperation of the patient and the specimen collection procedure. Address concerns about pain related to the procedure. Atropine is usually given before bronchoscopy examinations to reduce bronchial secretions and to prevent vagally induced bradycardia. Meperidine (Demerol) or morphine may be given as a sedative. Lidocaine is sprayed in the patient's throat to reduce discomfort caused by the presence of the tube.
▶ Reassure the patient that he or she will be able to breathe during the procedure if specimen is collected via suction method. Ensure that oxygen has been administered 20 to 30 min before the procedure if the specimen is to be obtained by tracheal suctioning.

▶ Assist in providing extra fluids, unless contraindicated, and proper humidification to loosen tenacious secretions. Inform the patient that increasing fluid intake before retiring on the night before the test aids in liquefying secretions and may make it easier to expectorate in the morning. Also explain that humidifying inspired air also helps to liquefy secretions.

▶ Assist with mouth care (brushing teeth or rinsing mouth with water), if needed, before collection so as not to contaminate the specimen by oral secretions.

▶ *Sensitivity to social and cultural issues,* as well as concern for modesty, is important in providing psychological support before, during and after the procedure.

▶ For specimens collected by suctioning or expectoration without bronchoscopy, there are no food, fluid, or medication restrictions unless by medical direction.

▶ Instruct the patient to fast and refrain from taking liquids from midnight the night before if bronchoscopy or biopsy is to be performed. Protocols may vary among facilities.

▶ *Make sure a written and informed consent has been signed prior to the bronchoscopy or biopsy procedure and before administering any medications.*

INTRATEST:

▶ Ensure that the patient has complied with dietary restrictions; assure that food and liquids have been restricted for at least 6 to 8 hr prior to the procedure.

▶ Have patient remove dentures, contact lenses, eyeglasses, and jewelry. Notify the HCP if the patient has permanent crowns on teeth. Have the patient remove clothing and change into a gown for the procedure.

▶ Have emergency equipment readily available. Keep resuscitation equipment on hand in the case of respiratory impairment or laryngospasm after the procedure.

▶ Avoid using morphine sulfate in those with asthma or other pulmonary disease. This drug can further exacerbate bronchospasms and respiratory impairment.

▶ If the patient has a history of allergic reaction to latex, avoid the use of equipment containing latex.

▶ Assist the patient to a comfortable position, and direct the patient to breathe normally during the beginning of the general anesthesia. Instruct the patient to cooperate fully and to follow directions. Direct the patient to breathe normally and to avoid unnecessary movement during the local anesthetic and the procedure.

▶ Observe standard precautions, and follow the general guidelines in Appendix A. Positively identify the patient, and label the appropriate collection container with the corresponding patient demographics, date and time of collection, and any medication the patient is taking that may interfere with test results (e.g., antibiotics). Cytology specimens may also be expressed onto a glass slide and sprayed with a fixative or 95% alcohol.

Bronchoscopy

▶ Record baseline vital signs.

▶ The patient is positioned in relation to the type of anesthesia being used. If local anesthesia is used, the patient is seated, and the tongue and oropharynx are sprayed and swabbed with anesthetic before the bronchoscope is inserted. For general anesthesia, the patient is placed in a supine position with the neck hyperextended. After anesthesia, the patient is kept in supine or shifted to side-lying position, and the bronchoscope is inserted. After inspection, the samples are collected from suspicious sites by bronchial brush or biopsy forceps.

Expectorated Specimen

▶ Ask the patient to sit upright, with assistance and support (e.g., with an overbed table) as needed.

▶ Ask the patient to take two or three deep breaths and cough deeply. Any sputum raised should be expectorated directly into a sterile sputum collection container.

- If the patient is unable to produce the desired amount of sputum, several strategies may be attempted. One approach is to have the patient drink two glasses of water, and then assume the position for postural drainage of the upper and middle lung segments. Effective coughing may be assisted by placing either the hands or a pillow over the diaphragmatic area and applying slight pressure.
- Another approach is to place a vaporizer or other humidifying device at the bedside. After sufficient exposure to adequate humidification, postural drainage of the upper and middle lung segments may be repeated before attempting to obtain the specimen.
- Other methods may include obtaining an order for an expectorant to be administered with additional water approximately 2 hr before attempting to obtain the specimen. Chest percussion and postural drainage of all lung segments may also be employed. If the patient is still unable to raise sputum, the use of an ultrasonic nebulizer ("induced sputum") may be necessary; this is usually done by a respiratory therapist.

Tracheal Suctioning

- Obtain the necessary equipment, including a suction device, suction kit, and Lukens tube or in-line trap.
- Position the patient with head elevated as high as tolerated.
- Put on sterile gloves. Maintain the dominant hand as sterile and the nondominant hand as clean.
- Using the sterile hand, attach the suction catheter to the rubber tubing of the Lukens tube or in-line trap. Then attach the suction tubing to the male adapter of the trap with the clean hand. Lubricate the suction catheter with sterile saline.
- Tell nonintubated patients to protrude the tongue and to take a deep breath as the suction catheter is passed through the nostril. When the catheter enters the trachea, a reflex cough is stimulated; immediately advance the catheter into the trachea and apply suction. Maintain suction for approximately 10 sec, but never longer than 15 sec. Withdraw the catheter without applying suction. Separate the suction catheter and suction tubing from the trap, and place the rubber tubing over the male adapter to seal the unit.

- For intubated patients or patients with a tracheostomy, the previous procedure is followed except that the suction catheter is passed through the existing endotracheal or tracheostomy tube rather than through the nostril. The patient should be hyperoxygenated before and after the procedure in accordance with standard protocols for suctioning these patients.
- Generally, a series of three to five early-morning sputum samples are collected in sterile containers.

General

- Monitor the patient for complications related to the procedure (e.g., allergic reaction, anaphylaxis, bronchospasm).
- Promptly transport the specimen to the laboratory for processing and analysis.

POST-TEST:

- A report of the results will be sent to the requesting HCP, who will discuss the results with the patient.
- Instruct the patient to resume usual diet, as directed by the HCP. Assess the patient's ability to swallow before allowing the patient to attempt liquids or solid foods.
- Inform the patient that he or she may experience some throat soreness and hoarseness. Instruct patient to treat throat discomfort with lozenges and warm gargles when the gag reflex returns.
- Monitor vital signs and compare with baseline values every 15 min for 1 hr, then every 2 hr for 4 hr, and then as ordered by the HCP. Monitor temperature every 4 hr for 24 hr. Notify the HCP if temperature is elevated. Protocols may vary among facilities.
- Emergency resuscitation equipment should be readily available if the

vocal cords become spastic after intubation.

- Observe/assess for delayed allergic reactions, such as rash, urticaria, tachycardia, hyperpnea, hypertension, palpitations, nausea, or vomiting.
- Observe/assess the patient for hemoptysis, difficulty breathing, cough, air hunger, excessive coughing, pain, or absent breathing sounds over the affected area. Report any symptoms to the HCP.
- Evaluate the patient for symptoms indicating the development of pneumothorax, such as dyspnea, tachypnea, anxiety, decreased breathing sounds, or restlessness. A chest x-ray may be ordered to check for the presence of this complication.
- Evaluate the patient for symptoms of empyema, such as fever, tachycardia, malaise, or elevated white blood cell count.
- Administer antibiotic therapy if ordered. Remind the patient of the importance of completing the entire course of antibiotic therapy, even if signs and symptoms disappear before completion of therapy.
- *Nutritional Considerations:* Malnutrition is commonly seen in patients with severe respiratory disease for numerous reasons including fatigue, lack of appetite, and gastrointestinal distress. Adequate intake of vitamins A and C are also important to prevent pulmonary infection and to decrease the extent of lung tissue damage.
- Recognize anxiety related to test results, and be supportive of impaired activity related to perceived loss of independence and fear of shortened life expectancy. Discuss the implications of abnormal test results on the patient's lifestyle. Provide teaching and information regarding the clinical implications of the test results, as appropriate. Educate the patient regarding access to counseling services. Provide contact information, if desired, for the American Lung Association (www.lungusa.org).
- Reinforce information given by the patient's HCP regarding further testing, treatment, or referral to another HCP. Inform the patient of smoking cessation programs, as appropriate. Inform the patient with abnormal findings of the importance of medical follow-up, and suggest ongoing support resources to assist in coping with chronic illness and possible early death. Answer any questions or address any concerns voiced by the patient or family.
- Instruct the patient in the use of any ordered medications. Explain the importance of adhering to the therapy regimen. As appropriate, instruct the patient in significant side effects and systemic reactions associated with the prescribed medication. Encourage him or her to review corresponding literature provided by a pharmacist.
- Depending on the results of this procedure, additional testing may be performed to evaluate or monitor progression of the disease process and determine the need for a change in therapy. Evaluate test results in relation to the patient's symptoms and other tests performed.

RELATED MONOGRAPHS:

- Related tests include arterial/alveolar oxygen ratio, biopsy lung, blood gases, bronchoscopy, CBC, CT thoracic, relevant cultures (fungal, mycobacteria, sputum, throat, viral), gallium scan, Gram/acid-fast stain, lung perfusion scan, lung ventilation scan, MRI chest, mediastinoscopy, pleural fluid analysis, pulmonary function tests, and TB tests.
- Refer to the Immune and Respiratory systems tables at the end of the book for related tests by body system.

Cytology, Urine

SYNONYM/ACRONYM: N/A.

COMMON USE: To identify the presence of neoplasms of the urinary tract and assist in the diagnosis of urinary tract infections.

SPECIMEN: Urine (180 mL for an adult; at least 10 mL for a child) collected in a clean wide-mouth plastic container.

REFERENCE VALUE: (Method: Microscopic examination) No abnormal cells or inclusions seen.

DESCRIPTION: Cytology is the study of the origin, structure, function, and pathology of cells. In clinical practice, cytological examinations are generally performed to detect cell changes resulting from neoplastic or inflammatory conditions. Cells from the epithelial lining of the urinary tract can be found in the urine. Examination of these cells for abnormalities is useful with suspected infection, inflammatory conditions, or malignancy.

It is essential that critical diagnoses be communicated immediately to the requesting health-care provider (HCP). A listing of these diagnoses varies among facilities.

INTERFERING FACTORS: N/A

INDICATIONS

- Assist in the diagnosis of urinary tract diseases, such as cancer, cytomegalovirus infection, and other inflammatory conditions

POTENTIAL DIAGNOSIS

Positive findings in
- Cancer of the urinary tract
- Cytomegalic inclusion disease
- Inflammatory disease of the urinary tract

Negative findings in: N/A

CRITICAL FINDINGS
- Identification of malignancy

NURSING IMPLICATIONS AND PROCEDURE

PRETEST:
- Positively identify the patient using at least two unique identifiers before providing care, treatment, or services.
- *Patient Teaching:* Inform the patient this test can assist in identification of the organism causing infection.
- Obtain a history of the patient's complaints, including a list of known allergens, especially allergies or sensitivities to latex.
- Obtain a history of the patient's genitourinary and immune systems, symptoms, and results of previously performed laboratory tests and diagnostic and surgical procedures.
- Obtain a list of the patient's current medications, including herbs, nutritional supplements, and nutraceuticals (see Appendix F).
- Note any recent procedures that can interfere with test results.

▶ Review the procedure with the patient. If a catheterized specimen is to be collected, explain this procedure to the patient and obtain a catheterization tray. Address concerns about pain and explain that there may be some discomfort during the catheterization.

▶ *Sensitivity to social and cultural issues,* as well as concern for modesty, is important in providing psychological support before, during, and after the procedure.

▶ There are no food, fluid, or medication restrictions, unless by medical direction.

▶ If the patient has a history of allergic reaction to latex, avoid the use of equipment containing latex.

▶ Instruct the patient to cooperate fully and to follow directions.

▶ Observe standard precautions, and follow the general guidelines in Appendix A. Positively identify the patient, and label the appropriate tubes with the corresponding patient demographics, date and time of collection, method of specimen collection, and any medications the patient has taken that may interfere with test results (e.g., antibiotics).

Clean-Catch Specimen

▶ Instruct the male patient to (1) thoroughly wash his hands, (2) cleanse the meatus, (3) void a small amount into the toilet, and (4) void directly into the specimen container.

▶ Instruct the female patient to (1) thoroughly wash her hands; (2) cleanse the labia from front to back; (3) while keeping the labia separated, void a small amount into the toilet; and (4) without interrupting the urine stream, void directly into the specimen container.

Pediatric Urine Collector

▶ Put on gloves. Appropriately cleanse the genital area, and allow the area to dry. Remove the covering over the adhesive strips on the collector bag and apply over the genital area. Diaper the child. After obtaining the specimen, place the entire collection bag in a sterile urine container.

Indwelling Catheter

▶ Put on gloves. Empty drainage tube of urine. It may be necessary to clamp off the catheter for 15 to 30 min before specimen collection. Cleanse specimen port with antiseptic swab, and then aspirate 5 mL of urine with a 21- to 25-gauge needle and syringe. Transfer urine to a sterile container.

Urinary Catheterization

▶ Place female patient in lithotomy position or male patient in supine position. Using sterile technique, open the straight urinary catheterization kit and perform urinary catheterization. Place the retained urine in a sterile specimen container.

Suprapubic Aspiration

▶ Place the patient in supine position. Cleanse the area with antiseptic, and drape with sterile drapes. A needle is inserted through the skin into the bladder. A syringe attached to the needle is used to aspirate the urine sample. The needle is then removed and a sterile dressing is applied to the site. Place the sterile sample in a sterile specimen container.

▶ Do not collect urine from the pouch from a patient with a urinary diversion (e.g., ileal conduit). Instead perform catheterization through the stoma.

General

▶ Promptly transport the specimen to the laboratory for processing and analysis. If a delay in transport is expected, add an equal volume of 50% alcohol to the specimen as a preservative.

▶ A report of the results will be sent to the requesting HCP, who will discuss the results with the patient.

▶ Instruct the patient to resume usual medication as directed by the HCP.

▶ Instruct the patient to report symptoms such as pain related to tissue inflammation, pain or irritation during void, bladder spasms, or alterations in urinary elimination.

▶ Observe for signs of inflammation if the specimen is obtained by suprapubic aspiration.

- Administer antibiotic therapy as ordered. Remind the patient of the importance of completing the entire course of antibiotic therapy, even if signs and symptoms disappear before completion of therapy.
- Recognize anxiety related to test results, and be supportive of fear of shortened life expectancy. Discuss the implications of abnormal test results on the patient's lifestyle. Provide teaching and information regarding the clinical implications of the test results, as appropriate. Educate the patient regarding access to counseling services.
- Reinforce information given by the patient's HCP regarding further testing, treatment, or referral to another HCP. Answer any questions or address any concerns voiced by the patient or family.
- Depending on the results of this procedure, additional testing may be performed to evaluate or monitor progression of the disease process and determine the need for a change in therapy. Evaluate test results in relation to the patient's symptoms and other tests performed.

RELATED MONOGRAPHS:

- Related tests include biopsy kidney, bladder cancer markers, cystoscopy, CMV IgG and IgM, Pap smear, UA, and US bladder.
- Refer to the Genitourinary and Immune systems tables at the end of the book for related tests by body system.

Cytomegalovirus, Immunoglobulin G and Immunoglobulin M

SYNONYM/ACRONYM: CMV.

COMMON USE: To assist in diagnosing cytomegalovirus infection.

SPECIMEN: Serum (1 mL) collected in a plain red-top tube.

REFERENCE VALUE: (Method: Indirect fluorescent antibody) Negative or less than a fourfold increase in titer.

DESCRIPTION: Cytomegalovirus (CMV) is a double-stranded DNA herpesvirus. The incubation period for primary infection is 4 to 8 wk. Transmission may occur by direct contact with oral, respiratory, or venereal secretions and excretions. CMV infection is of primary concern in pregnant or immunocompromised patients or patients who have recently received an organ transplant.

Blood units are sometimes tested for the presence of CMV if patients in these high-risk categories are the transfusion recipients. CMV serology is part of the TORCH (*t*oxoplasmosis, *o*ther [congenital syphilis and viruses], *r*ubella, *C*MV, and *h*erpes simplex type 2) panel used to test pregnant women. CMV, as well as these other infectious agents, can cross the placenta

and result in congenital malformations, abortion, or stillbirth. The
presence of immunoglobulin
(Ig) M antibodies indicates acute
infection. The presence of IgG
antibodies indicates current or
past infection.

INDICATIONS

• Assist in the diagnosis of congenital
  CMV infection in newborns
• Determine susceptibility, particularly in pregnant women, immunocompromised patients, and patients
  who recently have received an
  organ transplant
• Screen blood for high-risk-category
  transfusion recipients

POTENTIAL DIAGNOSIS

Positive findings in
• CMV infection

Negative findings in: N/A

CRITICAL FINDINGS: N/A

INTERFERING FACTORS

• False-positive results may occur in
  the presence of rheumatoid factor.
• False-negative results may occur if
  treatment was begun before antibodies developed or if the test was
  done less than 6 days after exposure to the virus.

NURSING IMPLICATIONS AND PROCEDURE

PRETEST:

▶ Positively identify the patient using at
least two unique identifiers before
providing care, treatment, or services.
▶ *Patient Teaching:* Inform the patient this
test can assist in identification of the
organism causing infection.
▶ Obtain a history of the patient's
complaints and history of exposure.
Obtain a list of known allergens,

especially allergies or sensitivities
to latex.
▶ Obtain a history of the patient's
immune and reproductive systems,
symptoms, and results of previously
performed laboratory tests and
diagnostic and surgical procedures.
▶ Obtain a list of the patient's current
medications, including herbs, nutritional
supplements, and nutraceuticals
(see Appendix F).
▶ Review the procedure with the patient.
Inform the patient that multiple
specimens may be required. Any
individual positive result should be
repeated in 7 to 14 days to monitor
a change in titer. Inform the patient
that specimen collection takes
approximately 5 to 10 min. Address
concerns about pain and explain that
there may be some discomfort during
the venipuncture.
▶ *Sensitivity to social and cultural issues,*
as well as concern for modesty, is
important in providing psychological
support before, during, and after the
procedure.
▶ There are no food, fluid, or medication
restrictions, unless by medical
direction.

INTRATEST:

▶ If the patient has a history of allergic
reaction to latex, avoid the use of
equipment containing latex.
▶ Instruct the patient to cooperate fully
and to follow directions. Direct the
patient to breathe normally and to
avoid unnecessary movement.
▶ Observe standard precautions, and
follow the general guidelines in
Appendix A. Positively identify the
patient, and label the appropriate
tubes with the corresponding patient
demographics, date, and time of
collection. Perform a venipuncture.
▶ Remove the needle and apply direct
pressure with dry gauze to stop
bleeding. Observe/assess venipuncture
site for bleeding or hematoma
formation and secure gauze with
adhesive bandage.
▶ Promptly transport the specimen to
the laboratory for processing and
analysis.

POST-TEST:

▶ A report of the results will be sent to the requesting health-care provider (HCP), who will discuss the results with the patient.

▶ Instruct the patient in isolation precautions during time of communicability or contagion.

▶ Emphasize the need to return to have a convalescent blood sample taken in 7 to 14 days.

▶ Warn the patient that there is a possibility of false-negative or false-positive results.

▶ Recognize anxiety related to test results if the patient is pregnant, and offer support. Discuss the implications of abnormal test results on the patient's lifestyle. Provide teaching and information regarding the clinical implications of the test results, as appropriate. Educate the patient regarding access to counseling services.

▶ Reinforce information given by the patient's HCP regarding further testing, treatment, or referral to another HCP. Answer any questions or address any concerns voiced by the patient or family.

▶ Depending on the results of this procedure, additional testing may be performed to evaluate or monitor progression of the disease process and determine the need for a change in therapy. Evaluate test results in relation to the patient's symptoms and other tests performed.

RELATED MONOGRAPHS:

▶ Related tests include β_2-microglobulin, bronchoscopy, *Chlamydia* group antibody, culture viral, cytology urine, HIV-1/2 antibodies, Pap smear, rubella antibody, and *Toxoplasma* antibody.

▶ Refer to the Immune and Reproductive systems tables at the end of the book for related tests by body system.

D-Dimer

SYNONYM/ACRONYM: Dimer, fibrin degradation fragment.

COMMON USE: To assist in diagnosing a diffuse state of hypercoagulation as seen in disseminated intravascular coagulation (DIC), acute myocardial infarction (MI), deep vein thrombosis (DVT), and pulmonary embolism (PE).

SPECIMEN: Plasma (1 mL) collected in a completely filled blue-top (3.2% sodium citrate) tube. If the patient's hematocrit exceeds 55%, the volume of citrate in the collection tube must be adjusted.

REFERENCE VALUE: (Method: Latex semiquantitative screen or quantitative enzyme-linked immunosorbent assay [ELISA])

Semiquantitative: No fragments detected
Quantitative: Less than 250 ng/mL

DESCRIPTION: The D-dimer is an asymmetric carbon compound formed by a cross-link between two identical fibrin molecules. The test is specific for secondary fibrinolysis because the cross-linkage occurs with fibrin and not fibrinogen. A positive test is presumptive evidence of disseminated intravascular coagulation (DIC) or pulmonary embolism (PE).

INDICATIONS

- Assist in the detection of DIC and deep venous thrombosis (DVT)
- Assist in the evaluation of myocardial infarction (MI) and unstable angina
- Assist in the evaluation of possible veno-occlusive disease associated with sequelae of bone marrow transplant
- Assist in the evaluation of pulmonary embolism

POTENTIAL DIAGNOSIS

The sensitivity and specificity of the assay varies among test kits and between test methods (e.g., latex vs. ELISA).

Increased in
D-Dimers are formed in inflammatory conditions where plasmin carries out its fibrinolytic action on a fibrin clot.

- Arterial or venous thrombosis
- DVT
- DIC
- Neoplastic disease
- Pre-eclampsia
- Pregnancy (late and postpartum)
- PE
- Recent surgery (within 2 days)
- Secondary fibrinolysis
- Thrombolytic or fibrinolytic therapy

Decreased in: N/A

CRITICAL FINDINGS: N/A

INTERFERING FACTORS

- High rheumatoid factor titers can cause a false-positive result.
- Increased CA 125 levels can cause a false-positive result.
- Drugs that may cause an increase in plasma D-dimer include those administered for antiplatelet therapy.
- Drugs that may cause a decrease in plasma D-dimer include pravastatin and warfarin.
- Placement of tourniquet for longer than 1 min can result in venous stasis and changes in the concentration of plasma proteins to be measured. Platelet activation may also occur under these conditions, causing erroneous results.

- Vascular injury during phlebotomy can activate platelets and coagulation factors, causing erroneous results.
- Hemolyzed specimens must be rejected because hemolysis is an indication of platelet and coagulation factor activation.
- Hematocrit greater than 55% may cause falsely prolonged results because of anticoagulant excess relative to plasma volume.
- Incompletely filled collection tubes, specimens contaminated with heparin, clotted specimens, or unprocessed specimens not delivered to the laboratory within 1 to 2 hr of collection should be rejected.
- Icteric or lipemic specimens interfere with optical testing methods, producing erroneous results.

NURSING IMPLICATIONS AND PROCEDURE

PRETEST:

▶ Positively identify the patient using at least two unique identifiers before providing care, treatment, or services.

▶ *Patient Teaching:* Inform the patient this test can assist in diagnosing and evaluating conditions affecting normal blood clot formation.

▶ Obtain a history of the patient's complaints, including a list of known allergens, especially allergies or sensitivities to latex.

▶ Obtain a history of hematological diseases and recent surgery.

▶ Obtain a history of the patient's cardiovascular, hematopoietic, and respiratory systems; symptoms; and results of previously performed laboratory tests and diagnostic and surgical procedures.

▶ Obtain a list of the patient's current medications, including herbs, nutritional supplements, and nutraceuticals (see Appendix F).

▶ Review the procedure with the patient. Inform the patient that specimen collection takes approximately 5 to 10 min. Address concerns about pain and explain that there may be some discomfort during the venipuncture.

▶ *Sensitivity to social and cultural issues,* as well as concern for modesty, is important in providing psychological support before, during, and after the procedure.

▶ There are no food, fluid, or medication restrictions unless by medical direction.

INTRATEST:

▶ If the patient has a history of allergic reaction to latex, avoid the use of equipment containing latex.

▶ Instruct the patient to cooperate fully and to follow directions. Direct the patient to breathe normally and to avoid unnecessary movement.

▶ Observe standard precautions, and follow the general guidelines in Appendix A. Positively identify the patient, and label the appropriate tubes with the corresponding patient demographics, date, and time of collection. Perform a venipuncture. Fill tube completely. Important note: Two different concentrations of sodium citrate preservative are currently added to blue-top tubes for coagulation studies: 3.2% and 3.8%. The Clinical and Laboratory Standards Institute/ CLSI (formerly the National Committee for Clinical Laboratory Standards/ NCCLS) guideline for sodium citrate is 3.2%. Laboratories establish reference ranges for coagulation testing based on numerous factors, including sodium citrate concentration, test equipment, and test reagents. It is important to ask the laboratory which concentration it recommends, because each concentration will have its own specific reference range. When multiple specimens are drawn, the blue-top tube should be collected after sterile (i.e., blood culture) tubes. Otherwise, when using a standard vacutainer system, the blue top is the first tube collected. When a butterfly is used and due to the added tubing, an

extra red-top tube should be collected before the blue-top tube to ensure complete filling of the blue-top tube.
▶ Remove the needle and apply direct pressure with dry gauze to stop bleeding. Observe/assess venipuncture site for bleeding or hematoma formation and secure gauze with adhesive bandage.
▶ Promptly transport the specimen to the laboratory for processing and analysis. The CLSI recommendation for processed and unprocessed samples stored in unopened tubes is that testing should be completed within 1 to 4 hr of collection. If the patient has a known hematocrit above 55%, adjust the amount of anticoagulant in the collection tube before drawing the blood according to the CLSI guidelines:

Anticoagulant vol. [x] = (100 – hematocrit)/(595 – hematocrit) × total vol. of anticoagulated blood required

Example:
Patient hematocrit = 60% = [(100 – 60)/(595 – 60) × 5.0] = 0.37 mL sodium citrate for a 5-mL standard drawing tube

POST-TEST:
▶ A report of the results will be sent to the requesting health-care provider

(HCP), who will discuss the results with the patient.
▶ Reinforce information given by the patient's HCP regarding further testing, treatment, or referral to another HCP. Answer any questions or address any concerns voiced by the patient or family.
▶ Depending on the results of this procedure, additional testing may be performed to evaluate or monitor progression of the disease process and determine the need for a change in therapy. Evaluate test results in relation to the patient's symptoms and other tests performed.

RELATED MONOGRAPHS:
▶ Related tests include aPTT, alveolar/arterial gradient, angiography pulmonary, antibodies anticardiolipin, AT-III, blood gases, coagulation factors, CBC platelet count, FDP, fibrinogen, lactic acid, lung perfusion scan, plasminogen, plethysmography, protein S, PT/INR, US venous Doppler extremity studies, and venography lower extremity studies.
▶ Refer to the Cardiovascular, Hematopoietic, and Respiratory systems tables at the end of the book for related tests by body system.

Dehydroepiandrosterone Sulfate

SYNONYM/ACRONYM: DHEAS.

COMMON USE: To assist in identifying the cause of infertility, amenorrhea, or hirsutism.

SPECIMEN: Serum (1 mL) collected in a red- or tiger-top tube. Plasma (1 mL) collected in a lavender-top (EDTA) tube is also acceptable.

REFERENCE VALUE: (Method: Immunochemiluminometric assay [ICMA])

Age	Conventional Units mcg/dL	SI Units micromol/L (Conventional Units × 0.027)
Newborn		
Male	18–254	0.5–6.9
Female	10–248	0.3–6.7
1 mo–5 yr male and female	1–55	0.03–1.5
6–9 yr male and female	2.5–145	0.07–3.9
10–11 yr		
Male	15–115	0.4–3.1
Female	15–260	0.4–7.0
12–17 yr male and female	20–555	0.5–15.0
19–30 yr		
Male	125–619	3.4–16.7
Female	45–380	1.2–10.3
31–50 yr		
Male	59–452	1.6–12.2
Female	12–379	0.3–10.2
51–60 yr male	20–413	0.5–11.1
61–83 yr male	10–285	0.3–7.7
Postmenopausal woman	30–260	0.8–7.0

Tanner Stage	Male Conventional Units mcg/dL	Male SI Units micromol/L	Female Conventional Units mcg/dL	Female SI Units micromol/L
I	5–265	0.1–7.2	5–125	0.1–3.4
II	15–380	0.4–10.3	15–150	0.4–4.0
III	60–505	1.6–13.6	20–535	0.5–14.4
IV	65–560	1.8–15.1	35–485	0.9–13.1
V	165–500	4.4–13.5	75–530	2.0–14.3

DESCRIPTION: Dehydroepiandrosterone sulfate (DHEAS) is the major precursor of 17-ketosteroids. DHEAS is a metabolite of DHEA, the principal adrenal androgen. DHEAS is primarily synthesized in the adrenal gland, with a small amount secreted by the testes. DHEAS is a weak androgen and can be converted into more potent androgens (e.g., testoster-one) as well as estrogens (e.g., estradiol). It is secreted in concert with cortisol, under the control of adrenocorticotropic hormone (ACTH) and prolactin. Excessive production causes masculinization in women and children. DHEAS has replaced measurement of urinary 17-ketosteroids in the estimation of adrenal androgen production.

INDICATIONS

- Assist in the evaluation of androgen excess, including congenital adrenal hyperplasia, adrenal tumor, and Stein-Leventhal syndrome
- Evaluate women with infertility, amenorrhea, or hirsutism

POTENTIAL DIAGNOSIS

Increased in
DHEAS is produced by the adrenal cortex and testis; therefore, any condition stimulating these organs or associated feedback mechanisms will result in increased levels.

- Anovulation
- Cushing's syndrome
- Ectopic ACTH-producing tumors
- Hirsutism
- Hyperprolactinemia
- Polycystic ovary (Stein-Leventhal syndrome)
- Virilizing adrenal tumors

Decreased in
DHEAS is produced by the adrenal cortex and testis; therefore, any condition suppressing the normal function of these organs or associated feedback mechanisms will result in decreased levels.

- Addison's disease
- Adrenal insufficiency (primary or secondary)
- Aging adults *(related to natural decline in production with age)*
- Hyperlipidemia
- Pregnancy *(related to DHEAS produced by fetal adrenals and converted to estrogens in the placenta)*
- Psoriasis *(some potent topical medications used for long periods of time can result in chronic adrenal insufficiency)*
- Psychosis *(related to acute adrenal insufficiency)*

CRITICAL FINDINGS: N/A

INTERFERING FACTORS

- Drugs that may increase DHEAS levels include aloin, benfluorex, clomiphene, corticotropin, danazol, exemestane, gemfibrozil, metformin, mifepristone, and nitrendipine.
- Drugs that may decrease DHEAS levels include aspirin, carbamazepine, dexamethasone, exemestane, finasteride, ketoconazole, leuprolide, oral contraceptives, phenobarbital, phenytoin, and tamoxifen.

NURSING IMPLICATIONS AND PROCEDURE

PRETEST:

- Positively identify the patient using at least two unique identifiers before providing care, treatment, or services.
- *Patient Teaching:* Inform the patient this test can assist in diagnosing the cause of hormonal fluctuations.
- Obtain a history of the patient's complaints, including a list of known allergens, especially allergies or sensitivities to latex.
- Obtain a history of the patient's endocrine system, symptoms, phase of menstrual cycle, and results of previously performed laboratory tests and diagnostic and surgical procedures.
- Obtain a list of the patient's current medications, including herbs, nutritional supplements, and nutraceuticals (see Appendix F).
- Review the procedure with the patient. Inform the patient that specimen collection takes approximately 5 to 10 min. Address concerns about pain and explain that there may be some discomfort during the venipuncture.
- *Sensitivity to social and cultural issues,* as well as concern for modesty, is important in providing psychological support before, during, and after the procedure.

There are no food, fluid, or medication restrictions unless by medical direction.

INTRATEST:

- If the patient has a history of allergic reaction to latex, avoid the use of equipment containing latex.
- Instruct the patient to cooperate fully and to follow directions. Direct the patient to breathe normally and to avoid unnecessary movement.
- Observe standard precautions, and follow the general guidelines in Appendix A. Positively identify the patient, and label the appropriate tubes with the corresponding patient demographics, date, and time of collection. Perform a venipuncture.
- Remove the needle and apply direct pressure with dry gauze to stop bleeding. Observe/assess venipuncture site for bleeding or hematoma formation and secure gauze with adhesive bandage.
- Promptly transport the specimen to the laboratory for processing and analysis.

POST-TEST:

- A report of the results will be sent to the requesting health-care provider (HCP), who will discuss the results with the patient.
- Reinforce information given by the patient's HCP regarding further testing, treatment, or referral to another HCP. Answer any questions or address any concerns voiced by the patient or family.
- Depending on the results of this procedure, additional testing may be performed to evaluate or monitor progression of the disease process and determine the need for a change in therapy. Evaluate test results in relation to the patient's symptoms and other tests performed.

RELATED MONOGRAPHS:

- Related tests include ACTH, cortisol, prolactin, and testosterone.
- Refer to the Endocrine System table at the end of the book for related tests by body system.

Drugs of Abuse

Amphetamines
Cannabinoids
Cocaine
Ethanol (Alcohol)
Opiates
Phencyclidine

SYNONYM/ACRONYM: Amphetamines, cannabinoids (THC), cocaine, ethanol (alcohol, ethyl alcohol, ETOH), phencyclidine (PCP), opiates (heroin).

COMMON USE: To assist in rapid identification of commonly abused drugs in suspected drug overdose or for workplace drug screening.

SPECIMEN: For ethanol, serum (1 mL) collected in a red-top tube; plasma (1 mL) collected in a gray-top (sodium fluoride/potassium oxalate) tube is also acceptable. For drug screen, urine (15 mL) collected in a clean plastic container. Gastric contents (20 mL) may also be submitted for testing.

Workplace drug-screening programs, because of the potential medicolegal consequences associated with them, require collection of urine and blood specimens using a *chain of custody protocol*. The protocol provides securing the sample in a sealed transport device in the presence of the donor and a representative of the donor's employer, such that tampering would be obvious. The protocol also provides a written document of specimen transfer from donor to specimen collection personnel, to storage, to analyst, and to disposal.

REFERENCE VALUE: (Method: Spectrophotometry for ethanol; immunoassay for drugs of abuse)

Ethanol: None detected
Drug screen: None detected

DESCRIPTION: Drug abuse continues to be one of the most significant social and economic problems in the United States. The Substance Abuse and Mental Health Services Administration (SAMHSA) has identified opiates, cocaine, cannabinoids, amphetamines, and phencyclidines (PCPs) as the most commonly abused illicit drugs. Alcohol is the most commonly encountered legal substance of abuse. Chronic alcohol abuse can lead to liver disease, high blood pressure, cardiac disease, and birth defects.

INDICATIONS

- Differentiate alcohol intoxication from diabetic coma, cerebral trauma, or drug overdose
- Investigate suspected drug abuse
- Investigate suspected drug overdose
- Investigate suspected noncompliance with drug or alcohol treatment program
- Monitor ethanol levels when administered to treat methanol intoxication
- Routine workplace screening

	Screening Cutoff Concentrations for Drugs of Abuse Recommended by SAMHSA	Confirmatory Cutoff Concentrations for Drugs of Abuse Recommended by SAMHSA	Detectable Duration After Last Single-Use Dose	Detectable Duration After Last Dose: Prolonged Use
Amphetamines	1,000 ng/mL	500 ng/mL	48 hr	7–10 days
Cannabinoids	50 ng/mL	15 ng/mL	2–7 days	1–2 mo
Cocaine	300 ng/mL	150 ng/mL	3 days	4 days
Opiates	2,000 ng/mL	2,000 ng/mL	1–3 days	1–3 days
Phencyclidine	25 ng/mL	25 ng/mL	1 wk	2–4 wk

POTENTIAL DIAGNOSIS

A urine screen merely identifies the presence of these substances in urine; it does not indicate time of exposure, amount used, quality of the source used, or level of impairment. Positive screens should be considered presumptive. Drug-specific confirmatory methods should be used to investigate questionable results of a positive urine screen.

CRITICAL FINDINGS

Note and immediately report to the health-care provider (HCP) any critically increased values and related symptoms.

The legal limit for ethanol intoxication varies by state, but in most states, greater than 80 mg/dL (0.08 G%) is considered impaired for driving. Levels greater than 300 mg/dL are associated with amnesia, vomiting, double vision, and hypothermia. Levels of 400 to 700 mg/dL are associated with coma and may be fatal. Possible interventions for ethanol toxicity include administration of tap water or 3% sodium bicarbonate lavage, breathing support, and hemodialysis (usually indicated only if levels exceed 300 mg/dL).

Amphetamine intoxication causes psychoses, tremors, convulsions, insomnia, tachycardia, dysrhythmias, impotence, cerebrovascular accident, and respiratory failure. Possible interventions include emesis (if orally ingested and if the patient has a gag reflex and normal central nervous system [CNS] function), administration of activated charcoal followed by magnesium citrate cathartic, acidification of the urine to promote excretion, and administration of liquids to promote urinary output.

Cocaine intoxication causes short-term symptoms of CNS stimulation, hypertension, tachypnea, mydriasis, and tachycardia. Possible interventions include emesis (if orally ingested and if the patient has a gag reflex and normal CNS function), gastric lavage (if orally ingested), whole-bowel irrigation (if packs of the drug were ingested), airway protection, cardiac support, and administration of diazepam or phenobarbital for convulsions. The use of beta blockers is contraindicated.

Heroin is an opiate that at toxic levels causes bradycardia, flushing, itching, hypotension, hypothermia, and respiratory depression. Possible interventions include airway protection and the administration of naloxone (Narcan).

PCP intoxication causes a variety of symptoms depending on the stage of intoxication. Stage I includes psychiatric signs, muscle spasms, fever, tachycardia, flushing, small pupils, salivation, nausea, and vomiting. Stage II includes stupor, convulsions, hallucinations, increased heart rate, and increased blood pressure. Stage III includes further increases of heart rate and blood pressure that may culminate in cardiac and respiratory failure. Possible interventions may include providing respiratory support, administration of activated charcoal with a cathartic such as sorbitol, gastric lavage and suction, administration of IV nutrition and electrolytes, and acidification of the urine to promote PCP excretion.

INTERFERING FACTORS

- Codeine-containing cough medicines and antidiarrheal preparations, as well as ingestion of large amounts of poppy seeds, may produce a false-positive opiate result.
- Adulterants such as bleach or other strong oxidizers can produce erroneous urine drug screen results.
- Alcohol is a volatile substance, and specimens should be stored in a tightly stoppered containers to avoid falsely decreased values.

NURSING IMPLICATIONS AND PROCEDURE

PRETEST:

▶ Positively identify the patient using at least two unique identifiers before providing care, treatment, or services.

▶ *Patient Teaching:* Inform the patient this test can assist with identification of drugs in the body.

▶ Obtain a history of the patient's complaints, including a list of known allergens, especially allergies or sensitivities to latex.

▶ Obtain a history of the patient's symptoms and previously performed laboratory tests and diagnostic and surgical procedures.

▶ Obtain a list of the patient's current medications, including herbs, nutritional supplements, and nutraceuticals (see Appendix F).

▶ Review the entire procedure with the patient, especially if the circumstances require collection of urine and blood specimens using a chain-of-custody protocol. Inform the patient that specimen collection takes approximately 5 to 10 min but may vary depending on the level of patient cooperation. Address concerns about pain and explain that there may be some discomfort during the venipuncture, but there should be no discomfort during urine specimen collection.

▶ *Sensitivity to social and cultural issues,* as well as concern for modesty, is important in providing psychological support before, during, and after the procedure.

▶ There are no food, fluid, or medication restrictions unless by medical direction.

▶ If appropriate or required: *Make sure a written and informed consent has been signed prior to the procedure.*

patient, and label the appropriate collection containers with the corresponding patient demographics, date, and time of collection. For alcohol level, use a non-alcohol-containing solution to cleanse the venipuncture site before specimen collection. Perform a venipuncture, as appropriate. Cadaver blood is taken from the aorta. For a urine drug screen, instruct the patient to obtain a clean-catch urine specimen.

▶ Remove the needle and apply direct pressure with dry gauze to stop bleeding. Observe/assess venipuncture site for bleeding or hematoma formation and secure gauze with adhesive bandage.

Clean-Catch Specimen

▶ Instruct the male patient to (1) thoroughly wash his hands, (2) cleanse the meatus, (3) void a small amount into the toilet, and (4) void directly into the specimen container.

▶ Instruct the female patient to (1) thoroughly wash her hands; (2) cleanse the labia from front to back; (3) while keeping the labia separated, void a small amount into the toilet; and (4) without interrupting the urine stream, void directly into the specimen container.

▶ Follow the chain-of-custody protocol, if required. Monitor specimen collection, labeling, and packaging to prevent tampering. This protocol may vary by institution.

▶ Promptly transport the specimen to the laboratory for processing and analysis.

INTRATEST:

▶ If the patient has a history of allergic reaction to latex, avoid the use of equipment containing latex.

▶ Instruct the patient to cooperate fully and to follow directions. Direct the patient receiving venipuncture to breathe normally and to avoid unnecessary movement.

▶ Observe standard precautions, and follow the general guidelines in Appendix A. Positively identify the

POST-TEST:

▶ A report of the results will be sent to the requesting HCP, who will discuss the results with the patient.

▶ Ensure that results are communicated to the proper individual, as indicated in the chain-of-custody protocol.

▶ Recognize anxiety related to test results. Discuss the implications of abnormal test results on the patient's lifestyle. Provide teaching and information regarding the clinical implications of the test results, as appropriate.

Educate the patient regarding access to counseling services. Provide support and information regarding detoxification programs, as appropriate. Provide contact information, if desired, for the National Institute on Drug Abuse (www.nida.nih.gov).

▶ Reinforce information given by the patient's HCP regarding further testing, treatment, or referral to another HCP. Answer any questions or address any concerns voiced by the patient or family.

▶ Depending on the results of this procedure, additional testing may be performed to evaluate or monitor progression of the disease process and determine the need for a change in therapy. Evaluate test results in relation to the patient's symptoms and other tests performed.

RELATED MONOGRAPHS:

▶ Refer to the Therapeutic/Toxicology table at the end of the book for related tests.

D

Ductography

SYNONYM/ACRONYM: Breast ductoscopy, fiberoptic ductoscopy, galactography.

COMMON USE: To visualize and assess the breast ducts for disease and malignancy in women with nipple discharge.

AREA OF APPLICATION: Breast.

CONTRAST: Iodine based contrast medium.

DESCRIPTION: Ductography is a procedure that outlines the ductal system and provides information on the reasons for production of a nipple discharge. It can locate the site within the duct where the nipple discharge is produced. Fiberoptic ductoscopy allows visualization of the breast ductal wall and sampling of the abnormal area for diagnostic purposes and provides specimens that are generally cellular. The majority of both benign and malignant breast disease originates from the cells that line the ductal-lobular unit. In ductography, the lactiferous duct is cannulated and a small amount of

contrast medium is injected into the duct. Mammographic radiographs are then taken. Ductography is not indicated in patients with bilateral discharge because this is generally caused by hormonal changes. Biopsy and ablation techniques can also be performed during ductoscopy with correlation between visual findings and histopathology.

INDICATIONS
- Breast cancer
- Normal breast examination with high risk of developing breast cancer
- Unilateral nipple discharge, bloody or clear and watery

POTENTIAL DIAGNOSIS

Normal findings in
• Normal breast tissue

Abnormal findings in
• Ductal thickening
• Papillary lesions

CRITICAL FINDINGS

• Ductal carcinoma in situ (DSIS)
• Invasive breast cancer

It is essential that critical diagnoses be communicated immediately to the appropriate health-care provider (HCP). A listing of these diagnoses varies among facilities. Note and immediately report to the HCP abnormal results and related symptoms.

INTERFERING FACTORS

This procedure is contraindicated for
• Patients who are pregnant or suspected of being pregnant, unless the potential benefits of the procedure far outweigh the risks to the fetus and mother.
• Patients younger than age 25, because the density of the breast tissue is such that diagnostic x-rays are of limited value.

Factors that may impair clear imaging
• Inability of the patient to cooperate or remain still during the procedure because of age, significant pain, or mental status.
• Metallic objects within the examination field (e.g., jewelry, body rings), which may inhibit organ visualization and can produce unclear images.
• Application of substances such as talcum powder, deodorant, or creams to the skin of breasts or underarms, which may alter test results.
• Previous breast surgery, breast augmentation, or the presence of breast implants, which may decrease the readability of the examination.

Other considerations
• Consultation with an HCP should occur before the procedure for radiation safety concerns regarding younger patients or patients who are lactating.
• Risks associated with radiologic overexposure can result from frequent x-ray procedures. Personnel in the room with the patient should stand behind a shield or leave the area while the examination is being done. Personnel working in the examination area should wear badges to record their level of radiation exposure.

NURSING IMPLICATIONS AND PROCEDURE

PRETEST:

▶ Positively identify the patient using at least two unique identifiers before providing care, treatment, or services.
▶ *Patient Teaching:* Inform the patient this procedure can assist in evaluating the breast and mammary ducts for disease.
▶ Obtain a history of the patient's complaints, including a list of known allergens, especially allergies or sensitivities to latex, iodine, seafood, contrast medium, or anesthetics.
▶ Obtain a history of the patient's reproductive system, symptoms, and results of previously performed laboratory tests and diagnostic and surgical procedures.
▶ Record the date of last menstrual period and determine the possibility of pregnancy in perimenopausal women.
▶ Obtain a list of the patient's current medications, including herbs, nutritional supplements, and nutraceuticals (see Appendix F).
▶ Review the procedure with the patient. Address concerns about pain and

explain that there may be moments of discomfort and some pain experienced during the test. Inform the patient that the procedure is usually performed in a mammography department by an HCP, with support staff, and takes approximately 30 min.

▶ *Sensitivity to social and cultural issues,* as well as concern for modesty, is important in providing psychological support before, during, and after the procedure.

▶ There are no food, fluid, or medication restrictions unless by medical direction.

▶ Inform the patient not to apply deodorant, body creams, or powders on the day of the procedure.

▶ Instruct the patient to remove jewelry and other metallic objects in the area to be examined.

▶ *Make sure a written and informed consent has been signed prior to the procedure and before administering any medications.*

INTRATEST:

▶ Ensure that the patient has removed external metallic objects prior to the procedure.

▶ Ensure that the patient has removed any deodorant and talcum powder.

▶ Have emergency equipment readily available for possible contrast reactions.

▶ Instruct the patient to change into the gown, robe, and foot coverings provided.

▶ Instruct the patient to cooperate fully and to follow directions. Instruct the patient to remain still throughout the procedure because movement produces unreliable results.

▶ Observe standard precautions, and follow the general guidelines in Appendix A.

▶ Place the patient in the supine position on an examination table.

▶ Stroke the breast with firm pressure to discharge a small amount of fluid from the duct.

▶ Cannulate the duct until it passes beyond the sphincter of the orifice.

▶ Inject a small amount of contrast into the duct, allowing gravity to move it.

▶ Tape the cannula to the breast and assist the patient to the mammography unit for two mammographic images.

▶ Remove the cannula and apply a dressing over the nipple.

▶ Observe/assess the cannula insertion site for bleeding, inflammation, or hematoma formation.

POST-TEST:

▶ A report of the results will be sent to the requesting HCP, who will discuss the results with the patient.

▶ Observe/assess the cannula insertion site for bleeding, inflammation, or hematoma formation.

▶ Instruct the patient in the care and assessment of the injection site.

▶ Recognize anxiety related to test results. Discuss the implications of abnormal test results on the patient's lifestyle. Provide teaching and information regarding the clinical implications of the test results, as appropriate. Educate the patient regarding access to counseling services.

▶ Reinforce information given by the patient's HCP regarding further testing, treatment, or referral to another HCP. Decisions regarding the need for and frequency of breast self-examination, mammography, MRI breast, or other cancer screening procedures should be made after consultation between the patient and HCP. The most current guidelines for breast cancer screening of the general population as well as individuals with increased risk are available from the American Cancer Society (www.cancer.org), the American College of Obstetricians and Gynecologists (ACOG) (www.acog.org), and the American College of Radiology (www.acr.org). Answer any questions or address any concerns voiced by the patient or family.

▶ Instruct the patient in the use of any ordered medications. Explain the importance of adhering to the therapy regimen. As appropriate, instruct the patient in significant side effects and systemic reactions associated with the prescribed medication. Encourage the patient to review corresponding literature provided by a pharmacist.

▶ Depending on the results of this procedure, additional testing may be needed to evaluate or monitor progression of the disease process and determine the need for a change in therapy. Evaluate test results in relation to the patient's symptoms and other tests performed.

RELATED MONOGRAPHS:

▶ Related tests include biopsy breast, cancer antigens, mammography, MRI breast, stereotactic biopsy breast, and US breast.
▶ Refer to the Reproductive System table at the end of the book for related tests by body system.

D-Xylose Tolerance Test

SYNONYM/ACRONYM: N/A.

COMMON USE: To assist in the differential diagnosis of small intestine malabsorption syndromes such as celiac, tropical sprue, and Crohn's diseases.

SPECIMEN: Plasma (1 mL) collected in a gray-top (fluoride/oxalate) tube and urine (10 mL from a 5-hr collection) in a clean amber plastic container.

REFERENCE VALUE: (Method: Spectrophotometry)

Dose by Age	Conventional Units	SI Units (Conventional Units × 0.0666)
Plasma		
Adult dose		
25 g	Greater than 25 mg/dL	Greater than 1.7 mmol/L
5 g	Greater than 20 mg/dL	Greater than 1.3 mmol/L
Pediatric dose		
0.5 g/kg (max. 25 g)	Greater than 30 mg/dL	Greater than 2.0 mmol/L
Urine		
Adult dose		
25 g	Greater than 4 g/5-hr collection	Greater than 26.6 mmol/5 hr
5 g	Greater than 1.2 g/5-hr collection	Greater than 8 mmol/5 hr
Pediatric dose		
0.5 g/kg (max. 25 g)	Greater than 16%–33% of dose	Greater than 16%–33% of dose

DESCRIPTION: The D-xylose tolerance test is used to screen for intestinal malabsorption of carbohydrates. D-Xylose is a pentose sugar not normally present in the blood in significant amounts. It is partially absorbed when ingested and normally passes unmetabolized in the urine.

INDICATIONS
Assist in the diagnosis of malabsorption syndromes

POTENTIAL DIAGNOSIS

Increased in: N/A

Decreased in
Conditions that involve defective mucosal absorption of carbohydrates and other nutrients.
- Amyloidosis
- Bacterial overgrowth *(sugar is consumed by bacteria)*
- Eosinophilic gastroenteritis
- Lymphoma
- Nontropical sprue (celiac disease, gluten-induced enteropathy)
- Parasitic infestations (Giardia, schistosomiasis, hookworm)
- Postoperative period after massive resection of the intestine
- Radiation enteritis
- Scleroderma
- Small bowel ischemia
- Tropical sprue
- Whipple's disease
- Zollinger-Ellison syndrome

CRITICAL FINDINGS: N/A

INTERFERING FACTORS
- Drugs that may increase urine D-xylose levels include phenazopyridine.
- Drugs and substances that may decrease urine D-xylose levels include acetylsalicylic acid, aminosalicylic acid, arsenicals, colchicine, digitalis, ethionamide, gold, indomethacin, isocarboxazid, kanamycin, monoamine oxidase inhibitors, neomycin, and phenelzine.
- Poor renal function or vomiting may cause low urine values.

NURSING IMPLICATIONS AND PROCEDURE

PRETEST:
- Positively identify the patient using at least two unique identifiers before providing care, treatment, or services.
- *Patient Teaching:* Inform the patient this test can assist in assessing the absorptive ability of the small intestine.
- Obtain a history of the patient's complaints, including a list of known allergens, especially allergies or sensitivities to latex.
- Obtain a history of the patient's gastrointestinal system, symptoms, and results of previously performed laboratory tests and diagnostic and surgical procedures.
- Obtain a list of the patient's current medications, including herbs, nutritional supplements, and nutraceuticals (see Appendix F).
- Review the procedure with the patient. Inform the patient that activity will be restricted during the test. Obtain the pediatric patient's weight to calculate dose of D-xylose to be administered. Inform the patient that blood specimen collection takes approximately 5 to 10 min. Address concerns about pain and explain that there may be some discomfort during the venipuncture.
- *Sensitivity to social and cultural issues,* as well as concern for modesty, is important in providing psychological support before, during, and after the procedure.
- Inform the patient that all urine for a 5-hr period must be saved. Provide a nonmetallic urinal, bedpan, or toilet-mounted collection device.

Instruct the patient not to void directly into the laboratory collection container. Instruct the patient to avoid defecating in the collection device and to keep toilet tissue out of the collection device to prevent contamination of the specimen. Place a sign in the bathroom to remind the patient to save all urine.

Instruct the patient to void all urine into the collection device and then to pour the urine into the laboratory collection container. Alternatively, the specimen can be left in the collection device for a health care staff member to add to the laboratory collection container.

Numerous medications (e.g., acetylsalicylic acid, indomethacin, neomycin) interfere with the test and should be withheld, by medical direction, for 24 hr before testing.

There are no fluid restrictions, unless by medical direction.

The patient should fast for at least 12 hr before the test. In addition, the patient should refrain from eating foods containing pentose sugars such as fruits, jams, jellies, and pastries. Protocols may vary among facilities.

INTRATEST:

Ensure that the patient has complied with dietary and medication restrictions; assure that food has been restricted for at least 12 hr prior to the procedure and medications have been withheld, by medical direction, for 24 hr prior to the procedure.

If the patient has a history of allergic reaction to latex, avoid the use of equipment containing latex.

Instruct the patient to cooperate fully and to follow directions. Direct the patient to breathe normally and to avoid unnecessary movement.

Observe standard precautions, and follow the general guidelines in Appendix A. Positively identify the patient, and label the appropriate tubes with the corresponding patient demographics, date, and time of collection. Perform a venipuncture.

Remove the needle and apply direct pressure with dry gauze to stop bleeding. Observe/assess venipuncture site for bleeding or hematoma formation

and secure gauze with adhesive bandage.

Timed Specimen

Obtain a clean 3-L urine specimen container, toilet-mounted collection device, and plastic bag (for transport of the specimen container). The specimen must be refrigerated or kept on ice throughout the entire collection period. If an indwelling urinary catheter is in place, the drainage bag must be kept on ice.

Begin the test between 6 a.m. and 8 a.m., if possible. Remind the patient to remain supine and at rest throughout the duration of the test. Instruct the patient to collect all urine for a 5-hr period after administration of the D-xylose.

Adults are given a 25-g dose of D-xylose dissolved in 250 mL of water to take orally. The dose for pediatric patients is calculated by weight up to a maximum of 25 g. The patient should drink an additional 250 mL of water as soon as the D-xylose solution has been taken. Some adult patients with severe symptoms may be given a 5-g dose, but the test results are less sensitive at the lower dose.

If an indwelling catheter is in place, replace the tubing and container system at the start of the collection time. Keep the container system on ice during the collection period or empty the urine into a larger container periodically during the collection period; monitor to ensure continued drainage.

Blood samples are collected 1 hr postdose for pediatric patients and 2 hr postdose for adults.

Direct the patient to breathe normally and to avoid unnecessary movement. Perform a venipuncture, and collect the specimen in a 5-mL gray-top tube.

Include on the collection container's label the amount of urine, test start and stop times, and ingestion of any foods or medications that could affect test results.

Promptly transport the specimens to the laboratory for processing and analysis.

POST-TEST:

▶ A report of the results will be sent to the requesting health-care provider (HCP), who will discuss the results with the patient.

▶ Instruct the patient to resume usual medications, as directed by the HCP.

▶ *Nutritional Considerations:* Decreased D-xylose levels may be associated with gastrointestinal disease. Nutritional therapy may be indicated in the presence of malabsorption disorders. Encourage the patient, as appropriate, to consult with a qualified nutrition specialist to plan a lactose- and gluten-free diet. This dietary planning is complex because patients are often malnourished and have related nutritional problems.

▶ Recognize anxiety related to test results. Discuss the implications of abnormal test results on the patient's lifestyle. Provide teaching and information regarding the clinical implications of the test results, as appropriate. Offer support to help the patient and/or caregiver cope with the long-term

implications of a chronic disorder and related lifestyle changes. Educate the patient regarding access to counseling services, as appropriate.

▶ Reinforce information given by the patient's HCP regarding further testing, treatment, or referral to another HCP. Answer any questions or address any concerns voiced by the patient or family.

▶ Depending on the results of this procedure, additional testing may be performed to evaluate or monitor progression of the disease process and determine the need for a change in therapy. Evaluate test results in relation to the patient's symptoms and other tests performed.

RELATED MONOGRAPHS:

▶ Related tests include biopsy intestine, chloride sweat, fecal analysis, fecal fat, gastric emptying scan, lactose tolerance, ova and parasite, and RAIU.

▶ Refer to the Gastrointestinal System table at the end of the book for related tests by body system.

Echocardiography

SYNONYM/ACRONYM: Doppler echo, Doppler ultrasound of the heart, echo.

COMMON USE: To assist in diagnosing cardiovascular disorders such as defect, failure, tumor, infection, and bleeding.

AREA OF APPLICATION: Chest/thorax.

CONTRAST: Can be done with or without noniodinated contrast medium (microspheres).

DESCRIPTION: Echocardiography, a noninvasive ultrasound (US) procedure, uses high-frequency sound waves of various intensities to assist in diagnosing cardiovascular disorders. The procedure records the echoes created by the deflection of an ultrasonic beam off the cardiac structures and allows visualization of the size, shape, position, thickness, and movement of all four valves, atria, ventricular and atria septa, papillary muscles, chordae tendineae, and ventricles. This study can also determine blood-flow velocity and direction and the presence of pericardial effusion during the movement of the transducer over areas of the chest. Electrocardiography and phonocardiography can be done simultaneously to correlate the findings with the cardiac cycle. These procedures can be done at the bedside or in a specialized department, health-care provider's (HPC's) office, or clinic.

Included in the study are the M-mode method, which produces a linear tracing of timed motions of the heart, its structures, and associated measurements over time; and the two-dimensional method, using real-time Doppler color-flow imaging with pulsed and continuous-wave Doppler spectral tracings, which produces a cross-section of the structures of the heart and their relationship to one another, including changes in the coronary vasculature, velocity and direction of blood flow, and areas of eccentric blood flow. Doppler color-flow imaging may also be helpful in depicting the function of biological and prosthetic valves.

Cardiac contrast medium is used to aid in the diagnosis of intracardiac shunt and tricuspid valve regurgitation. The contrast agent is injected IV and outlines the chambers of the heart.

INDICATIONS

- Detect atrial tumors (myxomas)
- Detect subaortic stenosis as evidenced either by displacement of the anterior atrial leaflet or by a reduction in aortic valve flow, depending on the obstruction
- Detect ventricular or atrial mural thrombi and evaluate cardiac wall motion after myocardial infarction
- Determine the presence of pericardial effusion, tamponade, and pericarditis
- Determine the severity of valvular abnormalities such as stenosis, prolapse, and regurgitation
- Evaluate congenital heart disorders
- Evaluate endocarditis
- Evaluate or monitor prosthetic valve function
- Evaluate the presence of shunt flow and continuity of the aorta and pulmonary artery

- Evaluate unexplained chest pain, electrocardiographic changes, and abnormal chest x-ray (e.g., enlarged cardiac silhouette)
- Evaluate ventricular aneurysms and/or thrombus
- Measure the size of the heart's chambers and determine if hypertrophic cardiomyopathy or congestive heart failure is present

POTENTIAL DIAGNOSIS

Normal findings in

- Normal appearance in the size, position, structure, and movements of the heart valves visualized and recorded in a combination of ultrasound modes; and normal heart muscle walls of both ventricles and left atrium, with adequate blood filling. Established values for the measurement of heart activities obtained by the study may vary by HCP and institution.

Abnormal findings in

- Aneurysm
- Aortic valve abnormalities
- Cardiac neoplasm
- Cardiomyopathy
- Congenital heart defect
- Congestive heart failure
- Coronary artery disease (CAD)
- Endocarditis
- Mitral valve abnormalities
- Myxoma
- Pericardial effusion, tamponade, and pericarditis
- Pulmonary hypertension
- Pulmonary valve abnormalities
- Septal defects
- Ventricular hypertrophy
- Ventricular or atrial mural thrombi

CRITICAL FINDINGS

- Aneurysm
- Infection
- Obstruction
- Tumor with significant mass effect (rare)

It is essential that critical diagnoses be communicated immediately to the appropriate HCP. A listing of these diagnoses varies among facilities. Note and immediately report to the HCP abnormal results and related symptoms.

INTERFERING FACTORS

Factors that may impair clear imaging

- Incorrect placement of the transducer over the desired test site.
- Retained barium from a previous radiological procedure.
- Patients who are dehydrated, resulting in failure to demonstrate the boundaries between organs and tissue structures.
- Metallic objects (e.g., jewelry, body rings) within the examination field, which may inhibit organ visualization and cause unclear images.
- The presence of chronic obstructive pulmonary disease or use of mechanical ventilation, which increases the air between the heart and chest wall (hyperinflation) and can attenuate the ultrasound waves.
- The presence of arrhythmias.
- Inability of the patient to cooperate or remain still during the procedure because of age, significant pain, or mental status.

NURSING IMPLICATIONS AND PROCEDURE

PRETEST:

- Positively identify the patient using at least two unique identifiers before providing care, treatment, or services.
- *Patient Teaching:* Inform the patient this procedure can assist in assessing cardiac (heart) function.
- Obtain a history of the patient's symptoms, including a list of known allergens, especially allergies or

sensitivities to latex, iodine, seafood, anesthetics, or contrast mediums.

▶ Obtain a history of the patient's cardiovascular system, symptoms, and results of previously performed laboratory tests and diagnostic and surgical procedures.

▶ Note any recent procedures that can interfere with test results (i.e., barium procedures, surgery, or biopsy). Ensure that barium studies were performed at least 24 hr before this test.

▶ Record the date of the last menstrual period and determine the possibility of pregnancy in perimenopausal women.

▶ Obtain a list of the patient's current medications, including herbs, nutritional supplements, and nutraceuticals (see Appendix F).

▶ Review the procedure with the patient. Address concerns about pain related to the procedure and explain that there should be no discomfort during the procedure. Inform the patient the procedure is performed in a US or car-diology department, usually by an HCP, and takes approximately 30 to 60 min.

▶ *Sensitivity to social and cultural issues,* as well as concern for modesty, is important in providing psychological support before, during, and after the procedure.

▶ Instruct the patient to remove jewelry, and other metallic objects from the area to be examined.

▶ There are no food or fluid restrictions unless by medical direction.

INTRATEST:

▶ Ensure the patient has removed all external metallic objects from the area to be examined prior to the procedure.

▶ Have emergency equipment readily available.

▶ Instruct the patient to void prior to the procedure and to change into the gown, robe, and foot coverings provided.

▶ Instruct the patient to cooperate fully and to follow directions. Instruct the patient to remain still throughout the procedure because movement produces unreliable results.

▶ Observe standard precautions, and fol-low the general guidelines in Appendix A.

▶ Place the patient in a supine position on a flat table with foam wedges to help maintain position and immobilization.

▶ Expose the chest, and attach electrocardiogram leads for simultaneous tracings, if desired.

▶ Apply conductive gel to the chest. Place the transducer on the chest surface along the left sternal border, the subxiphoid area, suprasternal notch, and supraclavicular areas to obtain views and tracings of the portions of the heart. Scan the areas by systematically moving the probe in a perpendicular position to direct the ultrasound waves to each part of the heart.

▶ To obtain different views or information about heart function, position the patient on the left side and/or sitting up, or request that the patient breathe slowly or hold the breath during the procedure. To evaluate heart function changes, the patient may be asked to inhale amyl nitrate (vasodilator).

▶ Administer contrast medium, if ordered. A second series of images is obtained.

POST-TEST:

▶ A report of the examination will be sent to the requesting HCP, who will discuss the results with the patient.

▶ When the study is completed, remove the gel from the skin.

▶ Recognize anxiety related to test results, and offer support. Discuss the implications of abnormal test results on the patient's lifestyle. Provide teaching and information regarding the clinical implications of the test results, as appropriate.

▶ *Nutritional Considerations:* Abnormal find-ings may be associated with cardio-vascular disease. The American Heart Association and National Heart, Lung, and Blood Institute (NHBLI) recom-mend nutritional therapy for individuals identified to be at high risk for develop-ing CAD or individuals who have specific risk factors and/or existing medical conditions (e.g., elevated LDL cholesterol levels, other lipid disorders, insulin-dependent diabetes, insulin resistance, or metabolic syndrome). If overweight, the patient should be encouraged to achieve a normal weight. The NHLBI's National Cholesterol Education Program (NCEP) revised its dietary guidelines for reducing CAD in 2001. Guidelines for the Therapeutic Lifestyle Changes (TLC) diet are outlined in the Third Report of the Expert Panel on Detection, Evaluation, and Treatment of High Blood Cholesterol in Adults (Adult Treatment Panel III [ATP III]). The TLC diet emphasizes a reduction in foods high in saturated fats and cholesterol. Red meats, eggs, and dairy products are the major sources of saturated fats and cholesterol. If triglycerides also are elevated, the patient should be advised to eliminate or reduce alcohol and simple carbohydrates from the diet. The TLC approach also includes the use of plant stanols or sterols and increased dissolved fiber as an option for lowering LDL cholesterol levels; nutritional recommendations for daily total caloric intake; recommendations for allowable percentage of calories derived from fat (saturated and unsaturated), carbohydrates, protein, and cholesterol; as well as recommendations for daily expenditure of energy.

▸ *Nutritional Considerations:* Overweight patients with high blood pressure should be encouraged to achieve a normal weight. Other changeable risk factors warranting patient education include strategies to safely decrease sodium intake, increase physical activity, decrease alcohol consumption, eliminate tobacco use, and decrease cholesterol levels.

▸ *Social and Cultural Considerations:* Numerous studies point to the prevalence of excess body weight in American children and adolescents. Experts estimate that obesity is present in 25% of the population ages 6 to 11 yr. The medical, social, and emotional consequences of excess body weight are significant. Special attention should be given to instructing the child and caregiver regarding health risks and weight control education.

▸ Recognize anxiety related to test results, and be supportive of fear of shortened life expectancy. Discuss the implications of abnormal test results on the patient's lifestyle. Provide teaching and information regarding the clinical implications of the test results, as appropriate. Educate the patient regarding access to counseling services. Provide contact information, if desired, for the American Heart Association (www.americanheart.org) or the NHLBI (www.nhlbi.nih.gov).

▸ Reinforce information given by the patient's HCP regarding further testing, treatment, or referral to another HCP. Answer any questions or address any concerns voiced by the patient or family.

▸ Depending on the results of this procedure, additional testing may be needed to evaluate or monitor progression of the disease process and determine the need for a change in therapy. Evaluate test results in relation to the patient's symptoms and other tests performed.

RELATED MONOGRAPHS:

▸ Related tests include antiarrhythmic drugs, apolipoprotein A and B, AST, atrial natriuretic peptide, BNP, blood gases, blood pool imaging, calcium, chest x-ray, cholesterol (total, HDL, LDL), CT cardiac scoring, CT thorax, CRP, CK and isoenzymes, echocardiography, echocardiography transesophageal, electrocardiogram, exercise stress test, glucose, glycated hemoglobin, Holter monitor, homocysteine, ketones, LDH and isos, lipoprotein electrophoresis, lung perfusion scan, magnesium, MRI chest, MI infarct scan, myocardial perfusion heart scan, myoglobin, PET heart, potassium, pulse oximetry, sodium, triglycerides, and troponin.

▸ Refer to the Cardiovascular System table at the end of the book for related tests by body system.

Echocardiography, Transesophageal

SYNONYM/ACRONYM: Echo, TEE.

COMMON USE: To assess and visualize cardiovascular structures to assist in diagnosing disorders such as tumors, congenital defects, valve disorders, chamber disorders, and bleeding.

AREA OF APPLICATION: Chest/thorax.

CONTRAST: Can be done with or without noniodinated contrast medium (microspheres).

DESCRIPTION: Transesophageal echocardiography (TEE) is performed to assist in the diagnosis of cardiovascular disorders when noninvasive echocardiography is contraindicated or does not reveal enough information to confirm a diagnosis. Noninvasive echocardiography may be an inadequate procedure for patients who are obese, have chest wall structure abnormalities, or have chronic obstructive pulmonary disease (COPD). TEE provides a better view of the posterior aspect of the heart, including the atrium and aorta. It is done with a transducer attached to a gastroscope that is inserted into the esophagus. The transducer and the ultrasound (US) instrument allow the beam to be directed to the back of the heart. The echoes are amplified and recorded on a screen for visualization and recorded on graph paper or videotape. The depth of the endoscope and movement of the transducer is controlled to obtain various images of the heart structures. TEE is usually performed during surgery; it is also used on patients who are in the intensive care unit, in whom the transmission of waves to and from the chest has been compromised and more definitive information is needed. The images obtained by TEE have better resolution than those obtained by routine transthoracic echocardiography because TEE uses higher frequency sound waves and offers closer proximity of the transducer to the cardiac structures. Cardiac contrast medium is used to improve the visualization of viable myocardial tissue within the heart.

INDICATIONS

- Confirm diagnosis if conventional echocardiography does not correlate with other findings
- Detect and evaluate congenital heart disorders
- Detect atrial tumors (myxomas)
- Detect or determine the severity of valvular abnormalities and regurgitation
- Detect subaortic stenosis as evidenced by displacement of the anterior atrial leaflet and reduction in aortic valve flow, depending on the obstruction

- Detect thoracic aortic dissection and coronary artery disease (CAD)
- Detect ventricular or atrial mural thrombi and evaluate cardiac wall motion after myocardial infarction
- Determine the presence of pericardial effusion
- Evaluate aneurysms and ventricular thrombus
- Evaluate or monitor biological and prosthetic valve function
- Evaluate septal defects
- Measure the size of the heart's chambers and determine if hypertrophic cardiomyopathy or congestive heart failure is present
- Monitor cardiac function during open heart surgery (most sensitive method for monitoring ischemia)
- Reevaluate after inadequate visualization with conventional echocardiography as a result of obesity, trauma to or deformity of the chest wall, or lung hyperinflation associated with COPD

POTENTIAL DIAGNOSIS

Normal findings in
- Normal appearance of the size, position, structure, movements of the heart valves and heart muscle walls, and chamber blood filling; no evidence of valvular stenosis or insufficiency, cardiac tumor, foreign bodies, or CAD. The established values for the measurement of heart activities obtained by the study may vary by health-care provider (HCP) and institution.

Abnormal findings in
- Aneurysm
- Aortic valve abnormalities
- CAD
- Cardiomyopathy
- Congenital heart defects
- Congestive heart failure
- Mitral valve abnormalities
- Myocardial infarction
- Myxoma˙

- Pericardial effusion
- Pulmonary hypertension
- Pulmonary valve abnormalities
- Septal defects
- Shunting of blood flow
- Thrombus
- Ventricular hypertrophy
- Ventricular or atrial mural thrombi

CRITICAL FINDINGS
- Aneurysm
- Aortic dissection

It is essential that critical diagnoses be communicated immediately to the appropriate HCP. A listing of these diagnoses varies among facilities. Note and immediately report to the HCP abnormal results and related symptoms.

INTERFERING FACTORS

This procedure is contraindicated for
- Patients with significant esophageal pathology (procedure may cause bleeding).

Factors that may impair clear imaging
- Incorrect placement of the transducer over the desired test site.
- Retained barium from a previous radiological procedure.
- Patients who are dehydrated, resulting in failure to demonstrate the boundaries between organs and tissue structures.
- Laryngospasm, dysrhythmias, or esophageal bleeding.
- Known upper esophageal pathology.
- Conditions such as esophageal dysphagia and irradiation of the mediastinum.
- The presence of COPD or use of mechanical ventilation, which increases the air between the heart and chest wall (hyperinflation) and can attenuate the US waves.
- The presence of arrhythmias.

- Inability of the patient to cooperate or remain still during the procedure because of age, significant pain, or mental status.

Other considerations
- Failure to follow dietary restrictions before the procedure may cause the procedure to be canceled or repeated.

NURSING IMPLICATIONS AND PROCEDURE

PRETEST:

▶ Positively identify the patient using at least two unique identifiers before providing care, treatment, or services.

▶ *Patient Teaching:* Inform the patient this procedure can assist in assessing cardiac (heart) function.

▶ Obtain a history of the patient's complaints, including a list of known allergens, especially allergies or sensitivities to latex, iodine, seafood, anesthetics, or contrast mediums.

▶ Obtain a history of the patient's cardiovascular system, symptoms, and results of previously performed laboratory tests and diagnostic and surgical procedures.

▶ Note any recent procedures that can interfere with test results (i.e., barium procedures, surgery, or biopsy). Ensure that barium studies were performed at least 24 hr before this test.

▶ Record the date of the last menstrual period and determine the possibility of pregnancy in perimenopausal women.

▶ Obtain a list of the patient's current medications, including anticoagulants, aspirin and other salicylates, herbs, nutritional supplements and nutraceuticals (see Appendix F). Note the last time and dose of medication taken.

▶ Review the procedure with the patient. Address concerns about pain related to the procedure. Explain that some pain may be experienced during the test, and there may be moments of discomfort during insertion of the scope. Lidocaine is sprayed in the patient's throat to reduce discomfort caused by the presence of the endoscope. Inform the patient that the procedure is performed in a US or cardiology department, usually by an HCP, and takes approximately 30 to 60 min.

▶ Explain that an IV line may be inserted to allow infusion of IV fluids, contrast medium, or sedatives.

▶ *Sensitivity to social and cultural issues,* as well as concern for modesty, is important in providing psychological support before, during, and after the procedure.

▶ Instruct the patient to remove jewelry and other metallic objects from the area to be examined.

▶ The patient should avoid food and fluids for 8 hr prior to the procedure. Protocols may vary among facilities.

▶ *Make sure a written and informed consent has been signed prior to the procedure and before administering any medications.*

INTRATEST:

▶ Ensure that the patient has complied with dietary and fluid restriction for at least 8 hr prior to the procedure.

▶ Ensure the patient has removed all external metallic objects from the area to be examined prior to the procedure.

▶ Have emergency equipment readily available.

▶ Instruct the patient to void prior to the procedure and to change into the gown, robe, and foot coverings provided.

▶ Obtain and record the patient's vital signs.

▶ Instruct the patient to cooperate fully and to follow directions. Instruct the patient to remain still throughout the procedure because movement produces unreliable results.

▶ Observe standard precautions, and follow the general guidelines in Appendix A.

▶ Ask the patient, as appropriate, to remove his or her dentures.

▶ Monitor pulse oximetry to determine oxygen saturation in sedated patients.

▶ Expose the chest, and attach electrocardiogram leads for simultaneous tracings, if desired.

▶ Spray or swab the patient's throat with a local anesthetic, and place the oral bridge device in the mouth to prevent biting of the endoscope.

▶ Place the patient in a left side-lying position on a flat table with foam wedges to help maintain position and immobilization. The pharyngeal area is anesthetized, and the endoscope with the ultrasound device attached to its tip is inserted 30 to 50 cm to the posterior area of the heart, as in any esophago-gastroduodenoscopy procedure.

▶ Ask the patient to swallow as the scope is inserted. When the transducer is in place, the scope is manipulated by controls on the handle to obtain scanning that provides real-time images of the heart motion and recordings of the images for viewing. Actual scanning is usually limited to 15 min or until the desired number of image planes is obtained at different depths of the scope.

▶ Administer contrast medium, if ordered. A second series of images is obtained.

POST-TEST:

▶ A report of the examination will be sent to the requesting HCP, who will discuss the results with the patient.

▶ Monitor vital signs and neurological status every 15 min for 1 hr, then every 2 hr for 4 hr, and as ordered. Take temperature every 4 hr for 24 hr. Monitor intake and output at least every 8 hr. Compare with baseline values. Notify the HCP if temperature is elevated. Protocols may vary among facilities.

▶ Instruct the patient to resume usual diet and activity 4 to 6 hr after the test, as directed by the HCP.

▶ Instruct the patient to treat throat discomfort with lozenges and warm gargles when the gag reflex returns.

▶ Recognize anxiety related to test results, and offer support. Discuss the implications of abnormal test results on the patient's lifestyle. Provide teaching and information regarding the clinical implications of the test results, as appropriate.

▶ *Nutritional Considerations:* Abnormal findings may be associated with cardiovascular disease. The American Heart Association and National Heart, Lung, and Blood Institute (NHBLI) recommend nutritional therapy for individuals identified to be at high risk for developing CAD or individuals who have specific risk factors and/or existing medical conditions (e.g., elevated LDL cholesterol levels, other lipid disorders, insulin-dependent diabetes, insulin resistance, or metabolic syndrome). If overweight, the patient should be encouraged to achieve a normal weight. The NHLBI's National Cholesterol Education Program (NCEP) revised its dietary guidelines for reducing CAD in 2001. Guidelines for the Therapeutic Lifestyle Changes (TLC) diet are outlined in the Third Report of the Expert Panel on Detection, Evaluation, and Treatment of High Blood Cholesterol in Adults (Adult Treatment Panel III [ATP III]). The TLC diet emphasizes a reduction in foods high in saturated fats and cholesterol. Red meats, eggs, and dairy products are the major sources of saturated fats and cholesterol. If triglycerides also are elevated, the patient should be advised to eliminate or reduce alcohol and simple carbohydrates from the diet. The TLC approach also includes the use of plant stanols or sterols and increased dissolved fiber as an option for lowering LDL cholesterol levels; nutritional recommendations for daily total caloric intake; recommendations for allowable percentage of calories derived from fat (saturated and unsaturated), carbohydrates, protein, and cholesterol; as well as recommendations for daily expenditure of energy.

▶ *Nutritional Considerations:* Overweight patients with high blood pressure should be encouraged to achieve a normal weight. Other changeable risk factors warranting patient education include strategies to safely decrease sodium intake, increase physical activity, decrease alcohol consumption, eliminate tobacco use, and decrease cholesterol levels.

▶ *Social and Cultural Considerations:* Numerous studies point to the prevalence of excess body weight in American children and adolescents. Experts estimate that obesity is present in 25% of the population ages 6 to 11 yr. The medical, social, and emotional consequences of excess body weight are significant. Special attention should be given to instructing the child and caregiver regarding health risks and weight control education.

▸ Recognize anxiety related to test results, and be supportive of fear of shortened life expectancy. Discuss the implications of abnormal test results on the patient's lifestyle. Provide teaching and information regarding the clinical implications of the test results, as appropriate. Educate the patient regarding access to counseling services. Provide contact information, if desired, for the American Heart Association (www.americanheart.org) or the NHLBI (www.nhlbi.nih.gov).

▸ Reinforce information given by the patient's HCP regarding further testing, treatment, or referral to another HCP. Answer any questions or address any concerns voiced by the patient or family.

▸ Depending on the results of this procedure, additional testing may be needed to evaluate or monitor progression of the disease process

and determine the need for a change in therapy. Evaluate test results in relation to the patient's symptoms and other tests performed.

RELATED MONOGRAPHS:

▸ Related tests include antiarrhythmic drugs, apolipoprotein A and B, AST, atrial natriuretic peptide, BNP, blood gases, blood pool imaging, calcium, chest x-ray, cholesterol (total, HDL, LDL), CT cardiac scoring, CT thorax, CRP, CK and isoenzymes, echocardiography, electrocardiogram, exercise stress test, glucose, glycated hemoglobin, Holter monitor, homocysteine, ketones, LDH and isos, lipoprotein electrophoresis, lung perfusion scan, magnesium, MRI chest, MI infarct scan, myocardial perfusion heart scan, myoglobin, PET heart, potassium, pulse oximetry, sodium, triglycerides, and troponin.

▸ Refer to the Cardiovascular System table at the end of the book for related tests by body system.

Electrocardiogram

SYNONYM/ACRONYM: ECG, EKG.

COMMON USE: To evaluate the electrical impulses generated by the heart during the cardiac cycle to assist with diagnosis of cardiac arrhythmias, blocks, damage, infection, or enlargement.

AREA OF APPLICATION: Heart.

CONTRAST: None.

DESCRIPTION: The cardiac muscle consists of three layers of cells: the inner layer called the *endocardium*, the middle layer called the *myocardium*, and the outer layer called the *epicardium*. The systolic phase of the cardiac cycle reflects the contraction of the myocardium, whereas the diastolic phase takes place when the heart relaxes to allow blood to rush in. All muscle cells have a characteristic rate of contraction called *depolarization*. Therefore, the heart will maintain a predetermined heart rate unless other stimuli are received.

The monitoring of pulse and blood pressure evaluates only the mechanical activity of the heart. The electrocardiogram (ECG), a noninvasive study, measures the electrical currents or impulses that the heart generates during a cardiac cycle (see figure of a normal ECG at end of monograph). Electrical impulses travel through a conduction system beginning with the sinoatrial (SA) node and moving to the atrioventricular (AV) node via internodal pathways. From the AV node, the impulses travel to the bundle of His and onward to the right and left bundle branches. These bundles are located within the right and left ventricles. The impulses continue to the cardiac muscle cells by terminal fibers called *Purkinje fibers*. The ECG is a graphic display of the electrical activity of the heart, which is analyzed by time intervals and segments. Continuous tracing of the cardiac cycle activities is captured as heart cells are electrically stimulated, causing depolarization and movement of the activity through the cells of the myocardium.

The ECG study is completed by using 12 electrodes attached to the skin surface to obtain the total electrical activity of the heart. Each lead records the electrical potential between the limbs or between the heart and limbs. The ECG machine records and marks the 12 leads on the strip of paper in the machine in proper sequence, usually 6 in. of the strip for each lead. The ECG pattern, called a *heart rhythm*, is recorded by a machine as a series of waves, intervals, and segments, each of which pertains to a specific occurrence during the contraction of the heart. The ECG tracings are recorded on graph paper using vertical and horizontal lines for analysis and calculations of time, measured by the vertical lines (1 mm apart and 0.04 sec per line), and of voltage, measured by the horizontal lines (1 mm apart and 0.5 mV per 5 squares). A pulse rate can be calculated from the ECG strip to obtain the beats per minute. The P wave represents the depolarization of the atrial myocardium; the QRS complex represents the depolarization of the ventricular myocardium; the P-R interval represents the time from beginning of the excitation of the atrium to the beginning of the ventricular excitation; and the ST segment has no deflection from baseline, but in an abnormal state may be elevated or depressed. An abnormal rhythm is called an *arrhythmia*.

INDICATIONS

- Assess the extent of congenital heart disease
- Assess the extent of myocardial infarction (MI) or ischemia, as indicated by abnormal ST segment, interval times, and amplitudes
- Assess the function of heart valves
- Assess global cardiac function
- Detect arrhythmias, as evidenced by abnormal wave deflections
- Detect pericarditis, shown by ST segment changes or shortened P-R interval
- Determine electrolyte imbalances, as evidenced by short or prolonged Q-T interval
- Determine hypertrophy of the chamber of the heart or heart hypertrophy, as evidenced by P or R wave deflections
- Evaluate and monitor cardiac pacemaker function
- Evaluate and monitor the effect of drugs, such as digitalis, antiarrhythmics, or vasodilating agents

- Monitor ECG changes during an exercise test
- Monitor rhythm changes during the recovery phase after an MI

POTENTIAL DIAGNOSIS

Normal findings in

- Normal heart rate according to age: range of 60 to 100 beats/min in adults
- Normal, regular rhythm and wave deflections with normal measurement of ranges of cycle components and height, depth, and duration of complexes as follows:

  P wave: 0.12 sec or three small blocks with amplitude of 2.5 mm

  Q wave: less than 0.04 mm

  R wave: 5 to 27 mm amplitude, depending on lead

  T wave: 1 to 13 mm amplitude, depending on lead

  QRS complex: 0.12 sec or three small blocks

  ST segment: 1 mm

Abnormal findings in

- Arrhythmias
- Atrial or ventricular hypertrophy
- Bundle branch block
- Electrolyte imbalances
- MI or ischemia
- Pericarditis
- Pulmonary infarction
- P wave: An enlarged P wave deflection could indicate atrial enlargement; an absent or altered P wave could suggest that the electrical impulse did not come from the SA node
- P-R interval: An increased interval could imply a conduction delay in the AV node
- QRS complex: An enlarged Q wave may indicate an old infarction; an enlarged deflection could indicate ventricular hypertrophy; increased time duration may indicate a bundle branch block

- ST segment: A depressed ST segment indicates myocardial ischemia; an elevated ST segment may indicate an acute MI or pericarditis; a prolonged ST segment may indicate hypocalcemia or hypokalemia (short segment)
- T wave: A flat or inverted T wave may indicate myocardial ischemia, infarction, or hypokalemia; a tall T wave may indicate hyperkalemia

CRITICAL FINDINGS

- Acute changes in ST elevation may indicate acute MI or pericarditis.
- Bradycardia (less than 40 beats per min)
- PVCs greater than three in a row, pauses greater than 3 sec, or identified blocks
- Tachycardia (greater than 120 beats per min), supraventricular tachycardia, and ventricular tachycardia

It is essential that critical diagnoses be communicated immediately to the appropriate health-care provider (HCP). A listing of these diagnoses varies among facilities. Note and immediately report to the HCP abnormal results and related symptoms.

INTERFERING FACTORS

Factors that may impair the results of the examination

- Anatomic ariation of the heart (i.e., the heart may be rotated in both the horizontal and frontal planes).
- Distortion of cardiac cycles due to age, gender, weight, or a medical condition (e.g., infants, women [may exhibit slight ST segment depression], obese patients, pregnant patients, patients with ascites).
- High intake of carbohydrates or electrolyte imbalances of potassium or calcium.
- Improper placement of electrodes or inadequate contact between

skin and electrodes because of insufficient conductive gel or poor placement, which can cause ECG tracing problems.

- ECG machine malfunction or interference from electromagnetic waves in the vicinity.
- Inability of the patient to remain still during the procedure, because movement, muscle tremor, or twitching can affect accurate test recording.
- Increased patient anxiety, causing hyperventilation or deep respirations.
- Medications such as barbiturates and digitalis.
- Strenuous exercise before the procedure.

NURSING IMPLICATIONS AND PROCEDURE

PRETEST:

▶ Positively identify the patient using at least two unique identifiers before providing care, treatment, or services.

▶ *Patient Teaching:* Inform the patient this procedure can assist in assessing cardiac (heart) function.

▶ Obtain a history of the patient's complaints, including a list of known allergens, especially allergies or sensitivities to latex, iodine, seafood, anesthetics, or contrast mediums. Ask if the patient has had a heart transplant or pacemaker implanted.

▶ Obtain a history of the patient's cardiovascular system, symptoms, and results of previously performed laboratory tests and diagnostic and surgical procedures.

▶ Obtain a list of the patient's current medications, including herbs, nutritional supplements and nutraceuticals (see Appendix F).

▶ Review the procedure with the patient. Address concerns about pain related to the procedure and explain that there should be no discomfort related to the procedure. Inform the patient that

the procedure is performed by an HCP and takes approximately 15 min.

▶ *Sensitivity to social and cultural issues,* as well as concern for modesty, is important in providing psychological support before, during, and after the procedure.

▶ Instruct the patient to remove jewelry and other metallic objects from the area to be examined.

▶ There are no food, fluid, or medication restrictions unless by medical direction.

INTRATEST:

▶ Ensure the patient has complied with pretesting preparations.

▶ Ensure the patient has removed all external metallic objects from the area to be examined prior to the procedure.

▶ Instruct the patient to void prior to the procedure and to change into the gown, robe, and foot coverings provided.

▶ Instruct the patient to cooperate fully and to follow directions. Instruct the patient to remain still throughout he procedure because movement produces unreliable results.

▶ Record baseline values.

▶ Observe standard precautions, and follow the general guidelines in Appendix A.

▶ Place patient in a supine position. Expose and appropriately drape the chest, arms, and legs.

▶ Prepare the skin surface with alcohol and remove excess hair. Shaving may be necessary. Dry skin sites.

▶ Apply the electrodes in the proper position. When placing the six unipolar chest leads, place V_1 at the fourth intercostal space at the border of the right sternum, V_2 at the fourth intercostal space at the border of the left sternum, V_3 between V_2 and V_4, V_4 at the fifth intercostal space at the midclavicular line, V_5 at the left anterior axillary line at the level of V_4 horizontally, and V_6 at the level of V_4 horizontally and at the left midaxillary line. The wires are connected to the matched electrodes and the ECG machine. Chest leads (V_1, V_2, V_3, V_4, V_5, and V_6) record data from the horizontal plane of the heart.

▶ Place three limb bipolar leads (two electrodes combined for each) on the arms and legs. Lead I is the

E

E

combination of two arm electrodes,
lead II is the combination of right arm
and left leg electrodes, and lead III is
the combination of left arm and left leg
electrodes. Limb leads (I, II, III, aVL,
aVF, and aVR) record data from the
frontal plane of the heart.

- The machine is set and turned on
after the electrodes, grounding,
connections, paper supply, computer,
and data storage device are checked.
- If the patient has any chest discomfort
or pain during the procedure, mark the
ECG strip indicating that occurrence.

POST-TEST:

- A report of the examination will
be sent to the requesting HCP, who
will discuss the results with the patient.
- When the procedure is complete,
remove the electrodes and clean the
skin where the electrode pads were
applied.
- Evaluate the results in relation to
previously performed ECGs.
Denote cardiac rhythm abnormalities
on the strip.
- Monitor vital signs and compare with
baseline values. Protocols may vary
among facilities.
- Instruct the patient to immediately
notify an HCP of chest pain, changes
in pulse rate, or shortness of breathe.
- Recognize anxiety related to the
test results and be supportive of
perceived loss of independence
and fear of shortened life expectancy.
Discuss the implications of abnormal
test results on the patient's lifestyle.
Provide teaching and information
regarding the clinical implications
of the test results, as appropriate.
- *Nutritional Considerations:* Abnormal
findings may be associated with
cardiovascular disease. The American
Heart Association and National Heart,
Lung, and Blood Institute (NHBLI) recommend nutritional therapy for individuals identified to be at high risk for
developing coronary artery disease
(CAD) or individuals who have specific
risk factors and/or existing medical
conditions (e.g., elevated LDL
cholesterol levels, other lipid
disorders, insulin-dependent diabetes,

insulin resistance, or metabolic syndrome). If overweight, the patient
should be encouraged to achieve a
normal weight. The NHLBI's National
Cholesterol Education Program
(NCEP) revised its dietary
guidelines for reducing CAD
in 2001. Guidelines for the
Therapeutic Lifestyle Changes
(TLC) diet are outlined in the
Third Report of the Expert Panel
on Detection, Evaluation, and
Treatment of High Blood Cholesterol
in Adults (Adult Treatment Panel III
[ATP III]). The TLC diet emphasizes
a reduction in foods high in
saturated fats and cholesterol.
Red meats, eggs, and dairy
products are the major sources of
saturated fats and cholesterol. If
triglycerides also are elevated, the
patient should be advised to
eliminate or reduce alcohol
and simple carbohydrates from the
diet. The TLC approach also
includes the use of plant stanols or
sterols and increased dissolved fiber
as an option for lowering LDL
cholesterol levels; nutritional
recommendations for daily total
caloric intake; recommendations for
allowable percentage of calories
derived from fat (saturated
and unsaturated), carbohydrates,
protein, and cholesterol; as well as
recommendations for daily
expenditure of energy.

- *Nutritional Considerations:* Overweight
patients with high blood pressure
should be encouraged to achieve a
normal weight. Other changeable risk
factors warranting patient education
include strategies to safely decrease
sodium intake, increase physical
activity, decrease alcohol consumption,
eliminate tobacco use, and decrease
cholesterol levels.
- *Social and Cultural Considerations:*
Numerous studies point to the
prevalence of excess body weight in
American children and adolescents.
Experts estimate that obesity is present
in 25% of the population ages 6 to 11 yr.
The medical, social, and emotional
consequences of excess body weight

are significant. Special attention should be given to instructing the child and caregiver regarding health risks and weight control education.

▶ Recognize anxiety related to test results, and be supportive of fear of shortened life expectancy. Discuss the implications of abnormal test results on the patient's lifestyle. Provide teaching and information regarding the clinical implications of the test results, as appropriate. Educate the patient regarding access to counseling services. Provide contact information, if desired, for the American Heart Association (www.americanheart.org) or the NHLBI (www.nhlbi.nih.gov).

▶ Reinforce information given by the patient's HCP regarding further testing, treatment, or referral to another HCP. Answer any questions or address any concerns voiced by the patient or family.

▶ Depending on the results of this procedure, additional testing may be performed to evaluate or monitor progression of the disease process and determine the need for a change in therapy. Evaluate test results in relation to the patient's symptoms and other tests performed.

RELATED MONOGRAPHS:

▶ Related tests include antiarrhythmic drugs, apolipoprotein A and B, AST, atrial natriuretic peptide, BNP, blood gases, blood pool imaging, calcium, chest x-ray, cholesterol (total, HDL, LDL), CT cardiac scoring, CT thorax, CRP, CK and isoenzymes, echocardiography, echocardiography transesophageal, exercise stress test, glucose, glycated hemoglobin, Holter monitor, homocysteine, ketones, LDH and isos, lipoprotein electrophoresis, lung perfusion scan, magnesium, MRI chest, MI infarct scan, myocardial perfusion heart scan, myoglobin, PET heart, potassium, pulse oximetry, sodium, triglycerides, and troponin.

▶ Refer to the Cardiovascular System table at the end of the book for related tests by body system.

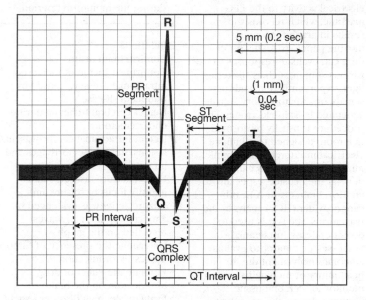

Electroencephalography

SYNONYM/ACRONYM: Electrical activity (for sleep disturbances), EEG.

COMMON USE: To assess the electrical activity in the brain to assist in diagnosis of brain death, injury, infection, and bleeding.

AREA OF APPLICATION: Brain.

CONTRAST: None.

E

DESCRIPTION: Electroencephalography (EEG) is a noninvasive study that measures the brain's electrical activity and records that activity on graph paper. These electrical impulses arise from the brain cells of the cerebral cortex. Electrodes, placed at 8 to 20 sites (or pairs of sites) on the patient's scalp, transmit the different frequencies and amplitudes of the brain's electrical activity to the EEG machine, which records the results in graph form on a moving paper strip. This procedure can evaluate responses to various stimuli, such as flickering light, hyperventilation, auditory signals, or somatosensory signals generated by skin electrodes. The procedure is usually performed in a room designed to eliminate electrical interference and minimize distractions. EEG can be done at the bedside, especially to confirm brain death. A healthcare provider (HCP) analyzes the waveforms. The test is used to detect epilepsy, intracranial abscesses, or tumors; to evaluate cerebral involvement due to head injury or meningitis; and to monitor for cerebral tissue ischemia during surgery when

cerebral vessels must be occluded. EEG is also used to confirm brain death, which can be defined as absence of electrical activity in the brain. To evaluate abnormal EEG waves further, the patient may be connected to an ambulatory EEG system similar to a Holter monitor for the heart. Patients keep a journal of their activities and any symptoms that occur during the monitoring period.

INDICATIONS
- Confirm brain death
- Confirm suspicion of increased intracranial pressure caused by trauma or disease
- Detect cerebral ischemia during endarterectomy
- Detect intracranial cerebrovascular lesions, such as hemorrhages and infarcts
- Detect seizure disorders and identify focus of seizure and seizure activity, as evidenced by abnormal spikes and waves recorded on the graph
- Determine the presence of tumors, abscesses, or infection
- Evaluate the effect of drug intoxication on the brain
- Evaluate sleeping disorders, such as sleep apnea and narcolepsy

- Identify area of abnormality in dementia

POTENTIAL DIAGNOSIS

Normal findings in
- Normal occurrences of alpha, beta, theta, and delta waves (rhythms varying depending on the patient's age)
- Normal frequency, amplitude, and characteristics of brain waves

Abnormal findings in
- Abscess
- Brain death
- Cerebral infarct
- Encephalitis
- Glioblastoma and other brain tumors
- Head injury
- Hypocalcemia or hypoglycemia
- Intracranial hemorrhage
- Meningitis
- Migraine headaches
- Narcolepsy
- Seizure disorders (grand mal, focal, temporal lobe, myoclonic, petit mal)
- Sleep apnea

CRITICAL FINDINGS

- Abscess
- Brain death
- Head injury
- Hemorrhage
- Intracranial hemorrhage

It is essential that critical diagnoses be communicated immediately to the appropriate HCP. A listing of these diagnoses varies among facilities. Note and immediately report to the HCP abnormal results and related symptoms.

INTERFERING FACTORS

Factors that may impair the results of the examination
- Inability of the patient to cooperate or remain still during the procedure because of age, significant pain, or mental status.
- Drugs and substances such as sedatives, anticonvulsants, anxiolytics, alcohol, and stimulants such as caffeine and nicotine.
- Hypoglycemic or hypothermic states.
- Hair that is dirty, oily, or sprayed or treated with hair preparations.

NURSING IMPLICATIONS AND PROCEDURE

PRETEST:

▶ Positively identify the patient using at least two unique identifiers before providing care, treatment, or services.

▶ *Patient Teaching:* Inform the patient/family this procedure can assist in measuring the electrical activity in the brain.

▶ Obtain a history of the patient's complaints, including a list of known allergens, especially allergies or sensitivities to latex, iodine, seafood, anesthetics, or contrast mediums.

▶ Obtain a history of the patient's musculoskeletal system, symptoms, and results of previously performed laboratory tests and diagnostic and surgical procedures.

▶ Obtain a list of the patient's current medications, including herbs, nutritional supplements, and nutraceuticals (see Appendix F).

▶ Review the procedure with the patient. Address concerns about pain related to the procedure and assure the patient there is no discomfort during the procedure, but if needle electrodes are used, a slight pinch may be felt. Explain that electricity flows from the patient's body, not into the body, during the procedure. Explain that the procedure reveals brain activity only, not thoughts, feelings, or intelligence. Inform the patient the procedure is performed in a neurodiagnostic department, usually by an HCP and support staff, and takes approximately 30 to 60 min.

E

- Inform the patient that he or she may be asked to alter breathing pattern; be asked to follow simple commands such as opening or closing eyes, blinking, or swallowing; be stimulated with bright light; or be given a drug to induce sleep during the study.
- *Sensitivity to social and cultural issues*, as well as concern for modesty, is important in providing psychological support before, during, and after the procedure.
- Instruct the patient to clean the hair and to refrain from using hair sprays, creams, or solutions before the test.
- Instruct the patient to limit sleep to 5 hr for an adult and 7 hr for a child the night before the study. Young infants and children should not be allowed to nap before the study.
- Instruct the patient to eat a meal before the study and to avoid stimulants such as caffeine and nicotine for 8 hr prior to the procedure. Under medical direction, the patient should avoid sedatives, anticonvulsants, anxiolytics, and alcohol for 24 to 48 hr before the test.
- *Make sure a written and informed consent has been signed prior to the procedure and before administering any medications.*

INTRATEST:

- Ensure the patient has complied with pretesting preparations. Ensure that caffeine-containing beverages were withheld for 8 hr before the procedure and that a meal was ingested before the study.
- Ensure that all substances with the potential to interfere with test results were withheld for 24 to 48 hr before the test.
- Ensure that the patient is able to relax; report any extreme anxiety or restlessness.
- Ensure that hair is clean and free of hair sprays, creams, or solutions.
- Observe standard precautions, and follow the general guidelines in Appendix A.
- Place the patient in the supine position in a bed or in a semi-Fowler's position on a recliner in a special room protected

from any noise or electrical interferences that could affect the tracings.
- Remind the patient to relax and not to move any muscles or parts of the face or head. The HCP should be able to observe the patient for movements or other interferences through a window into the test room.
- The electrodes are prepared and applied to the scalp. Electrodes are placed in as many as 20 locations over the frontal, temporal, parietal, and occipital areas, and amplifier wires are attached. An electrode is also attached to each earlobe as grounding electrodes. At this time, a baseline recording can be made with the patient at rest.
- Recordings are made with the patient at rest and with eyes closed. Recordings are stopped about every 5 min to allow the patient to move. Recordings are also made during a drowsy and sleep period, depending on the patient's clinical condition and symptoms.
- Procedures (e.g., stroboscopic light stimulation, hyperventilation to induce alkalosis, and sleep induction by administration of sedative to detect abnormalities that occur only during sleep) may be done to bring out abnormal electrical activity or other brain abnormalities.
- Observations for seizure activity are carried out during the study, and a description and time of activity is noted by the HCP.

POST-TEST:

- A report of the examination will be sent to the requesting HCP, who will discuss the results with the patient.
- When the procedure is complete, remove electrodes from the hair and remove paste by cleansing with oil or witch hazel.
- If a sedative was given during the test, allow the patient to recover. Bedside rails are put in the raised position for safety.
- Instruct the patient to resume medications, as directed by the HCP.
- Instruct the patient to report any seizure activity.

▶ Recognize anxiety related to test results, and be supportive of perceived loss of independent function. Discuss the implications of abnormal test results on the patient's lifestyle. Provide teaching and information regarding the clinical implications of the test results, as appropriate.

▶ Reinforce information given by the patient's HCP regarding further testing, treatment, or referral to another HCP. Answer any questions or address any concerns voiced by the patient or family.

▶ Depending on the results of this procedure, additional testing may be performed to evaluate or monitor progression of the disease process and determine the need for a change in therapy. Evaluate test results in relation to the patient's symptoms and other tests performed.

RELATED MONOGRAPHS:

▶ Related tests include CSF analysis, CT brain, evoked brain potentials (SER, VER), MRI brain, and PET brain.

▶ Refer to the Musculoskeletal System table at the end of the book for related tests by body system.

E

Electromyography

SYNONYM/ACRONYM: Electrodiagnostic study, EMG, neuromuscular junction testing.

COMMON USE: To assess the electrical activity within the skeletal muscles to assist in diagnosing diseases such as muscular dystrophy, Guillain-Barré, polio, and other myopathies.

AREA OF APPLICATION: Muscles.

CONTRAST: None.

DESCRIPTION: Electromyography (EMG) measures skeletal muscle activity during rest, voluntary contraction, and electrical stimulation. Percutaneous extracellular needle electrodes containing fine wires are inserted into selected muscle groups to detect neuromuscular abnormalities and measure nerve and electrical conduction properties of skeletal muscles. The electrical potentials are amplified, displayed on a screen in waveforms, and electronically recorded, similar to electrocardiography. Comparison and analysis of the amplitude, duration, number, and configuration of the muscle activity provide diagnostic information about the extent of nerve and muscle involvement in the detection of primary muscle diseases, including lower motor neuron, anterior horn cell, or neuromuscular junction diseases; defective transmission at the neuromuscular junction; and peripheral nerve damage or disease. Responses of a relaxed muscle are electrically silent, but spontaneous muscle movement such as fibrillation and fasciculation can be detected in a relaxed, denervated muscle. Muscle action potentials are detected with minimal or maximal muscle contractions. The differences in the size and numbers of activity potentials during voluntary contractions determine whether the muscle weakness is a disease of the striated muscle fibers or cell membranes (myogenic) or a disease of the lower motor neuron (neurogenic). Nerve conduction studies (electroneurography) are commonly done in conjunction with electromyelography; the combination of the procedures is known as electromyoneurography. The major use of the examination lies in differentiating among the following disease classes: primary myopathy, peripheral motor neuron disease, and disease of the neuromuscular junction.

INDICATIONS

- Assess primary muscle diseases affecting striated muscle fibers or cell membrane, such as muscular dystrophy or myasthenia gravis
- Detect muscle disorders caused by diseases of the lower motor neuron involving the motor neuron on the anterior horn of the spinal cord, such as anterior poliomyelitis, amyotrophic lateral sclerosis, amyotonia, and spinal tumors
- Detect muscle disorders caused by diseases of the lower motor neuron involving the nerve root, such as Guillain-Barré syndrome, herniated disk, or spinal stenosis
- Detect neuromuscular disorders, such as peripheral neuropathy caused by diabetes or alcoholism, and locate the site of the abnormality
- Determine if a muscle abnormality is caused by the toxic effects of drugs (e.g., antibiotics, chemotherapy) or toxins (e.g., *Clostridium botulinum*, snake venom, heavy metals)
- Differentiate between primary and secondary muscle disorders or between neuropathy and myopathy
- Differentiate secondary muscle disorders caused by polymyositis, sarcoidosis, hypocalcemia, thyroid toxicity, tetanus, and other disorders
- Monitor and evaluate progression of myopathies or neuropathies, including confirmation of diagnosis of carpal tunnel syndrome

POTENTIAL DIAGNOSIS

Normal findings in
- Normal muscle electrical activity during rest and contraction states

Abnormal findings in
- Evidence of neuromuscular disorders or primary muscle disease (*Note*: Findings must be correlated with the patient's history, clinical features, and results of other neurodiagnostic tests.):
  Amyotrophic lateral sclerosis
  Bell's palsy
  Beriberi
  Carpal tunnel syndrome
  Dermatomyositis
  Diabetic peripheral neuropathy
  Eaton-Lambert syndrome
  Guillain-Barré syndrome
  Multiple sclerosis
  Muscular dystrophy

Myasthenia gravis
Myopathy
Polymyositis
Radiculopathy
Traumatic injury

CRITICAL FINDINGS: N/A

INTERFERING FACTORS

This procedure is contraindicated for
- Patients with extensive skin infection.
- Patients receiving anticoagulant therapy.
- Patients with an infection at the sites of electrode placement.

Factors that may impair the results of the examination
- Inability of the patient to cooperate or remain still during the procedure because of age, significant pain, or mental status.
- Age-related decreases in electrical activity.
- Medications such as muscle relaxants, cholinergics, and anticholinergics.
- Improper placement of surface or needle electrodes.

NURSING IMPLICATIONS AND PROCEDURE

PRETEST:
- Positively identify the patient using at least two unique identifiers before providing care, treatment, or services.
- *Patient Teaching:* Inform the patient this procedure can assist in measuring the electrical activity of the muscles.
- Obtain a history of the patient's complaints, including a list of known allergens, especially allergies or sensitivities to latex, iodine, seafood, anesthetics, or contrast mediums.

- Obtain a history of the patient's musculoskeletal system, symptoms, and results of previously performed laboratory tests and diagnostic and surgical procedures.
- Obtain a list of the patient's current medications, including herbs, nutritional supplements, and nutraceuticals (see Appendix F).
- Review the procedure with the patient. Address concerns about pain related to the procedure and warn the patient the procedure may be uncomfortable, but an analgesic or sedative will be administered. Inform the patient that as many as 10 electrodes may be inserted at various locations on the body. Inform the patient the procedure is performed in a special laboratory by a health-care provider (HCP) and takes approximately 1 to 3 hr to complete, depending on the patient's condition.
- *Sensitivity to social and cultural issues,* as well as concern for modesty, is important in providing psychological support before, during, and after the procedure.
- Assess for the ability to comply with directions given for exercising during the test.
- Instruct the patient to remove jewelry and other metallic objects from the area to be examined.
- Under medical direction, the patient should avoid muscle relaxants, cholinergics, and anticholinergics for 3 to 6 days before the test.
- Instruct the patient to refrain from smoking and drinking caffeine-containing beverages for 3 hr before the procedure. Protocols may vary among facilities.
- *Make sure a written and informed consent has been signed prior to the procedure and before administering any medications.*

INTRATEST:
- Ensure the patient has refrained from smoking and drinking caffeine-containing beverages for 3 hr before the procedure.

- Ensure medications such as muscle relaxants, cholinergics, and anticholinergics have been withheld, as ordered.
- Ensure the patient has removed all external metallic objects from the area to be examined prior to the procedure.
- Instruct the patient to void prior to the procedure and to change into the gown, robe, and foot coverings provided.
- Ask the patient to remain very still and relaxed and to cooperate with instructions given to contract muscles during the procedure.
- Place the patient in a supine or sitting position depending on the location of the muscle to be tested. Ensure that the area or room is protected from noise or metallic interference that may affect the test results.
- Observe standard precautions, and follow the general guidelines in Appendix A.
- Administer mild analgesic (adult) or sedative (children), as ordered, to promote a restful state before the procedure.
- Cleanse the skin thoroughly with alcohol pads, as necessary.
- An electrode is applied to the skin to ground the patient, and then 24-gauge needles containing a fine-wire electrode are inserted into the muscle. The electrical potentials of the muscle are amplified, displayed on a screen, and electronically recorded.
- During the test, muscle activity is tested while the patient is at rest, during incremental needle insertion, and during varying degrees of muscle contraction.
- Ask the patient to alternate between a relaxed and a contracted muscle state or to perform progressive muscle contractions while the potentials are being measured.

POST-TEST:

- A report of the examination will be sent to the requesting HCP, who will discuss the results with the patient.
- When the procedure is complete, remove the electrodes and clean the skin where the electrode was applied.
- Monitor electrode sites for bleeding, hematoma, or inflammation.
- If residual pain is noted after the procedure, instruct the patient to apply warm compresses and to take analgesics, as ordered.
- Instruct the patient to resume usual diet, medication, and activity, as directed by the HCP.
- Reinforce information given by the patient's HCP regarding further testing, treatment, or referral to another HCP. Answer any questions or address any concerns voiced by the patient or family.
- Depending on the results of this procedure, additional testing may be performed to evaluate or monitor progression of the disease process and determine the need for a change in therapy. Evaluate test results in relation to the patient's symptoms and other tests performed.

RELATED MONOGRAPHS:

- Related tests include acetylcholine receptor antibody, biopsy muscle, CSF analysis, CT brain, CK, ENG, evoked brain potentials (SER, VER), MRI brain, plethysmography, and PET brain.
- Refer to the Musculoskeletal System table at the end of the book for related tests by body system.

Electromyography, Pelvic Floor Sphincter

SYNONYM/ACRONYM: Electrodiagnostic study, rectal electromyography.

COMMON USE: To assess urinary sphincter electrical activity to assist with diagnosis of urinary incontinence.

AREA OF APPLICATION: Sphincter muscles.

CONTRAST: None.

DESCRIPTION: Pelvic floor sphincter electromyography, also known as rectal electromyography, is performed to measure electrical activity of the external urinary sphincter. This procedure, often done in conjunction with cystometry and voiding urethrography as part of a full urodynamic study, helps to diagnose neuromuscular dysfunction and incontinence.

INDICATIONS

Evaluate neuromuscular dysfunction and incontinence

POTENTIAL DIAGNOSIS

Normal findings in
• Normal urinary and anal sphincter muscle function; increased electromyographic signals during the filling of the urinary bladder and at the conclusion of voiding; absence of signals during the actual voiding; no incontinence

Abnormal findings in
• Neuromuscular dysfunction of lower urinary sphincter, pelvic floor muscle dysfunction of the anal sphincter

CRITICAL FINDINGS: N/A

INTERFERING FACTORS

This procedure is contraindicated for
• Patients who are pregnant or suspected of being pregnant, unless the potential benefits of the procedure far outweigh the risks to the fetus and mother.

Factors that may impair the results of the examination
• Inability of the patient to cooperate or remain still during the procedure because of age, significant pain, or mental status.
• Age-related decreases in electrical activity.
• Medications such as muscle relaxants, cholinergics, and anticholinergics.

Other considerations
• Failure to follow dietary restrictions before the procedure may cause the procedure to be canceled or repeated.

NURSING IMPLICATIONS AND PROCEDURE

PRETEST:

▶ Positively identify the patient using at least two unique identifiers before providing care, treatment, or services.

E

▶ *Patient Teaching:* Inform the patient this procedure can assist in measuring the electrical activity of the pelvic floor muscles.

▶ Obtain a history of the patient's complaints, including a list of known allergens, especially allergies or sensitivities to latex, iodine, seafood, anesthetics, or contrast mediums.

▶ Obtain a history of the patient's genitourinary system, symptoms, and results of previously performed laboratory tests and diagnostic and surgical procedures.

▶ Obtain a list of the patient's current medications, including herbs, nutritional supplements, and nutraceuticals (see Appendix F).

▶ Review the procedure with the patient. Address concerns about pain related to the procedure. Warn the patient the procedure may be uncomfortable, but an analgesic or sedative will be administered. Assure the patient the pain is minimal during the catheter insertion. Inform the patient the procedure is performed in a special laboratory by a health-care provider (HCP) and takes about 30 min to complete.

▶ *Sensitivity to social and cultural issues,* as well as concern for modesty, is important in providing psychological support before, during, and after the procedure.

▶ Instruct the patient to remove jewelry and other metallic objects from the area to be examined.

▶ Assess for ability to comply with directions given for exercising during the test.

▶ Under medical direction, the patient should avoid muscle relaxants, cholinergics, and anticholinergics for 3 to 6 days before the test.

▶ Instruct the patient to refrain from smoking and drinking caffeine-containing beverages for 3 hr before the procedure. Protocols may vary among facilities.

▶ *Make sure a written and informed consent has been signed prior to the procedure and before administering any medications.*

INTRATEST:

▶ Ensure the patient has complied with dietary, fluid, tobacco, and medication restrictions and pretesting preparations.

▶ Record baseline vital signs.

▶ Instruct the patient to void prior to the procedure and to change into the gown, robe, and foot coverings provided.

▶ Place the patient in a supine position on the examining table and place a drape over the patient, exposing the perianal area.

▶ Ask the patient to remain very still and relaxed and to cooperate when instructed to contract muscles during the procedure.

▶ Observe standard precautions, and follow the general guidelines in Appendix A.

▶ Two skin electrodes are positioned slightly to the left and right of the perianal area and a grounding electrode is placed on the thigh.

▶ If needle electrodes are used, they are inserted into the muscle surrounding the urethra.

▶ Muscle activity signals are recorded as waves, which are interpreted for number and configurations in diagnosing urinary abnormalities.

▶ An indwelling urinary catheter is inserted, and the bulbocavernosus reflex is tested; the patient is instructed to cough while the catheter is gently pulled.

▶ Voluntary control is tested by requesting the patient to contract and relax the muscle. Electrical activity is recorded during this period of relaxation with the bladder empty.

▶ The bladder is filled with sterile water at a rate of 100 mL/min while the electrical activity during filling is recorded.

▶ The catheter is removed; the patient is then placed in a position to void and is asked to urinate and empty the full bladder. This voluntary urination is then recorded until completed. The complete procedure includes recordings of electrical signals before, during, and at the end of urination.

POST-TEST:

▶ A report of the examination will be sent to the requesting HCP, who will discuss the results with the patient.

- Instruct the patient to resume usual diet, fluids, medications, and activity, as directed by the HCP.
- Monitor vital signs and neurological status every 15 min for 1 hr, then every 2 hr for 4 hr, and as ordered. Take temperature every 4 hr for 24 hr. Monitor intake and output at least every 8 hr. Compare with baseline values. Protocols may vary among facilities.
- Instruct the patient to increase fluid intake unless contraindicated.
- If tested with needle electrodes, warn female patients to expect hematuria after the first voiding.
- Advise the patient to report symptoms of urethral irritation, such as dysuria, persistent or prolonged hematuria, and urinary frequency.
- Recognize anxiety related to test results, and be supportive of perceived loss of independent function. Discuss the implications of abnormal test results on the patient's lifestyle. Provide teaching and information regarding the clinical implications of the test results, as appropriate.
- Reinforce information given by the patient's HCP regarding further testing, treatment, or referral to another HCP. Answer any questions or address any concerns voiced by the patient or family.
- Depending on the results of this procedure, additional testing may be needed to evaluate or monitor progression of the disease process and determine the need for a change in therapy. Evaluate test results in relation to the patient's symptoms and other tests performed.

RELATED MONOGRAPHS:

- Related tests include CT pelvis, cystometry, cystoscopy, cystourethrography voiding, IVP, and US bladder.
- Refer to the Genitourinary System table at the end of the book for related tests by body system.

Electroneurography

SYNONYM/ACRONYM: Electrodiagnostic study, nerve conduction study, ENG.

COMMON USE: To assess peripheral nerve conduction to assist in the diagnosis of diseases such as diabetic neuropathy and muscular dystrophy.

AREA OF APPLICATION: Muscles.

CONTRAST: None.

DESCRIPTION: Electroneurography (ENG) is performed to identify peripheral nerve injury, to differentiate primary peripheral nerve pathology from muscular injury, and to monitor response of the nerve injury to treatment. A stimulus is applied through a surface electrode over a nerve. After a nerve is electrically stimulated proximally, the time for the impulse to travel to a second or distal site is measured. Because the conduction study of a nerve can vary from nerve to nerve, it is important to compare the results of the affected side to those of the contralateral side. The results of the stimulation are shown on a monitor, but the actual velocity must be calculated by dividing the distance in meters between the stimulation point and the response point by the time between the stimulus and response. Traumatic nerve transection, contusion, or neuropathy will usually cause maximal slowing of conduction velocity in the affected side compared with that in the normal side. A velocity greater than normal does not indicate a pathological condition. This test is usually performed in conjunction with electromyography in a combined test called *electromyoneurography.*

INDICATIONS

Confirm diagnosis of peripheral nerve damage or trauma

POTENTIAL DIAGNOSIS

Normal findings in

• No evidence of peripheral nerve injury or disease. Variable readings depend on the nerve being tested. For patients age 3 yr and older, the maximum conduction velocity is 40 to 80 milliseconds; for infants and the elderly, the values are divided by 2.

Abnormal findings in

• Carpal tunnel syndrome
• Diabetic neuropathy
• Guillain-Barré syndrome
• Herniated disk disease
• Muscular dystrophy
• Myasthenia gravis
• Poliomyelitis
• Tarsal tunnel syndrome
• Thoracic outlet syndrome

CRITICAL FINDINGS: N/A

INTERFERING FACTORS

Factors that may impair the results of the examination

• Inability of the patient to cooperate or remain still during the

procedure because of age, significant pain, or mental status.
• Age-related decreases in electrical activity.
• Poor electrode conduction or failure to obtain contralateral values for comparison.

NURSING IMPLICATIONS AND PROCEDURE

PRETEST:

▶ Positively identify the patient using at least two unique identifiers before providing care, treatment, or services.
▶ *Patient Teaching:* Inform the patient this procedure is performed to measure the electrical activity of the muscles.
▶ Obtain a history of the patient's complaints or symptoms, including a list of known allergens, especially allergies or sensitivities to latex, iodine, seafood, anesthetics, or contrast mediums.
▶ Obtain a history of the patient's neuromuscular system, symptoms, and results of previously performed laboratory tests and diagnostic and surgical procedures.
▶ Obtain a list of the patient's current medications, including herbs, nutritional supplements, and nutraceuticals (see Appendix F).
▶ Review the procedure with the patient. Address concerns about pain related to the procedure and inform the patient the procedure may be uncomfortable because of a mild electrical shock. Advise the patient that the electrical shock is brief and is not harmful. Inform the patient the procedure is performed in a special laboratory by a health-care provider (HCP) and takes approximately 15 min to complete but can take longer depending on the patient's condition.
▶ *Sensitivity to social and cultural issues,* as well as concern for modesty, is important in providing psychological support before, during, and after the procedure.
▶ There are no food, fluid, or medication restrictions unless by medical direction.

- Instruct the patient to remove jewelry and other metallic objects from the area to be examined.
- *Make sure a written and informed consent has been signed prior to the procedure and before administering any medications.*

INTRATEST:

- Ensure the patient has removed all external metallic objects from the area to be examined prior to the procedure.
- Instruct the patient to void prior to the procedure and to change into the gown, robe, and foot coverings provided.
- Place the patient in a supine or sitting position, depending on the location of the muscle to be tested.
- Observe standard precautions, and follow the general guidelines in Appendix A.
- Shave the extremity in the area to be stimulated, and cleanse the skin thoroughly with alcohol pads.
- Apply electrode gel and place a recording electrode at a known distance from the stimulation point. Measure the distance between the stimulation point and the site of the recording electrode in centimeters.
- Place a reference electrode nearby on the skin surface.
- The nerve is electrically stimulated by a shock-emitter device; the time between nerve impulse and electrical contraction, measured in milliseconds (distal latency), is shown on a monitor.
- The nerve is also electrically stimulated at a location proximal to the area of suspected injury or disease.
- The time required for the impulse to travel from the stimulation site to location of the muscle contraction (total latency) is recorded in milliseconds.
- Calculate the conduction velocity. The conduction velocity is converted to meters per second (m/sec) and computed using the following equation:

Conduction velocity (m/sec) = [distance (m)]/[total latency − distal latency]

POST-TEST:

- A report of the examination will be sent to the requesting HCP, who will discuss the results with the patient.
- When the procedure is complete, remove the electrodes and clean the skin where the electrodes were applied.
- Monitor electrode sites for inflammation.
- If residual pain is noted after the procedure, instruct the patient to apply warm compresses and to take analgesics, as ordered.
- Instruct the patient to resume usual diet, medication, and activity, as directed by the HCP.
- Recognize anxiety related to test results, and be supportive of perceived loss of independent function. Discuss the implications of abnormal test results on the patient's lifestyle. Provide teaching and information regarding the clinical implications of the test results, as appropriate.
- Reinforce information given by the patient's HCP regarding further testing, treatment, or referral to another HCP. Answer any questions or address any concerns voiced by the patient or family.
- Depending on the results of this procedure, additional testing may be performed to evaluate or monitor progression of the disease process and determine the need for a change in therapy. Evaluate test results in relation to the patient's symptoms and other tests performed.

RELATED MONOGRAPHS:

- Related tests include acetylcholine receptor antibody, biopsy muscle, CK, EMG, evoked brain potentials (SER, VER), fluorescein angiography, fundus photography, glucose, glycated hemoglobin, insulin, microalbumin, and plethysmography.
- Refer to the Musculoskeletal System table at the end of the book for related tests by body system.

Endoscopy, Sinus

SYNONYM/ACRONYM: N/A.

COMMON USE: To facilitate diagnosis and treatment of recurring sinus infections or infections resulting from unresolved sinus infection, including incursion into the brain, eye orbit, or eyeball.

AREA OF APPLICATION: Sinuses.

CONTRAST: N/A.

DESCRIPTION: Sinus endoscopy, done with a narrow flexible tube, is used to help diagnose damage to the sinuses, nose, and throat. The tube contains an optical device with a magnifying lens with a bright light; the tube is inserted through the nose and threaded through the sinuses to the throat. A camera, monitor, or other viewing device is connected to the endoscope to record areas being examined. Sinus endoscopy helps to diagnose structural defects, infection, damage to the sinuses, or structures in the nose and throat. It allows visualization of polyps and growths in the sinuses and can be used to investigate causes of recurrent inflammation of the sinuses (sinusitis). The procedure is usually done in a health-care provider's (HCP's) office, but if done as a surgical procedure, the endoscope may be used to remove polyps from the nose or throat.

INDICATIONS
- Nasal obstruction
- Recurrent sinusitis

POTENTIAL DIAGNOSIS

Normal findings in
- Normal soft tissue appearance

Abnormal findings in
- Foreign bodies in the nose
- Growths in the nasal passages
- Polyps
- Sinusitis

CRITICAL FINDINGS: N/A

INTERFERING FACTORS
- Inability of the patient to cooperate or remain still during the test because of age, significant pain, or mental status may interfere with the test results.

NURSING IMPLICATIONS AND PROCEDURE

PRETEST:
- Positively identify the patient using at least two unique identifiers before providing care, treatment, or services.
- *Patient Teaching:* Inform the patient this procedure can assist in locating and treating infection of the sinus or surrounding areas.
- Obtain a history of the patient's complaints, including a list of known allergens, especially allergies or sensitivities to latex.
- Obtain a history of the patient's respiratory system, symptoms, and results of

previously performed laboratory tests and diagnostic and surgical procedures.

- Obtain a list of the patient's current medications, including herbs, nutritional supplements, and nutraceuticals (see Appendix F).
- Instruct the patient to remove contact lenses or glasses, as appropriate.
- Review the procedure with the patient. Inform the patient that the procedure is usually done with the patient awake and seated upright in a chair. Address concerns about pain and explain that a local anesthetic spray or liquid may be applied to the throat to ease with insertion of the endoscope. Inform the patient that the procedure is usually performed in the office of an HCP and takes about 10 minutes.
- *Sensitivity to social and cultural issues*, as well as concern for modesty, is important in providing psychological support before, during, and after the procedure.
- There are no food, fluid, or medication restrictions unless by medical direction.
- *Make sure a written and informed consent has been signed prior to the procedure and before administering any medications.*

INTRATEST:

- Instruct the patient to cooperate fully and to follow directions. Instruct the patient to remain still throughout the procedure because movement produces unreliable results.
- Seat the patient comfortably. Instill ordered topical anesthetic in the throat, as ordered, and allow time for it to work.

- Observe standard precautions, and follow the general guidelines in Appendix A if cultures are to be obtained on aspirated sinus material.

POST-TEST:

- A report of the results will be sent to the requesting HCP, who will discuss the results with the patient.
- Instruct the patient to wait until the numbness in the throat wears off before attempting to eat or drink following the procedure.
- Recognize anxiety related to test results. Discuss the implications of abnormal test results on the patient's lifestyle. Provide teaching and information regarding the clinical implications of the test results, as appropriate.
- Reinforce information given by the patient's HCP regarding further testing, treatment, or referral to another HCP. Answer any questions or address any concerns voiced by the patient or family.
- Depending on the results of this procedure, additional testing may be needed to evaluate or monitor progression of the disease process and determine the need for a change in therapy. Evaluate test results in relation to the patient's symptoms and other tests performed.

RELATED MONOGRAPHS:

- Related tests include CT brain.
- Refer to the Respiratory System table at the end of the book for related tests by body system.

E

Eosinophil Count

SYNONYM/ACRONYM: Eos count, total eosinophil count.

COMMON USE: To assist in diagnosing conditions related to immune response such as asthma, dermatitis, hay fever, and Hodgkin's disease. Also used to assist in identification of parasitic infections.

SPECIMEN: Whole blood (1 mL) collected in a lavender-top (EDTA) tube.

REFERENCE VALUE: (Method: Manual count using eosinophil stain and hemocytometer or automated analyzer)

Absolute count: 50 to 500/mm^3
Relative percentage: 1% to 4%

DESCRIPTION: Eosinophils are white blood cells whose function is phagocytosis of antigen-antibody complexes and response to allergy-inducing substances and parasites. Eosinophils have granules that contain histamine used to kill foreign cells in the body. Eosinophils also contain proteolytic substances that damage parasitic worms. The binding of histamine to receptor sites on cells results in smooth muscle contraction in the bronchioles and upper respiratory tract, constriction of pulmonary vessels, increased mucus production, and secretion of acid by the cells that line the stomach. Eosinophil counts can increase to greater than 30% of normal in parasitic infections; however, a significant percentage of children with visceral larva migrans infestations have normal eosinophil counts.

INDICATIONS

Assist in the diagnosis of conditions such as allergies, parasitic infections, drug reactions, collagen diseases, Hodgkin's disease, and myeloproliferative disorders

POTENTIAL DIAGNOSIS

Increased in
Eosinophils are released and migrate to inflammatory sites in response to numerous environmental, chemical/drug, or immune-mediated triggers. T cells, mast cells, and macrophages release cytokines like interlukin-3 (IL3), interlukin-5 (IL5), granulocyte/macrophage colony–stimulating factor, and chemokines like the eotaxins, which can result in the activation of eosinophils.

- Addison's disease *(most commonly related to autoimmune destruction of adrenal glands)*
- Allergy
- Asthma
- Cancer
- Dermatitis
- Drug reactions
- Eczema
- Hay fever
- Hodgkin's disease
- Hypereosinophilic syndrome (rare and idiopathic)
- Löffler's syndrome *(pulmonary eosinophilia due to allergic reaction or infection from a fungus or parasite)*
- Myeloproliferative disorders *(related to abnormal changes in the bone marrow)*
- Parasitic infection (visceral larva migrans)
- Rheumatoid arthritis *(possibly related to medications used in therapy)*
- Rhinitis
- Sarcoidosis
- Splenectomy
- Tuberculosis

Decreased in
- Aplastic anemia *(bone marrow failure)*
- Eclampsia *(shift to the left; relative to significant production of neutrophils)*
- Infections *(shift to the left; relative to significant production of neutrophils)*

E

• Stress *(release of cortisol suppresses eosinophils)*

CRITICAL FINDINGS: N/A

INTERFERING FACTORS
• Numerous drugs and substances can cause an increase in eosinophil levels as a result of an allergic response or hypersensitivity reaction. These include acetophenazine, allopurinol, aminosalicylic acid, ampicillin, butaperazine, capreomycin, carisoprodol, cephaloglycin, cephaloridine, cephalosporins, cephapirin, cephradine, chloramphenicol, clindamycin, cloxacillin, dapsone, epicillin, erythromycin, fluorides, gold, imipramine, iodides, kanamycin, mefenamic acid, methicillin, methyldopa, minocycline, nalidixic acid, niridazole, nitrofurans (including nitrofurantoin), NSAIDs, nystatin, oxamniquine, penicillin, penicillin G, procainamide, ristocetin, streptokinase, streptomycin, tetracycline, triamterene, tryptophan, and viomycin.
• Drugs that can cause a decrease in eosinophil levels include acetylsalicylic acid, amphotericin B, corticotropin, desipramine, glucocorticoids, hydrocortisone, interferon, niacin, prednisone, and procainamide.
• Clotted specimens should be rejected for analysis.
• Specimens more than 4 hr old should be rejected for analysis.
• There is a diurnal variation in eosinophil counts. The count is lowest in the morning and continues to rise throughout the day until midnight. Therefore, serial measurements should be performed at the same time of day for purposes of continuity.

NURSING IMPLICATIONS AND PROCEDURE

PRETEST:
▶ Positively identify the patient using at least two unique identifiers before providing care, treatment, or services.
▶ *Patient Teaching:* Inform the patient this test can assist in diagnosing immune response conditions and parasitic infections.
▶ Obtain a history of the patient's complaints, including a list of known allergens, especially allergies or sensitivities to latex.
▶ Obtain a history of the patient's hematopoietic, immune, and respiratory systems; symptoms; and results of previously performed laboratory tests and diagnostic and surgical procedures.
▶ Obtain a list of the patient's current medications, including herbs, nutritional supplements, and nutraceuticals (see Appendix F).
▶ Review the procedure with the patient. Inform the patient that specimen collection takes approximately 5 to 10 min. Address concerns about pain and explain that there may be some discomfort during the venipuncture.
▶ *Sensitivity to social and cultural issues,* as well as concern for modesty, is important in providing psychological support before, during, and after the procedure.
▶ There are no food, fluid, or medication restrictions unless by medical direction.

INTRATEST:
▶ If the patient has a history of allergic reaction to latex, avoid the use of equipment containing latex.
▶ Instruct the patient to cooperate fully and to follow directions. Direct the patient to breathe normally and to avoid unnecessary movement.
▶ Observe standard precautions, and follow the general guidelines in Appendix A. Positively identify the patient, and label the appropriate tubes with the corresponding patient demographics, date, and time of collection. Perform a venipuncture.

- Remove the needle and apply direct pressure with dry gauze to stop bleeding. Observe/assess venipuncture site for bleeding or hematoma formation and secure gauze with adhesive bandage.
- Promptly transport the specimen to the laboratory for processing and analysis.

POST-TEST:

- A report of the results will be sent to the requesting health-care provider (HCP), who will discuss the results with the patient.
- *Nutritional Considerations:* Consideration should be given to diet if food allergies are present.
- Instruct the patient with an elevated eosinophil count to report any signs or symptoms of infection, such as fever.
- Instruct the patient with an elevated count to rest and take medications as prescribed, to increase fluid intake as appropriate, and to monitor temperature.

- Reinforce information given by the patient's HCP regarding further testing, treatment, or referral to another HCP. Answer any questions or address any concerns voiced by the patient or family.
- Depending on the results of this procedure, additional testing may be performed to evaluate or monitor progression of the disease process and determine the need for a change in therapy. Evaluate test results in relation to the patient's symptoms and other tests performed.

RELATED MONOGRAPHS:

- Related tests include allergen-specific immunoglobulin E, biopsy bone marrow, blood gases, CBC, culture stool, ESR, fecal analysis, hypersensitivity pneumonitis screen, IgE, lung perfusion scan, ova and parasites, plethysmography, and PFT.
- Refer to the Hematopoietic, Immune, and Respiratory systems tables at the end of the book for related tests by body system.

Erythrocyte Protoporphyrin, Free

SYNONYM/ACRONYM: Free erythrocyte protoporphyrin (FEP).

COMMON USE: To assist in diagnosing anemias related to chronic disease, hemolysis, iron deficiency, and lead toxicity.

SPECIMEN: Whole blood (1 mL) collected in a lavender-top (EDTA) or a green-top (heparin) tube.

REFERENCE VALUE: (Method: Fluorometry)

Conventional Units	SI Units (Conventional Units × 0.0178)
Adult	
Male	
Less than 30 mcg/dL	Less than 0.534 micromol/L
Female	
Less than 40 mcg/dL	Less than 0.712 micromol/L

DESCRIPTION: The free erythrocyte protoporphyrin (FEP) test measures the concentration of protoporphyrin in red blood cells. Protoporphyrin comprises the predominant porphyrin in red blood cells, which combines with iron to form the heme portion of hemoglobin. Protoporphyrin converts to bilirubin, combines with albumin, and remains unconjugated in the circulation after hemoglobin breakdown. Increased amounts of protoporphyrin can be detected in erythrocytes, urine, and stool in conditions interfering with heme synthesis. Protoporphyria is an autosomal dominant disorder in which increased amounts of protoporphyrin are secreted and excreted; the disorder is thought to be the result of an enzyme deficiency. Protoporphyria causes photosensitivity and may lead to cirrhosis of the liver and cholelithiasis as a result of protoporphyrin deposits. FEP is elevated in cases of lead toxicity or chronic exposure.

INDICATIONS
• Assist in the diagnosis of erythropoietic protoporphyrias
• Assist in the differential diagnosis of iron deficiency in pediatric patients
• Evaluate lead poisoning

POTENTIAL DIAGNOSIS

Increased in
• Anemia of chronic disease *(related to accumulation of protoporphyrin in the absence of available iron)*
• Conditions with marked erythropoiesis (e.g., hemolytic anemias)

(related to increased cell destruction)
• Erythropoietic protoporphyria *(related to abnormal increased secretion)*
• Iron-deficiency anemias *(related to accumulation of protoporphyrin in the absence of available iron)*
• Lead poisoning *(possibly related to inactivation of enzymes involved in iron binding or transfer)*
• Some sideroblastic anemias

Decreased in: N/A

CRITICAL FINDINGS: N/A

INTERFERING FACTORS
• Drugs that may increase FEP levels include erythropoietin.
• The test is unreliable in infants less than 6 mo of age.

NURSING IMPLICATIONS AND PROCEDURE

PRETEST:
▶ Positively identify the patient using at least two unique identifiers before providing care, treatment, or services.
▶ *Patient Teaching:* Inform the patient this test can assist in diagnosing specific types of anemias and lead toxicity as well as monitor chronic lead exposure.
▶ Obtain a history of the patient's complaints, including a list of known allergens, especially allergies or sensitivities to latex.
▶ Obtain a history of the patient's hematopoietic system, symptoms, and results of previously performed laboratory tests and diagnostic and surgical procedures.
▶ Obtain a list of the patient's current medications, including herbs, nutritional supplements, and nutraceuticals (see Appendix F).

E

▶ Review the procedure with the patient. Inform the patient that specimen collection takes approximately 5 to 10 min. Address concerns about pain and explain that there may be some discomfort during the venipuncture.

▶ *Sensitivity to social and cultural issues,* as well as concern for modesty, is important in providing psychological support before, during, and after the procedure.

▶ There are no food, fluid, or medication restrictions unless by medical direction.

INTRATEST:

▶ If the patient has a history of allergic reaction to latex, avoid the use of equipment containing latex.

▶ Instruct the patient to cooperate fully and to follow directions. Direct the patient to breathe normally and to avoid unnecessary movement.

▶ Observe standard precautions, and follow the general guidelines in Appendix A. Positively identify the patient, and label the appropriate tubes with the corresponding patient demographics, date, and time of collection. Perform a venipuncture. Specimens should be protected from light.

▶ Remove the needle and apply direct pressure with dry gauze to stop bleeding. Observe/assess venipuncture site for bleeding or hematoma formation and secure gauze with adhesive bandage.

▶ Promptly transport the specimen to the laboratory for processing and analysis.

POST-TEST:

▶ A report of the results will be sent to the requesting health-care provider (HCP), who will discuss the results with the patient.

▶ Reinforce information given by the patient's HCP regarding further testing, treatment, or referral to another HCP. Answer any questions or address any concerns voiced by the patient or family.

▶ Depending on the results of this procedure, additional testing may be performed to evaluate or monitor progression of the disease process and determine the need for a change in therapy. Evaluate test results in relation to the patient's symptoms and other tests performed.

RELATED MONOGRAPHS:

▶ Related tests include CBC hematocrit, CBC hemoglobin, iron/TIBC, lead, and urine porphyrins.

▶ Refer to the Hematopoietic System table at the end of the book for related tests by body system.

Erythrocyte Sedimentation Rate

SYNONYM/ACRONYM: Sed rate, ESR.

COMMON USE: To assist in diagnosing acute infection in diseases such as tissue necrosis, chronic infection, and acute inflammation.

SPECIMEN: Whole blood (5 mL) collected in a lavender-top (EDTA) tube for the modified Westergren method or a gray-top (3.8% sodium citrate) tube for the original Westergren method.

REFERENCE VALUE: (Method: Westergren)

Age	Male	Female
Newborn	0–2 mm/hr	0–2 mm/hr
Less than 50 yr	0–15 mm/hr	0–25 mm/hr
50 yr and older	0–20 mm/hr	0–30 mm/hr

DESCRIPTION: The erythrocyte sedimentation rate (ESR) is a measure of the rate of sedimentation of red blood cells (RBCs) in an anticoagulated whole blood sample over a specified period of time. The basis of the ESR test is the alteration of blood proteins by inflammatory and necrotic processes that cause the RBCs to stick together, become heavier, and rapidly settle at the bottom of a vertically held, calibrated tube over time. The most common promoter of rouleaux is an increase in circulating fibrinogen levels. In general, relatively little settling occurs in normal blood because normal RBCs do not form rouleaux (which increases their mass and rate of sedimentation) and would not stack together. The sedimentation rate is proportional to the size or mass of the falling RBCs and is inversely proportional to plasma viscosity. The test is a nonspecific indicator of disease but is fairly sensitive and is frequently the earliest indicator of widespread inflammatory reaction due to infection or autoimmune disorders. Prolonged elevations are also present in malignant disease. The ESR can also be used to monitor the course of a disease and the effectiveness of therapy. The most commonly used method to measure the ESR is the Westergren (or modified Westergren) method.

INDICATIONS

- Assist in the diagnosis of acute infection, such as tuberculosis or tissue necrosis
- Assist in the diagnosis of acute inflammatory processes
- Assist in the diagnosis of chronic infections
- Assist in the diagnosis of rheumatoid or autoimmune disorders
- Assist in the diagnosis of temporal arthritis and polymyalgia rheumatica
- Monitor inflammatory and malignant disease

POTENTIAL DIAGNOSIS

Increased in

Increased rouleaux formation is associated with increased levels of fibrinogen and/or production of cytokines and other acute-phase reactant proteins in response to inflammation. Anemia of chronic disease as well as acute anemia influence the ESR because the decreased number of RBCs falls faster with the relatively increased plasma volume.

- Acute myocardial infarction
- Anemia *(RBCs fall faster with increased plasma volume)*
- Carcinoma
- Cat scratch fever *(Bartonella henselae)*
- Collagen diseases, including systemic lupus erythematosus (SLE)
- Crohn's disease *(due to anemia or related to acute-phase reactant proteins)*
- Elevated blood glucose *(hyperglycemia in older patients can*

induce production of cytokines responsible for the inflammatory response; hyperglycemia related to insulin resistance can cause hepatocytes to shift protein synthesis from albumin to production of acute-phase reactant proteins)

- Endocarditis
- Heavy metal poisoning *(related to anemia affecting size and shape of RBCs)*
- Increased plasma protein level *(RBCs fall faster with increased plasma viscosity)*
- Infections (e.g., pneumonia, syphilis)
- Inflammatory diseases
- Lymphoma
- Lymphosarcoma
- Multiple myeloma *(RBCs fall faster with increased plasma viscosity)*
- Nephritis
- Pregnancy *(related to anemia)*
- Pulmonary embolism
- Rheumatic fever
- Rheumatoid arthritis
- Subacute bacterial endocarditis
- Temporal arteritis
- Toxemia
- Tuberculosis
- Waldenström's macroglobulinemia *(RBCs fall faster with increased plasma viscosity)*

Normal findings in
- Congestive heart failure
- Glucose-6-phosphate dehydrogenase deficiency
- Hemoglobin C disease
- Hypofibrinogenemia
- Polycythemia
- Sickle cell anemia
- Spherocytosis

Decreased in
- Conditions resulting in high hemoglobin and RBC count

CRITICAL FINDINGS: N/A

INTERFERING FACTORS

- Some drugs cause an SLE-like syndrome that results in a physiological increase in ESR. These include anticonvulsants, hydrazine derivatives, nitrofurantoin, procainamide, and quinidine. Other drugs that may cause an increased ESR include acetylsalicylic acid, cephalothin, cephapirin, cyclosporin A, dextran, and oral contraceptives.
- Drugs that may cause a decrease in ESR include aurothiomalate, corticotropin, cortisone, dexamethasone, methotrexate, minocycline, NSAIDs, penicillamine, prednisolone, prednisone, quinine, sulfasalazine, tamoxifen, and trimethoprim.
- Menstruation may cause falsely increased test results.
- Prolonged tourniquet constriction around the arm may cause hemoconcentration and falsely low values.
- The Westergren and modified Westergren methods are affected by heparin, which causes a false elevation in values.
- Bubbles in the Westergren tube or pipette, or tilting the measurement column more than 3° from vertical, will falsely increase the values.
- Movement or vibration of the surface on which the test is being conducted will affect the results.
- Inaccurate timing will invalidate test results.
- Specimens that are clotted, hemolyzed, or insufficient in volume should be rejected for analysis.
- The test should be performed within 4 hr of collection when the specimen has been stored at room temperature; delays in testing may result in decreased values. If a delay in testing is anticipated, refrigerate the sample at 2°C to 4°C; stability at refrigerated temperature is reported to be extended up to 12 hr. Refrigerated specimens should be brought to room temperature before testing.

NURSING IMPLICATIONS AND PROCEDURE

PRETEST:

- Positively identify the patient using at least two unique identifiers before providing care, treatment, or services.
- *Patient Teaching:* Inform the patient this test can assist in identification of inflammation.
- Obtain a history of the patient's complaints, including a list of known allergens, especially allergies or sensitivities to latex.
- Obtain a history of infectious, autoimmune, or neoplastic diseases.
- Obtain a history of the patient's cardiovascular, hematopoietic, immune, and respiratory systems; symptoms; and results of previously performed laboratory tests and diagnostic and surgical procedures.
- Obtain a list of the patient's current medications, including herbs, nutritional supplements, and nutraceuticals (see Appendix F).
- Review the procedure with the patient. Inform the patient that specimen collection takes approximately 5 to 10 min. Address concerns about pain and explain that there may be some discomfort during the venipuncture.
- *Sensitivity to social and cultural issues,* as well as concern for modesty, is important in providing psychological support before, during, and after the procedure.
- There are no food, fluid, or medication restrictions unless by medical direction.

INTRATEST:

- If the patient has a history of allergic reaction to latex, avoid the use of equipment containing latex.
- Instruct the patient to cooperate fully and to follow directions. Direct the patient to breathe normally and to avoid unnecessary movement.
- Observe standard precautions, and follow the general guidelines in Appendix A. Positively identify the patient, and label the appropriate tubes with the corresponding patient demographics, date, and time of collection. Perform a venipuncture; collect the specimen in a 5-mL gray-top (sodium citrate) tube if the Westergren method will be used. Collect the specimen in a 5-mL purple-top (EDTA) tube if the modified Westergren method will be used.
- Remove the needle and apply direct pressure with dry gauze to stop bleeding. Observe/assess venipuncture site for bleeding or hematoma formation and secure gauze with adhesive bandage.
- Promptly transport the specimen to the laboratory for processing and analysis.

POST-TEST:

- A report of the results will be sent to the requesting health-care provider (HCP), who will discuss the results with the patient.
- Reinforce information given by the patient's HCP regarding further testing, treatment, or referral to another HCP. Answer any questions or address any concerns voiced by the patient or family.
- Depending on the results of this procedure, additional testing may be performed to evaluate or monitor progression of the disease process and determine the need for a change in therapy. Evaluate test results in relation to the patient's symptoms and other tests performed.

RELATED MONOGRAPHS:

- Related tests include antibodies, anti-cyclic citrullinated peptide, ANA, arthroscopy, arthrogram, blood pool imaging, BMD, bone scan, CBC, CBC hematocrit, CBC hemoglobin, CBC RBC indices, CBC RBC morphology, CT cardiac scoring, copper, CRP, D-dimer, exercise stress test, fibrinogen, glucose, iron, lead, MRI musculoskeletal, microorganism-specific serologies and related cultures, myocardial perfusion heart scan, radiography bone, RF, synovial fluid analysis, and troponin.
- Refer to the Cardiovascular, Hematopoietic, Immune, and Respiratory systems tables at the end of the book for related tests by body system.

Erythropoietin

SYNONYM/ACRONYM: EPO.

COMMON USE: To evaluate the effectiveness of erythropoietin (EPO) administration as a treatment for anemia, especially related to chemotherapy and renal disease.

SPECIMEN: Serum (2 mL) collected in a red- or tiger-top tube.

REFERENCE VALUE: (Method: Immunochemiluminometric assay).

Age	Conventional Units	Conventional Units
	Male	*Female*
0–3 yr	1.7–17.9	2.1–15.9
4–6 yr	3.5–21.9	2.9–8.5
7–9 yr	1.0–13.5	2.1–8.2
10–12 yr	1.0–14.0	1.1–9.1
13–15 yr	2.2–14.4	3.8–20.5
16–18 yr	1.5–15.2	2.0–14.2
Adult	4.2–27.8	4.2–27.8

Based on normal hemoglobin and hematocrit. Values may be decreased in older adults due to the effects of medications and the presence of multiple chronic or acute diseases with or without muted symptoms.

DESCRIPTION: Erythropoietin (EPO) is a glycoprotein produced mainly by the kidney. Its function is to stimulate the bone marrow to make red blood cells (RBCs). EPO levels fall after removal of the kidney but do not disappear completely. It is thought that small amounts of EPO may be produced by the liver. Erythropoiesis is regulated by EPO and tissue Po_2. When Po_2 is normal, EPO levels decrease; when Po_2 falls, EPO secretion occurs and EPO levels increase.

INDICATIONS

- Assist in assessment of anemia of end-stage renal disease
- Assist in the diagnosis of EPO-producing tumors
- Evaluate the presence of rare anemias
- Monitor patients receiving EPO therapy

POTENTIAL DIAGNOSIS

Increased in

- After moderate bleeding in an otherwise healthy patient *(related to loss of RBCs, which stimulates production)*
- AIDS *(related to anemia, which stimulates production)*
- Anemias (e.g., hemolytic, iron deficiency, megaloblastic) *(related to low RBC count, which stimulates production)*
- Hepatoma *(related to EPO-producing tumors)*

- Kidney transplant rejection *(15% of cases respond with an exaggerated secretion of EPO and a transient post-transplantation erythrocytosis)*
- Nephroblastoma *(related to EPO-producing tumors)*
- Pheochromocytoma *(related to EPO-producing tumors)*
- Polycystic kidney disease *(related to EPO-producing tumors or cysts)*
- Pregnancy *(related to anemia of pregnancy, which stimulates production)*
- Secondary polycythemia where low oxygen levels stimulate production *(high-altitude hypoxia, chronic obstructive pulmonary disease, pulmonary fibrosis)*

Decreased in
- Chemotherapy *(related to therapy, which can be toxic to the kidney)*
- Primary polycythemia *(related to feedback loop response to elevated RBC count)*
- Renal failure *(related to decreased production and excessive loss through excretion by damaged kidneys)*

CRITICAL FINDINGS: N/A

INTERFERING FACTORS
- Drugs, hormones, and other substances that may increase EPO levels include adrenocorticotropic hormone (ACTH), anabolic steroids, androgens, angiotensin, epinephrine, daunorubicin, fenoterol, growth hormone, and thyroid-stimulating hormone (TSH).
- Phlebotomy may increase EPO levels.
- Drugs that may decrease EPO levels include amphotericin B, cisplatin, enalapril, estrogens, furosemide, and theophylline.
- Blood transfusions may also decrease EPO levels.

NURSING IMPLICATIONS AND PROCEDURE

PRETEST:
- Positively identify the patient using at least two unique identifiers before providing care, treatment, or services.
- *Patient Teaching:* Inform the patient this test can assist in evaluation of anemia.
- Obtain a history of the patient's complaints, including a list of known allergens, especially allergies or sensitivities to latex.
- Obtain a history of the patient's hematopoietic and genitourinary systems, symptoms, and results of previously performed laboratory tests and diagnostic and surgical procedures.
- Note any recent procedures that can interfere with test results.
- Obtain a list of the patient's current medications, including herbs, nutritional supplements, and nutraceuticals (see Appendix F).
- Review the procedure with the patient. Inform the patient that specimen collection takes approximately 5 to 10 min. Address concerns about pain and explain to the patient that there may be some discomfort during the venipuncture.
- *Sensitivity to social and cultural issues,* as well as concern for modesty, is important in providing psychological support before, during, and after the procedure.
- There are no food, fluid, or medication restrictions unless by medical direction.

INTRATEST:
- If the patient has a history of allergic reaction to latex, avoid the use of equipment containing latex.
- Instruct the patient to cooperate fully and to follow directions. Direct the patient to breathe normally and to avoid unnecessary movement.
- Observe standard precautions, and follow the general guidelines in Appendix A. Positively identify the patient, and label the appropriate tubes with the corresponding patient demographics, date, and time of collection. Perform a venipuncture.

▶ Remove the needle and apply direct pressure with dry gauze to stop bleeding. Observe/assess venipuncture site for bleeding or hematoma formation and secure gauze with adhesive bandage.

▶ Promptly transport the specimen to the laboratory for processing and analysis.

POST-TEST:

▶ A report of the results will be sent to the requesting health-care provider (HCP), who will discuss the results with the patient.

▶ Reinforce information given by the patient's HCP regarding further testing, treatment, or referral to another HCP. Answer any questions or address any concerns voiced by the patient or family.

▶ Depending on the results of this procedure, additional testing may be performed to evaluate or monitor progression of the disease process and determine the need for a change in therapy. Evaluate test results in relation to the patient's symptoms and other tests performed.

RELATED MONOGRAPHS:

▶ Related tests include biopsy bone marrow, BUN, CBC, CBC hematocrit, CBC hemoglobin, CBC RBC count, CBC RBC indices, CBC RBC morphology and inclusions, CT renal, creatinine, creatinine clearance, ferritin, iron/TIBC, microalbumin, retrograde ureteropyelography, US kidney, and vitamin B_{12}.

▶ Refer to the Hematopoietic and Genitourinary systems tables at the end of the book for related tests by body system.

Esophageal Manometry

SYNONYM/ACRONYM: Esophageal function study, esophageal acid study (Tuttle test), acid reflux test, Bernstein test (acid perfusion), esophageal motility study.

COMMON USE: To evaluate potential ineffectiveness of the esophageal muscle and structure in swallowing, vomiting, and regurgitation in diseases such as scleroderma, infection, and gastric esophageal reflux.

AREA OF APPLICATION: Esophagus.

CONTRAST: Done with or without nioniodinated contrast medium.

DESCRIPTION: Esophageal manometry (EM) consists of a group of invasive studies performed to assist in diagnosing abnormalities of esophageal muscle function and esophageal structure. These studies measure esophageal pressure, the effects of gastric acid in the esophagus, lower esophageal sphincter pressure, and motility patterns that result during swallowing. EM can be used to document and quantify gastroesophageal reflux (GER). It is indicated when a patient is experiencing difficulty swallowing, heartburn, regurgitation, or vomiting or has chest pain for which no diagnosis has been found. Tests performed in combination with EM include the acid reflux, acid clearing, and acid perfusion (Bernstein) tests.

INDICATIONS
- Aid in the diagnosis of achalasia, evidenced by increased pressure in EM
- Aid in the diagnosis of chalasia in children, evidenced by decreased pressure in EM
- Aid in the diagnosis of esophageal scleroderma, evidenced by decreased pressure in EM
- Aid in the diagnosis of esophagitis, evidenced by decreased motility
- Aid in the diagnosis of GER, evidenced by low pressure in EM, decreased pH in acidity test, and pain in acid reflux and perfusion tests
- Differentiate between esophagitis or cardiac condition as the cause of epigastric pain
- Evaluate pyrosis and dysphagia to determine if the cause is GER or esophagitis

POTENTIAL DIAGNOSIS

Normal findings in
- Acid clearing: fewer than 10 swallows
- Acid perfusion: no GER
- Acid reflux: no regurgitation into the esophagus
- Bernstein test: negative
- Esophageal secretions: pH 5 to 6
- Esophageal sphincter pressure: 10 to 20 mm Hg

Abnormal findings in
- Achalasia (sphincter pressure of 50 mm Hg)
- Chalasia
- Esophageal scleroderma
- Esophagitis
- GER (sphincter pressure of 0 to 5 mm Hg, pH of 1 to 3)

- Hiatal hernia
- Progressive systemic sclerosis (scleroderma)
- Spasms

CRITICAL FINDINGS: N/A

INTERFERING FACTORS

This procedure is contraindicated for
- Patients with unstable cardiopulmonary status, blood coagulation defects, recent gastrointestinal surgery, esophageal varices, or bleeding.

Factors that may impair the results of the examination
- Inability of the patient to cooperate or remain still during the procedure because of age, significant pain, or mental status.
- Administration of medications (e.g., sedatives, antacids, anticholinergics, cholinergics, corticosteroids) that can change pH or relax the sphincter muscle, causing inaccurate results.

Other considerations
- Failure to follow dietary restrictions before the procedure may cause the procedure to be canceled or repeated.

NURSING IMPLICATIONS AND PROCEDURE

PRETEST:
▶ Positively identify the patient using at least two unique identifiers before providing care, treatment, or services.
▶ *Patient Teaching:* Inform the patient this procedure can assist in assessing the esophagus.
▶ Obtain a history of the patient's complaints, including a list of known

allergens, especially allergies or sensitivities to latex, iodine, seafood, anesthetics, and contrast mediums.

▶ Obtain a history of the patient's gastrointestinal system, symptoms, and results of previously performed laboratory tests and diagnostic and surgical procedures.

▶ Note any recent barium or other radiological contrast procedures. Ensure that barium studies were performed more than 4 days before the EM.

▶ Record the date of the last menstrual period and determine the possibility of pregnancy in perimenopausal women.

▶ Obtain a list of the patient's current medications, including anticoagulants, aspirin and other salicylates, herbs, nutritional supplements, and nutraceuticals (see Appendix F). Note the last time and dose of medication taken.

▶ Review the procedure with the patient. Address concerns about pain related to the procedure and explain that some pain may be experienced during the test; there may be moments of discomfort and gagging when the scope is inserted, but there are no complications resulting from the procedure; and the throat will be anesthetized with a spray or swab. Inform the patient that he or she will not be able to speak during the procedure but breathing will not be affected. Inform the patient that the procedure is performed in an endoscopy suite by a health-care provider (HCP), under local anesthesia, and takes approximately 30 to 45 min.

▶ *Sensitivity to social and cultural issues,* as well as concern for modesty, is important in providing psychological support before, during, and after the procedure.

▶ Explain that an IV line may be started to allow for the infusion of a sedative or IV fluids.

▶ Instruct the patient to remove dentures and eyewear.

▶ Under medical direction, the patient should withhold medications for 24 hr before the study; special arrangements may be necessary for diabetic patients.

▶ Instruct the patient to fast and restrict fluids for 6 to 8 hr prior to the procedure. Protocols may vary among facilities.

▶ Obtain and record baseline vital signs.

▶ *Make sure a written and informed consent has been signed prior to the procedure and before administering any medications.*

INTRATEST:

▶ Ensure that the patient has complied with dietary, fluids, and medication restrictions and pretesting preparations for at least 6 to 8 hr prior to the procedure.

▶ Ensure the patient has removed dentures and eyewear prior to the procedure.

▶ Avoid using morphine sulfate in patients with asthma or other pulmonary disease. This drug can further exacerbate bronchospasms and respiratory impairment.

▶ Have emergency equipment readily available.

▶ Instruct the patient to void prior to the procedure and to change into the gown, robe, and foot coverings provided.

▶ Instruct the patient to cooperate fully and to follow directions. Instruct the patient to remain still throughout the procedure because movement produces unreliable results.

▶ Observe standard precautions, and follow the general guidelines in Appendix A.

▶ Insert an IV line and inject ordered sedation.

▶ Spray or swab the oropharynx with a topical local anesthetic.

▶ Provide an emesis basin for the increased saliva and encourage the patient to spit out saliva since the gag reflex may be impaired.

▶ Monitor the patient for complications related to the procedure (e.g., aspiration of stomach contents into the lungs, dyspnea, tachypnea, adventitious sounds).

▶ Suction the mouth, pharynx, and trachea, and administer oxygen as ordered.

Esophageal Manometry

▶ One or more small tubes are inserted through the nose into the esophagus and stomach.

▶ A small transducer is attached to the ends of the tubes to measure lower

esophageal sphincter pressure, intraluminal pressures, and regularity and duration of peristaltic contractions.
- Instruct the patient to swallow small amounts of water or flavored gelatin.

Esophageal Acid and Clearing (Tuttle Test)
- With the tube in place, a pH electrode probe is inserted into the esophagus with Valsalva maneuvers performed to stimulate reflux of stomach contents into the esophagus.
- If acid reflux is absent, 100 mL of 0.1% hydrochloric acid is instilled into the stomach during a 3-min period, and the pH measurement is repeated.
- To determine acid clearing, hydrochloric acid is instilled into the esophagus and the patient is asked to swallow while the probe measures the pH.

Acid Perfusion (Bernstein Test)
- A catheter is inserted through the nose into the esophagus, and the patient is asked to inform the HCP when pain is experienced.
- Normal saline solution is allowed to drip into the catheter at about 10 mL/min. Then hydrochloric acid is allowed to drip into the catheter.
- Pain experienced when the hydrochloric acid is instilled determines the presence of an esophageal abnormality. If no pain is experienced, symptoms are the result of some other condition.

POST-TEST:
- A report of the examination will be sent to the requesting HCP, who will discuss the results with the patient.
- Monitor the patient for signs of respiratory depression (less than 15 respirations/min) every 15 min for 2 hr. Resuscitation equipment should be available.
- Observe the patient for indications of perforation: painful swallowing with neck movement, substernal pain with respiration, shoulder pain, dyspnea, abdominal or back pain, cyanosis, and fever.

- Instruct the patient not to eat or drink until the gag reflex returns and then to eat lightly for 12 to 24 hr.
- Instruct the patient to resume usual activity, medication, and diet 24 hr after the examination or as tolerated, as directed by the HCP.
- Inform the patient to expect some throat soreness and possible hoarseness. Advise the patient to use warm gargles, lozenges, or ice packs to the neck and to drink cool fluids to alleviate throat discomfort.
- Emphasize that any severe pain, fever, difficulty breathing, or expectoration of blood must be reported to the HCP immediately.
- Recognize anxiety related to test results, and offer support. Discuss the implications of abnormal test results on the patient's lifestyle. Provide teaching and information regarding the clinical implications of the test results, as appropriate.
- Reinforce information given by the patient's HCP regarding further testing, treatment, or referral to another HCP. Answer any questions or address any concerns voiced by the patient or family.
- Depending on the results of this procedure, additional testing may be needed to evaluate or monitor progression of the disease process and determine the need for a change in therapy. Evaluate test results in relation to the patient's symptoms and other tests performed.

RELATED MONOGRAPHS:
- Related tests include ANA, barium swallow, biopsy skin, capsule endoscopy, chest x-ray, CT thoracic, esophagogastroduodenoscopy, fecal analysis, gastric emptying scan, GER scan, lung perfusion scan, mediastinoscopy, and upper GI series.
- Refer to the Gastrointestinal System table at the end of the book for related tests by body system.

Esophagogastroduodenoscopy

SYNONYM/ACRONYM: Esophagoscopy, gastroscopy, upper GI endoscopy, EGD.

COMMON USE: To visualize and assess the esophagus, stomach, and upper portion of the duodenum to assist in diagnosis of bleeding, ulcers, inflammation, tumor, and cancer.

AREA OF APPLICATION: Esophagus, stomach, and upper duodenum.

CONTRAST: Done without contrast.

DESCRIPTION: Esophagogastroduodenoscopy (EGD) allows direct visualization of the upper gastrointestinal (GI) tract mucosa, which includes the esophagus, stomach, and upper portion of the duodenum, by means of a flexible endoscope. The standard flexible fiberoptic endoscope contains three channels that allow passage of the instruments needed to perform therapeutic or diagnostic procedures, such as biopsies or cytology washings. The endoscope, a multichannel instrument, allows visualization of the GI tract linings, insufflation of air, aspiration of fluid, removal of foreign bodies by suction or by snare or forceps, and passage of a laser beam for obliteration of abnormal tissue or control of bleeding. Direct visualization yields greater diagnostic data than is possible through radiological procedures, and therefore EGD is rapidly replacing upper GI series as the diagnostic procedure of choice.

INDICATIONS
- Assist in differentiating between benign and neoplastic tumors
- Detect gastric or duodenal ulcers
- Detect upper GI inflammatory disease
- Determine the presence and location of acute upper GI bleeding
- Evaluate the extent of esophageal injury after ingestion of chemicals
- Evaluate stomach or duodenum after surgical procedures
- Evaluate suspected gastric outlet obstruction
- Identify tissue abnormalities and obtain biopsy specimens
- Investigate the cause of dysphagia, dyspepsia, and epigastric pain

POTENTIAL DIAGNOSIS

Normal findings in
- Esophageal mucosa is normally yellow-pink. At about 9 in. from the incisor teeth, a pulsation indicates the location of the aortic arch. The gastric mucosa is orange-red and contains rugae. The proximal duodenum is reddish and contains a few longitudinal folds, whereas the distal duodenum has circular folds lined with villi. No abnormal structures or functions are observed in the esophagus, stomach, or duodenum.

Abnormal findings in
- Acute and chronic gastric and duodenal ulcers
- Diverticular disease

- Duodenitis
- Esophageal varices
- Esophageal or pyloric stenosis
- Esophagitis or strictures
- Gastritis
- Hiatal hernia
- Mallory-Weiss syndrome
- Tumors (benign or malignant)

CRITICAL FINDINGS
- Presence and location of acute GI bleed

It is essential that critical diagnoses be communicated immediately to the appropriate health-care provider (HCP). A listing of these diagnoses varies among facilities. Note and immediately report to the HCP abnormal results and related symptoms.

INTERFERING FACTORS

This procedure is contraindicated for
- Patients who have had surgery involving the stomach or duodenum, which can make locating the duodenal papilla difficult.
- Patients with a bleeding disorder.
- Patients with unstable cardiopulmonary status, blood coagulation defects, or cholangitis, unless the patient received prophylactic antibiotic therapy before the test (otherwise the examination must be rescheduled).
- Patients with unstable cardiopulmonary status, blood coagulation defects, known aortic arch aneurysm, large esophageal Zenker's diverticulum, recent GI surgery, esophageal varices, or known esophageal perforation.

Factors that may impair clear imaging
- Gas or food in the GI tract resulting from inadequate cleansing or failure to restrict food intake before the study.

- Retained barium from a previous radiological procedure.
- Inability of the patient to cooperate or remain still during the procedure because of age, significant pain, or mental status.

Other considerations
- The procedure may be terminated if chest pain or severe cardiac arrhythmias occur.
- Failure to follow dietary restrictions and other pretesting preparations may cause the procedure to be canceled or repeated.

NURSING IMPLICATIONS AND PROCEDURE

PRETEST:
- Positively identify the patient using at least two unique identifiers before providing care, treatment, or services.
- *Patient Teaching:* Inform the patient this procedure can assist in assessing the esophagus and gastrointestinal tract.
- Obtain a history of the patient's complaints, including a list of known allergens, especially allergies or sensitivities to latex, iodine, seafood, anesthetics, or contrast mediums.
- Obtain a history of the patient's gastrointestinal system, symptoms, and results of previously performed laboratory tests and diagnostic and surgical procedures.
- Note any recent barium or other radiological contrast procedures ordered. Ensure that barium studies are performed after this study.
- Record the date of the last menstrual period and determine the possibility of pregnancy in perimenopausal women.
- Obtain a list of the patient's current medications including anticoagulants, aspirin and other salicylates, herbs, nutritional supplements, and nutraceuticals (see Appendix F). Note the last time and dose of medication taken.
- Review the procedure with the patient. Address concerns about pain related to the procedure and explain that some

pain may be experienced during the test, and there may be moments of discomfort, but the throat will be anesthetized with a spray or swab. Inform the patient that he or she will not be able to speak during the procedure, but breathing will not be affected. Inform the patient that the procedure is performed in a GI laboratory or radiology department, usually by an HCP and support staff, and takes approximately 30 to 60 min.

▶ *Sensitivity to social and cultural issues,* as well as concern for modesty, is important in providing psychological support before, during, and after the procedure.

▶ Explain that an IV line may be started to allow for the infusion of a sedative or IV fluids.

▶ Inform the patient that a laxative and cleansing enema may be needed the day before the procedure, with cleansing enemas on the morning of the procedure, depending on the institution's policy.

▶ Inform the patient that dentures and eyewear will be removed before the test.

▶ Instruct the patient to remove jewelry and other metallic objects from the area to be examined.

▶ Instruct the patient to fast and restrict fluids for 8 hr prior to the procedure. Protocols may vary among facilities.

▶ *Make sure a written and informed consent has been signed prior to the procedure and before administering any medications.*

INTRATEST:

▶ Ensure the patient has complied with dietary and medication restrictions and pretesting preparations for at least 8 hr prior to the procedure.

▶ Ensure the patient has removed all external metallic objects from the area to be examined prior to the procedure.

▶ Assess for completion of bowel preparation according to the institution's procedure.

▶ Have emergency equipment readily available.

▶ Instruct the patient to void prior to the procedure and to change into the gown, robe, and foot coverings provided.

▶ Instruct the patient to cooperate fully and to follow directions. Instruct the patient to remain still throughout the procedure because movement produces unreliable results.

▶ Observe standard precautions, and follow the general guidelines in Appendix A. Positively identify the patient, and label the appropriate collection container with the corresponding patient demographics, date, and time of collection.

▶ Obtain and record baseline vital signs.

▶ Start an IV line and administer ordered sedation.

▶ Spray or swab the oropharynx with a topical local anesthetic.

▶ Provide an emesis basin for the increased saliva and encourage the patient to spit out the saliva because the gag reflex may be impaired.

▶ Place the patient on an examination table in the left lateral decubitus position with the neck slightly flexed forward.

▶ The endoscope is passed through the mouth with a dental suction device in place to drain secretions. A sideviewing flexible, fiberoptic endoscope is advanced, and visualization of the GI tract is started.

▶ Air is insufflated to distend the upper GI tract, as needed. Biopsy specimens are obtained and/or endoscopic surgery is performed.

▶ Promptly transport the specimens to the laboratory for processing and analysis.

▶ At the end of the procedure, excess air and secretions are aspirated through the scope and the endoscope is removed.

▶ The needle or catheter is removed, and a pressure dressing is applied over the puncture site.

▶ Observe/assess the needle/catheter insertion site for bleeding, inflammation, or hematoma formation.

POST-TEST:

▶ A report of the examination will be sent to the requesting HCP, who will discuss the results with the patient.

▶ Observe the patient for indications of esophageal perforation (i.e., painful swallowing with neck movement, substernal pain with respiration, shoulder pain or dyspnea, abdominal or back pain, cyanosis, or fever).

- Do not allow the patient to eat or drink until the gag reflex returns; then allow the patient to eat lightly for 12 to 24 hr.
- Monitor vital signs and neurological status every 15 min for 1 hr, then every 2 hr for 4 hr, and as ordered by the HCP. Take temperature every 4 hr for 24 hr. Monitor intake and output at least every 8 hr. Compare with baseline values. Notify the HCP if temperature is elevated. Protocols may vary among facilities.
- Instruct the patient to resume usual activity and diet in 24 hr or as tolerated after the examination, as directed by the HCP.
- Observe/assess the needle/catheter insertion site for bleeding, inflammation, or hematoma formation.
- Instruct the patient in the care and assessment of the injection site.
- Inform the patient that he or she may experience some throat soreness and hoarseness. Instruct patient to treat throat discomfort with lozenges and warm gargles when the gag reflex returns.
- Inform the patient that any belching, bloating, or flatulence is the result of air insufflation and is temporary.
- Instruct the patient to report any severe pain, fever, difficulty breathing, or expectoration of blood. Immediately report symptoms to the appropriate HCP.
- Recognize anxiety related to test results, and offer support. Discuss the implications of abnormal test results on the patient's lifestyle. Provide teaching and information regarding the clinical implications of the test results, as appropriate.
- Reinforce information given by the patient's HCP regarding further testing, treatment, or referral to another HCP. Answer any questions or address any concerns voiced by the patient or family.
- Depending on the results of this procedure, additional testing may be needed to evaluate or monitor progression of the disease process and determine the need for a change in therapy. Evaluate test results in relation to the patient's symptoms and other tests performed.

RELATED MONOGRAPHS:

- Related tests include barium enema, barium swallow, capsule endoscopy, colonoscopy, CT abdomen, esophageal manometry, fecal analysis, gastric acid emptying scan, gastric fluid analysis and gastric acid stimulation test, gastrin and gastrin stimulation test, GI blood loss scan, *H. pylori,* MRI abdomen, proctosigmoidoscopy, US pelvis, and upper GI series.
- Refer to the Gastrointestinal System table at the end of the book for related tests by body system.

Estradiol

SYNONYM/ACRONYM: E_2.

COMMON USE: To assist in diagnosing female fertility problems that may occur from tumor or ovarian failure.

SPECIMEN: Serum (1 mL) collected in a red- or tiger-top tube. Plasma (1 mL) collected in green-top (heparin) tube is also acceptable.

REFERENCE VALUE: (Method: Immunoassay)

Age	Conventional Units	SI Units (Conventional Units × 3.67)
6 mo–10 yr	Less than 15 pg/mL	Less than 55 pmol/L
11–15 yr		
Male	Less than 40 pg/mL	Less than 147 pmol/L
Female	10–300 pg/mL	37–1,100 pmol/L
Adult male	10–50 pg/mL	37–184 pmol/L
Adult female		
Early follicular phase	20–150 pg/mL	73–551 pmol/L
Late follicular phase	40–350 pg/mL	147–1,285 pmol/L
Midcycle peak	150–750 pg/mL	551–2,753 pmol/L
Luteal phase	30–450 pg/mL	110–1,652 pmol/L
Postmenopause	Less than 20 pg/mL	Less than 73 pmol/L

POTENTIAL DIAGNOSIS

Increased in
- Adrenal tumors *(related to over-production by tumor cells)*
- Estrogen-producing tumors
- Feminization in children *(related to increased production)*
- Gynecomastia *(newborns may demonstrate swelling of breast tissue in response to maternal estrogens; somewhat common and transient in pubescent males)*
- Hepatic cirrhosis *(accumulation occurs due to lack of liver function)*
- Hyperthyroidism *(related to primary increases in estrogen or response to increased levels of sex hormone–binding globulin)*

Decreased in
- Ovarian failure *(resulting in lack of estrogen synthesis)*
- Primary and secondary hypogonadism *(related to lack of estrogen synthesis)*
- Turner's syndrome *(genetic abnormality in females in which there is only one X chromosome, resulting in varying degrees of underdeveloped sexual characteristics)*

CRITICAL FINDINGS: N/A

Find and print out the full monograph at DavisPlus (http://davisplus.fadavis.com, keyword Van Leeuwen).

Evoked Brain Potentials

SYNONYM/ACRONYM: Brainstem auditory evoked potentials (BAEP), brainstem auditory evoked responses (BAER), EP studies.

COMMON USE: To assist in diagnosing sensory deficits related to nervous system lesions manifested by visual defects, hearing defects, neuropathies, and cognitive disorders.

AREA OF APPLICATION: Brain.

CONTRAST: None.

DESCRIPTION: Evoked brain potentials, also known as evoked potential (EP) responses, are electrophysiological studies performed to measure the brain's electrical responses to various visual, auditory, and somatosensory stimuli. EP studies help diagnose lesions of the nervous system by evaluating the integrity of the visual, somatosensory, and auditory nerve pathways. Three response types are measured: visual evoked response (VER), auditory brainstem response (ABR), and somatosensory evoked response (SER). The stimuli activate the nerve tracts that connect the stimulated (receptor) area with the cortical (visual and somatosensory) or midbrain (auditory) sensory area. A number of stimuli are given, and then responses are electronically displayed in waveforms, recorded, and computer analyzed. Abnormalities are determined by a delay in time, measured in milliseconds, between the stimulus and the response. This is known as *increased latency.* VER provides information about visual pathway function to identify lesions of the optic nerves, optic tracts, and demyelinating diseases such as multiple sclerosis. ABR provides information about auditory pathways to identify hearing loss and lesions of the brainstem. SER provides information about the somatosensory pathways to identify lesions at various levels of the central nervous system (spinal cord and brain) and peripheral nerve disease. EP studies are especially useful in patients with problems and those unable to speak or respond to instructions during the test, because these studies do not require voluntary cooperation or participation in the activity. This allows collection of objective diagnostic information about visual or auditory disorders affecting infants and children and allows differentiation between organic brain and psychological disorders in adults. EP studies are also used to monitor the progression of or the effectiveness of treatment for deteriorating neurological diseases such as multiple sclerosis.

INDICATIONS

VER (potentials)
- Detect cryptic or past retrobulbar neuritis
- Detect lesions of the eye or optic nerves
- Detect neurological disorders such as multiple sclerosis, Parkinson's disease, and Huntington's chorea
- Evaluate binocularity in infants
- Evaluate optic pathway lesions and visual cortex defects

ABR (potentials)
- Detect abnormalities or lesions in the brainstem or auditory nerve areas
- Detect brainstem tumors and acoustic neuromas
- Screen or evaluate neonates, infants, children, and adults for auditory problems
- EP studies may be indicated when a child falls below growth chart norms

SER (potentials)
- Detect multiple sclerosis and Guillain-Barré syndrome
- Detect sensorimotor neuropathies and cervical pathology
- Evaluate spinal cord and brain injury and function
- Monitor sensory potentials to determine spinal cord function during a surgical procedure or medical regimen

ERP (potentials)
- Detect suspected psychosis or dementia
- Differentiate between organic brain disorder and cognitive function abnormality

POTENTIAL DIAGNOSIS

Normal findings in
- *VER and ABR:* Normal latency in recorded cortical and brainstem waveforms depending on age, gender, and stature
- *ERP:* Normal recognition and attention span
- *SER:* No loss of consciousness or presence of weakness

Abnormal findings in
- VER (potentials):

  P100 latencies (extended) confined to one eye suggest a lesion anterior to the optic chiasm.

  Bilateral abnormal P100 latencies indicate multiple sclerosis, optic neuritis, retinopathies, spinocerebellar degeneration, sarcoidosis, Parkinson's disease, adrenoleukodystrophy, Huntington's chorea, or amblyopias.

- ABR (potentials):

  Normal response at high intensities; wave V may occur slightly later. Earlier wave distortions suggest cochlear lesion.

  Absent or late waves at high intensities; increased amplitude of wave V suggests retrocochlear lesion.

- SER (potentials):

  Abnormal upper limb latencies suggest cervical spondylosis or intracerebral lesions.

  Abnormal lower limb latencies suggest peripheral nerve root disease such as Guillain-Barré syndrome, multiple sclerosis, transverse myelitis, or traumatic spinal cord injuries.

CRITICAL FINDINGS: N/A

INTERFERING FACTORS

Factors that may impair the results of the examination
- Inability of the patient to cooperate or remain still during the procedure because of age, significant pain, or mental status. (*Note:* Significant behavioral problems may limit the ability to complete the test.)
- Improper placement of electrodes.
- Patient stress, which can affect brain chemistry, thus making it difficult to distinguish whether the results are due to the patient's emotional reaction or to organic pathology.
- Extremely poor visual acuity, which can hinder accurate determination of VER.
- Severe hearing loss, which can interfere with accurate determination of ABR.

NURSING IMPLICATIONS AND PROCEDURE

PRETEST:
- Positively identify the patient using at least two unique identifiers before providing care, treatment, or services.
- *Patient Teaching:* Inform the patient this procedure measures electrical activity in the nervous system.
- Obtain a history of the patient's complaints or symptoms, including a list of known allergens, especially allergies or sensitivities to latex, iodine, seafood, anesthetics, or contrast mediums.
- Obtain a history of the patient's neuromuscular system, symptoms, and results of previously performed laboratory tests and diagnostic and surgical procedures.
- Obtain a list of the patient's current medications, including herbs, nutritional supplements, and nutraceuticals (see Appendix F).
- Review the procedure with the patient. Address concerns about pain related to the procedure and explain that the procedure is painless and harmless. Inform the patient that the procedure is performed in a special laboratory by a health-care provider (HCP) and takes approximately 30 min to 2 hr, depending on the type of studies required.
- *Sensitivity to social and cultural issues,* as well as concern for modesty, is important in providing psychological support before, during, and after the procedure.

- Instruct the patient to clean the hair and to refrain from using hair sprays, creams, or solutions before the test.
- Instruct the patient to remove jewelry and other metallic objects from the area to be examined.
- There are no food, fluid, or medication restrictions unless by medical direction.
- *Make sure a written and informed consent has been signed prior to the procedure and before administering any medications.*

INTRATEST:

- Ensure the patient is able to relax; report any extreme anxiety or restlessness.
- Ensure that hair is clean and free of hair sprays, creams, or solutions.
- Ensure the patient has removed all external metallic objects from the area to be examined prior to the procedure.
- Observe standard precautions, and follow the general guidelines in Appendix A.

Visual Evoked Potentials

- Place the patient in a comfortable position about 1 m from the stimulation source. Attach electrodes to the occipital and vertex lobe areas and a reference electrode to the ear. A light-emitting stimulation or a checkerboard pattern is projected on a screen at a regulated speed. This procedure is done for each eye (with the opposite eye covered) as the patient looks at a dot on the screen without any change in the gaze while the stimuli are delivered. A computer interprets the brain's responses to the stimuli and records them in waveforms.

Auditory Evoked Potentials

- Place the patient in a comfortable position, and place the electrodes on the scalp at the vertex lobe area and on each earlobe. Earphones are placed on the patient's ears, and a clicking noise stimulus is delivered into one ear while a continuous tone is delivered to the opposite ear. Responses to the stimuli are recorded as waveforms for analysis.

Somatosensory Evoked Potentials

- Place the patient in a comfortable position, and place the electrodes at the nerve sites of the wrist, knee, and ankle and on the scalp at the sensory cortex of the hemisphere on the opposite side (the electrode that picks up the response and delivers it to the recorder). Additional electrodes can be positioned at the cervical or lumbar vertebrae for upper or lower limb stimulation. The rate at which the electric shock stimulus is delivered to the nerve electrodes and travels to the brain is measured, computer analyzed, and recorded in waveforms for analysis. Both sides of the area being examined can be tested by switching the electrodes and repeating the procedure.

Event-Related Potentials

- Place the patient in a sitting position in a chair in a quiet room. Earphones are placed on the patient's ears and auditory cues administered. The patient is asked to push a button when the tones are recognized. Flashes of light are also used as visual cues, with the client pushing a button when cues are noted. Results are compared to normal EP waveforms for correct, incorrect, or absent responses.

POST-TEST:

- A report of the examination will be sent to the requesting HCP, who will discuss the results with the patient.
- When the procedure is complete, remove the electrodes and clean the skin where the electrodes were applied.
- Recognize anxiety related to test results, and be supportive of perceived loss of independent function. Discuss the implications of abnormal test results on the patient's lifestyle. Provide teaching and information regarding the clinical implications of the test results, as appropriate.
- Reinforce information given by the patient's HCP regarding further testing, treatment, or referral to another HCP. Answer any questions or address any concerns voiced by the patient or family.
- Depending on the results of this procedure, additional testing may be needed to evaluate or monitor progression of the disease process and determine the need for a change in therapy.

Evaluate test results in relation to the patient's symptoms and other tests performed.

RELATED MONOGRAPHS:

▸ Related tests include acetylcholine receptor antibody, Alzheimer's disease markers, biopsy muscle, CSF analysis, CT brain, CK, EEG, ENG, MRI brain, plethysmography, and PET brain.

▸ Refer to the Musculoskeletal System table at the end of the book for related tests by body system.

E

Exercise Stress Test

SYNONYM/ACRONYM: Exercise electrocardiogram, ECG, EKG, graded exercise tolerance test, stress testing, treadmill test.

COMMON USE: To assess cardiac function in relation to increased workload, evidenced by dysrhythmia or pain during exercise.

AREA OF APPLICATION: Heart.

CONTRAST: None.

DESCRIPTION: The exercise stress test is a noninvasive study to measure cardiac function during physical stress. Exercise electrocardiography is primarily useful in determining the extent of coronary artery occlusion by the heart's ability to meet the need for additional oxygen in response to the stress of exercising in a safe environment. The patient exercises on a treadmill or pedals a stationary bicycle to increase the heart rate to 80% to 90% of maximal heart rate determined by age and gender, known as the *target heart rate*. Every 2 to 3 min, the speed and/or grade of the treadmill is increased to yield an increment of stress. The patient's electrocardiogram (ECG) and blood pressure are monitored during the test. The test proceeds until the patient reaches the target heart rate or experiences chest pain or fatigue.

The risks involved in the procedure are possible myocardial infarction (1 in 500) and death (1 in 10,000) in patients experiencing frequent angina episodes before the test. Although useful, this procedure is not as accurate as cardiac nuclear scans for diagnosing coronary artery disease (CAD).

For patients unable to complete the test, pharmacological stress testing can be done. Medications used to pharmacologically exercise the patient's heart include vasodilators such as dipyridamole and adenosine or dobutamine (which stimulates heart rate and pumping force). The patient's electrocardiogram (ECG) and blood pressure are monitored during the test. The test proceeds until the stimulated exercise portion when a radiotracer, such as technetium-99m or sestamibi, is injected. Pictures are taken by a gamma camera during the stimulated portion and compared with images taken at rest.

INDICATIONS

- Detect dysrhythmias during exercising, as evidenced by ECG changes
- Detect peripheral arterial occlusive disease (intermittent claudication), as evidenced by leg pain or cramping during exercising
- Determine exercise-induced hypertension
- Evaluate cardiac function after myocardial infarction or cardiac surgery to determine safe exercise levels for cardiac rehabilitation as well as work limitations
- Evaluate effectiveness of medication regimens, such as antianginals or antiarrhythmics
- Evaluate suspected CAD in the presence of chest pain and other symptoms
- Screen for CAD in the absence of pain and other symptoms in patients at risk

POTENTIAL DIAGNOSIS

Normal findings in

- Normal heart rate during physical exercise. Heart rate and systolic blood pressure rise in direct proportion to workload and to metabolic oxygen demand, which is based on age and exercise protocol. Maximal heart rate for adults is normally 150 to 200 beats/min.

Abnormal findings in

- Activity intolerance related to oxygen supply and demand imbalance
- Bradycardia
- CAD
- Chest pain related to ischemia or inflammation
- Decreased cardiac output

- Dysrhythmias
- Hypertension
- Peripheral arterial occlusive disease
- ST segment depression of 1 mm (considered a positive test), indicating myocardial ischemia
- Tachycardia

CRITICAL FINDINGS: N/A

INTERFERING FACTORS

The following factors may impair interpretation of examination results because they create an artificial state that makes it difficult to determine true physiological function:

- Anxiety or panic attack.
- Drugs such as β-blockers, cardiac glycosides, calcium channel blockers, coronary vasodilators, and barbiturates.
- High food intake or smoking before testing.
- Hypertension, hypoxia, left bundle branch block, and ventricular hypertrophy.
- Improper electrode placement.
- Potassium or calcium imbalance.
- Viagra should not be taken in combination with nitroglycerin or other nitrates 24 hr prior to the procedure because it may result in a dangerously low blood pressure.
- Wolff-Parkinson-White syndrome (anomalous atrioventricular excitation).

NURSING IMPLICATIONS AND PROCEDURE

PRETEST:

- Positively identify the patient using at least two unique identifiers before providing care, treatment, or services.
- *Patient Teaching:* Inform the patient this procedure can assist in assessing the heart's ability to respond to an increasing workload.
- Obtain a history of the patient's cardiovascular system, symptoms, and results

of previously performed laboratory tests and diagnostic and surgical procedures.

▶ Inquire if the patient has had any chest pain within the past 48 hr or has a history of anginal attacks; if either of these has occurred, inform the health-care provider (HCP) immediately because the stress test may be too risky and should be rescheduled in 4 to 6 wk.

▶ Obtain a list of the patient's current medications, including herbs, nutritional supplements, and nutraceuticals (see Appendix F).

▶ Review the procedure with the patient. Address concerns about pain related to the procedure and explain that some discomfort may be experienced during the stimulated portion of the test. Inform the patient that the procedure is performed in a special department by an HCP specializing in this procedure and takes approximately 30 to 60 min.

▶ *Sensitivity to social and cultural issues,* as well as concern for modesty, is important in providing psychological support before, during, and after the procedure.

▶ Record a baseline 12-lead ECG and vital signs.

▶ Instruct the patient to wear comfortable shoes and clothing for the exercise.

▶ Instruct the patient to fast, restrict fluids, and avoid tobacco products for 4 hr prior to the procedure. Protocols may vary among facilities.

▶ *Make sure a written and informed consent has been signed prior to the procedure and before administering any medications.*

INTRATEST:

▶ Ensure the patient has complied with dietary and tobacco restrictions for at least 4 hr prior to the procedure.

▶ An IV access may be established for emergency use.

▶ Have emergency equipment readily available.

▶ Instruct the patient to void prior to the procedure and to change into the gown provided.

▶ Observe standard precautions, and follow the general guidelines in Appendix A.

▶ Place electrodes in appropriate positions on the patient and connect a blood pressure cuff to a monitoring device. If the patient's oxygen consumption is to be continuously monitored, connect the patient to a machine via a mouthpiece or to a pulse oximeter via a finger lead.

▶ Instruct the patient to walk on a treadmill (most commonly used) and use the handrails to maintain balance or to peddle a bicycle. As stress is increased, inform the patient to report any symptoms, such as chest or leg pain, dyspnea, or fatigue.

▶ Turn the treadmill on at a slow speed, and increase in speed and elevation to raise the patient's heart rate. Increase the stress until the patient's predicted target heart rate is reached.

▶ Instruct the patient to report symptoms such as dizziness, sweating, breathlessness, or nausea, which can be normal, as speed increases. The test is terminated if pain or fatigue is severe; maximum heart rate under stress is attained; signs of ischemia are present; maximum effort has been achieved; or dyspnea, hypertension (systolic blood pressure greater than 200 mm Hg, diastolic blood pressure greater than 110 mm Hg, or both), tachycardia (greater than 200 beats/min minus person's age), new dysrhythmias, chest pain that begins or worsens, faintness, extreme dizziness, or confusion develops.

▶ After the exercise period, allow a 3- to 15-min rest period with the patient in a sitting position. During this period, the ECG, blood pressure, and heart rate monitoring is continued.

▶ Remove the electrodes and cleanse the skin of any remaining gel or ECG electrode adhesive.

POST-TEST:

▶ A report of the examination will be sent to the requesting HCP, who will discuss the results with the patient.

▶ Instruct the patient to resume usual activity, as directed by the HCP.

▶ Instruct the patient to contact the HCP to report any anginal pain or other discomforts experienced after the test.

▶ *Nutritional Considerations:* Abnormal findings may be associated with cardiovascular disease. The American

Heart Association and National Heart, Lung, and Blood Institute (NHBLI) recommend nutritional therapy for individuals identified to be at high risk for developing CAD or individuals who have specific risk factors and/or existing medical conditions (e.g., elevated LDL cholesterol levels, other lipid disorders, insulin-dependent diabetes, insulin resistance, or metabolic syndrome). If overweight, the patient should be encouraged to achieve a normal weight. The NHLBI's National Cholesterol Education Program (NCEP) revised its dietary guidelines for reducing CAD in 2001. Guidelines for the Therapeutic Lifestyle Changes (TLC) diet are outlined in the Third Report of the Expert Panel on Detection, Evaluation, and Treatment of High Blood Cholesterol in Adults (Adult Treatment Panel III [ATP III]). The TLC diet emphasizes a reduction in foods high in saturated fats and cholesterol. Red meats, eggs, and dairy products are the major sources of saturated fats and cholesterol. If triglycerides also are elevated, the patient should be advised to eliminate or reduce alcohol and simple carbohydrates from the diet. The TLC approach also includes the use of plant stanols or sterols and increased dissolved fiber as an option for lowering LDL cholesterol levels; nutritional recommendations for daily total caloric intake; recommendations for allowable percentage of calories derived from fat (saturated and unsaturated), carbohydrates, protein, and cholesterol; as well as recommendations for daily expenditure of energy.

Nutritional Considerations: Overweight patients with high blood pressure should be encouraged to achieve a normal weight. Other changeable risk factors warranting patient education include strategies to safely decrease sodium intake, increase physical activity, decrease alcohol consumption, eliminate tobacco use, and decrease cholesterol levels.

Social and Cultural Considerations: Numerous studies point to the prevalence of excess body weight in American children and adolescents. Experts estimate that obesity is present in 25% of the population ages 6 to 11 yr. The medical, social, and emotional consequences of excess body weight are significant. Special attention should be given to instructing the child and caregiver regarding health risks and weight control education.

Recognize anxiety related to test results, and be supportive of fear of shortened life expectancy. Discuss the implications of abnormal test results on the patient's lifestyle. Provide teaching and information regarding the clinical implications of the test results, as appropriate. Educate the patient regarding access to counseling services. Provide contact information, if desired, for the American Heart Association (www.americanheart.org) or the NHLBI (www.nhlbi.nih.gov).

Reinforce information given by the patient's HCP regarding further testing, treatment, or referral to another HCP. Answer any questions or address any concerns voiced by the patient or family.

Depending on the results of this procedure, additional testing may be performed to evaluate or monitor progression of the disease process and determine the need for a change in therapy. Evaluate test results in relation to the patient's symptoms and other tests performed.

RELATED MONOGRAPHS:

Related tests include antiarrhythmic drugs, apolipoprotein A and B, AST, atrial natriuretic peptide, BNP, blood gases, blood pool imaging, calcium, chest x-ray, cholesterol (total, HDL, LDL), CT cardiac scoring, CT thorax, CRP, CK and isoenzymes, echocardiography, echocardiography transesophageal, electrocardiogram, glucose, glycated hemoglobin, Holter monitor, homocysteine, ketones, LDH and isos, lipoprotein electrophoresis, lung perfusion scan, magnesium, MRI chest, MI infarct scan, myocardial perfusion heart scan, myoglobin, PET heart, potassium, pulse oximetry, sodium, triglycerides, and troponin.

Refer to the Cardiovascular System table at the end of the book for related tests by body system.

Fecal Analysis

SYNONYM/ACRONYM: N/A.

COMMON USE: To assess for the presence of blood in the stool to assist in diagnosing gastrointestinal bleeding, cancer, inflammation, and infection.

SPECIMEN: Stool.

REFERENCE VALUE: (Method: Macroscopic examination, for appearance and color; microscopic examination, for cell count and presence of meat fibers; leukocyte esterase, for leukocytes; Clinitest [Bayer Corporation, Pittsburgh, Pennsylvania] for reducing substances; guaiac, for occult blood; x-ray paper, for trypsin.)

Characteristic	Normal Result
Appearance	Solid and formed
Color	Brown
Epithelial cells	Few to moderate
Fecal fat	See "Fecal Fat" monograph
Leukocytes (white blood cells)	Negative
Meat fibers	Negative
Occult blood	Negative
Reducing substances	Negative
Trypsin	2+ to 4+

DESCRIPTION: Feces consist mainly of cellulose and other undigested foodstuffs, bacteria, and water. Other substances normally found in feces include epithelial cells shed from the gastrointestinal (GI) tract, small amounts of fats, bile pigments in the form of urobilinogen, GI and pancreatic secretions, electrolytes, and trypsin. Trypsin is a proteolytic enzyme produced in the pancreas. The average adult excretes 100 to 300 g of fecal material per day, the residue of approximately 10 L of liquid material that enters the GI tract each day. The laboratory analysis of feces includes macroscopic examination (volume, odor, shape, color, consistency, presence of mucus), microscopic examination (leukocytes, epithelial cells, meat fibers), and chemical tests for specific substances (occult blood, trypsin, estimation of carbohydrate).

Detection of occult blood is the most common test performed on stool. The prevalence of colorectal adenoma is greater than 30% in people aged 60 and older. Progression from adenoma to carcinoma occurs over a period of 5 to 12 yr; from carcinoma to metastatic disease in 2 to 3 yr.

INDICATIONS

- Assist in diagnosing disorders associated with GI bleeding or drug therapy that leads to bleeding
- Assist in the diagnosis of pseudomembranous enterocolitis after use of broad-spectrum antibiotic therapy
- Assist in the diagnosis of suspected inflammatory bowel disorder
- Detect altered protein digestion
- Detect intestinal parasitic infestation, as indicated by diarrhea of unknown cause

- Investigate diarrhea of unknown cause
- Monitor effectiveness of therapy for intestinal malabsorption or pancreatic insufficiency
- Screen for cystic fibrosis

POTENTIAL DIAGNOSIS

Unusual Appearance
- Bloody: *Excessive intestinal wall irritation or malignancy*
- Bulky or frothy: *Malabsorption*
- Mucous: *Inflammation of intestinal walls*
- Slender or ribbonlike: *Obstruction*

Unusual Color
- Black: *Bismuth (antacid) or charcoal ingestion, iron therapy, upper GI bleeding*
- Grayish white: *Barium ingestion, bile duct obstruction*
- Green: *Antibiotics, biliverdin, green vegetables*
- Red: *Beets and food coloring, lower GI bleed, phenazopyridine hydrochloride compounds, rifampin*
- Yellow: *Rhubarb*

Increased
- Carbohydrates/reducing substances: *Malabsorption syndromes*
- Epithelial cells: *Inflammatory bowel disorders*
- Leukocytes: *Bacterial infections of the intestinal wall, salmonellosis, shigellosis, and ulcerative colitis*
- Meat fibers: *Altered protein digestion*
- Occult blood: *Anal fissure, diverticular disease, esophageal varices, esophagitis, gastritis, hemorrhoids, infectious diarrhea, inflammatory bowel disease, Mallory-Weiss tears, polyps, tumors, ulcers*

Decreased
- Leukocytes: *Amebic colitis, cholera, disorders resulting from toxins, parasites, viral diarrhea*

- Trypsin: *Cystic fibrosis, malabsorption syndromes, pancreatic deficiency*

CRITICAL FINDINGS: N/A

INTERFERING FACTORS
- Drugs that can cause positive results for occult blood include acetylsalicylic acid, anticoagulants, colchicine, corticosteroids, iron preparations, and phenylbutazone.
- Ingestion of a diet high in red meat, certain vegetables, and bananas can cause false-positive results for occult blood.
- Large doses of vitamin C can cause false-negative occult blood.
- Constipated stools may not indicate any trypsin activity owing to extended exposure to intestinal bacteria.

F

NURSING IMPLICATIONS AND PROCEDURE

PRETEST:
- Positively identify the patient using at least two unique identifiers before providing care, treatment, or services.
- *Patient Teaching:* Inform the patient this test can assist in the diagnosis of intestinal disorders.
- Obtain a history of the patient's complaints, including a list of known allergens, especially allergies or sensitivities to latex.
- Obtain a history of the patient's gastrointestinal system, symptoms, and results of previously performed laboratory tests and diagnostic and surgical procedures.
- Obtain a list of the patient's current medications, including herbs, nutritional supplements, and nutraceuticals (see Appendix F).
- Review the procedure with the patient. Inform the patient of the procedure for collecting a stool sample, including the importance of good hand-washing techniques. The patient should place the sample in a tightly covered container. Instruct the patient not to contaminate

the specimen with urine, water, or toilet tissue. Address concerns about pain and explain that there should be no discomfort during the procedure.

▶ *Sensitivity to social and cultural issues,* as well as concern for modesty, is important in providing psychological support before, during, and after the procedure.

▶ Instruct the patient not to use laxatives, enemas, or suppositories for 3 days before the test.

▶ Instruct the patient to follow a normal diet. If the test is being performed to identify blood, instruct the patient to follow a special diet that includes small amounts of chicken, turkey, and tuna (no red meats), raw and cooked vegetables and fruits, and bran cereal for several days before the test. Foods to avoid with the special diet include beets, turnips, cauliflower, broccoli, bananas, parsnips, and cantaloupe, because these foods can interfere with the occult blood test.

INTRATEST:

▶ Ensure that the patient has complied with medication restrictions; assure laxatives, enemas, or suppositories have been restricted for at least 3 days prior to the procedure.

▶ Instruct the patient to cooperate fully and to follow directions.

▶ Observe standard precautions, and follow the general guidelines in Appendix A. Positively identify the patient, and label the appropriate collection container with the corresponding patient demographics, date and time of collection, and suspected cause of enteritis; note any current or recent antibiotic therapy.

▶ Collect a stool specimen in a half-pint waterproof container with a tight-fitting lid; if the patient is not ambulatory, collect it in a clean, dry bedpan. Use a tongue blade to transfer the specimen to the container, and include any mucoid and bloody portions. Collect specimen from the first, middle, and last portion of the stool. The specimen should be refrigerated if it will not be transported to the laboratory within 4 hr after collection.

▶ To collect specimen by rectal swab, insert the swab past the anal sphincter, rotate gently, and withdraw. Place the swab in the appropriate container.

▶ Promptly transport the specimen to the laboratory for processing and analysis.

POST-TEST:

▶ A report of the results will be sent to the requesting health-care provider (HCP), who will discuss the results with the patient.

▶ Recognize anxiety related to test results. Discuss the implications of abnormal test results on the patient's lifestyle. Provide teaching and information regarding the clinical implications of the test results, as appropriate.

▶ Reinforce information given by the patient's HCP regarding further testing, treatment, or referral to another HCP. Decisions regarding the need for and frequency of occult blood testing, colonoscopy, or other cancer screening procedures should be made after consultation between the patient and HCP. The most current guidelines for colon cancer screening of the general population as well as of individuals with increased risk are available from the American Cancer Society (www.cancer .org) and the American College of Gastroenterology (www.gi.org). Answer any questions or address any concerns voiced by the patient or family.

▶ Depending on the results of this procedure, additional testing may be performed to evaluate or monitor progression of the disease process and determine the need for a change in therapy. Evaluate test results in relation to the patient's symptoms and other tests performed.

RELATED MONOGRAPHS:

▶ Related tests include α_1-antitrypsin/phenotyping, barium enema, biopsy intestine, capsule endoscopy, CEA and cancer antigens, chloride sweat, colonoscopy, CT colonoscopy, culture stool, D-xylose tolerance, fecal fat, gliadin antibody, lactose tolerance test, ova and parasites, and proctosigmoidoscopy.

▶ Refer to the Gastrointestinal System table at the end of the book for related tests by body system.

Fecal Fat

SYNONYM/ACRONYM: Stool fat, fecal fat stain.

COMMON USE: To assess for the presence of fat in the stool to assist in diagnosing malabsorption disorders such as Crohn's disease and cystic fibrosis.

SPECIMEN: Stool (80 mL) aliquot from an unpreserved and homogenized 24- to 72-hr timed collection. Random specimens may also be submitted.

REFERENCE VALUE: (Method: Stain with Sudan black or oil red O. Treatment with ethanol identifies neutral fats; treatment with acetic acid identifies fatty acids.)

	Random, Semiquantitative
Neutral fat	Less than 60 fat globules/hpf*
Fatty acids	Less than 100 fat globules/hpf
	72-hr, Quantitative
Age (normal diet)	
Infant (breast milk)	Less than 1 g/24 hr
0–6 yr	Less than 2 g/24 hr
Adult	2–7 g/24 hr; less than 20% of total solids
Adult (fat-free diet)	Less than 4 g/24 hr

*hpf = high-power field.

DESCRIPTION: Fecal fat primarily consists of triglycerides (neutral fats), fatty acids, and fatty acid salts. Through microscopic examination, the number and size of fat droplets can be determined as well as the type of fat present. Excretion of more than 7 g of fecal fat in a 24-hr period is abnormal but nonspecific for disease. Increases in excretion of neutral fats are associated with pancreatic exocrine insufficiency, whereas decreases are related to small bowel disease. An increase in triglycerides indicates that insufficient pancreatic enzymes are available to convert the triglycerides into fatty acids. Patients with malabsorption conditions have normal amounts of triglycerides but an increase in total fecal fat because the fats are not absorbed through the intestine. Malabsorption disorders (e.g., cystic fibrosis) cause blockage of the pancreatic ducts by mucus, which prevents the enzymes from reaching the duodenum and results in lack of fat digestion. Without digestion, the fats cannot be absorbed, and steatorrhea results. The appearance and odor of stool from patients with steatorrhea is typically foamy, greasy, soft, and foul-smelling. The semiquantitative test is used to screen for the presence of fecal fat. The quantitative method, which requires a 72-hr stool collection, measures the amount of fat present in grams.

INDICATIONS

- Assist in the diagnosis of malabsorption or pancreatic insufficiency, as indicated by elevated fat levels
- Monitor the effectiveness of therapy

POTENTIAL DIAGNOSIS

Increased in

- Abetalipoprotein deficiency *(related to lack of transport proteins for absorption)*
- Addison's disease *(related to impaired transport)*
- Amyloidosis *(increased rate of excretion related to malabsorption)*
- Bile salt deficiency *(related to lack of bile salts required for proper fat digestion)*
- Carcinoid syndrome *(increased rate of excretion related to malabsorption)*
- Celiac disease *(increased rate of excretion related to malabsorption)*
- Crohn's disease *(increased rate of excretion related to malabsorption)*
- Cystic fibrosis *(related to insufficient digestive enzymes)*
- Diabetes *(abnormal motility related to primary condition)*
- Enteritis *(increased rate of excretion related to malabsorption)*
- Malnutrition *(related to detrimental effects on organs and systems responsible for digestion, transport, and absorption)*
- Multiple sclerosis *(abnormal motility related to primary condition)*
- Pancreatic insufficiency or obstruction *(related to insufficient digestive enzymes)*
- Peptic ulcer disease *(related to improper digestion due to low pH)*
- Pernicious anemia *(related to bacterial overgrowth that decreases overall absorption and results in vitamin B_{12} deficiency)*
- Progressive systemic sclerosis *(abnormal motility related to primary condition)*
- Thyrotoxicosis *(abnormal motility related to primary condition)*
- Tropical sprue *(increased rate of excretion related to malabsorption)*
- Viral hepatitis *(related to insufficient production of digestive enzymes and bile)*
- Whipple's disease *(increased rate of excretion related to malabsorption)*
- Zollinger-Ellison syndrome *(related to improper digestion due to low pH)*

Decreased in: N/A

CRITICAL FINDINGS: N/A

INTERFERING FACTORS

- Cimetidine has been associated with decreased fecal fat in some patients with cystic fibrosis who are also receiving pancreatic enzyme therapy.
- Some drugs cause steatorrhea as a result of mucosal damage. These include colchicine, kanamycin, lincomycin, methotrexate, and neomycin. Other drugs that can cause an increase in fecal fat include aminosalicylic acid, bisacodyl and phenolphthalein (observed in laxative abusers), and cholestyramine (in high doses).
- Use of suppositories, oily lubricants, or mineral oil in the perianal area for 3 days before the test can falsely increase neutral fats.
- Use of herbals with laxative effects, including cascara, psyllium, and senna, for 3 days before the test can falsely increase neutral fats.

- Barium interferes with test results.
- Failure to collect all stools may reflect falsely decreased results.
- Ingestion of a diet too high or low in fats may alter the results.

NURSING IMPLICATIONS AND PROCEDURE

PRETEST:

▸ Positively identify the patient using at least two unique identifiers before providing care, treatment, or services.

▸ *Patient Teaching:* Inform the patient this test can assist in the diagnosis of intestinal disorders.

▸ Obtain a history of the patient's complaints that indicate a gastrointestinal (GI) disorder, diarrhea related to GI dysfunction, pain related to tissue inflammation or irritation, alteration in diet resulting from an inability to digest certain foods, or fluid volume deficit related to active loss. Obtain a history of known allergens.

▸ Obtain a history of the patient's gastrointestinal and respiratory systems, symptoms, and results of previously performed laboratory tests and diagnostic and surgical procedures.

▸ Note any recent procedures that can interfere with test results.

▸ Obtain a list of the patient's current medications, including herbs, nutritional supplements, and nutraceuticals (see Appendix F).

▸ Review the procedure with the patient. Stress the importance of collecting all stools for the quantitative test, including diarrhea, over the timed specimen-collection period. Inform the patient not to urinate in the stool-collection container and not to put toilet paper in the container. Address concerns about pain related to the procedure. Explain to the patient that there should be no discomfort during the procedure.

▸ *Sensitivity to social and cultural issues,* as well as concern for modesty, is important in providing psychological support before, during, and after the procedure.

▸ Instruct the patient not to use laxatives, enemas, or suppositories for 3 days before the test.

▸ There are no fluid restrictions unless by medical direction.

▸ Instruct the patient to ingest a diet containing 50 to 150 g of fat for at least 3 days before beginning specimen collection. This approach does not work well with children; instruct the caregiver to record the child's dietary intake to provide a basis from which an estimate of fat intake can be made.

INTRATEST:

▸ Ensure that the patient has complied with dietary and other pretesting preparations prior to the procedure.

▸ Instruct the patient to cooperate fully and to follow directions.

▸ Observe standard precautions, and follow the general guidelines in Appendix A. Positively identify the patient, and label the appropriate collection container with the corresponding patient demographics, date, and the start and stop times of collection.

▸ Obtain the appropriate-sized specimen container, toilet-mounted collection container to aid in specimen collection, and plastic bag for specimen transport. A large, clean, preweighed container should be used for the timed test. A smaller, clean container can be used for the collection of the random sample.

▸ For the quantitative procedure, instruct the patient to collect each stool and place it in the 500-mL container during the timed collection period. Keep the container refrigerated in the plastic bag throughout the entire collection period.

▸ Promptly transport the specimen to the laboratory for processing and analysis.

POST-TEST:

▸ A report of the results will be sent to the requesting health-care provider (HCP), who will discuss the results with the patient.

F

▸ Instruct the patient to resume usual diet and medication, as directed by the HCP.

▸ Recognize anxiety related to test results, and be supportive of impaired activity related to perceived loss of independence and fear of shortened life expectancy. Discuss the implications of abnormal test results on the patient's lifestyle. Instruct the patient with abnormal values on the importance of fluid intake and proper diet specific to his or her condition. Provide teaching and information regarding the clinical implications of the test results, as appropriate. Educate the patient regarding access to counseling services. Help the patient and caregiver cope with long-term implications. Recognize that anticipatory anxiety and grief may be expressed when someone is faced with a chronic disorder. Provide contact information, if desired and as appropriate, for the American Diabetes Association (www.diabetes.org), Celiac Disease Foundation (www.celiac.org), Crohn's and Colitis Foundation of America (www.ccfa.org), or the Cystic Fibrosis Foundation (www.cff.org).

▸ Reinforce information given by the patient's HCP regarding further testing, treatment, or referral to another HCP. Answer any questions or address any concerns voiced by the patient or family.

▸ Depending on the results of this procedure, additional testing may be performed to evaluate or monitor progression of the disease process and determine the need for a change in therapy. Evaluate test results in relation to the patient's symptoms and other tests performed.

RELATED MONOGRAPHS:

▸ Related tests include α_1-antitrypsin/phenotyping, biopsy intestine, chloride sweat, CBC, CBC RBC indices, CBC RBC morphology, D-xylose tolerance test, fecal analysis, folate, gastric acid stimulation test, gastric emptying scan, radioactive iodine uptake, and vitamin B_{12}.

▸ Refer to the Gastrointestinal and Respiratory systems tables at the end of the book for related tests by body system.

Ferritin

SYNONYM/ACRONYM: N/A.

COMMON USE: To assist in diagnosing and monitoring various forms of anemia related to ferritin levels such as iron-deficiency anemia, anemia of malnourishment related to alcoholism, hemolytic anemia, chronic anemia of inflammation, and anemia related to long-term kidney dialysis.

SPECIMEN: Serum (1 mL) collected in a red- or tiger-top tube.

REFERENCE VALUE: (Method: Immunoassay)

Age	Conventional Units	SI Units (Conventional Units × 1)
Newborn	25–200 ng/mL	25–200 mcg/L
1 mo	200–600 ng/mL	200–600 mcg/L
2–5 mo	50–200 ng/mL	50–200 mcg/L
6 mo–15 yr	7–140 ng/mL	7–140 mcg/L
Adult		
Males	20–250 ng/mL	20–250 mcg/L
Females (18–39 yr)	10–120 ng/mL	10–120 mcg/L
Females (40 yr and older)	12–263 ng/mL	12–263 mcg/L

DESCRIPTION: Ferritin, a protein manufactured in the liver, spleen, and bone marrow, consists of a protein shell, apoferritin, and an iron core. The amount of ferritin in the circulation is usually proportional to the amount of stored iron (ferritin and hemosiderin) in body tissues. Levels vary according to age and gender, but they are not affected by exogenous iron intake or subject to diurnal variations. Compared to iron and total iron-binding capacity, ferritin is a more sensitive and specific test for diagnosing iron-deficiency anemia. Iron-deficiency anemia in adults is indicated at ferritin levels less than 10 ng/mL; hemochromatosis or hemosiderosis is indicated at levels greater than 400 ng/mL.

INDICATIONS

- Assist in the diagnosis of iron-deficiency anemia
- Assist in the differential diagnosis of microcytic, hypochromic anemias
- Monitor hematological responses during pregnancy, when serum iron is usually decreased and ferritin may be decreased
- Support diagnosis of hemochromatosis or other disorders of iron metabolism and storage

POTENTIAL DIAGNOSIS

Increased in

- Alcoholism *(active abuse, as evidenced by release of ferritin into the circulation from damaged hepatocytes and red blood cells [RBCs])*
- Breast cancer *(acute, related to release of ferritin as an acute-phase reactant protein; chronic, pathophysiology is uncertain)*
- Hemochromatosis *(related to increased iron deposits in the liver, which stimulate ferritin production)*
- Hemolytic anemia *(related to increased iron levels from hemolyzed RBCs, which stimulate ferritin production)*
- Hemosiderosis *(related to increased iron levels, which stimulate ferritin production)*
- Hepatocellular disease *(acute, related to release of ferritin as an acute-phase reactant protein; chronic, related to release of ferritin into the circulation from damaged hepatocytes)*
- Hodgkin's disease *(acute, related to release of ferritin as an acute-phase reactant protein; chronic, pathophysiology is uncertain)*
- Hyperthyroidism *(possibly related to the stimulating effect of thyroid-stimulating hormone on ferritin production)*

F

- Infection *(acute, related to release of ferritin as an acute-phase reactant protein; chronic, pathophysiology is uncertain)*
- Inflammatory diseases *(related to release of ferritin as an acute-phase reactant protein)*
- Leukemias *(acute, related to release of ferritin as an acute-phase reactant protein; chronic, pathophysiology is uncertain)*
- Oral or parenteral administration of iron *(evidenced by an increased circulating iron level, which stimulates ferritin production)*
- Thalassemia *(related to increased iron levels from hemolyzed RBCs, which stimulate ferritin production)*

Decreased in
Conditions that decrease iron stores result in corresponding low levels of ferritin.
- Hemodialysis
- Iron-deficiency anemia

CRITICAL FINDINGS: N/A

INTERFERING FACTORS
- Drugs that may increase ferritin levels include ethanol, ferric polymaltose, iron, and oral contraceptives.
- Drugs that may decrease ferritin levels include erythropoietin and methimazole.
- Recent transfusion can elevate serum ferritin.

NURSING IMPLICATIONS AND PROCEDURE

PRETEST:
- Positively identify the patient using at least two unique identifiers before providing care, treatment, or services.
- *Patient Teaching:* Inform the patient this test can assist in the diagnosis of anemia.
- Obtain a history of the patient's complaints, including a list of known allergens, especially allergies or sensitivities to latex.
- Obtain a history of the patient's hematopoietic system, symptoms, and results of previously performed laboratory tests and diagnostic and surgical procedures.
- Note any recent procedures that can interfere with test results.
- Obtain a list of the patient's current medications, including herbs, nutritional supplements, and nutraceuticals (see Appendix F).
- Review the procedure with the patient. Inform the patient that specimen collection takes approximately 5 to 10 min. Address concerns about pain and explain that there may be some discomfort during the venipuncture.
- *Sensitivity to social and cultural issues,* as well as concern for modesty is important in providing psychological support before, during, and after the procedure.
- There are no food, fluid, or medication restrictions unless by medical direction.

INTRATEST:
- If the patient has a history of allergic reaction to latex, avoid the use of equipment containing latex.
- Instruct the patient to cooperate fully and to follow directions. Direct the patient to breathe normally and to avoid unnecessary movement.
- Observe standard precautions, and follow the general guidelines in Appendix A. Positively identify the patient, and label the appropriate tubes with the corresponding patient demographics, date, and time of collection. Perform a venipuncture.
- Remove the needle and apply direct pressure with dry gauze to stop bleeding. Observe/assess venipuncture site for bleeding or hematoma formation and secure gauze with adhesive bandage.
- Promptly transport the specimen to the laboratory for processing and analysis.

POST-TEST:
- A report of the results will be sent to the requesting health-care provider

(HCP), who will discuss the results with the patient.

- *Nutritional Considerations:* Nutritional therapy may be indicated for patients with decreased ferritin values because this may indicate corresponding iron deficiency. Instruct these patients in the dietary inclusion of iron-rich foods and in the administration of iron supplements, including side effects, as appropriate.
- Reinforce information given by the patient's HCP regarding further testing, treatment, or referral to another HCP. Answer any questions or address any concerns voiced by the patient or family.
- Depending on the results of this procedure, additional testing may be performed to evaluate or monitor progression of the disease process and determine the need for a change in therapy. Evaluate test results in relation to the patient's symptoms and other tests performed.

RELATED MONOGRAPHS:

- Related tests include biopsy bone marrow, biopsy liver, complement, CBC, CBC hematocrit, CBC hemoglobin, CBC platelet count, CBC RBC count, CBC RBC indices, CBC RBC morphology and inclusions, CBC WBC count and differential, Coomb's antiglobulin direct and indirect, erythropoietin, FEP, G6PD, Ham's test, Hgb electrophoresis, hemosiderin, iron/TIBC, osmotic fragility, PK, sickle cell screen, and transferrin.
- Refer to the Hematopoietic System table at the end of the book for related tests by body system.

Fetal Fibronectin

SYNONYM/ACRONYM: fFN.

COMMON USE: To assist in evaluating for premature labor.

SPECIMEN: Swab of vaginal secretions.

REFERENCE VALUE: (Method: Immunoassay) Negative.

DESCRIPTION: Fibronectin is a protein found in fetal connective tissue, amniotic fluid, and the placenta of pregnant women. Placental fFN is concentrated in the area where the placenta and its membranes are in contact with the uterine wall. It is first secreted early in pregnancy and is believed to help implantation of the fertilized egg to the uterus. Fibronectin is not detectable again until just before delivery, at approximately 37 wk. If it is detected in vaginal secretions at 22 to 34 wk of gestation, delivery may happen prematurely. The test is a useful marker for impending membrane rupture within 7 to 14 days if the level rises to greater than 0.05 mcg/mL.

INDICATIONS
- Investigate signs of premature labor

POTENTIAL DIAGNOSIS

Positive findings in
- Premature labor *(possibly initiated by mechanical or infectious*

processes, the membranes pull away from the uterine wall and amniotic fluid containing fFN leaks into endocervical fluid)

CRITICAL FINDINGS: N/A

INTERFERING FACTORS

If signs and symptoms persist in light of negative test results, repeat testing may be necessary.

NURSING IMPLICATIONS AND PROCEDURE

PRETEST:

▶ Positively identify the patient using at least two unique identifiers before providing care, treatment, or services.
▶ *Patient Teaching:* Inform the patient this test can assess for risk of preterm delivery.
▶ Obtain a history of the patient's complaints, including a list of known allergens, especially allergies or sensitivities to latex.
▶ Obtain a history of the patient's reproductive system, symptoms, and results of previously performed laboratory tests and diagnostic and surgical procedures.
▶ Ensure that the patient knows the symptoms of premature labor, which include uterine contractions (with or without pain) lasting 20 sec or longer or increasing in frequency, menstrual-like cramping (intermittent or continuous), pelvic pressure, lower back pain that does not dissipate with a change in position, persistent diarrhea, intestinal cramps, changes in vaginal discharge, or a feeling that something is wrong.
▶ The health-care provider (HCP) should be informed if contractions occur more frequently than four times per hour.
▶ Obtain a list of the patient's current medications, including herbs, nutritional supplements, and nutraceuticals (see Appendix F).
▶ Review the procedure with the patient. Inform the patient that specimen collection takes approximately 5 to 10 min and will be performed by an HCP specializing in this branch of medicine. Address concerns about pain related to the procedure. Explain to the patient that there should be minimal to no discomfort during the procedure.
▶ *Sensitivity to social and cultural issues,* as well as concern for modesty, is important in providing psychological support before, during, and after the procedure.
▶ There are no food, fluid, or medication restrictions unless by medical direction.

INTRATEST:

▶ If the patient has a history of allergic reaction to latex, avoid the use of equipment containing latex.
▶ Instruct the patient to cooperate fully and to follow directions. Direct the patient to breathe normally and to avoid unnecessary movement.
▶ Observe standard precautions, and follow the general guidelines in Appendix A. Positively identify the patient, and label the appropriate collection container with the corresponding patient demographics, date, and time of collection.
▶ Position the patient on the gynecological examination table with the feet up in stirrups. Drape the patient's legs to provide privacy and to reduce chilling. Collect a small amount of vaginal secretion using a special swab from a fetal fibronectin kit.
▶ Promptly transport the specimen to the laboratory for processing and analysis.

POST-TEST:

▶ A report of the results will be sent to the requesting HCP, who will discuss the results with the patient.
▶ Recognize anxiety related to test results. Discuss the implications of abnormal test results on the patient's

lifestyle. Provide teaching and information regarding the clinical implications of the test results, as appropriate. Educate the patient regarding access to counseling services.

Reinforce information given by the patient's HCP regarding further testing, treatment, or referral to another HCP. Explain the possible causes and increased risks associated with premature labor and delivery. Reinforce education on signs and symptoms of labor, as appropriate. Inform the patient that hospitalization or more frequent prenatal checks may be ordered. Other therapies may also be administered, such as antibiotics, corticosteroids, and IV tocolytics. Instruct the patient in the importance of completing the entire course of antibiotic therapy, if ordered, even if no symptoms are present. Answer any questions or address any concerns voiced by the patient or family.

Depending on the results of this procedure, additional testing may be performed to evaluate or monitor progression of the disease process and determine the need for a change in therapy. Evaluate test results in relation to the patient's symptoms and other tests performed.

RELATED MONOGRAPHS:

Related tests include amniotic fluid analysis (nitrazine and fern test), biopsy chorionic villus, chromosome analysis, estradiol, α₁-fetoprotein, HCG, LS ratio, progesterone, and US biophysical profile obstetric.

Refer to the Reproductive System table at the end of the book for related tests by body system.

α₁-Fetoprotein

SYNONYM/ACRONYM: AFP.

COMMON USE: To assist in the evaluation of fetal health related to neural tube defects and some forms of liver cancer.

SPECIMEN: Serum (1 mL for tumor marker in men and nonpregnant women; 3 mL for maternal triple- or quad-marker testing), collected in a red- or tiger-top tube. For maternal triple- or quad-marker testing, include human chorionic gonadotropin and free estriol measurement.

REFERENCE VALUE: (Method: Immunochemiluminometric assay)

Tumor Marker: Males, Females, and Children

α₁-Fetoprotein	
Males, nonpregnant females, and children	0–15 ng/mL

α_1-Fetoprotein (AFP) in Maternal Serum for Triple or Quad Marker			
	White AFP (Median)	Black AFP (Median)	Hispanic AFP (Median)	Asian AFP (Median)
Low risk	Less than 2 MoM	Less than 2 MoM	Less than 2 MoM	Less than 2 MoM
Gestational Age (wk)				
14	19.9 ng/mL	23.2 ng/mL	18.3 ng/mL	22.4 ng/mL
15	23.2 ng/mL	26.9 ng/mL	22.6 ng/mL	28.3 ng/mL
16	27.0 ng/mL	31.1 ng/mL	27.3 ng/mL	32.7 ng/mL
17	31.5 ng/mL	35.9 ng/mL	32.3 ng/mL	37.9 ng/mL
18	36.7 ng/mL	41.6 ng/mL	38.1 ng/mL	44.8 ng/mL
19	42.7 ng/mL	48.0 ng/mL	45.0 ng/mL	52.0 ng/mL
20	49.8 ng/mL	55.6 ng/mL	52.2 ng/mL	62.2 ng/mL
21	58.1 ng/mL	64.2 ng/mL	61.9 ng/mL	79.5 ng/mL
22	67.8 ng/mL	74.2 ng/mL	64.3 ng/mL	78.2 ng/mL

MoM = multiples of the median.

HCG and Estriol in Maternal Serum	HCG	Free Estriol
Gestational Age (wk)	*Median Value*	*Median Value*
14	41.5 international units/mL	0.5 ng/mL
15	36.0 international units/mL	0.7 ng/mL
16	31.0 international units/mL	0.9 ng/mL
17	27.0 international units/mL	1.1 ng/mL
18	24.0 international units/mL	1.4 ng/mL
19	21.0 international units/mL	1.8 ng/mL
20	18.0 international units/mL	2.3 ng/mL
21	16.0 international units/mL	2.8 ng/mL
22	14.0 international units/mL	3.6 ng/mL

Results vary widely among laboratories and methods.
HCG = human chorionic gonadotropin.

DESCRIPTION: α_1-Fetoprotein (AFP) is a glycoprotein produced in the fetal liver, gastrointestinal tract, and yolk sac. AFP is the major serum protein produced for 10 wk in early fetal life. (See "Amniotic Fluid Analysis" monograph for measurement of AFP levels in amniotic fluid.) After 10 wk of gestation, levels of fetal AFP can be detected in maternal blood, with peak levels occurring at 16 to 18 wk. Elevated maternal levels of AFP on two tests taken 1 wk apart suggest further investigation into fetal well-being by ultrasound or amniocentesis. Human chorionic gonadotropin (HCG), a hormone secreted by the placenta, stimulates secretion of progesterone by the corpus luteum. (The use of HCG as a triple marker is also discussed in the monograph titled "Human

Chorionic Gonadotropin.") During intrauterine development, the normal fetus and placenta produce estriol, a portion of which passes into maternal circulation. Decreased estriol levels are an independent indicator of neural tube defects. The incidence of neural tube defects is about 1 in 1,000 births. Dimeric inhibin-A (DIA) is the fourth biochemical marker used in prenatal quad screening. It is a glycoprotein secreted by the placenta. Maternal blood levels of DIA normally remain fairly stable during the 15th to 18th wk of pregnancy. Blood levels are twice as high in the second trimester of pregnancies affected by Down syndrome. The triple screen detection rate for Down syndrome is 67%. The Down syndrome detection rate increases to 76% and maintains a false-positive rate of 5% when DIA is included.

The presence of AFP in excessive amounts is abnormal in adults and children. AFP measurements are used as a tumor marker to assist in the diagnosis of cancer.

INDICATIONS

- Assist in the diagnosis of primary hepatocellular carcinoma or metastatic lesions involving the liver, as indicated by highly elevated levels (30% to 50% of Americans with liver cancer do not have elevated AFP levels)
- Investigate suspected hepatitis or cirrhosis, indicated by slightly to moderately elevated levels
- Monitor response to treatment for hepatic carcinoma, with successful treatment indicated by an immediate decrease in levels
- Monitor for recurrence of hepatic carcinoma, with elevated levels occurring 1 to 6 mo before the patient becomes symptomatic

- Investigate suspected intrauterine fetal death, as indicated by elevated levels
- Routine prenatal screening at 13 to 16 wk of pregnancy for fetal neural tube defects and other disorders, as indicated by elevated levels in maternal serum and amniotic fluid
- Support diagnosis of embryonal gonadal teratoblastoma, hepatoblastoma, and testicular or ovarian carcinomas

POTENTIAL DIAGNOSIS

Maternal serum AFP test results report actual values and multiples of the median (MoM) by gestational age (in weeks). MoM are calculated by dividing the patient's AFP by the midpoint (or median) of values expected for a large population of unaffected women at the same gestational age in weeks. MoM should be corrected for maternal weight. The MoM should also be corrected for maternal insulin requirement (achieved by dividing MoM by 1.1 for diabetic African American patients and by 0.8 for diabetic patients of other races) and multiple fetuses (multiply by 2.13 for twins). Some laboratories also provide additional statistical information regarding Down syndrome risk.

Increased in

- Pregnant women:

  Congenital nephrosis *(related to defective renal reabsorption)*

  Fetal abdominal wall defects *(related to release of AFP from open body wall defect)*

  Fetal distress

  Fetal neural tube defects (e.g., anencephaly, spina bifida, myelomeningocele) *(related to release of AFP from open body wall defect)*

  Low birth weight *(related to inaccurate estimation of gestational age)*

  Multiple pregnancy *(related to larger quantities from multiple fetuses)*

Polycystic kidneys *(related to defective renal reabsorption)*

Underestimation of gestational age *(related to the expectation of a lower value based on incorrect prediction of gestational age, i.e., AFP increases with age; therefore, if the age is believed to be less than it is actually, the expectation of the corresponding AFP value will be lower than it is actually, and the result appears to be elevated)*

• Men, nonpregnant women, and children (the cancer cells contain undifferentiated hepatocytes that produce glycoproteins of fetal origin):
Cirrhosis
Hepatic carcinoma
Hepatitis
Metastatic lesions involving the liver

Decreased in

• Pregnant women:
Down syndrome (trisomy 21)
Edwards' syndrome (trisomy 18)
Fetal demise (undetected over a lengthy period of time) *(related to cessation of AFP production)*
Hydatidiform moles *(partial mole may secrete some AFP)*
Overestimation of gestational age *(related to the expectation of a higher value based on incorrect prediction of gestational age; i.e., AFP increases with age; therefore, if the age is believed to be greater than it actually is, the expectation of the corresponding AFP value will be greater than it actually is, and the result appears to be decreased)*
Pseudopregnancy *(there is no fetus to produce AFP)*
Spontaneous abortion *(there is no fetus to produce AFP)*

CRITICAL FINDINGS: N/A

INTERFERING FACTORS

• Drugs that may decrease AFP levels in pregnant women include acetaminophen, acetylsalicylic acid, and phenacetin.

• Multiple fetuses can cause increased levels.

• Gestational age must be between 15 and 22 wk for initial and follow-up testing. The most common cause of an abnormal MoM is inaccurate estimation of gestational age (defined as weeks from the first day of the last menstrual period).

• Maternal AFP levels vary by race.

PRETEST:

▶ Positively identify the patient using at least two unique identifiers before providing care, treatment, or services.

▶ *Patient Teaching:* Inform the patient this test can assist in evaluating fetal health.

▶ Obtain a history of the patient's complaints and known or suspected malignancy. Obtain a list of known allergens, especially allergies or sensitivities to latex.

▶ Obtain a history of the patient's immune and reproductive systems, gestational age, symptoms, and results of previously performed laboratory tests and diagnostic and surgical procedures.

▶ Note any recent procedures that can interfere with test results.

▶ Provide required information to laboratory for triple-marker testing, including maternal birth date, weight, age, race, calculated gestational age, gestational age by ultrasound, gestational date by physical examination, first day of last menstrual period, estimated date of delivery, and whether the patient has insulin-dependent (type 1) diabetes.

▶ Obtain a list of the patient's current medications, including herbs, nutritional supplements, and nutraceuticals (see Appendix F).

▶ Review the procedure with the patient. Inform the patient that specimen collection takes approximately 5 to 10 min. Address concerns about pain and explain that there may be some discomfort during the venipuncture.

▶ There are no food, fluid, or medication restrictions unless by medical direction.

Make sure a written and informed consent has been signed prior to the procedure and before administering any medications.

INTRATEST:

- If the patient has a history of allergic reaction to latex, avoid the use of equipment containing latex.
- Instruct the patient to cooperate fully and to follow directions. Direct the patient to breathe normally and to avoid unnecessary movement.
- Observe standard precautions, and follow the general guidelines in Appendix A. Positively identify the patient, and label the appropriate tubes with the corresponding patient demographics, date, and time of collection. Perform a venipuncture.
- The sample may be collected directly from the cord using a syringe and transferred to a red-top tube.
- Remove the needle and apply direct pressure with dry gauze to stop bleeding. Observe/assess venipuncture site for bleeding or hematoma formation and secure gauze with adhesive bandage.
- Promptly transport the specimen to the laboratory for processing and analysis.

POST-TEST:

- A report of the results will be sent to the requesting health-care provider (HCP), who will discuss the results with the patient.
- *Nutritional Considerations:* Hyperhomocysteinemia resulting from folate deficiency in pregnant women is believed to increase the risk of neural tube defects. Elevated levels of homocysteine are thought to chemically damage the exposed neural tissue of the developing fetus. As appropriate, instruct pregnant patients to eat foods rich in folate, such as liver, salmon, eggs, asparagus, green leafy vegetables, broccoli, sweet potatoes, beans, and whole wheat.
- *Social and Cultural Considerations:* In pregnant patients, recognize anxiety related to test results, and encourage the family to seek counseling if concerned with pregnancy termination or to seek genetic counseling if a chromosomal abnormality is determined. Discuss the implications of abnormal test results on the patient's lifestyle. Provide teaching and information regarding the clinical implications of the test results, as appropriate. Decisions regarding elective abortion should take place in the presence of both parents. Provide a nonjudgmental, nonthreatening atmosphere for discussing the risks and difficulties of delivering and raising a developmentally challenged infant, as well as exploring other options (termination of pregnancy or adoption). It is also important to discuss feelings the mother and father may experience (e.g., guilt, depression, anger) if fetal abnormalities are detected. Educate the patient regarding access to counseling services.
- In patients with carcinoma, recognize anxiety related to test results, and offer support. Discuss the implications of abnormal test results on the patient's lifestyle. Provide teaching and information regarding the clinical implications of the test results, as appropriate. Educate the patient regarding access to counseling services, as appropriate.
- Reinforce information given by the patient's HCP regarding further testing, treatment, or referral to another HCP. Answer any questions or address any concerns voiced by the patient or family.
- Depending on the results of this procedure, additional testing may be performed to evaluate or monitor progression of the disease process and determine the need for a change in therapy. Inform the pregnant patient that an ultrasound may be performed and AFP levels in amniotic fluid may be analyzed if maternal blood levels are elevated in two samples obtained 1 wk apart. Evaluate test results in relation to the patient's symptoms and other tests performed.

RELATED MONOGRAPHS:

- Related tests include amniotic fluid analysis, biopsy chorionic villus, cancer antigens, estradiol, fetal fibronectin, folic acid, hexosaminidase, homocysteine, HCG, L/S ratio, and US biophysical profile obstetric.
- Refer to the Immune and Reproductive systems tables at the end of the book for related tests by body system.

Fetoscopy

SYNONYM/ACRONYM: Endoscopic fetal surgery, fetal endoscopy.

COMMON USE: To facilitate diagnosis and treatment of the fetus. Evaluate for disorders such as neural tube defects and congenital blood disorders, and assist with fetal karyotyping.

AREA OF APPLICATION: Fetus, uterus.

CONTRAST: N/A.

DESCRIPTION: Fetoscopy is usually performed around the 18th week of pregnancy or later when the fetus is developed sufficiently for diagnosis of potential problems. It is done to evaluate or treat the fetus during pregnancy. Fetoscopy can be accomplished externally using a stethoscope with an attached headpiece, which is placed on the mother's abdomen to assess the fetal heart tones. Endoscopic fetoscopy is accomplished using an instrument called a fetoscope, a thin, 1-mm flexible scope, which is placed with the aid of sonography. The fetoscope is inserted into the uterus through a thin incision in the abdominal wall (transabdominally) or through the cervix (transcervically) in earlier stages of pregnancy. Fetal tissue and blood samples can be obtained through the fetoscope. In addition, fetal surgery can be performed for such procedures as the repair of a fetal congenital diaphragmatic hernia, enlarged bladder, and spina bifida.

INDICATIONS
• Pregnancy

POTENTIAL DIAGNOSIS

Normal findings in
• Absence of birth defects

Abnormal findings in
• Acardiac twin
• Congenital diaphragmatic hernia (CDH)
• Hemophilia
• Neural tube defects
• Spinal bifida

CRITICAL FINDINGS: N/A

INTERFERING FACTORS

Factors that may impair clear imaging
• Activity of fetus.
• Amniotic fluid that is extremely cloudy.
• Inability of patient to remain still during the procedure.
• Obesity or very overweight patient.

NURSING IMPLICATIONS AND PROCEDURE

PRETEST:

▶ Positively identify the patient using at least two unique identifiers before providing care, treatment, or services.

Patient Teaching: Inform the patient this procedure can assist in locating and treating fetal abnormalities.

Obtain a history of the patient's complaints, including a list of known allergens, especially allergies or sensitivities to latex and anesthetics.

Obtain a history of the patient's reproductive system, symptoms, and results of previously performed laboratory tests and diagnostic and surgical procedures.

Note any recent procedures that can interfere with test results (i.e., barium procedures, surgery, or biopsy).

Record the date of last menstrual period and determine the age of the fetus.

Obtain a list of the patient's current medications, including herbs, nutritional supplements, and nutraceuticals (see Appendix F).

Instruct the patient to remove jewelry and other metallic objects in the area to be examined.

Review the procedure with the patient. Address concerns about pain and explain that a local anesthetic will be applied to the abdomen to ease with insertion of the fetoscope. Inform the patient that the procedure is performed in an ultrasound department, by a health-care provider (HCP) specializing in this procedure, with support staff, and takes approximately 60 min.

Sensitivity to social and cultural issues, as well as concern for modesty, is important in providing psychological support before, during, and after the procedure.

Food and fluid should be withheld for 8 hr prior to the procedure. There are no medication restrictions unless by medical direction.

Make sure a written and informed consent has been signed prior to the procedure and before administering any medications.

INTRATEST:

Ensure that the patient has complied with dietary restrictions; ensure that food and fluid has been restricted for at least 8 hr prior to the procedure.

Ensure that the patient has removed external metallic objects prior to the procedure.

Instruct the patient to void prior to the procedure and to change into the gown, robe, and foot coverings provided.

Instruct the patient to cooperate fully and to follow directions. Instruct the patient to remain still throughout the procedure because movement produces unreliable results.

Instruct the patient to lie on her back. The lower abdomen area is cleaned, and a local anesthetic is administered in the area where the incision will be made.

Observe standard precautions, and follow the general guidelines in Appendix A if cultures are to be obtained on aspirated amniotic fluid or fetal material.

Conductive gel is applied to the skin, and a Doppler transducer is moved over the skin to locate the position of the fetus.

Ask the patient to breathe normally during the examination. If necessary for better fetal visualization, ask the patient to inhale deeply and hold her breath.

POST-TEST:

A report of the results will be sent to the requesting HCP, who will discuss the results with the patient.

When the study is completed, remove the gel from the skin.

Observe/assess the incision for redness or leakage of fluid or blood.

Instruct the patient in the care of the incision and to contact her HCP immediately if she is experiencing chills, fever, dizziness, moderate or severe abdominal cramping, or fluid or blood loss from the vagina or incision.

Inform the patient that a follow-up ultrasound will be completed the next day to assess the fetus and placenta.

Recognize anxiety related to test results. Discuss the implications of abnormal test results on the patient's lifestyle. Provide teaching and information regarding the clinical implications of the test results, as appropriate.

Reinforce information given by the patient's HCP regarding further testing, treatment, or referral to another HCP. Answer any questions or address any concerns voiced by the patient or family.

F

▶ Depending on the results of this procedure, additional testing may be needed to evaluate or monitor progression of the disease process and determine the need for a change in therapy. Evaluate test results in relation to the patient's symptoms and other tests performed.

RELATED MONOGRAPHS:

▶ Related tests include amniotic fluid analysis, biopsy chorionic villus, blood groups and antibodies, chromosome analysis, culture bacterial anal/genital, culture viral, fetal fibronectin, α_1-fetoprotein, hexosaminidase A and B, human chorionic gonadotropin, KUB, Kleihauer-Betke test, lecithin/sphingomyelin ratio, prolactin, MRI abdomen, and ultrasound biophysical profile obstetric.

▶ Refer to the Reproductive System table at the end of the book for related tests by body system.

F **Fibrin Degradation Products**

SYNONYM/ACRONYM: Fibrin split products, fibrin breakdown products, FDP, FSP, FBP.

COMMON USE: To evaluate conditions associated with abnormal fibrinolytic and fibrinogenolytic activity such as DIC, DVT, and PE.

SPECIMEN: Plasma (1 mL) collected in a completely filled blue-top (3.2% sodium citrate) tube. If the patient's hematocrit exceeds 55%, the volume of citrate in the collection tube must be adjusted.

REFERENCE VALUE: (Method: Latex agglutination)

Conventional Units	SI Units (Conventional Units × 1)
Less than 5 mcg/mL	Less than 5 mg/dL

DESCRIPTION: This coagulation test evaluates fibrin split products or fibrin/fibrinogen degradation products that interfere with normal coagulation and formation of the hemostatic platelet plug. After a fibrin clot has formed, the fibrinolytic system prevents excessive clotting. In the fibrinolytic system, plasmin digests fibrin. Fibrinogen also can be degraded if there is a disproportion among plasmin, fibrin, and fibrinogen. Seven substances labeled *A, B, C, D, E, X,* and *Y* result from this degradation, which can indicate abnormal coagulation. Under normal conditions, the liver and reticuloendothelial system remove fibrin split products from the circulation.

INDICATIONS

* Assist in the diagnosis of suspected disseminated intravascular coagulation (DIC)
* Evaluate response to therapy with fibrinolytic drugs
* Monitor the effects on hemostasis of trauma, extensive surgery, obstetric complications, and disorders such as liver or renal disease

POTENTIAL DIAGNOSIS

Increased in

- DIC *(FDP can be positive in a number of conditions in which the coagulation system has been excessively stimulated as a result of tissue injury and fibrin and/or fibrinogen is being degraded by plasmin)*
- Excessive bleeding *(clot formation related to depletion of platelets and clotting factors will stimulate fibrinolysis and increase circulation of fibrin breakdown products)*
- Liver disease *(related to decreased hepatic clearance)*
- Myocardial infarction *(FDP can be positive in a number of conditions in which the coagulation system has been excessively stimulated as a result of tissue injury and fibrin and/or fibrinogen is being degraded by plasmin)*
- Obstetric complications, such as pre-eclampsia, abruptio placentae, intrauterine fetal death *(excessive stimulation of the coagulation system; microthrombi are formed and plasminogen is released to dissolve the fibrin clots)*
- Post–cardiothoracic surgery period *(FDP can be positive in a number of conditions in which the coagulation system has been excessively stimulated as a result of tissue injury and fibrin and/or fibrinogen is being degraded by plasmin)*
- Pulmonary embolism *(FDP can be positive in a number of conditions in which the coagulation system has been excessively stimulated as a result of tissue injury and fibrin and/or fibrinogen is being degraded by plasmin)*
- Renal disease *(FDP can be positive in a number of conditions in which the coagulation system has been excessively stimulated as a result of tissue injury and fibrin and/or fibrinogen is being degraded by plasmin)*
- Renal transplant rejection

Decreased in: N/A

CRITICAL FINDINGS: N/A

INTERFERING FACTORS

- Traumatic venipunctures and excessive agitation of the sample can alter test results.
- Drugs that may increase fibrin degradation product levels include heparin and fibrinolytic drugs such as streptokinase and urokinase.
- The presence of rheumatoid factor may falsely elevate results with some test kits.
- The test should not be ordered on patients receiving heparin therapy.
- Hematocrit greater than 55% may cause falsely prolonged results because of anticoagulant excess relative to plasma volume.
- Incompletely filled collection tubes, specimens contaminated with heparin, clotted specimens, or unprocessed specimens not delivered to the laboratory within 1 to 2 hr of collection should be rejected.

NURSING IMPLICATIONS AND PROCEDURE

PRETEST:

- Positively identify the patient using at least two unique identifiers before providing care, treatment, or services.
- *Patient Teaching:* Inform the patient this test can assist in diagnosing diseases associated with clotting disorders.

- Obtain a history of the patient's complaints, including a list of known allergens, especially allergies or sensitivities to latex.
- Obtain a history of the patient's hematopoietic system, any bleeding disorders, symptoms, and results of previously performed laboratory tests and diagnostic and surgical procedures.
- Note any recent procedures that can interfere with test results.
- Obtain a list of the patient's current medications, including anticoagulants, aspirin and other salicylates, herbs, nutritional supplements, and nutraceuticals (see Appendix F). Note the last time and dose of medication taken.
- Review the procedure with the patient. Inform the patient that specimen collection takes approximately 5 to 10 min. Address concerns about pain and explain that there may be some discomfort during the venipuncture.
- *Sensitivity to social and cultural issues,* as well as concern for modesty, is important in providing psychological support before, during, and after the procedure.
- There are no food, fluid, or medication restrictions unless by medical direction.

INTRATEST:

- If the patient has a history of allergic reaction to latex, avoid the use of equipment containing latex.
- Instruct the patient to cooperate fully and to follow directions. Direct the patient to breathe normally and to avoid unnecessary movement.
- Observe standard precautions, and follow the general guidelines in Appendix A. Positively identify the patient, and label the appropriate tubes with the corresponding patient demographics, date, and time of collection. Perform a venipuncture. Fill tube completely. *Important note:* Two different concentrations of sodium citrate preservative are currently added to blue-top tubes for coagulation studies: 3.2% and 3.8%. The Clinical and Laboratory Standards Institute (CLSI; formerly the National Committee for Clinical Laboratory Standards [NCCLS]) guideline for sodium citrate is 3.2%. Laboratories establish reference ranges for coagulation testing based on numerous factors, including sodium

citrate concentration, test equipment, and test reagents. It is important to ask the laboratory which concentration it recommends, because each concentration will have its own specific reference range. When multiple specimens are drawn, the blue-top tube should be collected after sterile (i.e., blood culture) tubes. Otherwise, when using a standard vacutainer system, the blue-top tube is the first tube collected. When a butterfly is used, due to the added tubing, an extra red-top tube should be collected before the blue-top tube to ensure complete filling of the blue top tube.
- Remove the needle and apply direct pressure with dry gauze to stop bleeding. Observe/assess venipuncture site for bleeding or hematoma formation and secure gauze with adhesive bandage.
- Promptly transport the specimen to the laboratory for processing and analysis. The CLSI recommendation for processed and unprocessed samples stored in unopened tubes is that testing should be completed within 1 to 4 hr of collection. If the patient has a known hematocrit above 55%, adjust the amount of anticoagulant in the collection tube before drawing the blood according to the CLSI guidelines:

Anticoagulant vol. [x] = (100 – hematocrit) / (595 – hematocrit) × total vol. of anticoagulated blood required

Example:

Patient hematocrit = 60% = (100 – 60) / (595 – 60) × 5.0 = 0.37 mL sodium citrate for a 5-mL standard drawing tube

POST-TEST:

- A report of the results will be sent to the requesting HCP, who will discuss the results with the patient.
- Instruct the patient to report bleeding from skin or mucous membranes, ecchymosis, petechiae, hematuria, and occult blood.
- Inform the patient with increased levels of fibrin degradation products of the importance of taking precautions against bruising and bleeding, including the use of a soft bristle toothbrush, use

of an electric razor, avoidance of constipation, avoidance of acetylsalicylic acid and similar products, and avoidance of intramuscular injections.

▶ Reinforce information given by the patient's HCP regarding further testing, treatment, or referral to another HCP. Answer any questions or address any concerns voiced by the patient or family.

▶ Depending on the results of this procedure, additional testing may be performed to evaluate or monitor progression of the disease process and determine the need for a change in therapy. Evaluate test results in relation to the patient's symptoms and other tests performed.

RELATED MONOGRAPHS:

▶ Related tests include aPTT, ALT, alveolar/arterial gradient, angiography pulmonary, AT-III, AST, bilirubin, biopsy liver, blood pool imaging, BUN, coagulation factors, CT cardiac scoring, creatinine, CBC, CK and isoenzymes, CRP, D-dimer, exercise stress test, FDP, fibrinogen, GGT, lung perfusion scan, lung ventilation scan, myoglobin, plasminogen, platelet count, PET heart, protein S, PT/INR, troponin, US venous Doppler extremity studies, and venography lower extremity studies.

▶ Refer to the Hematopoietic System table at the end of the book for related tests by body system.

F

Fibrinogen

SYNONYM/ACRONYM: Factor I.

COMMON USE: Commonly used to evaluate fibrinolytic activity as well as identify congenital deficiency, DIC, and severe liver disease.

SPECIMEN: Plasma (1 mL) collected in a completely filled blue-top (3.2% sodium citrate) tube. If the patient's hematocrit exceeds 55%, the volume of citrate in the collection tube must be adjusted.

REFERENCE VALUE: (Method: Photo-optical clot detection)

Age	Conventional Units	SI Units (Conventional Units × 0.01)
Newborn	125–300 mg/dL	1.25–3.00 g/L
Adult	200–400 mg/dL	2.00–4.00 g/L

DESCRIPTION: Fibrinogen (factor I) is synthesized in the liver. In the common final pathway of the coagulation sequence, thrombin converts fibrinogen to fibrin, which then clots blood as it combines with platelets. In healthy individuals, the serum should contain no residual fibrinogen after clotting has occurred.

INDICATIONS

• Assist in the diagnosis of suspected disseminated intravascular coagulation (DIC), as indicated by decreased fibrinogen levels
• Evaluate congenital or acquired dysfibrinogenemias
• Monitor hemostasis in disorders associated with low fibrinogen levels or elevated levels that can predispose patients to excessive thrombosis

POTENTIAL DIAGNOSIS

Increased in

Fibrinogen is an acute phase reactant protein and will be increased in inflammatory conditions.
- Acute myocardial infarction
- Cancer
- Eclampsia
- Hodgkin's disease
- Inflammation
- Multiple myeloma
- Nephrotic syndrome
- Pregnancy
- Tissue necrosis

Decreased in
- Congenital fibrinogen deficiency (rare) *(related to deficient synthesis)*
- DIC *(related to rapid consumption as fibrinogen is converted to fibrin)*
- Dysfibrinogenemia *(related to an inherited abnormality in fibrinogen synthesis)*
- Liver disease (severe) *(related to decreased synthesis)*
- Primary fibrinolysis *(related to rapid conversion during fibrinolysis; plasmin breaks down fibrinogen and fibrin)*

CRITICAL FINDINGS ✸
- Less than 80 mg/dL

Note and immediately report to the health-care provider (HCP) any critically decreased values and related symptoms. Signs and symptoms of microvascular thrombosis include cyanosis, ischemic tissue necrosis, hemorrhagic necrosis, tachypnea, dyspnea, pulmonary emboli, venous distention, abdominal pain, and oliguria. Possible interventions include identification and treatment of the underlying cause, support through administration of required blood products (platelets, cryoprecipitate, or fresh frozen plasma), and administration of heparin.

INTERFERING FACTORS
- Drugs that may increase fibrinogen levels include acetylsalicylic acid, norethandrolone, oral contraceptives, oxandrolone, and oxymetholone.
- Drugs that may decrease fibrinogen levels include anabolic steroids, asparaginase, bezafibrate, danazol, dextran, fenofibrate, fish oils, gemfibrozil, lovastatin, pentoxifylline, phosphorus, and ticlopidine.
- Transfusions of whole blood, plasma, or fractions within 4 wk of the test invalidate results.
- Placement of tourniquet for longer than 60 sec can result in venous stasis and changes in the concentration of plasma proteins to be measured. Platelet activation may also occur under these conditions, causing erroneous results.
- Vascular injury during phlebotomy can activate platelets and coagulation factors, causing erroneous results.
- Hemolyzed specimens must be rejected because hemolysis is an indication of platelet and coagulation factor activation.
- Hematocrit greater than 55% may cause falsely prolonged results because of anticoagulant excess relative to plasma volume.
- Incompletely filled collection tubes, specimens contaminated with heparin, clotted specimens, or unprocessed specimens not delivered to the laboratory within 1 to 2 hr of collection should be rejected.
- Icteric or lipemic specimens interfere with optical testing methods, producing erroneous results.
- Traumatic venipuncture and excessive agitation of the sample can alter test results.

NURSING IMPLICATIONS AND PROCEDURE

PRETEST:

- Positively identify the patient using at least two unique identifiers before providing care, treatment, or services.
- *Patient Teaching:* Inform the patient that this lab test can assist in diagnosing diseases associated with clotting disorders.
- Obtain a history of the patient's complaints, including a list of known allergens, especially allergies or sensitivities to latex.
- Obtain a history of the patient's hematopoietic and hepatobiliary systems, symptoms, and results of previously performed laboratory tests and diagnostic and surgical procedures.
- Note any recent procedures that can interfere with test results.
- Obtain a list of the patient's current medications, including herbs, nutritional supplements, and nutraceuticals (see Appendix F).
- Review the procedure with the patient. Inform the patient that specimen collection takes approximately 5 to 10 min. Address concerns about pain and explain that there may be some discomfort during the venipuncture.
- *Sensitivity to social and cultural issues,* as well as concern or modesty, is important in providing psychological support before, during, and after the procedure.
- There are no food, fluid, or medication restrictions unless by medical direction.

INTRATEST:

- If the patient has a history of allergic reaction to latex, avoid the use of equipment containing latex.
- Instruct the patient to cooperate fully and to follow directions. Direct the patient to breathe normally and to avoid unnecessary movement.
- Observe standard precautions, and follow the general guidelines in Appendix A. Positively identify the patient, and label the appropriate tubes with the corresponding patient demographics, date, and time of collection. Perform a venipuncture. Fill tube completely.

Important note: Two different concentrations of sodium citrate preservative are currently added to blue-top tubes for coagulation studies: 3.2% and 3.8%. The Clinical and Laboratory Standards Institute (CLSI; formerly the National Committee for Clinical Laboratory Standards [NCCLS]) guideline for sodium citrate is 3.2%. Laboratories establish reference ranges for coagulation testing based on numerous factors, including sodium citrate concentration, test equipment, and test reagents. It is important to ask the laboratory which concentration it recommends, because each concentration will have its own specific reference range. When multiple specimens are drawn, the blue-top tube should be collected after sterile (i.e., blood culture) tubes. Otherwise, when using a standard vacutainer system, the blue-top tube is the first tube collected. When a butterfly is used, due to the added tubing, an extra red-top tube should be collected before the blue-top tube to ensure complete filling of the blue top tube.

- Remove the needle and apply direct pressure with dry gauze to stop bleeding. Observe/assess venipuncture site for bleeding or hematoma formation and secure gauze with adhesive bandage.
- Promptly transport the specimen to the laboratory for processing and analysis. The CLSI recommendation for processed and unprocessed samples stored in unopened tubes is that testing should be completed within 1 to 4 hr of collection. If the patient has a known hematocrit above 55%, adjust the amount of anticoagulant in the collection tube before drawing the blood according to the CLSI guidelines:

Anticoagulant vol. [x] = (100 − hematocrit) / (595 − hematocrit) × total vol. of anticoagulated blood required

Example:

Patient hematocrit = 60% = (100 − 60) / (595 − 60) × 5.0 = 0.37 mL sodium citrate for a 5-mL standard drawing tube

POST-TEST:

- A report of the results will be sent to the requesting HCP, who will discuss the results with the patient.
- Instruct the patient to report bruising, petechiae, and bleeding from mucous membranes, hematuria, and occult blood.
- Inform the patient with a decreased fibrinogen level of the importance of taking precautions against bruising and bleeding, including the use of a soft bristle toothbrush, use of an electric razor, avoidance of constipation, avoidance of acetylsalicylic acid and similar products, and avoidance of intramuscular injections.
- Reinforce information given by the patient's HCP regarding further testing, treatment, or referral to another HCP. Answer any questions or address any concerns voiced by the patient or family.
- Depending on the results of this procedure, additional testing may be performed to evaluate or monitor progression of the disease process and determine the need for a change in therapy. Evaluate test results in relation to the patient's symptoms and other tests performed.

RELATED MONOGRAPHS:

- Related tests include ALT, albumin, ALP, AT-III, AST, bilirubin, biopsy bone, biopsy bone marrow, biopsy liver, clot retraction, coagulation factors, CBC platelet count, CT cardiac scoring, CK and isoenzymes, CRP, D-dimer, echocardiography, echocardiography transesophageal, ECG, ESR, exercise stress test, FDP, GGT, Holter monitor, IFE, immunoglobulins, myocardial perfusion heart scan, aPTT, plasminogen, protein S, and PT/INR.
- Refer to the Hematopoietic and Hepatobiliary systems tables at the end of the book for related tests by body system.

Fluorescein Angiography

SYNONYM/ACRONYM: FA.

COMMON USE: To assist in detecting vascular changes in the eyes affecting vision related to diseases such as diabetic retinopathy and macular degeneration.

AREA OF APPLICATION: Eyes.

CONTRAST: Fluorescein dye.

DESCRIPTION: Fluorescein angiography (FA) involves the color radiographic examination of the retinal vasculature following rapid IV injection of a sodium fluorescein contrast medium. A special camera allows images to be taken in sequence and manipulated by a computer to provide views of the retinal vessels during filling and emptying of the dye. The camera allows only light waves in the blue range to strike the fundus of the eye. When the fluorescein reaches the blood vessels in the eye, blue light excites the dye molecules to a higher state of activity and causes them to emit a greenish-yellow fluorescence that is recorded.

INDICATIONS

- Detect arterial or venous occlusion evidenced by the reduced, delayed, or absent flow of the contrast medium through the vessels or possible vessel leakage of the medium
- Detect possible vascular disorders affecting visual acuity
- Detect presence of microaneurysms caused by hypertensive retinopathy
- Detect the presence of tumors, retinal edema, or inflammation, as evidenced by abnormal patterns or degree of fluorescence
- Diagnose diabetic retinopathy
- Diagnose past reduced flow or patency of the vascular circulation of the retina, as evidenced by neovascularization
- Diagnose presence of macular degeneration and any other degeneration and any associated hemorrhaging
- Observe ocular effects resulting from the long-term use of high-risk medications

POTENTIAL DIAGNOSIS

Normal findings in
- No leakage of dye from retinal blood vessels
- Normal retina and retinal and choroidal vessels
- No evidence of vascular abnormalities, such as hemorrhage, retinopathy, aneurysms, or obstructions caused by stenosis and resulting in collateral circulation

Abnormal findings in
- Aneurysm
- Arteriovenous shunts
- Diabetic retinopathy
- Macular degeneration
- Neovascularization
- Obstructive disorders of the arteries or veins that lead to collateral circulation

CRITICAL FINDINGS: N/A

INTERFERING FACTORS

This procedure is contraindicated for
- Patients with a past history of hypersensitivity to radiographic dyes.
- Patients with narrow-angle glaucoma if pupil dilation is performed; dilation can initiate a severe and sight-threatening open-angle attack.
- Patients with allergies to mydriatics if pupil dilation using mydriatics is performed.

Factors that may impair the results of the examination
- Inability of the patient to cooperate or remain still during the test because of age, significant pain, or mental status may interfere with the test results.
- Presence of cataracts may interfere with fundal view.
- Ineffective dilation of the pupils may impair clear imaging.
- Allergic reaction to radiographic dye, including nausea and vomiting, may interrupt the procedure.
- Failure to follow medication restrictions before the procedure may cause the procedure to be canceled or repeated.

NURSING IMPLICATIONS AND PROCEDURE

PRETEST:
- Positively identify the patient using at least two unique identifiers before providing care, treatment, or services.
- *Patient Teaching:* Inform the patient this procedure can assist in detecting changes in the eye that affect vision.
- Obtain a history of the patient's complaints, including a list of known allergens, especially allergies or sensitivities to radiographic dyes, shellfish, and bee venom.
- Obtain a history of the patient's known or suspected vision loss; changes in visual acuity, including type and cause;

use of glasses or contact lenses; and eye conditions with treatment regimens.

▶ Obtain a history of the patient's symptoms and results of previously performed laboratory tests and diagnostic and surgical procedures.

▶ Obtain a list of the patient's current medications, including herbs, nutritional supplements, and nutraceuticals (see Appendix F).

▶ Instruct the patient to remove contact lenses or glasses, as appropriate. Instruct the patient regarding the importance of keeping the eyes open for the test.

▶ Review the procedure with the patient. Explain that the patient will be requested to fixate the eyes during the procedure. Address concerns about pain and explain that mydriatics, if used, may cause blurred vision and sensitivity to light. There may also be a brief stinging sensation when the drop is put in the eye. Explain to the patient that some discomfort may be experienced during the insertion of the IV. Inform the patient that when fluorescein dye is injected, it may cause facial flushing or nausea and vomiting. Inform the patient that a health-care provider (HCP) performs the test, in a quiet, darkened room, and that to dilate and evaluate both eyes, the test can take up 60 min.

▶ *Sensitivity to social and cultural issues,* as well as concern for modesty, is important in providing psychological support before, during, and after the procedure.

▶ Explain that an IV line will be inserted to allow intermittent infusion of dye.

▶ There are no food or fluid restrictions unless by medical direction.

▶ The patient should avoid eye medications (particularly mydriatic eyedrops if the patient has glaucoma) for at least 1 day prior to the test.

▶ Ensure that the patient understands that he or she must refrain from driving until the pupils return to normal (about 4 hr) after the test and has made arrangements to have someone else be responsible for transportation after the test.

▶ *Make sure a written and informed consent has been signed prior to the procedure and before administering any medications.*

INTRATEST:

▶ Ensure that the patient has complied with medication restrictions; ensure that eye medications, especially mydriatics, have been withheld for at least 1 day prior to the test.

▶ Have emergency equipment readily available.

▶ Instruct the patient to cooperate fully and to follow directions. Instruct the patient to remain still during the procedure because movement produces unreliable results.

▶ Seat the patient in a chair that faces the camera. Instruct the patient to look at a directed target while the eyes are examined.

▶ If dilation is to be performed, administer the ordered mydriatic to each eye and repeat in 5 to 15 min. Drops are placed in the eye with the patient looking up and the solution directed at the six o'clock position of the sclera (white of the eye) near the limbus (gray, semitransparent area of the eyeball where the cornea and sclera meet). Neither dropper nor bottle should touch the eyelashes.

▶ Insert an intermittent infusion device, as ordered, for subsequent injection of the contrast media or emergency medications.

▶ After the eyedrops are administered but before the dye is injected, color fundus photographs are taken.

▶ Instruct the patient to place the chin in the chin rest and gently press the forehead against the support bar. Instruct the patient to open his or her eyes wide and look at the desired target.

▶ Fluorescein dye is injected into the brachial vein using the intermittent infusion device, and a rapid sequence of photographs are taken and repeated after the dye has reached the retinal vascular system. Follow-up photographs are taken in 20 to 30 min.

▶ At the conclusion of the procedure, remove the IV needle and apply direct pressure with dry gauze to stop bleeding. Observe venipuncture site for bleeding or hematoma formation and secure gauze with adhesive bandage.

- Observe for hypersensitive reaction to the dye. The patient may become nauseous and vomit.

- A report of the results will be sent to the requesting HCP, who will discuss the results with the patient.
- Instruct the patient to resume usual medications, as directed by the HCP.
- *Nutritional Considerations:* Increased glucose levels may be associated with diabetes. There is no "diabetic diet"; however, many meal-planning approaches with nutritional goals are endorsed by the American Dietetic Association. Patients who adhere to dietary recommendations report a better general feeling of health, better weight management, greater control of glucose and lipid values, and improved use of insulin. Instruct the patient, as appropriate, in nutritional management of diabetes. In June 2006, the American Heart Association developed a Therapeutic Lifestyle Changes (TLC) diet with goals directed at people with specific risk factors and/or existing medical conditions (e.g., elevated LDL cholesterol levels, other lipid disorders, coronary artery disease, insulin-dependent diabetes, insulin resistance, or metabolic syndrome). The TLC approach also includes the use of plant stanols or sterols and increased dissolved fiber as an option for lowering LDL cholesterol levels; nutritional recommendations for daily total caloric intake; recommendations for allowable percentage of calories derived from fat (saturated and unsaturated), carbohydrates, protein, and cholesterol; as well as recommendations for daily expenditure of energy. The nutritional needs of each diabetic patient need to be determined individually (especially during pregnancy) with the appropriate HCPs, particularly professionals trained in nutrition.
- Recognize anxiety related to test results, and be supportive of impaired activity related to vision loss or anticipated loss of driving privileges. Discuss the implications of abnormal test results on the patient's lifestyle. Provide teaching and information regarding the clinical implications of the test results, as appropriate. Emphasize, as appropriate, that good glycemic control delays the onset of and slows the progression of diabetic retinopathy, nephropathy, and neuropathy. Provide education regarding smoking cessation, as appropriate. Provide contact information regarding vision aids, if desired, for ABLEDATA (sponsored by the National Institute on Disability and Rehabilitation Research [NIDRR], available at www.abledata.com). Information can also be obtained from the American Macular Degeneration Foundation (www.macular.org), the Glaucoma Research Foundation (www.glaucoma.org), the American Diabetes Association (www.diabetes.org), or the American Heart Association (www.americanheart.org).
- Reinforce information given by the patient's HCP regarding further testing, treatment, or referral to another HCP. Inform the patient that visual acuity and responses to light may change. Suggest that the patient wear dark glasses after the test until the pupils return to normal size. Inform the patient that yellow discoloration of the skin and urine from the radiographic dye is normally present for up to 2 days. Answer any questions or address any concerns voiced by the patient or family.
- Depending on the results of this procedure, additional testing may be performed to evaluate or monitor progression of the disease process and determine the need for a change in therapy. Evaluate test results in relation to the patient's symptoms and other tests performed.

- Related tests include fructosamine, fundus photography, glucagon, glucose, glycated hemoglobin, gonioscopy, insulin, intraocular pressure, microalbumin, plethysmography, refraction, slit-lamp biomicroscopy, and visual field testing.
- Refer to the Ocular System table at the end of the book for related tests by body system.

Folate

SYNONYM/ACRONYM: Folic acid, vitamin B_9.

COMMON USE: To assist in evaluation of diagnoses that are related to fluctuations in folate levels such as vitamin B_{12} deficiency and malabsorption.

SPECIMEN: Serum (1 mL) collected in a red- or tiger-top tube.

REFERENCE VALUE: (Method: Immunochemiluminometric assay [ICMA])

Age	Conventional Units	SI Units (Conventional Units × 2.265)
5–9 yr	Greater than 7.1 ng/mL	Greater than 16.1 nmol/L
10–17 yr	Greater than 8 ng/mL	Greater than 18.1 nmol/L
Adult		
Normal	Greater than 5.4 ng/mL	Greater than 12.2 nmol/L
Intermediate	3.4–5.4 ng/mL	7.7–12.2 nmol/L
Deficient	Less than 3.4 ng/mL	Less than 7.7 nmol/L

Values may be slightly decreased in older adults due to the effects of medications and the presence of multiple chronic or acute diseases with or without muted symptoms.

DESCRIPTION: Folate, a water-soluble vitamin, is produced by bacteria in the intestines and stored in small amounts in the liver. Dietary folate is absorbed through the intestinal mucosa and stored in the liver. Folate is necessary for normal red blood cell and white blood cell function, DNA replication, and cell division. Folate levels are often measured in association with serum vitamin B_{12} determinations because vitamin B_{12} is required for folate to enter tissue cells. Folate is an essential coenzyme in the conversion of homocysteine to methionine. Hyperhomocysteinemia resulting from folate deficiency in pregnant women is believed to increase the risk of neural tube defects. Hyperhomocyteinemia related to low folic acid levels is also associated with increased risk for cardiovascular disease.

INDICATIONS

- Assist in the diagnosis of megaloblastic anemia resulting from deficient folate intake or increased folate requirements, such as in pregnancy and hemolytic anemia
- Monitor the effects of prolonged parenteral nutrition
- Monitor response to disorders that may lead to folate deficiency or decreased absorption and storage

POTENTIAL DIAGNOSIS

Increased in

- Blind loop syndrome *(related to malabsorption in a segment of the intestine due to competition for absorption of folate produced by bacterial overgrowth)*
- Excessive dietary intake of folate or folate supplements
- Pernicious anemia *(related to inadequate levels of vitamin B_{12}, due to impaired absorption, resulting in increased circulating folate levels)*
- Vitamin B_{12} deficiency *(related to vitamin B_{12} levels inadequate to metabolize folate, resulting in increased circulating folate levels)*

Decreased in

- Chronic alcoholism *(related to insufficient intake combined with malabsorption)*
- Crohn's disease *(related to malabsorption)*
- Exfoliative dermatitis *(related to increased demand)*
- Hemolytic anemias *(related to increased demand due to shortened RBC life span caused by folate deficiency)*
- Liver disease *(related to increased excretion)*
- Malnutrition *(related to insufficient intake)*
- Megaloblastic anemia *(related to folate deficiency, which affects development of RBCs and results in anemia)*
- Myelofibrosis *(related to increased demand)*
- Neoplasms *(related to increased demand)*
- Pregnancy *(related to increased demand possibly combined with insufficient dietary intake)*
- Regional enteritis *(related to malabsorption)*
- Scurvy *(related to insufficient intake)*
- Sideroblastic anemias *(evidenced by an acquired anemia resulting from folate deficiency; iron enters and accumulates in the RBCs but cannot become incorporated in hemoglobin)*
- Sprue *(related to malabsorption)*
- Ulcerative colitis *(related to malabsorption)*
- Whipple's disease *(related to malabsorption)*

CRITICAL FINDINGS: N/A

INTERFERING FACTORS

- Drugs that may decrease folate levels include aminopterin, ampicillin, antacids, anticonvulsants, barbiturates, chloramphenicol, chloroguanide, erythromycin, ethanol, glutethimide, lincomycin, metformin, methotrexate, nitrofurans, oral contraceptives, penicillin, pentamidine, phenytoin, pyrimethamine, tetracycline, and triamterene.

NURSING IMPLICATIONS AND PROCEDURE

PRETEST:

- Positively identify the patient using at least two unique identifiers before providing care, treatment, or services.
- *Patient Teaching:* Inform the patient this test can assist in detecting folate deficiency and monitoring folate therapy.
- Obtain a history of the patient's complaints, including a list of known allergens, especially allergies or sensitivities to latex.
- Obtain a history of the patient's gastrointestinal and hematopoietic systems, symptoms, and results of previously performed laboratory tests and diagnostic and surgical procedures.

- Obtain a list of the patient's current medications, including herbs, nutritional supplements, and nutraceuticals (see Appendix F).
- Review the procedure with the patient. Inform the patient that specimen collection takes approximately 5 to 10 min. Address concerns about pain and explain that there may be some discomfort during the venipuncture.
- *Sensitivity to social and cultural issues,* as well as concern for modesty, is important in providing psychological support before, during, and after the procedure.
- There are no food, fluid, or medication restrictions unless by medical direction.

F

INTRATEST:

- If the patient has a history of allergic reaction to latex, avoid the use of equipment containing latex.
- Instruct the patient to cooperate fully and to follow directions. Direct the patient to breathe normally and to avoid unnecessary movement.
- Observe standard precautions, and follow the general guidelines in Appendix A. Positively identify the patient, and label the appropriate tubes with the corresponding patient demographics, date, and time of collection. Perform a venipuncture. Protect the specimen from light.
- Remove the needle and apply direct pressure with dry gauze to stop bleeding. Observe/assess venipuncture site for bleeding or hematoma formation and secure gauze with adhesive bandage.
- Promptly transport the specimen to the laboratory for processing and analysis.

POST-TEST:

- A report of the results will be sent to the requesting health-care provider (HCP), who will discuss the results with the patient.
- *Nutritional Considerations:* Instruct the folate-deficient patient (especially pregnant women), as appropriate, to eat foods rich in folate, such as liver, salmon, eggs, asparagus, green leafy vegetables, broccoli, sweet potatoes, beans, and whole wheat.
- Reinforce information given by the patient's HCP regarding further testing, treatment, or referral to another HCP. Answer any questions or address any concerns voiced by the patient or family.
- Depending on the results of this procedure, additional testing may be performed to evaluate or monitor progression of the disease process and determine the need for a change in therapy. Evaluate test results in relation to the patient's symptoms and other tests performed.

RELATED MONOGRAPHS:

- Related tests include antibodies antithyroglobulin, biopsy intestinal, capsule endoscopy, CBC, CBC RBC indices, complete blood count, RBC morphology, complete blood count, WBC count and differential, eosinophil count, fecal analysis, gastric acid emptying scan, gastric acid stimulation test, gastrin, G6PD, hemosiderin, homocysteine, intrinsic factor antibodies, thyroid, and vitamin B_{12}.
- Refer to the Gastrointestinal and Hematopoietic systems tables at the end of the book for related tests by body system.

Follicle-Stimulating Hormone

SYNONYM/ACRONYM: Follitropin, FSH.

COMMON USE: To distinguish primary causes of gonadal failure from secondary causes, evaluate menstrual disturbances, and assist in infertility evaluations.

SPECIMEN: Serum (1 mL) collected in a red- or tiger-top tube.

REFERENCE VALUE: (Method: Immunoassay)

Age	Conventional Units and SI Units
Child	
Prepuberty	Less than 10 international units/mL
Adult	
Male	1.4–15.5 international units/mL
Female	
Follicular phase	1.4–9.9 international units/mL
Ovulatory peak	6.2–17.2 international units/mL
Luteal phase	1.1–9.2 international units/mL
Postmenopause	19–100 international units/mL

DESCRIPTION: Follicle-stimulating hormone (FSH) is produced and stored in the anterior portion of the pituitary gland. In women, FSH promotes maturation of the graafian (germinal) follicle, causing estrogen secretion and allowing the ovum to mature. In men, FSH partially controls spermatogenesis, but the presence of testosterone is also necessary. Gonadotropin-releasing hormone secretion is stimulated by a decrease in estrogen and testosterone levels. Gonadotropin-releasing hormone secretion stimulates FSH secretion. FSH production is inhibited by an increase in estrogen and testosterone levels. FSH production is pulsatile, episodic, and cyclic and is subject to diurnal variation. Serial measurement is often required.

INDICATIONS

* Assist in distinguishing between primary and secondary (pituitary or hypothalamic) gonadal failure
* Define menstrual cycle phases as a part of infertility testing
* Evaluate ambiguous sexual differentiation in infants
* Evaluate early sexual development in girls younger than age 9 or boys younger than age 10 (precocious puberty associated with elevated levels)
* Evaluate failure of sexual maturation in adolescence
* Evaluate testicular dysfunction
* Investigate impotence, gynecomastia, and menstrual disturbances

POTENTIAL DIAGNOSIS

Increased in

* Alcoholism *(related to suppressed secretion from the pituitary gland)*

Access additional resources at davisplus.fadavis.com

- Castration *(oversecretion related to feedback mechanism involving decreased testosterone levels)*
- Gonadal failure *(oversecretion related to feedback mechanism involving decreased estrogen or testosterone levels)*
- Gonadotropin-secreting pituitary tumors *(related to oversecretion by tumor cells)*
- Klinefelter's syndrome *(oversecretion related to feedback mechanism involving decreased estrogen or testosterone levels)*
- Menopause *(oversecretion related to feedback mechanism involving decreased estrogen levels)*
- Orchitis *(oversecretion related to feedback mechanism involving decreased testosterone levels)*
- Precocious puberty in children *(related to oversecretion from the pituitary gland)*
- Primary hypogonadism *(oversecretion related to feedback mechanism involving decreased estrogen or testosterone levels; failure of testes or ovaries to produce sex hormones)*
- Reifenstein's syndrome *(oversecretion related to feedback mechanism involving familial partial resistance to testosterone levels)*
- Turner's syndrome *(oversecretion related to feedback mechanism involving decreased estrogen or testosterone levels)*

Decreased in
- Anorexia nervosa *(related to suppressive effects of severe caloric restriction on the hypothalmic-pituitary axis)*
- Anterior pituitary hypofunction *(underproduction resulting from dysfunctional pituitary gland)*
- Hemochromatosis *(hypogonadotropic hypogonadism related to absence of the gonadal stimulating pituitary hormones, estrogen, and testosterone; iron deposits in* pituitary may affect normal production of FSH)
- Hyperprolactinemia *(related to suppressive effect on estrogen production)*
- Hypothalamic disorders *(decreased production in response to lack of hypothalmic stimulators)*
- Polycystic ovary disease (Stein-Leventhal syndrome) *(suppressed secretion related to feedback mechanism involving increased estrogen levels)*
- Pregnancy *(related to elevated estrogen levels)*
- Sickle cell anemia *(although primary testicular dysfunction is mainly associated with sickle cell disease, related to testicular microinfarcts, hypogonadotropic hypogonadism has been reported in some men with sickle cell disease)*

CRITICAL FINDINGS: N/A

INTERFERING FACTORS
- Drugs that may increase FSH levels include bicalutamide, bombesin, cimetidine, clomiphene, digitalis, erythropoietin, exemestane, finasteride, gonadotropin-releasing hormone, ketoconazole, levodopa, metformin, nafarelin, naloxone, nilutamide, oxcarbazepine, pravastatin, and tamoxifen.
- Drugs that may decrease FSH levels include anabolic steroids, anticonvulsants, buserelin, estrogens, corticotropin-releasing hormone, danazol, diethylstilbestrol, goserelin, megestrol, mestranol, oral contraceptives, phenothiazine, pimozide, pravastatin, progesterone, stanozolol, tamoxifen, toremifene, and valproic acid.
- In menstruating women, values vary in relation to the phase of the menstrual cycle. Values are higher in postmenopausal women.

PRETEST:

▶ Positively identify the patient using at least two unique identifiers before providing care, treatment, or services.

▶ *Patient Teaching:* Inform the patient this test can assist in evaluating disturbances in hormone levels.

▶ Obtain a history of the patient's complaints, including a list of known allergens, especially allergies or sensitivities to latex.

▶ Obtain a history of the patient's endocrine and reproductive systems, as well as phase of menstrual cycle, symptoms, and results of previously performed laboratory tests and diagnostic and surgical procedures.

▶ Obtain a list of the patient's current medications, including herbs, nutritional supplements, and nutraceuticals (see Appendix F).

▶ Review the procedure with the patient. Inform the patient that specimen collection takes approximately 5 to 10 min. Address concerns about pain and explain that there may be some discomfort during the venipuncture.

▶ *Sensitivity to social and cultural issues,* as well as concern for modesty, is important in providing psychological support before, during, and after the procedure.

▶ There are no food, fluid, or medication restrictions unless by medical direction.

INTRATEST:

▶ If the patient has a history of allergic reaction to latex, avoid the use of equipment containing latex.

▶ Instruct the patient to cooperate fully and to follow directions. Direct the patient to breathe normally and to avoid unnecessary movement.

▶ Observe standard precautions, and follow the general guidelines in Appendix A. Positively identify the patient, and label the appropriate tubes with the corresponding patient demographics, date, and time of collection. Perform a venipuncture.

▶ Remove the needle and apply direct pressure with dry gauze to stop

bleeding. Observe/assess venipuncture site for bleeding or hematoma formation and secure gauze with adhesive bandage.

▶ Promptly transport the specimen to the laboratory for processing and analysis.

POST-TEST:

▶ A report of the results will be sent to the requesting health-care provider (HCP), who will discuss the results with the patient.

▶ Recognize anxiety related to test results and provide a supportive, non-judgmental environment when assisting a patient through the process of fertility testing. Discuss the implications of abnormal test results on the patient's lifestyle. Provide teaching and information regarding the clinical implications of the test results, as appropriate. Educate the patient and partner regarding access to counseling services, as appropriate.

▶ Reinforce information given by the patient's HCP regarding further testing, treatment, or referral to another HCP. Inform the patient that multiple specimens may be required. Answer any questions or address any concerns voiced by the patient or family.

▶ Depending on the results of this procedure, additional testing may be performed to evaluate or monitor progression of the disease process and determine the need for a change in therapy. Evaluate test results in relation to the patient's symptoms and other tests performed.

RELATED MONOGRAPHS:

▶ Related tests include antibodies antisperm, BMD, *Chlamydia* group antibody, chromosome analysis, CT pituitary, estradiol, laparoscopy gynecologic, LH, MRI pituitary, prolactin, testosterone, semen analysis, and US scrotal.

▶ Refer to the Endocrine and Reproductive systems tables at the end of the book for related tests by body system.

F

Fructosamine

SYNONYM/ACRONYM: Glycated albumin.

COMMON USE: To assist in assessing long-term glucose control in diabetes.

SPECIMEN: Serum (1 mL) collected in a red- or tiger-top tube.

REFERENCE VALUE: (Method: Spectrophotometry)

Status	Conventional Units	SI Units (Conventional Units × 0.01)
Normal	174–286 micromol/L	1.74–2.86 mmol/L
Diabetic (values vary with degree of controll)	210–563 micromol/L	2.10–5.63 mmol/L

DESCRIPTION: Fructosamine is the result of a covalent linkage between glucose and albumin or other proteins. Similar to glycated hemoglobin, fructosamine can be used to monitor long-term control of glucose in diabetics. It has a shorter half-life than glycated hemoglobin and is thought to be more sensitive to short-term fluctuations in glucose concentrations. Some glycated hemoglobin methods are affected by hemoglobin variants. Fructosamine is not subject to this interference.

INDICATIONS
• Evaluate diabetic control

POTENTIAL DIAGNOSIS

Increased in
• Diabetic patients with poor glucose control

Decreased in
• Severe hypoproteinemia

CRITICAL FINDINGS: N/A

INTERFERING FACTORS
• Drugs that may increase fructosamine levels include bendroflumethiazide and captopril.
• Drugs that may decrease fructosamine levels include ascorbic acid, pyridoxine, and terazosin.
• Decreased albumin levels may result in falsely decreased fructosamine levels.

NURSING IMPLICATIONS AND PROCEDURE

PRETEST:
▸ Positively identify the patient using at least two unique identifiers before providing care, treatment, or services.
▸ *Patient Teaching:* Inform the patient this test can assist in evaluating blood sugar control.
▸ Obtain a history of the patient's complaints, especially related to diabetic control. Obtain a list of known allergens, especially allergies or sensitivities to latex.

- Obtain a history of the patient's endocrine and gastrointestinal systems, symptoms, and results of previously performed laboratory tests and diagnostic and surgical procedures.
- Obtain a list of the patient's current medications, including herbs, nutritional supplements, and nutraceuticals (see Appendix F).
- Review the procedure with the patient. Inform the patient that specimen collection takes approximately 5 to 10 min. Address concerns about pain and explain that there may be some discomfort during the venipuncture.
- *Sensitivity to social and cultural issues,* as well as concern for modesty, is important in providing psychological support before, during, and after the procedure.
- There are no food, fluid, or medication restrictions unless by medical direction.

INTRATEST:

- If the patient has a history of allergic reaction to latex, avoid the use of equipment containing latex.
- Instruct the patient to cooperate fully and to follow directions. Direct the patient to breathe normally and to avoid unnecessary movement.
- Observe standard precautions, and follow the general guidelines in Appendix A. Positively identify the patient, and label the appropriate tubes with the corresponding patient demographics, date, and time of collection. Perform a venipuncture.
- Remove the needle and apply direct pressure with dry gauze to stop bleeding. Observe/assess venipuncture site for bleeding or hematoma formation and secure gauze with adhesive bandage.
- Promptly transport the specimen to the laboratory for processing and analysis.

POST-TEST:

- A report of the results will be sent to the requesting health-care provider (HCP), who will discuss the results with the patient.
- *Nutritional Considerations:* Abnormal fructosamine levels may be associated with conditions resulting from poor glucose

control. There is no "diabetic diet"; however, many meal-planning approaches with nutritional goals are endorsed by the American Dietetic Association. Patients who adhere to dietary recommendations report a better general feeling of health, better weight management, greater control of glucose and lipid values, and improved use of insulin. Instruct the patient, as appropriate, in nutritional management of diabetes. In June 2006, the American Heart Association developed a Therapeutic Lifestyle Changes (TLC) diet with goals directed at people with specific risk factors and/or existing medical conditions (e.g., elevated LDL cholesterol levels, other lipid disorders, coronary artery disease, insulin-dependent diabetes, insulin resistance, or metabolic syndrome). The TLC approach also includes the use of plant stanols or sterols and increased dissolved fiber as an option for lowering LDL cholesterol levels; nutritional recommendations for daily total caloric intake; recommendations for allowable percentage of calories derived from fat (saturated and unsaturated), carbohydrates, protein, and cholesterol; as well as recommendations for daily expenditure of energy. The nutritional needs of each diabetic patient need to be determined individually (especially during pregnancy) with the appropriate HCPs, particularly professionals trained in nutrition.

- Instruct the patient and caregiver to report signs and symptoms of hypoglycemia (weakness, confusion, diaphoresis, rapid pulse) or hyperglycemia (thirst, polyuria, hunger, lethargy).
- Recognize anxiety related to test results, and be supportive of perceived loss of independence and fear of shortened life expectancy. Discuss the implications of abnormal test results on the patient's lifestyle. Provide teaching and information regarding the clinical implications of the test results, as appropriate. Emphasize, if indicated, that good glycemic control delays the onset and slows the progression of diabetic retinopathy, nephropathy, and neuropathy. Educate the patient

regarding access to counseling services, as appropriate. Provide contact information, if desired, for the American Diabetes Association (www.diabetes.org) or the American Heart Association (www.americanheart.org).

▶ Reinforce information given by the patient's HCP regarding further testing, treatment, or referral to another HCP. Answer any questions or address any concerns voiced by the patient or family.

▶ Depending on the results of this procedure, additional testing may be performed to evaluate or monitor progression of the disease process and determine the need for a change in therapy. Evaluate test results in relation to the patient's symptoms and other tests performed.

RELATED MONOGRAPHS:

▶ Related tests include CT cardiac scoring, cortisol, C-peptide, fecal fat, fluorescein angiography, fundus photography, gastric emptying scan, glucagon, glucose, GTT, glycated hemoglobin, insulin, insulin antibodies, intraocular pressure, ketones, microalbumin, slit-lamp biomicroscopy, and visual fields testing.

▶ Refer to the Endocrine and Gastrointestinal systems tables at the end of the book for related tests by body system.

Fundus Photography

SYNONYM/ACRONYM: N/A.

COMMON USE: To evaluate vascular and structural changes in the eye in assessing the progression of diseases such as glaucoma, diabetic retinopathy, and macular degeneration.

AREA OF APPLICATION: Eyes.

CONTRAST: N/A.

DESCRIPTION: This test involves the photographic examination of the structures of the eye to document the condition of the eye, detect abnormalities, and assist in following the progress of treatment.

INDICATIONS
• Detect the presence of choroidal nevus
• Detect various types and stages of glaucoma
• Document the presence of diabetic retinopathy

• Document the presence of macular degeneration and any other degeneration and any associated hemorrhaging
• Observe ocular effects resulting from the long-term use of high-risk medications

POTENTIAL DIAGNOSIS

Normal findings in
• Normal optic nerve and vessels
• No evidence of other ocular abnormalities

Abnormal findings in
• Aneurysm
• Choroidal nevus

- Diabetic retinopathy
- Macular degeneration
- Obstructive disorders of the arteries or veins that lead to collateral circulation
- Retinal detachment or tear

CRITICAL FINDINGS
- Detached retina

Flashers, floaters, or a veil that moves across the field of vision may indicate detached retina or retinal tear. This condition requires immediate examination by an ophthalmologist. Untreated, full retinal detachment can result in irreversible and complete loss of vision in the affected eye.

It is essential that critical diagnoses be communicated immediately to the appropriate health-care provider (HCP). A listing of these diagnoses varies among facilities. Note and immediately report to the HCP abnormal results and related symptoms.

INTERFERING FACTORS

This procedure is contraindicated for
- Patients with narrow-angle glaucoma if pupil dilation is performed; dilation can initiate a severe and sight-threatening open-angle attack.
- Patients with allergies to mydriatics if pupil dilation using mydriatics is performed.

Factors that may impair the results of the examination
- Inability of the patient to cooperate or remain still during the test because of age, significant pain, or mental status may interfere with the test results.
- Presence of cataracts may interfere with fundal view.
- Ineffective dilation of the pupils may impair clear imaging.

- Rubbing or squeezing the eyes may affect results.
- Failure to follow medication restrictions before the procedure may cause the procedure to be canceled or repeated.

NURSING IMPLICATIONS AND PROCEDURE

PRETEST:
- Positively identify the patient using at least two unique identifiers before providing care, treatment, or services.
- *Patient Teaching:* Inform the patient this procedure assists in detecting changes in the eye that effect vision.
- Obtain a history of the patient's complaints, including a list of known allergens, especially mydriatics if dilation is to be performed.
- Obtain a history of the patient's known or suspected vision loss; changes in visual acuity, including type and cause; use of glasses or contact lenses; and eye conditions with treatment regimens.
- Obtain results of previously performed laboratory tests and diagnostic and surgical procedures.
- Obtain a list of the patient's current medications, including herbs, nutritional supplements, and nutraceuticals (see Appendix F).
- Instruct the patient to remove contact lenses or glasses, as appropriate. Instruct the patient regarding the importance of keeping the eyes open for the test.
- Review the procedure with the patient. Explain that the patient will be requested to fixate the eyes during the procedure. Address concerns about pain and explain that mydriatics, if used, may cause blurred vision and sensitivity to light. There may also be a brief stinging sensation when the drop is put in the eye, but no discomfort will be experienced during the examination. Inform the patient that an HCP performs the test, in a quiet, darkened room, and that to dilate and evaluate both eyes, the test can take up 60 min.

▶ *Sensitivity to social and cultural issues,* as well as concern for modesty, is important in providing psychological support before, during, and after the procedure.

▶ There are no food or fluid restrictions, unless by medical direction.

▶ The patient should avoid eye medications (particularly mydriatic eyedrops if the patient has glaucoma) for at least 1 day prior to the test.

▶ Ensure that the patient understands that he or she must refrain from driving until the pupils return to normal (about 4 hr) after the test and has made arrangements to have someone else be responsible for transportation after the test.

INTRATEST:

▶ Ensure that the patient has complied with medication restrictions; ensure that eye medications, especially mydriatics, have been restricted for at least 1 day prior to the test.

▶ Instruct the patient to cooperate fully and to follow directions. Instruct the patient to remain still during the procedure because movement produces unreliable results.

▶ Seat the patient in a chair that faces the camera. Instruct the patient to look at a directed target while the eyes are examined.

▶ If dilation is to be performed, administer the ordered mydriatic to each eye and repeat in 5 to 15 min. Drops are placed in the eye with the patient looking up and the solution directed at the six o'clock position of the sclera (white of the eye) near the limbus (gray, semitransparent area of the eyeball where the cornea and sclera meet). Neither dropper nor bottle should touch the eyelashes.

▶ Instruct the patient to place the chin in the chin rest and gently press the forehead against the support bar. Instruct the patient to open his or her eyes wide and look at desired target while a sequence of photographs are taken.

POST-TEST:

▶ A report of the results will be sent to the requesting HCP, who will discuss the results with the patient.

▶ Instruct the patient to resume usual medications, as directed by the HCP.

▶ *Nutritional Considerations:* Increased glucose levels may be associated with diabetes. There is no "diabetic diet"; however, many meal-planning approaches with nutritional goals are endorsed by the American Dietetic Association. Patients who adhere to dietary recommendations report a better general feeling of health, better weight management, greater control of glucose and lipid values, and improved use of insulin. Instruct the patient, as appropriate, in nutritional management of diabetes. In June 2006, the American Heart Association developed a Therapeutic Lifestyle Changes (TLC) diet with goals directed at people with specific risk factors and/or existing medical conditions (e.g., elevated LDL cholesterol levels, other lipid disorders, coronary artery disease, insulin-dependent diabetes, insulin resistance, or metabolic syndrome). The TLC approach also includes the use of plant stanols or sterols and increased dissolved fiber as an option for lowering LDL cholesterol levels; nutritional recommendations for daily total caloric intake; recommendations for allowable percentage of calories derived from fat (saturated and unsaturated), carbohydrates, protein, and cholesterol; as well as recommendations for daily expenditure of energy. The nutritional needs of each diabetic patient need to be determined individually (especially during pregnancy) with the appropriate health care professionals, particularly professionals trained in nutrition.

▶ Recognize anxiety related to test results, and be supportive of impaired activity related to vision loss or anticipated loss of driving privileges. Discuss the implications of abnormal test results on the patient's lifestyle. Provide teaching and information regarding the clinical implications of the test results, as appropriate. Emphasize, as appropriate, that good glycemic control delays the onset of and slows the progression of diabetic retinopathy, nephropathy, and neuropathy. Provide education regarding smoking cessation, as appropriate. Provide contact information regarding vision aids, if desired, for ABLEDATA (sponsored by the National Institute on Disability and Rehabilitation Research [NIDRR], available at www.abledata.com). Information can also be obtained from the American Macular Degeneration Foundation (www.macular.org), the American Diabetes Association (www .diabetes.org), or the American Heart Association (www.americanheart.org).

‣ Instruct the patient to avoid strenuous physical activities, like lifting heavy objects, that may increase pressure in the eye, as ordered.

‣ Reinforce information given by the patient's HCP regarding further testing, treatment, or referral to another HCP. Inform the patient that visual acuity and responses to light may change. Suggest that the patient wear dark glasses after the test until the pupils return to normal size. Answer any questions or address any concerns voiced by the patient or family.

‣ Depending on the results of this procedure, additional testing may be performed to evaluate or monitor progression of the disease process and determine the need for a change in therapy. Evaluate test results in relation to the patient's symptoms and other tests performed.

RELATED MONOGRAPHS:

‣ Related tests include fluorescein angiography, fructosamine, glucagon, glucose, glycated hemoglobin, gonioscopy, insulin, intraocular pressure, microalbumin, plethysmography, refraction, slit-lamp biomicroscopy, and visual field testing.

‣ Refer to the Ocular System table at the end of the book for related tests by body system.

Gallium Scan

SYNONYM/ACRONYM: Ga scan.

COMMON USE: To assist in diagnosing, evaluating, and staging tumors as well as in detecting areas of infection, inflammation, and abscess.

AREA OF APPLICATION: Whole body.

CONTRAST: IV radioactive gallium-67 citrate.

DESCRIPTION: Gallium imaging is a nuclear medicine study that assists in diagnosing neoplasm and inflammation activity. Gallium, which has 90% sensitivity for inflammatory disease, is readily distributed throughout plasma and body tissues. Gallium imaging is sensitive in detecting abscesses, pneumonia, pyelonephritis, active sarcoidosis, and active tuberculosis. In immunocompromised patients, such as patients with AIDS, gallium imaging can detect complications such as *Pneumocystis jiroveci* (formerly *P. carinii*) pneumonitis. Gallium imaging is useful but less commonly performed in the diagnosis and staging of some neoplasms, including Hodgkin's disease, lymphoma, melanoma, and leukemia. Imaging can be performed 6 to 72 hr after gallium injection. A gamma camera detects the radiation emitted from the injected radioactive material, and a representative image of the distribution of the radioactive material is obtained. The nonspecificity of gallium imaging requires correlation with other diagnostic studies, such as computed tomography, magnetic resonance imaging, and ultrasonography.

INDICATIONS
- Aid in the diagnosis of infectious or inflammatory diseases
- Evaluate lymphomas

- Evaluate recurrent lymphomas or tumors after radiation therapy or chemotherapy
- Perform as a screening examination for fever of undetermined origin

POTENTIAL DIAGNOSIS

Normal findings in
- Normal distribution of gallium; some localization of the radionuclide within the liver, spleen, bone, nasopharynx, lacrimal glands, breast, and bowel is expected

Abnormal findings in
- Abscess
- Infection
- Inflammation
- Lymphoma
- Tumor

CRITICAL FINDINGS: N/A

INTERFERING FACTORS

This procedure is contraindicated for
- Patients who are pregnant or suspected of being pregnant, unless the potential benefits of the procedure far outweigh the risks to the fetus and mother.

Factors that may impair clear imaging
- Inability of the patient to cooperate or remain still during the procedure because of age, significant pain, or mental status.
- Metallic objects (e.g., jewelry, body rings) within the examination field, which may

inhibit organ visualization and cause unclear images.

- Performance of other nuclear scans within the preceding 24 to 48 hr.
- Administration of certain medications (e.g., gastrin, cholecystokinin), which may interfere with gastric emptying.

Other considerations
- Improper injection of the radionuclide may allow the tracer to seep deep into the muscle tissue, producing erroneous hot spots.
- Consultation with a health-care provider (HCP) should occur before the procedure for radiation safety concerns regarding younger patients or patients who are lactating.
- Risks associated with radiation overexposure can result from frequent x-ray or radionuclide procedures. Personnel working in the examination area should wear badges to record their level of radiation.

NURSING IMPLICATIONS AND PROCEDURE

PRETEST:
- Positively identify the patient using at least two unique identifiers before providing care, treatment, or services.
- *Patient Teaching:* Inform the patient this procedure can assist in identifying infection or other disease.
- Obtain a history of the patient's complaints, including a list of known allergens, especially allergies or sensitivities to latex, iodine, seafood, contrast medium, anesthetics, or dyes.
- Obtain a history of the patient's immune system, symptoms, and results of previously performed laboratory tests and diagnostic and surgical procedures.
- Note any recent procedures that can interfere with test results, including examinations using iodine-based contrast medium.

- Record the date of the last menstrual period and determine the possibility of pregnancy in perimenopausal women.
- Obtain a list of the patient's current medications, including herbs, nutritional supplements, and nutraceuticals (see Appendix F).
- Review the procedure with the patient. Address concerns about pain related to the procedure and explain that some pain may be experienced during the test, or there may be moments of discomfort. Reassure the patient that the radionuclide poses no radioactive hazard and rarely produces side effects. Inform the patient that the procedure is performed in a nuclear medicine department by an HCP specializing in this procedure, with support staff, and takes approximately 60 min.
- *Sensitivity to social and cultural issues,* as well as concern for modesty, is important in providing psychological support before, during, and after the procedure.
- Instruct the patient to remove jewelry and other metallic objects from the area to be examined.
- There are no food, fluid, or medication restrictions unless by medical direction.
- *Make sure a written and informed consent has been signed prior to the procedure and before administering any medications.*

INTRATEST:
- Ensure that the patient has removed all external metallic objects from the area to be examined prior to the procedure.
- If the patient has a history of allergic reactions to any substance or drug, administer ordered prophylactic steroids or antihistamines before the procedure.
- Have emergency equipment readily available.
- Instruct the patient to void prior to the procedure and to change into the gown, robe, and foot coverings provided.
- Instruct the patient to cooperate fully and to follow directions. Instruct the patient to lie still during the procedure because movement produces unclear images.

- Observe standard precautions, and follow the general guidelines in Appendix A.
- Administer a sedative to a child or to an uncooperative adult, as ordered.
- Place the patient in a supine position on a flat table with foam wedges, which help maintain position and immobilization.
- IV radionuclide is administered, and the patient is instructed to return for scanning at a designated time after injection. Typical scanning occurs at 6, 24, 48, 72, 96, and/or 120 hr postinjection depending on diagnosis.
- If an abdominal abscess or infection is suspected, laxatives or enemas may be ordered before imaging at 48 or 72 hr after the injection.
- Monitor the patient for complications related to the procedure (e.g., allergic reaction, anaphylaxis, bronchospasm).
- The needle or catheter is removed, and a pressure dressing is applied over the puncture site.
- Observe the needle/catheter insertion site for bleeding, inflammation, or hematoma formation.

POST-TEST:

- A report of the results will be sent to the requesting HCP, who will discuss the results with the patient.
- Unless contraindicated, advise patient to drink increased amounts of fluids for 24 to 48 hr to eliminate the radionuclide from the body. Inform the patient that radionuclide is eliminated from the body within 6 to 24 hr.
- Instruct the patient to resume usual medication or activity, as directed by the HCP.
- Instruct the patient in the care and assessment of the injection site.
- If a woman who is breastfeeding must have a nuclear scan, she should not breastfeed the infant until the radionuclide has been eliminated. This could take as long as 3 days. She should be instructed to express the milk and discard it during the 3-day period to prevent cessation of milk production.

- Instruct the patient to immediately flush the toilet and to meticulously wash hands with soap and water after each voiding for 24 hr after the procedure.
- Instruct all caregivers to wear gloves when discarding urine for 48 hr after the procedure. Wash gloved hands with soap and water before removing gloves. Then wash ungloved hands after removing the gloves.
- Recognize anxiety related to test results, and be supportive of perceived loss of independent function. Discuss the implications of abnormal test results on the patient's lifestyle. Provide teaching and information regarding the clinical implications of the test results, as appropriate.
- Reinforce information given by the patient's HCP regarding further testing, treatment, or referral to another HCP. Answer any questions or address any concerns voiced by the patient or family.
- Depending on the results of this procedure, additional testing may be needed to evaluate or monitor progression of the disease process and determine the need for a change in therapy. Evaluate test results in relation to the patient's symptoms and other tests performed.

RELATED MONOGRAPHS:

- Related tests include angiotensin converting enzyme, biopsy bone marrow, biopsy kidney, biopsy lung, blood gases, bronchoscopy, CBC, CBC WBC and differential, chest x-ray, CT abdomen, CT pelvis, CT thoracic, culture blood, culture and smear mycobacteria, culture viral, cytology sputum, cytology urine, ESR, HIV-1/2 antibodies, IVP, lung perfusion scan, MRI chest, MRI abdomen, mediastinoscopy, pleural fluid analysis, plethysmography, PFT, pulse oximetry, renogram, US kidney, and US lymph node.
- Refer to the Immune System table at the end of the book for related tests by body system.

γ-Glutamyltranspeptidase

SYNONYM/ACRONYM: Serum γ-glutamyltransferase, γ-glutamyl transpeptidase, GGT, SGGT.

COMMON USE: To assist in diagnosing and monitoring liver disease.

SPECIMEN: Serum (1 mL) collected in a red- or tiger-top tube. Plasma (1 mL) collected in a green-top (heparin) tube is also acceptable.

REFERENCE VALUE: (Method: Enzymatic spectrophotometry)

Gender	Conventional & SI Units
6 mo and older	
Male	0–30 units/L
Female	0–24 units/L

Values are higher in infants. Values are higher in adult males than in adult females. Values may be elevated in older adults due to the effects of medications and the presence of multiple chronic or acute diseases with or without muted symptoms.

DESCRIPTION: Glutamyltransferase (GGT) assists with the reabsorption of amino acids and peptides from the glomerular filtrate and intestinal lumen. Hepatobiliary, renal tubular, and pancreatic tissues contain large amounts of GGT. Other sources include the prostate gland, brain, and heart. GGT is elevated in all types of liver disease and is more responsive to biliary obstruction, cholangitis, or cholecystitis than any of the other enzymes used as markers for liver disease.

INDICATIONS

- Assist in the diagnosis of obstructive jaundice in neonates
- Detect the presence of liver disease
- Evaluate and monitor patients with known or suspected alcohol abuse

(levels rise after ingestion of small amounts of alcohol)

POTENTIAL DIAGNOSIS

Increased in

GGT is released from any damaged cell in which it is stored, so conditions that affect the liver, kidneys, or pancreas and cause cellular destruction demonstrate elevated GGT levels.

- Cirrhosis
- Diabetes with hypertension
- Hepatitis
- Hepatobiliary tract disorders
- Hepatocellular carcinoma
- Hyperthyroidism *(there is a strong association with concurrent liver abnormalities)*
- Infectious mononucleosis
- Obstructive liver disease
- Pancreatitis
- Renal transplantation
- Significant alcohol ingestion

Decreased in
- Hypothyroidism *(related to decreased enzyme production by the liver)*

CRITICAL FINDINGS: N/A

INTERFERING FACTORS
- Drugs and substances that may increase GGT levels include acetaminophen, alcohol, aminoglutethimide, anticonvulsants, aurothioglucose, barbiturates, captopril, cetirizine, dactinomycin, dantrolene, dexfenfluramine, estrogens, flucytosine, halothane, labetalol, medroxyprogesterone, meropenem, methyldopa, naproxen, niacin, nortriptyline, oral contraceptives, pegaspargase, phenothiazines, piroxicam, probenecid, rifampin, streptokinase, tocainide, and trifluoperazine.
- Drugs that may decrease GGT levels include clofibrate conjugated estrogens and ursodiol.

NURSING IMPLICATIONS AND PROCEDURE

PRETEST:
- Positively identify the patient using at least two unique identifiers before providing care, treatment, or services.
- *Patient Teaching:* Inform the patient this test can assist in assessing liver function.
- Obtain a history of the patient's complaints, including a list of known allergens, especially allergies or sensitivities to latex.
- Obtain a history of the patient's hepatobiliary system, symptoms, and results of previously performed laboratory tests and diagnostic and surgical procedures.
- Obtain a history of IV drug use, alcohol use, high-risk sexual activity, and occupational exposure.
- Obtain a list of the patient's current medications, including herbs, nutritional supplements, and nutraceuticals (see Appendix F).

- Review the procedure with the patient. Inform the patient that specimen collection takes approximately 5 to 10 min. Address concerns about pain and explain that there may be some discomfort during the venipuncture.
- *Sensitivity to social and cultural issues,* as well as concern for modesty, is important in providing psychological support before, during, and after the procedure.
- There are no food, fluid, or medication restrictions unless by medical direction.

INTRATEST:
- If the patient has a history of allergic reaction to latex, avoid the use of equipment containing latex.
- Instruct the patient to cooperate fully and to follow directions. Direct the patient to breathe normally and to avoid unnecessary movement.
- Observe standard precautions, and follow the general guidelines in Appendix A. Positively identify the patient, and label the appropriate tubes with the corresponding patient demographics, date, and time of collection. Perform a venipuncture.
- Remove the needle and apply direct pressure with dry gauze to stop bleeding. Observe/assess venipuncture site for bleeding or hematoma formation and secure gauze with adhesive bandage.
- Promptly transport the specimen to the laboratory for processing and analysis.

POST-TEST:
- A report of the results will be sent to the requesting health-care provider (HCP), who will discuss the results with the patient.
- *Nutritional Considerations:* Increased GGT levels may be associated with liver disease. Dietary recommendations may be indicated and vary depending on the condition and its severity. Currently, there are no specific medications that can be given to cure hepatitis, but elimination of alcohol ingestion and a diet optimized for convalescence are commonly included in the treatment plan. A high-calorie, high-protein, moderate-fat diet with a high fluid intake is often recommended for patients with hepatitis. Treatment of cirrhosis is different because a

G

low-protein diet may be in order if the patient's liver has lost the ability to process the end products of protein metabolism. A diet of soft foods also may be required if esophageal varices have developed. Ammonia levels may be used to determine whether protein should be added to or reduced from the diet. The patient should be encouraged to eat simple carbohydrates and emulsified fats (as in homogenized milk or eggs) rather than complex carbohydrates (e.g., starch, fiber, and glycogen [animal carbohydrates]) and complex fats, which require additional bile to emulsify them so that they can be used. The cirrhotic patient should also be carefully observed for the development of ascites, in which case fluid and electrolyte balance requires strict attention. The alcoholic patient should be encouraged to avoid alcohol and to seek appropriate counseling for substance abuse.

▶ Recognize anxiety related to test results, and be supportive of impaired activity related to lack of neuromuscular control, perceived loss of independence, and fear of shortened life expectancy. Discuss the implications of abnormal test results on the patient's lifestyle. Provide teaching and information regarding the clinical implications of the test results, as appropriate. Educate the patient regarding access to counseling services.

▶ Reinforce information given by the patient's HCP regarding further testing, treatment, or referral to another HCP. Answer any questions or address any concerns voiced by the patient or family.

▶ Depending on the results of this procedure, additional testing may be performed to evaluate or monitor progression of the disease process and determine the need for a change in therapy. Evaluate test results in relation to the patient's symptoms and other tests performed.

RELATED MONOGRAPHS:

▶ Related tests include ALT, ALP ammonia, AST, bilirubin, cholangiography percutaneous transhepatic, electrolytes, HAV antibody, HBV antigen and antibody, HCV antibody, hepatobiliary scan, infectious mono screen, KUB studies, liver and spleen scan, MRI liver, TSH, and US liver.

▶ Refer to the Hepatobiliary System table at the end of the book for related tests by body system.

Gastric Analysis and Gastric Acid Stimulation Test

SYNONYM/ACRONYM: N/A.

COMMON USE: To evaluate gastric fluid and the amount of gastric acid secreted to assist in diagnosing gastrointestinal disorders such as ulcers, cancers, and inflammation.

SPECIMEN: Gastric fluid collected in eight plastic tubes at 15-min intervals.

REFERENCE VALUE: (Method: Volume measurement and pH by ion-selective electrode)

Basal acid output (BAO)	Male: 0–10.5 mmol/hr
	Female: 0–5.6 mmol/hr
Peak acid output (PAO)	Male: 12–60 mmol/hr
	Female: 8–40 mmol/hr
Peak response time	Pentagastrin, intramuscular: 15–45 min
	Pentagastrin, subcutaneous: 10–30 min
BAO/PAO ratio	Less than 0.20

DESCRIPTION: Gastric fluid is evaluated macroscopically for general physical and chemical characteristics such as color, presence of mucus or blood, and pH; gastric fluid is also evaluated microscopically for the presence of organisms and abnormal cells. The normal appearance of gastric fluid is a translucent, pale gray, slightly viscous fluid containing some mucus but not usually blood. pH is usually less than 2.0 and not greater than 6.0. Organisms are usually absent in gastric fluid owing to the acidic pH.

The gastric acid stimulation test is performed to determine the response to substances administered to induce increased gastric acid production. Pentagastrin is the usual drug of choice to induce gastric secretion because it has no major side effects. The samples obtained from gastric acid stimulation tests are examined for volume, pH, and amount of acid secreted. First, basal acid output (BAO) is determined by averaging the results of gastric samples collected before the administration of a gastric stimulant. Then a gastric stimulant is administered and peak acid output (PAO) is determined by adding together the gastric acid output of the highest two consecutive 15-min stimulation samples. Finally, BAO and PAO are compared as a ratio, which is normally less than 0.20.

INDICATIONS

- Detect duodenal ulcer
- Detect gastric carcinoma
- Detect pernicious anemia
- Detect Zollinger-Ellison syndrome
- Evaluate effectiveness of vagotomy in the treatment of peptic ulcer disease

POTENTIAL DIAGNOSIS

Increased in
Any alteration in the balance between the digestive and protective functions of the stomach that increases gastric acidity, such as hypersecretion of gastrin, use of NSAIDs, or Helicobacter pylori infection.

Appearance
- Color
  Yellow to green indicates the presence of bile. *(related to obstruction in the small intestine distal to the ampulla of Vater)*
  Pink, red, brown indicates the presence of blood. *(related to some type of gastric lesion evidenced by ulcer, gastritis, or carcinoma)*
- Microscopic evaluation
  Red blood cells *(related to trauma or active bleeding)*
  White blood cells *(related to inflammation of the gastric mucosa, mouth, paranasal sinuses, or respiratory tract)*

Epithelial cells *(related to inflammation of the gastric mucosa)*

Malignant cells *(related to gastric carcinoma)*

Bacteria and yeast *(related to conditions such as pyloric obstruction, pulmonary tuberculosis)*

Parasites *(related to parasitic infestation such as Giardia, H. pylori, hookworm, or Strongyloides)*

Increased Gastric Acid Output
- BAO
  Basophilic leukemia
  Duodenal ulcer
  G-cell hyperplasia
  Recurring peptic ulcer
  Retained antrum syndrome
  Systemic mastocytosis
  Vagal hyperfunction
  Zollinger-Ellison syndrome
- PAO
  Duodenal ulcer
  Zollinger-Ellison syndrome

Decreased in
Conditions that result in the gradual loss of function of the antrum and G cells, where gastrin is produced, will reflect decreased gastrin levels.

Decreased Gastric Acid Output
- BAO
  Gastric ulcer
- PAO
  Chronic gastritis
  Gastric cancers
  Gastric polyps
  Gastric ulcer
  Myxedema
  Pernicious anemia

CRITICAL FINDINGS: N/A

INTERFERING FACTORS
- Drugs that may increase gastric volume include atropine, diazepam, ganglionic blocking agents, and insulin.

- Drugs and substances that may increase gastric pH include caffeine, calcium salts, corticotropin, ethanol, rauwolfia, reserpine, and tolazoline.
- Drugs and substances that may decrease gastric pH include atropine, cimetidine, diazepam, famotidine, ganglionic blocking agents, glucagon, nizatidine, omeprazole, oxmetidine, propranolol, prostaglandin F_{2a}, ranitidine, and secretin.
- Gastric intubation is contraindicated in patients with esophageal varices, diverticula, stenosis, malignant neoplasm of the esophagus, aortic aneurysm, severe gastric hemorrhage, and congenital heart failure.
- The use of histamine diphosphate is contraindicated in patients with a history of asthma, paroxysmal hypertension, urticaria, or other allergic conditions.
- Failure to follow dietary restrictions may result in stimulation of gastric secretions.
- Failure to follow dietary restrictions before the procedure may cause the procedure to be canceled or repeated.
- Exposure to the sight, smell, or thought of food immediately before and during the test may result in stimulation of gastric secretions.

NURSING IMPLICATIONS AND PROCEDURE

PRETEST:

- Positively identify the patient using at least two unique identifiers before providing care, treatment, or services.
- *Patient Teaching:* Inform the patient this procedure can assist in diagnosing disease and inflammation in the stomach and upper intestine.
- Obtain a history of the patient's complaints, including a list of known

allergens, especially allergies or sensitivities to latex.

- Obtain a history of the patient's gastrointestinal system, symptoms, and results of previously performed laboratory tests and diagnostic and surgical procedures.
- Obtain a list of the patient's current medications, including herbs, nutritional supplements, and nutraceuticals (see Appendix F).
- Review the procedure with the patient. Inform the patient that specimen collection takes approximately 60 to 120 min. Address concerns about pain and explain that some discomfort is experienced from insertion of the nasogastric tube.
- *Sensitivity to social and cultural issues,* as well as concern for modesty, is important in providing psychological support before, during, and after the procedure.
- Drugs and substances that may alter gastric secretions (e.g., alcohol, histamine, nicotine, adrenocorticotropic steroids, insulin, parasympathetic agents, belladonna alkaloids, anticholinergic drugs, histamine receptor antagonists) should be restricted by medical direction for 72 hr before the test.
- Instruct the patient to fast from food after the evening meal the night before the test and not to drink water for 1 hr before the test. Instruct the patient to refrain from the use of chewing gum or tobacco products for at least 12 hr prior to and for the duration of the test. Protocols may vary among facilities.
- *Make sure a written and informed consent has been signed prior to the procedure and before administering any medications.*

INTRATEST:

- Ensure that the patient has complied with dietary restrictions and other pretesting preparations; ensure that food has been restricted for at least 12 hr prior to the procedure.
- If the patient has a history of allergic reaction to latex, avoid the use of equipment containing latex.
- Ensure that the patient does not have a history of asthma, paroxysmal hypertension, urticaria, or other allergic

conditions if histamine diphosphate is being considered for use in the test.

- Record baseline vital signs.
- If the patient is wearing dentures, have him or her remove them.
- Ask the patient to sit, or help the patient recline on the left side.
- Instruct the patient to cooperate fully and to follow directions. Direct the patient to breathe normally and to avoid unnecessary movement.
- Observe standard precautions, and follow the general guidelines in Appendix A. Positively identify the patient, and label the appropriate collection containers with the corresponding patient demographics, date, and time of collection.
- A cold lubricated gastric (Levine) tube is inserted orally. Alternatively, if the patient has a hyperactive gag reflex, the tube can be inserted nasally. The tube must have a radiopaque tip.
- Fluoroscopy or x-ray is used to confirm proper position of the tube before the start of the test.
- Using a constant but gentle suction, gastric contents are collected. Do not use specimens obtained from the first 15 to 30 min of suctioning.
- The gastric stimulant is administered, and the peak basal specimens are collected over a 60-min period as four 15-min specimens. Number the specimen tubes in the order in which they were collected.
- Promptly transport the specimen to the laboratory for processing and analysis.

POST-TEST:

- A report of the results will be sent to the requesting health-care provider (HCP), who will discuss the results with the patient.
- Instruct the patient to resume usual diet and medication, as directed by the HCP.
- Monitor vital signs and neurological status every 15 min for 1 hr, then every 2 hr for 4 hr, and then as ordered by the HCP for evaluation. Protocols may vary among facilities.
- Instruct the patient to report any chest pain, upper abdominal pain, pain on swallowing, difficulty breathing, or expectoration of blood. Report these to the HCP immediately.

Monitor for side effects of drugs administered to induce gastric secretion (e.g., flushing, headache, nasal stuffiness, dizziness, faintness, nausea).

Nutritional Considerations: Nutritional support with calcium, iron, and vitamin B_{12} supplementation may be ordered, as appropriate. Dietary modifications may include encouraging liquids and low-residue foods, eating multiple small meals throughout the day, and avoidance of foods that slow digestion such as foods high in fat and fiber. Severe cases of gastroparesis may require temporary treatments that include total parenteral nutrition or use of jejunostomy tubes.

Recognize anxiety related to test results. Discuss the implications of abnormal test results on the patient's lifestyle. Provide teaching and information regarding the clinical implications of the test results, as appropriate.

Reinforce information given by the patient's HCP regarding further testing, treatment, or referral to another HCP. Answer any questions or address any concerns voiced by the patient or family.

Instruct the patient in the use of any ordered medications. Explain the importance of adhering to the therapy regimen. As appropriate, instruct the patient in significant side effects and systemic reactions associated with the prescribed medication. Encourage him or her to review corresponding literature provided by a pharmacist.

Depending on the results of this procedure, additional testing may be performed to evaluate or monitor progression of the disease process and determine the need for a change in therapy. Evaluate test results in relation to the patient's symptoms and other tests performed.

RELATED MONOGRAPHS:

Related tests include capsule endoscopy, CBC, CBC RBC indices, CBC RBC morphology, CBC WBC count and differential, endoscopy sinus, esophagogastroduodenoscopy, fecal analysis, folate, gastric emptying scan, gastrin, *H. pylori* antibody, intrinsic factor antibodies, upper GI series, and vitamin B_{12}.

Refer to the Gastrointestinal System table at the end of the book for related tests by body system.

Gastric Emptying Scan

SYNONYM/ACRONYM: Gastric emptying quantitation, gastric emptying scintigraphy.

COMMON USE: To visualize and assess the time frame for gastric emptying to assist in the diagnosis of diseases such as gastroenteritis and dumping syndrome.

AREA OF APPLICATION: Esophagus, stomach, small bowel.

CONTRAST: Oral radioactive technetium-99m sulfur colloid.

DESCRIPTION: A gastric emptying scan quantifies gastric emptying physiology. The procedure is indicated for patients with gastric motility symptoms, including diabetic gastroparesis, anorexia nervosa, gastric outlet obstruction syndromes, postvagotomy and postgastrectomy syndromes, and assessment of medical and surgical treatments for diseases known to affect gastric motility. A radionuclide is administered, and the clearance of solids and liquids may be evaluated. The images are recorded electronically, showing the gastric emptying function over time.

INDICATIONS

- Investigate the cause of rapid or slow rate of gastric emptying
- Measure gastric emptying rate

POTENTIAL DIAGNOSIS

Normal findings in

- Mean time emptying of liquid phase: 30 min (range, 11 to 49 min)
- Mean time emptying of solid phase: 40 min (range, 28 to 80 min)
- No delay in gastric emptying rate

Abnormal findings in

- Decreased rate:
  Dumping syndrome
  Duodenal ulcer
  Malabsorption syndromes
  Zollinger-Ellison syndrome
- Increased rate:
  Amyloidosis
  Anorexia nervosa
  Diabetes
  Gastric outlet obstruction
  Gastric ulcer
  Gastroenteritis
  Gastroesophageal reflux
  Hypokalemia, hypomagnesemia
  Post–gastric surgery period
  Postoperative ileus
  Post–radiation therapy period
  Scleroderma

CRITICAL FINDINGS: N/A

INTERFERING FACTORS

This procedure is contraindicated for

- Patients who are pregnant or suspected of being pregnant, unless the potential benefits of the procedure far outweigh the risks to the fetus and mother.
- Patients with esophageal motor disorders or swallowing difficulties.

Factors that may impair clear imaging

- Inability of the patient to cooperate or remain still during the procedure because of age, significant pain, or mental status.
- Metallic objects (e.g., jewelry, body rings) within the examination field, which may inhibit organ visualization and cause unclear images.
- Retained barium from a previous radiological procedure.
- Other nuclear scans done within the previous 24 to 48 hr.
- Administration of certain medications (e.g., gastrin, cholecystokinin), which may interfere with gastric emptying.

Other considerations

- Failure to follow dietary restrictions before the procedure may cause the procedure to be canceled or repeated.
- Consultation with a health-care provider (HCP) should occur before the procedure for radiation safety concerns regarding younger patients or patients who are lactating.
- Risks associated with radiation overexposure can result from frequent x-ray or radionuclide

procedures. Personnel working in the examination area should wear badges to record their level of radiation.

NURSING IMPLICATIONS AND PROCEDURE

PRETEST:

- Positively identify the patient using at least two unique identifiers before providing care, treatment, or services.
- *Patient Teaching:* Inform the patient this procedure can assist in evaluating the time it takes for the stomach to empty.
- Obtain a history of the patient's complaints, including a list of known allergens, especially allergies or sensitivities to latex, iodine, seafood, contrast medium, anesthetics, or dyes.
- Obtain a history of the patient's gastrointestinal system, symptoms, and results of previously performed laboratory tests and diagnostic and surgical procedures.
- Note any recent procedures that can interfere with test results, including examinations using barium- or iodine-based contrast medium.
- Record the date of the last menstrual period and determine the possibility of pregnancy in perimenopausal women.
- Obtain a list of the patient's current medications, including herbs, nutritional supplements, and nutraceuticals (see Appendix F).
- Review the procedure with the patient. Address concerns about pain related to the procedure and explain that some pain may be experienced during the test, and there may be moments of discomfort. Reassure the patient that the radionuclide poses no radioactive hazard and rarely produces side effects. Inform the patient that the procedure is performed in a nuclear medicine department by an HCP specializing in this procedure, with support staff, and takes approximately 30 to 120 min.
- *Sensitivity to social and cultural issues,* as well as concern for modesty, is important in providing psychological support before, during and after the procedure.

- Instruct the patient to restrict food and fluids for 8 hr before the scan. Protocols may vary among facilities.
- Instruct the patient to remove jewelry and other metallic objects from the area to be examined.
- *Make sure a written and informed consent has been signed prior to the procedure and before administering any medications.*

INTRATEST:

- Ensure the patient has complied with dietary and fluid restrictions for 8 hr before the scan.
- Ensure that the patient has removed all external metallic objects from the area to be examined prior to the procedure.
- Instruct the patient to void prior to the procedure and to change into the gown, robe, and foot coverings provided.
- Record baseline vital signs and neurological status. Protocols may vary among facilities.
- Instruct the patient to cooperate fully and to follow directions. Instruct the patient to lie still during the procedure because movement produces unclear images.
- Observe standard precautions, and follow the general guidelines in Appendix A.
- Administer sedative to a child or to an uncooperative adult, as ordered.
- Place the patient in an upright position in front of the gamma camera.
- Ask the patient to take the radionuclide mixed with water or other liquid orally, or combined with eggs for a solid study.
- Images are recorded over a period of time (30 to 60 min) and evaluated with regard to the amount of time the stomach takes to empty its contents.

POST-TEST:

- A report of the results will be sent to the requesting HCP, who will discuss the results with the patient.
- Advise the patient to drink increased amounts of fluids for 24 to 48 hr to eliminate the radionuclide from the body, unless contraindicated. Tell the patient that radionuclide is eliminated from the body within 6 to 24 hr.
- Monitor vital signs every 15 min for 1 hr, then every 2 hr for 4 hr, and then

as ordered by the HCP. Monitor intake and output at least every 8 hr. Compare with baseline values. Protocols may vary among facilities.

▶ Instruct the patient to resume usual diet, fluids, medication, and activity, as directed by the HCP.

▶ If a woman who is breastfeeding must have a nuclear scan, she should not breastfeed the infant until the radionuclide has been eliminated. This could take as long as 3 days. She should be instructed to express the milk and discard it during the 3-day period to prevent cessation of milk production.

▶ Instruct the patient to immediately flush the toilet and to meticulously wash hands with soap and water after each voiding for 24 hr after the procedure.

▶ Instruct all caregivers to wear gloves when discarding urine for 24 hr after the procedure. Wash gloved hands with soap and water before removing gloves. Then wash hands after removing the gloves.

▶ Recognize anxiety related to test results, and be supportive of perceived loss of independent function. Discuss the implications of abnormal test results on the patient's lifestyle. Provide teaching and information regarding the clinical implications of the test results, as appropriate.

▶ Reinforce information given by the patient's HCP regarding further testing, treatment, or referral to another HCP. Answer any questions or address any concerns voiced by the patient or family.

▶ Depending on the results of this procedure, additional testing may be needed to evaluate or monitor progression of the disease process and determine the need for a change in therapy. Evaluate test results in relation to the patient's symptoms and other tests performed.

RELATED MONOGRAPHS:

▶ Related tests include barium swallow, biopsy kidney, biopsy liver, biopsy lung, calcitonin stimulation, calcium, capsule endoscopy, CT abdomen, esophageal manometry, EGD, fecal analysis, gastric fluid analysis and gastric acid stimulation test, gastrin and gastrin stimulation test, GI blood loss scan, glucose, glycated hemoglobin, *H. pylori* antibodies, liver and spleen scan, magnesium, PTH, UGI and small bowel series, and vitamin B_{12}.

▶ Refer to the Gastrointestinal System table at the end of the book for related tests by body system.

Gastrin and Gastrin Stimulation Test

SYNONYM/ACRONYM: N/A.

COMMON USE: To evaluate gastric production to assist in diagnosis of gastric disease such as Zollinger-Ellison syndrome and gastric cancer.

SPECIMEN: Serum (1 mL) collected in a red- or tiger-top tube.

REFERENCE VALUE: (Method: Radioimmunoassay)

Age	Conventional Units	SI Units (Conventional Units × 1)
Infant	120–183 pg/mL	120–183 ng/L
Child	Less than 10–125 pg/mL	Less than 10–125 ng/L
Adult		
Up to 60 yr	25–90 pg/mL	25–90 ng/L
60 yr and older	Less than 100 pg/mL	Less than 100 ng/L

Stimulation Tests

Gastrin stimulation test with calcium or secretin	No response or slight increase over baseline

DESCRIPTION: Gastrin is a hormone secreted by the stomach and duodenum in response to vagal stimulation; the presence of food, alcohol, or calcium in the stomach; and the alkalinity of gastric secretions. After its absorption into the circulation, gastrin returns to the stomach and acts as a stimulant for acid, insulin, pepsin, and intrinsic factor secretion. Gastrin stimulation tests can be performed after a test meal or IV infusion of calcium or secretin.

INDICATIONS

- Assist in the diagnosis of gastric carcinoma, pernicious anemia, or G-cell hyperplasia
- Assist in the diagnosis of Zollinger-Ellison syndrome
- Assist in the differential diagnosis of ulcers from other gastrointestinal (GI) peptic disorders

POTENTIAL DIAGNOSIS

Increased in

- Chronic gastritis *(related to hypersecretion of gastrin, use of NSAIDs, or Helicobacter pylori infection)*
- Chronic renal failure *(related to inadequate renal excretion)*
- Gastric and duodenal ulcers *(related to hypersecretion of gastrin, use of NSAIDs, or H. pylori infection)*
- Gastric carcinoma *(related to disturbance in pH favoring alkalinity, which stimulates gastrin production)*
- G-cell hyperplasia *(hyperplastic G cells produce excessive amounts of gastrin)*
- Hyperparathyroidism *(related to hypercalcemia; calcium is a potent stimulator for the release of gastrin)*
- Pernicious anemia *(related to antibodies against gastric intrinsic factor [66% of cases] and parietal cells [80% of cases that affect the stomach's ability to secrete acid; achlorhydria is a strong stimulator of gastrin production])*
- Pyloric obstruction *(related to gastric distention, which stimulates gastrin production)*
- Retained antrum *(remaining tissue stimulates gastrin production)*

- Zollinger-Ellison syndrome *(gastrin-producing tumor)*

Decreased in
- Hypothyroidism *(related to hypocalcemia)*
- Vagotomy *(vagus nerve impulses stimulate secretion of digestive secretions; interruptions in these nerve impulses result in decreased gastrin levels)*

CRITICAL FINDINGS: N/A

INTERFERING FACTORS
- Drugs and substances that may increase gastrin levels include amino acids, catecholamines, cimetidine, insulin, morphine, omeprazole, pantoprazole, sufotidine, terbutaline, calcium products, and coffee.
- Drugs that may decrease gastrin levels include atropine, enprostil, glucagon, secretin, streptozocin, and tolbutamide.
- In some cases, protein ingestion elevates serum gastrin levels.
- Recent radioactive scans or radiation within 1 wk before the test can interfere with test results when radioimmunoassay is the test method.
- Failure to follow dietary and medication restrictions before the procedure may cause the procedure to be canceled or repeated.

NURSING IMPLICATIONS AND PROCEDURE

PRETEST:
- Positively identify the patient using at least two unique identifiers before providing care, treatment, or services.
- *Patient Teaching:* Inform the patient this test can assist in diagnosing stomach disease.

- Obtain a history of the patient's complaints, including a list of known allergens, especially allergies or sensitivities to latex.
- Obtain a history of the patient's endocrine and gastrointestinal systems, symptoms, and results of previously performed laboratory tests and diagnostic and surgical procedures.
- Note any recent procedures that can interfere with test results.
- Obtain a list of the patient's current medications, including herbs, nutritional supplements, and nutraceuticals (see Appendix F).
- Review the procedure with the patient. Inform the patient that specimen collection takes approximately 5 to 10 min. Address concerns about pain and explain that there may be some discomfort during the venipuncture.
- *Sensitivity to social and cultural issues,* as well as concern for modesty, is important in providing psychological support before, during, and after the procedure.
- Instruct the patient to fast for 12 hr before the test. Instruct the patient to refrain from the use of chewing gum or tobacco products for at least 4 hr prior to and for the duration of the test. Protocols may vary among facilities.
- Instruct the patient to withhold medications and alcohol for 12 to 24 hr, as ordered by the health-care provider (HCP).
- There are no fluid restrictions unless by medical direction.
- *Make sure a written and informed consent has been signed prior to the procedure and before administering any medications.*

INTRATEST:
- Ensure that the patient has complied with dietary and medication restrictions and other pretesting preparations; ensure that food and medications have been withheld for at least 4 and 12 hr, respectively, prior to the procedure. The patient should be reminded to refrain from use of chewing gum or

tobacco products during the test.

- If the patient has a history of allergic reaction to latex, avoid the use of equipment containing latex.
- Instruct the patient to cooperate fully and to follow directions. Direct the patient to breathe normally and to avoid unnecessary movement.
- Administer gastrin stimulators as appropriate.
- Observe standard precautions, and follow the general guidelines in Appendix A. Positively identify the patient, and label the appropriate tubes with the corresponding patient demographics, date, and time of collection. Perform a venipuncture.
- Remove the needle and apply direct pressure with dry gauze to stop bleeding. Observe/assess venipuncture site for bleeding or hematoma formation and secure gauze with adhesive bandage.
- Promptly transport the specimen to the laboratory for processing and analysis.

POST-TEST:

- A report of the results will be sent to the requesting HCP, who will discuss the results with the patient.
- Instruct the patient to resume usual diet and medications, as directed by the HCP.
- *Nutritional Considerations:* Nutritional support with calcium, iron, and vitamin B_{12} supplementation may be ordered, as appropriate. Dietary modifications may include encouraging liquids and low-residue foods, eating multiple small meals throughout the day, and avoidance of foods that slow digestion such as foods high in fat and fiber. Severe cases of

gastroparesis may require temporary treatments that include total parenteral nutrition or use of jejunostomy tubes.

- Reinforce information given by the patient's HCP regarding further testing, treatment, or referral to another HCP. Answer any questions or address any concerns voiced by the patient or family.
- Instruct the patient in the use of any ordered medications. Explain the importance of adhering to the therapy regimen. As appropriate, instruct the patient in the significant side effects and systemic reactions associated with the prescribed medication. Encourage him or her to review corresponding literature provided by a pharmacist.
- Depending on the results of this procedure, additional testing may be performed to evaluate or monitor progression of the disease process and determine the need for a change in therapy. Evaluate test results in relation to the patient's symptoms and other tests performed.

RELATED MONOGRAPHS:

- Related tests include capsule endoscopy, CBC, CBC RBC indices, CBC RBC morphology, CBC WBC count and differential, esophagogastroduodenoscopy, fecal analysis, folate, gastric acid stimulation test, gastric emptying scan, *H. pylori* antibody, intrinsic factor antibodies, upper GI series, and vitamin B_{12}.
- Refer to the Endocrine and Gastrointestinal systems tables at the end of the book for related tests by body system.

Gastroesophageal Reflux Scan

SYNONYM/ACRONYM: Aspiration scan, GER scan, GERD scan.

COMMON USE: To assess for gastric reflux in relation to heartburn, difficulty swallowing, vomiting, and aspiration.

AREA OF APPLICATION: Esophagus and stomach.

CONTRAST: Oral radioactive technetium-99m sulfur colloid.

DESCRIPTION: The gastroesophageal reflux (GER) scan assesses gastric reflux across the esophageal sphincter. Symptoms of GER include heartburn, regurgitation, vomiting, dysphagia, and a bitter taste in the mouth. This procedure may be used to evaluate the medical or surgical treatment of patients with GER and to detect aspiration of gastric contents into the lungs. A radionuclide such as technetium-99m sulfur colloid is ingested orally in orange juice. Scanning studies are done immediately to assess the amount of liquid that has reached the stomach. An abdominal binder is applied and then tightened gradually to obtain images at increasing degrees of abdominal pressure: 0, 20, 40, 60, 80, and 100 mm Hg. Computer calculation determines the amount of reflux into the esophagus at each of these abdominal pressures as recorded on the images. For aspiration scans, images are taken over the lungs to detect tracheoesophageal aspiration of the radionuclide.

In infants, the study distinguishes between vomiting and reflux. Reflux occurs predominantly in infants younger than age 2 who are mainly on a milk diet. This procedure is indicated when an infant has symptoms such as failure to thrive, feeding problems, and episodes of wheezing with chest infection. The radionuclide is added to the infant's milk, images are obtained of the gastric and esophageal area, and the images are evaluated visually and by computer.

INDICATIONS

- Aid in the diagnosis of GER in patients with unexplained nausea and vomiting
- Distinguish between vomiting and reflux in infants with failure to thrive, feeding problems, and wheezing combined with chest infection

POTENTIAL DIAGNOSIS

Normal findings in
- Reflux less than or equal to 4% across the esophageal sphincter

Abnormal findings in
- Reflux of greater than 4% at any pressure level
- Pulmonary aspiration

CRITICAL FINDINGS: N/A

INTERFERING FACTORS

This procedure is contraindicated for
- Patients who are pregnant or suspected of being pregnant, unless the potential benefits of the procedure far outweigh the risks to the fetus and mother.
- Patients with hiatal hernia, esophageal motor disorders, or swallowing difficulties.

Factors that may impair clear imaging
- Inability of the patient to cooperate or remain still during the procedure because of age, significant pain, or mental status.
- Metallic objects (e.g., jewelry, body rings, dentures) within the examination field, which may inhibit organ visualization and cause unclear images.
- Retained barium from a previous radiological procedure.
- Other nuclear scans done within the previous 24 to 48 hr.

Other considerations
- Failure to follow dietary restrictions before the procedure may cause the procedure to be canceled or repeated.
- Consultation with a health-care provider (HCP) should occur before the procedure for radiation safety concerns regarding younger patients or patients who are lactating.
- Risks associated with radiation overexposure can result from frequent x-ray or radionuclide procedures. Personnel working in the examination area should wear badges to record their level of radiation.

NURSING IMPLICATIONS AND PROCEDURE

PRETEST:
- Positively identify the patient using at least two unique identifiers before providing care, treatment, or services.
- *Patient Teaching:* Inform the patient this procedure can assist in evaluating stomach reflux.
- Obtain a history of the patient's complaints, including a list of known allergens (especially allergies or sensitivities to latex, iodine, seafood, contrast medium, anesthetics, or dyes).
- Obtain a history of the patient's gastrointestinal system, symptoms, and results of previously performed laboratory tests and diagnostic and surgical procedures.
- Note any recent procedures that can interfere with test results, including examinations using barium- or iodine-based contrast medium.
- Record the date of the last menstrual period and determine the possibility of pregnancy in perimenopausal women.
- Obtain a list of the patient's current medications, including herbs, nutritional supplements, and nutraceuticals (see Appendix F).
- Review the procedure with the patient. Address concerns about pain related to the procedure and explain that some pain may be experienced during the test, or there may be moments of discomfort. Reassure the patient that the radionuclide poses no radioactive hazard and rarely produces side effects. Inform the patient that the procedure is performed in a nuclear medicine department by an HCP specializing in this procedure, with support staff, and takes approximately 30 to 60 min.
- *Sensitivity to social and cultural issues,* as well as concern for modesty, is important in providing psychological support before, during, and after the procedure.
- Instruct the patient to remove jewelry and other metallic objects from the area to be examined.
- There are no food or fluid restrictions unless by medical direction.

G

Make sure a written and informed consent has been signed prior to the procedure and before administering any medications.

INTRATEST:

▸ Ensure that the patient has removed all external metallic objects from the area to be examined prior to the procedure.

▸ Have emergency equipment readily available.

▸ Instruct the patient to void prior to the procedure and to change into the gown, robe, and foot coverings provided.

▸ Record baseline vital signs and assess neurological status. Protocols may vary among facilities.

▸ Instruct the patient to cooperate fully and to follow directions. Instruct the patient to remain still throughout the procedure because movement produces unreliable results.

▸ Observe standard precautions, and follow the general guidelines in Appendix A.

▸ Administer a sedative to a child or to an uncooperative adult, as ordered.

▸ Place the patient in an upright position and instruct him or her to ingest the radionuclide combined with orange juice.

▸ Place the patient in a supine position on a flat table 15 min after ingestion

▸ An abdominal binder with an attached sphygmomanometer is applied, and scans are taken as the binder is tightened at various pressures.

▸ If reflux occurs at lower pressures, an additional 30 mL of water may be given to clear the esophagus.

▸ Instruct the patient to take slow, deep breaths if nausea occurs during the procedure. Monitor and administer an antiemetic agent if ordered. Ready an emesis basin for use.

▸ Monitor the patient for complications related to the procedure (e.g., allergic reaction, anaphylaxis, bronchospasm).

POST-TEST:

▸ A report of the results will be sent to the requesting HCP, who will discuss the results with the patient.

▸ Advise the patient to drink increased amounts of fluids for 24 to 48 hr to

eliminate the radionuclide from the body unless contraindicated. Tell the patient that radionuclide is eliminated from the body within 6 to 24 hr.

▸ Monitor vital signs and neurological status every 15 min for 1 hr, then every 2 hr for 4 hr, and then as ordered by the HCP. Monitor intake and output at least every 8 hr. Compare with baseline values. Protocols may vary among facilities.

▸ Instruct the patient to resume usual diet, fluids, medication, and activity, as directed by the HCP.

▸ No other radionuclide tests should be scheduled for 24 to 48 hr after this procedure.

▸ If a woman who is breastfeeding must have a nuclear scan, she should not breastfeed the infant until the radionuclide has been eliminated. This could take as long as 3 days. She should be instructed to express the milk and discard it during the 3-day period to prevent cessation of milk production.

▸ Instruct the patient to immediately flush the toilet and to meticulously wash hands with soap and water after each voiding for 24 hr after the procedure.

▸ Instruct all caregivers to wear gloves when discarding urine for 24 hr after the procedure. Wash gloved hands with soap and water before removing gloves. Then wash hands after the gloves are removed.

▸ *Nutritional Considerations:* A low-fat, low-cholesterol, and low-sodium diet should be consumed to reduce current disease processes. High fat consumption increases the amount of bile acids in the colon and should be avoided.

▸ Recognize anxiety related to test results, and be supportive of expected changes in lifestyle. Discuss the implications of abnormal test results on the patient's lifestyle. Provide teaching and information regarding the clinical implications of the test results, as appropriate.

▸ Reinforce information given by the patient's HCP regarding further testing, treatment, or referral to another HCP. Answer any questions or address any concerns voiced by the patient or family.

◗ Depending on the results of this procedure, additional testing may be needed to evaluate or monitor progression of the disease process and determine the need for a change in therapy. Evaluate test results in relation to the patient's symptoms and other tests performed.

RELATED MONOGRAPHS:

◗ Related tests include CT abdomen, esophageal manometry, gastric emptying scan, and upper GI series.
◗ Refer to the Gastrointestinal System table at the end of the book for related tests by body system.

Gastrointestinal Blood Loss Scan

SYNONYM/ACRONYM: Gastrointestinal bleed localization study, GI scintigram, GI bleed scintigraphy, lower GI blood loss scan.

COMMON USE: To detect areas of active gastrointestinal bleeding or hemorrhage to facilitate surgical intervention or medical treatment. Usefulness is limited in emergency situations because of time constraints in performing the scan.

AREA OF APPLICATION: Abdomen.

CONTRAST: IV radioactive technetium-99m–labeled red blood cells.

DESCRIPTION: Gastrointestinal (GI) blood loss scan is a nuclear medicine study that assists in detecting and localizing active GI tract bleeding (2 or 3 mL/min) for the purpose of better directing endoscopic or angiographic studies. This procedure can detect bleeding if the rate is greater than 0.5 mL/min, but it is not specific for site localization or cause of bleeding. Endoscopy is the procedure of choice for diagnosing upper GI bleeding. After injection of technetium-99m–labeled red blood cells, immediate and delayed images of various views of the abdomen are obtained. The radionuclide remains in the circulation long enough to extravasate and accumulate within the bowel lumen at the site of active bleeding. This procedure is valuable for the detection and localization of recent non-GI intra-abdominal hemorrhage. Images may be taken over an extended period to show intermittent bleeding.

INDICATIONS
• Diagnose unexplained abdominal pain and GI bleeding

POTENTIAL DIAGNOSIS

Normal findings in
• Normal distribution of radionuclide in the large vessels with no extravascular activity

Abnormal findings in
• Angiodysplasia
• Aortoduodenal fistula

- Diverticulosis
- GI bleeding
- Inflammatory bowel disease
- Polyps
- Tumor
- Ulcer

CRITICAL FINDINGS

- Acute GI bleed

It is essential that critical diagnoses be communicated immediately to the appropriate health-care provider (HCP). A listing of these diagnoses varies among facilities. Note and immediately report to the HCP abnormal results and related symptoms.

INTERFERING FACTORS

This procedure is contraindicated for

- Patients who are pregnant or suspected of being pregnant, unless the potential benefits of the procedure far outweigh the risks to the fetus and mother.

Factors that may impair clear imaging

- Inability of the patient to cooperate or remain still during the procedure because of age, significant pain, or mental status.
- Retained barium from a previous radiological procedure.
- Metallic objects (e.g., jewelry, body rings) within the examination field, which may inhibit organ visualization and cause unclear images.
- Other nuclear scans done within the previous 24 to 48 hr.
- Inaccurate timing of imaging after the radionuclide injection.

Other considerations

- The examination detects only active or intermittent bleeding.
- The procedure is of little value in patients with chronic anemia or slowly decreasing hematocrit.

- The scan is less accurate for localization of bleeding sites in the upper GI tract.
- Improper injection of the radionuclide allows the tracer to seep deep into the muscle tissue, producing erroneous hot spots.
- The test is not specific, does not indicate the exact pathological condition causing the bleeding, and may miss small sites of bleeding (less than 0.5 mL/min) caused by diverticular disease or angiodysplasia.
- Physiologically unstable patients may be unable to be scanned over long periods or may need to go to surgery before the procedure is complete.
- Consultation with an HCP should occur before the procedure for radiation safety concerns regarding younger patients or patients who are lactating.
- Risks associated with radiation overexposure can result from frequent x-ray or radionuclide procedures. Personnel working in the examination area should wear badges to record their level of radiation exposure.

NURSING IMPLICATIONS AND PROCEDURE

PRETEST:

- Positively identify the patient using at least two unique identifiers before providing care, treatment, or services.
- *Patient Teaching:* Inform the patient this procedure can assist in evaluating for stomach and intestinal bleeding.
- Obtain a history of the patient's complaints, including a list of known allergens, especially allergies or sensitivities to latex, iodine, seafood, contrast medium, anesthetics, or dyes.
- Obtain a history of the patient's gastrointestinal system, symptoms, and results of previously performed

laboratory tests and diagnostic and surgical procedures.

- Note any recent procedures that can interfere with test results, including examinations using barium- or iodine-based contrast medium.
- Record the date of the last menstrual period and determine the possibility of pregnancy in perimenopausal women.
- Obtain a list of the patient's current medications, including herbs, nutritional supplements, and nutraceuticals (see Appendix F).
- Review the procedure with the patient. Address concerns about pain related to the procedure and explain that some pain may be experienced during the test, or there may be moments of discomfort. Reassure the patient that the radionuclide poses no radioactive hazard and rarely produces side effects. Inform the patient that the procedure is performed in a nuclear medicine department by an HCP specializing in this procedure, with support staff, and takes approximately 60 min to complete, with additional images taken periodically over 24 hr.
- Explain that an IV line may be inserted to allow infusion of IV fluids, contrast medium, or sedatives. Usually normal saline is infused.
- *Sensitivity to social and cultural issues, as well as concern for modesty, is important in providing psychological support before, during, and after the procedure.*
- Instruct the patient to remove jewelry and other metallic objects from the area to be examined.
- There are no food or fluid restrictions unless by medical direction.
- *Make sure a written and informed consent has been signed prior to the procedure and before administering any medications.*

- Ensure that the patient has removed all external metallic objects from the area to be examined prior to the procedure.
- Instruct the patient to void prior to the procedure and to change into the gown, robe, and foot coverings provided.

- Record baseline vital signs and assess neurological status. Protocols may vary among facilities.
- Have emergency equipment readily available.
- Instruct the patient to cooperate fully and to follow directions. Instruct the patient to remain still throughout the procedure because movement produces unreliable results.
- Observe standard precautions, and follow the general guidelines in Appendix A.
- Administer a sedative to a child or to an uncooperative adult, as ordered.
- Establish IV fluid line for the injection of emergency drugs, radionuclide, and sedatives.
- Place the patient in a supine position on a flat table with foam wedges to help maintain position and immobilization.
- The radionuclide is administered IV, and images are recorded immediately and every 5 min over a period of 60 min in various positions.
- The needle or catheter is removed, and a pressure dressing is applied over the puncture site.
- Observe/assess the needle/catheter insertion site for bleeding, inflammation, or hematoma formation.

POST-TEST:

- A report of the results will be sent to the requesting HCP, who will discuss the results with the patient.
- Advise the patient to drink increased amounts of fluids for 24 to 48 hr to eliminate the radionuclide from the body, unless contraindicated. Tell the patient that radionuclide is eliminated from the body within 6 to 24 hr.
- Monitor vital signs and neurological status every 15 min for 1 hr, then every 2 hr for 4 hr, and then as ordered by the HCP. Monitor intake and output at least every 8 hr. Compare with baseline values. Protocols may vary among facilities.
- No other radionuclide tests should be scheduled for 24 to 48 hr after this procedure.
- Instruct the patient to resume usual diet, fluids, medication, and activity, as directed by the HCP.

▶ Instruct the patient in the care and assessment of the injection site.

▶ If a woman who is breastfeeding must have a nuclear scan, she should not breastfeed the infant until the radionuclide has been eliminated. This could take as long as 3 days. She should be instructed to express the milk and discard it during the 3-day period to prevent cessation of milk production.

▶ Instruct the patient to immediately flush the toilet and to meticulously wash hands with soap and water after each voiding for 24 hr after the procedure.

▶ Instruct all caregivers to wear gloves when discarding urine for 24 hr after the procedure. Wash gloved hands with soap and water before removing gloves. Then wash hands after the gloves are removed.

▶ *Nutritional Considerations:* A low-fat, low-cholesterol, and low-sodium diet should be consumed to reduce current disease processes. High fat consumption increases the amount of bile acids in the colon and should be avoided.

▶ Recognize anxiety related to test results, and be supportive of perceived loss of independent function. Discuss the implications of abnormal test results on the patient's lifestyle. Provide teaching and information regarding the clinical implications of the test results, as appropriate.

▶ Reinforce information given by the patient's HCP regarding further testing, treatment, or referral to another HCP. Answer any questions or address any concerns voiced by the patient or family.

▶ Depending on the results of this procedure, additional testing may be needed to evaluate or monitor progression of the disease process and determine the need for a change in therapy. Evaluate test results in relation to the patient's symptoms and other tests performed.

RELATED MONOGRAPHS:

▶ Related tests include antibodies antineutrophilic cytoplasmic, angiography abdomen, barium enema, barium swallow, cancer antigens, capsule endoscopy, colonoscopy, CBC, CBC hematocrit, CBC hemoglobin, CT abdomen, EGD, fecal analysis, IgA, MRI abdomen, Meckel's diverticulum scan, proctosigmoidoscopy, upper GI series, and WBC scan.

▶ Refer to the Gastrointestinal System table at the end of the book for related tests by body system.

Glucagon

SYNONYM/ACRONYM: N/A.

COMMON USE: To evaluate the amount of circulating glucagon to assist in diagnosing diseases such as hypoglycemia, pancreatic cancer, or inflammation.

SPECIMEN: Plasma (1 mL) collected in chilled, lavender-top (EDTA) tube. Specimen should be transported tightly capped and in an ice slurry.

REFERENCE VALUE: (Method: Radioimmunoassay)

Age	Conventional Units	SI Units (Conventional Units × 1)
Cord blood	0–215 pg/mL	0–215 ng/L
1–3 days	0–1,750 pg/mL	0–1,750 ng/L
4–14 yr	0–148 pg/mL	0–148 ng/L
Adult	20–100 pg/mL	20–100 ng/L

DESCRIPTION: Glucagon is a hormone secreted by the alpha cells of the islets of Langerhans in the pancreas in response to hypoglycemia. This hormone acts primarily on the liver to promote glucose production from glycogen stores and to control glycogen storage. Glucagon also produces glucose from the oxidation of fatty acids like triglycerides to basic glycerol components. The coordinated release of insulin, glucagon, and somatostatin ensures an adequate fuel supply while maintaining stable blood glucose. Patients with glucagonoma have values greater than 500 ng/L. Values greater than 1,000 ng/L are diagnostic for this condition. Glucagonoma causes three different syndromes:

Syndrome 1: A characteristic skin rash, diabetes or impaired glucose tolerance, weight loss, anemia, and venous thrombosis
Syndrome 2: Severe diabetes
Syndrome 3: Multiple endocrine neoplasia

A dramatic increase in glucagon occurring soon after renal transplant may indicate organ rejection. In the case of kidney transplant rejection, glucagon levels increase several days before an increase in creatinine levels.

Glucagon deficiency can be confirmed by measuring glucagon levels before and after IV infusion of arginine 0.5 g/kg. Glucagon deficiency is confirmed when levels fail to rise 30 to 60 min after infusion. Newborn infants of diabetic mothers have impaired glucagon secretion, which may play a role in their hypoglycemia.

INDICATIONS
• Assist in confirming glucagon deficiency
• Assist in the diagnosis of suspected glucagonoma (alpha islet-cell neoplastic tumor)
• Assist in the diagnosis of suspected renal failure or renal transplant rejection

POTENTIAL DIAGNOSIS

Increased in
Glucagon is produced in the pancreas and excreted by the kidneys; conditions that affect the pancreas and cause cellular destruction or conditions that impair the ability of the kidneys to remove glucagon from circulation will result in elevated glucagon levels.
• Acromegaly *(related to stimulated production of glucagon in response to growth hormone)*
• Acute pancreatitis *(related to decreased pancreatic function)*
• Burns *(related to stress-induced release of catecholamines, which stimulates glucagon production)*
• Cirrhosis *(pathophysiology is not well established)*
• Cushing's syndrome *(evidenced by overproduction of cortisol, which stimulates glucagon production)*

- Diabetes (uncontrolled) *(pathophysiology is not well established)*
- Glucagonoma *(related to excessive production by the tumor)*
- Hyperlipoproteinemia *(pathophysiology is not well established)*
- Hypoglycemia *(related to response to decreased glucose level)*
- Infection *(related to feedback loop in response to stress)*
- Kidney transplant rejection *(related to decreased renal excretion)*
- Pheochromocytoma *(excessive production of catecholamines stimulates increased glucagon levels)*
- Renal failure *(related to decreased renal excretion)*
- Stress *(related to stress-induced release of catecholamines, which stimulates glucagon production)*
- Trauma *(related to stress-induced release of catecholamines, which stimulates glucagon production)*

Decreased in
Low glucagon levels are related to decreased pancreatic function.
- Chronic pancreatitis
- Cystic fibrosis
- Postpancreatectomy period

CRITICAL FINDINGS: N/A

INTERFERING FACTORS
- Drugs that may increase glucagon levels include amino acids (e.g., arginine), cholecystokinin, danazol, gastrin, glucocorticoids, insulin, and nifedipine.
- Drugs that may decrease glucagon levels include atenolol, pindolol, propranolol, secretin, and verapamil.
- Recent radioactive scans or radiation within 1 wk before the test can interfere with test results when radioimmunoassay is the test method.

- Failure to follow dietary restrictions before the procedure may cause the procedure to be canceled or repeated.

NURSING IMPLICATIONS AND PROCEDURE

PRETEST:
- Positively identify the patient using at least two unique identifiers before providing care, treatment, or services.
- *Patient Teaching:* Inform the patient this test can assist in evaluating the hormone that participates in regulating blood sugar.
- Obtain a history of the patient's complaints, including a list of known allergens, especially allergies or sensitivities to latex.
- Obtain a history of the patient's endocrine system, symptoms, and results of previously performed laboratory tests and diagnostic and surgical procedures.
- Note any recent procedures that can interfere with test results.
- Obtain a list of the patient's current medications, including herbs, nutritional supplements, and nutraceuticals (see Appendix F).
- Review the procedure with the patient. Inform the patient that specimen collection takes approximately 5 to 10 min. Address concerns about pain and explain that there may be some discomfort during the venipuncture.
- *Sensitivity to social and cultural issues,* as well as concern for modesty, is important in providing psychological support before, during, and after the procedure.
- Instruct the patient to fast for at least 12 hr before specimen collection for baseline values. Diabetic patients should be in good glycemic control before testing.
- Prepare an ice slurry in a cup or plastic bag to have ready for immediate transport of the specimen to the laboratory. Prechill the lavender-top tube in the ice slurry.

INTRATEST:

▶ Ensure that the patient has complied with dietary restrictions; ensure that food has been restricted for at least 12 hr prior to the procedure.

▶ If the patient has a history of allergic reaction to latex, avoid the use of equipment containing latex.

▶ Instruct the patient to cooperate fully and to follow directions. Direct the patient to breathe normally and to avoid unnecessary movement.

▶ Observe standard precautions, and follow the general guidelines in Appendix A. Positively identify the patient, and label the appropriate tubes with the corresponding patient demographics, date, and time of collection. Perform a venipuncture; collect the specimen in a chilled tube. The sample should be placed in an ice slurry immediately after collection. Information on the specimen label should be protected from water in the ice slurry by first placing the specimen in a protective plastic bag.

▶ Remove the needle and apply direct pressure with dry gauze to stop bleeding. Observe/assess venipuncture site for bleeding or hematoma formation and secure gauze with adhesive bandage.

▶ Promptly transport the specimen to the laboratory for processing and analysis.

POST-TEST:

▶ A report of the results will be sent to the requesting health-care provider (HCP), who will discuss the results with the patient.

▶ Instruct the patient to resume usual diet, as directed by the HCP.

▶ *Nutritional Considerations:* Abnormal results may be associated with diabetes. There is no "diabetic diet"; however, many meal-planning approaches with nutritional goals are endorsed by the American Dietetic Association. Patients who adhere to dietary recommendations report a better general feeling of health, better weight management, greater control of glucose and lipid values, and improved use of insulin. Instruct the patient, as

appropriate, in nutritional management of diabetes. In June 2006, the American Heart Association developed a Therapeutic Lifestyle Changes (TLC) diet with goals directed at people with specific risk factors and/or existing medical conditions (e.g., elevated LDL cholesterol levels, other lipid disorders, coronary artery disease, insulin-dependent diabetes, insulin resistance, or metabolic syndrome). The TLC approach also includes the use of plant stanols or sterols and increased dissolved fiber as an option for lowering LDL cholesterol levels; nutritional recommendations for daily total caloric intake; recommendations for allowable percentage of calories derived from fat (saturated and unsaturated), carbohydrates, protein, and cholesterol; as well as recommendations for daily expenditure of energy. The nutritional needs of each diabetic patient need to be determined individually (especially during pregnancy) with the appropriate HCPs, particularly professionals trained in nutrition.

▶ Increased glucagon levels may be associated with diabetes. Instruct the patient and caregiver to report signs and symptoms of hypoglycemia (weakness, confusion, diaphoresis, rapid pulse) or hyperglycemia (thirst, polyuria, hunger, lethargy).

▶ Recognize anxiety related to test results, and be supportive of perceived loss of independence and fear of shortened life expectancy. Discuss the implications of abnormal test results on the patient's lifestyle. Provide teaching and information regarding the clinical implications of the test results, as appropriate. Emphasize, if indicated, that good glycemic control delays the onset and slows the progression of diabetic retinopathy, nephropathy, and neuropathy. Educate the patient regarding access to counseling services, as appropriate. Provide contact information, if desired, for the American Diabetes Association (www.diabetes.org) or the American Heart Association (www.americanheart.org).

▶ Reinforce information given by the patient's HCP regarding further testing, treatment, or referral to another HCP. Answer any questions or address any concerns voiced by the patient or family.

▶ Depending on the results of this procedure, additional testing may be performed to evaluate or monitor progression of the disease process and determine the need for a change in therapy. Evaluate test results in relation to the patient's symptoms and other tests performed.

RELATED MONOGRAPHS:

▶ Related tests include angiography adrenal, catecholamines, cholangio-pancreatography endoscopic retrograde, CT cardiac scoring, CT pancreas, CT renal, C peptide, gastric emptying scan, glucose, GTT, glycated hemoglobin, GH, HVA, insulin, insulin antibodies, MRI pancreas, metanephrines, microalbumin, peritoneal fluid analysis, and US pancreas.

▶ Refer to the Endocrine System table at the end of the book for related tests by body system.

Glucose

SYNONYM/ACRONYM: Blood sugar, fasting blood sugar (FBS), postprandial glucose, 2-hr PC.

COMMON USE: To assist in the diagnosis of diabetes and to evaluate disorders of carbohydrate metabolism such as malabsorption syndrome.

SPECIMEN: Serum (1 mL) collected in a red- or tiger-top tube, although plasma is recommended for diagnosis of diabetes. Plasma (1 mL) collected in a gray-top (sodium fluoride) or a green-top (heparin) tube.

REFERENCE VALUE: (Method: Spectrophotometry)

Age	Conventional Units	SI Units (Conventional Units × 0.0555)
Fasting		
Cord blood	45–96 mg/dL	2.5–5.3 mmol/L
Premature infant	20–60 mg/dL	1.1–3.3 mmol/L
Neonate	30–60 mg/dL	1.7–3.3 mmol/L
Newborn 1 day	40–60 mg/dL	2.2–3.3 mmol/L
Newborn 2 days–2 yr	50–80 mg/dL	2.8–4.4 mmol/L
Child	60–100 mg/dL	3.3–5.6 mmol/L
Adult–older adult	Less than 110 mg/dL	Less than 6.1 mmol/L
Prediabetes or impaired fasting glucose	111–125 mg/dL	6.2–6.9 mmol/L
2-hr postprandial	65–139 mg/dL	3.61–7.71 mmol/L
Random	Less than 200 mg/dL	Less than 11.1 mmol/L

American Diabetes Association–recommended treatment goal for fasting blood glucose is less than 120 mg/dL.

DESCRIPTION: Glucose, a simple six-carbon sugar (monosaccharide), enters the diet as part of the sugars sucrose, lactose, and maltose and as the major constituent of the complex polysaccharide called dietary starch. The body acquires most of its energy from the oxidative metabolism of glucose. Excess glucose is stored in the liver or in muscle tissue as glycogen.

Diabetes is a group of diseases characterized by hyperglycemia, or elevated glucose levels. Hyperglycemia results from a defect in insulin secretion (type 1 diabetes), a defect in insulin action, or a combination of defects in secretion and action (type 2 diabetes). The chronic hyperglycemia of diabetes may result over time in damage, dysfunction, and eventually failure of the eyes, kidneys, nerves, heart, and blood vessels. The American Diabetes Association's criteria for diagnosing diabetes include any combination of the following findings or confirmation of any of the individual findings by repetition on a subsequent day:

Symptoms of diabetes (e.g., polyuria, polydipsia, unexplained weight loss) in addition to a random glucose level greater than 200 mg/dL

Fasting blood glucose greater than 126 mg/dL after a minimum of an 8-hr fast

Glucose level greater than 200 mg/dL 2 hr after glucose challenge with standardized 75-mg load

INDICATIONS
- Assist in the diagnosis of insulinoma
- Determine insulin requirements
- Evaluate disorders of carbohydrate metabolism
- Identify hypoglycemia
- Screen for diabetes

POTENTIAL DIAGNOSIS

Increased in
- Acromegaly, gigantism *(growth hormone [GH] stimulates the release of glucagon, which in turn increases glucose levels)*
- Acute stress reaction *(hyperglycemia is stimulated by the release of catecholamines and glucagon)*
- Cerebrovascular accident *(possibly related to stress)*
- Cushing's syndrome *(related to elevated cortisol)*
- Diabetes *(glucose intolerance and elevated glucose levels define diabetes)*
- Glucagonoma *(glucagon releases stored glucose; glucagon-secreting tumors will increase glucose levels)*
- Hemochromatosis *(related to iron deposition in the pancreas; subsequent damage to pancreatic tissue releases cell contents, including glucagon, resulting in hyperglycemia)*
- Liver disease (severe) *(damaged liver tissue releases cell contents, including stored glucose, into circulation)*
- Myocardial infarction *(related to stress and/or pre-existing diabetes)*
- Pancreatic adenoma *(damage to pancreatic tissue releases cell contents, including glucagon, resulting in hyperglycemia)*
- Pancreatitis (acute and chronic) *(damage to pancreatic tissue releases cell contents, including glucagon, resulting in hyperglycemia)*
- Pancreatitis due to mumps *(damage to pancreatic tissue releases*

cell contents, including glucagon, resulting in hyperglycemia)
- Pheochromocytoma *(related to increased catecholamines, which increase glucagon; glucagon increases glucose levels)*
- Renal disease (severe) *(glucagon is degraded by the kidneys; when damaged kidneys cannot metabolize glucagon, glucagon levels in blood rise and result in hyperglycemia)*
- Shock, trauma *(hyperglycemia is stimulated by the release of catecholamines and glucagon)*
- Somatostatinoma *(somatostatin-producing tumor of pancreatic delta cells, associated with diabetes)*
- Strenuous exercise *(hyperglycemia is stimulated by the release of catecholamines and glucagon)*
- Syndrome X (metabolic syndrome) *(related to the development of diabetes)*
- Thyrotoxicosis *(related to loss of kidney function)*
- Vitamin B_1 deficiency *(thiamine is involved in the metabolism of glucose; deficiency results in accumulation of glucose)*

Decreased in
- Acute alcohol ingestion *(most glucose metabolism occurs in the liver; alcohol inhibits the liver from making glucose)*
- Addison's disease *(cortisol affects glucose levels; insufficient levels of cortisol result in diminished glucose levels)*
- Ectopic insulin production from tumors (adrenal carcinoma, carcinoma of the stomach, fibrosarcoma)
- Excess insulin by injection
- Galactosemia *(inherited enzyme disorder that results in accumulation of galactose in excessive proportion to glucose levels)*

- Glucagon deficiency *(glucagon controls glucose levels; hypoglycemia occurs in the absence of glucagon)*
- Glycogen storage diseases *(deficiencies in enzymes involved in conversion of glycogen to glucose)*
- Hereditary fructose intolerance *(inherited disorder of fructose metabolism; phosphates needed for intermediate steps in gluconeogenesis are trapped from further action by the enzyme deficiency responsible for fructose metabolism)*
- Hypopituitarism *(decreased levels of hormones such as adrenocorticotropin hormone [ACTH] and GH result in decreased glucose levels)*
- Hypothyroidism *(thyroid hormones affect glucose levels; decreased thyroid hormone levels result in decreased glucose levels)*
- Insulinoma *(the function of insulin is to decrease glucose levels)*
- Malabsorption syndromes *(insufficient absorption of carbohydrates)*
- Maple syrup urine disease *(inborn error of amino acid metabolism; accumulation of leucine is believed to inhibit the rate of gluconeogenesis, independently of insulin, and thereby diminish release of hepatic glucose stores)*
- Poisoning resulting in severe liver disease *(decreased liver function correlates with decreased glucose metabolism)*
- Postgastrectomy *(insufficient intake of carbohydrates)*
- Starvation *(insufficient intake of carbohydrates)*
- von Gierke's disease *(most common glycogen storage disease; G6PD deficiency)*

CRITICAL FINDINGS ◈

- Less than 40 mg/dL
- Greater than 400 mg/dL

Note and immediately report to the health-care provider (HCP) any critically increased or decreased values and related symptoms.

Glucose monitoring is an important measure in achieving tight glycemic control. The enzymatic GDH-PQQ test method may produce falsely elevated results in patients who are receiving products that contain other sugars (e.g., oral xylose, parenterals containing maltose or galactose, and peritoneal dialysis solutions that contain icodextrin). The GDH-NAD, glucose oxidase, and glucose hexokinase methods can distinguish between glucose and other sugars.

Symptoms of decreased glucose levels include headache, confusion, hunger, irritability, nervousness, restlessness, sweating, and weakness. Possible interventions include oral or IV administration of glucose, IV or intramuscular injection of glucagon, and continuous glucose monitoring.

Symptoms of elevated glucose levels include abdominal pain, fatigue, muscle cramps, nausea, vomiting, polyuria, and thirst. Possible interventions include subcutaneous or IV injection of insulin with continuous glucose monitoring.

INTERFERING FACTORS

- Drugs that may increase glucose levels include acetazolamide, alanine, albuterol, anesthetic agents, antipyrine, atenolol, betamethasone, cefotaxime, chlorpromazine, chlorprothixene, clonidine, clorexolone, corticotropin, cortisone, cyclic AMP, cyclopropane, dexamethasone, dextroamphetamine, diapamide, epinephrine, enflurane, ethacrynic acid, ether, fludrocortisone, fluoxymesterone, furosemide, glucagon, glucocorticoids, homoharringtonine, hydrochlorothiazide, hydroxydione, isoniazid, maltose, meperidine, meprednisone, methyclothiazide, metolazone, niacin, nifedipine, nortriptyline, octreotide, oral contraceptives, oxyphenbutazone, pancreozymin, phenelzine, phenylbutazone, piperacetazine, polythiazide, prednisone, quinethazone, reserpine, rifampin, ritodrine, salbutamol, secretin, somatostatin, thiazides, thyroid hormone, and triamcinolone.
- Drugs that may decrease glucose levels include acarbose, acetylsalicylic acid, acipimox, alanine, allopurinol, antimony compounds, arsenicals, ascorbic acid, benzene, buformin, cannabis, captopril, carbutamide, chloroform, clofibrate, dexfenfluramine, enalapril, enprostil, erythromycin, fenfluramine, gemfibrozil, glibornuride, glyburide, guanethidine, niceritrol, nitrazepam, oral contraceptives, oxandrolone, oxymetholone, phentolamine, phosphorus, promethazine, ramipril, rotenone, sulfonylureas, thiocarlide, tolbutamide, tromethamine, and verapamil.
- Elevated urea levels and uremia can lead to falsely elevated glucose levels.
- Extremely elevated white blood cell counts can lead to falsely decreased glucose values.
- Failure to follow dietary restrictions before the fasting test can lead to falsely elevated glucose values.
- Administration of insulin or oral hypoglycemic agents within 8 hr of a fasting blood glucose can lead to falsely decreased values.
- Specimens should never be collected above an IV line because of the potential for dilution when the specimen and the IV solution

combine in the collection container, falsely decreasing the result. There is also the potential of contaminating the sample with the substance of interest, if it is present in the IV solution, falsely increasing the result.
• Failure to follow dietary restrictions before the procedure may cause the procedure to be canceled or repeated.

NURSING IMPLICATIONS AND PROCEDURE

PRETEST:

▶ Positively identify the patient using at least two unique identifiers before providing care, treatment, or services.
▶ *Patient Teaching:* Inform the patient this test can assist in evaluating blood sugar levels.
▶ Obtain a history of the patient's complaints, including a list of known allergens, especially allergies or sensitivities to latex.
▶ Obtain a history of the patient's endocrine system, symptoms, and results of previously performed laboratory tests and diagnostic and surgical procedures.
▶ Obtain a list of medications the patient is taking, including herbs, nutritional supplements, nutraceuticals (see Appendix F), insulin, and any other substances used to regulate glucose levels.
▶ Review the procedure with the patient. Inform the patient that specimen collection takes approximately 5 to 10 min. Address concerns about pain and explain that there may be some discomfort during the venipuncture.
▶ *Sensitivity to social and cultural issues,* as well as concern for modesty, is important in providing psychological support before, during, and after the procedure.
▶ For the fasting glucose test, the patient should fast for at least 12 hr before specimen collection.

▶ The patient should follow the instructions given for 2-hr postprandial glucose test. Some HCPs may order administration of a standard glucose solution, whereas others may instruct the patient to eat a meal with a known carbohydrate composition.

INTRATEST:

▶ Ensure that the patient has complied with dietary restrictions and other pretesting preparations; assure that food has been restricted for at least 12 hr prior to the fasting procedure.
▶ If the patient has a history of allergic reaction to latex, avoid the use of equipment containing latex.
▶ Instruct the patient to cooperate fully and to follow directions. Direct the patient to breathe normally and to avoid unnecessary movement.
▶ Observe standard precautions, and follow the general guidelines in Appendix A. Positively identify the patient, and label the appropriate tubes with the corresponding patient demographics, date, and time of collection. Perform a venipuncture.
▶ Remove the needle and apply direct pressure with dry gauze to stop bleeding. Observe/assess venipuncture site for bleeding or hematoma formation and secure gauze with adhesive bandage.
▶ Promptly transport the specimen to the laboratory for processing and analysis.

POST-TEST:

▶ A report of the results will be sent to the requesting HCP, who will discuss the results with the patient.
▶ Instruct the patient to resume usual diet, as directed by the HCP.
▶ *Nutritional Considerations:* Increased glucose levels may be associated with diabetes. There is no "diabetic diet"; however, many meal-planning approaches with nutritional goals are endorsed by the American Dietetic Association. Patients who adhere to dietary recommendations report a better general feeling of health, better weight management, greater control of glucose and lipid values, and

improved use of insulin. Instruct the patient, as appropriate, in nutritional management of diabetes. In June 2006, the American Heart Association developed a Therapeutic Lifestyle Changes (TLC) diet with goals directed at people with specific risk factors and/or existing medical conditions (e.g., elevated LDL cholesterol levels, other lipid disorders, coronary artery disease, insulin-dependent diabetes, insulin resistance, or metabolic syndrome). The TLC approach also includes the use of plant stanols or sterols and increased dissolved fiber as an option for lowering LDL cholesterol levels; nutritional recommendations for daily total caloric intake; recommendations for allowable percentage of calories derived from fat (saturated and unsaturated), carbohydrates, protein, and cholesterol; as well as recommendations for daily expenditure of energy. The nutritional needs of each diabetic patient need to be determined individually (especially during pregnancy) with the appropriate health-care professionals, particularly professionals trained in nutrition.

Social and Cultural Considerations:
Numerous studies point to the prevalence of excess body weight in American children and adolescents. Experts estimate that obesity is present in 25% of the population ages 6 to 11 yr. The medical, social, and emotional consequences of excess body weight are significant. Special attention should be given to instructing the child and caregiver regarding health risks and weight control education.

Instruct the patient and caregiver to report signs and symptoms of hypoglycemia (weakness, confusion, diaphoresis, rapid pulse) or hyperglycemia (thirst, polyuria, hunger, lethargy).

Recognize anxiety related to test results, and be supportive of perceived loss of independence and fear of shortened life expectancy. Discuss the implications of abnormal test results on the patient's lifestyle. Provide teaching and information regarding the clinical implications of the test results, as appropriate. Emphasize, if indicated,

that good glycemic control delays the onset and slows the progression of diabetic retinopathy, nephropathy, and neuropathy. Educate the patient regarding access to counseling services, as appropriate. Provide contact information, if desired, for the American Diabetes Association (ADA; www.diabetes.org) or the American Heart Association (www.americanheart .org) or the NHLBI (www.nhlbi.nih.gov). The ADA recommends A_{1C} testing 4 times a year for insulin-dependent type 1 or type 2 diabetes and twice a year for non-insulin-dependent type 2 diabetes.

Reinforce information given by the patient's HCP regarding further testing, treatment, or referral to another HCP. Instruct the patient in the use of home test kits approved by the U.S. Food and Drug Administration, if prescribed. Answer any questions or address any concerns voiced by the patient or family.

Depending on the results of this procedure, additional testing may be performed to evaluate or monitor progression of the disease process and determine the need for a change in therapy. Evaluate test results in relation to the patient's symptoms and other tests performed.

RELATED MONOGRAPHS:

Related tests include ACTH, angiography adrenal, BUN, calcium, catecholamines, cholesterol (HDL, LDL, total), cortisol, C-peptide, CT cardiac scoring, CRP, CK and isoenzymes, creatinine, DHEA, echocardiography, fecal analysis, fecal fat, fluorescein angiography, fructosamine, fundus photography, gastric emptying scan, GTT, glycated hemoglobin A_{1C}, gonioscopy, Holter monitor, HVA, insulin, insulin antibodies, ketones, LDH and isoenzymes, lipoprotein electrophoresis, MRI chest, metanephrines, microalbumin, myoglobin, MI infarct scan, myocardial perfusion heart scan, PET heart, renin, sodium, troponin, and visual fields test.

Refer to the Endocrine System table at the end of the book for related tests by body system.

Glucose-6-Phosphate Dehydrogenase

SYNONYM/ACRONYM: G6PD.

COMMON USE: To identify an enzyme deficiency that can result in hemolytic anemia.

SPECIMEN: Whole blood (1 mL) collected in a lavender-top (EDTA) tube.

REFERENCE VALUE: (Method: Fluorescent) Qualitative assay—enzyme activity detected; quantitative assay—the following table reflects enzyme activity in units per gram of hemoglobin:

Age	Conventional Units (× 0.0645)	SI Units
Newborn	7.8–14.4 international units/g hemoglobin	0.5–0.93 micro units/mol hemoglobin
Adult–older adult	5.5–9.3 international units/g hemoglobin	0.35–0.60 micro units/mol hemoglobin

DESCRIPTION: Glucose-6-phosphate dehydrogenase (G6PD) is a red blood cell (RBC) enzyme. It is involved in the hexose monophosphate shunt, and its function is to protect hemoglobin from oxidation. G6PD deficiency is an inherited X-linked abnormality; approximately 20% of female carriers are heterozygous. This deficiency results in hemolysis of varying degrees and acuity depending on the severity of the abnormality. There are three G6PD variants of high frequency in different ethnic groups. G6PD A– is more common in African Americans (10% of males). G6PD Mediterranean is especially common in Iraqis, Kurds, Sephardic Jews, and Lebanese and less common in Greeks, Italians, Turks, North Africans, Spaniards, Portuguese, and Ashkenazi Jews. G6PD Mahidol is common in Southeast Asians (22% of males).

INDICATIONS

- Assist in identifying the cause of hemolytic anemia resulting from drug sensitivity, metabolic disorder, or infection
- Assist in identifying the cause of hemolytic anemia resulting from enzyme deficiency

POTENTIAL DIAGNOSIS

Increased in

The pathophysiology is not well understood but release of the enzymes from hemolyzed cells increases blood levels.

- Chronic blood loss *(related to reticulocytosis; replacement of RBCs)*
- Hepatic coma *(pathophysiology is unclear)*

- Hyperthyroidism *(possible response to increased basal metabolic rate and role of G6PD in glucose metabolism)*
- Idiopathic thrombocytopenic purpura
- Megaloblastic anemia *(related to reticulocytosis; replacement of RBCs)*
- Myocardial infarction *(medications [e.g., salicylates] may aggravate or stimulate a hemolytic crisis in G6PD-deficient patients)*
- Pernicious anemia *(related to reticulocytosis; replacement of RBCs)*
- Viral hepatitis *(pathophysiology is unclear)*

Decreased in
- Congenital nonspherocytic anemia
- G6PD deficiency
- Nonimmunological hemolytic disease of the newborn

CRITICAL FINDINGS: N/A

INTERFERING FACTORS
- Drugs that may increase G6PD levels include fluorouracil.
- Drugs that may precipitate hemolysis in G6PD deficient individuals include acetanilid, acetylsalicylic acid, ascorbic acid, chloramphenicol (Chloromycetin), dapsone, doxorubicin, furazolidone, isobutyl nitrate, methylene blue, nalidixic acid, naphthalene, niridazole, nitrofurantoin, para-aminosalicylic acid, pentaquine, phenacetin, phenazopyridine, phenylhydrazine, primaquine, quinidine, quinine, sulfacetamide, sulfamethoxazole, sulfanilamide, sulfapyridine, sulfisoxazole, thiazolsulfone, toluidine blue, trinitrotoluene, urate oxidase, and vitamin K.
- G6PD levels are increased in reticulocytes; the test results may be falsely positive when a patient is in a period of acute hemolysis. G6PD

levels can also be affected by the presence of large numbers of platelets and white blood cells, which also contain significant amounts of the enzyme.

NURSING IMPLICATIONS AND PROCEDURE

PRETEST:

- Positively identify the patient using at least two unique identifiers before providing care, treatment, or services.
- *Patient Teaching:* Inform the patient this test can assist in diagnosing anemia.
- Obtain a history of the patient's complaints, including a list of known allergens, especially allergies or sensitivities to latex.
- Obtain a history of the patient's hematopoietic system, symptoms, and results of previously performed laboratory tests and diagnostic and surgical procedures.
- Obtain a list of the patient's current medications, including herbs, nutritional supplements, and nutraceuticals (see Appendix F).
- Review the procedure with the patient. Inform the patient that specimen collection takes approximately 5 to 10 min. Address concerns about pain and explain that there may be some discomfort during the venipuncture.
- *Sensitivity to social and cultural issues,* as well as concern for modesty, is important in providing psychological support before, during, and after the procedure.
- There are no food, fluid, or medication restrictions unless by medical direction.

INTRATEST:

- If the patient has a history of allergic reaction to latex, avoid the use of equipment containing latex.
- Instruct the patient to cooperate fully and to follow directions. Direct the patient to breathe normally and to avoid unnecessary movement.
- Observe standard precautions, and follow the general guidelines in Appendix A. Positively identify the patient, and label

the appropriate tubes with the corresponding patient demographics, date, and time of collection. Perform a venipuncture.

▶ Remove the needle and apply direct pressure with dry gauze to stop bleeding. Observe/assess venipuncture site for bleeding or hematoma formation and secure gauze with adhesive bandage.

▶ Promptly transport the specimen to the laboratory for processing and analysis.

POST-TEST:

▶ A report of the results will be sent to the requesting health-care provider (HCP), who will discuss the results with the patient.

▶ *Nutritional Considerations:* Educate the patient with G6PD deficiency, as appropriate, to avoid certain foods, vitamins, and drugs that may precipitate an acute episode of intravascular hemolysis, including fava beans, ascorbic acid (large doses), acetanilid, antimalarials, furazolidone, isobutyl nitrate, methylene blue, nalidixic acid, naphthalene, niridazole, nitrofurantoin, phenazopyridine, phenylhydrazine, primaquine, sulfacetamide, sulfamethoxazole, sulfanilamide, sulfapyridine, thiazolsulfone, toluidine blue, trinitrotoluene, and urate oxidase.

▶ Reinforce information given by the patient's HCP regarding further testing, treatment, or referral to another HCP. Answer any questions or address any concerns voiced by the patient or family.

▶ Depending on the results of this procedure, additional testing may be performed to evaluate or monitor progression of the disease process and determine the need for a change in therapy. Evaluate test results in relation to the patient's symptoms and other tests performed.

RELATED MONOGRAPHS:

▶ Related tests include biopsy bone marrow, bilirubin, CBC, CBC RBC morphology (including examination of peripheral smear for the presence of Heinz bodies), direct antiglobulin test, folate, Ham's test, haptoglobin, hemosiderin, osmotic fragility, reticulocyte count, UA, and vitamin B_{12}.

▶ Refer to the Hematopoietic System table at the end of the book for related tests by body system.

Glucose Tolerance Tests

SYNONYM/ACRONYM: Standard oral tolerance test, standard gestational screen, standard gestational tolerance test, GTT.

COMMON USE: To evaluate blood glucose levels to assist in diagnosing diseases such as diabetes.

SPECIMEN: Plasma (1 mL) collected in a gray-top (sodium fluoride) tube. Serum (1 mL) collected in a red- or tiger-top tube or plasma collected in a green-top (heparin) tube is also acceptable, but plasma is recommended for diagnosis. It is important to use the same type of collection container throughout the entire test.

REFERENCE VALUE: (Method: Spectrophotometry)

	Conventional Units	SI Units (Conventional Units × 0.0555)
Standard Oral Glucose Tolerance (up to 75-g glucose load)		
Fasting sample	Less than 110 mg/dL	Less than 7.0 mmol/L
Prediabetes or impaired fasting sample	Greater than 110 mg/dL and less than 126 mg/dL	Greater than 6.11 mmol/L and less than 6.99 mmol/L
2-hr sample	Less than 200 mg/dL	Less than 11.1 mmol/L
Tolerance Tests for Gestational Diabetes		
Standard gestational screen (50-g glucose load)	Less than 141 mg/dL	Less than 7.8 mmol/L
Standard gestational tolerance (100-g glucose load)	ADA and ACOG Threshold Recommendations for Gestational Diabetes (1979)	Alternate Threshold Recommendations from the Fourth International Conference on Gestational Diabetes (1998)
Fasting sample	Less than 105 mg/dL	Less than 95 mg/dL
1-hr sample	Less than 190 mg/dL	Less than 180 mg/dL
2-hr sample	Less than 165 mg/dL	Less than 155 mg/dL
3-hr sample	Less than 145 mg/dL	Less than 140 mg/dL

Plasma glucose values are reported to be 10% to 20% higher than serum values. According to recommendations of the ADA and ACOG, the diagnosis of gestational diabetes is made if any two of the four thresholds are met or exceeded.
ACOG = American Congress of Obstetricians and Gynecologists; ADA = American Diabetes Association.

DESCRIPTION: The glucose tolerance test (GTT) measures glucose levels after administration of an oral or IV carbohydrate challenge. Patients with diabetes are unable to metabolize glucose at a normal rate. The oral GTT is used for individuals who are able to eat and who are not known to have problems with gastrointestinal malabsorption. The IV GTT is used for individuals who are unable to tolerate oral glucose.

Diabetes is a group of diseases characterized by hyperglycemia or elevated glucose levels.

Hyperglycemia results from a defect in insulin secretion (type 1 diabetes), a defect in insulin action, or a combination of dysfunction secretion and action (type 2 diabetes). The chronic hyperglycemia of diabetes over time results in damage, dysfunction, and eventually failure of the eyes, kidneys, nerves, heart, and blood vessels. The American Diabetes Association's criteria for diagnosing diabetes include any combination of the following findings or confirmation of any of the individual findings by repetition on a subsequent day:

Symptoms of diabetes (e.g.,
polyuria, polydipsia, and unexplained weight loss) in addition to
a random glucose level greater than
200 mg/dL
Fasting blood glucose greater than
126 mg/dL, after a minimum of an
8-hr fast
Glucose level greater than 200 mg/dL
2 hr after glucose challenge with
standardized 75-mg load

INDICATIONS

- Evaluate abnormal fasting or
  postprandial blood glucose
  levels that do not clearly indicate
  diabetes
- Evaluate glucose metabolism in
  women of childbearing age, especially women who are pregnant
  and have (1) a history of previous
  fetal loss or birth of infants weighing 9 lb or more and/or (2) a
  family history of diabetes
- Identify abnormal renal tubular
  function if glycosuria occurs without hyperglycemia
- Identify impaired glucose metabolism without overt diabetes
- Support the diagnosis of hyperthyroidism and alcoholic liver disease,
  which are characterized by a sharp
  rise in blood glucose followed by a
  decline to subnormal levels

POTENTIAL DIAGNOSIS

Tolerance Increased in

- Decreased absorption of
  glucose:
  Adrenal insufficiency (Addison's disease,
    hypopituitarism)
  Hypothyroidism
  Intestinal diseases, such as celiac disease
    and tropical sprue
  Whipple's disease
- Increased insulin secretion:
  Pancreatic islet cell tumor

Tolerance Impaired in

- Increased absorption of glucose:
  Excessive intake of glucose
  Gastrectomy
  Gastroenterostomy
  Hyperthyroidism
  Vagotomy
- Decreased usage of glucose:
  Central nervous system lesions
  Cushing's syndrome
  Diabetes
  Hemochromatosis
  Hyperlipidemia
- Decreased glycogenesis:
  Hyperthyroidism
  Infections
  Liver disease (severe)
  Pheochromocytoma
  Pregnancy
  Stress
  Von Gierke disease

CRITICAL FINDINGS

- Less than 40 mg/dL
- Greater than 400 mg/dL

Note and immediately report to the
health-care provider (HCP) any critically increased or decreased values and
related symptoms.

Symptoms of decreased glucose
levels include headache, confusion,
hunger, irritability, nervousness, restlessness, sweating, and weakness.
Possible interventions include oral
or IV administration of glucose, IV or
intramuscular injection of glucagon,
and continuous glucose monitoring.

Symptoms of elevated glucose levels include abdominal pain, fatigue,
muscle cramps, nausea, vomiting, polyuria, and thirst. Possible interventions
include subcutaneous or IV injection
of insulin with continuous glucose
monitoring.

INTERFERING FACTORS

- Drugs and substances that may
  increase GTT values include

acetylsalicylic acid, atenolol, bendroflumethiazide, caffeine, clofibrate, fenfluramine, fluoxymesterone, glyburide, guanethidine, lisinopril, methandrostenolone, metoprolol, nandrolone, niceritrol, nifedipine, nitrendipine, norethisterone, phenformin, phenobarbital, prazosin, and terazosin.

- Drugs and substances that may decrease GTT values include acebutolol, beclomethasone, bendroflumethiazide, betamethasone, calcitonin, catecholamines, chlorothiazide, chlorpromazine, chlorthalidone, cimetidine, corticotropin, cortisone, danazol, deflazacort, dexamethasone, diapamide, diethylstilbestrol, ethacrynic acid, fludrocortisone, furosemide, glucagon, glucocorticosteroids, heroin, hydrochlorothiazide, mephenytoin, mestranol, methadone, methandrostenolone, methylprednisolone, muzolimine, niacin, nifedipine, norethindrone, norethynodrel, oral contraceptives, paramethasone, perphenazine, phenolphthalein, phenothiazine, phenytoin, pindolol, prednisolone, prednisone, propranolol, quinethazone, thiazides, triamcinolone, triamterene, and verapamil.
- The test should be performed on ambulatory patients. Impaired physical activity can lead to falsely increased values.
- Excessive physical activity before or during the test can lead to falsely decreased values.
- Failure of the patient to ingest a diet with sufficient carbohydrate content (e.g., 150 g/day) for at least 3 days before the test can result in falsely decreased values.
- The patient may have difficulty drinking the extremely sweet glucose beverage and become nauseous. Vomiting during the course of the test will cause the test to be canceled.

- Smoking before or during the test can lead to falsely increased values.
- The patient should not be under recent or current physiological stress during the test. If the patient has had recent surgery (less than 2 wk previously), an infectious disease, or a major illness (e.g., myocardial infarction), the test should be delayed or rescheduled.
- Failure to follow dietary restrictions before the procedure may cause the procedure to be canceled or repeated.

NURSING IMPLICATIONS AND PROCEDURE

PRETEST:

- Positively identify the patient using at least two unique identifiers before providing care, treatment, or services.
- *Patient Teaching:* Inform the patient this test can assist in evaluating blood sugar levels.
- Obtain a history of the patient's complaints, including a list of known allergens, especially allergies or sensitivities to latex.
- Obtain a history of the patient's endocrine system, symptoms, and results of previously performed laboratory tests and diagnostic and surgical procedures.
- Obtain a list of the patient's current medications, including herbs, nutritional supplements, and nutraceuticals (see Appendix F).
- Review the procedure with the patient. Inform the patient that specimen collection takes approximately 5 to 10 min. Inform the patient that multiple specimens may be required. Address concerns about pain and explain that there may be some discomfort during the venipuncture.
- *Sensitivity to social and cultural issues,* as well as concern for modesty, is important in providing psychological support before, during, and after the procedure.

- The patient should fast for at least 8 to 16 hr before the standard oral and standard gestational GTTs.
- There are no fluid or medication restrictions unless by medical direction prior to the gestational screen.

INTRATEST:

- Ensure that the patient has complied with dietary and activity restrictions as well as other pretesting preparations; ensure that food has been restricted for at least 8 to 12 hr prior to the procedure.
- If the patient has a history of allergic reaction to latex, avoid the use of equipment containing latex.
- Instruct the patient to cooperate fully and to follow directions. Direct the patient to breathe normally and to avoid unnecessary movement.
- Observe standard precautions, and follow the general guidelines in Appendix A. Positively identify the patient, and label the appropriate tubes with the corresponding patient demographics, date, and time of collection. Perform a venipuncture.
- Remove the needle and apply direct pressure with dry gauze to stop bleeding. Observe/assess venipuncture site for bleeding or hematoma formation and secure gauze with adhesive bandage.
- Promptly transport the specimen to the laboratory for processing and analysis. Do not wait until all specimens have been collected to transport.

Standard Oral GTT

- The standard oral GTT takes 2 hr. A fasting blood glucose is determined before administration of an oral glucose load. If the fasting blood glucose is less than 126 mg/dL, the patient is given an oral glucose load.
- An oral glucose load should not be administered before the value of the fasting specimen has been received. If the fasting blood glucose is greater than 126 mg/dL, the standard glucose load is not administered and the test is canceled. The laboratory will follow its protocol as far as notifying the patient of his or her glucose level and the reason why the test was canceled.

The requesting HCP will then be issued a report indicating the glucose level and the cancellation of the test. A fasting glucose greater than 126 mg/dL indicates diabetes; therefore, the glucose load would never be administered before allowing the requesting HCP to evaluate the clinical situation.

- Adults receive 75 g and children receive 1.75 g/kg ideal weight, not to exceed 75 g. The glucose load should be consumed within 5 min, and time 0 begins as soon as the patient begins to ingest the glucose load. A second specimen is collected at 2 hr, concluding the test. The test is discontinued if the patient vomits before the second specimen has been collected.

Standard Gestational Screen

- The standard gestational screen is performed on pregnant women. If results from the screen are abnormal, a full gestational GTT is performed. The gestational screen does not require a fast. The patient is given a 50-g oral glucose load. The glucose load should be consumed within 5 min, and time 0 begins as soon as the patient begins to ingest the glucose load. A specimen is collected 1 hr after ingestion. The test is discontinued if the patient vomits before the 1-hr specimen has been collected. If the result is normal, the test may be repeated between 24 and 28 wk gestation.

Standard Gestational GTT

- The standard gestational GTT takes 3 hr. A fasting blood glucose is determined before administration of a 100-g oral glucose load. If the fasting blood glucose is less than 126 mg/dL, the patient is given an oral glucose load.
- An oral glucose load should not be administered before the value of the fasting specimen has been received. *If the fasting blood glucose is greater than 126 mg/dL, the Glucola is not administered and the test is canceled* (see previous explanation).
- The glucose load should be consumed within 5 min, and time 0 begins as soon as the patient begins to ingest the glucose load. Subsequent specimens are collected at 1, 2, and 3 hr, concluding the test. The test is discontinued if the

patient vomits before all specimens have been collected.

POST-TEST:

▶ A report of the results will be sent to the requesting HCP, who will discuss the results with the patient.

▶ Instruct the patient to resume usual diet and activity, as directed by the HCP.

▶ *Nutritional Considerations:* Increased glucose levels may be associated with diabetes. There is no "diabetic diet"; however, many meal-planning approaches with nutritional goals are endorsed by the American Dietetic Association. Patients who adhere to dietary recommendations report a better general feeling of health, better weight management, greater control of glucose and lipid values, and improved use of insulin. Instruct the patient, as appropriate, in nutritional management of diabetes. In June 2006, the American Heart Association developed a Therapeutic Lifestyle Changes (TLC) diet with goals directed at people with specific risk factors and/or existing medical conditions (e.g., elevated LDL cholesterol levels, other lipid disorders, coronary artery disease, insulin-dependent diabetes, insulin resistance, or metabolic syndrome). The TLC approach also includes the use of plant stanols or sterols and increased dissolved fiber as an option for lowering LDL cholesterol levels; nutritional recommendations for daily total caloric intake; recommendations for allowable percentage of calories derived from fat (saturated and unsaturated), carbohydrates, protein, and cholesterol; as well as recommendations for daily expenditure of energy. The nutritional needs of each diabetic patient need to be determined individually (especially during pregnancy) with the appropriate HCPs, particularly professionals trained in nutrition.

▶ Impaired glucose tolerance may be associated with diabetes. Instruct the patient and caregiver to report signs and symptoms of hypoglycemia (weakness, confusion, diaphoresis, rapid pulse) or hyperglycemia (thirst, polyuria, hunger, lethargy).

▶ Recognize anxiety related to test results, and be supportive of perceived

loss of independence and fear of shortened life expectancy. Discuss the implications of abnormal test results on the patient's lifestyle. Provide teaching and information regarding the clinical implications of the test results, as appropriate. Emphasize, if indicated, that good glycemic control delays the onset and slows the progression of diabetic retinopathy, nephropathy, and neuropathy. Educate the patient regarding access to counseling services, as appropriate. Provide contact information, if desired, for the American Diabetes Association (www.diabetes.org) or the American Heart Association (www.americanheart.org).

▶ Reinforce information given by the patient's HCP regarding further testing, treatment, or referral to another HCP. Instruct the patient in the use of home test kits approved by the U.S. Food and Drug Administration, if prescribed. Answer any questions or address any concerns voiced by the patient or family.

▶ Depending on the results of this procedure, additional testing may be performed to evaluate or monitor progression of the disease process and determine the need for a change in therapy. Evaluate test results in relation to the patient's symptoms and other tests performed.

RELATED MONOGRAPHS:

▶ Related tests include ACTH, ALP, antibodies gliadin, angiography adrenal, biopsy intestinal, biopsy thyroid, BUN, C-peptide, capsule endoscopy, catecholamines, cholesterol (total and HDL), cortisol, creatinine, DHEAS, fecal fat, fluorescein angiography, folate, fructosamine, fundus photography, gastric acid stimulation, gastrin stimulation, glucagon, glucose, glycated hemoglobin, gonioscopy, 5-HIAA, insulin, insulin antibodies, ketones, metanephrines, microalbumin, oxalate, RAIU, thyroid scan, TSH, thyroxine, triglycerides, VMA, and visual fields test.

▶ Refer to the Endocrine System table at the end of the book for related tests by body system.

Glycated Hemoglobin

SYNONYM/ACRONYM: Hemoglobin A_{1C}, A_{1C}.

COMMON USE: To monitor treatment in individuals with diabetes by evaluating their long-term glycemic control.

SPECIMEN: Whole blood (1 mL) collected in a lavender-top (EDTA) tube.

REFERENCE VALUE: (Method: Chromatography)

Total A_1	4.0–7.0%
A_{1c}	4.0–5.5%

Values vary widely by method. American Diabetes Association (ADA)—recommended treatment goal for hemoglobin A_{1C} is less than 7%.

DESCRIPTION: *Glycosylated* or *glycated hemoglobin* is the combination of glucose and hemoglobin into a ketamine; the rate at which this occurs is proportional to glucose concentration. The average life span of a red blood cell (RBC) is approximately 120 days; measurement of glycated hemoglobin is a way to monitor long-term diabetic management. The average plasma glucose can be estimated using the formula:

Average plasma glucose (mg/dL) = $[(A_{1C} \times 35.6) - 77.3]$ For example, an A_{1C} value of 6% would reflect an average plasma glucose of 136.3 mg/dL or $[(6 \times 35.6) - 77.3]$.

Diabetes is a group of diseases characterized by hyperglycemia or elevated glucose levels. Hyperglycemia results from a defect in insulin secretion (type 1 diabetes), a defect in insulin action, or a combination of dysfunctional secretion and action (type 2 diabetes). The chronic hyperglycemia of diabetes over time results in damage, dysfunction, and eventually failure of the eyes, kidneys, nerves, heart, and blood vessels. Hemoglobin A_{1C} levels are not age dependent and are not affected by exercise, diabetic medications, or nonfasting state before specimen collection.

INDICATIONS

Assess long-term glucose control in individuals with diabetes

POTENTIAL DIAGNOSIS

Increased in
- Diabetes (poorly controlled or uncontrolled) *(related to and evidenced by elevated glucose levels)*
- Pregnancy *(evidenced by gestational diabetes)*
- Splenectomy *(related to prolonged RBC survival, which extends the amount of time hemoglobin is available for glycosylation)*

Decreased in
- Chronic blood loss *(related to decreased concentration of RBC-bound glycated hemoglobin due to blood loss)*

- Chronic renal failure *(low RBC count associated with this condition reflects corresponding decrease in RBC-bound glycated hemoglobin)*
- Conditions that decrease RBC life span *(evidenced by anemia and low RBC count, reflecting a corresponding decrease in RBC-bound glycated hemoglobin)*
- Hemolytic anemia *(evidenced by low RBC count due to hemolysis, reflecting a corresponding decrease in RBC-bound glycated hemoglobin)*
- Pregnancy *(evidenced by anemia and low RBC count, reflecting a corresponding decrease in RBC-bound glycated hemoglobin)*

CRITICAL FINDINGS: N/A

INTERFERING FACTORS
- Drugs that may increase glycated hemoglobin A_{1C} values include insulin and sulfonylureas.
- Drugs that may decrease glycated hemoglobin A_{1C} values include cholestyramine and metformin.
- Conditions involving abnormal hemoglobins (hemoglobinopathies) affect the reliability of glycated hemoglobin A_{1C} values, causing (1) falsely increased values, (2) falsely decreased values, or (3) discrepancies in either direction depending on the method.

NURSING IMPLICATIONS AND PROCEDURE

PRETEST:
- Positively identify the patient using at least two unique identifiers before providing care, treatment, or services.
- *Patient Teaching:* Inform the patient this test can assist in evaluating blood sugar control over approximately the past 3 mo.

- Obtain a history of the patient's complaints, including a list of known allergens, especially allergies or sensitivities to latex.
- Obtain a history of the patient's endocrine system, symptoms, and results of previously performed laboratory tests and diagnostic and surgical procedures.
- Obtain a list of the patient's current medications, including herbs, nutritional supplements, and nutraceuticals (see Appendix F).
- Review the procedure with the patient. Inform the patient that specimen collection takes approximately 5 to 10 min. Address concerns about pain and explain that there may be some discomfort during the venipuncture.
- *Sensitivity to social and cultural issues,* as well as concern for modesty, is important in providing psychological support before, during, and after the procedure.
- There are no food, fluid, or medication restrictions unless by medical direction.

INTRATEST:
- If the patient has a history of allergic reaction to latex, avoid the use of equipment containing latex.
- Instruct the patient to cooperate fully and to follow directions. Direct the patient to breathe normally and to avoid unnecessary movement.
- Observe standard precautions, and follow the general guidelines in Appendix A. Positively identify the patient, and label the appropriate tubes with the corresponding patient demographics, date, and time of collection. Perform a venipuncture.
- Remove the needle and apply direct pressure with dry gauze to stop bleeding. Observe/assess venipuncture site for bleeding or hematoma formation and secure gauze with adhesive bandage.
- Promptly transport the specimen to the laboratory for processing and analysis.

POST-TEST:
- A report of the results will be sent to the requesting health-care provider (HCP), who will discuss the results with the patient.

Nutritional Considerations: Increased glycated hemoglobin A_{1C} levels may be associated with diabetes. There is no "diabetic diet"; however, many meal-planning approaches with nutritional goals are endorsed by the American Dietetic Association. Patients who adhere to dietary recommendations report a better general feeling of health, better weight management, greater control of glucose and lipid values, and improved use of insulin. Instruct the patient, as appropriate, in nutritional management of diabetes. In June 2006, the American Heart Association developed a Therapeutic Lifestyle Changes (TLC) diet with goals directed at people with specific risk factors and/or existing medical conditions (e.g., elevated LDL cholesterol levels, other lipid disorders, coronary artery disease, insulin-dependent diabetes, insulin resistance, or metabolic syndrome). The TLC approach also includes the use of plant stanols or sterols and increased dissolved fiber as an option for lowering LDL cholesterol levels; nutritional recommendations for daily total caloric intake; recommendations for allowable percentage of calories derived from fat (saturated and unsaturated), carbohydrates, protein, and cholesterol; as well as recommendations for daily expenditure of energy. The nutritional needs of each diabetic patient need to be determined individually (especially during pregnancy) with the appropriate HCPs, particularly professionals trained in nutrition.

Social and Cultural Considerations: Numerous studies point to the prevalence of excess body weight in American children and adolescents. Experts estimate that obesity is present in 25% of the population ages 6 to 11 yr. The medical, social, and emotional consequences of excess body weight are significant. Special attention should be given to instructing the child and caregiver regarding health risks and weight control education.

Instruct the patient and caregiver to report signs and symptoms of hypoglycemia (weakness, confusion, diaphoresis, rapid pulse) or hyperglycemia (thirst, polyuria, hunger, lethargy).

Recognize anxiety related to test results, and be supportive of perceived loss of independence and fear of shortened life expectancy. Discuss the implications of abnormal test results on the patient's lifestyle. Provide teaching and information regarding the clinical implications of the test results, as appropriate. Emphasize, if indicated, that good glycemic control delays the onset and slows the progression of diabetic retinopathy, nephropathy, and neuropathy. Educate the patient regarding access to counseling services, as appropriate. Provide contact information, if desired, for the American Diabetes Association (ADA; www.diabetes.org) or the American Heart Association (www.americanheart.org) or the NHLBI (www.nhlbi.nih.gov). The ADA recommends A_{1C} testing 4 times a year for insulin-dependent type 1 or type 2 diabetes and twice a year for non–insulin-dependent type 2 diabetes.

Reinforce information given by the patient's HCP regarding further testing, treatment, or referral to another HCP. Instruct the patient in the use of home test kits approved by the U.S. Food and Drug Administration, if prescribed. Answer any questions or address any concerns voiced by the patient or family.

Depending on the results of this procedure, additional testing may be performed to evaluate or monitor progression of the disease process and determine the need for a change in therapy. Evaluate test results in relation to the patient's symptoms and other tests performed.

RELATED MONOGRAPHS:

Related tests include C-peptide, cholesterol (total and HDL), CT cardiac scoring, creatinine/eGFR, EMG, ENG, fluorescein angiography, fructosamine, fundus photography, gastric emptying scan, glucagon, glucose, glucose tolerance tests, insulin, insulin antibodies, ketones, microalbumin, plethysmography, slit-lamp biomicroscopy, triglycerides, and visual fields test.

Refer to the Endocrine System table at the end of the book for related tests by body system.

Gonioscopy

SYNONYM/ACRONYM: N/A.

COMMON USE: To detect abnormalities in the structure of the anterior chamber of the eye such as in glaucoma.

AREA OF APPLICATION: Eyes.

CONTRAST: N/A.

DESCRIPTION: Gonioscopy is a technique used for examination of the anterior chamber structures of the eye (i.e., the trabecular meshwork and the anatomical relationship of the trabecular meshwork to the iris). The trabecular meshwork is the drainage system of the eye, and gonioscopy is performed to determine if the drainage angle is damaged, blocked, or clogged. Gonioscopy in combination with biomicroscopy is considered to be the most thorough basis to confirm a diagnosis of glaucoma and to differentiate between open-angle and angle-closure glaucoma. The angle structures of the anterior chamber are normally not visible because light entering the eye through the cornea is reflected back into the anterior chamber. Placement of a special contact lens (goniolens) over the cornea allows reflected light to pass back through the cornea and onto a reflective mirror in the contact lens. It is in this way that the angle structures can be visualized. There are two types of gonioscopy: indirect and direct. The more commonly used indirect technique employs a mirrored goniolens and biomicroscope.

Direct gonioscopy is performed with a gonioscope containing a dome-shaped contact lens known as a gonioprism. The gonioprism eliminates internally reflected light, allowing direct visualization of the angle. Interpretation of visual examination is usually documented in a colored hand-drawn diagram. Scheie's classification is used to standardize definition of angles based on appearance by gonioscopy. Shaffer's classification is based on the angular width of the angle recess.

INDICATIONS

- Assessment of peripheral anterior synechiae (PAS)
- Conditions affecting the ciliary body
- Degenerative conditions of the anterior chamber
- Evaluation of glaucoma (confirmation of normal structures and estimation of angle width)
- Growth or tumor in the angle
- Hyperpigmentation
- Post-trauma evaluation for angle recession
- Suspected neovascularization of the angle
- Uveitis

POTENTIAL DIAGNOSIS

Scheie's Classification Based on Visible Angle Structures

Classification	Appearance
Wide open	All angle structures seen
Grade I narrow	Difficult to see over the iris root
Grade II narrow	Ciliary band obscured
Grade III narrow	Posterior trabeculum hazy
Grade IV narrow	Only Schwalbe's line visible

Shaffer's Classification Based on Angle Width

Classification	Appearance
Wide open (20°–45°)	Closure improbable
Moderately narrow (10°–20°)	Closure possible
Extremely narrow (less than 10°)	Closure possible
Partially/totally closed	Closure present

Normal findings in
- Normal appearance of anterior chamber structures and wide, unblocked, normal angle

Abnormal findings in
- Corneal endothelial disorders (Fuchs' endothelial dystrophy, iridocorneal endothelial syndrome)
- Glaucoma
- Lens disorders (cataract, displaced lens)
- Malignant ocular neoplasm in angle
- Neovascularization in angle
- Ocular hemorrhage
- PAS
- Schwartz's syndrome
- Trauma
- Tumors
- Uveitis

CRITICAL FINDINGS: N/A

INTERFERING FACTORS
- Inability of the patient to cooperate or remain still during the test because of age, significant pain, or mental status may interfere with the test results.

NURSING IMPLICATIONS AND PROCEDURE

PRETEST:

- Positively identify the patient using at least two unique identifiers before providing care, treatment, or services.
- *Patient Teaching:* Inform the patient this procedure can assist in evaluating the eye for disease.
- Obtain a history of the patient's complaints, including a list of known allergens, especially allergies or sensitivities to latex.
- Obtain a history of the patient's known or suspected vision loss; changes in visual acuity, including type and cause, use of glasses or contact lenses, eye conditions with treatment regimens, and eye surgery; as well as results of previously performed laboratory tests and diagnostic and surgical procedures.
- Obtain a list of the patient's current medications, including herbs, nutritional supplements, and nutraceuticals (see Appendix F).
- Instruct the patient to remove contact lenses or glasses, as appropriate. Instruct the patient regarding the importance of keeping the eyes open for the test.
- Review the procedure with the patient. Explain that the patient will be requested to fixate the eyes during the

procedure. Address concerns about pain related to the procedure. Explain that no pain will be experienced during the test, but there may be moments of discomfort. Explain that some discomfort may be experienced after the test when the numbness wears off from anesthetic drops administered prior to the test. Inform the patient that the test is performed by a health-care provider (HCP) or optometrist specially trained to perform this procedure and takes about 5 min to complete.

▶ *Sensitivity to social and cultural issues,* as well as concern for modesty, is important in providing psychological support before, during, and after the procedure.

▶ There are no food, fluid, or medication restrictions unless by medical direction.

INTRATEST:

▶ Instruct the patient to cooperate fully and to follow directions. Ask the patient to remain still during the procedure because movement produces unreliable results.

▶ Seat the patient comfortably. Instill topical anesthetic in each eye, as ordered, and allow time for it to work. Topical anesthetic drops are placed in the eye with the patient looking up and the solution directed at the six o'clock position of the sclera (white of the eye) near the limbus (gray, semitransparent area of the eyeball where the cornea and sclera meet). Neither the dropper nor the bottle should touch the eyelashes.

▶ Ask the patient to place the chin in the chin rest and gently press the forehead against the support bar. Ask the patient

to open his or her eyes wide and look at desired target. Explain that the HCP or optometrist will place a lens on the eye while a narrow beam of light is focused on the eye.

POST-TEST:

▶ A report of the results will be sent to the requesting HCP, who will discuss the results with the patient.

▶ Recognize anxiety related to test results, and be supportive of impaired activity related to vision loss or anticipated loss of driving privileges. Discuss the implications of abnormal test results on the patient's lifestyle. Provide teaching and information regarding the clinical implications of the test results, as appropriate.

▶ Reinforce information given by the patient's HCP regarding further testing, treatment, or referral to another HCP. Answer any questions or address any concerns voiced by the patient or family.

▶ Depending on the results of this procedure, additional testing may be performed to evaluate or monitor progression of the disease process and determine the need for a change in therapy. Evaluate test results in relation to the patient's symptoms and other tests performed.

RELATED MONOGRAPHS:

▶ Related tests include fundus photography, pachymetry, slit-lamp biomicroscopy, and visual field testing.

▶ Refer to the Ocular System table at the end of the book for related tests by body system.

G

Gram Stain

SYNONYM/ACRONYM: N/A.

COMMON USE: To provide a quick reference for gram-negative or gram-positive organisms to assist in medical management.

SPECIMEN: Blood, biopsy specimen, or body fluid as collected for culture.

REFERENCE VALUE: N/A.

DESCRIPTION: Gram stain is a technique commonly used to identify bacterial organisms on the basis of their specific staining characteristics. The method involves smearing a small amount of specimen on a slide, and then exposing it to gentian or crystal violet, iodine, alcohol, and safranin O. Gram-positive bacteria retain the gentian or crystal violet and iodine stain complex after a decolorization step and appear purple-blue in color. Gram-negative bacteria do not retain the stain after decolorization but can pick up the pink color of the safranin O counterstain. Gram stains provide information regarding the adequacy of a sample. For example, a sputum Gram stain showing greater than 25 squamous epithelial cells per low-power field, regardless of the number of polymorphonuclear white blood cells, indicates contamination of the specimen with saliva, and the specimen should be rejected for subsequent culture. Gram stains are reviewed over a number of fields for an impression of the quantity of organisms present, which reflects the extent of infection. For example, a Gram stain of unspun urine showing the occasional presence of bacteria per low-power field suggests a correlating colony count of 10,000 bacteria/mL, while the presence of bacteria in most fields is clinically significant and suggests greater than 100,000 bacteria/mL of urine. Gram stain results should be correlated with culture and sensitivity results to interpret the significance of isolated organisms and to select appropriate antibiotic therapy.

INDICATIONS

- Provide a rapid determination of the acceptability of the specimen for further analysis
- Provide rapid, presumptive information about the type of potential pathogen present in the specimen (i.e., gram-positive bacteria, gram-negative bacteria, or yeast)

POTENTIAL DIAGNOSIS

Gram Positive				
Actinomadura	Actinomyces	Bacillus	Clostridium	Corynebacterium
Enterococcus	Erysipelothrix	Lactobacillus	Listeria	Micrococcus
Mycobacterium (gram variable)	Peptostreptococcus	Propionibacterium	Rhodococcus	Staphylococcus
Streptococcus				

Gram Negative				
Acinetobacter	Aeromonas	Alcaligenes	Bacteroides	Bordetella
Borrelia	Brucella	Campylobacter	Citrobacter	Chlamydia
Enterobacter	Escherichia	Flavobacterium	Francisella	Fusobacterium

Gram Negative				
Gardnerella	Haemophilus	Helicobacter	Klebsiella	Legionella
Leptospira	Moraxella	Neisseria	Pasteurella	Plesiomonas
Porphy-romonas	Prevotella	Proteus	Pseudomonas	Rickettsia
Salmonella	Serratia	Shigella	Vibrio	Xanthomonas
Yersinia				

Acid Fast or Partial Acid Fast	
Nocardia	Mycobacterium

Note: *Treponema* species are classified as gram-negative spirochetes, but they are most often visualized using dark-field or silver-staining techniques.

CRITICAL FINDINGS

- Any positive results in blood, cerebrospinal fluid, or any body cavity fluid.

Note and immediately report to the requesting health-care provider (HCP) any positive results and related symptoms.

INTERFERING FACTORS

- Very young, very old, or dead cultures may react atypically to the Gram stain technique.

NURSING IMPLICATIONS AND PROCEDURE

PRETEST:

- Positively identify the patient using at least two unique identifiers before providing care, treatment, or services.
- *Patient Teaching:* Inform the patient this test can assist in identifying the presence of pathogenic organisms.
- Obtain a history of the patient's complaints, including a list of known allergens, especially allergies or sensitivities to latex.
- Obtain a history of the patient's gastrointestinal, genitourinary, immune, reproductive, and respiratory systems; symptoms; and results of previously performed laboratory tests and diagnostic and surgical procedure.
- Obtain a list of the patient's current medications, including herbs, nutritional supplements, and nutraceuticals (see Appendix F).
- Review the procedure with the patient. Inform the patient that the time it takes to collect a proper specimen varies according to the patient's level of cooperation as well as the specimen collection site. Address concerns about pain and explain that there may be some discomfort during the procedure.
- *Sensitivity to social and cultural issues,* as well as concern for modesty, is important in providing psychological support before, during, and after the procedure.
- There are no food, fluid, or medication restrictions unless by medical direction.

INTRATEST:

- Instruct the patient to cooperate fully and to follow directions.
- Observe standard precautions, and follow the general guidelines in Appendix A. Positively identify the patient, and label the appropriate collection container with the corresponding patient demographics, date, and time of collection.
- Specific collection instructions are found in the associated culture monographs.
- Promptly transport the specimen to the laboratory for processing and analysis.

POST-TEST:

▶ A report of the results will be sent to the requesting HCP, who will discuss the results with the patient.

▶ Administer antibiotics as ordered, and instruct the patient in the importance of completing the entire course of antibiotic therapy even if no symptoms are present.

▶ Recognize anxiety related to test results. Discuss the implications of abnormal test results on the patient's lifestyle. Provide teaching and information regarding the clinical implications of the test results, as appropriate.

▶ Reinforce information given by the patient's HCP regarding further testing, treatment, or referral to another HCP. Answer any questions or address any concerns voiced by the patient or family.

▶ Depending on the results of this procedure, additional testing may be performed to evaluate or monitor progression of the disease process and determine the need for a change in therapy. Evaluate test results in relation to the patient's symptoms and other tests performed.

RELATED MONOGRAPHS:

▶ Related tests include amniotic fluid analysis, relevant biopsies, bronchoscopy, cultures bacterial and viral, CSF analysis, CBC, pericardial fluid analysis, peritoneal fluid analysis, pleural fluid analysis, synovial fluid analysis, and UA.

▶ Refer to the Gastrointestinal, Genitourinary, Immune, Reproductive, and Respiratory systems tables at the end of the book for related tests by body system.

Group A Streptococcal Screen

SYNONYM/ACRONYM: Strep screen, rapid strep screen, direct strep screen.

COMMON USE: To detect a group A streptococcal infection such as strep throat.

SPECIMEN: Throat swab (two swabs should be submitted so that a culture can be performed if the screen is negative).

REFERENCE VALUE: (Method: Enzyme immunoassay or latex agglutination) Negative.

DESCRIPTION: Rheumatic fever is a possible sequela to an untreated streptococcal infection. Early diagnosis and treatment appear to lessen the seriousness of symptoms during the acute phase and overall duration of the infection and sequelae. The onset of strep throat is sudden and includes symptoms such as chills, headache, sore throat, malaise, and exudative gray-white patches on the tonsils or pharynx. The group A streptococcal screen should not be ordered unless the results would be available within 1 to 2 hr of specimen collection to make rapid, effective therapeutic decisions. A positive result can be a reliable basis for the initiation of therapy. A negative result is presumptive for infection and should be backed up by culture results. In general, specimens showing growth of less than 10 colonies on culture yield negative results by the rapid screening method. Evidence of group A streptococci disappears rapidly after the initiation of antibiotic therapy. A nucleic acid probe method has also been developed for rapid detection of group A streptococci.

INDICATIONS

• Assist in the rapid determination of the presence of group A streptococci

POTENTIAL DIAGNOSIS

Positive findings in
• Rheumatic fever
• Scarlet fever
• Strep throat
• Streptococcal glomerulonephritis
• Tonsillitis

CRITICAL FINDINGS: N/A

INTERFERING FACTORS

• Polyester (rayon or Dacron) swabs are favored over cotton for best chance of detection. Fatty acids are created on cotton fibers during the sterilization process. Detectable target antigens on the streptococcal cell wall are destroyed without killing the organism when there is contact between the specimen and the fatty acids on the cotton collection swab. False-negative test results can be obtained on specimens collected with cotton tip swabs. Negative strep screens should always be followed with a traditional culture.
• Sensitivity of the method varies among manufacturers.
• Adequate specimen collection in children may be difficult to achieve,

which explains the higher percentage of false-negative results in this age group.

NURSING IMPLICATIONS AND PROCEDURE

PRETEST:

▶ Positively identify the patient using at least two unique identifiers before providing care, treatment, or services.
▶ *Patient Teaching:* Inform the patient this test can assist in identifying a streptococcal infection.
▶ Obtain a history of the patient's complaints, including a list of known allergens, especially allergies or sensitivities to latex.
▶ Obtain a history of the patient's immune and respiratory systems, symptoms, and results of previously performed laboratory tests and diagnostic and surgical procedures.
▶ Obtain a history of prior antibiotic therapy.
▶ Obtain a list of the patient's current medications, including herbs, nutritional supplements, and nutraceuticals (see Appendix F).
▶ Before specimen collection, verify with the laboratory whether wet or dry swabs are preferred for collection.
▶ Review the procedure with the patient. Inform the patient that specimen collection takes approximately 5 to 10 min. Address concerns about pain and explain that there may be some discomfort during the swabbing procedure.
▶ *Sensitivity to social and cultural issues,* as well as concern for modesty, is important in providing psychological support before, during, and after the procedure.
▶ There are no food, fluid, or medication restrictions unless by medical direction.

INTRATEST:

▶ Instruct the patient to cooperate fully and to follow directions. Direct the patient to breathe normally and to avoid unnecessary movement.
▶ Observe standard precautions, and follow the general guidelines in

G

Appendix A. Positively identify the patient, and label the appropriate specimen container with the corresponding patient demographics, date, and time of collection. Vigorous swabbing of both tonsillar pillars and the posterior throat enhances the probability of streptococcal antigen detection.

▶ Promptly transport the specimen to the laboratory for processing and analysis.

POST-TEST:

▶ A report of the results will be sent to the requesting health-care provider (HCP), who will discuss the results with the patient.

▶ Administer antibiotics as ordered, and emphasize to the patient or caregiver the importance of completing the entire course of antibiotic therapy even if no symptoms are present.

▶ Reinforce information given by the patient's HCP regarding further testing, treatment, or referral to another HCP. Answer any questions or address any concerns voiced by the patient or family.

▶ Depending on the results of this procedure, additional testing may be performed to evaluate or monitor progression of the disease process and determine the need for a change in therapy. Evaluate test results in relation to the patient's symptoms and other tests performed.

RELATED MONOGRAPHS:

▶ Related laboratory tests include analgesic and antipyretic drugs, antibiotic drugs, ASO, chest x-ray, CBC, culture (throat, viral), and Gram stain.

▶ Refer to the Immune and Respiratory systems tables at the end of the book for related tests by body system.

Growth Hormone, Stimulation and Suppression Tests

SYNONYM/ACRONYM: Somatotropic hormone, somatotropin, GH, hGH.

COMMON USE: To assess pituitary function and evaluate the amount of secreted growth hormone to assist in diagnosing diseases such as giantism and dwarfism.

SPECIMEN: Serum (1 mL) collected in a red- or tiger-top tube.

REFERENCE VALUE: (Method: Radioimmunoassay)

Growth Hormone

Age	Conventional Units	SI Units (Conventional Units × 1)
Cord blood	8–40 ng/mL	8–40 mcg/L
1 day	5–50 ng/mL	5–50 mcg/L
1 wk	5–25 ng/mL	5–25 mcg/L
Child	2–10 ng/mL	2–10 mcg/L

Age	Conventional Units	SI Units (Conventional Units × 1)
Adult		
Male	0–5 ng/mL	0–5 mcg/L
Female	0–10 ng/mL	0–10 mcg/L
Male older than 60 yr	0–10 ng/mL	0–10 mcg/L
Female older than 60 yr	0–14 ng/mL	0–14 mcg/L
Stimulation Tests		
Rise above baseline	Greater than 5 ng/mL	Greater than 5 mcg/L
Peak response	Greater than 10 ng/mL	Greater than 10 mcg/L
Suppression Tests		
	0–2 ng/mL	0–2 mcg/L

DESCRIPTION: Human growth hormone (GH) is secreted in episodic bursts by the anterior pituitary gland; the highest level is usually secreted during deep sleep. Release of GH is modulated by three hypothalmic factors: GH-releasing hormone, GH-releasing peptide-6, and GH inhibitory hormone (also known as somatostatin). The effects of GH are carried out by insulin-like growth factors, formerly called somatomedins. GH plays an integral role in growth from birth to puberty. GH promotes skeletal growth by stimulating hepatic production of proteins; it also affects lipid and glucose metabolism. Random levels are rarely useful because secretion of GH is episodic and pulsatile. Stimulation tests with arginine, glucagon, insulin, or L-dopa, as well as suppression tests with glucose, provide useful information.

INDICATIONS

- Assist in the diagnosis of acromegaly in adults
- Assist in establishing a diagnosis of dwarfism or growth retardation in children with decreased GH levels, indicative of a pituitary cause
- Assist in establishing a diagnosis of gigantism in children with GH increased levels, indicative of a pituitary cause
- Detect suspected disorder associated with decreased GH
- Monitor response to treatment of growth retardation

POTENTIAL DIAGNOSIS

Increased in
Production of GH is modulated by numerous factors, including stress, exercise, sleep, nutrition, and response to circulating levels of GH.
- Acromegaly
- Anorexia nervosa
- Cirrhosis
- Diabetes (uncontrolled)
- Ectopic GH secretion (neoplasms of stomach, lung)
- Exercise
- Gigantism (pituitary)
- Hyperpituitarism
- Laron dwarfism
- Malnutrition
- Renal failure
- Stress

Decreased in
- Adrenocortical hyperfunction *(inhibits secretion of GH)*
- Dwarfism (pituitary) *(related to GH deficiency)*

• Hypopituitarism *(related to lack of production)*

CRITICAL FINDINGS: N/A

INTERFERING FACTORS
• Drugs that may increase GH levels include alanine, anabolic steroids, angiotensin II, apomorphine, arginine, clonidine, corticotropin, cyclic AMP, desipramine, dexamethasone, dopamine, fenfluramine, galanin, glucagon, GH-releasing hormone, hydrazine, levodopa, methamphetamine, methyldopa, metoclopramide, midazolam, niacin, oral contraceptives, phenytoin, propranolol, and vasopressin.
• Drugs that may decrease GH levels include corticosteroids, corticotropin, hydrocortisone, octreotide, and pirenzepine.
• Recent radioactive scans or radiation within 1 wk before the test can interfere with test results when radioimmunoassay is the test method.
• Failure to follow dietary and activity restrictions before the procedure may cause the procedure to be canceled or repeated.

NURSING IMPLICATIONS AND PROCEDURE

PRETEST:
▶ Positively identify the patient using at least two unique identifiers before providing care, treatment, or services.
▶ *Patient Teaching:* Inform the patient this test can assist in assessing the amount of growth hormone secreted.
▶ Obtain a history of the patient's complaints, including a list of known allergens, especially allergies or sensitivities to latex.
▶ Obtain a history of the patient's endocrine system, symptoms, and results of previously performed laboratory tests and diagnostic and surgical procedures.

▶ Record pertinent information related to diet, sleep pattern, and activity at the time of the test.
▶ Note any recent procedures that can interfere with test results.
▶ Obtain a list of the patient's current medications, including herbs, nutritional supplements, and nutraceuticals (see Appendix F).
▶ Review the procedure with the patient. Protocols may vary depending on the type of induction used. Patients may be allowed to walk around, or they may be required to be recumbent. Inform the patient that multiple specimens may be required. Inform the patient that specimen collection takes approximately 5 to 10 min. Address concerns about pain and explain that there may be some discomfort during the venipuncture.
▶ *Sensitivity to social and cultural issues,* as well as concern for modesty, is important in providing psychological support before, during, and after the procedure.
▶ The patient should fast and avoid strenuous exercise for 12 hr before specimen collection. Protocols may vary among facilities.

INTRATEST:
▶ Ensure that the patient has complied with dietary and activity restrictions; ensure that food and strenuous activity have been restricted for at least 12 hr prior to the procedure.
▶ If the patient has a history of allergic reaction to latex, avoid the use of equipment containing latex.
▶ Instruct the patient to cooperate fully and to follow directions. Direct the patient to breathe normally and to avoid unnecessary movement.
▶ Observe standard precautions, and follow the general guidelines in Appendix A. Positively identify the patient, and label the appropriate tubes with the corresponding patient demographics, date, and time of collection. Perform a venipuncture. Test samples may be requested at baseline and 30-, 60-, 90-, and 120-min intervals after stimulation and at baseline and 60- and 120-min intervals after suppression.

- Remove the needle and apply direct pressure with dry gauze to stop bleeding. Observe/assess venipuncture site for bleeding or hematoma formation and secure gauze with adhesive bandage.
- Promptly transport the specimen to the laboratory for processing and analysis.

POST-TEST:

- A report of the results will be sent to the requesting health-care provider (HCP), who will discuss the results with the patient.
- Instruct the patient to resume usual diet, fluids, medications, and activity, as directed by the HCP.
- Reinforce information given by the patient's HCP regarding further testing, treatment, or referral to another HCP. Answer any questions or address any concerns voiced by the patient or family.
- Depending on the results of this procedure, additional testing may be performed to evaluate or monitor progression of the disease process and determine the need for a change in therapy. Evaluate test results in relation to the patient's symptoms and other tests performed.

RELATED MONOGRAPHS:

- Related tests include ACTH and insulin.
- Refer to the Endocrine System table at the end of the book for related tests by body system.

Ham's Test for Paroxysmal Nocturnal Hemoglobinuria

SYNONYM/ACRONYM: Acid hemolysis test for PNH.

COMMON USE: To assist in diagnosing a rare condition called paroxysmal nocturnal hemoglobinuria (PNH), wherein red blood cells undergo lysis during and after sleep with hemoglobin excreted in the urine.

SPECIMEN: Whole blood (5 mL) collected in lavender-top (EDTA) tube and serum (3 mL) collected in red-top tube.

REFERENCE VALUE: (Method: Acidified hemolysis) No hemolysis seen.

POTENTIAL DIAGNOSIS

Increased in
- Congenital dyserythropoietic anemia, type II
- PNH

Decreased in: N/A

CRITICAL FINDINGS: N/A

Find and print out the full monograph at DavisPlus (http://davisplus.fadavis.com, keyword Van Leeuwen).

Haptoglobin

SYNONYM/ACRONYM: Hapto, HP, Hp.

COMMON USE: To assist in evaluating for intravascular hemolysis related to transfusion reactions, chronic liver disease, hemolytic anemias, and tissue inflammation or destruction.

SPECIMEN: Serum (1 mL) collected in a red- or tiger-top tube.

REFERENCE VALUE: (Method: Nephelometry)

Age	Conventional Units	SI Units (Conventional Units × 0.01)
Newborn	5–48 mg/dL	0.05–0.48 g/L
6 mo–16 yr	25–138 mg/dL	0.25–1.38 g/L
Adult	15–200 mg/dL	0.15–2.00 g/L

DESCRIPTION: Haptoglobin is an α_2-globulin produced in the liver. It binds with the free hemoglobin released when red blood cells (RBCs) are lysed. If left unchecked, free hemoglobin in the plasma can cause renal damage; haptoglobin prevents it from accumulating. In conditions such as hemolytic anemia, so many hemolyzed RBCs are available for binding that the liver cannot compensate by producing additional haptoglobin fast enough, resulting in low serum levels.

INDICATIONS

- Assist in the investigation of suspected transfusion reaction
- Evaluate known or suspected chronic liver disease, as indicated by decreased levels of haptoglobin
- Evaluate known or suspected disorders characterized by excessive RBC hemolysis, as indicated by decreased levels of haptoglobin
- Evaluate known or suspected disorders involving a diffuse inflammatory process or tissue destruction, as indicated by elevated levels of haptoglobin

POTENTIAL DIAGNOSIS

Increased in

Haptoglobin is an acute-phase reactant protein, and any condition that stimulates an acute-phase response will result in elevations of haptoglobin.

- Biliary obstruction
- Disorders involving tissue destruction, such as cancers, burns, and acute myocardial infarction
- Infection or inflammatory diseases, such as ulcerative colitis, arthritis, and pyelonephritis
- Neoplasms
- Steroid therapy

Decreased in

- Autoimmune hemolysis *(related to increased excretion rate of haptoglobin bound to free hemoglobin; rate of excretion exceeds the liver's immediate ability to replenish)*
- Hemolysis due to drug reaction *(related to increased excretion rate of haptoglobin bound to free hemoglobin; rate of excretion exceeds the liver's immediate ability to replenish)*
- Hemolysis due to mechanical destruction (e.g., artificial heart valves, contact sports, subacute bacterial endocarditis) *(related to*

increased excretion rate of haptoglobin bound to free hemoglobin; rate of excretion exceeds the liver's immediate ability to replenish)
- Hemolysis due to RBC membrane or metabolic defects *(related to increased excretion rate of haptoglobin bound to free hemoglobin; rate of excretion exceeds the liver's immediate ability to replenish)*
- Hemolysis due to transfusion reaction *(related to increased excretion rate of haptoglobin bound to free hemoglobin; rate of excretion exceeds the liver's immediate ability to replenish)*
- Hypersplenism *(related to increased excretion rate of haptoglobin bound to free hemoglobin due to increased red blood cell destruction; rate of excretion exceeds the liver's immediate ability to replenish)*
- Ineffective hematopoiesis due to conditions such as folate deficiency or hemoglobinopathies *(related to decreased numbers of RBCs or dysfunctional binding in the presence of abnormal hemoglobins)*
- Liver disease *(related to decreased production)*
- Pregnancy *(related to effect of estrogen)*

CRITICAL FINDINGS: N/A

INTERFERING FACTORS

- Drugs that may increase haptoglobin levels include anabolic steroids, danazol, ethylestrenol, fluoxymesterone, methandrostenolone, norethandrolone, oxandrolone, oxymetholone, and stanozolol.
- Drugs that may decrease haptoglobin levels include acetanilid, aminosalicylic acid, chlorpromazine, dapsone, dextran, diphenhydramine,

furadaltone, furazolidone, isoniazid, nitrofurantoin, norethindrone, oral contraceptives, quinidine, resorcinol, stibophen, tamoxifen, thiazolsulfone, and tripelennamine.

NURSING IMPLICATIONS AND PROCEDURE

PRETEST:

▶ Positively identify the patient using at least two unique identifiers before providing care, treatment, or services.

▶ *Patient Teaching:* Inform the patient this test can assist with evaluating causes of red blood cell loss.

▶ Obtain a history of the patient's complaints, including a list of known allergens, especially allergies or sensitivities to latex.

▶ Obtain a history of the patient's hematopoietic, hepatobiliary, and immune systems; symptoms; and results of previously performed laboratory tests and diagnostic and surgical procedures.

▶ Obtain a list of the patient's current medications, including herbs, nutritional supplements, and nutraceuticals (see Appendix F).

▶ Review the procedure with the patient. Inform the patient that specimen collection takes approximately 5 to 10 min. Address concerns about pain and explain that there may be some discomfort during the venipuncture.

▶ There are no food, fluid, or medication restrictions unless by medical direction.

INTRATEST:

▶ If the patient has a history of allergic reaction to latex, avoid the use of equipment containing latex.

▶ Instruct the patient to cooperate fully and to follow directions. Direct the patient to breathe normally and to avoid unnecessary movement.

▶ Observe standard precautions, and follow the general guidelines in Appendix A. Positively identify the patient, and label the appropriate tubes with the corresponding patient demographics, date, and time of collection. Perform a venipuncture.

▶ Remove the needle and apply direct pressure with dry gauze to stop bleeding. Observe/assess venipuncture site for bleeding or hematoma formation and secure gauze with adhesive bandage.

▶ Promptly transport the specimen to the laboratory for processing and analysis.

POST-TEST:

▶ A report of the results will be sent to the requesting health-care provider (HCP), who will discuss the results with the patient.

▶ Instruct the patient to immediately report symptoms of hemolysis, including chills, fever, flushing, back pain, and fast heartbeat, to the HCP.

▶ Reinforce information given by the patient's HCP regarding further testing, treatment, or referral to another HCP. Answer any questions or address any concerns voiced by the patient or family.

▶ Depending on the results of this procedure, additional testing may be performed to evaluate or monitor progression of the disease process and determine the need for a change in therapy. Evaluate test results in relation to the patient's symptoms and other tests performed.

RELATED MONOGRAPHS:

▶ Related tests include ALT, AST, bilirubin, blood group and type, CBC, CBC RBC count, CBC RBC indices, CBC RBC morphology, Coombs' antiglobulin, folate, G6PD, GGT, Ham's test, hepatobiliary scan, and osmotic fragility.

▶ Refer to the Hematopoietic, Hepatobiliary, and Immune systems tables at the end of the book for related tests by body system.

Helicobacter Pylori Antibody

SYNONYM/ACRONYM: *H. pylori.*

COMMON USE: To test blood for findings that would indicate past or current *Helicobacter pylori* infection.

SPECIMEN: Serum (1 mL) collected in a plain red-top tube.

REFERENCE VALUE: (Method: Enzyme-linked immunosorbent assay [ELISA]) Negative.

DESCRIPTION: There is a strong association between *Helicobacter pylori* infection and gastric cancer, duodenal and gastric ulcer, and chronic gastritis. Immunoglobulin G (IgG) antibodies can be detected for up to 1 yr after treatment. The presence of *H. pylori* can also be demonstrated by a positive urea breath test, positive stool culture, or positive endoscopic biopsy. Patients with symptoms and evidence of *H. pylori* infection are considered to be infected with the organism; patients who demonstrate evidence of *H. pylori* but are without symptoms are said to be colonized.

INDICATIONS

• Assist in differentiating between *H. pylori* infection and NSAID use as the cause of gastritis or peptic or duodenal ulcer
• Assist in establishing a diagnosis of gastritis, gastric carcinoma, or peptic or duodenal ulcer

POTENTIAL DIAGNOSIS

Positive findings in
• *H. pylori* infection
• *H. pylori* colonization:

Negative findings in: N/A

CRITICAL FINDINGS: N/A

INTERFERING FACTORS: N/A

NURSING IMPLICATIONS AND PROCEDURE

PRETEST:
▶ Positively identify the patient using at least two unique identifiers before providing care, treatment, or services.
▶ Inform the patient that the test is used to assist in the diagnosis of *H. pylori* infection in patients with duodenal and gastric disease.
▶ Obtain a history of the patient's complaints, including a list of known allergens, especially allergies or sensitivities to latex.
▶ Obtain a history of the patient's gastrointestinal system, symptoms, and results of previously performed laboratory tests and diagnostic and surgical procedures.
▶ Obtain a list of the patient's current medications, including herbs, nutritional supplements, and nutraceuticals (see Appendix F).
▶ Review the procedure with the patient. Inform the patient that specimen collection takes approximately 5 to 10 min. Address concerns about pain and explain that there may be some discomfort during the venipuncture.
▶ *Sensitivity to social and cultural issues,* as well as concern for modesty, is

important in providing psychological support before, during, and after the procedure.

▶ There are no food, fluid, or medication restrictions unless by medical direction.

INTRATEST:

▶ If the patient has a history of allergic reaction to latex, avoid the use of equipment containing latex.

▶ Instruct the patient to cooperate fully and to follow directions. Direct the patient to breathe normally and to avoid unnecessary movement.

▶ Observe standard precautions, and follow the general guidelines in Appendix A. Positively identify the patient, and label the appropriate tubes with the corresponding patient demographics, date, and time of collection. Perform a venipuncture.

▶ Remove the needle and apply direct pressure with dry gauze to stop bleeding. Observe/assess venipuncture site for bleeding or hematoma formation and secure gauze with adhesive bandage.

▶ Promptly transport the specimen to the laboratory for processing and analysis.

POST-TEST:

▶ A report of the results will be sent to the requesting health-care provider (HCP), who will discuss the results with the patient.

▶ Reinforce information given by the patient's HCP regarding further testing, treatment, or referral to another HCP. Inform the patient that a positive test result constitutes an independent risk factor for gastric cancer. Answer any questions or address any concerns voiced by the patient or family.

▶ Depending on the results of this procedure, additional testing may be performed to evaluate or monitor progression of the disease process and determine the need for a change in therapy. Evaluate test results in relation to the patient's symptoms and other tests performed.

RELATED MONOGRAPHS:

▶ Related tests include capsule endoscopy, EGD, gastric acid stimulation, gastric emptying scan, gastrin, and upper GI series.

▶ Refer to the Gastrointestinal System table at the end of the book for related test by body system.

Hemoglobin Electrophoresis

SYNONYM/ACRONYM: N/A.

COMMON USE: To assist in evaluating hemolytic anemias and identifying hemoglobin variants, diagnose thalassemias, and sickle cell anemia.

SPECIMEN: Whole blood (1 mL) collected in a lavender-top (EDTA) tube.

REFERENCE VALUE: (Method: Electrophoresis)

	Hgb A
Adult	Greater than 95%
	Hgb A$_2$
Adult	1.5–3.7%

Hgb F	
Newborns and infants	
1 day–3 wk	70–77%
6–9 wk	42–64%
3–4 mo	7–39%
6 mo	3–7%
8–11 mo	0.6–2.6%
Adult–older adult	Less than 2%

DESCRIPTION: Hemoglobin (Hgb) electrophoresis is a separation process used to identify normal and abnormal forms of Hgb. Hgb A is the main form of Hgb in the normal adult. Hgb F is the main form of Hgb in the fetus, the remainder being composed of Hgb A_1 and A_2. Small amounts of Hgb F are normal in the adult. Hgb D, E, H, S, and C result from abnormal amino acid substitutions during the formation of Hgb and are inherited hemoglobinopathies.

INDICATIONS

• Assist in the diagnosis of Hgb C disease
• Assist in the diagnosis of thalassemia, especially in patients with a family history positive for the disorder
• Differentiate among thalassemia types
• Evaluate hemolytic anemia of unknown cause
• Evaluate a positive sickle cell screening test to differentiate sickle cell trait from sickle cell disease

POTENTIAL DIAGNOSIS

Increased in

Hgb A_2
• Hyperthyroidism
• Megaloblastic anemia
• β-Thalassemias
• Sickle trait

Hgb F
• Anemia (aplastic, associated with chronic disease or due to blood loss)
• Erythropoietic porphyria
• Hereditary elliptocytosis or spherocytosis
• Hereditary persistence of fetal Hgb
• Hyperthyroidism
• Leakage of fetal blood into maternal circulation
• Leukemia (acute or chronic)
• Myeloproliferative disorders
• Paroxysmal nocturnal hemoglobinuria
• Pernicious anemia
• Sickle cell disease
• Thalassemias
• Unstable hemoglobins

Hgb C
• Hgb C disease (second most common variant in the United States; has a higher prevalence among African Americans)

Hgb D
• Hgb D (rare hemoglobinopathy that may also be found in combination with Hgb S or thalassemia)

Hgb E
• Hgb E disease; thalassemia-like condition (second most common hemoglobinopathy in the world; occurs with the highest frequency in Southeast Asians and African Americans)

Hgb S
• Sickle cell trait or disease (most common variant in the United

States; occurs with a frequency of about 8% among African Americans)

Hgb H
• α -Thalassemias
• Hgb Bart' s hydrops fetalis syndrome

Decreased in

Hgb A$_2$
• Erythroleukemia
• Hgb H disease
• Iron-deficiency anemia (untreated)
• Sideroblastic anemia

CRITICAL FINDINGS: N/A

INTERFERING FACTORS
• High altitude and dehydration may increase values.
• Iron deficiency may decrease Hgb A$_2$, C, and S.
• In patients less than 3 mo of age, false-negative results for Hgb S occur in coincidental polycythemia.
• Red blood cell transfusion within 4 mo of test can mask abnormal Hgb levels.

NURSING IMPLICATIONS AND PROCEDURE

PRETEST:
▶ Positively identify the patient using at least two unique identifiers before providing care, treatment, or services.
▶ *Patient Teaching:* Inform the patient this test can assist in diagnosing various types of anemias.
▶ Obtain a history of the patient's complaints, including a list of known allergens, especially allergies or sensitivities to latex.
▶ Obtain a history of the patient's hematopoietic system, symptoms, and results of previously performed laboratory tests and diagnostic and surgical procedures.
▶ Note any recent procedures that can interfere with test results.
▶ Obtain a list of the patient's current medications, including herbs, nutritional supplements, and nutraceuticals (see Appendix F).
▶ Review the procedure with the patient. Inform the patient that specimen collection takes approximately 5 to 10 min. Address concerns about pain and explain that there may be some discomfort during the venipuncture.
▶ *Sensitivity to social and cultural issues,* as well as concern for modesty, is important in providing psychological support before, during, and after the procedure.
▶ There are no food, fluid, or medication restrictions unless by medical direction.

INTRATEST:
▶ If the patient has a history of allergic reaction to latex, avoid the use of equipment containing latex.
▶ Instruct the patient to cooperate fully and to follow directions. Direct the patient to breathe normally and to avoid unnecessary movement.
▶ Observe standard precautions, and follow the general guidelines in Appendix A. Positively identify the patient, and label the appropriate tubes with the corresponding patient demographics, date, and time of collection. Perform a venipuncture.
▶ Remove the needle and apply direct pressure with dry gauze to stop bleeding. Observe/assess venipuncture site for bleeding or hematoma formation and secure gauze with adhesive bandage.
▶ Promptly transport the specimen to the laboratory for processing and analysis.

POST-TEST:
▶ A report of the results will be sent to the requesting health-care provider (HCP), who will discuss the results with the patient.
▶ Reinforce information given by the patient's HCP regarding further testing, treatment, or referral to another HCP. Answer any questions or address any concerns voiced by the patient or family.
▶ Depending on the results of this procedure, additional testing may be performed to evaluate or monitor progression of the disease process and determine the need for a change in therapy. Evaluate test results in relation to the patient's symptoms and other tests performed.

▶ Related tests include biopsy bone marrow, blood gases, CBC, CBC hematocrit, CBC hemoglobin, CBC RBC morphology, methemoglobin, osmotic fragility, and sickle cell screen.
▶ Refer to the Hematopoietic System table at the end of the book for related tests by body system.

Hemosiderin

SYNONYM/ACRONYM: Hemosiderin stain, Pappenheimer body stain, iron stain.

COMMON USE: To assist in investigating recent intravascular hemolysis and to assist in the diagnosis of unexplained anemias, hemochromatosis, and renal tube damage.

SPECIMEN: Urine (5 mL) from a random first morning sample, collected in a clean plastic collection container.

REFERENCE VALUE: (Method: Microscopic examination of Prussian blue–stained specimen) None seen.

DESCRIPTION: Hemosiderin stain is used to indicate the presence of iron storage granules called *hemosiderin* by microscopic examination of urine sediment. Granules of hemosiderin stain blue when potassium ferrocyanide is added to the sample. Hemosiderin is normally found in the liver, spleen, and bone marrow, but not in the urine. Under normal conditions, hemosiderin is absorbed by the renal tubules; however, in extensive hemolysis, renal tubule damage, or an iron metabolism disorder, hemosiderin filters its way into the urine. The Prussian blue stain may also be used to identify siderocytes (iron-containing red blood cells [RBCs]) in peripheral blood. The presence of siderocytes in circulating RBCs is abnormal.

INDICATIONS
• Assist in the diagnosis of hemochromatosis (tissue damage caused by iron toxicity)
• Detect excessive RBC hemolysis within the systemic circulation
• Evaluate renal tubule dysfunction

POTENTIAL DIAGNOSIS

Increased in
Any condition that involves hemolysis will release hemoglobin from RBCs into circulation. Hemoglobin is converted to hemosiderin in the renal tubular epithelial cells.
• Burns
• Cold hemagglutinin disease
• Hemochromatosis
• Hemolytic transfusion reactions
• Mechanical trauma to RBCs
• Megaloblastic anemia
• Microangiopathic hemolytic anemia
• Paroxysmal nocturnal hemoglobinuria
• Pernicious anemia

- Sickle cell anemia
- Thalassemia major

Decreased in: N/A

CRITICAL FINDINGS: N/A

INTERFERING FACTORS: N/A

NURSING IMPLICATIONS AND PROCEDURE

PRETEST:

- Positively identify the patient using at least two unique identifiers before providing care, treatment, or services.
- *Patient Teaching:* Inform the patient this test can assist in diagnosing various types of anemias.
- Obtain a history of the patient's complaints, including a list of known allergens, especially allergies or sensitivities to latex.
- Obtain a history of the patient's hematopoietic system, especially a history of hemolytic anemia; symptoms; and results of previously performed laboratory tests and diagnostic and surgical procedures.
- Obtain a list of the patient's current medications, including herbs, nutritional supplements, and nutraceuticals (see Appendix F).
- Review the procedure with the patient. Inform the patient that specimen collection takes approximately 5 to 10 min. Address concerns about pain and explain that there should be no discomfort during the procedure.
- *Sensitivity to social and cultural issues*, as well as concern for modesty, is important in providing psychological support before, during, and after the procedure.
- There are no food, fluid, or medication restrictions unless by medical direction.

INTRATEST:

- If the patient has a history of allergic reaction to latex, avoid the use of equipment containing latex.
- Instruct the patient to cooperate fully and to follow directions.

- Observe standard precautions, and follow the general guidelines in Appendix A. Positively identify the patient, and label the appropriate collection container with the corresponding patient demographics, date, and time of collection.

Clean-Catch Specimen
- Instruct the male patient to (1) thoroughly wash his hands, (2) cleanse the meatus, (3) void a small amount into the toilet, and (4) void directly into the specimen container.
- Instruct the female patient to (1) thoroughly wash her hands; (2) cleanse the labia from front to back; (3) while keeping the labia separated, void a small amount into the toilet; and (4) without interrupting the urine stream, void directly into the specimen container.

Indwelling Catheter
- Put on gloves. Empty drainage tube of urine. It may be necessary to clamp off the catheter for 15 to 30 min before specimen collection. Cleanse specimen port with antiseptic swab, and then aspirate 5 mL of urine with a 21- to 25-gauge needle and syringe. Transfer urine to a collection container.

General
- Promptly transport the specimen to the laboratory for processing and analysis.

POST-TEST:

- A report of the results will be sent to the requesting health-care provider (HCP), who will discuss the results with the patient.
- Recognize anxiety related to test results. Discuss the implications of abnormal test results on the patient's lifestyle. Provide teaching and information regarding the clinical implications of the test results, as appropriate.
- Reinforce information given by the patient's HCP regarding further testing, treatment, or referral to another HCP. Answer any questions or address any concerns voiced by the patient or family.
- Depending on the results of this procedure, additional testing may be

performed to evaluate or monitor progression of the disease process and determine the need for a change in therapy. Evaluate test results in relation to the patient's symptoms and other tests performed.

RELATED MONOGRAPHS:

▸ Related tests include biopsy bone marrow, biopsy kidney, BUN, CBC, CBC

hematocrit, CBC hemoglobin, CBC RBC count, CBC RBC morphology, CBC WBC count and differential, CT renal, creatinine, creatinine clearance, D-dimer, ferritin, iron/total iron-binding capacity, lead, aPTT, PT/INR, and transferrin.

▸ Refer to the Hematopoietic System table at the end of the book for related tests by body system.

Hepatitis A Antibody

SYNONYM/ACRONYM: HAV serology.

COMMON USE: To test blood for the presence of antibodies that would indicate a past or current hepatitis A infection.

SPECIMEN: Serum (1 mL) collected in a red- or tiger-top tube.

REFERENCE VALUE: (Method: Enzyme immunoassay) Negative.

DESCRIPTION: The hepatitis A virus (HAV) is classified as a picornavirus. Its primary mode of transmission is by the fecal-oral route under conditions of poor personal hygiene or inadequate sanitation. The incubation period is about 28 days, with a range of 15 to 50 days. Onset is usually abrupt, with the acute disease lasting about 1 wk. Therapy is supportive, and there is no development of chronic or carrier states. Assays for total (immunoglobulin G and immunoglobulin M [IgM]) hepatitis A antibody and IgM-specific hepatitis A antibody assist in differentiating recent infection from prior exposure. If results from the IgM-specific or from both assays are positive, recent infection is suspected. If the IgM-specific test results are negative and the total antibody test results are positive, past

infection is indicated. The clinically significant assay—IgM-specific antibody—is often the only test requested. Jaundice occurs in 70% to 80% of adult cases of HAV infection and in 70% of pediatric cases.

INDICATIONS

- Screen individuals at high risk of exposure, such as those in long-term residential facilities or correctional facilities
- Screen individuals with suspected HAV infection

POTENTIAL DIAGNOSIS

Positive findings in
- Individuals with current HAV infection
- Individuals with past HAV infection

CRITICAL FINDINGS: N/A

INTERFERING FACTORS: N/A

NURSING IMPLICATIONS AND PROCEDURE

PRETEST:

▶ Positively identify the patient using at least two unique identifiers before providing care, treatment, or services.
▶ *Patient Teaching:* Inform the patient this test can assist in evaluating for hepatitis infection.
▶ Obtain a history of the patient's complaints, including a list of known allergens, especially allergies or sensitivities to latex.
▶ Obtain a history of the patient's hepatobiliary and immune systems, symptoms, and results of previously performed laboratory tests and diagnostic and surgical procedures.
▶ Obtain a list of the patient's current medications, including herbs, nutritional supplements, and nutraceuticals (see Appendix F).
▶ Review the procedure with the patient. Inform the patient that specimen collection takes approximately 5 to 10 min. Address concerns about pain and explain that there may be some discomfort during the venipuncture.
▶ There are no food, fluid, or medication restrictions unless by medical direction.

INTRATEST:

▶ If the patient has a history of allergic reaction to latex, avoid the use of equipment containing latex.
▶ Instruct the patient to cooperate fully and to follow directions. Direct the patient to breathe normally and to avoid unnecessary movement.
▶ Observe standard precautions, and follow the general guidelines in Appendix A . Positively identify the patient, and label the appropriate tubes with the corresponding patient demographics, date, and time of collection. Perform a venipuncture.
▶ Remove the needle and apply direct pressure with dry gauze to stop bleeding. Observe/assess venipuncture site for bleeding or hematoma formation and secure gauze with adhesive bandage.
▶ Promptly transport the specimen to the laboratory for processing and analysis.

POST-TEST:

▶ A report of the results will be sent to the requesting health-care provider (HCP), who will discuss the results with the patient.
▶ *Nutritional Considerations:* Dietary recommendations may be indicated and will vary depending on the type and severity of the condition. Elimination of alcohol ingestion and a diet optimized for convalescence are commonly included in the treatment plan.
▶ *Social and Cultural Considerations:* Recognize anxiety related to test results, and offer support. Discuss the implications of abnormal test results on the patient's lifestyle. Provide teaching and information regarding the clinical implications of the test results, as appropriate. Counsel the patient, as appropriate, regarding risk of transmission and proper prophylaxis. Immune globulin can be given before exposure (in the case of individuals who may be traveling to a location where the disease is endemic) or after exposure, during the incubation period. Prophylaxis is most effective when administered 2 wk after exposure.
▶ Reinforce information given by the patient's HCP regarding further testing, treatment, or referral to another HCP. Provide information regarding vaccine-preventable diseases where indicated (e.g., encephalitis, hepatitis A and B, human papillomavirus, influenza, measles, mumps, polio, rubella, smallpox, varicella, yellow fever). Answer any questions or address any concerns voiced by the patient or family.
▶ Depending on the results of this procedure, additional testing may be performed to evaluate or monitor progression of the disease process and determine the need for a change in therapy. Evaluate test results in relation to the patient's symptoms and other tests performed.

RELATED MONOGRAPHS:

▶ Related tests include ALT, ALP, AST, bilirubin, GGT, and HBV and HBC antigens and antibodies.
▶ Refer to the Hepatobiliary and Immune systems tables at the end of the book for related tests by body system.

Hepatitis B Antigen and Antibody

SYNONYM/ACRONYM: HBeAg, HBeAb, HBcAb, HBsAb, HBsAg.

COMMON USE: To test blood for the presence of antibodies that would indicate a past or current hepatitis B infection.

SPECIMEN: Serum (1 mL) collected in a red- or tiger-top tube.

REFERENCE VALUE: (Method: Enzyme immunoassay) Negative.

DESCRIPTION: The hepatitis B virus (HBV) is classified as a double-stranded DNA retrovirus of the Hepadnaviridae family. Its primary modes of transmission are parenteral, perinatal, and sexual contact. Serological profiles vary with different scenarios (i.e., asymptomatic infection, acute/resolved infection, coinfection, and chronic carrier state). The formation and detectability of markers is also dose dependent. The following description refers to HBV infection that becomes resolved. The incubation period is generally 6 to 16 wk. The hepatitis B surface antigen (HBsAg) is the first marker to appear after infection. It is detectable 8 to 12 wk after exposure and often precedes symptoms. At about the time liver enzymes fall back to normal levels, the HBsAg titer has fallen to nondetectable levels. If the HBsAg remains detectable after 6 mo, the patient will likely become a chronic carrier who can transmit the virus. Hepatitis Be antigen (HBeAg) appears in the serum 10 to 12 wk after exposure. HBeAg can be found in the serum of patients with acute or chronic HBV infection and is a sign of active viral replication and infectivity. Levels of hepatitis Be antibody (HBeAb) appear about 14 wk after exposure, suggesting resolution of the infection and reduction of the patient's ability to transmit the disease. The more quickly HBeAg disappears, the shorter the acute phase of the infection. Immunoglobulin M–specific hepatitis B core antibody (HBcAb) appears 6 to 14 wk after exposure to HBsAg and continues to be detectable either until the infection is resolved or over the life span in patients who are in a chronic carrier state. In some cases, HBcAb may be the only detectable marker; hence, its lone appearance has sometimes been referred to as the *core window*. HBcAb is not an indicator of recovery or immunity; however, it does indicate current or previous infection. Hepatitis B surface antibody (HBsAb) appears 2 to 16 wk after HBsAg disappears. Appearance of HBsAb represents clinical recovery and immunity to the virus.

Onset of HBV infection is usually insidious. Most children and half of infected adults are asymptomatic. During the acute phase of infection, symptoms range from mild to

H

severe. Chronicity decreases with age. HBsAg and HBcAb tests are used to screen donated blood before transfusion. HBsAg testing is often part of the routine prenatal screen. Vaccination of infants, children, and young adults is becoming a standard of care and in some cases a requirement.

INDICATIONS
- Detect exposure to HBV
- Detect possible carrier status
- Pre- and postvaccination testing
- Routine prenatal testing
- Screen donated blood before transfusion
- Screen for individuals at high risk of exposure, such as hemodialysis patients, persons with multiple sex partners, persons with a history of other sexually transmitted diseases, IV drug abusers, infants born to infected mothers, individuals residing in long-term residential facilities or correctional facilities, recipients of blood- or plasma-derived products, allied health-care workers, and public service employees who come in contact with blood and blood products

POTENTIAL DIAGNOSIS

Positive findings in
- Patients currently infected with HBV
- Patients with a past HBV infection

CRITICAL FINDINGS: N/A

INTERFERING FACTORS
- Drugs that may decrease HBeAb and HBsAb include interferon.

NURSING IMPLICATIONS AND PROCEDURE

PRETEST:
- Positively identify the patient using at least two unique identifiers before providing care, treatment, or services.
- *Patient Teaching:* Inform the patient this test can assist in evaluating for hepatitis infection.
- Obtain a history of the patient's complaints, including a list of known allergens, especially allergies or sensitivities to latex.
- Obtain a history of the patient's hepatobiliary and immune systems, symptoms, and results of previously performed laboratory tests and diagnostic and surgical procedures.
- Obtain a history of IV drug use, high-risk sexual activity, or occupational exposure.
- Obtain a list of the patient's current medications, including herbs, nutritional supplements, and nutraceuticals (see Appendix F).
- Review the procedure with the patient. Inform the patient that specimen collection takes approximately 5 to 10 min. Address concerns about pain and explain that there may be some discomfort during the venipuncture.
- *Sensitivity to social and cultural issues,* as well as concern for modesty, is important in providing psychological support before, during, and after the procedure.
- There are no food, fluid, or medication restrictions unless by medical direction.

INTRATEST:
- If the patient has a history of allergic reaction to latex, avoid the use of equipment containing latex.
- Instruct the patient to cooperate fully and to follow directions. Direct the patient to breathe normally and to avoid unnecessary movement.
- Observe standard precautions, and follow the general guidelines in Appendix A. Positively identify the patient, and label the appropriate tubes with the corresponding patient demographics, date, and time of collection. Perform a venipuncture.

- Remove the needle and apply direct pressure with dry gauze to stop bleeding. Observe/assess venipuncture site for bleeding or hematoma formation and secure gauze with adhesive bandage.
- Promptly transport the specimen to the laboratory for processing and analysis.

POST-TEST:

- A report of the results will be sent to the requesting health-care provider (HCP), who will discuss the results with the patient.
- *Nutritional Considerations:* Dietary recommendations may be indicated and will vary depending on the type and severity of the condition. Elimination of alcohol ingestion and a diet optimized for convalescence are commonly included in the treatment plan. A high-calorie, high-protein, moderate-fat diet with a high fluid intake is often recommended for patients with hepatitis.
- *Cultural and Social Considerations:* Recognize anxiety related to test results, and be supportive of impaired activity related to lack of neuromuscular control, perceived loss of independence, and fear of shortened life expectancy. Discuss the implications of abnormal test results on the patient's lifestyle. Provide teaching and information regarding the clinical implications of the test results, as appropriate. Educate the patient regarding access to counseling services. Counsel the patient, as appropriate, regarding risk of transmission and proper prophylaxis. Hepatitis B immune globulin (HBIG) vaccination should be given immediately after situations in which there is a potential for HBV exposure (e.g., accidental needle stick, perinatal period, sexual contact) for temporary, passive protection. Some studies have indicated that interferon alfa may be useful in the treatment of chronic hepatitis B.
- Counsel the patient and significant contacts, as appropriate, that HBIG immunization is available and has in fact become a requirement in many places as part of childhood immunization and employee health programs. Parents may choose to sign a waiver preventing their newborns from

receiving the vaccine; they may choose not to vaccinate on the basis of philosophical, religious, or medical reasons. Vaccination regulations vary by state.
- Inform the patient that positive findings must be reported to local health department officials, who will question him or her regarding sexual partners.
- *Sensitivity to Social and Cultural Considerations:* Offer support, as appropriate, to patients who may be the victims of rape or other forms of sexual assault, including children and elderly individuals. Educate the patient regarding access to counseling services. Provide a nonjudgmental, nonthreatening atmosphere for a discussion during which the risks of sexually transmitted diseases are explained. It is also important to discuss the problems that the patient may experience (e.g., guilt, depression, anger).
- Reinforce information given by the patient's HCP regarding further testing, treatment, or referral to another HCP. Provide information regarding vaccine-preventable diseases where indicated (e.g., encephalitis, hepatitis A and B, human papillomavirus, influenza, measles, mumps, polio, rubella, smallpox, varicella, yellow fever). Answer any questions or address any concerns voiced by the patient or family.
- Depending on the results of this procedure, additional testing may be performed to evaluate or monitor progression of the disease process and determine the need for a change in therapy. Evaluate test results in relation to the patient's symptoms and other tests performed.

RELATED MONOGRAPHS:

- Related tests include ALT, ALP, antibodies, antimitochondrial, AST, bilirubin, biopsy liver, *Chlamydia* group antibody, cholangiography percutaneous transhepatic, culture anal, GGT, hepatitis C serology, HIV serology, liver and spleen scan, syphilis serology, and US liver.
- Refer to the Hepatobiliary and Immune systems tables at the end of the book for related tests by body system.

Hepatitis C Antibody

SYNONYM/ACRONYM: HCV serology, hepatitis non-A/non-B.

COMMON USE: To test blood for the presence of antibodies that would indicate a past or current hepatitis C infection.

SPECIMEN: Serum (1 mL) collected in a red- or tiger-top tube.

REFERENCE VALUE: (Method: Enzyme immunoassay, branched chain DNA [bDNA], polymerase chain reaction [PCR], recombinant immunoblot assay [RIBA]) Negative.

DESCRIPTION: The hepatitis C virus (HCV) causes the majority of bloodborne non-A/non-B hepatitis cases. Its primary modes of transmission are parenteral, perinatal, and sexual contact. The virus is thought to be a flavivirus and contains a single-stranded RNA core. The incubation period varies widely, from 2 to 52 wk. Onset is insidious, and the risk of chronic liver disease after infection is high. On average, antibodies to hepatitis C are detectable in approximately 45% of infected individuals within 6 wk of infection. The remaining 55% produce antibodies within the next 6 to 12 mo. Once infected with HCV, 50% of patients will become chronic carriers. Infected individuals and carriers have a high frequency of chronic liver diseases such as cirrhosis and chronic active hepatitis, and they have a higher risk of developing hepatocellular cancer. The transmission of hepatitis C by blood transfusion has decreased dramatically since it became part of the routine screening panel for blood donors. The possibility of prenatal transmission exists, especially in the presence of HIV coinfection. Therefore, this test is often included in prenatal testing packages. Currently, nucleic acid amplification testing (NAT) is the only way to document the presence of ongoing infection. PCR and bDNA methods are recognized by the Centers for Disease Control and Prevention (CDC) as appropriate supplemental testing for the confirmation of anti-HCV antibody.

INDICATIONS
- Assist in the diagnosis of non-A/non-B viral hepatitis infection
- Monitor patients suspected of HCV infection but who have not yet produced antibody
- Routine prenatal testing
- Screen donated blood before transfusion

POTENTIAL DIAGNOSIS

Positive findings in
- Patients currently infected with HCV
- Patients with a past HCV infection

Negative findings in: N/A

CRITICAL FINDINGS: N/A

INTERFERING FACTORS
- Drugs that may decrease hepatitis C antibody levels include interferon.

NURSING IMPLICATIONS AND PROCEDURE

PRETEST:

- Positively identify the patient using at least two unique identifiers before providing care, treatment, or services.
- *Patient Teaching:* Inform the patient this test can assist in evaluating for hepatitis infection.
- Obtain a history of the patient's complaints, including a list of known allergens, especially allergies or sensitivities to latex.
- Obtain a history of the patient's hepatobiliary and immune systems, symptoms, and results of previously performed laboratory tests and diagnostic and surgical procedures.
- Obtain a history of IV drug use, high-risk sexual activity, and occupational exposure.
- Obtain a list of the patient's current medications, including herbs, nutritional supplements, and nutraceuticals (see Appendix F).
- Review the procedure with the patient. Inform the patient that specimen collection takes approximately 5 to 10 min. Address concerns about pain and explain that there may be some discomfort during the venipuncture.
- *Sensitivity to social and cultural issues,* as well as concern for modesty, is important in providing psychological support before, during, and after the procedure.
- There are no food, fluid, or medication restrictions unless by medical direction.

INTRATEST:

- If the patient has a history of allergic reaction to latex, avoid the use of equipment containing latex.
- Instruct the patient to cooperate fully and to follow directions. Direct the patient to breathe normally and to avoid unnecessary movement.
- Observe standard precautions, and follow the general guidelines in Appendix A. Positively identify the patient, and label the appropriate tubes with the corresponding patient

demographics, date, and time of collection. Perform a venipuncture.
- Remove the needle and apply direct pressure with dry gauze to stop bleeding. Observe/assess venipuncture site for bleeding or hematoma formation and secure gauze with adhesive bandage.
- Promptly transport the specimen to the laboratory for processing and analysis.

POST-TEST:

- A report of the results will be sent to the requesting health-care provider (HCP), who will discuss the results with the patient.
- *Nutritional Considerations:* Dietary recommendations may be indicated and will vary depending on the type and severity of the condition. Currently, for example, there are no specific medications that can be given to cure hepatitis; however, bedrest, elimination of alcohol ingestion, and a diet optimized for convalescence are commonly included in the treatment plan. A high-calorie, high-protein, moderate-fat diet with a high fluid intake is often recommended for patients with hepatitis.
- *Cultural and Social Considerations:* Recognize anxiety related to test results, and be supportive of impaired activity related to lack of neuromuscular control, perceived loss of independence, and fear of shortened life expectancy. Discuss the implications of abnormal test results on the patient's lifestyle. Provide teaching and information regarding the clinical implications of the test results, as appropriate. Educate the patient regarding access to counseling services. Counsel the patient, as appropriate, regarding the risk of transmission and proper prophylaxis. Interferon alfa was approved in 1991 by the U.S. Food and Drug Administration for use as a therapeutic agent in the treatment of chronic HCV infection.
- Inform the patient that positive findings must be reported to local health department officials, who will question him or her regarding sexual partners.

▶ *Sensitivity to Social and Cultural Considerations:* Offer support, as appropriate, to patients who may be the victims of rape or other forms of sexual assault, including children and elderly individuals. Educate the patient regarding access to counseling services. Provide a nonjudgmental, nonthreatening atmosphere for a discussion during which the risks of sexually transmitted diseases are explained. It is also important to discuss the problems that the patient may experience (e.g., guilt, depression, anger).

▶ Reinforce information given by the patient's HCP regarding further testing, treatment, or referral to another HCP. Answer any questions or address any concerns voiced by the patient or family.

▶ Depending on the results of this procedure, additional testing may be performed to evaluate or monitor progression of the disease process and determine the need for a change in therapy. Evaluate test results in relation to the patient's symptoms and other tests performed.

RELATED MONOGRAPHS:

▶ Related tests include ALT, ALP, antibodies, antimitochondrial, AST, bilirubin, biopsy liver, *Chlamydia* group antibody, cholangiography percutaneous transhepatic, culture anal, GGT, hepatitis B serology, hepatobiliary scan, HIV serology, liver and spleen scan, syphilis serology, and US liver.

▶ Refer to the Hepatobiliary and Immune systems tables at the end of the book for related tests by body system.

H

Hepatitis D Antibody

SYNONYM/ACRONYM: Delta hepatitis.

COMMON USE: To test blood for the presence of antibodies that would indicate a past or current hepatitis D infection.

SPECIMEN: Serum (1 mL) collected in a red- or tiger-top tube.

REFERENCE VALUE: (Method: Enzyme immunoassay, EIA) Negative.

POTENTIAL DIAGNOSIS

Positive findings in
• Individuals currently infected with HDV

• Individuals with a past HDV infection

CRITICAL FINDINGS: N/A

Find and print out the full monograph at DavisPlus (http://davisplus.fadavis.com, keyword Van Leeuwen).

Hepatobiliary Scan

SYNONYM/ACRONYM: Biliary tract radionuclide scan, cholescintigraphy, hepatobiliary imaging, hepatobiliary scintigraphy, gallbladder scan, HIDA (a technetium-99m diisopropyl analogue) scan.

COMMON USE: To visualize and assess the cystic and common bile ducts of the gall bladder to assist in diagnosing obstructions, stones, inflammation, and tumor.

AREA OF APPLICATION: Bile ducts.

CONTRAST: IV contrast medium (aminodiacetic acid compounds), usually combined with technetium-99m.

DESCRIPTION: The hepatobiliary scan is a nuclear medicine study of the hepatobiliary excretion system. It is primarily used to determine the patency of the cystic and common bile ducts, but it can also be used to determine overall hepatic function, gallbladder function, presence of gallstones (indirectly), and sphincter of Oddi dysfunction. Technetium (Tc-99m) HIDA (tribromoethyl, an aminodiacetic acid) is injected IV and excreted into the bile duct system. A gamma camera detects the radiation emitted from the injected contrast medium, and a representative image of the duct system is obtained. The results are correlated with other diagnostic studies, such as IV cholangiography, computed tomography (CT) scan of the gallbladder, and ultrasonography. Gallbladder emptying or ejection fraction can be determined by administering a fatty meal or cholecystokinin to the patient. This procedure can be used before and after surgery to determine the extent of bile reflux.

INDICATIONS
- Aid in the diagnosis of acute and chronic cholecystitis
- Aid in the diagnosis of suspected gallbladder disorders, such as inflammation, perforation, or calculi
- Assess enterogastric reflux
- Assess obstructive jaundice when done in combination with radiography or ultrasonography
- Determine common duct obstruction caused by tumors or choledocholithiasis
- Evaluate biliary enteric bypass patency
- Postoperatively evaluate gastric surgical procedures and abdominal trauma

POTENTIAL DIAGNOSIS

Normal findings in
- Normal shape, size, and function of the gallbladder with patent cystic and common bile ducts

Abnormal findings in
- Cholecystitis (acalculous, acute, chronic)

- Common bile duct obstruction secondary to gallstones, tumor, or stricture
- Congenital biliary atresia or chole-dochal cyst
- Postoperative biliary leak, fistula, or obstruction
- Trauma-induced bile leak or cyst

CRITICAL FINDINGS: N/A

INTERFERING FACTORS

This procedure is contraindicated for

- Patients who are pregnant or suspected of being pregnant, unless the potential benefits of the procedure far outweigh the risks to the fetus and mother.

Factors that may impair clear imaging

- Inability of the patient to cooperate or remain still during the procedure because of age, significant pain, or mental status.
- Retained barium from a previous radiological procedure.
- Metallic objects (e.g., jewelry, body rings) within the examination field, which may inhibit organ visualization and cause unclear images.
- Bilirubin levels greater than or equal to 30 mg/dL, depending on the radionuclide used, which may decrease hepatic uptake.
- Other nuclear scans done within the previous 24 to 48 hr.
- Fasting for more than 24 hr before the procedure, total parenteral nutrition, and alcoholism.
- Ingestion of food or liquids within 2 to 4 hr before the scan.

Other considerations

- Failure to follow dietary restrictions before the procedure may cause the procedure to be canceled or repeated.
- Improper injection of the radionuclide that allows the tracer to seep deep into the muscle tissue can produce erroneous hot spots.
- Inaccurate timing of imaging after the radionuclide injection can affect the results.
- Consultation with a health-care provider (HCP) should occur before the procedure for radiation safety concerns regarding younger patients or patients who are lactating.
- Risks associated with radiation overexposure can result from frequent x-ray or radionuclide procedures. Personnel working in the examination area should wear badges to record their level of radiation exposure.

NURSING IMPLICATIONS AND PROCEDURE

PRETEST:

- Positively identify the patient using at least two unique identifiers before providing care, treatment, or services.
- *Patient Teaching:* Inform the patient this procedure can assist in detecting inflammation or obstruction of the gallbladder or ducts.
- Obtain a history of the patient's complaints, including a list of known allergens, especially allergies or sensitivities to latex, iodine, seafood, contrast medium, anesthetics, or dyes.
- Obtain a history of the patient's hepatobiliary system, symptoms, and results of previously performed laboratory tests and diagnostic and surgical procedures.
- Note any recent procedures that can interfere with test results, including examinations using iodine-based contrast medium.

- Record the date of the last menstrual period and determine the possibility of pregnancy in perimenopausal women.
- Obtain a list of the patient's current medications, including herbs, nutritional supplements, and nutraceuticals (see Appendix F).
- Review the procedure with the patient. Address concerns about pain and explain that some pain may be experienced during the test, or there may be moments of discomfort. Reassure the patient that the radionuclide poses no radioactive hazard and rarely produces side effects. Inform the patient the procedure is performed in a nuclear medicine department by an HCP specializing in this procedure, with support staff, and takes approximately 30 to 60 min.
- Inform the patient that the HCP will place him or her in a supine position on a flat table.
- *Sensitivity to social and cultural issues,* as well as concern for modesty, is important in providing psychological support before, during, and after the procedure.
- Instruct the patient to remove jewelry and other metallic objects from the area to be examined prior to the procedure.
- Instruct the patient to restrict food and fluids for 4 to 6 hr prior to the procedure. Protocols may vary among facilities.
- *Make sure a written and informed consent has been signed prior to the procedure and before administering any medications.*

INTRATEST:

- Ensure that the patient has complied with dietary, fluids, and medication restrictions for 4 to 6 hr prior to the procedure.
- Ensure that the patient has removed all external metallic objects prior to the procedure.
- If the patient has a history of allergic reactions to any substance or drug, administer ordered prophylactic steroids or antihistamines before the procedure.
- Have emergency equipment readily available.
- Instruct the patient to void prior to the procedure and to change into the gown, robe, and foot coverings provided.
- Instruct the patient to cooperate fully and to follow directions. Instruct the patient to lie still during the procedure because movement produces unclear images.
- Observe standard precautions, and follow the general guidelines in Appendix A.
- Administer sedative to a child or to an uncooperative adult, as ordered.
- Place the patient in a supine position on a flat table with foam wedges to help maintain position and immobilization.
- IV radionuclide is administered, and the upper right quadrant of the abdomen is scanned immediately, with images then taken every 5 min for the first 30 min and every 10 min for the next 30 min. If the gallbladder cannot be visualized, delayed views are taken in 2, 4, and 24 hr in order to differentiate acute from chronic cholecystitis or to detect the degree of obstruction.
- IV morphine may be administered during the study to initiate spasms of the sphincter of Oddi, forcing the radionuclide into the gallbladder, if the organ is not visualized within 1 hr of injection of the radionuclide. Imaging is then done 20 to 50 min later to determine delayed visualization or nonvisualization of the gallbladder.
- If gallbladder function or bile reflux is being assessed, the patient will be given a fatty meal or cholecystokinin 60 min after the injection.
- Remove the needle or catheter and apply a pressure dressing over the puncture site.

H

▶ Observe the needle/catheter insertion site for bleeding, inflammation, or hematoma formation.

POST-TEST:

▶ A report of the results will be sent to the requesting HCP, who will discuss the results with the patient.
▶ Unless contraindicated, advise patient to drink increased amounts of fluids for 24 to 48 hr to eliminate the radionuclide from the body. Inform the patient that radionuclide is eliminated from the body within 6 to 24 hr.
▶ No other radionuclide tests should be scheduled for 24 to 48 hr after this procedure.
▶ Instruct the patient to resume usual diet, fluids, medications, and activity as directed by the HCP.
▶ Instruct the patient in the care and assessment of the injection site.
▶ If a woman who is breastfeeding must have a nuclear scan, she should not breastfeed the infant until the radionuclide has been eliminated. This could take as long as 3 days. She should be instructed to express the milk and discard it during the 3-day period to prevent cessation of milk production.
▶ Instruct the patient to immediately flush the toilet and to meticulously wash hands with soap and water after each voiding for 24 hr after the procedure.

▶ Instruct all caregivers to wear gloves when discarding urine for 24 hr after the procedure. Wash gloved hands with soap and water before removing gloves. Then wash ungloved hands after the gloves are removed.
▶ Recognize anxiety related to test results, and be supportive of perceived loss of independent function. Discuss the implications of abnormal test results on the patient's lifestyle. Provide teaching and information regarding the clinical implications of the test results, as appropriate.
▶ Reinforce information given by the patient's HCP regarding further testing, treatment, or referral to another HCP. Answer any questions or address any concerns voiced by the patient or family.
▶ Depending on the results of this procedure, additional testing may be needed to evaluate or monitor progression of the disease process and determine the need for a change in therapy. Evaluate test results in relation to the patient's symptoms and other tests performed.

RELATED MONOGRAPHS:

▶ Related tests include amylase, bilirubin, CT abdomen, lipase, liver and spleen scan, MRI abdomen, radiofrequency ablation liver, and US liver and bile ducts.
▶ Refer to the Hepatobiliary System table at the end of the book for related tests by body system.

Hexosaminidase A and B

SYNONYM/ACRONYM: N/A.

COMMON USE: To assist in diagnosing Tay-Sachs disease by identifying a hexosaminidase enzyme deficiency.

SPECIMEN: Serum (3 mL) collected in a red-top tube. After the specimen is collected, it must be brought *immediately* to the laboratory. Once in the laboratory, the specimen must be allowed to clot for 1 to 1.5 hr in the refrigerator. The serum should then be removed and frozen immediately.

REFERENCE VALUE: (Method: Fluorometry)

Total Hexosaminidase	Conventional Units	SI Units (Conventional Units × 0.0167)
Noncarrier	589–955 nmol/hr/mL	9.83–15.95 units/L
Heterozygote	465–675 nmol/hr/mL	3.30–5.39 units/L
Tay-Sachs homozygote	Greater than 1,027 nmol/hr/mL	Greater than 17.15 units/L

Hexosaminidase A	Conventional Units	SI Units (Conventional Units × 0.0167)
Noncarrier	456–592 nmol/hr/mL	7.2–9.88 units/L
Heterozygote	197–323 nmol/hr/mL	3.3–5.39 units/L
Tay-Sachs homozygote	0 nmol/hr/mL	0 units/L

Hexosaminidase B	Conventional Units	SI Units (Conventional Units × 0.0167)
Noncarrier	12–32 nmol/hr/mL	0.2–0.54 units/L
Heterozygote	21–81 nmol/hr/mL	0.35–1.35 units/L
Tay-Sachs homozygote	Greater than 305 nmol/hr/mL	Greater than 5.09 units/L

DESCRIPTION: Hexosaminidase is a lysosomal enzyme. There are three predominant isoenzymes: hexosaminidase A, B, and S. Deficiency results in the accumulation of complex sphingolipids and gangliosides in the brain. There are more than 70 lysozymal enzyme disorders. Testing for hexosaminidase A is done to determine the presence of Tay-Sachs disease, a genetic autosomal recessive condition characterized by early and progressive retardation of physical and mental development. This enzyme deficiency is most common among Ashkenazi Jews. Genetic testing by DNA polymerase chain reaction analysis can identify as many as 94% of the gene mutations associated with Tay-Sachs disease in persons with Ashkenazi Jewish heritage, 80% of the mutations in persons with French-Canadian ancestry, and 25% of mutations in non-Jewish Caucasians. Genetic testing combined with enzyme screening analysis and correlation of clinical information provides the most reliable means of determining carrier status. Patients who are homozygous for this trait have no hexosaminidase A and have greatly elevated levels of hexosaminidase B; signs and symptoms include red spot in the retina, blindness, and muscular weakness. Tay-Sachs disease results in early death, usually by age 3 or 4.

INDICATIONS
- Assist in the diagnosis of Tay-Sachs disease
- Identify carriers with hexosaminidase deficiency

POTENTIAL DIAGNOSIS

Increased in
Alterations in lysosomal enzymes metabolism are associated with various conditions.
- Total
  Gastric cancer
  Hepatic disease
  Myeloma
  Myocardial infarction
  Pregnancy
  Symptomatic porphyria
  Vascular complications of diabetes

- Hexosaminidase A
  Diabetes
  Pregnancy
- Hexosaminidase B
  Tay-Sachs disease

Decreased in
- Total
  Sandhoff's disease *(inherited disorder of enzyme metabolism lacking both essential enzymes for metabolizing gangliosides)*
- Hexosaminidase A
  Tay-Sachs disease *(inherited disorder of enzyme metabolism lacking only the hexosaminidase A enzyme for metabolizing gangliosides)*
- Hexosaminidase B
  Sandhoff's disease

CRITICAL FINDINGS: N/A

INTERFERING FACTORS
- Drugs that may increase hexosaminidase levels include ethanol, isoniazid, oral contraceptives, and rifampin.
- The serum specimen hexosaminidase assay should not be performed on women who are pregnant or who are taking oral contraceptives. Increases in enzyme activity during pregnancy occur in carriers and noncarriers of the Tay-Sachs gene. Enzyme activity is also notably increased in women taking oral contraceptives regardless of carrier status.

NURSING IMPLICATIONS AND PROCEDURE

PRETEST:
- Positively identify the patient using at least two unique identifiers before providing care, treatment, or services.
- *Patient Teaching:* Inform the patient this test can assist in diagnosing or

identifying carrier status for Tay-Sachs disease.

- Obtain a history of the patient's complaints, including a list of known allergens, especially allergies or sensitivities to latex.
- Obtain a history of the patient's reproductive system, symptoms, and results of previously performed laboratory tests and diagnostic and surgical procedures.
- Obtain a list of the patient's current medications, including herbs, nutritional supplements, and nutraceuticals (see Appendix F).
- Review the procedure with the patient. Inform the patient that specimen collection takes approximately 5 to 10 min. Address concerns about pain and explain that there may be some discomfort during the venipuncture.
- *Sensitivity to social and cultural issues,* as well as concern for modesty, is important in providing psychological support before, during, and after the procedure.
- There are no food, fluid, or medication restrictions unless by medical direction.

INTRATEST:

- If the patient has a history of allergic reaction to latex, avoid the use of equipment containing latex.
- Instruct the patient to cooperate fully and to follow directions. Direct the patient to breathe normally and to avoid unnecessary movement.
- Observe standard precautions, and follow the general guidelines in Appendix A. Positively identify the patient, and label the appropriate tubes with the corresponding patient demographics, date, and time of collection. Perform a venipuncture.
- Remove the needle and apply direct pressure with dry gauze to stop bleeding. Observe/assess venipuncture site for bleeding or hematoma formation and secure gauze with adhesive bandage.

- *Immediately* transport the specimen to the laboratory for processing and analysis.

POST-TEST:

- A report of the results will be sent to the requesting health-care provider (HCP), who will discuss the results with the patient.
- Recognize anxiety related to test results, and be supportive of fear of shortened life expectancy. Discuss the implications of abnormal test results on the patient's lifestyle. Provide teaching and information regarding the clinical implications of the test results, as appropriate. Encourage the family to seek genetic counseling if results are abnormal. It is also important to discuss feelings the mother and father may experience (e.g., guilt, depression, anger) if abnormalities are detected. Educate the patient regarding access to counseling services. Provide contact information, if desired, for the National Tay Sachs and Allied Diseases Association (www.ntsad.org).
- Reinforce information given by the patient's HCP regarding further testing, treatment, or referral to another HCP. Answer any questions or address any concerns voiced by the patient or family.
- Depending on the results of this procedure, additional testing may be performed to evaluate or monitor progression of the disease process and determine the need for a change in therapy. Evaluate test results in relation to the patient's symptoms and other tests performed.

RELATED MONOGRAPHS:

- Related tests include ALT, amniotic fluid analysis, bilirubin, biopsy chorionic villus, biopsy liver, chromosome analysis, GGT, liver and spleen scan, and protein total and fractions.
- Refer to the Reproductive System table at the end of the book for related tests by body system.

H

Holter Monitor

SYNONYM/ACRONYM: Ambulatory electrocardiography, ambulatory monitoring, event recorder, Holter electrocardiography.

COMMON USE: To evaluate cardiac symptoms associated with activity to assist with diagnosis of arrhythmias and cardiomegaly.

AREA OF APPLICATION: Heart.

CONTRAST: None.

DESCRIPTION: The Holter monitor records electrical cardiac activity on a continuous basis for 24 to 48 hr. This noninvasive study includes the use of a portable device worn around the waist or over the shoulder that records cardiac electrical impulses on a magnetic tape. The recorder has a clock that allows accurate time markings on the tape. The patient is asked to keep a log or diary of daily activities and to record any occurrence of cardiac symptoms. When the client pushes a button indicating that symptoms (e.g., pain, palpitations, dyspnea, syncope) have occurred, an event marker is placed on the tape for later comparison with the cardiac activity recordings and the daily activity log. Some recorders allow the data to be transferred to the physician's office by telephone, where the tape is interpreted by a computer to detect any significantly abnormal variations in the recorded waveform patterns.

- Evaluate activity intolerance related to oxygen supply and demand imbalance
- Evaluate chest pain, dizziness, syncope, and palpitations
- Evaluate the effectiveness of antiarrhythmic medications for dosage adjustment, if needed
- Evaluate pacemaker function
- Monitor for ischemia and arrhythmias after myocardial infarction or cardiac surgery before changing rehabilitation and other therapy regimens

POTENTIAL DIAGNOSIS

Normal findings in
- Normal sinus rhythm

Abnormal findings in
- Arrhythmias such as premature ventricular contractions, bradyarrhythmias, tachyarrhythmias, conduction defects, and bradycardia
- Cardiomyopathy
- Hypoxic or ischemic changes
- Mitral valve abnormality
- Palpitations

CRITICAL FINDINGS: N/A

INTERFERING FACTORS

Factors that may impair the results of the examination
- Improper placement of the electrodes or movement of the electrodes.

INDICATIONS
- Detect arrhythmias that occur during normal daily activities and correlate them with symptoms experienced by the patient

• Failure of the patient to maintain a daily log of symptoms or to push the button to produce a mark on the strip when experiencing a symptom.

NURSING IMPLICATIONS AND PROCEDURE

PRETEST:

▶ Positively identify the patient using at least two unique identifiers before providing care, treatment, or services.

▶ *Patient Teaching:* Inform the patient this procedure can assist in evaluating the heart's response to exercise or medication.

▶ Obtain a history of the patient's complaints or symptoms, including a list of known allergens, especially allergies or sensitivities to latex, iodine, seafood, anesthetics, or contrast mediums.

▶ Obtain a history of the patient's cardiovascular system, symptoms, and results of previously performed laboratory tests and diagnostic and surgical procedures.

▶ Obtain a list of the patient's current medications, including herbs, nutritional supplements, and nutraceuticals (see Appendix F).

▶ Review the procedure with the patient. Address concerns about pain related to the procedure and explain that no electricity is delivered to the body during this procedure and no discomfort is experienced during monitoring. Inform the patient that the electrocardiography (ECG) recorder is worn for 24 to 48 hr, at which time the patient is to return to the laboratory with an activity log to have the monitor and strip removed for interpretation.

▶ *Sensitivity to social and cultural issues,* as well as concern for modesty, is important in providing psychological support before, during, and after the procedure.

▶ Instruct the patient to wear loose-fitting clothing over the electrodes and not to disturb or disconnect the electrodes or wires.

▶ Advise the patient to avoid contact with electrical devices that can affect the strip tracings (e.g., shavers, toothbrush, massager, blanket) and to avoid showers and tub bathing.

▶ Instruct the patient to perform normal activities, such as walking, sleeping, climbing stairs, sexual activity, bowel or urinary elimination, cigarette smoking, emotional upsets, and medications, and to record them in an activity log.

▶ Instruct the patient regarding recording and pressing the button upon experiencing pain or discomfort.

▶ Advise the patient to report a light signal on the monitor, which indicates equipment malfunction or that an electrode has come off.

▶ There are no food, fluid, or medication restrictions unless by medical direction.

INTRATEST:

▶ Instruct the patient to void prior to the procedure and to change into the gown, robe, and foot coverings provided.

▶ Instruct the patient to cooperate fully and to follow directions.

▶ Observe standard precautions, and follow the general guidelines in Appendix A.

▶ Place the patient in a supine position.

▶ Expose the chest. Shave excessive hair at the skin sites; cleanse thoroughly with alcohol and rub until red in color.

▶ Apply electropaste to the skin sites to provide conduction between the skin and electrodes, or apply prelubricated disposable disk electrodes.

▶ Apply two electrodes (negative electrodes) on the manubrium, one in the V_1 position (fourth intercostal space at the border of the right sternum), and one at the V_5 position (level of the fifth intercostal space at the midclavicular line, horizontally and at the left axillary line). A ground electrode is also placed and secured to the skin of the chest or abdomen.

▶ After checking to ensure that the electrodes are secure, attach the electrode cable to the monitor and the lead wires to the electrodes.

▶ Check the monitor for paper supply and battery, insert the tape, and turn on the recorder. Tape all wires to the chest, and place the belt or shoulder strap in the proper position.

H

POST-TEST:

▶ After the patient has worn the monitor for the required 24 to 48 hr, gently remove the tape and other items securing the electrodes to him or her.

▶ The activity log and tape recording are compared for changes during the monitoring period.

▶ A report of the examination will be sent to the requesting health-care provider (HCP), who will discuss the results with the patient.

▶ Advise the patient to immediately report symptoms such as fast heart rate or difficulty breathing.

▶ Recognize anxiety related to test results, and be supportive of perceived loss of independence and fear of shortened life expectancy. Discuss the implications of abnormal test results on the patient's lifestyle. Provide teaching and information regarding the clinical implications of the test results, as appropriate. Educate the patient regarding access to counseling services.

▶ Reinforce information given by the patient's HCP regarding further testing, treatment, or referral to another HCP. Answer any questions or address any concerns voiced by the patient or family.

▶ Depending on the results of this procedure, additional testing may be needed to evaluate or monitor progression of the disease process and determine the need for a change in therapy. Evaluate test results in relation to the patient's symptoms and other tests performed.

RELATED MONOGRAPHS:

▶ Related tests include antiarrhythmic drugs, blood pool imaging, calcium, chest x-ray, echocardiography, echocardiography transesophageal, electrocardiogram, exercise stress test, magnesium, myocardial perfusion heart scan, PET heart, and potassium.

▶ Refer to the Cardiovascular System table at the end of the book for related tests by body system.

Homocysteine and Methylmalonic Acid

SYNONYM/ACRONYM: N/A.

COMMON USE: To assist in evaluating increased risk for blood clots, plaque formation, and platelet aggregations associated with atherosclerosis and stroke risk.

SPECIMEN: Serum (4 mL) collected in a red- or tiger-top tube if methylmalonic acid and homocysteine are to be measured together. Alternatively, plasma collected in a lavender-top (EDTA) tube may be acceptable for the homocysteine measurement. The laboratory should be consulted before specimen collection because specimen type may be method dependent. Care must be taken to use the same type of collection container if serial measurements are to be taken.

REFERENCE VALUE: (Method: Chromatography) Homocysteine: 4.6–11.2 micromol/L; methylmalonic acid: 70–270 nmol/L.

DESCRIPTION: Homocysteine is an amino acid formed from methionine. Normally, homocysteine is rapidly remetabolized in a biochemical pathway that requires vitamin B_{12} and folate, preventing the buildup of homocysteine in the blood. Excess levels damage the endothelial lining of blood vessels; change coagulation factor levels, increasing the risk of blood clot formation and stroke; prevent smaller arteries from dilating, increasing the risk of plaque formation; cause platelet aggregation; and cause smooth muscle cells lining the arterial wall to multiply, promoting atherosclerosis.

Approximately one-third of patients with hyperhomocystinuria have normal fasting levels. Patients with a heterozygous biochemical enzyme defect in cystathionine B synthase or with a nutritional deficiency in vitamin B_6 can be identified through the administration of a methionine challenge or loading test. Specimens are collected while fasting and 2 hr later. An increase in homocysteine after 2 hr is indicative of hyperhomocystinuria. In patients with vitamin B_{12} deficiency, elevated levels of methylmalonic acid and homocysteine develop fairly early in the course of the disease. Unlike vitamin B_{12} levels, homocysteine levels will remain elevated for at least 24 hr after the start of vitamin therapy. This may be useful if vitamin therapy is inadvertently begun before specimen collection. Patients with folate deficiency, for the most part, will only develop elevated homocysteine levels. A methylmalonic acid level can differentiate between vitamin B_{12} and folate deficiency, since it is increased in vitamin B_{12} deficiency, but not in folate deficiency. Hyperhomocysteinemia due to folate deficiency in pregnant women is believed to increase the risk of neural tube defects. Elevated levels of homocysteine are thought to chemically damage the exposed neural tissue of the developing fetus.

INDICATIONS
- Evaluate inherited enzyme deficiencies that result in homocystinuria
- Evaluate the risk for cardiovascular disease
- Evaluate the risk for venous thrombosis

POTENTIAL DIAGNOSIS

Increased in
- Cerebrovascular disease (CVD) *(there is a relationship, but the pathophysiology is unclear)*
- Chronic renal failure *(pathophysiology is unclear)*
- Coronary artery disease (CAD) *(there is a relationship, but the pathophysiology is unclear)*
- Folic acid deficiency *(folate is required for completion of biochemical reactions involved in homocysteine metabolism)*
- Homocystinuria *(inherited disorder of methionine metabolism that results in accumulation of homocysteine)*
- Peripheral vascular disease *(related to vascular wall damage and formation of occlusive plaque)*
- Vitamin B_{12} deficiency *(vitamin B_{12} is required for completion of biochemical reactions involved in homocysteine metabolism)*

H

Decreased in: N/A

CRITICAL FINDINGS: N/A

INTERFERING FACTORS
- Drugs that may increase plasma homocysteine levels include anticonvulsants, cycloserine, hydralazine, isoniazid, methotrexate, penicillamine, phenelzine, and procarbazine.
- Drugs that may decrease plasma homocysteine levels include folic acid.
- Specimens should be kept at a refrigerated temperature and delivered immediately to the laboratory for processing.

H

NURSING IMPLICATIONS AND PROCEDURE

PRETEST:
- ▶ Positively identify the patient using at least two unique identifiers before providing care, treatment, or services.
- ▶ *Patient Teaching:* Inform the patient this test can assist in screening for risk of cardiovascular disease and stroke.
- ▶ Obtain a history of the patient's complaints, including a list of known allergens, especially allergies or sensitivities to latex.
- ▶ Obtain a history of the patient's cardiovascular and hematopoietic systems, symptoms, and results of previously performed laboratory tests and diagnostic and surgical procedures.
- ▶ Obtain a list of the patient's current medications, including herbs, nutritional supplements, and nutraceuticals (see Appendix F).
- ▶ Review the procedure with the patient. Inform the patient that specimen collection takes approximately 5 to 10 min. Address concerns about pain and explain that there may be some discomfort during the venipuncture.
- ▶ *Sensitivity to social and cultural issues,* as well as concern for modesty, is important

in providing psychological support before, during, and after the procedure.
- ▶ There are no food, fluid, or medication restrictions unless by medical direction.

INTRATEST:
- ▶ If the patient has a history of allergic reaction to latex, avoid the use of equipment containing latex.
- ▶ Instruct the patient to cooperate fully and to follow directions. Direct the patient to breathe normally and to avoid unnecessary movement.
- ▶ Observe standard precautions, and follow the general guidelines in Appendix A. Positively identify the patient, and label the appropriate tubes with the corresponding patient demographics, date, and time of collection. Perform a venipuncture; collect the specimen for combined methylmalonic acid and homocysteine studies in two 5-mL red- or tiger-top tubes. If only homocysteine is to be measured, a 5-mL lavender-top tube is acceptable.
- ▶ Remove the needle and apply direct pressure with dry gauze to stop bleeding. Observe/assess venipuncture site for bleeding or hematoma formation and secure gauze with adhesive bandage.
- ▶ Promptly transport the specimen to the laboratory for processing and analysis.

POST-TEST:
- ▶ A report of the results will be sent to the requesting health-care provider (HCP), who will discuss the results with the patient.
- ▶ *Nutritional Considerations:* Increased homocysteine levels may be associated with atherosclerosis and CAD. Nutritional therapy is recommended for individuals identified to be at high risk for developing CAD. The American Heart Association and National Heart, Lung, and Blood Institute (NHBLI) recommend nutritional therapy for individuals identified to be at high risk for developing CAD or individuals who have specific risk factors and/or existing medical conditions (e.g., elevated LDL cholesterol levels, other lipid disorders, insulin-dependent diabetes, insulin resistance, or metabolic syndrome).

If overweight, the patient should be encouraged to achieve a normal weight. The NHLBI's National Cholesterol Education Program (NCEP) revised its dietary guidelines for reducing CAD in 2001. Guidelines for the Therapeutic Lifestyle Changes (TLC) diet are outlined in the Third Report of the Expert Panel on Detection, Evaluation, and Treatment of High Blood Cholesterol in Adults (Adult Treatment Panel III [ATP III]). The TLC diet emphasizes a reduction in foods high in saturated fats and cholesterol. Red meats, eggs, and dairy products are the major sources of saturated fats and cholesterol. If triglycerides also are elevated, the patient should be advised to eliminate or reduce alcohol and simple carbohydrates from the diet. The TLC approach also includes the use of plant stanols or sterols and increased dissolved fiber as an option for lowering LDL cholesterol levels; nutritional recommendations for daily total caloric intake; recommendations for allowable percentage of calories derived from fat (saturated and unsaturated), carbohydrates, protein, and cholesterol; as well as recommendations for daily expenditure of energy.

▶ *Nutritional Considerations:* Overweight patients with high blood pressure should be encouraged to achieve a normal weight. Other changeable risk factors warranting patient education include strategies to safely decrease sodium intake, increase physical activity, decrease alcohol consumption, eliminate tobacco use, and decrease cholesterol levels.

▶ *Nutritional Considerations:* Diets rich in fruits, grains, and cereals, in addition to a multivitamin containing B_{12} and folate, may be recommended for patients with elevated homocysteine levels. Processed and refined foods should be kept to a minimum.

▶ *Social and Cultural Considerations:* Numerous studies point to the prevalence of excess body weight in American children and adolescents. Experts estimate that obesity is present in 25% of the population ages 6 to 11 yr.

The medical, social, and emotional consequences of excess body weight are significant. Special attention should be given to instructing the child and caregiver regarding health risks and weight-control education.

▶ Recognize anxiety related to test results, and be supportive of fear of shortened life expectancy. Discuss the implications of abnormal test results on the patient's lifestyle. Provide teaching and information regarding the clinical implications of the test results, as appropriate. Educate the patient regarding access to counseling services. Provide contact information, if desired, for the American Heart Association (www.americanheart.org) or the NHLBI (www.nhlbi.nih.gov).

▶ Reinforce information given by the patient's HCP regarding further testing, treatment, or referral to another HCP. Answer any questions or address any concerns voiced by the patient or family.

▶ Depending on the results of this procedure, additional testing may be performed to evaluate or monitor progression of the disease process and determine the need for a change in therapy. Evaluate test results in relation to the patient's symptoms and other tests performed.

RELATED MONOGRAPHS:

▶ Related tests include antiarrhythmic drugs, apolipoprotein A and B, AST, ANP, blood gases, BMD, BNP, BUN, calcitonin, calcium, cholesterol (total, HDL, and LDL), CBC, CBC RBC count, CBC RBC indices, CBC RBC morphology, CBC WBC count and differential, CRP, CK and isoenzymes, creatinine, folate, glucose, glycated hemoglobin, ketones, LDH and isoenzymes, lipoprotein electrophoresis, magnesium, myoglobin, osteocalcin, PTH, pericardial fluid analysis, potassium, prealbumin, renogram, triglycerides, troponin, US kidney, UA, and vitamin B_{12}.

▶ Refer to the Cardiovascular and Hematopoietic systems tables at the end of the book for related tests by body system.

H

Homovanillic Acid

SYNONYM/ACRONYM: HVA.

COMMON USE: To assist in diagnosis of neuroblastoma, pheochromocytoma, and ganglioblastoma and to monitor therapy.

SPECIMEN: Urine (10 mL) from a timed specimen collected in a clean plastic collection container with 6N HCl as a preservative.

REFERENCE VALUE: (Method: Chromatography)

Age	Conventional Units	SI Units
Homovanillic Acid		*(Conventional Units × 5.49)*
3–6 yr	1.4–4.3 mg/24 hr	8–24 micromol/24 hr
7–10 yr	2.1–4.7 mg/24 hr	12–26 micromol/24 hr
11–16 yr	2.4–8.7 mg/24 hr	13–48 micromol/24 hr
Adult–older adult	1.4–8.8 mg/24 hr	8–48 micromol/24 hr
Vanillylmandelic Acid		*(Conventional Units × 5.05)*
3–6 yr	1.0–2.6 mg/24 hr	5–13 micromol/24 hr
7–10 yr	2.0–3.2 mg/24 hr	10–16 micromol/24 hr
11–16 yr	2.3–5.2 mg/24 hr	12–26 micromol/24 hr
Adult–older adult	1.4–6.5 mg/24 hr	7–33 micromol/24 hr

DESCRIPTION: Homovanillic acid (HVA) is the main terminal metabolite of dopamine. Vanillylmandelic acid is a major metabolite of epinephrine and norepinephrine. Both of these tests should be evaluated together for the diagnosis of neuroblastoma. Excretion may be intermittent; therefore, a 24-hr specimen is preferred. Creatinine is usually measured simultaneously to ensure adequate collection and to calculate an excretion ratio of metabolite to creatinine.

INDICATIONS
• Assist in the diagnosis of pheochromocytoma, neuroblastoma, and ganglioblastoma
• Monitor the course of therapy

POTENTIAL DIAGNOSIS

Increased in
HVA is excreted in excessive amounts in the following conditions:
• Ganglioblastoma
• Neuroblastoma
• Pheochromocytoma
• Riley-Day syndrome

Decreased in
• Schizotypal personality disorders

CRITICAL FINDINGS: N/A

INTERFERING FACTORS
- Drugs that may increase HVA levels include acetylsalicylic acid, disulfiram, levodopa, pyridoxine, and reserpine.
- Drugs that may decrease HVA levels include moclobemide.
- All urine voided for the timed collection period must be included in the collection, or else falsely decreased values may be obtained. Compare output records with volume collected to verify that all voids were included in the collection.

NURSING IMPLICATIONS AND PROCEDURE

PRETEST:
▶ Positively identify the patient using at least two unique identifiers before providing care, treatment, or services.
▶ *Patient Teaching:* Inform the patient this test can assist in screening for presence of a tumor.
▶ Obtain a history of the patient's complaints, including a list of known allergens, especially allergies or sensitivities to latex.
▶ Obtain a history of the patient's endocrine system, symptoms, and results of previously performed laboratory tests and diagnostic and surgical procedures.
▶ Obtain a list of the patient's current medications, including herbs, nutritional supplements, and nutraceuticals (see Appendix F).
▶ Review the procedure with the patient. Provide a nonmetallic urinal, bedpan, or toilet-mounted collection device. Address concerns about pain and explain that there should be no discomfort during the procedure.
▶ Usually a 24-hr time frame for urine collection is ordered. Inform the patient

that all urine must be saved during that 24-hr period. Instruct the patient not to void directly into the laboratory collection container. Instruct the patient to avoid defecating in the collection device and to keep toilet tissue out of the collection device to prevent contamination of the specimen. Place a sign in the bathroom to remind the patient to save all urine.
▶ Instruct the patient to void all urine into the collection device and then to pour the urine into the laboratory collection container. Alternatively, the specimen can be left in the collection device for a health-care staff member to add to the laboratory collection container.
▶ *Sensitivity to social and cultural issues,* as well as concern for modesty, is important in providing psychological support before, during, and after the procedure.
▶ If possible, and with medical direction, patients should withhold acetylsalicylic acid, disulfiram, pyridoxine, and reserpine for 2 days before specimen collection. Levodopa should be withheld for 2 wk before specimen collection.
▶ There are no food or fluid restrictions unless by medical direction.

INTRATEST:
▶ Ensure that the patient has complied with medication restrictions; assure that specified medications, with medical direction, have been restricted for at least 2 days prior to the procedure.
▶ If the patient has a history of allergic reaction to latex, avoid the use of equipment containing latex.
▶ Instruct the patient to cooperate fully and to follow directions.
▶ Observe standard precautions, and follow the general guidelines in Appendix A. Positively identify the patient, and label the appropriate tubes with the corresponding patient demographics, date, and time of collection.

Timed Specimen

▶ Obtain a clean 3-L urine specimen container, toilet-mounted collection device, and plastic bag (for transport of the specimen container). The specimen must be refrigerated or kept on ice throughout the entire collection period. If an indwelling urinary catheter is in place, the drainage bag must be kept on ice.

▶ Begin the test between 6 and 8 a.m. if possible. Collect first voiding and discard. Record the time the specimen was discarded as the beginning of the timed collection period. The next morning, ask the patient to void at the same time the collection was started and add this last voiding to the container. Urinary output should be recorded throughout the collection time.

▶ If an indwelling catheter is in place, replace the tubing and container system at the start of the collection time. Keep the container system on ice during the collection period, or empty the urine into a larger refrigerated container periodically during the collection period; monitor to ensure continued drainage, and conclude the test the next morning at the same hour the collection was begun.

▶ At the conclusion of the test, compare the quantity of urine with the urinary output record for the collection; if the specimen contains less than what was recorded as output, some urine may have been discarded, invalidating the test.

▶ Include on the collection container's label the amount of urine, test start and stop times, and ingestion of any foods or medications that can affect test results.

▶ Promptly transport the specimen to the laboratory for processing and analysis.

POST-TEST:

▶ A report of the results will be sent to the requesting health-care provider (HCP), who will discuss the results with the patient.

▶ Instruct the patient to resume usual medications, as directed by the HCP.

▶ Recognize anxiety related to test results. Discuss the implications of abnormal test results on the patient's lifestyle. Provide teaching and information regarding the clinical implications of the test results, as appropriate. Educate the patient regarding access to counseling services.

▶ Reinforce information given by the patient's HCP regarding further testing, treatment, or referral to another HCP. Answer any questions or address any concerns voiced by the patient or family.

▶ Depending on the results of this procedure, additional testing may be performed to evaluate or monitor progression of the disease process and determine the need for a change in therapy. Evaluate test results in relation to the patient's symptoms and other tests performed.

RELATED MONOGRAPHS:

▶ Related tests include angiography adrenal, CEA, catecholamines, CT renal, metanephrines, renin, and VMA.

▶ Refer to the Endocrine System table at the end of the book for related tests by body system.

Human Chorionic Gonadotropin

SYNONYM/ACRONYM: Chorionic gonadotropin, pregnancy test, HCG, hCG, α-HCG, β-subunit HCG.

COMMON USE: To assist in verification of pregnancy, screen for neural tube defects, and evaluate human chorionic gonadotropin (HCG)–secreting tumors.

SPECIMEN: Serum (1 mL) collected in a red- or tiger-top tube. Plasma (1 mL) collected in a green-top (heparin) tube is also acceptable.

REFERENCE VALUE: (Method: Immunoassay)

	Conventional Units	SI Units (Conventional Units × 1)
Males and nonpregnant females	Less than 5 milli international units/mL	Less than 5 international units/L
Pregnant females by week of gestation:		
Less than 1 wk	5–50 milli international units/mL	5–50 international units/L
2 wk	50–500 milli international units/mL	50–500 international units/L
3 wk	100–10,000 milli international units/mL	100–10,000 international units/L
4 wk	1,000–30,000 milli international units/mL	1,000–30,000 international units/L
5 wk	3,500–115,000 milli international units/mL	3,500–115,000 international units/L
6–8 wk	12,000–270,000 milli international units/mL	12,000–270,000 international units/L
12 wk	15,000–220,000 milli international units/mL	15,000–220,000 international units/L

DESCRIPTION: Human chorionic gonadotropin (HCG) is a hormone secreted by the placenta beginning 8 to 10 days after conception, which coincides with implantation of the fertilized ovum. It stimulates secretion of progesterone by the corpus luteum. HCG levels peak at 8 to 12 wk of gestation and then fall to less than 10% of first trimester levels by the end of pregnancy. By postpartum week 2, levels are undetectable. HCG levels increase at a slower rate in ectopic pregnancy and spontaneous abortion than in normal pregnancy; a low rate of change between serial specimens is predictive of a nonviable fetus. As assays improve in sensitivity over time, ectopic pregnancies are increasingly being identified before rupture. HCG is used along with α-fetoprotein, dimeric inhibin-A, and estriol in prenatal screening for neural tube defects. These prenatal measurements are also known as *triple* or *quad markers*, depending on which tests are included. Serial measurements are needed for an accurate estimate of gestational stage and determination of fetal viability. Triple- and quad-marker testing has also been used to screen for trisomy 21 (Down syndrome). (To compare HCG to other tests in the triple- and quad-marker screening procedure, see monograph titled "α$_1$-Fetoprotein.") HCG is also produced by some germ cell tumors. Most assays measure both the intact and free β-HCG subunit, but if HCG is to be used as a tumor marker, the assay must be capable of detecting both intact and free β-HCG.

INDICATIONS

- Assist in the diagnosis of suspected HCG-producing tumors, such as choriocarcinoma, germ cell tumors of the ovary and testes, or hydatidiform moles
- Confirm pregnancy, assist in the diagnosis of suspected ectopic pregnancy, or determine threatened or incomplete abortion
- Determine adequacy of hormonal levels to maintain pregnancy
- Monitor effects of surgery or chemotherapy
- Monitor ovulation induction treatment
- Prenatally detect neural tube defects and trisomy 21 (Down syndrome)

POTENTIAL DIAGNOSIS

Increased in

- Choriocarcinoma *(related to HCG-producing tumor)*
- Ectopic HCG-producing tumors (stomach, lung, colon, pancreas, liver, breast) *(related to HCG-producing tumor)*
- Erythroblastosis fetalis *(hemolytic anemia as a result of fetal sensitization by incompatible maternal blood group antigens such as Rh, Kell, Kidd, and Duffy is associated with increased HCG levels)*
- Germ cell tumors (ovary and testes) *(related to HCG-producing tumors)*
- Hydatidiform mole *(related to HCG-secreting mole)*
- Islet cell tumors *(related to HCG-producing tumors)*
- Multiple gestation pregnancy *(related to increased levels produced by the presence of multiple fetuses)*
- Pregnancy *(related to increased production by placenta)*

Decreased in

Any condition associated with diminished viability of the placenta will reflect decreased levels.

- Ectopic pregnancy *(HCG levels increase slower than in viable intrauterine pregnancies, plateau, and then decrease prior to rupture)*
- Incomplete abortion
- Intrauterine fetal demise
- Spontaneous abortion
- Threatened abortion

CRITICAL FINDINGS: N/A

INTERFERING FACTORS

- Drugs that may decrease HCG levels include epostane and mifepristone.

- Results may vary widely depending on the sensitivity and specificity of the assay. Performance of the test too early in pregnancy may cause false-negative results. HCG is composed of an α and a β subunit. The structure of the α subunit is essentially identical to the β subunit of follicle-stimulating hormone, luteinizing hormone, and thyroid-stimulating hormone. The structure of the β subunit differentiates HCG from the other hormones. False-positive results can therefore be obtained if the HCG assay does not detect β subunit.

NURSING IMPLICATIONS AND PROCEDURE

PRETEST:

- Positively identify the patient using at least two unique identifiers before providing care, treatment, or services.
- *Patient Teaching:* Inform the patient this test can assist in screening for pregnancy, identifying tumors, and evaluating fetal health.
- Obtain a history of the patient's complaints, including a list of known allergens, especially allergies or sensitivities to latex.
- Obtain a history of the patient's endocrine, immune, and reproductive systems; symptoms; and results of previously performed laboratory tests and diagnostic and surgical procedures.
- Record the date of the last menstrual period and determine the possibility of pregnancy in perimenopausal women.
- Obtain a list of the patient's current medications, including herbs, nutritional supplements, and nutraceuticals (see Appendix F).
- Review the procedure with the patient. Inform the patient that specimen collection takes approximately 5 to 10 min. Address concerns about pain and explain that there may be some discomfort during the venipuncture.

- *Sensitivity to social and cultural issues,* as well as concern for modesty, is important in providing psychological support before, during, and after the procedure.
- There are no food, fluid, or medication restrictions unless by medical direction.

INTRATEST:

- If the patient has a history of allergic reaction to latex, avoid the use of equipment containing latex.
- Instruct the patient to cooperate fully and to follow directions. Direct the patient to breathe normally and to avoid unnecessary movement.
- Observe standard precautions, and follow the general guidelines in Appendix A. Positively identify the patient, and label the appropriate tubes with the corresponding patient demographics, date, and time of collection. Perform a venipuncture.
- Remove the needle and apply direct pressure with dry gauze to stop bleeding. Observe/assess venipuncture site for bleeding or hematoma formation and secure gauze with adhesive bandage.
- Promptly transport the specimen to the laboratory for processing and analysis.

POST-TEST:

- A report of the results will be sent to the requesting health-care provider (HCP), who will discuss the results with the patient.
- *Social and Cultural Considerations:* Recognize anxiety related to abnormal test results, and encourage the family to seek counseling if concerned with pregnancy termination or to seek genetic counseling if a chromosomal abnormality is determined. Provide teaching and information regarding the clinical implications of the test results, as appropriate. Decisions regarding elective abortion should take place in the presence of both parents. Provide a nonjudgmental, nonthreatening atmosphere for discussing the risks and difficulties of delivering and raising a developmentally challenged infant, as well as exploring other options (termination of pregnancy or adoption). It is

H

also important to discuss feelings the mother and father may experience (e.g., guilt, depression, anger) if fetal abnormalities are detected.

▶ *Social and Cultural Considerations:* Offer support, as appropriate, to patients who may be the victims of rape or sexual assault. Educate the patient regarding access to counseling services. Provide a nonjudgmental, nonthreatening atmosphere for a discussion during which risks of sexually transmitted diseases are explained. It is also important to discuss problems the victim of sexual assault may experience (e.g., guilt, depression, anger) if there is possibility of pregnancy related to the assault.

▶ *Social and Cultural Considerations:* In patients with carcinoma, recognize anxiety related to test results and offer support. Provide teaching and information regarding the clinical implications of abnormal test results, as appropriate. Educate the patient regarding access to counseling services, as appropriate.

▶ Reinforce information given by the patient's HCP regarding further testing, treatment, or referral to another HCP.

Instruct the patient in the use of home test kits for pregnancy approved by the U.S. Food and Drug Administration, as appropriate. Answer any questions or address any concerns voiced by the patient or family.

▶ Depending on the results of this procedure, additional testing may be performed to evaluate or monitor the patient's condition and determine the need for a change in therapy. Evaluate test results in relation to the patient's symptoms and other tests performed.

RELATED MONOGRAPHS:

▶ Related laboratory tests include biopsy chorionic villus, *Chlamydia* group antibody, chromosome analysis, CMV, estradiol, fetal fibronectin, α_1-fetoprotein, CBC, hematocrit, CBC hemoglobin, CBC WBC count and differential, progesterone, rubella antibody, rubeola antibody, syphilis serology, toxoplasma antibody, and US biophysical profile obstetric.

▶ Refer to the Endocrine, Immune, and Reproductive systems tables at the end of the book for related tests by body system.

Human Immunodeficiency Virus Type 1 and Type 2 Antibodies

SYNONYM/ACRONYM: HIV-1/HIV-2.

COMMON USE: Test blood for the presence of antibodies that would indicate an HIV infection.

SPECIMEN: Serum (1 mL) collected in a red-top tube.

REFERENCE VALUE: (Method: Enzyme immunoassay) Negative.

DESCRIPTION: Human immunodeficiency virus (HIV) is the etiological agent of AIDS and is transmitted through bodily secretions, especially by blood or sexual contact. The virus preferentially binds to the T4 helper lymphocytes and replicates within the cells. Current assays detect several viral proteins. Positive results should be confirmed by Western blot assay. This test is routinely recommended as part of a prenatal work-up and is required for evaluating donated blood units before release for transfusion. The Centers for Disease Control and Prevention (CDC) has structured its recommendations to increase identification of HIV-infected patients as early as possible; early identification increases treatment options, increases frequency of successful treatment, and can decrease further spread of disease. The reports "Advancing HIV Prevention: New Strategies for a Changing Epidemic 2003" (a report by the CDC available at www.cdc.gov) and "Revised Recommendations for HIV Screening of Pregnant Women" (*Morbidity and Mortality Weekly Report* 2001;50 [No. RR-19]:63–85) recommend the following:

- Include HIV testing in routine medical care; screening of all patients between the ages of 13 and 64 years of age as part of routine medical care.
- Implement new models to diagnose HIV infections outside medical settings; promote availability of rapid waived testing kits like OraQuick.
- Prevent new infections by working with persons diagnosed with HIV and their partners; adapt a voluntary opt-out approach that includes elimination of pretest counseling and written consent requirements.
- Further decrease prenatal transmission of HIV by incorporating HIV testing as a routine part of prenatal medical care and third-trimester testing in areas with elevated rates of HIV infection among pregnant women.

INDICATIONS

- Evaluate donated blood units before transfusion
- Perform as part of prenatal screening
- Screen organ transplant donors
- Test individuals who have documented and significant exposure to other infected individuals
- Test exposed high-risk individuals for detection of antibody (e.g., persons with multiple sex partners, persons with a history of other sexually transmitted diseases, IV drug users, infants born to infected mothers, allied health-care workers, public service employees who have contact with blood and blood products)

POTENTIAL DIAGNOSIS

Positive findings in
- HIV-1 or HIV-2 infection

CRITICAL FINDINGS: N/A

INTERFERING FACTORS

- Drugs that may decrease HIV antibody levels include didanosine, dideoxycytidine, zalcitabine, and zidovudine.
- Nonreactive HIV test results occur during the acute stage of the disease, when the virus is present but antibodies have not sufficiently developed to be detected. It may

take up to 6 mo for the test to become positive. During this stage, the test for HIV antigen may not confirm an HIV infection.

• Test kits for HIV are very sensitive. As a result, nonspecific reactions may occur, leading to a false-positive result.

NURSING IMPLICATIONS AND PROCEDURE

PRETEST:

▶ Positively identify the patient using at least two unique identifiers before providing care, treatment, or services.

▶ *Patient Teaching:* Inform the patient that this laboratory test can assist in evaluating for HIV infection.

▶ Obtain a history of the patient's complaints, including a list of known allergens, especially allergies or sensitivities to latex.

▶ Obtain a history of the patient's immune system, a history of high-risk behaviors, symptoms, and results of previously performed laboratory tests and diagnostic and surgical procedures.

▶ Obtain a list of the patient's current medications, including herbs, nutritional supplements, and nutraceuticals (see Appendix F).

▶ Review the procedure with the patient. Inform the patient that specimen collection takes approximately 5 to 10 min. Address concerns about pain and explain that there may be some discomfort during the venipuncture.

▶ There are no food, fluid, or medication restrictions unless by medical direction.

▶ *Make sure a written and informed consent has been signed prior to the procedure if required.*

INTRATEST:

▶ If the patient has a history of allergic reaction to latex, avoid the use of equipment containing latex.

▶ Instruct the patient to cooperate fully and to follow directions. Direct the

patient to breathe normally and to avoid unnecessary movement.

▶ Observe standard precautions, and follow the general guidelines in Appendix A. Positively identify the patient, and label the appropriate tubes with the corresponding patient demographics, date, and time of collection. Perform a venipuncture.

▶ Remove the needle and apply direct pressure with dry gauze to stop bleeding. Observe/assess venipuncture site for bleeding or hematoma formation and secure gauze with adhesive bandage.

▶ Promptly transport the specimen to the laboratory for processing and analysis.

POST-TEST:

▶ A report of the results will be sent to the requesting health-care provider (HCP), who will discuss the results with the patient.

▶ Warn the patient that false-positive results occur and that the absence of antibody does not guarantee absence of infection, because the virus may be latent or may not have produced detectable antibody at the time of testing.

▶ *Social and Cultural Considerations:* Recognize anxiety related to test results, and be supportive of impaired activity related to weakness, perceived loss of independence, and fear of shortened life expectancy. Discuss the implications of abnormal test results on the patient's lifestyle. Provide teaching and information regarding the clinical implications of the test results, as appropriate. Educate the patient regarding access to counseling services. Provide contact information, if desired, for AIDS information provided by the National Institutes of Health (www.aidsinfo.nih.gov) or the CDC (www.cdc.gov).

▶ *Social and Cultural Considerations:* Counsel the patient, as appropriate, regarding risk of transmission and proper prophylaxis, and reinforce the importance of strict adherence to the treatment regimen, including consultation with a pharmacist.

• *Social and Cultural Considerations:* Inform patient that positive findings must be reported to local health department officials, who will question him or her regarding sexual partners.

• *Social and Cultural Considerations:* Offer support, as appropriate, to patients who may be the victims of rape or sexual assault. Educate the patient regarding access to counseling services. Provide a nonjudgmental, nonthreatening atmosphere for a discussion during which risks of sexually transmitted diseases are explained. It is also important to discuss problems the patient may experience (e.g., guilt, depression, anger).

• Inform the patient that retesting may be necessary.

• Reinforce information given by the patient's HCP regarding further testing, treatment, or referral to another HCP. Answer any questions or address any concerns voiced by the patient or family.

• Depending on the results of this procedure, additional testing may be performed to evaluate or monitor progression of the disease process and determine the need for a change in therapy. Evaluate test results in relation to the patient's symptoms and other tests performed.

RELATED MONOGRAPHS:

• Related tests include biopsy bone marrow, bronchoscopy, CD4/CD8 enumeration, *Chlamydia* group antibody, CBC, CBC platelet count, CBC WBC count and differential, culture and smear mycobacteria, culture viral, cytology sputum, CMV, culture skin, gallium scan, HBV antibody and antigen, HCV antibody, human T-cell lymphotropic virus types I and II, laparoscopy abdominal, LAP, lymphangiogram, MRI musculoskeletal, mediastinoscopy, β_2-microglobulin, and syphilis serology.

• Refer to the Immune System table at the end of the book for related tests by body system.

Human Leukocyte Antigen B27

SYNONYM/ACRONYM: HLA-B27.

COMMON USE: To assist in diagnosing juvenile rheumatoid arthritis, psoriac arthritis, ankylosing spondylitis, and Reiter's syndrome.

SPECIMEN: Whole blood (5 mL) collected in a green-top (heparin) or a yellow-top (acid-citrate-dextrose [ACD]) tube.

REFERENCE VALUE: (Method: Flow cytometry) Negative (indicating absence of the antigen).

DESCRIPTION: The human leukocyte antigens (HLAs) are gene products of the major histocompatibility complex, derived from their respective loci on the short arm of chromosome 6. There are more than 27 identified HLAs.

HLA-B27 is an allele (one of two or more genes for an inheritable trait that occupy the same location on each chromosome, paternal and maternal) of the HLA-B locus. The antigens are present on the surface of nucleated tissue cells as well as on white blood cells. HLA testing is used in determining histocompatibility for organ and tissue transplantation. Another application for HLA testing is in paternity investigations. The presence of HLA-B27 is associated with several specific conditions, but HLA-B27 should not be used as a screening test for these conditions.

INDICATIONS
• Assist in diagnosing ankylosing spondylitis and Reiter's syndrome
• Determine compatibility for organ and tissue transplantation

POTENTIAL DIAGNOSIS

Positive findings in
• Ankylosing spondylitis
• Juvenile rheumatoid arthritis
• Psoriatic arthritis
• Reiter's syndrome
• Sacroiliitis

CRITICAL FINDINGS: N/A

INTERFERING FACTORS
• The specimen should be stored at room temperature and should be received by the laboratory performing the assay within 24 hr of collection. It is highly recommended that the laboratory be contacted before specimen collection to avoid specimen rejection.

NURSING IMPLICATIONS AND PROCEDURE

PRETEST:
▶ Positively identify the patient using at least two unique identifiers before providing care, treatment, or services.
▶ *Patient Teaching:* Inform the patient this test can assist with investigation of

specific leukocyte disorders and determine compatibility for organ and tissue transplantation.
▶ Obtain a history of the patient's complaints, including a list of known allergens, especially allergies or sensitivities to latex.
▶ Obtain a history of the patient's immune system, symptoms, and results of previously performed laboratory tests and diagnostic and surgical procedures.
▶ Obtain a list of the patient's current medications, including herbs, nutritional supplements, and nutraceuticals (see Appendix F).
▶ Review the procedure with the patient. Inform the patient that specimen collection takes approximately 5 to 10 min. Address concerns about pain and explain that there may be some discomfort during the venipuncture.
▶ *Sensitivity to social and cultural issues,* as well as concern for modesty, is important in providing psychological support before, during, and after the procedure.
▶ There are no food, fluid, or medication restrictions unless by medical direction.

INTRATEST:
▶ If the patient has a history of allergic reaction to latex, avoid the use of equipment containing latex.
▶ Instruct the patient to cooperate fully and to follow directions. Direct the patient to breathe normally and to avoid unnecessary movement.
▶ Observe standard precautions, and follow the general guidelines in Appendix A. Positively identify the patient, and label the appropriate tubes with the corresponding patient demographics, date, and time of collection. Perform a venipuncture.
▶ Remove the needle and apply direct pressure with dry gauze to stop bleeding. Observe/assess venipuncture site for bleeding or hematoma formation and secure gauze with adhesive bandage.
▶ Promptly transport the specimen to the laboratory for processing and analysis.

- A report of the results will be sent to the requesting health-care provider (HCP), who will discuss the results with the patient.
- Recognize anxiety related to test results, and be supportive of perceived loss of independence and fear of short-ened life expectancy. These diseases can be moderately to severely debilitat-ing, resulting in significant lifestyle changes. Discuss the implications of abnormal test results on the patient's lifestyle. Provide teaching and informa-tion regarding the clinical implications of the test results, as appropriate. Educate the patient regarding access to counseling services.
- Reinforce information given by the patient's HCP regarding further testing, treatment, or referral to another HCP.

Inform the patient that false-positive test results occur and that retesting may be required. Answer any questions or address any concerns voiced by the patient or family.
- Depending on the results of this procedure, additional testing may be performed to evaluate or monitor pro-gression of the disease process and determine the need for a change in therapy. Evaluate test results in relation to the patient's symptoms and other tests performed.

RELATED MONOGRAPHS:

- Related tests include ANA, CBC, CT spine, ESR, MRI musculoskeletal, radiography bone, and RF.
- Refer to the Immune System table at the end of the book for related tests by body system.

Human T-Lymphotropic Virus Type I and Type II Antibodies

SYNONYM/ACRONYM: HTLV-I/HTLV-II.

COMMON USE: To test the blood for the presence of antibodies that would indi-cate past or current human T-lymphocyte virus (HTLV) infection. Helpful in diagnosing certain types of leukemia.

SPECIMEN: Serum (1 mL) collected in a red-top tube.

REFERENCE VALUE: (Method: Enzyme immunoassay) Negative.

DESCRIPTION: Human T-lympho-tropic virus type I (HTLV-I) and type II (HTLV-II) are two closely related retroviruses known to remain latent for extended peri-ods before becoming reactive. The viruses are transmitted by sexual contact, contact with blood, placental transfer from mother to fetus, or ingestion of breast milk. As with HIV-1 and HIV-2, HTLV targets the T4 lym-phocytes. HTLV-I has been associated with adult T-cell leukemia/lymphoma (ATL) and myelopathy/tropical spastic para-paresis (HAM/TSP). While it is believed HTLV-II may affect the immune system, it has been not been associated clearly with any particular disease or condition. Retrospective studies conducted by the American Red Cross demonstrated that a small percentage of transfusion recipients became infected by HTLV-positive blood. The results of this study led to a requirement that all donated blood units be tested for HTLV-I/HTLV-II before release for transfusion.

INDICATIONS

- Distinguish HTLV-I/HTLV-II infection from spastic myelopathy
- Establish HTLV-I as the causative agent in adult lymphoblastic (T-cell) leukemia
- Evaluate donated blood units before transfusion
- Evaluate HTLV-II as a contributing cause of chronic neuromuscular disease

POTENTIAL DIAGNOSIS

Positive findings in
- HTLV-I/HTLV-II infection

CRITICAL FINDINGS: N/A

INTERFERING FACTORS: N/A

NURSING IMPLICATIONS AND PROCEDURE

PRETEST:

- Positively identify the patient using at least two unique identifiers before providing care, treatment, or services.
- *Patient Teaching:* Inform the patient this test can assist with indicating a past or present HTLV infection.
- Obtain a history of the patient's complaints, including a list of known allergens, especially allergies or sensitivities to latex.

- Obtain a history of the patient's immune system, a history of high-risk behaviors, symptoms, and results of previously performed laboratory tests and diagnostic and surgical procedures.
- Obtain a list of the patient's current medications, including herbs, nutritional supplements, and nutraceuticals (see Appendix F).
- Review the procedure with the patient. Inform the patient that specimen collection takes approximately 5 to 10 min. Address concerns about pain and explain that there may be some discomfort during the venipuncture.
- *Sensitivity to social and cultural issues,* as well as concern for modesty, is important in providing psychological support before, during, and after the procedure.
- There are no food, fluid, or medication restrictions unless by medical direction.

INTRATEST:

- If the patient has a history of allergic reaction to latex, avoid the use of equipment containing latex.
- Instruct the patient to cooperate fully and to follow directions. Direct the patient to breathe normally and to avoid unnecessary movement.
- Observe standard precautions, and follow the general guidelines in Appendix A. Positively identify the patient, and label the appropriate tubes with the corresponding patient demographics, date, and time of collection. Perform a venipuncture.
- Remove the needle and apply direct pressure with dry gauze to stop bleeding. Observe/assess venipuncture site for bleeding or hematoma formation and secure gauze with adhesive bandage.
- Promptly transport the specimen to the laboratory for processing and analysis.

POST-TEST:

- A report of the results will be sent to the requesting health-care provider (HCP), who will discuss the results with the patient.
- Warn the patient that false-positive results occur and that the absence of antibody does not guarantee absence

of infection, because the virus may be latent or not have produced detectable antibody at the time of testing.

- Recognize anxiety related to test results, and be supportive of impaired activity related to weakness, perceived loss of independence, and fear of shortened life expectancy. Discuss the implications of positive test results on the patient's lifestyle. Provide teaching and information regarding the clinical implications of the test results, as appropriate. Educate the patient regarding access to counseling services.

- *Social and Cultural Considerations:* Counsel the patient, as appropriate, regarding risk of transmission and proper prophylaxis, and reinforce the importance of strict adherence to the treatment regimen, including consultation with a pharmacist.

- Inform the patient that the presence of HTLV-I/HTLV-II antibodies precludes blood donation, but it does not mean that leukemia or a neurological disorder is present or will develop.

- Inform the patient that subsequent retesting may be necessary.

- Reinforce information given by the patient's HCP regarding further testing, treatment, or referral to another HCP. Answer any questions or address any concerns voiced by the patient or family.

- Depending on the results of this procedure, additional testing may be performed to evaluate or monitor progression of the disease process and determine the need for a change in therapy. Evaluate test results in relation to the patient's symptoms and other tests performed.

RELATED MONOGRAPHS:

- Related tests include CBC; hepatitis B, C, and D antigens and antibodies; and HIV-1/HIV-2.
- Refer to the Immune System table at the end of the book for related tests by body system.

H

5-Hydroxyindoleacetic Acid

SYNONYM/ACRONYM: 5-HIAA.

COMMON USE: To assist in diagnosing carcinoid tumors.

SPECIMEN: Urine (10 mL) from a timed specimen collected in a clean plastic collection container with boric acid as a preservative.

REFERENCE VALUE: (Method: High-pressure liquid chromatography)

Conventional Units	SI Units (Conventional Units × 5.23)
2–7 mg/24 hr	10.5–36.6 micromol/24 hr

DESCRIPTION: Because 5-hydroxyindoleacetic acid (5-HIAA) is a metabolite of serotonin, 5-HIAA levels reflect plasma serotonin concentrations. 5-HIAA is excreted in the urine. Increased urinary excretion occurs in the presence of carcinoid tumors. This test, which replaces serotonin measurement, is most accurate when obtained from a 24-hr urine specimen.

INDICATIONS

Detect early, small, or intermittently secreting carcinoid tumors

POTENTIAL DIAGNOSIS

Increased in

Serotonin is produced by the entero-chromaffin cells of the small intestine and secreted ectopically by tumor cells. It is converted to 5-HIAA in the liver and excreted in the urine. Increased values are associated with malabsorption conditions, but the relationship is unclear.

- Celiac and tropical sprue
- Cystic fibrosis
- Foregut and midgut carcinoid tumors
- Oat cell carcinoma of the bronchus
- Ovarian carcinoid tumors
- Whipple's disease

Decreased in

The documented relationship between decreased levels of serotonin, defective amino acid metabolism, and mental illness is not well understood.

- Depressive illnesses
- Hartnup's disease
- Mastocytosis
- Phenylketonuria
- Renal disease *(related to decreased renal excretion)*
- Small intestine resection *(related to a decrease in enterochromaffin-producing cells)*

CRITICAL FINDINGS: N/A

INTERFERING FACTORS

- Drugs that may increase 5-HIAA levels include cisplatin, fluorouracil, cough syrups containing glyceryl guaiacolate, melphalan, rauwolfia alkaloids, and reserpine.
- Drugs that may decrease 5-HIAA levels include chlorophenylalanine, corticotropin, ethanol, imipramine, isocarboxazid, isoniazid, levodopa, methyldopa, monoamine oxidase inhibitors, and octreotide.
- Foods containing serotonin, such as avocados, bananas, chocolate, eggplant, pineapples, plantains, red plums, tomatoes, and walnuts, can falsely elevate levels if ingested within 4 days of specimen collection.
- Severe gastrointestinal disturbance or diarrhea can interfere with test results.
- Failure to collect all the urine and store the specimen properly during the 24-hr test period invalidates the results.
- Failure to follow dietary restrictions before the procedure may cause the procedure to be canceled or repeated.

NURSING IMPLICATIONS AND PROCEDURE

PRETEST:

- Positively identify the patient using at least two unique identifiers before providing care, treatment, or services.
- *Patient Teaching:* Inform the patient this test can assist in diagnosing tumor.
- Obtain a history of the patient's complaints, including a list of known allergens, especially allergies or sensitivities to latex.
- Obtain a history of the patient's endocrine, gastrointestinal, and immune systems; symptoms; and results of previously performed laboratory tests and diagnostic and surgical procedures.
- Obtain a list of the patient's current medications, including herbs, nutritional supplements, and nutraceuticals (see Appendix F).
- Review the procedure with the patient. Provide a nonmetallic urinal, bedpan, or toilet-mounted collection device. Address concerns about pain and explain to the patient that there

should be no discomfort during the procedure.

- Inform the patient that all urine collected over a 24-hr period must be saved; if a preservative has been added to the container, instruct the patient not to discard the preservative. Instruct the patient not to void directly into the container. Instruct the patient to avoid defecating in the collection device and to keep toilet tissue out of the collection device to prevent contamination of the specimen. Place a sign in the bathroom as a reminder to save all urine.
- Instruct the patient to void all urine into the collection device, then pour the urine into the laboratory collection container. Alternatively, the specimen can be left in the collection device for a health-care staff member to add to the laboratory collection container.
- *Sensitivity to social and cultural issues,* as well as concern for modesty, is important in providing psychological support before, during, and after the procedure.
- There are no fluid restrictions unless by medical direction.
- Inform the patient that foods and medications listed under "Interfering Factors" should be restricted by medical direction for at least 4 days before specimen collection.

INTRATEST:

- Ensure that the patient has complied with dietary and medication restrictions; assure foods and medications listed under "Interfering Factors" have been restricted for at least 4 days prior to the procedure.
- If the patient has a history of allergic reaction to latex, avoid the use of equipment containing latex.
- Instruct the patient to cooperate fully and to follow directions.
- Observe standard precautions, and follow the general guidelines in Appendix A. Positively identify the patient, and label the appropriate collection container with the corresponding patient demographics, date, and time of collection.

Timed Specimen

- Obtain a clean 3-L urine specimen container, toilet-mounted collection device, and plastic bag (for transport of the specimen container). The specimen must be refrigerated or kept on ice throughout the entire collection period. If an indwelling urinary catheter is in place, the drainage bag must be kept on ice.
- Begin the test between 6 and 8 a.m. if possible. Collect first voiding and discard. Record the time the specimen was discarded as the beginning of the timed collection period. The next morning, ask the patient to void at the same time the collection was started, and add this last voiding to the container. Urinary output should be recorded throughout the collection time.
- If an indwelling catheter is in place, replace the tubing and container system at the start of the collection time. Keep the container system on ice during the collection period, or empty the urine into a larger container periodically during the collection period; monitor to ensure continued drainage. Conclude the test the next morning at the same hour the collection was begun.
- At the conclusion of the test, compare the quantity of urine with the urinary output record for the collection; if the specimen contains less than what was recorded as output, some urine may have been discarded, invalidating the test.
- Include on the specimen collection container's label the amount of urine, test start and stop times, and ingestion of any foods or medications that can affect test results. Promptly transport the specimen to the laboratory for processing and analysis.

POST-TEST:

- A report of the results will be sent to the requesting health-care provider (HCP), who will discuss the results with the patient.
- Instruct the patient to resume usual diet, as directed by the HCP. Consideration may be given to niacin

supplementation and increased protein, if appropriate, for patients with abnormal findings. In some cases, the tumor may divert dietary tryptophan to serotonin, resulting in pellagra.

▶ Recognize anxiety related to test results. Discuss the implications of abnormal test results on the patient's lifestyle. Provide teaching and information regarding the clinical implications of the test results, as appropriate.

▶ Reinforce information given by the patient's HCP regarding further testing, treatment, or referral to another HCP. Answer any questions or address any concerns voiced by the patient or family.

Depending on the results of this procedure, additional testing may be performed to evaluate or monitor progression of the disease process and determine the need for a change in therapy. Evaluate test results in relation to the patient's symptoms and other tests performed.

RELATED MONOGRAPHS:

▶ Related tests include ALP, amino acid screen, antibodies gliadin, biopsy intestine, biopsy lung, calcium, cancer antigens, capsule endoscopy, chloride sweat, fecal fat, and folate.

▶ Refer to the Endocrine, Gastrointestinal, and Immune systems tables at the end of the book for related tests by body system.

H

Hypersensitivity Pneumonitis Serology

SYNONYM/ACRONYM: Farmer's lung disease serology, extrinsic allergic alveolitis.

COMMON USE: To assist in identification of pneumonia related to inhaled allergens containing *Aspergillus* or actinomycetes (dust, mold, or chronic exposure to moist organic materials).

SPECIMEN: Serum (2 mL) collected in a red-top tube.

REFERENCE VALUE: (Method: Immunodiffusion) Negative.

POTENTIAL DIAGNOSIS

Increased in
Hypersensitivity pneumonitis

CRITICAL FINDINGS: N/A

Find and print out the full monograph at DavisPlus (http://davisplus.fadavis .com, keyword Van Leeuwen).

Hysterosalpingography

SYNONYM/ACRONYM: Hysterogram, uterography, uterosalpingography.

COMMON USE: To visualize and assess the uterus and fallopian tubes to assess for obstruction, adhesions, malformations, or injuries that may be related to infertility.

AREA OF APPLICATION: Uterus and fallopian tubes.

CONTRAST: Iodinated contrast medium.

DESCRIPTION: Hysterosalpingography is performed as part of an infertility study to identify anatomical abnormalities of the uterus or occlusion of the fallopian tubes. The procedure allows visualization of the uterine cavity, fallopian tubes, and peritubal area after the injection of contrast medium into the cervix. The contrast medium should flow through the uterine cavity, through the fallopian tubes, and into the peritoneal cavity, where it is absorbed if no obstruction exists. Passage of the contrast medium through the tubes may clear mucous plugs, straighten kinked tubes, or break up adhesions, thus restoring fertility. This procedure is also used to evaluate the fallopian tubes after tubal ligation and to evaluate the results of reconstructive surgery. Risks include uterine perforation, exposure to radiation, infection, allergic reaction to contrast medium, bleeding, and pulmonary embolism.

INDICATIONS
- Confirm the presence of fistulas or adhesions
- Confirm tubal abnormalities such as adhesions and occlusions
- Confirm uterine abnormalities such as congenital malformation, traumatic injuries, or the presence of foreign bodies
- Detect bicornate uterus
- Evaluate adequacy of surgical tubal ligation and reconstructive surgery

POTENTIAL DIAGNOSIS

Normal findings in
- Contrast medium flowing freely into the fallopian tubes and from the uterus into the peritoneal cavity
- Normal position, shape, and size of the uterine cavity

Abnormal findings in
- Bicornate uterus
- Developmental abnormalities
- Extrauterine pregnancy
- Internal scarring
- Kinking of the fallopian tubes due to adhesions
- Partial or complete blockage of fallopian tube(s)
- Tumors
- Uterine cavity anomalies
- Uterine fistulas
- Uterine masses or foreign body
- Uterine fibroid tumors (leiomyomas)

H

CRITICAL FINDINGS: N/A

INTERFERING FACTORS

This procedure is contraindicated for

- Patients with allergies to shellfish or iodinated dye. The contrast medium used may cause a life-threatening allergic reaction. Patients with a known hypersensitivity to the contrast medium may benefit from premedication with corticosteroids or the use of nonionic contrast medium.
- Patients with bleeding disorders.
- Patients who are chronically dehydrated before the test, because of their risk of contrast-induced renal failure.
- Patients who are in renal failure.
- Patients with menses, undiagnosed vaginal bleeding, or pelvic inflammatory disease.
- Young patients (17 yr and younger), unless the benefits of the x-ray diagnosis outweigh the risks of exposure to high levels of radiation.

Factors that may impair clear imaging

- Gas or feces in the gastrointestinal tract resulting from inadequate cleansing or failure to restrict food intake before the study.
- Retained barium from a previous radiological procedure.
- Metallic objects (e.g., jewelry, body rings) within the examination field, which may inhibit organ visualization and cause unclear images.
- Inability of the patient to cooperate or remain still during the procedure because of age, significant pain, or mental status.
- Insufficient injection of contrast medium.
- Excessive traction during the test or tubal spasm, which may cause

the appearance of a stricture in an otherwise normal fallopian tube.

Other considerations

- Excessive traction during the test may displace adhesions, making the fallopian tubes appear normal.
- The procedure may be terminated if chest pain or severe cardiac arrhythmias occur.
- Failure to follow pretesting preparations may cause the procedure to be canceled or repeated.
- Risks associated with radiation overexposure can result from frequent x-ray procedures. Personnel in the room with the patient should wear a protective lead apron, stand behind a shield, or leave the area while the examination is being done. Personnel working in the examination area should wear badges to record their level of radiation exposure.

NURSING IMPLICATIONS AND PROCEDURE

PRETEST:

- Positively identify the patient using at least two unique identifiers before providing care, treatment, or services.
- *Patient Teaching:* Inform the patient this procedure can assist in assessing the uterus and fallopian tubes.
- Obtain a history of the patient's complaints, including a list of known allergens, especially allergies or sensitivities to latex, iodine, seafood, anesthetics, and contrast mediums.
- Obtain a history of the patient's reproductive system, symptoms, and results of previously performed laboratory tests and diagnostic and surgical procedures.
- Note any recent barium or other radiological contrast procedures. Ensure that barium studies were performed more than 4 days before the hysterosalpingography.

- Record the date of the last menstrual period and determine the possibility of pregnancy in perimenopausal women.
- Obtain a list of the patient's current medications, including anticoagulants, aspirin and other salicylates, herbs, nutritional supplements, and nutraceuticals, especially those known to affect coagulation (see Appendix F). Such products should be discontinued by medical direction for the appropriate number of days prior to a surgical procedure. Note the last time and dose of medication taken.
- Review the procedure with the patient. Address concerns about pain related to the procedure and explain that some pain may be experienced during the test, and there may be moments of discomfort. Explain to the patient that she may feel temporary sensations of nausea, dizziness, slow heartbeat, and menstrual-like cramping during the procedure, as well as shoulder pain from subphrenic irritation from the contrast medium as it spills into the peritoneal cavity. Inform the patient that the procedure is performed in a radiology department by a health-care provider (HCP), with support staff, and takes approximately 30 to 60 min.
- *Sensitivity to social and cultural issues,* as well as concern for modesty, is important in providing psychological support before, during and after the procedure.
- Instruct the patient to take a laxative or a cathartic, as ordered, on the evening before the examination.
- Instruct the patient to remove jewelry and other metallic objects from the area to be examined.
- There are no food, fluid, or medication restrictions unless by medical direction or department protocol.
- *Make sure a written and informed consent has been signed prior to the procedure and before administering any medications.*

INTRATEST:

- Ensure the patient has complied with pretesting preparations prior to the procedure.

- Ensure the patient has removed all external metallic objects from the area to be examined prior to the procedure.
- Assess for completion of bowel preparation according to the institution's procedure. Administer enemas or suppositories on the morning of the test, as ordered.
- Have emergency equipment readily available.
- Instruct the patient to void prior to the procedure and to change into the gown, robe, and foot coverings provided.
- Instruct the patient to cooperate fully and to follow directions. Instruct the patient to remain still throughout the procedure because movement produces unreliable results.
- Observe standard precautions, and follow the general guidelines in Appendix A.
- Place the patient in a lithotomy position on the fluoroscopy table.
- A kidney, ureter, and bladder film is taken to ensure that no stool, gas, or barium will obscure visualization of the uterus and fallopian tubes.
- A speculum is inserted into the vagina, and contrast medium is introduced into the uterus through the cervix via a cannula, after which both fluoroscopic and radiographic images are taken.

POST-TEST:

- A report of the examination will be sent to the requesting HCP, who will discuss the results with the patient.
- Instruct the patient to resume usual medications and activity, as directed by the HCP.
- Observe for delayed reaction to iodinated contrast medium, including rash, urticaria, tachycardia, hyperpnea, hypertension, palpitations, nausea, or vomiting.
- Instruct the patient to immediately report symptoms such as fast heart rate, difficulty breathing, skin rash, itching, chest pain, persistent right shoulder pain, or abdominal pain. Immediately report symptoms to the appropriate HCP.

H

◗ Inform the patient that a vaginal discharge is common and that it may be bloody, lasting 1 to 2 days after the test.

◗ Inform the patient that dizziness and cramping may follow this procedure, and that analgesia may be given if there is persistent cramping. Instruct the patient to contact the HCP in the event of severe cramping or profuse bleeding.

◗ Recognize anxiety related to test results. Discuss the implications of abnormal test results on the patient's lifestyle. Provide teaching and information regarding the clinical implications of the test results, as appropriate.

◗ Reinforce information given by the patient's HCP regarding further testing, treatment, or referral to another HCP.

Answer any questions or address any concerns voiced by the patient or family.

◗ Depending on the results of this procedure, additional testing may be needed to evaluate or monitor progression of the disease process and determine the need for a change in therapy. Evaluate test results in relation to the patient's symptoms and other tests performed.

RELATED MONOGRAPHS:

◗ Related tests include CT abdomen, laparoscopy gynecological, MRI abdomen, US obstetric, US pelvis, and uterine fibroid embolization.

◗ Refer to the Reproductive System table at the end of the book for related tests by body system.

H

Hysteroscopy

SYNONYM/ACRONYM: N/A.

COMMON USE: To visualize and assess the endometrial lining of the uterus to assist in diagnosing disorders such as fibroids, cancer, and polyps.

AREA OF APPLICATION: Uterus.

CONTRAST: Carbon dioxide, saline.

DESCRIPTION: Hysteroscopy is a diagnostic or surgical procedure of the uterus done using a thin telescope (hysteroscope), which is inserted through the cervix with minimal or no dilation. Normal saline, glycine, or carbon dioxide is used to fill and distend the uterus. The inner surface of the uterus is examined, and laser beam or electrocautery can be accomplished

during the procedure. Diagnostic hysteroscopy is used to diagnose uterine abnormalities and may be completed in conjunction with a dilatation and curettage (D & C). This minor surgical procedure is generally done to assess abnormal uterine bleeding or repeated miscarriages. An operative hysteroscopy is done instead of abdominal surgery to treat many uterine conditions such as septums or fibroids (myomas). A resectoscope (a hysteroscope that uses high-frequency electrical current to cut or coagulate tissue) may be used to remove any localized myomas. Local, regional, or general anesthesia can be used, but usually general anesthesia is needed. The procedure may done in a health-care practitioner's office, but if done as an outpatient surgical procedure, it is usually completed in a hospital setting.

INDICATIONS

POTENTIAL DIAGNOSIS

Normal findings in
• Normal uterine appearance

Abnormal findings in
• Areas of active bleeding
• Adhesions
• Displaced intrauterine devices
• Fibroid tumors
• Polyps
• Uterine septum

CRITICAL FINDINGS: N/A

INTERFERING FACTORS

• Inability of the patient to cooperate or remain still during the test because of age, significant pain, or mental status may interfere with the test results.
• Patients with bleeding disorders.
• Failure to follow dietary restrictions and other pretesting preparations may cause the procedure to be canceled or repeated.

NURSING IMPLICATIONS AND PROCEDURE

PRETEST:

▶ Positively identify the patient using at least two unique identifiers before providing care, treatment, or services.

▶ *Patient Teaching:* Inform the patient that this procedure can assist in assessing uterine health.
▶ Obtain a history of the patient's complaints, including a list of known allergens, especially allergies or sensitivities to latex.
▶ Obtain a history of the patient's reproductive system, symptoms, and results of previously performed laboratory tests and diagnostic and surgical procedures.
▶ Record the date of last menstrual period and determine the possibility of pregnancy in perimenopausal women.
▶ Obtain a list of the patient's current medications, including herbs, nutritional supplements, and nutraceuticals (see Appendix F).
▶ Review the procedure with the patient. Address concerns about pain and explain that a local anesthetic spray or liquid may be applied to the cervix to ease with insertion of the hysteroscope if general anesthesia is not used. Inform the patient that the procedure is usually performed in the office of a health-care provider (HCP) or a surgery suite and takes about 30 to 45 min.
▶ *Sensitivity to social and cultural issues,* as well as concern for modesty, is important in providing psychological support before, during, and after the procedure.
▶ Explain that an IV line may be inserted to allow infusion of IV fluids, anesthetics, or sedatives. Usually normal saline is infused.
▶ Instruct the patient to fast and restrict fluids for 8 hr prior to the procedure. Protocols may vary among facilities.
▶ Instruct the patient not to douche or use tampons or vaginal medications for 24 hr prior to the procedure.
▶ *Make sure a written and informed consent has been signed prior to the procedure and before administering any medications.*

INTRATEST:

▶ Ensure the patient has complied with dietary and fluid restrictions for 8 hr prior to the procedure.

- Instruct the patient to void prior to the procedure and to change into the gown, robe, and foot coverings provided.
- Instruct the patient to cooperate fully and to follow directions.
- Record baseline vital signs, and continue to monitor throughout the procedure. Protocols may vary among facilities.
- Observe standard precautions, and follow the general guidelines in Appendix A.
- Establish an IV fluid line for the injection of emergency drugs and of sedatives.
- Place the patient in the supine position on an exam table. Cleanse the vaginal area, and cover with a sterile drape.
- Monitor the patient for complications related to the procedure.

POST-TEST:

- A report of the results will be sent to the requesting HCP, who will discuss the results with the patient.
- Instruct the patient to resume usual diet, fluids, medications, and activity as directed by the HCP.

- Instruct the patient to immediately report symptoms such as excessive uterine bleeding or fever.
- Recognize anxiety related to test results. Discuss the implications of abnormal test results on the patient's lifestyle. Provide teaching and information regarding the clinical implications of the test results, as appropriate.
- Reinforce information given by the patient's HCP regarding further testing, treatment, or referral to another HCP. Answer any questions or address any concerns voiced by the patient or family.
- Depending on the results of this procedure, additional testing may be needed to evaluate or monitor progression of the disease process and determine the need for a change in therapy. Evaluate test results in relation to the patient's symptoms and other tests performed.

RELATED MONOGRAPHS:

- Related tests include CBC hematocrit, CBC hemoglobin, CT abdomen, HCG, KUB, and US pelvis.
- Refer to the Reproductive System table at the end of the book for related tests by body system.

Immunofixation Electrophoresis, Blood and Urine

SYNONYM/ACRONYM: IFE.

COMMON USE: To identify the individual types of immunoglobulins, to assist in diagnosis of diseases such as multiple myeloma, and to evaluate effectiveness of chemotherapy.

SPECIMEN: Serum (1 mL) collected in a red-top tube. Urine (10 mL) from a random or timed collection in a clean plastic container.

REFERENCE VALUE: (Method: Immunoprecipitation combined with electrophoresis) Test results are interpreted by a pathologist. Normal placement and intensity of staining provide information about the immunoglobulin bands.

DESCRIPTION: Immunofixation electrophoresis (IFE) is a qualitative technique that provides a detailed separation of individual immunoglobulins according to their electrical charges. Abnormalities are revealed by changes produced in the individual bands, such as displacement, color, or absence of color. Urine IFE has replaced the Bence Jones screening test for light chains. IFE has replaced immunoelectrophoresis because it is more sensitive and easier to interpret.

INDICATIONS

- Assist in the diagnosis of multiple myeloma and amyloidosis
- Assist in the diagnosis of suspected immunodeficiency
- Assist in the diagnosis of suspected immunoproliferative disorders, such as multiple myeloma and Waldenström's macroglobulinemia
- Identify biclonal or monoclonal gammopathies
- Identify cryoglobulinemia
- Monitor the effectiveness of chemotherapy or radiation therapy

POTENTIAL DIAGNOSIS

See monograph titled "Immunoglobulins A, D, G, and M."

CRITICAL FINDINGS: N/A

INTERFERING FACTORS

- Drugs that may increase immunoglobulin levels include asparaginase, cimetidine, and narcotics.
- Drugs that may decrease immunoglobulin levels include dextran, oral contraceptives, methylprednisolone (high doses), and phenytoin.
- Chemotherapy and radiation treatments may alter the width of the bands and make interpretation difficult.

NURSING IMPLICATIONS AND PROCEDURE

PRETEST:

- Positively identify the patient using at least two unique identifiers before providing care, treatment, or services.
- *Patient Teaching:* Inform the patient this test can assist in assessing the immune system.
- Obtain a history of the patient's complaints, including a list of known allergens, especially allergies or sensitivities to latex.
- Obtain a history of the patient's hematopoietic and immune systems, symptoms, and results of previously performed laboratory tests and diagnostic and surgical procedures.
- Note any recent procedures that can interfere with test results. Assess whether the patient received any vaccinations or immunizations within the last 6 mo or any blood or blood components within the last 6 wk.

▶ Obtain a list of the patient's current medications, including herbs, nutritional supplements, and nutraceuticals (see Appendix F).

▶ Review the procedure with the patient. Inform the patient that specimen collection takes approximately 5 to 10 min. Address concerns about pain and explain that there may be some discomfort during the venipuncture.

▶ Provide a nonmetallic urinal, bedpan, or toilet-mounted collection device.

▶ Usually a 24-hr time frame for urine collection is ordered. Inform the patient that all urine must be saved during that 24-hr period. Instruct the patient not to void directly into the laboratory collection container. Instruct the patient to avoid defecating in the collection device and to keep toilet tissue out of the collection device to prevent contamination of the specimen. Place a sign in the bathroom to remind the patient to save all urine.

▶ Instruct the patient to void all urine into the collection device and then to pour the urine into the laboratory collection container. Alternatively the specimen can be left in the collection device for a health-care staff member to add to the laboratory collection container.

▶ *Sensitivity to social and cultural issues,* as well as concern for modesty, is important in providing psychological support before, during, and after the procedure.

▶ There are no food, fluid, or medication restrictions unless by medical direction.

INTRATEST:

▶ If the patient has a history of allergic reaction to latex, avoid the use of equipment containing latex.

▶ Instruct the patient to cooperate fully and to follow directions. Direct the patient to breathe normally and to avoid unnecessary movement.

▶ Observe standard precautions, and follow the general guidelines in Appendix A. Positively identify the patient, and label the appropriate specimen containers with the corresponding patient demographics, date, and time of collection.

Blood
▶ Perform a venipuncture.

▶ Remove the needle and apply direct pressure with dry gauze to stop bleeding. Observe/assess venipuncture site for bleeding or hematoma formation and secure gauze with adhesive bandage.

Urine

Clean-Catch Specimen
▶ Instruct the male patient to (1) thoroughly wash his hands, (2) cleanse the meatus, (3) void a small amount into the toilet, and (4) void directly into the specimen container.

▶ Instruct the female patient to (1) thoroughly wash her hands; (2) cleanse the labia from front to back; (3) while keeping the labia separated, void a small amount into the toilet; and (4) without interrupting the urine stream, void directly into the specimen container.

Blood or Urine
▶ Promptly transport the specimen to the laboratory for processing and analysis.

POST-TEST:

▶ A report of the results will be sent to the requesting health-care provider (HCP), who will discuss the results with the patient.

▶ Reinforce information given by the patient's HCP regarding further testing, treatment, or referral to another HCP. Answer any questions or address any concerns voiced by the patient or family.

▶ Depending on the results of this procedure, additional testing may be performed to evaluate or monitor progression of the disease process and determine the need for a change in therapy. Evaluate test results in relation to the patient's symptoms and other tests performed.

RELATED MONOGRAPHS:

▶ Related tests include anion gap, biopsy bone, biopsy bone marrow, biopsy liver, biopsy lymph node, cold agglutinin, CBC, CBC WBC count and differential, cryoglobulin, ESR, fibrinogen, quantitative immunoglobulin levels, LAP, liver and spleen scan, β-2-microglobulin, platelet antibodies, protein total and fractions, and UA.

▶ Refer to the Hematopoietic and Immune systems tables at the end of the book for related tests by body system.

Immunoglobulin E

SYNONYM/ACRONYM: IgE.

COMMON USE: To assess immunoglobulin E (IgE) levels in order to identify the presence of an allergic or inflammatory immune response.

SPECIMEN: Serum (1 mL) collected in a red- or tiger-top tube.

REFERENCE VALUE: (Method: Immunoassay)

Age	Conventional Units
Newborn	Less than 12 kU/L
Less than 1 yr	Less than 50 kU/L
2–4 yr	Less than 100 kU/L
5 yr and older	Less than 300 kU/L

DESCRIPTION: Immunoglobulin E (IgE) is an antibody whose primary response is to allergic reactions and parasitic infections. Most of the body's IgE is bound to specialized tissue cells; little is available in the circulating blood. IgE binds to the membrane of special granulocytes called *basophils* in the circulating blood and *mast cells* in the tissues. Basophil and mast cell membranes have receptors for IgE. Mast cells are abundant in the skin and the tissues lining the respiratory and alimentary tracts. When IgE antibody becomes cross-linked with antigen/allergen, the release of histamine, heparin, and other chemicals from the granules in the cells is triggered. A sequence of events follows activation of IgE that affects smooth muscle contraction, vascular permeability, and inflammatory reactions. The inflammatory response allows proteins from the bloodstream to enter the tissues.

Helminths (worm parasites) are especially susceptible to immunoglobulin-mediated cytotoxic chemicals. The inflammatory reaction proteins attract macrophages from the circulatory system and granulocytes, such as eosinophils, from circulation and bone marrow. Eosinophils also contain enzymes effective against the parasitic invaders.

INDICATIONS

Assist in the evaluation of allergy and parasitic infection

POTENTIAL DIAGNOSIS

Increased in
Conditions involving allergic reactions or infections that stimulate production of IgE.
- Alcoholism *(alcohol may play a role in the development of environmentally instigated IgE mediated hypersensitivity)*
- Allergy
- Asthma
- Bronchopulmonary aspergillosis
- Dermatitis
- Eczema
- Hay fever
- IgE myeloma
- Parasitic infestation

- Rhinitis
- Sinusitis
- Wiskott-Aldrich syndrome

Decreased in
- Advanced carcinoma *(related to generalized decrease in immune system response)*
- Agammaglobulinemia *(related to decreased production)*
- Ataxia-telangiectasia *(evidenced by familial immunodeficiency disorder)*
- IgE deficiency

CRITICAL FINDINGS: N/A

INTERFERING FACTORS
- Drugs that may cause a decrease in IgE levels include phenytoin and tryptophan.
- Penicillin G has been associated with increased IgE levels in some patients with drug-induced acute interstitial nephritis.
- Normal IgE levels do not eliminate allergic disorders as a possible diagnosis.

NURSING IMPLICATIONS AND PROCEDURE

PRETEST:
▶ Positively identify the patient using at least two unique identifiers before providing care, treatment, or services.
▶ *Patient Teaching:* Inform the patient this test can assist in identification of an allergic or inflammatory response.
▶ Obtain a history of the patient's complaints, including a list of known allergens, especially allergies or sensitivities to latex.
▶ Obtain a history of the patient's immune and respiratory systems, symptoms, and results of previously performed laboratory tests and diagnostic and surgical procedures.
▶ Obtain a list of the patient's current medications, including herbs, nutritional supplements, and nutraceuticals (see Appendix F).

▶ Review the procedure with the patient. Inform the patient that specimen collection takes approximately 5 to 10 min. Address concerns about pain and explain that there may be some discomfort during the venipuncture.
▶ *Sensitivity to social and cultural issues,* as well as concern for modesty, is important in providing psychological support before, during, and after the procedure.
▶ There are no food, fluid, or medication restrictions unless by medical direction.

INTRATEST:
▶ If the patient has a history of allergic reaction to latex, avoid the use of equipment containing latex.
▶ Instruct the patient to cooperate fully and to follow directions. Direct the patient to breathe normally and to avoid unnecessary movement.
▶ Observe standard precautions, and follow the general guidelines in Appendix A. Positively identify the patient, and label the appropriate tubes with the corresponding patient demographics, date, and time of collection. Perform a venipuncture.
▶ Remove the needle and apply direct pressure with dry gauze to stop bleeding. Observe/assess venipuncture site for bleeding or hematoma formation and secure gauze with adhesive bandage.
▶ Promptly transport the specimen to the laboratory for processing and analysis.

POST-TEST:
▶ A report of the results will be sent to the requesting health-care provider (HCP), who will discuss the results with the patient.
▶ *Nutritional Considerations:* Increased IgE levels may be associated with allergy. Consideration should be given to diet if the patient has food allergies.
▶ Reinforce information given by the patient's HCP regarding further testing, treatment, or referral to another HCP. Answer any questions or address any concerns voiced by the patient or family.
▶ Depending on the results of this procedure, additional testing may be performed to evaluate or monitor

progression of the patient's condition and determine the need for a change in therapy. Evaluate test results in relation to the patient's symptoms and other tests performed.

RELATED MONOGRAPHS:

▶ Related tests include allergen-specific IgE, alveolar/arterial gradient, biopsy intestine, biopsy liver, biopsy muscle, blood gases, carbon dioxide, CBC, CBC platelet count, CBC WBC count and differential, eosinophil count, fecal analysis, hypersensitivity pneumonitis, lung perfusion scan, and PFT.

▶ Refer to the Immune and Respiratory systems tables at the end of the book for related tests by body system.

Immunoglobulins A, D, G, and M

SYNONYM/ACRONYM: IgA, IgD, IgG, and IgM.

COMMON USE: To quantitate immunoglobulins A, D, G, and M as an indicator of immune system function, to assist in the diagnosis of immune system disorders such as multiple myeloma, and to investigate transfusion anaphylaxis.

SPECIMEN: Serum (1 mL) collected in a red-top tube.

REFERENCE VALUE: (Method: Nephelometry)

Age	Conventional Units	SI Units
Immunoglobulin A		*(Conventional Units × 0.01)*
Newborn	1–4 mg/dL	0.01–0.04 g/L
1–9 mo	2–80 mg/dL	0.02–0.80 g/L
10–12 mo	15–90 mg/dL	0.15–0.90 g/L
2–3 yr	18–150 mg/dL	0.18–1.50 g/L
4–5 yr	25–160 mg/dL	0.25–1.60 g/L
6–8 yr	35–200 mg/dL	0.35–2.00 g/L
9–12 yr	45–250 mg/dL	0.45–2.50 g/L
Older than 12 yr	40–350 mg/dL	0.40–3.50 g/L
Immunoglobulin D		*(Conventional Units × 10)*
Newborn	Greater than 2 mg/dL	Greater than 20 mg/L
Adult	Less than 15 mg/dL	Less than 150 mg/L
Immunoglobulin G		*(Conventional Units × 0.01)*
Newborn	650–1,600 mg/dL	6.5–16 g/L
1–9 mo	250–900 mg/dL	2.5–9 g/L
10–12 mo	290–1,070 mg/dL	2.9–10.7 g/L
2–3 yr	420–1,200 mg/dL	4.2–12 g/L
4–6 yr	460–1,240 mg/dL	4.6–12.4 g/L
Greater than 6 yr	650–1,600 mg/dL	6.5–16 g/L

(table continues on page 820)

Age	Conventional Units	SI Units
Immunoglobulin M		*(Conventional Units × 0.01)*
Newborn	Less than 25 mg/dL	Less than 0.25 g/L
1–9 mo	20–125 mg/dL	0.2–1.25 g/L
10–12 mo	40–150 mg/dL	0.4–1.5 g/L
2–8 yr	45–200 mg/dL	0.45–2.0 g/L
9–12 yr	50–250 mg/dL	0.5–2.5 g/L
Greater than 12 yr	50–300 mg/dL	0.5–3.0 g/L

DESCRIPTION: Immunoglobulins A, D, E, G, and M are made by plasma cells in response to foreign particles. Immunoglobulins neutralize toxic substances, support phagocytosis, and destroy invading microorganisms. They are made up of heavy and light chains. Immunoglobulins produced by the proliferation of a single plasma cell (clone) are called *monoclonal*. Polyclonal increases result when multiple cell lines produce antibody. IgA is found mainly in secretions such as tears, saliva, and breast milk. It is believed to protect mucous membranes from viruses and bacteria. The function of IgD is not well understood. For details on IgE, see the monograph titled "Immunoglobulin E." IgG is the predominant serum immunoglobulin and is important in long-term defense against disease. It is the only antibody that crosses the placenta. IgM is the largest immunoglobulin, and it is the first antibody to react to an antigenic stimulus. IgM also forms natural antibodies, such as ABO blood group antibodies. The presence of IgM in cord blood is an indication of congenital infection.

INDICATIONS

• Assist in the diagnosis of multiple myeloma

• Evaluate humoral immunity status
• Monitor therapy for multiple myeloma
• IgA: Evaluate patients suspected of IgA deficiency prior to transfusion. Evaluate anaphylaxis associated with the transfusion of blood and blood products (anti-IgA antibodies may develop in patients with low levels of IgA, possibly resulting in anaphylaxis when donated blood is transfused)

POTENTIAL DIAGNOSIS

Increased in

IgA
Polyclonal
• Chronic liver disease *(pathophysiology is unclear)*
• Immunodeficiency states, such as Wiskott-Aldrich syndrome *(inherited condition of lymphocytes characterized by increased IgA and IgE)*
• Inflammatory bowel disease *(IgG and/or IgA antibody positive for Saccharomyces cerevisiae with negative perinuclear-anti-neutrophil cytoplasmic antibody is indicative of Crohn's disease)*
• Lower gastrointestinal (GI) cancer *(pathophysiology is unclear)*
• Rheumatoid arthritis *(pathophysiology is unclear)*

Monoclonal
• IgA-type multiple myeloma *(related to excessive production by a single clone of plasma cells)*

IgD
Polyclonal *(pathophysiology is unclear, but increases are associated with increases in IgM)*

- Certain liver diseases
- Chronic infections
- Connective tissue disorders

Monoclonal
- IgD-type multiple myeloma (related to excessive production by a single clone of plasma cells)

IgG

(Conditions that involve inflammation and/or development of an infection stimulate production of IgG.)

Polyclonal
- Autoimmune diseases, such as systemic lupus erythematosus, rheumatoid arthritis, and Sjögren's syndrome
- Chronic liver disease
- Chronic or recurrent infections
- Intrauterine devices (the IUD creates a localized inflammatory reaction that stimulates production of IgG)
- Sarcoidosis

Monoclonal
- IgG-type multiple myeloma (related to excessive production by a single clone of plasma cells)
- Leukemias
- Lymphomas

IgM

Polyclonal (humoral response to infections and inflammation; both acute and chronic)
- Active sarcoidosis
- Chronic hepatocellular disease
- Collagen vascular disease
- Early response to bacterial or parasitic infection
- Hyper-IgM dysgammaglobulinemia
- Rheumatoid arthritis
- Variable in nephrotic syndrome
- Viral infection (hepatitis or mononucleosis)

Monoclonal
- Cold agglutinin hemolysis disease
- Malignant lymphoma
- Neoplasms (especially in GI tract)
- Reticulosis
- Waldenström's macroglobulinemia (related to excessive production by a single clone of plasma cells)

Decreased in

IgA
- Ataxia-telangiectasia
- Chronic sinopulmonary disease
- Genetic IgA deficiency

IgD
- Genetic IgD deficiency
- Malignant melanoma of the skin
- Pre-eclampsia

IgG
- Burns
- Genetic IgG deficiency
- Nephrotic syndrome
- Pregnancy

IgM
- Burns
- Secondary IgM deficiency associated with IgG or IgA gammopathies

CRITICAL FINDINGS: N/A

INTERFERING FACTORS
- Drugs that may increase immunoglobulin levels include asparaginase, cimetidine, and narcotics.
- Drugs that may decrease immunoglobulin levels include dextran, oral contraceptives, methylprednisolone (high doses), and phenytoin.
- Chemotherapy, immunosuppressive therapy, and radiation treatments decrease immunoglobulin levels.
- Specimens with macroglobulins, cryoglobulins, or cold agglutinins tested at cold temperatures may give falsely low values.

NURSING IMPLICATIONS AND PROCEDURE

PRETEST:
- Positively identify the patient using at least two unique identifiers before providing care, treatment, or services.
- *Patient Teaching:* Inform the patient this test can assess the immune system by

evaluating the levels of immunoglobulins in the blood.

▶ Obtain a history of the patient's complaints, including a list of known allergens, especially allergies or sensitivities to latex.

▶ Obtain a history of the patient's hematopoietic and immune systems, symptoms, and results of previously performed laboratory tests and diagnostic and surgical procedures.

▶ Obtain a list of the patient's current medications, including herbs, nutritional supplements, and nutraceuticals (see Appendix F).

▶ Note any recent procedures that can interfere with test results.

▶ Review the procedure with the patient. Inform the patient that specimen collection takes approximately 5 to 10 min. Address concerns about pain and explain to the patient that there may be some discomfort during the venipuncture.

▶ *Sensitivity to social and cultural issues,* as well as concern for modesty, is important in providing psychological support before, during, and after the procedure.

▶ There are no food, fluid, or medication restrictions unless by medical direction.

INTRATEST:

▶ If the patient has a history of allergic reaction to latex, avoid the use of equipment containing latex.

▶ Instruct the patient to cooperate fully and to follow directions. Direct the patient to breathe normally and to avoid unnecessary movement.

▶ Observe standard precautions, and follow the general guidelines in Appendix A. Positively identify the patient, and label the appropriate tubes with the corresponding patient demographics, date, and time of collection. Perform a venipuncture.

▶ Remove the needle and apply direct pressure with dry gauze to stop bleeding. Observe/assess venipuncture site for bleeding or hematoma formation and secure gauze with adhesive bandage.

▶ Promptly transport the specimen to the laboratory for processing and analysis.

POST-TEST:

▶ A report of the results will be sent to the requesting health-care provider (HCP), who will discuss the results with the patient.

▶ Reinforce information given by the patient's HCP regarding further testing, treatment, or referral to another HCP. Answer any questions or address any concerns voiced by the patient or family.

▶ Depending on the results of this procedure, additional testing may be performed to evaluate or monitor progression of the disease process and determine the need for a change in therapy. Evaluate test results in relation to the patient's symptoms and other tests performed.

RELATED MONOGRAPHS:

▶ Related tests include ALT, anion gap, ANA, bilirubin, biopsy bone, biopsy bone marrow, biopsy liver, biopsy lymph node, blood groups and antibodies, cold agglutinin, CBC, CBC WBC count and differential, Coomb's antiglobulin (direct and indirect), cryoglobulin, ESR, fibrinogen, IFE, quantitative immunoglobulin levels, GGT, LAP, liver and spleen scan, beta-2-microglobulin, platelet antibodies, protein total and fractions, RF, and uric acid.

▶ Refer to the Hematopoietic and Immune systems tables at the end of the book for related tests by body system.

Immunosuppressants: Cyclosporine, Methotrexate

SYNONYM/ACRONYM: Cyclosporine (Sandimmune), methotrexate (MTX, amethopterin, Folex, Rheumatrex), methotrexate sodium (Mexate).

COMMON USE: To monitor appropriate drug dosage of cyclosporine and methotrexate related to organ transplant maintenance.

SPECIMEN: Whole blood (1 mL) collected in lavender-top tube for cyclosporine. Serum (1 mL) collected in a red-top tube for methotrexate.

Immunosuppressant	Route of Administration	Recommended Collection Time
Cyclosporine	Oral or Intravenous	12 hr after dose or immediately prior to next dose
Methotrexate	Oral	Varies according to dosing protocol
	Intramuscular	Varies according to dosing protocol

Leucovorin therapy, also called leucovorin rescue, is used in conjunction with administration of methotrexate. Leucovorin, a fast-acting form of folic acid, protects healthy cells from the toxic effects of methotrexate.

Important note: This information must be clearly and accurately communicated to avoid misunderstanding of the dose time in relation to the collection time. Miscommunication between the individual administering the medication and the individual collecting the specimen is the most frequent cause of subtherapeutic levels, toxic levels, and misleading information used in calculation of future doses.

REFERENCE VALUE: (Method: Immunoassay)

	Therapeutic Dose		Half-Life	Volume of Distribution	Protein Binding	Excretion
	Conventional Units	*SI Units (Conventional Units × 0.832)*				
Cyclosporine	100–300 ng/mL renal transplant	83–250 nmol/L	8–24 hr	4–6 L/kg	90%	Renal

(*table continues on page 824*)

	Therapeutic Dose		Half-Life	Volume of Distribution	Protein Binding	Excretion
	Conventional Units	*SI Units (Conventional Units × 0.832)*				
	200–350 ng/mL cardiac, hepatic, pancreatic transplant	166–291 nmol/L	8–24 hr	4–6 L/kg	90%	Renal
	100–300 ng/mL bone marrow transplant	83–250 nmol/L	8–24 hr	4–6 L/kg	90%	Renal
Methotrexate	Dependent on therapeutic approach		0.5–1 hr; 5–9 hr for elimination	0.4–1.0 L/kg	50–70%	Renal

DESCRIPTION: Cyclosporine is an immunosuppressive drug used in the management of organ rejection, especially rejection of heart, liver, pancreas, and kidney transplants. Its most serious side effect is renal impairment or renal failure. Cyclosporine is often administered in conjunction with corticosteroids (e.g., prednisone) for its anti-inflammatory or immune-suppressing properties and with other drugs (e.g., tacrolimus) to reduce graft-versus-host disease. Methotrexate is a highly toxic drug that causes cell death by disrupting DNA synthesis. Methotrexate is also used in the treatment of rheumatoid arthritis, psoriasis, polymyositis, and Reiter's syndrome.

Many factors must be considered in effective dosing and monitoring of therapeutic drugs, including patient age; weight; interacting medications; electrolyte balance; protein levels; water balance; conditions that affect absorption and excretion; as well as foods, herbals, vitamins, and minerals that can either potentiate or inhibit the intended target concentration.

INDICATIONS

Cyclosporine
- Assist in the management of treatments to prevent organ rejection
- Monitor for toxicity

Methotrexate
- Monitor effectiveness of treatment of cancer and some autoimmune disorders
- Monitor for toxicity

POTENTIAL DIAGNOSIS

Normal levels	Therapeutic effect
Toxic levels	Adjust dose as indicated
Cyclosporine	Renal impairment
Methotrexate	Renal impairment

CRITICAL FINDINGS

It is important to note the adverse effects of toxic and subtherapeutic levels. Care must be taken to investigate signs and symptoms of too little and too much medication.

Note and immediately report to the health-care provider (HCP) any critically increased values and related symptoms.

Cyclosporine: Greater Than 400 ng/mL

Signs and symptoms of cyclosporine toxicity include increased severity of expected side effects, which include nausea, stomatitis, vomiting, anorexia, hypertension, infection, fluid retention, hypercalcemic metabolic acidosis, tremor, seizures, headache, and flushing. Possible interventions include close monitoring of blood levels to make dosing adjustments, inducing emesis (if orally ingested), performing gastric lavage (if orally ingested), withholding the drug, and initiating alternative therapy for a short time until the patient is stabilized.

Methotrexate: Greater Than 1.00 micromol/L After 48 hr With High-Dose Therapy; Greater Than 0.02 micromol/L After 48 hr With Low-Dose Therapy

Signs and symptoms of methotrexate toxicity include increased severity of expected side effects, which include nausea, stomatitis, vomiting, anorexia, bleeding, infection, bone marrow depression, and, over a prolonged period of use, hepatotoxicity. The effect of methotrexate on normal cells can be reversed by administration of 5-formyltetrahydrofolate (citrovorum or leucovorin). 5-Formyltetrahydrofolate allows higher doses of methotrexate to be given.

INTERFERING FACTORS

- Numerous drugs interact with cyclosporine and either increase cyclosporine levels or increase the risk of toxicity. These drugs include acyclovir, aminoglycosides, amiodarone, amphotericin B, anabolic steroids, cephalosporins, cimetidine, danazol, erythromycin, furosemide, ketoconazole, melphalan, methylprednisolone, miconazole, NSAIDs, oral contraceptives, and trimethoprimsulfamethoxazole.
- Drugs that may decrease cyclosporine levels include carbamazepine, ethotoin, mephenytoin, phenobarbital, phenytoin, primidone, and rifampin.
- Drugs that may increase methotrexate levels or increase the risk of toxicity include NSAIDs, probenecid, salicylate, and sulfonamides.
- Antibiotics may decrease the absorption of methotrexate.

NURSING IMPLICATIONS AND PROCEDURE

PRETEST:

▶ Positively identify the patient using at least two unique identifiers before providing care, treatment, or services.
▶ *Patient Teaching:* Inform the patient this test can assess in monitoring therapeutic and toxic drug levels.
▶ Obtain a history of the patient's complaints, including a list of known allergens, especially allergies or sensitivities to latex.

Obtain a history of the patient's genito-urinary and immune systems, symptoms, and results of previously performed laboratory tests and diagnostic and surgical procedures. Some considerations prior to the administration of methotrexate include documentation of adequate renal function with creatinine and BUN levels, documentation of adequate hepatic function with alanine aminotransferase (ALT) and bilirubin levels, and documentation of adequate hematological and immune function with platelet and white blood cell (WBC) count. Patients must be well hydrated and, depending on the therapy, may be treated with sodium bicarbonate for urinary alkalinization to enhance drug excretion. Leucovorin calcium rescue therapy may also be part of the protocol.

Obtain a list of the patient's current medications, including herbs, nutritional supplements, and nutraceuticals (see Appendix F).

Review the procedure with the patient. Inform the patient that specimen collection takes approximately 5 to 10 min. Address concerns about pain and explain that there may be some discomfort during the venipuncture.

Sensitivity to social and cultural issues, as well as concern for modesty, is important in providing psychological support before, during, and after the procedure.

There are no food, fluid, or medication restrictions unless by medical direction.

INTRATEST:

If the patient has a history of allergic reaction to latex, avoid the use of equipment containing latex.

Instruct the patient to cooperate fully and to follow directions. Direct the patient to breathe normally and to avoid unnecessary movement.

Observe standard precautions, and follow the general guidelines in Appendix A. Consider recommended collection time with regard to dosing schedule. Positively identify the patient, and label the appropriate tubes with the corresponding patient demographics, date, and time of collection. Perform a venipuncture.

Remove the needle and apply direct pressure with dry gauze to stop bleeding.

Observe/assess venipuncture site for bleeding or hematoma formation and secure gauze with adhesive bandage.

Promptly transport the specimen to the laboratory for processing and analysis.

POST-TEST:

A report of the results will be sent to the requesting HCP, who will discuss the results with the patient.

Nutritional Considerations: Patients taking immunosuppressant therapy tend to have decreased appetites due to the side effects of the medication. Instruct patients to consume a variety of foods within the basic food groups, maintain a healthy weight, be physically active, limit salt intake, limit alcohol intake, and be a nonsmoker.

Recognize anxiety related to test results, and offer support. Patients receiving these drugs usually have conditions that can be intermittently moderately to severely debilitating, resulting in significant lifestyle changes. Educate the patient regarding access to counseling services, as appropriate.

Reinforce information given by the patient's HCP regarding further testing, treatment, or referral to another HCP. Explain to the patient the importance of following the medication regimen and give instructions regarding drug interactions. Answer any questions or address any concerns voiced by the patient or family.

Instruct the patient to be prepared to provide the pharmacist with a list of other medications he or she is already taking in the event that the requesting HCP prescribes a medication.

Depending on the results of this procedure, additional testing may be performed to evaluate or monitor progression of the disease process and determine the need for a change in therapy. Evaluate test results in relation to the patient's symptoms and other tests performed.

RELATED MONOGRAPHS:

Related tests include ALT, bilirubin, BUN, CBC platelet count, CBC WBC count and differential, and creatinine.

Refer to the Genitourinary and Immune systems tables at the end of the book for related tests by body system.

Infectious Mononucleosis Screen

SYNONYM/ACRONYM: Monospot, heterophil antibody test, IM serology.

COMMON USE: To assess for Epstein-Barr virus and assist with diagnosis of infectious mononucleosis.

SPECIMEN: Serum (1 mL) collected in a red-top tube.

REFERENCE VALUE: (Method: Agglutination) Negative.

DESCRIPTION: Infectious mononucleosis is caused by the Epstein-Barr virus (EBV). The incubation period is 10 to 50 days, and the symptoms last 1 to 4 wk after the infection has fully developed. The hallmark of EBV infection is the presence of heterophil antibodies, also called *Paul-Bunnell-Davidsohn antibodies*, which are immunoglobulin M (IgM) antibodies that agglutinate sheep or horse red blood cells. The disease induces formation of abnormal lymphocytes in the lymph nodes; stimulates increased formation of heterophil antibodies; and is characterized by fever, cervical lymphadenopathy, tonsillopharyngitis, and hepatosplenomegaly. EBV is also thought to play a role in Burkitt's lymphoma, nasopharyngeal carcinoma, and chronic fatigue syndrome. If the results of the heterophil antibody screening test are negative and infectious mononucleosis is highly suspected, EBV-specific serology should be requested.

INDICATIONS
• Assist in confirming infectious mononucleosis

POTENTIAL DIAGNOSIS

Positive findings in
• Infectious mononucleosis

Negative findings in: N/A

CRITICAL FINDINGS: N/A

INTERFERING FACTORS
• False-positive results may occur in the presence of narcotic addiction, serum sickness, lymphomas, hepatitis, leukemia, cancer of the pancreas, and phenytoin therapy.
• A false-negative result may occur if treatment was begun before antibodies developed or if the test was done less than 6 days after exposure to the virus.

NURSING IMPLICATIONS AND PROCEDURE

PRETEST:

• Positively identify the patient using at least two unique identifiers before providing care, treatment, or services.
• *Patient Teaching:* Inform the patient this test can assist with diagnosing a mononucleosis infection.
• Obtain a history of the patient's complaints, including a list of known allergens, especially allergies or sensitivities to latex. Obtain a history of exposure.
• Obtain a history of the patient's hepatobiliary and immune systems, symptoms,

and results of previously performed laboratory tests and diagnostic and surgical procedures.

- Note any recent therapies that can interfere with test results.
- Obtain a list of the patient's current medications, including herbs, nutritional supplements, and nutraceuticals (see Appendix F).
- Review the procedure with the patient. Inform the patient that specimen collection takes approximately 5 to 10 min. Address concerns about pain and explain that there may be some discomfort during the venipuncture.
- *Sensitivity to social and cultural issues,* as well as concern for modesty, is important in providing psychological support before, during, and after the procedure.
- There are no food, fluid, or medication restrictions unless by medical direction.

INTRATEST:

- If the patient has a history of allergic reaction to latex, avoid the use of equipment containing latex.
- Instruct the patient to cooperate fully and to follow directions. Direct the patient to breathe normally and to avoid unnecessary movement.
- Observe standard precautions, and follow the general guidelines in Appendix A. Positively identify the patient, and label the appropriate tubes with the corresponding patient demographics, date, and time of collection. Perform a venipuncture.
- Remove the needle and apply direct pressure with dry gauze to stop bleeding. Observe/assess venipuncture site for bleeding or hematoma formation and secure gauze with adhesive bandage.

- Promptly transport the specimen to the laboratory for processing and analysis.

POST-TEST:

- A report of the results will be sent to the requesting health-care provider (HCP), who will discuss the results with the patient.
- Inform the patient that approximately 10% of all results are false-negative or false-positive. Inform the patient that signs and symptoms of infection include fever, chills, sore throat, enlarged lymph nodes, and fatigue. Self-care while the disease runs its course includes adequate fluid and nutritional intake along with sufficient rest. Activities that cause fatigue or stress should be avoided.
- Reinforce information given by the patient's HCP regarding further testing, treatment, or referral to another HCP. Advise the patient to refrain from direct contact with others because the disease is transmitted through saliva. Answer any questions or address any concerns voiced by the patient or family.
- Depending on the results of this procedure, additional testing may be performed to evaluate or monitor progression of the disease process and determine the need for a change in therapy. Evaluate test results in relation to the patient's symptoms and other tests performed.

RELATED MONOGRAPHS:

- Related tests include CBC with peripheral blood smear evaluation.
- Refer to the Hepatobiliary and Immune systems tables at the end of the book for related tests by body system.

Insulin and Insulin Response to Glucose

SYNONYM/ACRONYM: N/A.

COMMON USE: To assess the amount of insulin secreted in response to blood glucose to assist in diagnosis of types of hypoglycemia and insulin resistant pathologies.

SPECIMEN: Serum (1 mL) collected in a red-top tube.

REFERENCE VALUE: (Method: Immunoassay)

75-g Glucose Load	Insulin	SI Units (Conventional Units × 6.945)	Tolerance for Glucose (Hypoglycemia)
Fasting	Less than 17 micro international units/L	Less than 118.1 pmol/L	Less than 110 mg/dL
30 min	6–86 micro international units/L	41.7–597.3 pmol/L	Less than 200 mg/dL
1 hr	8–118 micro international units/L	55.6–819.5 pmol/L	Less than 200 mg/dL
2 hr	5–55 micro international units/L	34.7–382.0 pmol/L	Less than 140 mg/dL
3 hr	Less than 25 micro international units/L	Less than 174 pmol/L	65–120 mg/dL
4 hr	Less than 15 micro international units/L	Less than 104.2 pmol/L	65–120 mg/dL
5 hr	Less than 8 micro international units/L	Less than 55.6 pmol/L	65–115 mg/dL

DESCRIPTION: Insulin is secreted in response to elevated blood glucose, and its overall effect is to promote glucose use and energy storage. The insulin response test measures the rate of insulin secreted by the beta cells of the islets of Langerhans in the pancreas; it may be performed simultaneously with a 5-hr glucose tolerance test for hypoglycemia.

INDICATIONS

- Assist in the diagnosis of early or developing non-insulin-dependent (type 2) diabetes, as indicated by excessive production of insulin in relation to blood glucose levels (best shown with glucose tolerance tests or 2-hr postprandial tests)
- Assist in the diagnosis of insulinoma, as indicated by sustained high levels of insulin and absence of blood glucose–related variations

- Confirm functional hypoglycemia, as indicated by circulating insulin levels appropriate to changing blood glucose levels
- Differentiate between insulin-resistant diabetes, in which insulin levels are high, and non-insulin-resistant diabetes, in which insulin levels are low
- Evaluate fasting hypoglycemia of unknown cause
- Evaluate postprandial hypoglycemia of unknown cause
- Evaluate uncontrolled insulin-dependent (type 1) diabetes

POTENTIAL DIAGNOSIS

Increased in
- Acromegaly *(related to excess production of growth hormone, which increases insulin levels)*
- Alcohol use *(related to stimulation of insulin production)*
- Cushing's syndrome *(related to overproduction of cortisol, which increases insulin levels)*
- Excessive administration of insulin
- Insulin- and proinsulin-secreting tumors (insulinomas)
- Obesity *(related to development of insulin resistance; body does not respond to insulin being produced)*
- Persistent hyperinsulinemic hypoglycemia *(collection of hypoglycemic disorders of infants and children)*
- Reactive hypoglycemia in developing diabetes
- Severe liver disease

Decreased in
- Beta cell failure *(pancreatic beta cells produce insulin; therefore, damage to these cells will decrease insulin levels)*
- Insulin-dependent diabetes *(related to lack of endogenous insulin)*

CRITICAL FINDINGS: N/A

INTERFERING FACTORS
- Drugs and substances that may increase insulin levels include acetohexamide, albuterol, amino acids, beclomethasone, betamethasone, broxaterol, calcium gluconate, cannabis, chlorpropamide, glibornuride, glipizide, glisoxepide, glucagon, glyburide, ibopamine, insulin, oral contraceptives, pancreozymin, prednisolone, prednisone, rifampin, terbutaline, tolazamide, tolbutamide, trichlormethiazide, and verapamil.
- Drugs that may decrease insulin levels include acarbose, calcitonin, cimetidine, clofibrate, dexfenfluramine, diltiazem, doxazosin, enalapril, enprostil, ether, hydroxypropyl methylcellulose, metformin (Glucophage), niacin, nifedipine, nitrendipine, octreotide, phenytoin, propranolol, and psyllium.
- Administration of insulin or oral hypoglycemic agents within 8 hr of the test can lead to falsely elevated levels.
- Hemodialysis destroys insulin and affects test results.

NURSING IMPLICATIONS AND PROCEDURE

PRETEST:
- Positively identify the patient using at least two unique identifiers before providing care, treatment, or services.
- *Patient Teaching:* Inform the patient this test can assist in the evaluation of low blood sugar.
- Obtain a history of the patient's complaints, including a list of known allergens, especially allergies or sensitivities to latex.
- Obtain a history of the patient's endocrine system, symptoms, and results of previously performed laboratory tests and diagnostic and surgical procedures.
- Note any recent procedures that can interfere with test results.

- Obtain a list of the patient's current medications, including herbs, nutritional supplements, and nutraceuticals (see Appendix F). Note the last time and dose of medication taken.
- Review the procedure with the patient. Inform the patient that multiple specimens may be required. Inform the patient that specimen collection takes approximately 5 to 10 min. Address concerns about pain and explain that there may be some discomfort during the venipuncture.
- *Sensitivity to social and cultural issues,* as well as concern for modesty, is important in providing psychological support before, during, and after the procedure.
- If a single sample is to be collected, the patient should have fasted and refrained, with medical direction, from taking insulin or other oral hypoglycemic agents for at least 8 hr before specimen collection. Protocols may vary among facilities.
- *Hypoglycemia:* Serial specimens for insulin levels are collected in conjunction with glucose levels after administration of a 75-g glucose load. The patient should be prepared as for a standard oral glucose tolerance test over a 5-hr period. Protocols may vary among facilities.
- There are no fluid restrictions unless by medical direction.

INTRATEST:

- Ensure that the patient has complied with dietary and medication restrictions and other pretesting preparations; assure that food or medications have been restricted as instructed prior to the specific procedure's protocol.
- If the patient has a history of allergic reaction to latex, avoid the use of equipment containing latex.
- Instruct the patient to cooperate fully and to follow directions. Direct the patient to breathe normally and to avoid unnecessary movement.
- Observe standard precautions, and follow the general guidelines in Appendix A. Positively identify the patient, and label the appropriate tubes with the corresponding patient demographics, date,

and time of collection. Perform a venipuncture.
- Remove the needle and apply direct pressure with dry gauze to stop bleeding. Observe/assess venipuncture site for bleeding or hematoma formation and secure gauze with adhesive bandage.
- Promptly transport the specimen to the laboratory for processing and analysis.

POST-TEST:

- A report of the results will be sent to the requesting health-care provider (HCP), who will discuss the results with the patient.
- Instruct the patient to resume usual diet and medication, as directed by the HCP.
- *Nutritional Considerations:* Increased insulin levels may be associated with diabetes. There is no "diabetic diet"; however, many meal-planning approaches with nutritional goals are endorsed by the American Dietetic Association. Patients who adhere to dietary recommendations report a better general feeling of health, better weight management, greater control of glucose and lipid values, and improved use of insulin. Instruct the patient, as appropriate, in nutritional management of diabetes. In June 2006, the American Heart Association developed a Therapeutic Lifestyle Changes (TLC) diet with goals directed at people with specific risk factors and/or existing medical conditions (e.g., elevated LDL cholesterol levels, other lipid disorders, coronary artery disease [CAD], insulin-dependent diabetes, insulin resistance, or metabolic syndrome). The TLC approach also includes the use of plant stanols or sterols and increased dissolved fiber as an option for lowering LDL cholesterol levels; nutritional recommendations for daily total caloric intake; recommendations for allowable percentage of calories derived from fat (saturated and unsaturated), carbohydrates, protein, and cholesterol; as well as recommendations for daily expenditure of energy. The nutritional needs of each diabetic patient need to be determined individually (especially during

I

pregnancy) with the appropriate HCPs, particularly professionals trained in nutrition.

- Impaired glucose tolerance may be associated with diabetes. Instruct the patient and caregiver to report signs and symptoms of hypoglycemia (weakness, confusion, diaphoresis, rapid pulse) or hyperglycemia (thirst, polyuria, hunger, lethargy).

- *Social and Cultural Considerations:* Numerous studies point to the prevalence of excess body weight in American children and adolescents. Experts estimate that obesity is present in 25% of the population ages 6 to 11 yr. The medical, social, and emotional consequences of excess body weight are significant. Special attention should be given to instructing the child and caregiver regarding health risks and weight control education.

- Recognize anxiety related to test results, and be supportive of perceived loss of independence and fear of shortened life expectancy. Discuss the implications of abnormal test results on the patient's lifestyle. Provide teaching and information regarding the clinical implications of the test results, as appropriate. Emphasize, if indicated, that good glycemic control delays the onset and slows the progression of diabetic retinopathy, nephropathy, and neuropathy. Educate the patient regarding access to counseling services, as appropriate. Provide contact information, if desired, for the American Diabetes Association (www.diabetes.org), the American Heart Association (www.americanheart .org), or the NHLBI (www.nhlbi.nih.gov).

- Reinforce information given by the patient's HCP regarding further testing, treatment, or referral to another HCP. Instruct the patient in the use of home test kits approved by the U.S. Food and Drug Administration, if prescribed. Answer any questions or address any concerns voiced by the patient or family.

- Depending on the results of this procedure, additional testing may be performed to evaluate or monitor progression of the disease process and determine the need for a change in therapy. Evaluate test results in relation to the patient's symptoms and other tests performed.

RELATED MONOGRAPHS:

- Related tests include ACTH, ALT, angiography adrenal, bilirubin, BUN, calcium, catecholamines, cholesterol (HDL, LDL, total), cortisol, C-peptide, DHEA, creatinine, fecal analysis, fecal fat, fructosamine, GGT, gastric emptying scan, glucagon, glucose, GTT, glycated hemoglobin, GH, HVA, insulin antibodies, ketones, lipoprotein electrophoresis, metanephrines, microalbumin, and myoglobin.

- Refer to the Endocrine System table at the end of the book for related tests by body system.

Insulin Antibodies

SYNONYM/ACRONYM: N/A.

COMMON USE: To assist in the prediction, diagnosis, and management of type 1 diabetes as well as insulin resistance and insulin allergy.

SPECIMEN: Serum (1 mL) collected in a red-top tube.

REFERENCE VALUE: (Method: Radioimmunoassay) Less than 3%; includes binding of human, beef, and pork insulin to antibodies in patient's serum.

DESCRIPTION: The most common anti-insulin antibody is immunoglobulin (Ig) G, but IgA, IgM, IgD, and IgE antibodies also have anti-insulin properties. These antibodies usually do not cause clinical problems, but they may complicate insulin assay testing. IgM is thought to participate in insulin resistance and IgE in insulin allergy. Improvements in the purity of animal insulin and increased use of human insulin have resulted in a significant decrease in the incidence of insulin antibody formation.

INDICATIONS

• Assist in confirming insulin resistance
• Assist in determining if hypoglycemia is caused by insulin abuse
• Assist in determining insulin allergy

POTENTIAL DIAGNOSIS

Increased in

• Factitious hypoglycemia *(assists in differentiating lack of response due to the presence of insulin antibodies from secretive self-administration of insulin)*
• Insulin allergy or resistance *(antibodies bind to insulin and decrease amount of free insulin available for glucose metabolism)*
• Polyendocrine autoimmune syndromes
• Steroid-induced diabetes *(a side effect of treatment for systemic lupus erythematosus)*

Decreased in: N/A

CRITICAL FINDINGS: N/A

INTERFERING FACTORS

• Recent radioactive scans or radiation can interfere with test results when radioimmunoassay is the test method.

NURSING IMPLICATIONS AND PROCEDURE

PRETEST:

▶ Positively identify the patient using at least two unique identifiers before providing care, treatment, or services.
▶ *Patient Teaching:* Inform the patient this test can assist in the diagnosis and management of type 1 diabetes.
▶ Obtain a history of the patient's complaints, including a list of known allergens, especially allergies or sensitivities to latex.
▶ Obtain a history of the patient's endocrine and immune systems, symptoms, and results of previously performed laboratory tests and diagnostic and surgical procedures.
▶ Note any recent procedures that can interfere with test results.
▶ Obtain a list of the patient's current medications, including herbs, nutritional supplements, and nutraceuticals (see Appendix F). Note the last time and dose of medication taken.
▶ Review the procedure with the patient. Inform the patient that specimen collection takes approximately 5 to 10 min. Address concerns about pain and explain that there may be some discomfort during the venipuncture.
▶ *Sensitivity to social and cultural issues,* as well as concern for modesty, is important in providing psychological support before, during, and after the procedure.
▶ There are no food, fluid, or medication restrictions unless by medical direction.

INTRATEST:

▶ If the patient has a history of allergic reaction to latex, avoid the use of equipment containing latex.
▶ Instruct the patient to cooperate fully and to follow directions. Direct the patient to breathe normally and to avoid unnecessary movement.

- Observe standard precautions, and follow the general guidelines in Appendix A. Positively identify the patient, and label the appropriate tubes with the corresponding patient demographics, date, and time of collection. Perform a venipuncture.
- Remove the needle and apply direct pressure with dry gauze to stop bleeding. Observe/assess venipuncture site for bleeding or hematoma formation and secure gauze with adhesive bandage.
- Promptly transport the specimen to the laboratory for processing and analysis.

POST-TEST:

- A report of the results will be sent to the requesting health-care provider (HCP), who will discuss the results with the patient.
- Instruct the patient to resume usual diet and medication, as directed by the HCP.
- *Nutritional Considerations:* Abnormal findings may be associated with diabetes. There is no "diabetic diet"; however, many meal-planning approaches with nutritional goals are endorsed by the American Dietetic Association. Patients who adhere to dietary recommendations report a better general feeling of health, better weight management, greater control of glucose and lipid values, and improved use of insulin. Instruct the patient, as appropriate, in nutritional management of diabetes. In June 2006, the American Heart Association developed a Therapeutic Lifestyle Changes (TLC) diet with goals directed at people with specific risk factors and/or existing medical conditions (e.g., elevated LDL cholesterol levels, other lipid disorders, coronary artery disease [CAD], insulin-dependent diabetes, insulin resistance, or metabolic syndrome). The TLC approach also includes the use of plant stanols or sterols and increased dissolved fiber as an option for lowering LDL cholesterol levels; nutritional recommendations for daily total caloric intake; recommendations for allowable percentage of calories derived from fat (saturated and unsaturated), carbohydrates, protein, and cholesterol; as well as recommendations for daily expenditure of energy. The nutritional needs of each diabetic patient need to be determined individually (especially during pregnancy) with the appropriate HCPs, particularly professionals trained in nutrition.

- Impaired glucose tolerance may be associated with diabetes. Instruct the patient and caregiver to report signs and symptoms of hypoglycemia (weakness, confusion, diaphoresis, rapid pulse) or hyperglycemia (thirst, polyuria, hunger, lethargy).
- Recognize anxiety related to test results, and be supportive of perceived loss of independence and fear of shortened life expectancy. Discuss the implications of abnormal test results on the patient's lifestyle. Provide teaching and information regarding the clinical implications of the test results, as appropriate. Emphasize, if indicated, that good glycemic control delays the onset and slows the progression of diabetic retinopathy, nephropathy, and neuropathy. Educate the patient regarding access to counseling services, as appropriate. Provide contact information, if desired, for the American Diabetes Association (www.diabetes.org) or the American Heart Association (www.americanheart.org).
- Reinforce information given by the patient's HCP regarding further testing, treatment, or referral to another HCP. Answer any questions or address any concerns voiced by the patient or family.
- Depending on the results of this procedure, additional testing may be performed to evaluate or monitor progression of the disease process and determine the need for a change in therapy. Evaluate test results in relation to the patient's symptoms and other tests performed.

RELATED MONOGRAPHS:

- Related tests include C-peptide, glucose, GTT, and insulin.
- Refer to the Endocrine and Immune systems tables at the end of the book for related tests by body system.

Intraocular Muscle Function

SYNONYM/ACRONYM: IOM function.

COMMON USE: To assess the function of the extraocular muscle to assist with diagnosis of strabismus, amblyopia, and other ocular disorders.

AREA OF APPLICATION: Eyes.

CONTRAST: N/A.

DESCRIPTION: Evaluation of ocular motility is performed to detect and measure muscle imbalance in conditions classified as heterophorias or heterotropias. This evaluation is performed in a manner to assess fixation of each eye, alignment of both eyes in all directions, and the ability of both eyes to work together binocularly. Heterophorias are latent ocular deviations kept in check by the binocular power of fusion and made intermittent by disrupting fusion. Heterotropias are conditions that manifest constant ocular deviations. The prefixes *eso-* (tendency for the eye to turn in), *exo-* (tendency for the eye to turn out), and *hyper-* (tendency for one eye to turn up) indicate the direction in which the affected eye moves spontaneously. *Strabismus* is the failure of both eyes to spontaneously fixate on the same object because of a muscular imbalance (crossed eyes). *Amblyopia*, or lazy eye, is a term used for loss of vision in one or both eyes that cannot be attributed to an organic pathological condition of the eye or optic nerve. There are six extraocular muscles in each eye; their movement is controlled by three nerves. The actions of the muscles

vary depending on the position of the eye when they become innervated. The cover test is commonly used because it is reliable, easy to perform, and does not require special equipment. The cover test method is described in this monograph. Another method for evaluation of ocular muscle function is the corneal light reflex test. It is useful with patients who cannot cooperate for prism cover testing or for patients who have poor fixation.

INDICATIONS
• Detection and evaluation of extraocular muscle imbalance

POTENTIAL DIAGNOSIS
The examiner should determine the range of ocular movements in all gaze positions, usually to include up and out, in, down and out, up and in, down and in, and out. Limited movements in gaze position can be recorded semiquantitatively as −1 (minimal), −2 (moderate), −3 (severe), or −4 (total).

Normal findings in
• Normal range of ocular movements in all gaze positions.

Abnormal findings in
- Amblyopia
- Heterophorias
- Heterotropias
- Strabismus

CRITICAL FINDINGS: N/A

INTERFERING FACTORS

Factors that may impair the results of the examination
- Inability of the patient to cooperate and remain still during the test because of age, significant pain, or mental status may interfere with the test results.
- Rubbing or squeezing the eyes may affect results.

NURSING IMPLICATIONS AND PROCEDURE

PRETEST:

- Positively identify the patient using at least two unique identifiers before providing care, treatment, or services.
- *Patient Teaching:* Inform the patient this procedure can assist in evaluating eye muscle function.
- Obtain a history of the patient's complaints, including a list of known allergens, especially latex.
- Obtain a history of the patient's known or suspected vision loss, changes in visual acuity, including type and cause; use of glasses or contact lenses; eye conditions with treatment regimens; eye surgery; and other tests and procedures to assess and diagnose visual deficit.
- Obtain a history of symptoms and results of previously performed laboratory tests and diagnostic and surgical procedures.
- Obtain a list of the patient's current medications, including herbs, nutritional supplements, and nutraceuticals (see Appendix F).
- Review the procedure with the patient. Address concerns about pain and explain that no discomfort will be

experienced during the test. Inform the patient that a health-care provider (HCP) performs the test in a quiet room and that to evaluate both eyes, the test can take 2 to 4 min.
- Instruct the patient to remove contact lenses or glasses, as appropriate. Instruct the patient regarding the importance of keeping the eyes open for the test.
- *Sensitivity to social and cultural issues,* as well as concern for modesty, is important in providing psychological support before, during, and after the procedure.
- There are no food, fluid, or medication restrictions unless by medical direction.

INTRATEST:

- Instruct the patient to cooperate fully and to follow directions. Ask the patient to remain still during the procedure because movement produces unreliable results.
- One eye is tested at a time. The patient is given a fixation point, usually the testing personnel's index finger. An object, such as a small toy, can be used to ensure fixation in pediatric patients. The patient is asked to follow the fixation point with his or her gaze in the direction the fixation point moves. When testing is completed, the procedure is repeated using the other eye. The procedure is performed at a distance and near, first with and then without corrective lenses.

POST-TEST:

- A report of the results will be sent to the requesting HCP, who will discuss the results with the patient.
- Recognize anxiety related to test results, and be supportive of impaired activity related to vision loss, anticipated loss of driving privileges, or the possibility of requiring corrective lenses (self-image).
- Reinforce information given by the patient's HCP regarding further testing, treatment, or referral to another HCP. Educate the patient, as appropriate, that he or she may be referred for special therapy to correct the anomaly, which may include glasses, prisms, eye exercises, eye patches, or chemical

patching with drugs that modify the focusing power of the eye. The patient and family should be educated that the chosen therapy involves a process of mental retraining. The mode of therapy in itself does not correct vision. It is the process by which the brain becomes readapted to accept, receive, and store visual images received by the eye that results in vision correction. Therefore, the patient must be prepared to be alert, cooperative, and properly motivated. Answer any questions or address any concerns voiced by the patient or family.

▶ Depending on the results of this procedure, additional testing may be performed to evaluate or monitor progression of the disease process and determine the need for a change in therapy. Evaluate test results in relation to the patient's symptoms and other tests performed.

RELATED MONOGRAPHS:

▶ Related tests include refraction and slit-lamp biomicroscopy.
▶ Refer to the Ocular System table at the end of the book for related tests by body system.

Intraocular Pressure

SYNONYM/ACRONYM: IOP.

COMMON USE: To evaluate changes in ocular pressure to assist in diagnosis of disorders such as glaucoma.

AREA OF APPLICATION: Eyes.

CONTRAST: N/A.

DESCRIPTION: The intraocular pressure (IOP) of the eye depends on a number of factors. The two most significant are the amount of aqueous humor present in the eye and the circumstances by which it leaves the eye. Other physiological variables that affect IOP include respiration, pulse, and the degree of hydration of the body. Individual eyes respond to IOP differently. Some can tolerate high pressures (20 to 30 mm Hg), and some will incur optic nerve damage at lower pressures. With respiration, variations of up to 4 mm Hg in IOP can occur, and changes of 1 to 2 mm Hg occur with every

pulsation of the central retinal artery. IOP is measured with a tonometer; normal values indicate the pressure at which no damage is done to the intraocular contents. The rate of fluid leaving the eye, or its ability to leave the eye unimpeded, is the most important factor regulating IOP. There are three primary conditions that result in occlusion of the outflow channels for fluid. The most common condition is open-angle glaucoma, in which the diameter of the openings of the trabecular meshwork becomes narrowed, resulting in an increased IOP due to an increased resistance of fluid moving out of the eye. In secondary glaucoma, the trabecular meshwork becomes occluded by tumor cells, pigment, red blood cells in hyphema, or other material. Additionally, the obstructing material may cover parts of the meshwork itself, as with scar tissue or other types of adhesions that form after severe iritis, an angle-closure glaucoma attack, or a central retinal vein occlusion. The third condition impeding fluid outflow in the trabecular channels occurs with pupillary block, most commonly associated with primary angle-closure glaucoma. In eyes predisposed to this condition, dilation of the pupil causes the iris to fold up like an accordion against the narrow-angle structures of the eye. Fluid in the posterior chamber has difficulty circulating into the anterior chamber; therefore, pressure in the posterior chamber increases, causing the iris to bow forward and obstruct the outflow channels even more. Angle-closure attacks occur quite suddenly and therefore do not give the eye a chance to adjust itself to the sudden increase in pressure. The eye becomes very red, the cornea edematous (patient may report seeing halos), and the pupil fixed and dilated, accompanied by a complaint of moderate pain. Pupil dilation can be initiated by emotional arousal or fear, conditions in which the eye must adapt to darkness (movie theaters), or mydriatics. Angle-closure glaucoma is an ocular emergency resolved by a peripheral iridectomy to allow movement of fluid between the anterior and posterior chambers. This procedure constitutes removal of a portion of the peripheral iris either by surgery or by use of an argon or yttrium-aluminum-garnet (YAG) laser.

INDICATIONS

- Diagnosis or ongoing monitoring of glaucoma
- Screening test included in a routine eye examination

POTENTIAL DIAGNOSIS

Normal findings in
- Normal IOP is between 13 and 22 mm Hg

Abnormal findings in
- Open-angle glaucoma
- Primary angle-closure glaucoma
- Secondary glaucoma

CRITICAL FINDINGS: N/A

INTERFERING FACTORS

- Inability of the patient to remain still and cooperative during the test may interfere with the test results.

NURSING IMPLICATIONS AND PROCEDURE

PRETEST:

- Positively identify the patient using at least two unique identifiers before providing care, treatment, or services.
- *Patient Teaching:* Inform the patient this procedure can assist in measuring eye pressure.
- Obtain a history of the patient's complaints, including a list of known allergens, especially allergies or sensitivities to topical anesthetic eyedrops.
- Obtain a history of the patient's known or suspected vision loss, changes in visual acuity, including type and cause; use of glasses or contact lenses; eye conditions with treatment regimens; eye surgery; and other tests and procedures to assess and diagnose visual deficit.
- Obtain a history of symptoms and results of previously performed laboratory tests and diagnostic and surgical procedures.
- Obtain a list of the patient's current medications, including herbs, nutritional

supplements, and nutraceuticals (see Appendix F).

▶ Review the procedure with the patient. Explain that the patient will be requested to fixate the eyes during the procedure. Address concerns about pain and explain that he or she may feel coldness or a slight sting when the anesthetic drops are instilled at the beginning of the procedure but that no discomfort will be experienced during the test. Instruct the patient as to what should be expected with the use of the tonometer. The patient will experience less anxiety if he or she understands that the tonometer tip will touch the tear film and not the eye directly. Inform the patient that a health-care provider (HCP) performs the test in a quiet, darkened room and that to evaluate both eyes, the test can take 1 to 3 min.

▶ Instruct the patient to remove contact lenses or glasses, as appropriate. Instruct the patient regarding the importance of keeping the eyes open for the test.

▶ *Sensitivity to social and cultural issues,* as well as concern for modesty, is important in providing psychological support before, during, and after the procedure.

▶ There are no food, fluid, or medication restrictions unless by medical direction.

INTRATEST:

▶ Instruct the patient to cooperate fully and to follow directions. Ask the patient to remain still during the procedure because any movement, such as coughing, breath-holding, or wandering eye movements, produces unreliable results.

▶ Seat the patient comfortably. Instruct the patient to look at directed target while the eyes are examined.

▶ Instill ordered topical anesthetic in each eye, as ordered, and allow time for it to work. Topical anesthetic drops are placed in the eye with the patient looking up and the solution directed at the six o'clock position of the sclera (white of the eye) near the limbus (gray, semitransparent area of the eyeball where the cornea and sclera meet). Neither dropper nor bottle should touch the eyelashes.

▶ Instruct the patient to look straight ahead, keeping the eyes open and unblinking.

▶ A number of techniques are used to measure IOP. It can be measured at the slit lamp or with a miniaturized, handheld applanation tonometer or an airpuff tonometer.

▶ When the applanation tonometer is positioned on the patient's cornea, the instrument's headrest is placed against the patient's forehead. The tonometer should be held at an angle with the handle slanted away from the patient's nose. The tonometer tip should not touch the eyelids.

▶ When the tip is properly aligned and in contact with the fluorescein-stained tear film, force is applied to the tip using an adjustment control to the desired endpoint. The tonometer is removed from the eye. The reading is taken a second time, and if the pressure is elevated, a third reading is taken. The procedure is repeated on the other eye.

▶ With the airpuff tonometer, an air pump blows air onto the cornea, and the time it takes for the air puff to flatten the cornea is detected by infrared light and photoelectric cells. This time is directly related to the IOP.

POST-TEST:

▶ A report of the results will be sent to the requesting HCP, who will discuss the results with the patient.

▶ Recognize anxiety related to test results, and be supportive of impaired activity related to vision loss or anticipated loss of driving privileges. Discuss the implications of abnormal test results on the patient's lifestyle. Provide teaching and information regarding the clinical implications of the test results, as appropriate. Provide contact information, if desired, for the Glaucoma Research Foundation (www.glaucoma.org).

▶ Reinforce information given by the patient's HCP regarding further testing, treatment, or referral to another HCP. Answer any questions or address any concerns voiced by the patient or family.

▶ Instruct the patient in the use of any ordered medications, usually eyedrops, that are intended to decrease IOP. Explain the importance of adhering to the therapy regimen, especially since increased IOP does not present symptoms. Instruct the patient in both the ocular side effects and systemic reactions associated with the prescribed medication. Encourage him or her to review corresponding literature provided by a pharmacist.

▶ Depending on the results of this procedure, additional testing may be performed to evaluate or monitor progression of the disease process and determine the need for a change in therapy. Evaluate test results in relation to the patient's symptoms and other tests performed.

RELATED MONOGRAPHS:

▶ Related tests include fundus photography, gonioscopy, nerve fiber analysis, pachymetry, slit-lamp biomicroscopy, and visual field testing.

▶ Refer to the Ocular System table at the end of the book for related tests by body system.

Intravenous Pyelography

SYNONYM/ACRONYM: Antegrade pyelography, excretory urography (EUG), intravenous urography (IVU, IUG), IVP.

COMMON USE: To assess urinary tract dysfunction or evaluate progression of renal disease such as stones, bleeding, and congenital anomalies.

AREA OF APPLICATION: Kidneys, ureters, bladder, and renal pelvis.

CONTRAST: IV radiopaque iodine-based contrast medium.

DESCRIPTION: Intravenous pyelography (IVP) is the most commonly performed test to determine urinary tract dysfunction or renal disease. IVP uses IV radiopaque contrast medium to visualize the kidneys, ureters, bladder, and renal pelvis. The contrast medium concentrates in the blood and is filtered out by the glomeruli; it passes out through the renal tubules and is concentrated in the urine. Renal function is reflected by the length of time it takes the contrast medium to appear and to be excreted by each kidney. A series of images is performed during a 30-min period to view passage of the contrast through the kidneys and ureters into the bladder.

Tomography may be employed during the examination to permit the examination of an individual layer or plane of the organ that may be obscured by surrounding overlying structures.

INDICATIONS
• Aid in the diagnosis of renovascular hypertension
• Evaluate the cause of blood in the urine
• Evaluate the effects of urinary system trauma
• Evaluate function of the kidneys, ureters, and bladder
• Evaluate known or suspected ureteral obstruction
• Evaluate the presence of renal, ureter, or bladder calculi

- Evaluate space-occupying lesions or congenital anomalies of the urinary system

POTENTIAL DIAGNOSIS

Normal findings in
- Normal size and shape of kidneys, ureters, and bladder
- Normal bladder and absence of masses or renal calculi, with prompt visualization of contrast medium through the urinary system

Abnormal findings in
- Absence of a kidney (congenital malformation)
- Benign and malignant kidney tumors
- Bladder tumors
- Congenital renal or urinary tract abnormalities
- Glomerulonephritis
- Hydronephrosis
- Prostatic enlargement
- Pyelonephritis
- Renal cysts
- Renal hematomas
- Renal or ureteral calculi
- Soft tissue masses
- Tumors of the collecting system

CRITICAL FINDINGS: N/A

INTERFERING FACTORS

This procedure is contraindicated for
- Patients with allergies to shellfish or iodinated dye. The contrast medium used may cause a life-threatening allergic reaction. Patients with a known hypersensitivity to the contrast medium may benefit from pre-medication with corticosteroids or the use of nonionic contrast medium.
- Patients with bleeding disorders.
- Patients who are pregnant or suspected of being pregnant, unless the potential benefits of the procedure far outweigh the risks to the fetus and mother.

- ❄ Elderly and other patients who are chronically dehydrated before the test, because of their risk of contrast-induced renal failure.
- ❄ Patients who are in renal failure.
- Patients with renal insufficiency, indicated by a blood urea nitrogen (BUN) value greater than 40 mg/dL or creatinine value greater than 1.5 mg/dL, because contrast medium can complicate kidney function.
- Young patients (17 yr and younger), unless the benefits of the x-ray diagnosis outweigh the risks of exposure to high levels of radiation.
- Patients with multiple myeloma, who may experience decreased kidney function subsequent to administration of contrast medium.

Factors that may impair clear imaging
- Gas or feces in the gastrointestinal (GI) tract resulting from inadequate cleansing or failure to restrict food intake before the study.
- Retained barium from a previous radiological procedure.
- Metallic objects (e.g., jewelry, body rings) within the examination field, which may inhibit organ visualization and cause unclear images.
- Inability of the patient to cooperate or remain still during the procedure because of age, significant pain, or mental status.

Other considerations
- The procedure may be terminated if chest pain or severe cardiac arrhythmias occur.
- Failure to follow dietary restrictions and other pretesting preparations may cause the procedure to be canceled or repeated.
- Consultation with a health-care provider (HCP) should occur before the procedure for radiation safety concerns regarding younger

patients or patients who are lactating.

• Risks associated with radiation overexposure can result from frequent x-ray procedures. Personnel in the room with the patient should wear a protective lead apron, stand behind a shield, or leave the area while the examination is being done. Personnel working in the examination area should wear badges to record their level of radiation exposure.

NURSING IMPLICATIONS AND PROCEDURE

PRETEST:

▶ Positively identify the patient using at least two unique identifiers before providing care, treatment, or services.

▶ *Patient Teaching:* Inform the patient this procedure can assist in assessing the kidneys, ureters, and bladder.

▶ Obtain a history of the patient's complaints or symptoms, including a list of known allergens, especially allergies or sensitivities to latex, iodine, seafood, anesthetics, or contrast mediums.

▶ Obtain a history of the patient's genitourinary system, symptoms, and results of previously performed laboratory tests and diagnostic and surgical procedures. Ensure that the results of blood tests, especially BUN and creatinine, are obtained and recorded before the procedure.

▶ Note any recent barium or other radiological contrast procedures. Ensure that barium studies were performed more than 4 days before the IVP.

▶ Record the date of the last menstrual period and determine the possibility of pregnancy in perimenopausal women.

▶ Obtain a list of the patient's current medications including anticoagulants, aspirin and other salicylates, herbs, nutritional supplements, and nutraceuticals (see Appendix F). Note the last time and dose of medication taken.

▶ If contrast media is scheduled to be used, patients receiving metformin (Glucophage) for non-insulin-dependent (type 2) diabetes should discontinue the drug on the day of the test and continue to withhold it for 48 hr after the test. Failure to do so may result in lactic acidosis.

▶ Review the procedure with the patient. Address concerns about pain related to the procedure and explain that some pain may be experienced during the test, and there may be moments of discomfort. Inform the patient that the procedure is performed in a radiology department by an HCP and takes approximately 30 to 60 min.

▶ *Sensitivity to social and cultural issues, as well as concern for modesty, is important in providing psychological support before, during, and after the procedure.*

▶ Instruct the patient to take a laxative or a cathartic, as ordered, on the evening before the examination.

▶ Instruct the patient to remove jewelry and other metallic objects from the area to be examined.

▶ Instruct the patient to fast and restrict fluids for 8 hr prior to the procedure. Protocols may vary among facilities.

▶ *Make sure a written and informed consent has been signed prior to the procedure and before administering any medications.*

INTRATEST:

▶ Ensure the patient has complied with dietary, fluid, and medication restrictions for 8 hr prior to the procedure.

▶ Ensure the patient has removed all external metallic objects from the area to be examined prior to the procedure.

▶ Assess for completion of bowel preparation according to the institution's procedure. Administer enemas or suppositories on the morning of the test, as ordered.

▶ If the patient has a history of allergic reactions to any substance or drug, administer ordered prophylactic steroids or antihistamines before the procedure. Use nonionic contrast medium for the procedure.

- Have emergency equipment readily available.
- Instruct the patient to void prior to the procedure and to change into the gown, robe, and foot coverings provided.
- Instruct the patient to cooperate fully and to follow directions. Instruct the patient to remain still throughout the procedure because movement produces unreliable results.
- Observe standard precautions, and follow the general guidelines in Appendix A.
- Place the patient in the supine position on an examination table.
- A kidney, ureter, and bladder (KUB) or plain film is taken to ensure that no barium or stool obscures visualization of the urinary system.
- Insert an IV line, if one is not already in place, and inject the contrast medium.
- Instruct the patient to take slow, deep breaths if nausea occurs during the procedure.
- Monitor the patient for complications related to the procedure (e.g., allergic reaction, anaphylaxis, bronchospasm).
- Images are taken at 1, 5, 10, 15, 20, and 30 min following injection of the contrast medium into the urinary system. Instruct the patient to exhale deeply and to hold his or her breath while each image is taken.
- Remove the needle or catheter and apply a pressure dressing over the puncture site.
- Instruct the patient to void if a post-voiding exposure is required to visualize the empty bladder.

POST-TEST:

- A report of the examination will be sent to the requesting HCP, who will discuss the results with the patient.
- Instruct the patient to resume usual diet, fluids, medications, and activity, as directed by the HCP. Renal function should be assessed before metformin is resumed if contrast was used.
- Observe for delayed reaction to iodinated contrast medium, including rash, urticaria, tachycardia, hyperpnea, hypertension, palpitations, nausea, or vomiting.
- Observe/assess the needle/catheter insertion site for bleeding, inflammation, or hematoma formation.
- Instruct the patient in the care and assessment of the injection site.
- Instruct the patient to apply cold compresses to the puncture site as needed, to reduce discomfort or edema.
- Monitor urinary output after the procedure. Decreased urine output may indicate impending renal failure.
- Recognize anxiety related to test results, and offer support. Discuss the implications of abnormal test results on the patient's lifestyle. Provide teaching and information regarding the clinical implications of the test results, as appropriate.
- Reinforce information given by the patient's HCP regarding further testing, treatment, or referral to another HCP. Answer any questions or address any concerns voiced by the patient or family.
- Depending on the results of this procedure, additional testing may be needed to evaluate or monitor progression of the disease process and determine the need for a change in therapy. Evaluate test results in relation to the patient's symptoms and other tests performed.

RELATED MONOGRAPHS:

- Related tests include biopsy bladder, biopsy kidney, biopsy prostate, BUN, CT abdomen, CT pelvis, creatinine, cystometry, cystoscopy, gallium scan, KUB, MRI abdomen, renogram, retrograde ureteropyelography, US bladder, US kidney, US prostate, urine markers of bladder cancer, urinalysis, urine cytology, and voiding cystourethrography.
- Refer to the Genitourinary System table at the end of the book for related tests by body system.

Intrinsic Factor Antibodies

SYNONYM/ACRONYM: IF antibodies.

COMMON USE: To assist in the investigation of suspected pernicious anemia.

SPECIMEN: Serum (1 mL) collected in a red- or tiger-top tube.

REFERENCE VALUE: (Method: Radioimmunoassay) None detected.

DESCRIPTION: Intrinsic factor (IF) is produced by the parietal cells of the gastric mucosa and is required for the normal absorption of vitamin B_{12}. Intrinsic factor antibodies are found in 50% to 75% of adults and also in a high percentage of pediatric patients with juvenile pernicious anemia. In some diseases, antibodies are produced that bind to the cobalamin-IF complex, prevent the complex from binding to ileum receptors, and prevent vitamin B_{12} absorption. There are two types of antibodies: type 1, the more commonly present blocking antibody, and type 2, the binding antibody. The blocking antibody inhibits uptake of vitamin B_{12} at the binding site of IF. Binding antibody combines with either free or complexed IF.

INDICATIONS
• Assist in the diagnosis of pernicious anemia
• Evaluate patients with decreased vitamin B_{12} levels

POTENTIAL DIAGNOSIS

Increased in
Conditions that involve the production of these blocking and binding autoantibodies

• Megaloblastic anemia
• Pernicious anemia
• Some patients with hyperthyroidism
• Some patients with insulin-dependent (type 1) diabetes

Decreased in: N/A

CRITICAL FINDINGS: N/A

INTERFERING FACTORS
• Recent treatment with methotrexate or another folic acid antagonist can interfere with test results.
• Vitamin B_{12} injected or ingested within 48 hr of the test invalidates results.
• Recent radioactive scans or radiation can interfere with test results when radioimmunoassay is the test method.
• Failure to follow dietary restrictions before the procedure may cause the procedure to be canceled or repeated.

NURSING IMPLICATIONS AND PROCEDURE

PRETEST:
▶ Positively identify the patient using at least two unique identifiers before providing care, treatment, or services.
▶ *Patient Teaching:* Inform the patient this test can assist in assessing for anemia.
▶ Obtain a history of the patient's complaints, including a list of known

allergens, especially allergies or sensitivities to latex.

▶ Obtain a history of the patient's gastrointestinal and hematopoietic systems, symptoms, and results of previously performed laboratory tests and diagnostic and surgical procedures.

▶ Note any recent procedures that can interfere with test results.

▶ Obtain a list of the patient's current medications, including herbs, nutritional supplements, and nutraceuticals (see Appendix F).

▶ Review the procedure with the patient. Inform the patient that specimen collection takes approximately 5 to 10 min. Address concerns about pain and explain that there may be some discomfort during the venipuncture.

▶ *Sensitivity to social and cultural issues,* as well as concern for modesty, is important in providing psychological support before, during, and after the procedure.

▶ There are no food or fluid restrictions unless by medical direction. Administration of vitamin B_{12} should be withheld within 48 hr before testing.

INTRATEST:

▶ Ensure that vitamin B_{12} has been withheld within 48 hr before testing.

▶ If the patient has a history of allergic reaction to latex, avoid the use of equipment containing latex.

▶ Instruct the patient to cooperate fully and to follow directions. Direct the patient to breathe normally and to avoid unnecessary movement.

▶ Observe standard precautions, and follow the general guidelines in Appendix A.

Positively identify the patient, and label the appropriate tubes with the corresponding patient demographics, date, and time of collection. Perform a venipuncture.

▶ Remove the needle and apply direct pressure with dry gauze to stop bleeding. Observe/assess venipuncture site for bleeding or hematoma formation and secure gauze with adhesive bandage.

▶ Promptly transport the specimen to the laboratory for processing and analysis.

POST-TEST:

▶ A report of the results will be sent to the requesting health-care provider (HCP), who will discuss the results with the patient.

▶ Reinforce information given by the patient's HCP regarding further testing, treatment, or referral to another HCP. Answer any questions or address any concerns voiced by the patient or family.

▶ Depending on the results of this procedure, additional testing may be performed to evaluate or monitor progression of the disease process and determine the need for a change in therapy. Evaluate test results in relation to the patient's symptoms and other tests performed.

RELATED MONOGRAPHS:

▶ Related tests include antibodies antithyroglobulin and antithyroid peroxidase, biopsy bone marrow, CBC, CBC RBC indices, folic acid, and vitamin B_{12}.

▶ Refer to the Gastrointestinal and Hematopoietic systems tables at the end of the book for related tests by body system.

Iron

SYNONYM/ACRONYM: Fe.

COMMON USE: To monitor and assess blood iron levels related to treatment, blood loss, metabolism, anemia, and storage disorders.

SPECIMEN: Serum (1 mL) collected in a red- or tiger-top tube.

REFERENCE VALUE: (Method: Spectrophotometry)

Age	Conventional Units	SI Units (Conventional Units × 0.179)
Newborn	100–250 mcg/dL	17.9–44.8 micromol/L
Infant–9 yr	20–105 mcg/dL	3.6–18.8 micromol/L
10–14 yr	20–145 mcg/dL	3.6–26.0 micromol/L
Adult		
Male	65–175 mcg/dL	11.6–31.3 micromol/L
Female	50–170 mcg/dL	9–30.4 micromol/L

DESCRIPTION: Iron plays a principal role in erythropoiesis. Iron is necessary for the proliferation and maturation of red blood cells (RBCs) and is required for hemoglobin (Hgb) synthesis. Of the body's normal 4 g of iron, approximately 65% resides in Hgb and 3% in myoglobin. A small amount is also found in cellular enzymes that catalyze the oxidation and reduction of iron. The remainder of iron is stored in the liver, bone marrow, and spleen as ferritin or hemosiderin. Any iron present in the serum is in transit among the alimentary tract, the bone marrow, and available iron storage forms. Iron travels in the bloodstream bound to transferrin, a protein manufactured by the liver. Normally, iron enters the body by oral ingestion; only 10% is absorbed, but up to 20% can be absorbed in patients with iron-deficiency anemia. Unbound iron is highly toxic, but there is generally an excess of transferrin available to prevent the buildup of unbound iron in the circulation. Iron overload is as clinically significant as iron deficiency, especially in the accidental poisoning of children caused by excessive intake of iron-containing multivitamins.

INDICATIONS

• Assist in the diagnosis of blood loss, as evidenced by decreased serum iron
• Assist in the diagnosis of hemochromatosis or other disorders of iron metabolism and storage
• Determine the differential diagnosis of anemia
• Determine the presence of disorders that involve diminished protein synthesis or defects in iron absorption
• Evaluate accidental iron poisoning
• Evaluate iron overload in dialysis patients or patients with transfusion-dependent anemias
• Evaluate thalassemia and sideroblastic anemia
• Monitor hematological responses during pregnancy, when serum iron is usually decreased
• Monitor response to treatment for anemia

POTENTIAL DIAGNOSIS

Increased in
• Acute iron poisoning (children) *(related to excessive intake)*
• Acute leukemia
• Acute liver disease *(possibly related to decrease in synthesis of iron storage proteins by damaged liver; iron accumulates and levels increase)*
• Aplastic anemia *(related to repeated blood transfusions)*

- Excessive iron therapy *(related to excessive intake)*
- Hemochromatosis *(inherited disorder of iron overload; the iron is not excreted in proportion to the rate of accumulation)*
- Hemolytic anemias *(related to release of iron from lysed RBCs)*
- Lead toxicity *(lead can biologically mimic iron, displace it, and release it into circulation where its concentration increases)*
- Nephritis *(related to decreased renal excretion; accumulation in blood)*
- Pernicious anemias (PA) *(achlorhydria associated with PA prevents absorption of dietary iron, and it accumulates in the blood)*
- Sideroblastic anemias *(enzyme disorder prevents iron from being incorporated into Hgb, and it accumulates in the blood)*
- Thalassemia *(treatment for some types of thalassemia include blood transfusions, which can lead to iron overload)*
- Transfusions (repeated)
- Vitamin B$_6$ deficiency *(this vitamin is essential to Hgb formation; deficiency prevents iron from being incorporated into Hgb, and it accumulates in the blood)*

Decreased in

- Acute and chronic infection *(iron is a nutrient for invading organisms)*
- Carcinoma *(related to depletion of iron stores)*
- Chronic blood loss (gastrointestinal, uterine) *(blood contains iron incorporated in Hgb)*
- Dietary deficiency
- Hypothyroidism *(pathophysiology is unclear)*
- Intestinal malabsorption
- Iron-deficiency anemia *(related to depletion of iron stores)*
- Nephrosis *(anemia is common in people with kidney disease; fewer RBCs are made because of a deficiency of erythropoietin related to the damaged kidneys, blood can be lost in dialysis, and iron intake may be lower due to lack of appetite)*
- Postoperative state
- Pregnancy *(related to depletion of iron stores by developing fetus)*
- Protein malnutrition (kwashiorkor) *(protein is required to form transport proteins, RBCs, and Hgb)*

CRITICAL FINDINGS

- Mild toxicity: greater than 350 mcg/dL
- Serious toxicity: greater than 400 mcg/dL
- Lethal: greater than 1,000 mcg/dL

Note and immediately report to the health-care provider (HCP) any critically increased values and related symptoms. Intervention may include chelation therapy by administration of deferoxamine mesylate (Desferal).

INTERFERING FACTORS

- Drugs that may increase iron levels include blood transfusions, chemotherapy drugs, iron (intramuscular), iron dextran, iron-protein-succinylate, methimazole, methotrexate, oral contraceptives, and rifampin.
- Drugs that may decrease iron levels include acetylsalicylic acid, allopurinol, cholestyramine, corticotropin, cortisone, deferoxamine, and metformin.
- Gross hemolysis can interfere with test results.
- Failure to withhold iron-containing medications 24 hr before the test may falsely increase values.
- Failure to follow dietary restrictions before the procedure may cause the procedure to be canceled or repeated.

NURSING IMPLICATIONS AND PROCEDURE

PRETEST:

- Positively identify the patient using at least two unique identifiers before providing care, treatment, or services.
- *Patient Teaching:* Inform the patient this test can assist in evaluating the amount of iron in the blood.
- Obtain a history of the patient's complaints, including a list of known allergens, especially allergies or sensitivities to latex.
- Obtain a history of the patient's gastrointestinal and hematopoietic systems, symptoms, and results of previously performed laboratory tests and diagnostic and surgical procedures.
- Note any recent therapies that can interfere with test results. Specimen collection should be delayed for several days after blood transfusion.
- Obtain a list of the patient's current medications, including herbs, nutritional supplements, and nutraceuticals (see Appendix F).
- Review the procedure with the patient. Inform the patient that specimen collection takes approximately 5 to 10 min. Address concerns about pain and explain that there may be some discomfort during the venipuncture.
- *Sensitivity to social and cultural issues,* as well as concern for modesty, is important in providing psychological support before, during, and after the procedure.
- Instruct the patient to fast for at least 12 hr before testing and, with medical direction, to refrain from taking iron-containing medicines before specimen collection. Protocols may vary among facilities.
- There are no fluid restrictions unless by medical direction.

INTRATEST:

- Ensure that the patient has complied with dietary and medication restrictions; ensure that food has been restricted for at least 12 hr prior to the procedure.
- If the patient has a history of allergic reaction to latex, avoid the use of equipment containing latex.
- Instruct the patient to cooperate fully and to follow directions. Direct the patient to breathe normally and to avoid unnecessary movement.
- Observe standard precautions, and follow the general guidelines in Appendix A. Positively identify the patient, and label the appropriate tubes with the corresponding patient demographics, date, and time of collection. Perform a venipuncture.
- Remove the needle and apply direct pressure with dry gauze to stop bleeding. Observe/assess venipuncture site for bleeding or hematoma formation and secure gauze with adhesive bandage.
- Promptly transport the specimen to the laboratory for processing and analysis.

POST-TEST:

- A report of the results will be sent to the requesting HCP, who will discuss the results with the patient.
- Instruct the patient to resume usual diet, fluids, medications, or activity, as directed by the HCP.
- *Nutritional Considerations:* Educate the patient with abnormally elevated iron values, as appropriate, on the importance of reading food labels. Foods high in iron include meats (especially liver), eggs, grains, and green leafy vegetables. It is also important to explain that iron levels in foods can be increased if foods are cooked in cookware containing iron.
- *Nutritional Considerations:* Educate the patient with abnormal iron values that numerous factors affect the absorption of iron, enhancing or decreasing absorption regardless of the original content of the iron-containing dietary source. Patients must be educated to either increase or avoid intake of iron and iron-rich foods depending on their specific condition; for example, a patient with hemochromatosis or acute pernicious anemia should be educated to avoid foods rich in iron. Consumption of large amounts of alcohol damages the intestine and allows increased absorption of iron. A high intake of calcium and ascorbic acid also increases iron absorption.

Iron absorption after a meal is also increased by factors in meat, fish, and poultry. Iron absorption is decreased by the absence (gastric resection) or diminished presence (use of antacids) of gastric acid. Phytic acids from cereals, tannins from tea and coffee, oxalic acid from vegetables, and minerals such as copper, zinc, and manganese interfere with iron absorption.

▶ Reinforce information given by the patient's HCP regarding further testing, treatment, or referral to another HCP. Answer any questions or address any concerns voiced by the patient or family.

▶ Depending on the results of this procedure, additional testing may be performed to evaluate or monitor progression of the disease process and determine the need for a change in therapy. Evaluate test results in relation to the patient's symptoms and other tests performed.

RELATED MONOGRAPHS:

▶ Related tests include biopsy bone marrow, biopsy liver, CBC, CBC RBC count, CBC RBC indices, CBC RBC morphology, CBC WBC count and differential, erythropoietin, ferritin, folate, FEP, gallium scan, hemosiderin, iron binding/transferrin, lead, porphyrins, reticulocyte count, and vitamin B_{12}.

▶ Refer to the Gastrointestinal and Hematopoietic systems tables at the end of the book for related tests by body system.

Iron-Binding Capacity (Total), Transferrin, and Iron Saturation

SYNONYM/ACRONYM: TIBC, Fe Sat.

COMMON USE: To monitor iron replacement therapy and assess blood iron levels to assist in diagnosing types of anemia such as iron deficiency.

SPECIMEN: Serum (1 mL) collected in a red- or tiger-top tube.

REFERENCE VALUE: (Method: Spectrophotometry for TIBC and nephelometry for transferrin)

Test	Conventional Units	SI Units
TIBC	250–350 mcg/dL	(Conventional Units × 0.179) 45–63 micromol/L
Transferrin	215–380 mg/dL	(Conventional Units × 0.01) 2.15–3.80 g/L
Iron saturation	20–50%	

TIBC = total iron-binding capacity.

DESCRIPTION: Iron plays a principal role in erythropoiesis. It is necessary for proliferation and maturation of red blood cells and for hemoglobin (Hgb) synthesis. Of the body's normal 4 g of iron (less in women), about 65% is present in Hgb and about 3% in myoglobin. A small amount is also found in cellular enzymes that catalyze the oxidation and reduction of iron. The remainder of iron is stored in the liver, bone marrow, and spleen as ferritin or hemosiderin. Any iron present in the serum is in transit among the alimentary tract, the bone marrow, and available iron storage forms. Iron travels in the bloodstream bound to transport proteins. Transferrin is the major iron-transport protein, carrying 60% to 70% of the body's iron. (See monograph titled "Transferrin" for more detailed information.) For this reason, total iron-binding capacity (TIBC) and transferrin are sometimes referred to interchangeably, even though other proteins carry iron and contribute to the TIBC. Unbound iron is highly toxic, but there is generally an excess of transferrin available to prevent the buildup of unbound iron in the circulation. The percentage of iron saturation is calculated by dividing the serum iron value by the TIBC value and multiplying by 100.

INDICATIONS

- Assist in the diagnosis of iron-deficiency anemia
- Differentiate between iron-deficiency anemia and anemia secondary to chronic disease
- Monitor hematological response to therapy during pregnancy and iron-deficiency anemias

- Provide support for diagnosis of hemochromatosis or diseases of iron metabolism and storage

POTENTIAL DIAGNOSIS

Increased in
- Acute liver disease
- Hypochromic (iron-deficiency) anemias *(insufficient circulating iron levels to saturate binding sites)*
- Late pregnancy

Decreased in
- Chronic infections *(transferrin is a negative acute-phase reactant protein and during periods of inflammation will demonstrate decreased levels)*
- Cirrhosis *(transferrin is a negative acute-phase reactant protein and during periods of inflammation will demonstrate decreased levels)*
- Hemochromatosis *(occurs early in the disease as intestinal absorption of iron available for binding increases)*
- Hemolytic anemias *(transferrin becomes saturated, and the iron-binding capacity is significantly decreased)*
- Neoplastic diseases *(transferrin is a negative acute-phase reactant protein and during periods of inflammation will demonstrate decreased levels)*
- Protein depletion *(transferrin contributes to the total protein concentration and will reflect a decrease in protein depletion)*
- Renal disease *(transferrin is a negative acute-phase reactant protein and during periods of inflammation will demonstrate decreased levels)*
- Sideroblastic anemias *(transferrin becomes saturated, and the iron-binding capacity is significantly decreased)*

- Thalassemia *(transferrin becomes saturated, and the iron-binding capacity is significantly decreased)*

CRITICAL FINDINGS: N/A

INTERFERING FACTORS

- Drugs that may increase TIBC levels include mestranol and oral contraceptives.
- Drugs that may decrease TIBC levels include asparaginase, chloramphenicol, corticotropin, cortisone, and testosterone.

NURSING IMPLICATIONS AND PROCEDURE

PRETEST:

- Positively identify the patient using at least two unique identifiers before providing care, treatment, or services.
- *Patient Teaching:* Inform the patient this test can assist in diagnosing anemia.
- Obtain a history of the patient's complaints, including a list of known allergens, especially allergies or sensitivities to latex.
- Obtain a history of the patient's hematopoietic system, symptoms, and results of previously performed laboratory tests and diagnostic and surgical procedures.
- Obtain a list of the patient's current medications, including herbs, nutritional supplements, and nutraceuticals (see Appendix F).
- Review the procedure with the patient. Inform the patient that specimen collection takes approximately 5 to 10 min. Address concerns about pain and explain that there may be some discomfort during the venipuncture.
- *Sensitivity to social and cultural issues,* as well as concern for modesty, is important in providing psychological support before, during, and after the procedure.
- There are no food, fluid, or medication restrictions unless by medical direction.

INTRATEST:

- If the patient has a history of allergic reaction to latex, avoid the use of equipment containing latex.
- Instruct the patient to cooperate fully and to follow directions. Direct the patient to breathe normally and to avoid unnecessary movement.
- Observe standard precautions, and follow the general guidelines in Appendix A. Positively identify the patient, and label the appropriate tubes with the corresponding patient demographics, date, and time of collection. Perform a venipuncture.
- Remove the needle and apply direct pressure with dry gauze to stop bleeding. Observe/assess venipuncture site for bleeding or hematoma formation and secure gauze with adhesive bandage.
- Promptly transport the specimen to the laboratory for processing and analysis.

POST-TEST:

- A report of the results will be sent to the requesting health-care provider (HCP), who will discuss the results with the patient.
- Reinforce information given by the patient's HCP regarding further testing, treatment, or referral to another HCP. Answer any questions or address any concerns voiced by the patient or family.
- Depending on the results of this procedure, additional testing may be performed to evaluate or monitor progression of the disease process and determine the need for a change in therapy. Evaluate test results in relation to the patient's symptoms and other tests performed.

RELATED MONOGRAPHS:

- Related tests include biopsy bone marrow, biopsy liver, CBC, CBC RBC count, CBC RBC indices, CBC RBC morphology, CBC WBC count and differential, erythropoietin, ferritin, folate, FEP, gallium scan, hemosiderin, lead, porphyrins, reticulocyte count, and vitamin B_{12}.
- Refer to the Hematopoietic System table at the end of the book for related tests by body system.

Ketones, Blood and Urine

SYNONYM/ACRONYM: Ketone bodies, acetoacetate, acetone.

COMMON USE: To investigate diabetes as the cause of ketoacidosis and monitor therapeutic interventions.

SPECIMEN: Serum (1 mL) collected from red- or tiger-top tube. Urine (5 mL), random or timed specimen, collected in a clean plastic collection container.

REFERENCE VALUE: (Method: Colorimetric nitroprusside reaction) Negative.

DESCRIPTION: Ketone bodies refer to the three intermediate products of metabolism: acetone, acetoacetic acid, and β-hydroxybutyrate. Even though β-hydroxybutyrate is not a ketone, it is usually listed with the ketone bodies. In healthy individuals, ketones are produced and completely metabolized by the liver so that measurable amounts are not normally present in serum. Ketones appear in the urine before a significant serum level is detectable. If the patient has excessive fat metabolism, ketones are found in blood and urine. Excessive fat metabolism may occur if the patient has impaired ability to metabolize carbohydrates, inadequate carbohydrate intake, inadequate insulin levels, excessive carbohydrate loss, or increased carbohydrate demand. A strongly positive acetone result without severe acidosis, accompanied by normal glucose, electrolyte, and bicarbonate levels, is strongly suggestive of isopropyl alcohol poisoning. A low-carbohydrate or high-fat diet may cause a positive acetone test. Ketosis in people with diabetes is usually accompanied by increased glucose and decreased bicarbonate and pH. Extremely elevated levels of ketone bodies can result in coma. This situation is particularly life-threatening in children younger than 10 yr.

INDICATIONS
- Assist in the diagnosis of starvation, stress, alcoholism, suspected isopropyl alcohol ingestion, glycogen storage disease, and other metabolic disorders
- Detect and monitor treatment of diabetic ketoacidosis
- Monitor the control of diabetes
- Screen for ketonuria due to acute illness or stress in nondiabetic patients
- Screen for ketonuria to assist in the assessment of inborn errors of metabolism
- Screen for ketonuria to assist in the diagnosis of suspected isopropyl alcohol poisoning

POTENTIAL DIAGNOSIS

Increased in

Ketones are generated in conditions that involve the metabolism of carbohydrates, fatty acids, and protein.
- Acidosis
- Branched-chain ketonuria
- Carbohydrate deficiency
- Eclampsia
- Fasting or starvation
- Gestational diabetes
- Glycogen storage diseases
- High-fat or high-protein diet
- Hyperglycemia
- Ketoacidosis of alcoholism and diabetes
- Illnesses with marked vomiting and diarrhea

K

- Isopropyl alcohol ingestion
- Methylmalonic aciduria
- Postanesthesia period
- Propionyl coenzyme A carboxylase deficiency

Decreased in: N/A

CRITICAL FINDINGS ✦

Strongly positive test results for glucose and ketones

Note and immediately report to the health-care provider (HCP) strongly positive results in urine and related symptoms. An elevated level of ketone bodies is evidenced by fruity-smelling breath, acidosis, ketonuria, and decreased level of consciousness. Administration of insulin and frequent blood glucose measurement may be indicated.

INTERFERING FACTORS

- Drugs that may cause an increase in serum ketone levels include acetylsalicylic acid (if therapy results in acidosis, especially in children), albuterol, fenfluramine, nifedipine, and rimiterol.
- Drugs that may cause a decrease in serum ketone levels include acetylsalicylic acid and valproic acid. Increases have been shown in hyperthyroid patients receiving propranolol and propylthiouracil.
- Drugs that may increase urine ketone levels include acetylsalicylic acid (if therapy results in acidosis, especially in children), ether, metformin, and niacin.
- Drugs that may decrease urine ketone levels include acetylsalicylic acid.
- Urine should be checked within 60 min of collection.
- Bacterial contamination of urine can cause false-negative results.
- Failure to keep reagent strip container tightly closed can cause false-negative results. Light and

moisture affect the ability of the chemicals in the strip to perform as expected.
- False-negative or weakly false-positive test results can be obtained when β-hydroxybutyrate is the predominating ketone body in cases of lactic acidosis.

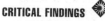

NURSING IMPLICATIONS AND PROCEDURE

PRETEST:

▶ Positively identify the patient using at least two unique identifiers before providing care, treatment, or services.

▶ *Patient Teaching:* Inform the patient this test can assist in diagnosing metabolic disorders such as diabetes.

▶ Obtain a history of the patient's complaints, including a list of known allergens, especially allergies or sensitivities to latex.

▶ Obtain a history of the patient's endocrine system, symptoms, and results of previously performed laboratory tests and diagnostic and surgical procedures.

▶ Obtain a list of the patient's current medications, including herbs, nutritional supplements, and nutraceuticals (see Appendix F).

▶ Review the procedure with the patient. Inform the patient that blood specimen collection takes approximately 5 to 10 min. The amount of time required to collect a urine specimen depends on the level of cooperation from the patient. Address concerns about pain and explain that there may be some discomfort during the venipuncture.

▶ *Sensitivity to social and cultural issues,* as well as concern for modesty, is important in providing psychological support before, during, and after the procedure.

▶ There are no food, fluid, or medication restrictions, unless by medical direction.

K

INTRATEST:

▶ Observe standard precautions, and follow the general guidelines in Appendix A.

Blood

▶ If the patient has a history of allergic reaction to latex, avoid the use of equipment containing latex.

▶ Instruct the patient to cooperate fully and to follow directions. Direct the patient to breathe normally and to avoid unnecessary movement.

▶ Positively identify the patient, and label the appropriate tubes with the corresponding patient demographics, date, and time of collection. Perform a venipuncture. Alternatively, a finger-stick- or heel-stick method of specimen collection can be used.

▶ Remove the needle and apply direct pressure with dry gauze to stop bleeding. Observe/assess venipuncture site for bleeding or hematoma formation and secure gauze with adhesive bandage.

Urine

▶ Review the procedure with the patient. Explain to the patient how to collect a second-voided midstream void, then drink a glass of water, wait 30 min, and then try to void again.

▶ Instruct the patient to avoid excessive exercise and stress before specimen collection.

Clean-Catch Specimen

▶ Instruct the male patient to (1) thoroughly wash his hands, (2) cleanse the meatus, (3) void a small amount into the toilet, and (4) void directly into the specimen container.

▶ Instruct the female patient to (1) thoroughly wash her hands; (2) cleanse the labia from front to back; (3) while keeping the labia separated, void a small amount into the toilet; and (4) without interrupting the urine stream, void directly into the specimen container.

Blood or Urine

▶ Promptly transport the specimen to the laboratory for processing and analysis.

POST-TEST:

▶ A report of the results will be sent to the requesting HCP, who will discuss the results with the patient.

▶ *Nutritional Considerations:* Increased levels of ketone bodies may be associated with diabetes. There is no "diabetic diet"; however, many meal-planning approaches with nutritional goals are endorsed by the American Dietetic Association. Patients who adhere to dietary recommendations report a better general feeling of health, better weight management, greater control of glucose and lipid values, and improved use of insulin. Instruct the patient, as appropriate, in nutritional management of diabetes. In June 2006, the American Heart Association developed a Therapeutic Lifestyle Changes (TLC) diet with goals directed at people with specific risk factors and/or existing medical conditions, (e.g., elevated LDL cholesterol levels, other lipid disorders, coronary artery disease [CAD], insulin-dependent diabetes, insulin resistance, or metabolic syndrome). The TLC approach also includes the use of plant stanols or sterols and increased dissolved fiber as an option for lowering LDL cholesterol levels; nutritional recommendations for daily total caloric intake; recommendations for allowable percentage of calories derived from fat (saturated and unsaturated), carbohydrates, protein, and cholesterol; as well as recommendations for daily expenditure of energy. The nutritional needs of each diabetic patient need to be determined individually (especially during pregnancy) with the appropriate HCPs, particularly professionals trained in nutrition.

▶ Impaired glucose tolerance may be associated with diabetes. Instruct the patient and caregiver to report signs and symptoms of hypoglycemia (weakness, confusion, diaphoresis, rapid pulse) or hyperglycemia (thirst, polyuria, hunger, lethargy).

▶ *Nutritional Considerations:* Increased levels of ketone bodies may be associated with poor carbohydrate intake; therefore, the body breaks down fat instead of carbohydrate for energy. Increasing carbohydrate intake in the patient's diet reduces the levels of ketone bodies.

Carbohydrates can be found in starches and sugars. Starch is a complex carbohydrate that can be found in foods such as grains (breads, cereals, pasta, rice) and starchy vegetables (corn, peas, potatoes). Sugar is a simple carbohydrate that can be found in natural foods (fruits and natural honey) and processed foods (desserts and candy).

▶ Recognize anxiety related to test results, and be supportive of perceived loss of independence and fear of shortened life expectancy. Discuss the implications of abnormal test results on the patient's lifestyle. Provide teaching and information regarding the clinical implications of the test results, as appropriate. Emphasize, if indicated, that good glycemic control delays the onset and slows the progression of diabetic retinopathy, nephropathy, and neuropathy. Educate the patient regarding access to counseling services, as appropriate. Provide contact information, if desired, for the American Diabetes Association (www.diabetes.org) or the American Heart Association (www.americanheart.org).

▶ Reinforce information given by the patient's HCP regarding further testing, treatment, or referral to another HCP. Answer any questions or address any concerns voiced by the patient or family.

▶ Depending on the results of this procedure, additional testing may be performed to evaluate or monitor progression of the disease process and determine the need for a change in therapy. Evaluate test results in relation to the patient's symptoms and other tests performed.

RELATED MONOGRAPHS:

▶ Related tests include ACTH, angiography adrenal, anion gap, blood gases, BUN, calcium, catecholamines, cholesterol (HDL, LDL, total), cortisol, C-peptide, DHEA, electrolytes, fecal analysis, fecal fat, fluorescein angiography, fructosamine, fundus photography, gastric emptying scan, GTT, glycated hemoglobin A_{1C}, HVA, insulin, insulin antibodies, lactic acid, lipoprotein electrophoresis, metanephrines, microalbumin, osmolality, phosphorus, UA, and visual fields test.

▶ Refer to the Endocrine System table at the end of the book for related tests by body system.

K

Kidney, Ureter, and Bladder Study

SYNONYM/ACRONYM: Flat plate of the abdomen, KUB, plain film of the abdomen.

COMMON USE: To visualize and assess the abdominal organs for obstruction or abnormality related to mass, trauma, bleeding, stones, or congenital anomaly.

AREA OF APPLICATION: Kidneys, ureters, bladder, and abdomen.

CONTRAST: None.

DESCRIPTION: A kidney, ureter, and bladder (KUB) x-ray examination provides information regarding the structure, size, and position of the abdominal organs; it also indicates whether there is any obstruction or abnormality of the abdomen caused by disease or congenital malformation. Calcifications of the renal calyces, renal pelvis, and any radiopaque calculi present in the urinary tract or surrounding organs may be visualized. Normal air and gas patterns are visualized within the intestinal tract. Perforation of the intestinal tract or an intestinal obstruction can be visualized on erect KUB images. KUB x-rays are among the first examinations done to diagnose intra-abdominal diseases such as intestinal obstruction, masses, tumors, ruptured organs, abnormal gas accumulation, and ascites.

K

INDICATIONS
- Determine the cause of acute abdominal pain or palpable mass
- Evaluate the effects of lower abdominal trauma, such as internal hemorrhage
- Evaluate known or suspected intestinal obstructions
- Evaluate the presence of renal, ureter, or other organ calculi
- Evaluate the size, shape, and position of the liver, kidneys, and spleen
- Evaluate suspected abnormal fluid, air, or metallic objects in the abdomen

POTENTIAL DIAGNOSIS

Normal findings in
- Normal size and shape of kidneys
- Normal bladder, absence of masses and renal calculi, and no abnormal accumulation of air or fluid

Abnormal findings in
- Abnormal accumulation of bowel gas
- Ascites
- Bladder distention
- Congenital renal anomaly
- Hydronephrosis
- Intestinal obstruction
- Organomegaly
- Renal calculi
- Renal hematomas
- Ruptured viscus
- Soft tissue masses
- Trauma to liver, spleen, kidneys, and bladder
- Vascular calcification

CRITICAL FINDINGS
- Bowel obstruction
- Ischemic bowel
- Visceral injury

It is essential that critical diagnoses be communicated immediately to the appropriate health-care provider (HCP). A listing of these diagnoses varies among facilities. Note and immediately report to the HCP abnormal results and related symptoms.

INTERFERING FACTORS

This procedure is contraindicated for
- Patients who are pregnant or suspected of being pregnant, unless the potential benefits of the procedure far outweigh the risks to the fetus and mother.

Factors that may impair clear imaging
- Inability of the patient to cooperate or remain still during the procedure because of age, significant pain, or mental status.
- Metallic objects (e.g., jewelry, body rings) within the examination field, which may inhibit organ visualization and cause unclear images.

- Improper adjustment of the radiographic equipment to accommodate obese or thin patients, which can cause overexposure or underexposure and a poor-quality study.
- Incorrect positioning of the patient, which may produce poor visualization of the area to be examined, for images done by portable equipment.
- Retained barium from a previous radiological procedure.

Other considerations

- Consultation with an HCP should occur before the procedure for radiation safety concerns regarding patients younger than 17.
- Risks associated with radiation overexposure can result from frequent x-ray procedures. Personnel in the room with the patient should wear a protective lead apron, stand behind a shield, or leave the area while the examination is being done. Personnel working in the examination area should wear badges to record their level of radiation exposure.

NURSING IMPLICATIONS AND PROCEDURE

PRETEST:

- Positively identify the patient using at least two unique identifiers before providing care, treatment, or services.
- *Patient Teaching:* Inform the patient this procedure can assist in assessing the status of the abdomen.
- Obtain a history of the patient's complaints, including a list of known allergens, especially allergies and sensitivities to latex.
- Obtain a history of the patient's gastrointestinal and genitourinary systems, symptoms, and results of previously performed laboratory tests and diagnostic and surgical procedures.
- Record the date of the last menstrual period and determine the possibility of pregnancy in perimenopausal women.
- Obtain a list of the patient's current medications, including herbs, nutritional supplements, and nutraceuticals (see Appendix F).
- Review the procedure with the patient. Address concerns about pain and explain that little to no pain is expected during the test, but there may be moments of discomfort. Inform the patient that the procedure is performed in the radiology department or at the bedside by a registered radiologic technologist and takes approximately 5 to 15 min to complete.
- *Sensitivity to social and cultural issues,* as well as concern for modesty, is important in providing psychological support before, during, and after the procedure.
- Instruct the patient to remove all metallic objects from the area to be examined.
- There are no food, fluid, or medication restrictions unless by medical direction.

INTRATEST:

- Ensure the patient has removed all metallic objects from the area to be examined prior to the procedure.
- Instruct the patient to void prior to the procedure and to change into the gown, robe, and foot coverings provided.
- Instruct the patient to cooperate fully and follow directions. Instruct the patient to remain still throughout the procedure because movement produces unreliable results.
- Place the patient on the table in a supine position with hands relaxed at the side.
- Instruct the patient to inhale deeply and hold his or her breath while the x-ray images are taken, and then to exhale after the images are taken.
- Observe standard precautions, and follow the general guidelines in Appendix A.

POST-TEST:

- A report will be sent to the requesting HCP, who will discuss the results with the patient.
- Reinforce information given by the patient's HCP regarding further testing,

treatment, or referral to another HCP. Answer any questions or address any concerns voiced by the patient or family.
- Depending on the results of this procedure, additional testing may be performed to evaluate or monitor progression of the disease process and determine the need for a change in therapy. Evaluate test results in relation to the patient's symptoms and other tests performed.

RELATED MONOGRAPHS:
- Related tests include angiography renal, calculus kidney stone panel, CT abdomen, CT pelvis, CT renal, IVP, and MRI abdomen, retrograde ureteropyelography, US abdomen, US kidney, US pelvis, and UA.
- Refer to the Gastrointestinal and Genitourinary systems tables at the end of the book for related tests by body system.

Kleihauer-Betke Test

SYNONYM/ACRONYM: Fetal hemoglobin, hemoglobin F, acid elution slide test.

COMMON USE: To assist in assessing occurrence and extent of fetal maternal hemorrhage and calculate the amount of Rh immune globulin to be administered.

SPECIMEN: Whole blood (1 mL) collected in a lavender-top (EDTA) tube. Freshly prepared blood smears are also acceptable. Cord blood may be requested for use as a positive control.

REFERENCE VALUE: (Method: Microscopic examination of treated and stained peripheral blood smear) Less than 1%.

DESCRIPTION: The Kleihauer-Betke test is used to determine the degree of fetal-maternal hemorrhage (FMH) and to help calculate the dosage of Rh immune globulin (RhIG)—Rh$_o$(D) RhoGAM IM or Rhophylac IM or IV—to be given in some cases of Rh-negative mothers. A single dose of RhIG inhibits formation of Rh antibodies in the mother to prevent Rh disease in future pregnancies with Rh-positive children. The test is also used to

resolve the question of whether FMH was the cause of fetal death in the case of stillbirth. A sample of maternal blood should be collected within 1 hr of delivery. A blood film of maternal red blood cells (RBCs) is prepared, treated with an acid buffer, and stained. The acid solution causes hemoglobin to be leached from the maternal cells, giving them a ghostlike appearance. Fetal cells containing hemoglobin F retain their hemoglobin and are stained bright red. Approximately 2,000 cells are examined microscopically and counted. The ratio between maternal cells and fetal cells is determined. A percentage of fetal cells is reported. Enumeration of a total of 2,000 cells is important to achieve the accuracy and precision to detect an FMH of 15 mL of fetal RBCs or 30 mL of fetal whole blood, which is the amount of FMH that corresponds to a 300-mcg dose of RhIG. Recommendations for initial RhIG doses range from 100 to 300 mcg to cover 10 to 30 mL of fetal blood volumes. Many manufacturers recommend additional 50 mcg doses for each 2.5 mL of fetal blood. Calculation of RhIG dosage is based on the calculated size of FMH and *should only be done after reviewing the information in the manufacturer's package insert.* The formula to calculate quantity of fetal bleed in milliliters of fetal blood is to multiply the percentage of fetal cells in maternal circulation by 50, based on the assumption that maternal blood volume is 5 liters. For example, if the percentage of fetal cells counted is 0.6%, then FMH = 0.6 × 50 = 30 mL. The formula to calculate FMH in relation to fetal blood cell volume is to multiply the percentage of fetal cells in maternal circulation by 2, based on the assumption that the hematocrit of fetal whole blood is 50%. For example, if the quantity of fetal bleed is 30 mL of fetal whole blood, then FMH = (30/2) = 15 mL fetal RBCs. Postpartum RhIG should be given within 72 hr of delivery. The test can also be used to distinguish some forms of thalassemia from the hereditary persistence of fetal hemoglobin, but hemoglobin electrophoresis and flow cytometry methods are more commonly used for this purpose.

INDICATIONS
- Assist in the diagnosis of certain types of anemia
- Calculating dosage of RhoGAM
- Determine whether FMH was a potential cause of death in stillborn delivery
- Screening postpartum maternal blood for the presence of FMH

POTENTIAL DIAGNOSIS
Positive findings in
- Fetal-maternal hemorrhage *(related to leakage of fetal RBCs into maternal circulation)*
- Hereditary persistence of fetal hemoglobin *(the test does not differentiate fetal hemoglobin from neonate and adult)*

Negative findings in: N/A

CRITICAL FINDINGS: N/A

INTERFERING FACTORS
Specimens must be obtained before transfusion.

NURSING IMPLICATIONS AND PROCEDURE

PRETEST:
- Positively identify the patient using at least two unique identifiers before providing care, treatment, or services.
- *Patient Teaching:* Inform the patient this test can assist in identifying how much medication should be given after delivery.

▶ Obtain a history of the patient's complaints, including a list of known allergens, especially allergies or sensitivities to latex.

▶ Obtain a history of the patient's hematopoietic and reproductive systems, symptoms, and results of previously performed laboratory tests and diagnostic and surgical procedures.

▶ Note any recent procedures that can interfere with test results.

▶ Obtain a list of the patient's current medications, including herbs, nutritional supplements, and nutraceuticals (see Appendix F).

▶ Review the procedure with the patient. Inform the patient that specimen collection takes approximately 5 to 10 min. Address concerns about pain and explain that there may be some discomfort during the venipuncture.

▶ *Sensitivity to social and cultural issues,* as well as concern for modesty, is important in providing psychological support before, during, and after the procedure.

▶ There are no food, fluid, or medication restrictions unless by medical direction.

INTRATEST:

▶ If the patient has a history of allergic reaction to latex, avoid the use of equipment containing latex.

▶ Instruct the patient to cooperate fully and to follow directions. Direct the patient to breathe normally and to avoid unnecessary movement.

▶ Observe standard precautions, and follow the general guidelines in Appendix A. Positively identify the patient, and label the appropriate tubes with the corresponding patient demographics, date, and time of collection. Perform a venipuncture.

▶ Remove the needle and apply direct pressure with dry gauze to stop bleeding. Observe/assess venipuncture site for bleeding or hematoma formation and secure gauze with adhesive bandage.

▶ Promptly transport the specimen to the laboratory for processing and analysis. Sample must be less than 6 hr old.

POST-TEST:

▶ A report of the results will be sent to the requesting health-care provider (HCP), who will discuss the results with the patient.

▶ Reinforce information given by the patient's HCP regarding further testing, treatment, or referral to another HCP. Answer any questions or address any concerns voiced by the patient or family.

▶ Depending on the results of this procedure, additional testing may be performed to evaluate or monitor progression of the disease process and determine the need for a change in therapy. Evaluate test results in relation to the patient's symptoms and other tests performed.

RELATED MONOGRAPHS:

▶ Related tests include amniotic fluid analysis, blood group and type, hemoglobin electrophoresis, and US biophysical profile obstetric.

▶ Refer to the Hematopoietic and Reproductive systems tables at the end of the book for related tests by body system.

Lactate Dehydrogenase and Isoenzymes

SYNONYM/ACRONYM: LDH and isos, LD and isos.

COMMON USE: To assess myocardial or skeletal muscle damage to assist in diagnosis of disorders such as myocardial infarction or damage to brain, liver, kidneys, and skeletal muscle.

SPECIMEN: Serum (1 mL) collected in a red- or tiger-top tube.

REFERENCE VALUE: (Method: Enzymatic [L to P] for lactate dehydrogenase, electrophoretic analysis for isoenzymes) Reference ranges are method dependent and may vary among laboratories.

Age	Conventional & SI Units
0–2 yr	125–275 units/L
2–3 yr	166–232 units/L
4–6 yr	104–206 units/L
7–12 yr	90–203 units/L
13–14 yr	90–199 units/L
15–43 yr	90–156 units/L
Greater than 43 yr	90–176 units/L

LDH Fraction	% of Total	Fraction of Total
LDH_1	14–26	0.14–0.26
LDH_2	29–39	0.29–0.39
LDH_3	20–26	0.20–0.26
LDH_4	8–16	0.08–0.16
LDH_5	6–16	0.06–0.16

POTENTIAL DIAGNOSIS

Total LDH Increased In

LDH is released from any damaged cell in which it is stored so conditions that affect the heart, liver, kidneys, red blood cells, skeletal muscle, or other tissue source and cause cellular destruction demonstrate elevated LDH levels.

- Carcinoma of the liver
- Chronic alcoholism
- Cirrhosis
- Congestive heart failure
- Hemolytic anemias
- Hypoxia
- Leukemias
- Megaloblastic and pernicious anemia
- MI or pulmonary infarction
- Musculoskeletal disease
- Obstructive jaundice
- Pancreatitis
- Renal disease (severe)
- Shock
- Viral hepatitis

Total LDH Decreased In: N/A

LDH Isoenzymes

- LDH_1 fraction increased over LDH_2 can be seen in acute MI, anemias (pernicious, hemolytic, acute sickle cell, megaloblastic, hemolytic), and

acute renal cortical injury due to any cause. The LDH$_1$ fraction in particular is elevated in cases of germ cell tumors.
• Increases in the middle fractions are associated with conditions in which massive platelet destruction has occurred (e.g., pulmonary embolism, post-transfusion period) and in lymphatic system disorders (e.g., infectious mononucleosis, lymphomas, lymphocytic leukemias).
• An increase in LDH$_5$ occurs with musculoskeletal damage and many types of liver damage (e.g., cirrhosis, cancer, hepatitis).

CRITICAL FINDINGS: N/A

Find and print out the full monograph at DavisPlus (http://davisplus.fadavis .com, keyword Van Leeuwen)

Lactic Acid

SYNONYM/ACRONYM: Lactate.

COMMON USE: To assess for lactic acid acidosis related to poor organ perfusion and liver failure. May also be used to differentiate between lactic acid acidosis and ketoacidosis by evaluating blood glucose levels.

SPECIMEN: Plasma (1 mL) collected in a gray-top (sodium fluoride) or a green-top (lithium heparin) tube. Specimen should be transported tightly capped and in an ice slurry.

REFERENCE VALUE: (Method: Spectrophotometry/enzymatic analysis)

Conventional Units	SI Units (Conventional Units × 0.111)
3–23 mg/dL	0.3–2.6 mmol/L

DESCRIPTION: Lactic acid (present in blood as lactate) is a by-product of carbohydrate metabolism. Normally metabolized in the liver, lactate concentration is based on the rate of production and metabolism. Levels increase during strenuous exercise, which results in insufficient oxygen delivery to the tissues. Pyruvate, the normal end product of glucose metabolism, is converted to lactate in emergency situations when energy is needed but there is insufficient oxygen in the system to favor the aerobic and customary energy cycle. When hypoxia or circulatory collapse increases production of lactate, or when the hepatic system does not metabolize lactate sufficiently, lactate levels become elevated. The lactic acid test can be performed in conjunction with pyruvic acid testing to monitor tissue oxygenation. Lactic acidosis can be differentiated from ketoacidosis by the absence of ketosis and grossly elevated glucose levels.

INDICATIONS
• Assess tissue oxygenation
• Evaluate acidosis

POTENTIAL DIAGNOSIS

Increased in
The liver is the major organ responsible for the breakdown of lactic acid. Any condition affecting normal liver function may also reflect increased blood levels of lactic acid.
• Cardiac failure *(decreased blood flow and insufficient oxygen in tissues result in accumulation of lactic acid from anaerobic glycolysis)*
• Diabetes *(inefficient aerobic glycolysis and decreased blood flow caused by diabetes result in accumulation of lactic acid from anaerobic glycolysis)*
• Hemorrhage *(decreased blood circulation and insufficient oxygen in tissues result in accumulation of lactic acid from anaerobic glycolysis)*
• Hepatic coma *(related to liver damage and decreased tissue oxygenation)*
• Ingestion of large doses of alcohol or acetaminophen *(related to liver damage)*
• Lactic acidosis *(related to strenuous exercise that results in accumulations in metabolic by-products of anaerobic breakdown of sugars for energy)*
• Pulmonary embolism *(decreased blood flow and insufficient oxygen in tissues result in accumulation of lactic acid from anaerobic glycolysis)*
• Pulmonary failure *(decreased blood flow and insufficient*

oxygen in tissues result in accumulation of lactic acid from anaerobic glycolysis)
• Reye's syndrome *(related to liver damage)*
• Shock *(decreased blood flow and insufficient oxygen in tissues result in accumulation of lactic acid from anaerobic glycolysis)*
• Strenuous exercise *(related to lactic acidosis)*

Decreased in: N/A

CRITICAL FINDINGS

Greater Than or Equal to 31 mg/dL
Note and immediately report to the health-care provider (HCP) any critically increased values and related symptoms.

Observe the patient for signs and symptoms of elevated levels of lactate, such as Kussmaul's breathing and increased pulse rate. In general, there is an inverse relationship between critically elevated lactate levels and survival.

INTERFERING FACTORS
• Drugs that may increase lactate levels include albuterol, aspirin, anticonvulsants (long-term use), isoniazid, metformin (Glucophage), oral contraceptives, sodium bicarbonate, and sorbitol.
• Falsely low lactate levels are obtained in samples with elevated levels of the enzyme lactate dehydrogenase because this enzyme reacts with the available lactate substrate.
• Using a tourniquet or instructing the patient to clench his or her fist during a venipuncture can cause elevated levels.
• Engaging in strenuous physical activity (i.e., activity in which blood flow and oxygen distribution

cannot keep pace with increased energy needs) before specimen collection can cause an elevated result.

• Delay in transport of the specimen to the laboratory must be avoided. Specimens not processed by centrifugation in a tightly stoppered collection container within 15 min of collection should be rejected for analysis. It is preferable to transport specimens to the laboratory in an ice slurry to further retard cellular metabolism that might shift lactate levels in the sample before analysis.

• Failure to follow dietary restrictions before the procedure may cause the procedure to be canceled or repeated.

NURSING IMPLICATIONS AND PROCEDURE

PRETEST:

▶ Positively identify the patient using at least two unique identifiers before providing care, treatment, or services.

▶ *Patient Teaching:* Inform the patient this test can assist with assessing organ function.

▶ Obtain a history of the patient's complaints, including a list of known allergens, especially allergies or sensitivities to latex.

▶ Obtain a history of the patient's cardiovascular, endocrine, hepatobiliary, musculoskeletal, and respiratory systems; symptoms; and results of previously performed laboratory tests and diagnostic and surgical procedures.

▶ Obtain a list of the patient's current medications, including herbs, nutritional supplements, and nutraceuticals (see Appendix F).

▶ Review the procedure with the patient. Instruct the patient to rest for 1 hr before specimen collection. Inform the patient that specimen collection takes approximately 5 to 10 min. Address concerns about pain and explain that there may be some discomfort during the venipuncture.

▶ Instruct the patient to fast and to restrict fluids overnight. Instruct the patient not to ingest alcohol for 12 hr

before the test. Protocols may vary among facilities.

▶ *Sensitivity to social and cultural issues,* as well as concern for modesty, is important in providing psychological support before, during, and after the procedure.

▶ There are no medication restrictions unless by medical direction.

▶ Prepare an ice slurry in a cup or plastic bag to have on hand for immediate transport of the specimen to the laboratory.

INTRATEST:

▶ Ensure that the patient has complied with dietary restrictions and other pretesting preparations; ensure that food and liquids have been restricted for at least 12 hr prior to the procedure.

▶ If the patient has a history of allergic reaction to latex, avoid the use of equipment containing latex.

▶ Instruct the patient to cooperate fully and to follow directions. Direct the patient to breathe normally and to avoid unnecessary movement.

▶ Observe standard precautions, and follow the general guidelines in Appendix A. Positively identify the patient, and label the appropriate tubes with the corresponding patient demographics, date, and time of collection. Instruct the patient *not* to clench and unclench fist immediately before or during specimen collection. Do not use a tourniquet. Perform a venipuncture. The tightly capped sample should be placed in an ice slurry immediately after collection. Information on the specimen label should be protected from water in the ice slurry by first placing the specimen in a protective plastic bag.

▶ Remove the needle and apply direct pressure with dry gauze to stop bleeding. Observe/assess venipuncture site for bleeding or hematoma formation and secure gauze with adhesive bandage.

▶ Promptly transport the specimen to the laboratory for processing and analysis.

POST-TEST:

▶ A report of the results will be sent to the requesting HCP, who will discuss the results with the patient.

▶ Instruct the patient to resume usual diet and fluids, as directed by the HCP.

● **Nutritional Considerations:** Instruct patients to consume water when exercising. Dehydration may occur when the body loses water during exercise. Early signs of dehydration include dry mouth, thirst, and concentrated dark yellow urine. If replacement fluids are not consumed at this time, the patient may become moderately dehydrated and exhibit symptoms of extreme thirst, dry oral mucus membranes, inability to produce tears, decreased urinary output, and lightheadedness. Severe dehydration manifests as confusion, lethargy, vertigo, tachycardia, anuria, diaphoresis, and loss of consciousness.
● Reinforce information given by the patient's HCP regarding further testing, treatment, or referral to another HCP. Answer any questions or address any concerns voiced by the patient or family.

● Depending on the results of this procedure, additional testing may be performed to evaluate or monitor progression of the disease process and determine the need for a change in therapy. Evaluate test results in relation to the patient's symptoms and other tests performed.

RELATED MONOGRAPHS:

● Related laboratory tests include ALT, alveolar/arterial oxygen ratio, ammonia, analgesic and antipyretic drugs, anion gap, AST, biopsy liver, blood gases, CK, glucose, ketones, plethysmography, potassium, pulse oximetry, and sodium.
● Refer to the Cardiovascular, Endocrine, Hepatobiliary, Musculoskeletal, and Respiratory systems tables at the end of the book for related tests by body system.

Lactose Tolerance Test

SYNONYM/ACRONYM: LTT.

COMMON USE: To assess for lactose intolerance or other metabolic disorders.

SPECIMEN: Plasma (1 mL) collected in a gray-top (fluoride/oxalate) tube.

REFERENCE VALUE: (Method: Spectrophotometry)

Change in Glucose Value*	Conventional Units	SI Units (Conventional Units × 0.0555)
Normal	Greater than 30 mg/dL	Greater than 1.7 mmol/L
Inconclusive	20–30 mg/dL	1.1–1.7 mmol/L
Abnormal	Less than 20 mg/dL	Less than 1.1 mmol/L

*Compared to fasting sample.

DESCRIPTION: Lactose is a disaccharide found in dairy products. When ingested, lactose is broken down in the intestine by the sugar-splitting enzyme

lactase, into glucose and galactose. When sufficient lactase is not available, intestinal bacteria metabolize the lactose, resulting in abdominal bloating, pain, flatus, and diarrhea. The lactose tolerance test screens for lactose intolerance by monitoring glucose levels after ingestion of a dose of lactose.

INDICATIONS
• Evaluate patients for suspected lactose intolerance

POTENTIAL DIAGNOSIS

Glucose Levels Increased In
• Normal response

Glucose Levels Decreased In
• Lactose intolerance (lactase is insufficient to break down ingested lactose into glucose)

CRITICAL FINDINGS
• Less than 40 mg/dL
• Greater than 400 mg/dL

Note and immediately report to the health-care provider (HCP) any critically increased or decreased values and symptoms.

Symptoms of decreased glucose levels include headache, confusion, hunger, irritability, nervousness, restlessness, sweating, and weakness. Possible interventions include oral or IV administration of glucose, IV or intramuscular injection of glucagon, and continuous glucose monitoring.

Symptoms of elevated glucose levels include abdominal pain, fatigue, muscle cramps, nausea, vomiting, polyuria, and thirst. Possible interventions include subcutaneous or IV injection of insulin with continuous glucose monitoring.

INTERFERING FACTORS
• Numerous medications may alter glucose levels (see monograph titled "Glucose").

• Delayed gastric emptying may decrease glucose levels.
• Smoking may falsely increase glucose levels.
• Failure to follow dietary and activity restrictions before the procedure may cause the procedure to be canceled or repeated.

NURSING IMPLICATIONS AND PROCEDURE

PRETEST:
▶ Positively identify the patient using at least two unique identifiers before providing care, treatment, or services.
▶ *Patient Teaching:* Inform the patient this test can assist with evaluating tolerance to dairy products which contain lactose.
▶ Obtain a history of the patient's complaints, including a list of known allergens, especially allergies or sensitivities to latex.
▶ Obtain a history of the patient's gastrointestinal system, symptoms, and results of previously performed laboratory tests and diagnostic and surgical procedures.
▶ Obtain a list of the patient's current medications, including herbs, nutritional supplements, and nutraceuticals (see Appendix F).
▶ Review the procedure with the patient. Obtain the pediatric patient's weight to calculate dose of lactose to be administered. Inform the patient that multiple samples will be collected over a 90-min interval. Inform the patient that each specimen collection takes approximately 5 to 10 min. Address concerns about pain related to the procedure. Inform the patient that the test may produce symptoms such as cramps and diarrhea. Instruct the patient not to smoke cigarettes or chew gum during the test. Explain that there may be some discomfort during the venipuncture.
▶ *Sensitivity to social and cultural issues,* as well as concern for modesty, is important in providing psychological support before, during, and after the procedure.
▶ Inform the patient that fasting for at least 12 hr before the test is required and that strenuous activity should also be avoided for at least 12 hr before the test. Protocols may vary among facilities.

◆There are no medication restrictions unless by medical direction.

INTRATEST:

◆Ensure that the patient has complied with dietary and activity restrictions as well as other pretesting preparations; ensure that food has been restricted for at least 12 hr prior to the procedure.

◆If the patient has a history of allergic reaction to latex, avoid the use of equipment containing latex.

◆Administer lactose dissolved in a small amount of water over a 5- to 10-min period. Adult dosage is 1 g/kg body weight to a maximum of 50 g. Pediatric dosage is based on weight: 0.6 to 1.3 g lactose per kilogram of body weight for infants less than 12 mo old; 1.7 g lactose per kilogram of body weight for children 1 to 12 yr with a minimum of 10 g and a maximum of 50 g. One pound is equal to 0.45 kg; therefore, a weight of 50 lb is equal to 22 kg. The appropriate dosage of lactose in this example would be 38 g. Record time of ingestion. Encourage the patient to drink one to two glasses of water during the test.

◆Instruct the patient to cooperate fully and to follow directions. Direct the patient to breathe normally and to avoid unnecessary movement.

◆Observe standard precautions, and follow the general guidelines in Appendix A. Positively identify the patient, and label the appropriate tubes with the corresponding patient demographics, date, and time of collection. Perform a venipuncture; collect the specimen in the appropriate tube or in a red pediatric Microtainer. Samples should be collected at baseline, 15, 30, 60, 90, and 120 min. Record any symptoms the patient reports throughout the course of the test.

◆Remove the needle and apply direct pressure with dry gauze to stop bleeding. Observe/assess venipuncture site for bleeding or hematoma formation and secure gauze with adhesive bandage.

◆Promptly transport the specimen to the laboratory for processing and analysis. Glucose values change rapidly in an unprocessed, unpreserved specimen; therefore, if a Microtainer is used, each sample should be transported immediately after collection.

POST-TEST:

◆A report of the results will be sent to the requesting HCP, who will discuss the results with the patient.

◆Instruct the patient that resuming his or her usual diet may not be possible if lactose intolerance is identified. Educate patients on the importance of following the dietary advice of a nutritionist to ensure proper nutritional balance.

◆*Nutritional Considerations:* Instruct the patient with lactose intolerance to avoid milk products and to carefully read labels on prepared products. Yogurt, which contains inactive lactase enzyme, may be ingested. The lactase in yogurt is activated by the temperature and pH of the duodenum and substitutes for the lack of endogenous lactase. Advise the patient that products such as Lactaid tablets or drops may allow ingestion of milk products without sequelae. Many lactose-free food products are now available in grocery stores.

◆Recognize anxiety related to test results, and be supportive of concerns related to a perceived change in lifestyle. Discuss the implications of abnormal test results on the patient's lifestyle. Provide teaching and information regarding the clinical implications of the test results, as appropriate.

◆Reinforce information given by the patient's HCP regarding further testing, treatment, or referral to another HCP. Answer any questions or address any concerns voiced by the patient or family.

◆Depending on the results of this procedure, additional testing may be performed to evaluate or monitor progression of the disease process and determine the need for a change in therapy. Evaluate test results in relation to the patient's symptoms and other tests performed.

RELATED MONOGRAPHS:

◆Related tests include D-xylose absorption, fecal analysis, and glucose.

◆Refer to the Gastrointestinal System table at the end of the book for related tests by body system.

L

Laparoscopy, Abdominal

SYNONYM/ACRONYM: Abdominal peritoneoscopy.

COMMON USE: To visualize and assess the liver, gallbladder, and spleen to assist with surgical interventions, staging tumor, and performing diagnostic biopsies.

AREA OF APPLICATION: Pelvis.

CONTRAST: Carbon dioxide (CO_2).

DESCRIPTION: Abdominal or gastrointestinal (GI) laparoscopy provides direct visualization of the liver, gallbladder, spleen, and stomach after insufflation of carbon dioxide (CO_2). In this procedure, a rigid laparoscope is introduced into the body cavity through a 1- to 2-cm abdominal incision. The endoscope has a microscope to allow visualization of the organs, and it can be used to insert instruments for performing certain procedures, such as biopsy and tumor resection. Under general anesthesia, the peritoneal cavity is inflated with 2 to 3 L of CO_2. The gas distends the abdominal wall so that the instruments can be inserted safely. Advantages of this procedure compared to an open laparotomy include reduced pain, reduced length of stay at the hospital or surgical center, and reduced time off from work.

INDICATIONS
- Assist in performing surgical procedures such as cholecystectomy, appendectomy, hernia repair, hiatal hernia repair, and bowel resection
- Detect cirrhosis of the liver
- Detect pancreatic disorders
- Evaluate abdominal pain or abdominal mass of unknown origin
- Evaluate abdominal trauma in an emergency
- Evaluate and treat appendicitis
- Evaluate the extent of splenomegaly due to portal hypertension
- Evaluate jaundice of unknown origin
- Obtain biopsy specimens of benign or cancerous tumors
- Stage neoplastic disorders such as lymphomas, Hodgkin's disease, and hepatic carcinoma

POTENTIAL DIAGNOSIS

Normal findings in
- Normal appearance of the liver, spleen, gallbladder, pancreas, and other abdominal contents

Abnormal findings in
- Abdominal adhesions
- Appendicitis
- Ascites
- Cancer of any of the organs
- Cirrhosis of the liver
- Gangrenous gallbladder
- Intra-abdominal bleeding
- Portal hypertension
- Splenomegaly

CRITICAL FINDINGS
- Appendicitis

It is essential that critical diagnoses be communicated immediately to the appropriate health-care provider (HCP). A listing of these diagnoses varies among facilities. Note and immediately report to the HCP abnormal results and related symptoms.

INTERFERING FACTORS

This procedure is contraindicated for

- Patients who are pregnant or suspected of being pregnant, unless the potential benefits of the procedure far outweigh the risk of radiation exposure to the fetus.
- Patients with bleeding disorders, especially those associated with uremia and cytotoxic chemotherapy.
- Patients with cardiac conditions or dysrhythmias.
- Patients with advanced respiratory or cardiovascular disease.
- Patients with intestinal obstruction, abdominal mass, abdominal hernia, or suspected intra-abdominal hemorrhage.
- Patients with a history of peritonitis or multiple abdominal operations causing dense adhesions.

Factors that may impair clear visualization

- Gas or feces in the GI tract resulting from inadequate cleansing or failure to restrict food intake before the study.
- Retained barium from a previous radiological procedure.
- Inability of the patient to cooperate or remain still during the procedure because of age, significant pain, or mental status.
- Metallic objects (e.g., jewelry, body rings) within the examination field, which may inhibit organ visualization and cause unclear images.

Other considerations

- The procedure may be terminated if chest pain or severe cardiac arrhythmias occur.
- Failure to follow dietary restrictions and other pretesting preparations may cause the procedure to be canceled or repeated.
- Patients who are in a hypoxemic or hypercapnic state will require continuous oxygen administration.
- Patients with acute infection or advanced malignancy involving the abdominal wall are at increased risk because organisms may be introduced into the normally sterile peritoneal cavity.

NURSING IMPLICATIONS AND PROCEDURE

PRETEST:

- Positively identify the patient using at least two unique identifiers before providing care, treatment, or services.
- *Patient Teaching:* Inform the patient this procedure can assist in assessing the abdominal organs.
- Obtain a history of the patient's complaints, including a list of known allergens, especially allergies or sensitivities to latex and anesthetics.
- Obtain a history of the patient's gastrointestinal and hepatobiliary systems, symptoms, and results of previously performed laboratory tests and diagnostic and surgical procedures.
- Ensure that this procedure is performed before any barium studies.
- Record the date of the last menstrual period and determine the possibility of pregnancy in perimenopausal women.
- Obtain a list of the patient's current medications, including anticoagulants, aspirin and other salicylates, herbs, nutritional supplements, and nutraceuticals, especially those known to affect coagulation (see Appendix F). Such products should be discontinued by medical direction for the appropriate number of days prior to a surgical procedure. Note the last time and dose of medication taken.

▶ Review the procedure with the patient. Address concerns about pain related to the procedure and explain that some pain may be experienced during the test, and there may be moments of discomfort. Inform the patient that the procedure is performed in a surgery department, by an HCP, with support staff, and takes approximately 30 to 60 min.

▶ *Sensitivity to social and cultural issues,* as well as concern for modesty, is important in providing psychological support before, during, and after the procedure.

▶ Explain that an IV line may be inserted to allow infusion of IV fluids, anesthetics, analgesics, or IV sedation.

▶ Inform the patient that a laxative and cleansing enema may be needed the day before the procedure, with cleansing enemas on the morning of the procedure, depending on the institution's policy.

▶ Instruct the patient to remove jewelry and other metallic objects from the area to be examined prior to the procedure.

▶ Instruct the patient to fast and restrict fluids for 8 hr prior to the procedure. Protocols may vary among facilities.

▶ *Make sure a written and informed consent has been signed prior to the procedure and before administering any medications.*

INTRATEST:

▶ Ensure that the patient has complied with dietary, fluid, and medication restrictions for at least 8 hr prior to the procedure.

▶ Ensure the patient has removed all external metallic objects from the area to be examined.

▶ Ensure that nonallergy to anesthesia is confirmed before the procedure is performed under general anesthesia.

▶ Assess for completion of bowel preparation according to the institution's procedure.

▶ Have emergency equipment readily available.

▶ Instruct the patient to void prior to the procedure and to change into the gown, robe, and foot coverings provided.

▶ Instruct the patient to cooperate fully and to follow directions. Instruct the patient to remain still throughout the procedure because movement produces unreliable results.

▶ Obtain and record baseline vital signs.

▶ Observe standard precautions, and follow the general guidelines in Appendix A.

▶ Insert an IV line or venous access device at a low "keep open" rate.

▶ Administer medications, as ordered, to reduce discomfort and to promote relaxation and sedation.

▶ Place the patient on the laparoscopy table. If general anesthesia is to be used, it is administered at this time. Place the patient in a modified lithotomy position with the head tilted downward. Cleanse the abdomen with an antiseptic solution, and drape and catheterize the patient, if ordered.

▶ The HCP identifies the site for the scope insertion and administers local anesthesia if that is to be used. After deeper layers are anesthetized, a pneumoperitoneum needle is placed between the visceral and parietal peritoneum.

▶ CO_2 is insufflated through the pneumoperitoneum needle to separate the abdominal wall from the viscera and to aid in visualization of the abdominal structures. The pneumoperitoneum needle is removed, and the trocar and laparoscope are inserted through the incision.

▶ After the examination, collection of tissue samples, and performance of therapeutic procedures, the scope is withdrawn. All possible CO_2 is evacuated via the trocar, which is then removed. The skin incision is closed with sutures, clips, or sterile strips, and a small dressing or adhesive strip is applied.

▶ Observe/assess the incision site for bleeding, inflammation, or hematoma formation.

POST-TEST:

▶ A report of the examination will be sent to the requesting HCP, who will discuss the results with the patient.

▶ Instruct the patient to resume usual diet, fluids, and medication, as directed by the HCP.

- Monitor vital signs and neurological status every 15 min for 1 hr, then every 2 hr for 4 hr, and as ordered. Take temperature every 4 hr for 24 hr. Monitor intake and output at least every 8 hr. Compare with baseline values. Notify the HCP if temperature is elevated. Protocols may vary among facilities.
- Instruct the patient to restrict activity for 2 to 7 days after the procedure.
- Instruct the patient in the care and assessment of the incision site.
- If indicated, inform the patient of a follow-up appointment for the removal of sutures.
- Inform the patient that shoulder discomfort may be experienced for 1 or 2 days after the procedure as a result of abdominal distention caused by insufflation of CO_2 into the abdomen and that mild analgesics and cold compresses, as ordered, can be used to relieve the discomfort.
- Emphasize that any persistent shoulder pain, abdominal pain, vaginal bleeding, fever, redness, or swelling of the incisional area must be reported to the HCP immediately.
- Recognize anxiety related to test results. Discuss the implications of abnormal test results on the patient's lifestyle. Provide teaching and information regarding the clinical implications of the test results, as appropriate.
- Reinforce information given by the patient's HCP regarding further testing, treatment, or referral to another HCP. Answer any questions or address any concerns voiced by the patient or family.
- Depending on the results of this procedure, additional testing may be needed to evaluate or monitor progression of the disease process and determine the need for a change in therapy. Evaluate test results in relation to the patient's symptoms and other tests performed.

RELATED MONOGRAPHS:

- Related tests include amylase, barium swallow, biopsy bone marrow, CBC, CBC WBC count and differential, CT abdomen, CT biliary tract and liver, CT pancreas, CRP, ESR, gallium scan, hepatobiliary scan, KUB, lipase, liver and spleen scan, lymphangiogram, MRI abdomen, MRI pelvis, peritoneal fluid analysis, US abdomen, and US pelvis.
- Refer to the Gastrointestinal and Hepatobiliary systems tables at the end of the book for related tests by body system.

Laparoscopy, Gynecologic

SYNONYM/ACRONYM: Gynecologic pelviscopy, gynecologic laparoscopy, pelvic endoscopy, peritoneoscopy.

COMMON USE: To visualize and assess the ovaries, fallopian tubes, and uterus to assist in diagnosing inflammation, malformations, cysts, and fibroids and to evaluate causes of infertility.

AREA OF APPLICATION: Pelvis.

CONTRAST: Carbon dioxide (CO_2).

DESCRIPTION: Gynecologic laparoscopy provides direct visualization of the internal pelvic contents, including the ovaries, fallopian tubes, and uterus, after insufflation of carbon dioxide (CO_2). It is done to diagnose and treat pelvic organ disorders as well as to perform surgical procedures on the organs. In this procedure, a rigid laparoscope is introduced into the body cavity through a 1- to 2-cm periumbilical incision. The endoscope has a microscope to allow visualization of the organs, and it can be used to insert instruments for performing procedures such as biopsy and tumor resection. Under general or local anesthesia, the peritoneal cavity is inflated with 2 to 3 L of CO_2. The gas distends the abdominal wall so that the instruments can be inserted safely. Advantages of this procedure compared to an open laparotomy include reduced pain, reduced length of stay at the hospital or surgical center, and reduced time off from work.

INDICATIONS

- Detect ectopic pregnancy and determine the need for surgery
- Detect pelvic inflammatory disease or abscess
- Detect uterine fibroids, ovarian cysts, and uterine malformations (ovarian cysts may be aspirated during the procedure)
- Evaluate amenorrhea and infertility
- Evaluate fallopian tubes and anatomic defects to determine the cause of infertility
- Evaluate known or suspected endometriosis, salpingitis, and hydrosalpinx
- Evaluate pelvic pain or masses of unknown cause

- Evaluate reproductive organs after therapy for infertility
- Obtain biopsy specimens to confirm suspected pelvic malignancies or metastasis
- Perform tubal sterilization and ovarian biopsy
- Perform vaginal hysterectomy
- Remove adhesions or foreign bodies such as intrauterine devices
- Treat endometriosis through electrocautery or laser vaporization

POTENTIAL DIAGNOSIS

Normal findings in
- Normal appearance of uterus, ovaries, fallopian tubes, and other pelvic contents

Abnormal findings in
- Ectopic pregnancy
- Endometriosis
- Ovarian cyst
- Ovarian tumor
- Pelvic adhesions
- Pelvic inflammatory disease
- Pelvic tumor
- Salpingitis
- Uterine fibroids

CRITICAL FINDINGS
- Ectopic pregnancy
- Foreign body
- Tumor with significant mass effect

It is essential that critical diagnoses be communicated immediately to the appropriate health-care provider (HCP). A listing of these diagnoses varies among facilities. Note and immediately report to the HCP abnormal results and related symptoms.

INTERFERING FACTORS

This procedure is contraindicated for
- Patients who are pregnant or suspected of being pregnant, unless the potential benefits of

the procedure far outweigh the risks to the fetus and mother.

- Patients with bleeding disorders, especially those associated with uremia and cytotoxic chemotherapy.
- Patients with cardiac conditions or dysrhythmias.
- Patients with advanced respiratory or cardiovascular disease.
- Patients with intestinal obstruction, abdominal mass, abdominal hernia, or suspected intra-abdominal hemorrhage.

Factors that may impair clear visualization

- Gas or feces in the gastrointestinal (GI) tract resulting from inadequate cleansing or failure to restrict food intake before the study.
- Retained barium from a previous radiological procedure.
- Inability of the patient to cooperate or remain still during the procedure because of age, significant pain, or mental status.
- Metallic objects (e.g., jewelry, body rings) within the examination field, which may inhibit organ visualization and cause unclear images.

Other considerations

- The procedure may be terminated if chest pain or severe cardiac arrhythmias occur.
- Failure to follow dietary restrictions and other pretesting preparations may cause the procedure to be canceled or repeated.
- Patients who are in a hypoxemic or hypercapnic state will require continuous oxygen administration.
- Patients with acute infection or advanced malignancy involving the abdominal wall are at increased risk because organisms may be introduced into the normally sterile peritoneal cavity.

NURSING IMPLICATIONS AND PROCEDURE

PRETEST:

- Positively identify the patient using at least two unique identifiers before providing care, treatment, or services.
- *Patient Teaching:* Inform the patient this procedure can assist in assessing the abdominal and pelvic organs.
- Obtain a history of the patient's complaints, including a list of known allergens, especially allergies or sensitivities to latex and anesthetics.
- Obtain a history of the patient's reproductive system, symptoms, and results of previously performed laboratory tests and diagnostic and surgical procedures.
- Ensure that this procedure is performed before any barium studies.
- Record the date of the last menstrual period and determine the possibility of pregnancy in perimenopausal women.
- Obtain a list of the patient's current medications, including anticoagulants, aspirin and other salicylates, herbs, nutritional supplements, and nutraceuticals, especially those known to affect coagulation (see Appendix F). Such products should be discontinued by medical direction for the appropriate number of days prior to a surgical procedure. Note the last time and dose of medication taken.
- Review the procedure with the patient. Address concerns about pain related to the procedure and explain that some pain may be experienced during the test, and there may be moments of discomfort. Inform the patient that the procedure is performed in a surgery department by an HCP and support staff and takes approximately 30 to 60 min.
- *Sensitivity to social and cultural issues,* as well as concern for modesty, is important in providing psychological support before, during, and after the procedure.
- Explain that an IV line may be inserted to allow infusion of IV fluids, anesthetics, analgesics, or IV sedation.
- Inform the patient that a laxative and cleansing enema may be needed the day before the procedure, with

cleansing enemas on the morning of the procedure, depending on the institution's policy.

▶ Instruct the patient to remove jewelry and other metallic objects from the area to be examined prior to the procedure.

▶ Instruct the patient to fast and restrict fluids for 8 hr prior to the procedure. Protocols may vary among facilities.

▶ *Make sure a written and informed consent has been signed prior to the procedure and before administering any medications.*

INTRATEST:

▶ Ensure that the patient has complied with dietary, fluid, and medication restrictions for at least 8 hr prior to the procedure.

▶ Ensure the patient has removed all external metallic objects from the area to be examined.

▶ Ensure that nonallergy to anesthesia is confirmed before the procedure is performed under general anesthesia.

▶ Assess for completion of bowel preparation according to the institution's procedure.

▶ Have emergency equipment readily available.

▶ Instruct the patient to void prior to the procedure and to change into the gown, robe, and foot coverings provided.

▶ Instruct the patient to cooperate fully and to follow directions. Instruct the patient to remain still throughout the procedure because movement produces unreliable results.

▶ Obtain and record baseline vital signs.

▶ Observe standard precautions, and follow the general guidelines in Appendix A.

▶ Insert an IV line or venous access device at a low "keep open" rate.

▶ Administer medications, as ordered, to reduce discomfort and to promote relaxation and sedation.

▶ Place the patient on the laparoscopy table. If general anesthesia is to be used, it is administered at this time. Place the patient in a modified lithotomy position with the head tilted downward. Cleanse the abdomen with an antiseptic solution, and drape and catheterize the patient, if ordered.

▶ The HCP identifies the site for the scope insertion and administers local anesthesia if that is to be used. After deeper layers are anesthetized, a pneumoperitoneum needle is placed between the visceral and parietal peritoneum.

▶ CO_2 is insufflated through the pneumoperitoneum needle to separate the abdominal wall from the viscera and to aid in visualization of the abdominal structures. The pneumoperitoneum needle is removed, and the trocar and laparoscope are inserted through the incision.

▶ The HCP inserts a uterine manipulator through the vagina and cervix and into the uterus so that the uterus, fallopian tubes, and ovaries can be moved to permit better visualization.

▶ After the examination, collection of tissue samples, and performance of therapeutic procedures (e.g., tubal ligation), the scope is withdrawn. All possible CO_2 is evacuated via the trocar, which is then removed. The skin incision is closed with sutures, clips, or sterile strips and a small dressing or adhesive strip is applied. After the perineum is cleansed, the uterine manipulator is removed and a sterile pad applied.

▶ Observe/assess the incision site for bleeding, inflammation, or hematoma formation.

POST-TEST:

▶ A report of the examination will be sent to the requesting HCP, who will discuss the results with the patient.

▶ Instruct the patient to resume usual diet, fluids, and medication, as directed by the HCP.

▶ Monitor vital signs and neurological status every 15 min for 1 hr, then every 2 hr for 4 hr, and as ordered. Take temperature every 4 hr for 24 hr. Monitor intake and output at least every 8 hr. Compare with baseline values. Notify the HCP if temperature is elevated. Protocols may vary among facilities.

▶ Instruct the patient to restrict activity for 2 to 7 days after the procedure.

- Instruct the patient in the care and assessment of the incision site.
- If indicated, inform the patient of a follow-up appointment for the removal of sutures.
- Inform the patient that shoulder discomfort may be experienced for 1 or 2 days after the procedure as a result of abdominal distention caused by insufflation of CO_2 into the abdomen and that mild analgesics and cold compresses, as ordered, can be used to relieve the discomfort.
- Emphasize that any persistent shoulder pain, abdominal pain, vaginal bleeding, fever, redness, or swelling of the incisional area must be reported to the HCP immediately.
- Recognize anxiety related to test results. Discuss the implications of abnormal test results on the patient's lifestyle. Provide teaching and information regarding the clinical implications of the test results, as appropriate.

- Reinforce information given by the patient's HCP regarding further testing, treatment, or referral to another HCP. Answer any questions or address any concerns voiced by the patient or family.
- Depending on the results of this procedure, additional testing may be needed to evaluate or monitor progression of the disease process and determine the need for a change in therapy. Evaluate test results in relation to the patient's symptoms and other tests performed.

RELATED MONOGRAPHS:

- Related tests include cancer antigens, *Chlamydia* group antibody, CT abdomen, CT pelvis, HCG, MRI pelvis, Pap smear, progesterone, US pelvis, and uterine fibroid embolization.
- Refer to the Reproductive System table at the end of the book for related tests by body system.

L

Latex Allergy

SYNONYM/ACRONYM: N/A.

COMMON USE: To assess for allergic reaction to products containing latex.

SPECIMEN: Serum (1 mL) collected in a red-top tube.

REFERENCE VALUE: (Method: Immunoassay) Negative.

POTENTIAL DIAGNOSIS

Positive findings in
Latex allergy

Negative findings in: N/A

CRITICAL FINDINGS: N/A

Find and print out the full monograph at DavisPlus (http://davisplus.fadavis.com, keyword Van Leeuwen).

Lead

SYNONYM/ACRONYM: Pb.

COMMON USE: To assess for lead toxicity and monitor exposure to lead to assist in diagnosing lead poisoning.

SPECIMEN: Whole blood (1 mL) collected in a special lead-free royal blue– or tan-top tube. Plasma (1 mL) collected in a lavender-top (EDTA) tube is also acceptable.

REFERENCE VALUE: (Method: Atomic absorption spectrophotometry)

	Conventional Units	SI Units (Conventional Units × 0.0483)
Children and adults (WHO environmental exposure)	Less than 10 mcg/dL	Less than 0.48 micromol/L
OSHA (occupational exposure standard)	Less than 40 mcg/dL	Less than 1.93 micromol/L

OSHA = Occupational Safety and Health Administration; WHO = World Health Organization.

DESCRIPTION: Lead is a heavy metal and trace element. It is absorbed through the respiratory and gastrointestinal systems. It can also be transported from mother to fetus through the placenta. When there is frequent exposure to lead-containing items (e.g., paint, batteries, gasoline, pottery, bullets, printing materials) or occupations (mining, automobile, printing, and welding industries), many organs of the body are affected. Lead poisoning can cause severe behavioral and neurological effects. The blood test is considered the best indicator of lead poisoning, and confirmation is made by the lead mobilization test performed on a 24-hr urine specimen.

INDICATIONS
Assist in the diagnosis and treatment of lead poisoning

POTENTIAL DIAGNOSIS

Increased in
Heme synthesis involves the conversion of D-amino levulinic acid to porphobilinogen. Lead interferes with the enzyme that is responsible for this critical step in heme synthesis, amino levulinic acid dehydrase.
• Anemia of lead intoxication
• Lead encephalopathy
• Metal poisoning

Decreased in: N/A

CRITICAL FINDINGS
• Levels greater than 30 mcg/dL indicate significant exposure

• Levels greater than 60 mcg/dL require chelation therapy

Note and immediately report to the health-care provider (HCP) any critically increased values and related symptoms.

INTERFERING FACTORS

Contamination of the collection site and/or specimen with lead in dust can be avoided by taking special care to have the surfaces surrounding the collection location cleaned. Extra care should also be used to avoid contamination during the actual venipuncture.

NURSING IMPLICATIONS AND PROCEDURE

PRETEST:

▶ Positively identify the patient using at least two unique identifiers before providing care, treatment, or services.
▶ *Patient Teaching:* Inform the patient this test can assist in detecting lead exposure.
▶ Obtain a history of the patient's complaints, including a list of known allergens, especially allergies or sensitivities to latex.
▶ Obtain a history of the patient's hematopoietic system, symptoms, and results of previously performed laboratory tests and diagnostic and surgical procedures.
▶ Obtain a history of the patient's exposure to lead.
▶ Obtain a list of the patient's current medications, including herbs, nutritional supplements, and nutraceuticals (see Appendix F).
▶ Review the procedure with the patient. Inform the patient that specimen collection takes approximately 5 to 10 min. Address concerns about pain and explain that there may be some discomfort during the venipuncture.
▶ *Sensitivity to social and cultural issues,* as well as concern for modesty, is important in providing psychological support before, during, and after the procedure.

▶ There are no food, fluid, or medication restrictions unless by medical direction.

INTRATEST:

▶ If the patient has a history of allergic reaction to latex, avoid the use of equipment containing latex.
▶ Instruct the patient to cooperate fully and to follow directions. Direct the patient to breathe normally and to avoid unnecessary movement.
▶ Observe standard precautions, and follow the general guidelines in Appendix A. Positively identify the patient, and label the appropriate tubes with the corresponding patient demographics, date, and time of collection. Perform a venipuncture.
▶ Remove the needle and apply direct pressure with dry gauze to stop bleeding. Observe/assess venipuncture site for bleeding or hematoma formation and secure gauze with adhesive bandage.
▶ Promptly transport the specimen to the laboratory for processing and analysis.

POST-TEST:

▶ A report of the results will be sent to the requesting HCP, who will discuss the results with the patient.
▶ Reinforce information given by the patient's HCP regarding further testing, treatment, or referral to another HCP. Answer any questions or address any concerns voiced by the patient or family.
▶ Depending on the results of this procedure, additional testing may be performed to evaluate or monitor progression of the disease process and determine the need for a change in therapy. Evaluate test results in relation to the patient's symptoms and other tests performed.

RELATED MONOGRAPHS:

▶ Related tests include δ-aminolevulinic acid, CBC, CBC RBC morphology, erythrocyte protoporphyrin, and urine porphyrins.
▶ Refer to the Hematopoietic System table at the end of the book for related tests by body system.

Lecithin/Sphingomyelin Ratio

SYNONYM/ACRONYM: L/S ratio.

COMMON USE: To assess for preterm infant fetal lung maturity to assist in evaluating for potential diagnosis of respiratory distress syndrome (RDS).

SPECIMEN: Amniotic fluid (10 mL) collected in a sterile amber glass or plastic tube or bottle protected from light.

REFERENCE VALUE: (Method: Thin-layer chromatography)
Mature (nondiabetic): Greater than 2:1 in the presence of phosphatidyl glycerol
Borderline: 1.5 to 1.9:1
Immature: Less than 1.5:1

DESCRIPTION: Respiratory distress syndrome (RDS) is the most common problem encountered in the care of premature infants. RDS, also called hyaline membrane disease, results from a deficiency of phospholipid lung surfactants. The phospholipids in surfactant are produced by specialized alveolar cells and stored in granular lamellar bodies in the lung. In normally developed lungs, surfactant coats the surface of the alveoli. Surfactant reduces the surface tension of the alveolar wall during breathing. When there is an insufficient quantity of surfactant, the alveoli are unable to expand normally and gas exchange is inhibited. Amniocentesis, a procedure by which fluid is removed from the amniotic sac, is used to assess fetal lung maturity.

Lecithin is the primary surfactant phospholipid, and it is a stabilizing factor for the alveoli. It is produced at a low but constant rate until the 35th wk of gestation, after which its production sharply increases.

Sphingomyelin, another phospholipid component of surfactant, is also produced at a constant rate after the 26th wk of gestation. Before the 35th wk, the lecithin/sphingomyelin (L/S) ratio is usually less than 1.6:1. The ratio increases to 2.0 or greater when the rate of lecithin production increases after the 35th wk of gestation. Other phospholipids, such as phosphatidyl glycerol (PG) and phosphatidyl inositol (PI), increase over time in amniotic fluid as well. The presence of PG indicates that the fetus is within 2 to 6 wk of lung maturity (i.e., at full term). Simultaneous measurement of PG with the L/S ratio improves diagnostic accuracy. Production of phospholipid surfactant is delayed in diabetic mothers. Therefore, caution must be used when interpreting the results obtained from a diabetic patient, and a higher ratio is expected to predict maturity.

INDICATIONS
• Assist in the evaluation of fetal lung maturity
• Determine the optimal time for obstetric intervention in cases of threatened fetal survival caused by stresses related to maternal diabetes, toxemia, hemolytic diseases of the newborn, or postmaturity
• Identify fetuses at risk of developing RDS

POTENTIAL DIAGNOSIS

Increased in
Evidenced by conditions that increase production of surfactant.
• Hypertension
• Intrauterine growth retardation
• Malnutrition
• Maternal diabetes
• Placenta previa
• Placental infarction
• Premature rupture of the membranes

Decreased in
Evidenced by conditions that decrease production of surfactant.
• Advanced maternal age
• Immature fetal lungs
• Multiple gestation
• Polyhydramnios

CRITICAL FINDINGS
• An L/S ratio less than 1.5:1 is predictive of RDS at the time of delivery.

Note and immediately report to the health-care provider (HCP) any critically increased or decreased values and related symptoms. Infants known to be at risk for RDS can be treated with surfactant by intratracheal administration at birth.

INTERFERING FACTORS
• Fetal blood falsely elevates the L/S ratio.
• Exposing the specimen to light may cause falsely decreased values.
• There is some risk to having an amniocentesis performed, and this should be weighed against the need to obtain the desired diagnostic information. A small percentage (0.5%) of patients have experienced complications including premature rupture of the membranes, premature labor, spontaneous abortion, and stillbirth.

NURSING IMPLICATIONS AND PROCEDURE

PRETEST:
▶ Positively identify the patient using at least two unique identifiers before providing care, treatment, or services.
▶ *Patient Teaching:* Inform the parent this test can assist in obtaining an estimate of fetal lung maturity.
▶ Obtain a history of the patient's complaints, including a list of known allergens, especially allergies or sensitivities to latex.
▶ Obtain a history of the patient's reproductive and respiratory systems, symptoms, and results of previously performed laboratory tests and diagnostic and surgical procedures. Include any family history of genetic disorders such as cystic fibrosis, Duchenne's muscular dystrophy, hemophilia, sickle cell disease, Tay-Sachs disease, thalassemia, and trisomy 21. Obtain maternal Rh type. If Rh-negative, check for prior sensitization. A standard RhoGAM dose is indicated after amniocentesis; repeat doses should be considered if repeated amniocentesis is performed.
▶ Record the date of the last menstrual period, and determine that the pregnancy is in the third trimester between the 28th and 40th wk.
▶ Obtain a list of the patient's current medications, including herbs, nutritional supplements, and nutraceuticals (see Appendix F).
▶ Review the procedure with the patient. Warn the patient that normal results do not guarantee a normal fetus. Assure the patient that precautions to avoid injury to the fetus will be taken by localizing the fetus with ultrasound. Address

concerns about pain and explain that during the transabdominal procedure, any discomfort with a needle biopsy will be minimized with local anesthetics. Patients who are at 20 wk gestation or beyond should void before the test, because an empty bladder is less likely to be accidentally punctured during specimen collection. Encourage relaxation and controlled breathing during the procedure to aid in reducing any mild discomfort. Inform the patient that specimen collection is performed by an HCP specializing in this procedure and usually takes approximately 20 to 30 min to complete.

▶ *Sensitivity to social and cultural issues,* as well as concern for modesty, is important in providing psychological support before, during, and after the procedure.

▶ There are no food, fluid, or medication restrictions unless by medical direction.

▶ *Make sure a written and informed consent has been signed prior to the procedure and before administering any medications.*

INTRATEST:

▶ Ensure that the patient has voided before the procedure if gestation is 21 wk or more.

▶ Have emergency equipment readily available.

▶ Have patient remove clothes below the waist. Assist the patient to a supine position on the examination table with abdomen exposed. Drape the patient's legs, leaving the abdomen exposed. Raise her head or legs slightly to promote comfort and to relax abdominal muscles. If the uterus is large, place a pillow or rolled blanket under the patient's right side to prevent hypertension caused by great-vessel compression.

▶ Instruct the patient to cooperate fully and to follow directions. Direct the patient to breathe normally and to avoid unnecessary movement during administration of the local anesthetic and the procedure.

▶ Record maternal and fetal baseline vital signs and continue to monitor throughout the procedure. Monitor for uterine contractions. Monitor fetal vital signs

using ultrasound. Protocols may vary among facilities.

▶ Observe standard precautions, and follow the general guidelines in Appendix A. Positively identify the patient, and label the appropriate collection containers with the corresponding patient demographics, date and time of collection, and site location.

▶ Assess the position of the amniotic fluid, fetus, and placenta using ultrasound.

▶ Assemble the necessary equipment, including an amniocentesis tray with solution for skin preparation, local anesthetic, 10- or 20-mL syringe, needles of various sizes (including a 22-gauge, 5-in. spinal needle), sterile drapes, sterile gloves, and foil-covered or amber specimen collection containers.

▶ Cleanse suprapubic area with an antiseptic solution and protect with sterile drapes. A local anesthetic is injected. Explain that this may cause a stinging sensation.

▶ A 22-gauge, 5-in. spinal needle is inserted through the abdominal and uterine walls. Explain that a sensation of pressure may be experienced when the needle is inserted. Explain to the patient how to use focusing and controlled breathing for relaxation during the procedure.

▶ After the fluid is collected and the needle withdrawn, apply slight pressure to the site. Apply a sterile adhesive bandage to the site.

▶ Monitor the patient for complications related to the procedure (e.g., premature labor, allergic reaction, anaphylaxis).

▶ Place samples in properly labeled specimen container and promptly transport the specimen to the laboratory for processing and analysis.

POST-TEST:

▶ A report of the results will be sent to the requesting HCP, who will discuss the results with the patient.

▶ Fetal heart rate and maternal vital signs (i.e., heart rate, blood pressure, pulse, and respiration) must be compared to baseline values and closely monitored every 15 min for 30 to 60 min after the amniocentesis procedure. Protocols may vary among facilities.

- Observe/assess for delayed allergic reactions, such as rash, urticaria, tachycardia, hyperpnea, hypertension, palpitations, nausea, or vomiting.
- Observe/assess the amniocentesis site for bleeding, inflammation, or hematoma formation.
- Instruct the patient to report any redness, edema, bleeding, or pain at the site.
- Instruct the patient in the care and assessment of the amniocentesis site.
- Instruct the patient to expect mild cramping, leakage of small amount of amniotic fluid, and vaginal spotting for up to 2 days following the procedure. Instruct the patient to immediately report moderate to severe abdominal pain or cramps, change in fetal activity, increased or prolonged leaking of amniotic fluid from abdominal needle site, vaginal bleeding that is heavier than spotting, and either chills or fever to the HCP.
- Instruct the patient to rest until all symptoms have disappeared before resuming normal levels of activity.
- Administer standard dose of $Rh_o(D)$ immune globulin RhoGAM IM or Rhophylac IM or IV to maternal Rh-negative patients to prevent maternal Rh sensitization should the fetus be Rh-positive.
- Administer mild analgesic and antibiotic therapy as ordered. Remind the patient of the importance of completing the entire course of antibiotic therapy, even if signs and symptoms disappear before completion of therapy.
- Recognize anxiety related to test results, and offer support. Provide teaching and information regarding the clinical implications of the test results, as appropriate. Encourage the family to seek counseling if concerned with pregnancy termination or to seek genetic counseling if a chromosomal

abnormality is determined. Decisions regarding elective abortion should take place in the presence of both parents. Provide a nonjudgmental, nonthreatening atmosphere for discussing the risks and difficulties of delivering and raising a developmentally challenged infant as well as for exploring other options (termination of pregnancy or adoption). It is also important to discuss feelings the mother and father may experience (e.g., guilt, depression, anger) if fetal abnormalities are detected.
- Reinforce information given by the patient's HCP regarding further testing, treatment, or referral to another HCP. Answer any questions or address any concerns voiced by the patient or family.
- Instruct the patient in the use of any ordered medications. Explain the importance of adhering to the therapy regimen. As appropriate, instruct the patient in significant side effects and systemic reactions associated with the prescribed medication. Encourage her to review corresponding literature provided by a pharmacist.
- Depending on the results of this procedure, additional testing may be performed to evaluate or monitor progression of the disease process and determine the need for a change in therapy. Evaluate test results in relation to the patient's symptoms and other tests performed.

RELATED MONOGRAPHS:
- Related tests include amniotic fluid analysis, antibodies anticardiolipin, blood groups and antibodies, chromosome analysis, fetal fibronectin, α-fetoprotein, glucose, ketones, Kleihauer-Betke test, potassium, US biophysical profile obstetric, and UA.
- Refer to the Reproductive and Respiratory systems tables at the end of the book for related tests by body system.

Leukocyte Alkaline Phosphatase

SYNONYM/ACRONYM: LAP, LAP score, LAP smear.

COMMON USE: To monitor response to therapy in Hodgkin's disease and diagnose other disorders of the hematological system such as aplastic anemia.

SPECIMEN: Whole blood (1 mL) collected in a lavender-top (EDTA) tube.

REFERENCE VALUE: (Method: Microscopic evaluation of specially stained blood smears) 25 to 130 (score based on 0 to 4+ rating of 100 neutrophils).

DESCRIPTION: Alkaline phosphatase is an enzyme important for intracellular metabolic processes. It is present in the cytoplasm of neutrophilic granulocytes from the metamyelocyte to the segmented stage. Leukocyte alkaline phosphatase (LAP) concentrations may be altered by the presence of infection, stress, chronic inflammatory diseases, Hodgkin's disease, and hematological disorders. Levels are low in leukemic leukocytes and high in normal white blood cells (WBCs), making this test useful as a supportive test in the differential diagnosis of leukemia. It should be noted that test results must be correlated with the patient's condition because LAP levels increase toward normal in response to therapy.

INDICATIONS
- Differentiate chronic myelocytic leukemia from other disorders that increase the WBC count
- Monitor response of Hodgkin's disease to therapy

POTENTIAL DIAGNOSIS

Increased in
Conditions that result in an increase in leukocytes in all stages of maturity will reflect a corresponding increase in LAP.
- Aplastic leukemia
- Chronic inflammation
- Down's syndrome
- Hairy cell leukemia
- Hodgkin's disease
- Leukemia (acute and chronic lymphoblastic)
- Myelofibrosis with myeloid metaplasia
- Multiple myeloma
- Polycythemia vera *(increase in all blood cell lines, including leukocytes)*
- Pregnancy
- Stress
- Thrombocytopenia

Decreased in
- Chronic myelogenous leukemia
- Hereditary hypophosphatemia *(insufficient phosphorus levels)*
- Idiopathic thrombocytopenia purpura
- Nephrotic syndrome *(excessive loss of phosphorus)*
- Paroxysmal nocturnal hemoglobinuria *(possibly related to the absence of LAP and other proteins anchored to the red blood cell wall, resulting in complement-mediated hemolysis)*
- Sickle cell anemia
- Sideroblastic anemia

CRITICAL FINDINGS: N/A

INTERFERING FACTORS

Drugs that may increase the LAP score include steroids.

NURSING IMPLICATIONS AND PROCEDURE

PRETEST:

▸ Positively identify the patient using at least two unique identifiers before providing care, treatment, or services.

▸ *Patient Teaching:* Inform the patient this test can assist in evaluating for blood disorders.

▸ Obtain a history of the patient's complaints, including a list of known allergens, especially allergies or sensitivities to latex.

▸ Obtain a history of the patient's hematopoietic and immune systems, symptoms, and results of previously performed laboratory tests and diagnostic and surgical procedures.

▸ Obtain a list of the patient's current medications, including herbs, nutritional supplements, and nutraceuticals (see Appendix F).

▸ Review the procedure with the patient. Inform the patient that specimen collection takes approximately 5 to 10 min. Address concerns about pain and explain that there may be some discomfort during the venipuncture.

▸ *Sensitivity to social and cultural issues,* as well as concern for modesty, is important in providing psychological support before, during, and after the procedure.

▸ There are no food, fluid, or medication restrictions unless by medical direction.

INTRATEST:

▸ If the patient has a history of allergic reaction to latex, avoid the use of equipment containing latex.

▸ Instruct the patient to cooperate fully and to follow directions. Direct the patient to breathe normally and to avoid unnecessary movement.

▸ Observe standard precautions, and follow the general guidelines in Appendix A. Positively identify the patient, and label the appropriate tubes with the corresponding patient demographics, date, and time of collection. Perform a venipuncture.

▸ Remove the needle and apply direct pressure with dry gauze to stop bleeding. Observe/assess venipuncture site for bleeding or hematoma formation and secure gauze with adhesive bandage.

▸ Promptly transport the specimen to the laboratory for processing and analysis.

POST-TEST:

▸ A report of the results will be sent to the requesting health-care provider (HCP), who will discuss the results with the patient.

▸ Instruct the patient to avoid exposure to infection if WBC count is decreased.

▸ Recognize anxiety related to test results, and be supportive of perceived loss of independence and fear of shortened life expectancy. Discuss the implications of abnormal test results on the patient's lifestyle. Provide teaching and information regarding the clinical implications of the test results, as appropriate. Educate the patient regarding access to counseling services.

▸ Reinforce information given by the patient's HCP regarding further testing, treatment, or referral to another HCP. Answer any questions or address any concerns voiced by the patient or family.

▸ Depending on the results of this procedure, additional testing may be performed to evaluate or monitor progression of the disease process and determine the need for a change in therapy. Evaluate test results in relation to the patient's symptoms and other tests performed.

RELATED MONOGRAPHS:

▸ Related tests include biopsy bone marrow, calcium, CBC, CBC platelet count, CBC WBC count and differential, CT thoracic, gallium scan, Ham's test, Hgb electrophoresis, hemosiderin, IFE, immunoglobulins, iron, laparoscopy abdominal, liver and spleen scan, lymphangiogram, mediastinoscopy, phosphorus, and sickle cell screen.

▸ Refer to the Hematopoietic and Immune systems tables at the end of the book for related tests by body system.

Lipase

SYNONYM/ACRONYM: Triacylglycerol acylhydrolase.

COMMON USE: To assess for pancreatic disease related to inflammation, tumor, or cyst, specific to the diagnosis of pancreatitis.

SPECIMEN: Serum (1 mL) collected in a red- or tiger-top tube. Plasma (1 mL) collected in a green-top (heparin) tube is also acceptable.

REFERENCE VALUE: (Method: Enzymatic Spectrophotometry)

Conventional & SI Units
3–73 units/L

DESCRIPTION: Lipases are digestive enzymes secreted by the pancreas into the duodenum. Different lipolytic enzymes have specific substrates, but overall activity is collectively described as lipase. Lipase participates in fat digestion by breaking down triglycerides into fatty acids and glycerol. Lipase is released into the bloodstream when damage occurs to the pancreatic acinar cells. Its presence in the blood indicates pancreatic disease because the pancreas is the only organ that secretes this enzyme.

INDICATIONS
• Assist in the diagnosis of acute and chronic pancreatitis
• Assist in the diagnosis of pancreatic carcinoma

POTENTIAL DIAGNOSIS

Increased in
Lipase is contained in pancreatic tissue and is released into the serum when cell damage or necrosis occurs.

• Acute cholecystitis
• Obstruction of the pancreatic duct
• Pancreatic carcinoma (early)
• Pancreatic cyst or pseudocyst
• Pancreatic inflammation
• Pancreatitis (acute and chronic)
• Renal failure *(related to decreased renal excretion)*

Decreased in: N/A

CRITICAL FINDINGS: N/A

INTERFERING FACTORS
• Drugs that may increase lipase levels include acetaminophen, asparaginase, azathioprine, calcitriol, cholinergics, codeine, deoxycholate, diazoxide, didanosine, felbamate, glycocholate, hydrocortisone, indomethacin, meperidine, methacholine, methylprednisolone, metolazone, morphine, narcotics, nitrofurantoin, pancreozymin, pegaspargase, pentazocine, and taurocholate.
• Drugs that may decrease lipase levels include protamine and saline (IV infusions).
• Endoscopic retrograde cholangiopancreatography may increase lipase levels.
• Serum lipase levels increase with hemodialysis. Therefore, predialysis specimens should be collected for lipase analysis.

NURSING IMPLICATIONS AND PROCEDURE

PRETEST:

▶ Positively identify the patient using at least two unique identifiers before providing care, treatment, or services.

▶ *Patient Teaching:* Inform the patient this test can assist in diagnosing pancreatitis.

▶ Obtain a history of the patient's complaints, including a list of known allergens, especially allergies or sensitivities to latex.

▶ Obtain a history of the patient's gastrointestinal and hepatobiliary systems, symptoms, and results of previously performed laboratory tests and diagnostic and surgical procedures.

▶ Note any recent procedures that can interfere with test results.

▶ Obtain a list of the patient's current medications, including herbs, nutritional supplements, and nutraceuticals (see Appendix F).

▶ Review the procedure with the patient. Inform the patient that specimen collection takes approximately 5 to 10 min. Address concerns about pain and explain that there may be some discomfort during the venipuncture.

▶ *Sensitivity to social and cultural issues,* as well as concern for modesty, is important in providing psychological support before, during, and after the procedure.

▶ There are no food, fluid, or medication restrictions unless by medical direction.

INTRATEST:

▶ If the patient has a history of allergic reaction to latex, avoid the use of equipment containing latex.

▶ Instruct the patient to cooperate fully and to follow directions. Direct the patient to breathe normally and to avoid unnecessary movement.

▶ Observe standard precautions, and follow the general guidelines in Appendix A. Positively identify the patient, and label the appropriate tubes with the corresponding patient demographics, date, and time of collection. Perform a venipuncture.

▶ Remove the needle and apply direct pressure with dry gauze to stop bleeding. Observe/assess venipuncture site

for bleeding or hematoma formation and secure gauze with adhesive bandage.

▶ Promptly transport the specimen to the laboratory for processing and analysis.

POST-TEST:

▶ A report of the results will be sent to the requesting health-care provider (HCP), who will discuss the results with the patient.

▶ *Nutritional Considerations:* Instruct the patient to ingest small, frequent meals if he or she has a gastrointestinal disorder; advise the patient to consider other dietary alterations as well. After acute symptoms subside and bowel sounds return, patients are usually prescribed a clear liquid diet, progressing to a low-fat, high-carbohydrate diet.

▶ Administer vitamin B_{12}, as ordered, to the patient with decreased lipase levels, especially if his or her disease prevents adequate absorption of the vitamin.

▶ Encourage the alcoholic patient to avoid alcohol and to seek appropriate counseling for substance abuse.

▶ Reinforce information given by the patient's HCP regarding further testing, treatment, or referral to another HCP. Answer any questions or address any concerns voiced by the patient or family.

▶ Depending on the results of this procedure, additional testing may be performed to evaluate or monitor progression of the disease process and determine the need for a change in therapy. Evaluate test results in relation to the patient's symptoms and other tests performed.

RELATED MONOGRAPHS:

▶ Related tests include ALT, ALP, amylase, AST, bilirubin, calcitonin stimulation, calcium, cancer antigens, cholangiography percutaneous transhepatic, cholesterol, CBC, CBC WCB count and diff, ERCP, fecal fat, GGT, hepatobiliary scan, magnesium, MRI pancreas, mumps serology, pleural fluid analysis, peritoneal fluid analysis, triglycerides, and US pancreas.

▶ Refer to the Gastrointestinal and Hepatobiliary systems tables at the end of the book for related tests by body system.

Lipoprotein Electrophoresis

SYNONYM/ACRONYM: Lipid fractionation; lipoprotein phenotyping; 3ga₁-lipoprotein cholesterol, high-density lipoprotein (HDL); β-lipoprotein cholesterol, low-density lipoprotein (LDL); pre-β-lipoprotein cholesterol, very-low-density lipoprotein (VLDL).

COMMON USE: To assist in categorizing lipoprotein as an indicator of cardiac health.

SPECIMEN: Serum (3 mL) collected in a red- or tiger-top tube.

REFERENCE VALUE: (Method: Electrophoresis and 4°C test for specimen appearance) There is no quantitative interpretation of this test. The specimen appearance and electrophoretic pattern is visually interpreted.

Hyperlipoproteinemia: Fredrickson Type	Specimen Appearance	Electrophoretic Pattern
Type I	Clear with creamy top layer	Heavy chylomicron band
Type IIa	Clear	Heavy β band
Type IIb	Clear or faintly turbid	Heavy β and pre-β bands
Type III	Slightly to moderately turbid	Heavy β band
Type IV	Slightly to moderately turbid	Heavy pre-β band
Type V	Slightly to moderately turbid with creamy top layer	Intense chylomicron band and heavy β and pre-β bands

POTENTIAL DIAGNOSIS

• *Type I:* Hyperlipoproteinemia, or increased chylomicrons, can be primary, *resulting from an inherited deficiency of lipoprotein lipase,* or secondary, *caused by uncontrolled diabetes, systemic lupus erythematosus, and dysgammaglobulinemia.* Total cholesterol is normal to moderately elevated, and triglycerides (mostly exogenous chylomicrons) are grossly elevated. If the condition is inherited, symptoms will appear in childhood.

• *Type IIa:* Hyperlipoproteinemia can be primary, *resulting from*

inherited characteristics, or secondary, *caused by uncontrolled hypothyroidism, nephrotic syndrome, and dysgammaglobulinemia.* Total cholesterol is elevated, triglycerides are normal, and LDLC is elevated. If the condition is inherited, symptoms will appear in childhood.

• *Type IIb:* Hyperlipoproteinemia *can occur for the same reasons as in type IIa.* Total cholesterol, triglycerides, and LDLC are all elevated.

• *Type III:* Hyperlipoproteinemia can be primary, *resulting from inherited characteristics,* or secondary, *caused by hypothyroidism, uncontrolled diabetes, alcoholism, and dysgammaglobulinemia.* Total cholesterol and triglycerides are elevated, whereas LDLC is normal.

- *Type IV:* Hyperlipoproteinemia can be primary, *resulting from inherited characteristics,* or secondary, *caused by poorly controlled diabetes, alcoholism, nephrotic syndrome, chronic renal failure, and dysgammaglobulinemia.*

Total cholesterol is normal to moderately elevated, triglycerides are moderately to grossly elevated, and LDLC is normal.

- *Type V:* Hyperlipoproteinemia can be primary, *resulting from inherited characteristics,* or secondary, *caused by uncontrolled diabetes, alcoholism, nephrotic syndrome, and dysgammaglobulinemia.* Total cholesterol is normal to moderately elevated, triglycerides are grossly elevated, and LDLC is normal.

CRITICAL FINDINGS: N/A

Find and print out the full monograph at DavisPlus (http://davisplus.fadavis .com, keyword Van Leeuwen).

Liver and Spleen Scan

SYNONYM/ACRONYM: Liver and spleen scintigraphy, radionuclide liver scan, spleen scan.

COMMON USE: To visualize and assess the liver and spleen related to tumors, inflammation, cysts, abscess, trauma, and portal hypertension.

AREA OF APPLICATION: Abdomen.

CONTRAST: IV radioactive technetium-99m sulfur colloid.

DESCRIPTION: The liver and spleen scan is performed to help diagnose abnormalities in the function and structure of the liver and spleen. It is often performed in combination with lung scanning to help diagnose masses or inflammation in the diaphragmatic area. This procedure is useful for evaluating right-upper-quadrant pain, metastatic disease, jaundice, cirrhosis, ascites, traumatic infarction, and radiation-induced organ cellular necrosis. Technetium-99m (Tc-99m) sulfur colloid is injected IV and rapidly taken up through phagocytosis by the reticuloendothelial cells, which normally function to remove particulate matter, including radioactive colloids in the liver and spleen. False-negative results may occur in patients with space-occupying lesions (e.g., tumors, cysts, abscesses) smaller than 2 cm. This scan can detect portal hypertension, demonstrated by a greater uptake of the radionuclide in the spleen than in the liver. Single-photon emission computed tomography (SPECT) has significantly improved the resolution and accuracy of liver scanning. SPECT enables images to be recorded from multiple angles around the body and reconstructed by a computer to produce images or "slices" representing the organ at different levels. For evaluation of a suspected hemangioma, the patient's red blood cells are combined with Tc-99m and images are recorded over the liver. To confirm the diagnosis, liver and spleen scans are done in conjunction with computed tomography (CT), magnetic resonance imaging (MRI), ultrasonography (US), and SPECT scans and interpreted in light of the results of liver function tests.

INDICATIONS

- Assess the condition of the liver and spleen after abdominal trauma
- Detect a bacterial or amebic abscess
- Detect and differentiate between primary and metastatic tumor focal disease
- Detect benign tumors, such as adenoma and cavernous hemangioma
- Detect cystic focal disease
- Detect diffuse hepatocellular disease, such as hepatitis and cirrhosis
- Detect infiltrative processes that affect the liver, such as sarcoidosis and amyloidosis
- Determine superior vena cava obstruction or Budd-Chiari syndrome
- Differentiate between splenomegaly and hepatomegaly
- Evaluate the effects of lower abdominal trauma, such as internal hemorrhage
- Evaluate jaundice
- Evaluate liver and spleen damage caused by radiation therapy or toxic drug therapy
- Evaluate palpable abdominal masses

POTENTIAL DIAGNOSIS

Normal findings in
- Normal size, contour, position, and function of the liver and spleen

Abnormal findings in
- Abscesses
- Cirrhosis
- Cysts
- Hemangiomas
- Hematomas
- Hepatitis
- Hodgkin's disease
- Infarction
- Infection
- Infiltrative process (amyloidosis and sarcoidosis)
- Inflammation of the diaphragmatic area
- Metastatic tumors
- Nodular hyperplasia
- Portal hypertension
- Primary benign or malignant tumors
- Traumatic lesions

CRITICAL FINDINGS

- Visceral injury

INTERFERING FACTORS

This procedure is contraindicated for
- Patients who are pregnant or suspected of being pregnant, unless the potential benefits of the procedure far outweigh the risks to the fetus and mother.

Factors that may impair clear imaging
- Inability of the patient to cooperate or remain still during the procedure because of age, significant pain, or mental status.
- Metallic objects (e.g., jewelry, body rings) within the examination field, which may inhibit organ visualization and cause unclear images.
- Other nuclear scans done within the preceding 24 to 48 hr.

Other considerations

- The scan may fail to detect focal lesions smaller than 2 cm in diameter.
- Improper injection of the radionuclide may allow the tracer to seep deep into the muscle tissue, producing erroneous hot spots.
- Consultation with a health-care provider (HCP) should occur before the procedure for radiation safety concerns regarding younger patients or patients who are lactating.
- Risks associated with radiation overexposure can result from frequent x-ray or radionuclide procedures. Personnel working in the examination area should wear badges to record their level of radiation exposure.

NURSING IMPLICATIONS AND PROCEDURE

PRETEST:

▶ Positively identify the patient using at least two unique identifiers before providing care, treatment, or services.

▶ *Patient Teaching:* Inform the patient this procedure can assist in evaluating liver and spleen function.

▶ Obtain a history of the patient's complaints, including a list of known allergens, especially allergies or sensitivities to latex, iodine, seafood, anesthetics, or contrast medium.

▶ Obtain a history of the patient's hematopoietic, hepatobiliary, and immune systems; symptoms; and results of previously performed laboratory tests and diagnostic and surgical procedures.

▶ Note any recent procedures that can interfere with test results, including examinations using iodine-based contrast medium.

▶ Record the date of the last menstrual period and determine the possibility of pregnancy in perimenopausal women.

▶ Obtain a list of the patient's current medications, including herbs, nutritional supplements, and nutraceuticals (see Appendix F).

▶ Review the procedure with the patient. Address concerns about pain related to the procedure and explain that some pain may be experienced during the test, or there may be moments of discomfort. Reassure the patient that the radionuclide poses no radioactive hazard and rarely produces side effects. Inform the patient the procedure is performed in a nuclear medicine department by an HCP specializing in this procedure, with support staff, and takes approximately 30 to 60 min.

▶ *Sensitivity to social and cultural issues,* as well as concern for modesty, is important in providing psychological support before, during, and after the procedure.

▶ Instruct the patient to remove jewelry and other metallic objects from the area to be examined.

▶ There are no food, fluid, or medication restrictions unless by medical direction.

▶ *Make sure a written and informed consent has been signed prior to the procedure and before administering any medications.*

INTRATEST:

▶ Ensure that the patient has removed all external metallic objects from the area to be examined prior to the procedure.

▶ If the patient has a history of allergic reactions to any substance or drug, administer ordered prophylactic steroids or antihistamines before the procedure.

▶ Have emergency equipment readily available.

▶ Instruct the patient to void prior to the procedure and to change into the gown, robe, and foot coverings provided.

▶ Instruct the patient to cooperate fully and to follow directions. Instruct the patient to remain still throughout the procedure because movement produces unreliable results.

▶ Observe standard precautions, and follow the general guidelines in Appendix A.

• Administer sedative to a child or to an uncooperative adult, as ordered.
• Place the patient in a supine position on a flat table with foam wedges, which help maintain position and immobilization.
• IV radionuclide is administered, and the abdomen is scanned immediately to screen for vascular lesions with images taken in various positions.
• Monitor the patient for complications related to the procedure (e.g., allergic reaction, anaphylaxis, bronchospasm).
• Remove the needle or catheter and apply a pressure dressing over the puncture site.
• Observe/assess the needle/catheter insertion site for bleeding, inflammation, or hematoma formation.
• The patient may be imaged by SPECT techniques to further clarify areas of suspicious radionuclide localization.

POST-TEST:

• A report of the results will be sent to the requesting HCP, who will discuss the results with the patient.
• Instruct the patient to resume usual medication and activity, as directed by the HCP.
• Unless contraindicated, advise patient to drink increased amounts of fluids for 24 to 48 hr to eliminate the radionuclide from the body. Inform the patient that radionuclide is eliminated from the body within 6 to 24 hr.
• No other radionuclide tests should be scheduled for 24 to 48 hr after this procedure.
• Instruct the patient in the care and assessment of the injection site.
• If a woman who is breastfeeding must have a nuclear scan, she should not breastfeed the infant until the radionuclide has been eliminated. This could take as long as 3 days. She should be instructed to express the milk and discard it during the 3-day period to prevent cessation of milk production.

• Instruct the patient to immediately flush the toilet and to meticulously wash hands with soap and water after each voiding for 24 hr after the procedure.
• Instruct all caregivers to wear gloves when discarding urine for 24 hr after the procedure. Wash gloved hands with soap and water before removing gloves. Then wash hands after the gloves are removed.
• *Nutritional Considerations:* A low-fat, low-cholesterol, and low-sodium diet should be consumed to reduce current disease processes. High fat consumption increases the amount of bile acids in the colon and should be avoided.
• Recognize anxiety related to test results, and be supportive of perceived loss of independent function. Discuss the implications of abnormal test results on the patient's lifestyle. Provide teaching and information regarding the clinical implications of the test results, as appropriate.
• Reinforce information given by the patient's HCP regarding further testing, treatment, or referral to another HCP. Answer any questions or address any concerns voiced by the patient or family.
• Depending on the results of this procedure, additional testing may be needed to evaluate or monitor progression of the disease process and determine the need for a change in therapy. Evaluate test results in relation to the patient's symptoms and other tests performed.

RELATED MONOGRAPHS:

• Related tests include ALT, antibodies antimitochondrial, AST, bilirubin, biopsy liver, CT abdomen, CT biliary tract and liver, GGT, HAV, HBV, HCV, hepatobiliary scan, MRI abdomen, and US liver.
• Refer to the Hematopoietic, Hepatobiliary, and Immune systems tables at the end of the book for related tests by body system.

Lung Perfusion Scan

SYNONYM/ACRONYM: Lung perfusion scintigraphy, lung scintiscan, pulmonary scan, radioactive perfusion scan, radionuclide lung scan, ventilation-perfusion scan, V/Q scan.

COMMON USE: To assess pulmonary blood flow to assist in diagnosis of pulmonary embolism.

AREA OF APPLICATION: Chest/thorax.

CONTRAST: IV radioactive material, usually macroaggregated albumin (MAA).

DESCRIPTION: The lung perfusion scan is a nuclear medicine study performed to evaluate a patient for pulmonary embolus (PE) or other pulmonary disorders. Technetium (Tc-99m) is injected IV and distributed throughout the pulmonary vasculature because of the gravitational effect on perfusion. The scan, which produces a visual image of pulmonary blood flow, is useful in diagnosing or confirming pulmonary vascular obstruction. The diameter of the IV-injected macroaggregated albumin (MAA) is larger than that of the pulmonary capillaries; therefore, the MAA temporarily becomes lodged in the pulmonary vasculature. A gamma camera detects the radiation emitted from the injected radioactive material, and a representative image of the lung is obtained. This procedure is often done in conjunction with the lung ventilation scan to obtain clinical information that assists in differentiating among the many possible pathological conditions revealed by the procedure. The results are correlated with other diagnostic studies, such as pulmonary function, chest x-ray, pulmonary angiography, and arterial blood gases. A recent chest x-ray is essential for accurate interpretation of the lung perfusion scan. An area of nonperfusion seen in the same area as a pulmonary parenchymal abnormality on the chest x-ray indicates that a PE is not present; the defect may represent some other pathological condition, such as pneumonia.

INDICATIONS
- Aid in the diagnosis of PE in a patient with a normal chest x-ray
- Detect malignant tumor
- Differentiate between PE and other pulmonary diseases, such as pneumonia, pulmonary effusion, atelectasis, asthma, bronchitis, emphysema, and tumors
- Evaluate perfusion changes associated with congestive heart failure and pulmonary hypertension
- Evaluate pulmonary function preoperatively in a patient with pulmonary disease

L

POTENTIAL DIAGNOSIS

Normal findings in
• Diffuse and homogeneous uptake of the radioactive material by the lungs

Abnormal findings in
• Asthma
• Atelectasis
• Bronchitis
• Chronic obstructive pulmonary disease
• Emphysema
• Left atrial or pulmonary hypertension
• Lung displacement by fluid or chest masses
• Pneumonia
• Pneumonitis
• PE
• Tuberculosis

CRITICAL FINDINGS

• PE

It is essential that critical diagnoses be communicated immediately to the appropriate health-care provider (HCP). A listing of these diagnoses varies among facilities. Note and immediately report to the HCP abnormal results and related symptoms.

INTERFERING FACTORS

This procedure is contraindicated for
• Patients who are pregnant or suspected of being pregnant, unless the potential benefits of the procedure far outweigh the risks to the fetus and mother.
• Patients with atrial and ventricular septal defects, because the MAA particles will not reach the lungs.
• Patients with pulmonary hypertension.

Factors that may impair clear imaging:
• Inability of the patient to cooperate or remain still during the procedure because of age, significant pain, or mental status.
• Metallic objects (e.g., jewelry, body rings) within the examination field, which may inhibit organ visualization and cause unclear images.
• Other nuclear scans done on the same day.

Other considerations
• Improper injection of the radionuclide may allow the tracer to seep deep into the muscle tissue, producing erroneous hot spots.
• Consultation with an HCP should occur before the procedure for radiation safety concerns regarding younger patients or patients who are lactating.
• Risks associated with radiation overexposure can result from frequent x-ray or radionuclide procedures. Personnel working in the examination area should wear badges to record their level of radiation.

NURSING IMPLICATIONS AND PROCEDURE

PRETEST:

▸ Positively identify the patient using at least two unique identifiers before providing care, treatment, or services.
▸ *Patient Teaching:* Inform the patient this procedure can assist in assessing blood flow to the lungs.
▸ Obtain a history of the patient's complaints, including a list of known allergens, especially allergies or sensitivities to latex, iodine, seafood, contrast medium, anesthetics, or dyes.
▸ Obtain a history of the patient's respiratory system, symptoms, and results of previously performed laboratory tests and diagnostic and surgical procedures.
▸ Note any recent procedures that can interfere with test results, including examinations using iodine-based contrast medium.

- Record the date of the last menstrual period and determine the possibility of pregnancy in perimenopausal women.
- Obtain a list of the patient's current medications, including herbs, nutritional supplements, and nutraceuticals (see Appendix F).
- Review the procedure with the patient. Address concerns about pain related to the procedure and explain that some pain may be experienced during the test, or there may be moments of discomfort. Reassure the patient that the radionuclide poses no radioactive hazard and rarely produces side effects. Inform the patient that the procedure is performed in a nuclear medicine department, by an HCP specializing in this procedure, with support staff, and takes approximately 60 min.
- *Sensitivity to social and cultural issues,* as well as concern for modesty, is important in providing psychological support before, during, and after the procedure.
- Instruct the patient to remove jewelry and other metallic objects from the area to be examined prior to the procedure.
- There are no food, fluid or medication restrictions unless by medical direction.
- *Make sure a written and informed consent has been signed prior to the procedure and before administering any medications.*

INTRATEST:

- Ensure that the patient has removed all external metallic objects from the area to be examined prior to the procedure.
- If the patient has a history of allergic reactions to any substance or drug, administer ordered prophylactic steroids or antihistamines before the procedure.
- Have emergency equipment readily available.
- Instruct the patient to void prior to the procedure and to change into the gown, robe, and foot coverings provided.
- Record baseline vital signs and assess neurological status. Protocols may vary among facilities.
- Instruct the patient to cooperate fully and to follow directions. Instruct the patient to remain still throughout the procedure because movement produces unreliable results.
- Observe standard precautions, and follow the general guidelines in Appendix A.
- Administer a sedative to a child or to an uncooperative adult, as ordered.
- Place the patient in a supine position on a flat table with foam wedges, which help maintain position and immobilization.
- IV radionuclide is administered, and the abdomen is scanned immediately to screen for vascular lesions with images taken in various positions.
- Monitor the patient for complications related to the procedure (e.g., allergic reaction, anaphylaxis, bronchospasm).
- Remove the needle or catheter and apply a pressure dressing over the puncture site.
- Observe/assess the needle/catheter insertion site for bleeding, inflammation, or hematoma formation.

POST-TEST:

- A report of the results will be sent to the requesting HCP, who will discuss the results with the patient.
- Unless contraindicated, advise patient to drink increased amounts of fluids for 24 to 48 hr to eliminate the radionuclide from the body. Inform the patient that radionuclide is eliminated from the body within 6 to 24 hr.
- No other radionuclide tests should be scheduled for 24 to 48 hr after this procedure.
- Monitor vital signs and neurological status every 15 min for 1 hr, then every 2 hr for 4 hr, and then as ordered by the HCP. Compare with baseline values. Protocols may vary among facilities.
- Instruct the patient to resume usual medication and activity, as directed by the HCP.
- Observe for delayed allergic reactions, such as rash, urticaria, tachycardia, hyperpnea, hypertension, palpitations, nausea, or vomiting.
- Instruct the patient to immediately report symptoms such as fast heart rate, difficulty breathing, skin rash, itching, chest pain, persistent right shoulder pain, or abdominal pain.

Immediately report symptoms to the appropriate HCP.

‣ Observe/assess the needle/catheter insertion site for bleeding, inflammation, or hematoma formation.

‣ Instruct the patient in the care and assessment of the injection site.

‣ If a woman who is breastfeeding must have a nuclear scan, she should not breastfeed the infant until the radionuclide has been eliminated. This could take as long as 3 days. She should be instructed to express the milk and discard it during the 3-day period to prevent cessation of milk production.

‣ Instruct the patient to immediately flush the toilet and to meticulously wash hands with soap and water after each voiding for 24 hr after the procedure.

‣ Instruct all caregivers to wear gloves when discarding urine for 24 hr after the procedure. Wash gloved hands with soap and water before removing gloves. Then wash hands after the gloves are removed.

‣ Recognize anxiety related to test results, and be supportive of perceived loss of independent function. Discuss the implications of abnormal test results on the patient's lifestyle. Provide teaching and information regarding the clinical implications of the test results, as appropriate.

‣ Reinforce information given by the patient's HCP regarding further testing, treatment, or referral to another HCP. Answer any questions or address any concerns voiced by the patient or family.

‣ Depending on the results of this procedure, additional testing may be needed to evaluate or monitor progression of the disease process and determine the need for a change in therapy. Evaluate test results in relation to the patient's symptoms and other tests performed.

RELATED MONOGRAPHS:

‣ Related tests include α-1 AT, eosinophil count, ACE, alveolar/arterial gradient, angiography pulmonary, biopsy lung, blood gases, blood pool imaging, bronchoscopy, carbon dioxide, chest x-ray, CBC, CBC WCB count and differential, CT thoracic, culture and smear mycobacteria, culture blood, culture throat, culture sputum, culture viral, cytology sputum, ESR, IgE, gallium scan, lung ventilation scan, MRI chest, mediastinoscopy, plethysmography, pleural fluid analysis, PET heart, PFT, pulse oximetry, and TB skin tests.

‣ Refer to the Respiratory System table at the end of the book for related tests by body system.

Lung Ventilation Scan

SYNONYM/ACRONYM: Aerosol lung scan, radioactive ventilation scan, ventilation scan, VQ lung scan, xenon lung scan.

COMMON USE: To assess pulmonary ventilation to assist in diagnosis of pulmonary embolism.

AREA OF APPLICATION: Chest/thorax.

CONTRAST: Done with inhaled radioactive material (xenon gas or technetium-DTPA).

DESCRIPTION: The lung ventilation scan is a nuclear medicine study performed to evaluate a patient for pulmonary embolus (PE) or other pulmonary disorders. It can evaluate respiratory function (i.e., demonstrating areas of the lung that are patent and capable of ventilation) and dysfunction (e.g., parenchymal abnormalities affecting ventilation, such as pneumonia). The procedure is performed after the patient inhales air mixed with a radioactive gas through a face mask and mouthpiece. The radioactive gas delineates areas of the lung during ventilation. The distribution of the gas throughout the lung is measured in three phases:

- *Wash-in phase:* Phase during buildup of the radioactive gas
- *Equilibrium phase:* Phase after the patient rebreathes from a closed delivery system
- *Wash-out phase:* Phase after the radioactive gas has been removed

This procedure is usually performed along with a lung perfusion scan. When PE is present, ventilation scans display a normal wash-in and wash-out of radioactivity from the lung areas. Parenchymal disease responsible for perfusion abnormalities will produce abnormal wash-in and wash-out phases. This test can be used to quantify regional ventilation in patients with pulmonary disease.

INDICATIONS

- Aid in the diagnosis of PE
- Differentiate between PE and other pulmonary diseases, such as pneumonia, pulmonary effusion, atelectasis, asthma, bronchitis, emphysema, and tumors
- Evaluate regional respiratory function

- Identify areas of the lung that are capable of ventilation
- Locate hypoventilation (regional), which can result from chronic obstructive pulmonary disease (COPD) or excessive smoking

POTENTIAL DIAGNOSIS

Normal findings in
- Equal distribution of radioactive gas throughout both lungs and a normal wash-out phase

Abnormal findings in
- Atelectasis
- Bronchitis
- Bronchogenic carcinoma
- COPD
- Emphysema
- PE
- Pneumonia
- Regional hypoventilation
- Sarcoidosis
- Tuberculosis
- Tumor

CRITICAL FINDINGS
- PE

It is essential that critical diagnoses be communicated immediately to the appropriate health-care provider (HCP). A listing of these diagnoses varies among facilities. Note and immediately report to the HCP abnormal results and related symptoms.

INTERFERING FACTORS

This procedure is contraindicated for
- Patients who are pregnant or suspected of being pregnant, unless the potential benefits of the procedure far outweigh the risks to the fetus and mother.

Factors that may impair clear imaging
- Inability of the patient to cooperate or remain still during the procedure

because of age, significant pain, or mental status.
- Metallic objects (e.g., jewelry, body rings) within the examination field, which may inhibit organ visualization and cause unclear images.
- Other nuclear scans done within the preceding 24 to 48 hr.

Other considerations
- The presence of conditions that affect perfusion or ventilation (e.g., tumors that obstruct the pulmonary artery, vasculitis, pulmonary edema, sickle cell disease, parasitic disease, emphysema, effusion, infection) can simulate a perfusion defect similar to PE.
- Consultation with a health-care provider (HCP) should occur before the procedure for radiation safety concerns regarding younger patients or patients who are lactating.
- Risks associated with radiation overexposure can result from frequent x-ray or radionuclide procedures. Personnel working in the examination area should wear badges to record their level of radiation exposure.

NURSING IMPLICATIONS AND PROCEDURE

PRETEST:
- Positively identify the patient using at least two unique identifiers before providing care, treatment, or services.
- *Patient Teaching:* Inform the patient this procedure can assist in assessing air flow to the lungs.
- Obtain a history of the patient's complaints, including a list of known allergens, especially allergies or sensitivities to latex, iodine, seafood, contrast medium, anesthetics, or dyes.
- Obtain a history of the patient's respiratory system, symptoms, and results of previously performed laboratory tests and diagnostic and surgical procedures.

- Note any recent procedures that can interfere with test results, including examinations using iodine-based contrast medium.
- Record the date of the last menstrual period and determine the possibility of pregnancy in perimenopausal women.
- Obtain a list of the patient's current medications, including herbs, nutritional supplements, and nutraceuticals (see Appendix F).
- Review the procedure with the patient. Address concerns about pain related to the procedure and explain that some pain may be experienced during the test, and there may be moments of discomfort. Reassure the patient that the radionuclide poses no radioactive hazard and rarely produces side effects. Inform the patient that the procedure is performed in a nuclear medicine department, usually by an HCP who specializes in this procedure, with support staff, and takes approximately 30 to 60 min.
- *Sensitivity to social and cultural issues,* as well as concern for modesty, is important in providing psychological support before, during, and after the procedure.
- Instruct the patient to remove jewelry and other metallic objects from the area to be examined.
- There are no food, fluid, or medication restrictions unless by medical direction.
- *Make sure a written and informed consent has been signed prior to the procedure and before administering any medications.*

INTRATEST:
- Ensure that the patient has removed all external metallic objects from the area to be examined prior to the procedure.
- If the patient has a history of allergic reactions to any substance or drug, administer ordered prophylactic steroids or antihistamines before the procedure.
- Have emergency equipment readily available.
- Instruct the patient to void prior to the procedure and to change into the gown, robe, and foot coverings provided.
- Record baseline vital signs and assess neurological status. Protocols may vary among facilities.

▶ Instruct the patient to cooperate fully and to follow directions. Direct the patient to remain still throughout the procedure because movement produces unreliable results.

▶ Observe standard precautions, and follow the general guidelines in Appendix A.

▶ Administer sedative to a child or to an uncooperative adult, as ordered.

▶ Place the patient in a supine position on a flat table with foam wedges, which help maintain position and immobilization.

▶ The radionuclide is administered through a mask, which is placed over the patient's nose and mouth. The patient is asked to hold his or her breath for a short period of time while the scan is taken.

▶ Monitor the patient for complications related to the procedure (e.g., allergic reaction, anaphylaxis, bronchospasm).

POST-TEST:

▶ A report of the results will be sent to the requesting HCP, who will discuss the results with the patient.

▶ Unless contraindicated, advise patient to drink increased amounts of fluids for 24 to 48 hr to eliminate the radionuclide from the body. Inform the patient that radionuclide is eliminated from the body within 6 to 24 hr.

▶ No other radionuclide tests should be scheduled for 24 to 48 hr after this procedure.

▶ Evaluate the patient's vital signs. Monitor vital signs and neurological status every 15 min for 1 hr, then every 2 hr for 4 hr, and then as ordered by the HCP. Compare with baseline values. Protocols may vary among facilities.

▶ Instruct the patient to resume medication or activity, as directed by the HCP.

▶ If a woman who is breastfeeding must have a nuclear scan, she should not breastfeed the infant until the radionuclide has been eliminated. This could take as long as 3 days. She should be instructed to express the milk and discard it during the 3-day period to prevent cessation of milk production.

▶ Instruct the patient to immediately flush the toilet and to meticulously wash hands with soap and water after each voiding for 24 hr after the procedure.

▶ Instruct all caregivers to wear gloves when discarding urine for 24 hr after the procedure. Wash gloved hands with soap and water before removing gloves. Then wash hands after the gloves are removed.

▶ *Nutritional Considerations:* A low-fat, low-cholesterol, and low-sodium diet should be consumed to reduce current disease processes and/or decrease risk of hypertension and coronary artery disease.

▶ Recognize anxiety related to test results, and be supportive of perceived loss of independent function. Discuss the implications of abnormal test results on the patient's lifestyle. Provide teaching and information regarding the clinical implications of the test results, as appropriate.

▶ Reinforce information given by the patient's HCP regarding further testing, treatment, or referral to another HCP. Answer any questions or address any concerns voiced by the patient or family.

▶ Depending on the results of this procedure, additional testing may be needed to evaluate or monitor progression of the disease process and determine the need for a change in therapy. Evaluate test results in relation to the patient's symptoms and other tests performed.

RELATED MONOGRAPHS:

▶ Related tests include α-1 antitrypsin, alveolar/arterial ratio, ACE, angiography pulmonary, biopsy lung, blood gases, blood pool imaging, bronchoscopy, carbon dioxide, chest x-ray, CBC, CBC WBC count and differential, CT thorax, culture and smear mycobacteria, culture blood, culture sputum, culture throat, culture viral, cytology sputum, D-dimer, gallium scan, lung perfusion scan, MRI chest, mediastinoscopy, plethysmography, pleural fluid analysis, PET heart, PFT, TB skin tests, US venous Doppler extremity studies, and venography.

▶ Refer to the Respiratory System table at the end of the book for related tests by body system.

L

Lupus Anticoagulant Antibodies

SYNONYM/ACRONYM: Lupus inhibitor phospholipid type, lupus antiphospholipid antibodies, LA.

COMMON USE: To assess for systemic dysfunction related to anticoagulation and assist in diagnosing conditions such as lupus erythematosus and fetal loss.

SPECIMEN: Plasma (1 mL) collected in a completely filled blue-top (3.2% sodium citrate) tube. If the patient's hematocrit exceeds 55%, the volume of citrate in the collection tube must be adjusted.

REFERENCE VALUE: (Method: Dilute Russell viper venom test time) Negative.

DESCRIPTION: Lupus anticoagulant antibodies (LA) are immunoglobulins, usually of the immunoglobulin G class. They are also called lupus antiphospholipid antibodies because they interfere with phospholipid-dependent coagulation tests such as activated partial thromboplastin time (aPTT) by reacting with the phospholipids in the test system. They are not associated with a bleeding disorder unless thrombocytopenia or antiprothrombin antibodies are already present. They are associated with an increased risk of thrombosis.

INDICATIONS
• Evaluate prolonged aPTT
• Investigate reasons for fetal death

POTENTIAL DIAGNOSIS

Positive findings in
• Fetal loss *(thrombosis associated with LA can form clots that lodge in the placenta and disrupt nutrition to the fetus)*
• Raynaud's disease *(LA can be detected with this condition and can cause vascular inflammation)*
• Rheumatoid arthritis *(LA can be detected with this condition and can cause vascular inflammation)*
• Systemic lupus erythematosus *(related to formation of thrombi as a result of LA binding to phospholipids on cell walls)*
• Thromboembolism *(related to formation of thrombi as a result of LA binding to phospholipids on cell walls)*

Negative findings in: N/A

CRITICAL FINDINGS: N/A

INTERFERING FACTORS
• Drugs that may cause a positive LA test result include calcium channel blockers, chlorpromazine, heparin, hydralazine, hydantoin, isoniazid, methyldopa, phenytoin, phenothiazine, procainamide, quinine, quinidine, and Thorazine.
• Placement of a tourniquet for longer than 1 min can result in venous stasis and changes in the concentration of plasma proteins to be measured. Platelet activation may also occur under these conditions, causing erroneous results.

L

- Vascular injury during phlebotomy can activate platelets and coagulation factors, causing erroneous results.
- Hemolyzed specimens must be rejected because hemolysis is an indication of platelet and coagulation factor activation.
- Icteric or lipemic specimens interfere with optical testing methods, producing erroneous results.
- Hematocrit greater than 55% may cause falsely prolonged results because of anticoagulant excess relative to plasma volume.
- Incompletely filled collection tubes, specimens contaminated with heparin, clotted specimens, or unprocessed specimens not delivered to the laboratory within 1 to 2 hr of collection should be rejected.

NURSING IMPLICATIONS AND PROCEDURE

PRETEST:

- Positively identify the patient using at least two unique identifiers before providing care, treatment, or services.
- *Patient Teaching:* Inform the patient that this test can assist in evaluation of clotting disorders.
- Obtain a history of the patient's complaints, including a list of known allergens, especially allergies or sensitivities to latex.
- Obtain a history of the patient's hematopoietic, immune, musculoskeletal, and reproductive systems; symptoms; and results of previously performed laboratory tests and diagnostic and surgical procedures.
- Obtain a list of the patient's current medications, including herbs, nutritional supplements, and nutraceuticals (see Appendix F).
- Review the procedure with the patient. Inform the patient that specimen

collection takes approximately 5 to 10 min. Address concerns about pain and explain that there may be some discomfort during the venipuncture.
- *Sensitivity to social and cultural issues,* as well as concern for modesty, is important in providing psychological support before, during, and after the procedure.
- Heparin therapy should be discontinued 2 days before specimen collection, with medical direction. Coumarin therapy should be discontinued 2 wk before specimen collection, with medical direction.
- There are no food or fluid restrictions unless by medical direction.

INTRATEST:

- Ensure that the patient has complied with pretesting preparations; assure that anticoagulant therapy has been restricted as required prior to the procedure.
- If the patient has a history of allergic reaction to latex, avoid the use of equipment containing latex.
- Instruct the patient to cooperate fully and to follow directions. Direct the patient to breathe normally and to avoid unnecessary movement.
- Observe standard precautions, and follow the general guidelines in Appendix A. Positively identify the patient, and label the appropriate tubes with the corresponding patient demographics, date, and time of collection. Perform a venipuncture. Fill tube completely. *Important note:* Two different concentrations of sodium citrate preservative are currently added to blue-top tubes for coagulation studies: 3.2% and 3.8%. The Clinical and Laboratory Standards Institute (CLSI; formerly the National Committee for Clinical Laboratory Standards [NCCLS]) guideline for sodium citrate is 3.2%. Laboratories establish reference ranges for coagulation testing based on numerous factors, including sodium citrate concentration, test equipment, and test reagents. It is important to ask the laboratory which concentration it

recommends, because each concentration will have its own specific reference range. When multiple specimens are drawn, the blue-top tube should be collected after sterile (i.e., blood culture) tubes. Otherwise, when using a standard vacutainer system, the blue-top tube is the first tube collected. When a butterfly is used, due to the added tubing, an extra red-top tube should be collected before the blue-top tube to ensure complete filling of the blue-top tube.

▶ Remove the needle and apply direct pressure with dry gauze to stop bleeding. Observe/assess venipuncture site for bleeding or hematoma formation and secure gauze with adhesive bandage.

▶ Promptly transport the specimen to the laboratory for processing and analysis. The CLSI recommendation for processed and unprocessed samples stored in unopened tubes is that testing should be completed within 1 to 4 hr of collection. If the patient has a known hematocrit above 55%, adjust the amount of anticoagulant in the collection tube before drawing the blood according to the CLSI guidelines:

Anticoagulant vol. [x] = (100 – hematocrit)/(595 – hematocrit) × total vol. of anticoagulated blood required

Example:

Patient hematocrit = 60% = [(100 – 60)/(595 – 60) × 5.0] = 0.37 mL sodium citrate for a 5-mL standard drawing tube

POST-TEST:

▶ A report of the results will be sent to the requesting health-care provider (HCP), who will discuss the results with the patient.

▶ Instruct the patient to resume usual medications, as directed by the HCP.

▶ Recognize anxiety related to test results, and offer support. Provide teaching and information regarding the clinical implications of the test results, as appropriate. It is also important to discuss feelings the mother and father may experience (e.g., guilt, depression, anger) if test results are abnormal. Educate the patient regarding access to counseling services. Provide contact information, if desired, for the Lupus Foundation of America (www.lupus.org).

▶ Reinforce information given by the patient's HCP regarding further testing, treatment, or referral to another HCP. Answer any questions or address any concerns voiced by the patient or family.

▶ Depending on the results of this procedure, additional testing may be performed to evaluate or monitor progression of the disease process and determine the need for a change in therapy. Evaluate test results in relation to the patient's symptoms and other tests performed.

RELATED MONOGRAPHS:

▶ Related tests include antibody, anticardiolipin antibodies, anticyclic citrullinated peptide, ANA, arthroscopy, BMD, bone scan, CRP, ESR, FDP, MRI musculoskeletal, aPTT, protein S, PT/INR and mixing studies, radiography bone, RF, synovial fluid analysis, and US obstetric.

▶ Refer to the Hematopoietic, Immune, Musculoskeletal, and Reproductive systems tables at the end of the book for related tests by body system.

Luteinizing Hormone

SYNONYM/ACRONYM: LH, luteotropin, interstitial cell–stimulating hormone (ICSH).

COMMON USE: To assess gonadal function related to fertility issues and response to therapy.

SPECIMEN: Serum (1 mL) collected in a red- or tiger-top tube. Plasma (1 mL) collected in a green-top (heparin) tube is also acceptable.

REFERENCE VALUE: (Method: Immunoassay)

Concentration by Gender and by Phase (in Females)	Conventional and SI Units
	Male
Less than 2 yr	0.5–1.9 international units/mL
2–10 yr	Less than 0.5 international units/mL
11–20 yr	0.5–5.3 international units/mL
Adult	1.2–7.8 international units/mL
	Female
Less than 2–10 yr	Less than 0.5 international units/mL
11–20 yr	0.5–9.0 international units/mL
	Phase in Females
Follicular	1.7–15.0 international units/mL
Ovulatory	21.9–80.0 international units/mL
Luteal	0.6–16.3 international units/mL
Postmenopausal	14.2–52.3 international units/mL

DESCRIPTION: Luteinizing hormone (LH) is secreted by the anterior pituitary gland in response to stimulation by gonadotropin-releasing hormone, the same hypothalamic-releasing factor that stimulates follicle-stimulating hormone release. LH affects gonadal function in both men and women. In women, a surge of LH normally occurs at the midpoint of the menstrual cycle (ovulatory phase); this surge is believed to be induced by high estrogen levels. LH causes the ovum to be expelled from the ovary and stimulates development of the corpus luteum and progesterone production. As progesterone levels rise, LH production decreases. In males, LH stimulates the interstitial cells of Leydig, located in the testes, to produce testosterone. For this reason, in reference to males, LH is sometimes called interstitial cell–stimulating hormone. Secretion of LH is pulsatile and follows a circadian rhythm in response to the normal intermittent secretion of gonadotropin-releasing hormone. Serial specimens may be required to accurately demonstrate blood levels.

INDICATIONS
- Distinguish between primary and secondary causes of gonadal failure
- Evaluate children with precocious puberty
- Evaluate male and female infertility, as indicated by decreased LH levels
- Evaluate response to therapy to induce ovulation
- Support diagnosis of infertility caused by anovulation, as evidenced by lack of LH surge at the midpoint of the menstrual cycle

POTENTIAL DIAGNOSIS

Increased in
Conditions of decreased gonadal function cause a feedback response that stimulates LH secretion.
- Anorchia
- Gonadal failure
- Menopause
- Primary gonadal dysfunction

Decreased in
- Anorexia nervosa *(pathophysiology is unclear)*

- Kallmann's syndrome *(pathophysiology is unclear)*
- Malnutrition *(pathophysiology is unclear)*
- Pituitary or hypothalamic dysfunction *(these organs control production of LH; failure of the pituitary to produce LH or of the hypothalamus to produce gonadotropin-releasing hormone results in decreased LH levels)*
- Severe stress *(pathophysiology is unclear)*

CRITICAL FINDINGS: N/A

INTERFERING FACTORS
- Drugs and hormones that may increase LH levels include clomiphene, gonadotropin-releasing hormone, goserelin, ketoconazole, leuprolide, mestranol, nafarelin, naloxone, nilutamide, spironolactone, and tamoxifen.
- Drugs and hormones that may decrease LH levels include anabolic steroids, anticonvulsants, conjugated estrogens, cyproterone, danazol, digoxin, D-Trp-6-LHRH, estradiol valerate, estrogen/progestin therapy, finasteride, ganirelix, goserelin, ketoconazole, leuprolide, Marvelon, medroxyprogesterone, megestrol, metformin, methandrostenolone, norethindrone, octreotide, oral contraceptives, phenothiazine, pimozide, pravastatin, progesterone, stanozolol, and tamoxifen.
- In menstruating women, values vary in relation to the phase of the menstrual cycle.
- LH secretion follows a circadian rhythm, with higher levels occurring during sleep.

NURSING IMPLICATIONS AND PROCEDURE

PRETEST:

- Positively identify the patient using at least two unique identifiers before providing care, treatment, or services.
- *Patient Teaching:* Inform the patient this test can assist in assessing hormone and fertility disorders.
- Obtain a history of the patient's complaints, including a list of known allergens, especially allergies or sensitivities to latex.
- Obtain a history of the patient's endocrine and reproductive systems, symptoms, and results of previously performed laboratory tests and diagnostic and surgical procedures.
- Record the date of the last menstrual period and determine the possibility of pregnancy in perimenopausal women.
- Obtain a list of the patient's current medications, including herbs, nutritional supplements, and nutraceuticals (see Appendix F).
- Review the procedure with the patient. If the test is being performed to detect ovulation, inform the patient that it may be necessary to obtain a series of samples over a period of several days to detect peak LH levels. Inform the patient that specimen collection takes approximately 5 to 10 min. Address concerns about pain and explain that there may be some discomfort during the venipuncture.
- *Sensitivity to social and cultural issues,* as well as concern for modesty, is important in providing psychological support before, during, and after the procedure.
- There are no food, fluid, or medication restrictions unless by medical direction.

INTRATEST:

- If the patient has a history of allergic reaction to latex, avoid the use of equipment containing latex.

- Instruct the patient to cooperate fully and to follow directions. Direct the patient to breathe normally and to avoid unnecessary movement.
- Observe standard precautions, and follow the general guidelines in Appendix A. Positively identify the patient, and label the appropriate tubes with the corresponding patient demographics, date, and time of collection. Perform a venipuncture.
- Remove the needle and apply direct pressure with dry gauze to stop bleeding. Observe/assess venipuncture site for bleeding or hematoma formation and secure gauze with adhesive bandage.
- Promptly transport the specimen to the laboratory for processing and analysis.

POST-TEST:

- A report of the results will be sent to the requesting health-care provider (HCP), who will discuss the results with the patient.
- Reinforce information given by the patient's HCP regarding further testing, treatment, or referral to another HCP. Instruct the patient in the use of home ovulation test kits approved by the U.S. Food and Drug Administration, as appropriate. Answer any questions or address any concerns voiced by the patient or family.
- Depending on the results of this procedure, additional testing may be performed to evaluate or monitor progression of the disease process and determine the need for a change in therapy. Evaluate test results in relation to the patient's symptoms and other tests performed.

RELATED MONOGRAPHS:

- Related tests include ACTH, antisperm antibody, estradiol, FSH, progesterone, prolactin, and testosterone.
- Refer to the Endocrine and Reproductive systems tables at the end of the book for related tests by body system.

L

Lyme Antibody

SYNONYM/ACRONYM: N/A.

COMMON USE: To detect antibodies to the organism that causes Lyme disease.

SPECIMEN: Serum (1 mL) collected in a red-top tube.

REFERENCE VALUE: (Method: Indirect immunofluorescence) Negative.

DESCRIPTION: *Borrelia burgdorferi*, a deer tick–borne spirochete, is the organism that causes Lyme disease. Lyme disease affects multiple systems and is characterized by fever, arthralgia, and arthritis. The circular, red rash characterizing erythema migrans can appear 3 to 30 days after the tick bite. About one-half of patients in the early stage of Lyme disease (stage 1) and generally all of those in the advanced stage (stage 2—with cardiac, neurological, and rheumatoid manifestations) will have a positive test result. Patients in remission will also have a positive test response. The presence of immunoglobulin M (IgM) antibodies indicates acute infection. The presence of IgG antibodies indicates current or past infection. The Centers for Disease Control and Prevention (CDC) recommends a two-step testing process that begins with an immunofluoresence or enzyme-linked immunosorbent assay (ELISA) and is confirmed by using a Western blot test.

INDICATIONS

Assist in establishing a diagnosis of Lyme disease

POTENTIAL DIAGNOSIS

Positive findings in
Lyme disease

Negative findings in: N/A

CRITICAL FINDINGS: N/A

INTERFERING FACTORS

- High rheumatoid-factor titers as well as cross-reactivity with Epstein-Barr virus and other spirochetes (e.g., *Rickettsia, Treponema*) may cause false-positive results.
- Positive test results should be confirmed by the Western blot method.

NURSING IMPLICATIONS AND PROCEDURE

PRETEST:

- Positively identify the patient using at least two unique identifiers before providing care, treatment, or services.
- *Patient Teaching:* Inform the patient this test can assist in diagnosing Lyme disease.
- Obtain a history of the patient's complaints, including a list of known allergens, especially allergies or sensitivities to latex.
- Obtain a history of the patient's immune and musculoskeletal systems, symptoms, a history of exposure, and results of previously performed laboratory tests and diagnostic and surgical procedures.

- Obtain a list of the patient's current medications, including herbs, nutritional supplements, and nutraceuticals (see Appendix F).
- Review the procedure with the patient. Inform the patient that several tests may be necessary to confirm diagnosis. Inform the patient that specimen collection takes approximately 5 to 10 min. Address concerns about pain and explain that there may be some discomfort during the venipuncture.
- *Sensitivity to social and cultural issues,* as well as concern for modesty, is important in providing psychological support before, during, and after the procedure.
- There are no food, fluid, or medication restrictions unless by medical direction.

INTRATEST:

- If the patient has a history of allergic reaction to latex, avoid the use of equipment containing latex.
- Instruct the patient to cooperate fully and to follow directions. Direct the patient to breathe normally and to avoid unnecessary movement.
- Observe standard precautions, and follow the general guidelines in Appendix A. Positively identify the patient, and label the appropriate tubes with the corresponding patient demographics, date, and time of collection. Perform a venipuncture.
- Remove the needle and apply direct pressure with dry gauze to stop bleeding. Observe/assess venipuncture site for bleeding or hematoma formation and secure gauze with adhesive bandage.
- Promptly transport the specimen to the laboratory for processing and analysis.

POST-TEST:

- A report of the results will be sent to the requesting health-care provider (HCP), who will discuss the results with the patient.
- Advise the patient to wear light-colored clothing that covers extremities when in areas infested by deer ticks and to check body for ticks after returning from infested areas.
- Recognize anxiety related to test results, and be supportive of impaired activity related to perceived loss of independence and fear of shortened life expectancy. Lyme disease can be debilitating and can result in significant changes in lifestyle. Discuss the implications of abnormal test results on the patient's lifestyle. Provide teaching and information regarding the clinical implications of the test results, as appropriate. Educate the patient regarding access to counseling services.
- Reinforce information given by the patient's HCP regarding further testing, treatment, or referral to another HCP. Warn the patient that false-positive test results can occur and that false-negative test results frequently occur. Answer any questions or address any concerns voiced by the patient or family.
- Depending on the results of this procedure, additional testing may be performed to evaluate or monitor progression of the disease process and determine the need for a change in therapy. Evaluate test results in relation to the patient's symptoms and other tests performed.

RELATED MONOGRAPHS:

- A related test is synovial fluid analysis.
- Refer to the Immune and Musculoskeletal systems tables at the end of the book for related tests by body system.

Lymphangiography

SYNONYM/ACRONYM: Lymphangiogram.

COMMON USE: To visualize and assess the lymphatic system related to diagnosis of lymphomas such as Hodgkin's disease.

AREA OF APPLICATION: Lymphatic system.

CONTRAST: IV iodine based contrast medium.

DESCRIPTION: Lymphangiography involves visualization of the lymphatic system after the injection of an iodinated oil–based contrast medium into a lymphatic vessel in the hand or foot. The lymphatic system consists of lymph vessels and nodes. Assessment of this system is important because cancer (lymphomas and Hodgkin's disease) often spreads via the lymphatic system. When the lymphatic system becomes obstructed, painful edema of the extremities usually results. The procedure is usually performed for cancer staging in patients with an established diagnosis of lymphoma or metastatic tumor. Injection into the hand allows visualization of the axillary and supraclavicular nodes. Injection into the foot allows visualization of the lymphatics of the leg, inguinal and iliac regions, and retroperitoneum up to the thoracic duct. Less commonly, injection into the foot can be used to visualize the cervical region (retroauricular area). This procedure can assess progression of the disease, assist in planning surgery, and monitor the effectiveness of chemotherapy or radiation treatment.

INDICATIONS

- Determine the extent of adenopathy
- Determine lymphatic cancer staging
- Distinguish primary from secondary lymphedema
- Evaluate edema of an extremity without known cause
- Evaluate effects of chemotherapy or radiation therapy
- Plan surgical treatment or evaluate effectiveness of chemotherapy or radiation therapy in controlling malignant tumors

POTENTIAL DIAGNOSIS

Normal findings in

- Normal lymphatic vessels and nodes that fill completely with contrast medium on the initial films. On 24-hr images, the lymph nodes are fully opacified and well circumscribed. The lymphatic channels are emptied a few hours after injection of the contrast medium

Abnormal findings in

- Abnormal lymphatic vessels
- Hodgkin's disease
- Metastatic tumor involving the lymph glands
- Nodal lymphoma
- Retroperitoneal lymphomas associated with Hodgkin's disease

CRITICAL FINDINGS: N/A

INTERFERING FACTORS

This procedure is contraindicated for

- ❋ Patients with pulmonary insufficiencies, cardiac diseases, or severe renal or hepatic disease.
- Patients with allergies to shellfish or iodinated dye. The contrast medium used may cause a life-threatening allergic reaction. Patients with a known hypersensitivity to the contrast medium may benefit from premedication with corticosteroids or the use of nonionic contrast medium.
- Patients who are pregnant or suspected of being pregnant, unless the potential benefits of the procedure far outweigh the risks to the fetus and mother.
- ❋ Elderly and other patients who are chronically dehydrated before the test, because of their risk of contrast-induced renal failure.
- ❋ Patients who are in renal failure.
- Young patients (17 yr and younger), unless the benefits of the x-ray diagnosis outweigh the risks of exposure to high levels of radiation.

Factors that may impair clear imaging

- Gas or feces in the gastrointestinal tract resulting from inadequate cleansing or failure to restrict food intake before the study.
- Retained barium from a previous radiological procedure.
- Metallic objects (e.g., jewelry, body rings) within the examination field, which may inhibit organ visualization and cause unclear images.
- Inability of the patient to cooperate or remain still during the procedure because of age, significant pain, or mental status.

- Inability to cannulate the lymphatic vessels.

Other considerations

- ❋ Be aware of risks associated with the contrast medium. The oil-based contrast medium may embolize into the lungs and will temporarily diminish pulmonary function. This can produce lipid pneumonia, which is a life-threatening complication.
- Consultation with a health-care provider (HCP) should occur before the procedure for radiation safety concerns regarding younger patients or patients who are lactating.
- Risks associated with radiation overexposure can result from frequent x-ray procedures. Personnel in the room with the patient should wear a protective lead apron, stand behind a shield, or leave the area while the examination is being done. Personnel working in the examination area should wear badges to record their level of radiation exposure.
- Failure to follow dietary restrictions and other pretesting preparations may cause the procedure to be canceled or repeated.

NURSING IMPLICATIONS AND PROCEDURE

PRETEST:

- Positively identify the patient using at least two unique identifiers before providing care, treatment, or services.
- *Patient Teaching:* Inform the patient this procedure can assist in assessing the lymphatic system.
- Obtain a history of the patient's complaints, including a list of known allergens, especially allergies or sensitivities to iodine, latex, seafood, anesthetics, or contrast mediums.
- Obtain a history of the patient's endocrine and immune systems, symptoms,

L

and results of previously performed laboratory tests and diagnostic and surgical procedures.

▶ Note any recent procedures that can interfere with test results, including examinations using barium- or iodine-based contrast medium. Ensure that barium studies were performed more than 4 days before lymphangiography.

▶ Record the date of the last menstrual period and determine the possibility of pregnancy in perimenopausal women.

▶ Obtain a list of the patient's current medications, including herbs, nutritional supplements, and nutraceuticals (see Appendix F).

▶ Review the procedure with the patient. Address concerns about pain and explain there may be moments of discomfort and some pain experienced during the test. Inform the patient that the procedure is performed by an HCP, with support staff, and takes approximately 1 to 2 hr. Inform the patient that he or she will have to return the next day, and the set of images taken upon return will take only 30 min.

▶ *Sensitivity to social and cultural issues,* as well as concern for modesty, is important in providing psychological support before, during, and after the procedure.

▶ Instruct the patient to remove jewelry and other metallic objects from the area to be examined prior to the procedure.

▶ Instruct patient to withhold anticoagulant medication or to reduce dosage before the procedure, as ordered by the HCP.

▶ There are no food or fluid restrictions unless by medical direction.

▶ *Make sure a written and informed consent has been signed prior to the procedure and before administering any medications.*

INTRATEST:

▶ Ensure the patient has complied with medication restrictions and pretesting preparations.

▶ Ensure the patient has removed all external metallic objects from the area to be examined.

▶ If the patient has a history of allergic reactions to any substance or drug,

administer ordered prophylactic steroids or antihistamines before the procedure. Use nonionic contrast medium for the procedure.

▶ Have emergency equipment readily accessible.

▶ Instruct the patient to void prior to the procedure and to change into the gown, robe, and foot coverings provided.

▶ Instruct the patient to cooperate fully and to follow directions. Direct the patient to remain still throughout the procedure because movement produces unreliable results.

▶ Obtain and record baseline vital signs, and assess neurological status.

▶ Observe standard precautions, and follow the general guidelines in Appendix A.

▶ Administer a mild sedative, as ordered.

▶ Place the patient in a supine position on an x-ray table. Cleanse the selected area and cover with a sterile drape.

▶ A local anesthetic is injected at the site, and a small incision is made or a needle inserted. A blue dye is injected intradermally into the area between the toes or fingers. The lymphatic vessels are identified as the dye moves. A local anesthetic is then injected into the dorsum of each foot or hand, and a small incision is made and cannulated for injection of the contrast medium.

▶ The contrast medium is then injected, and the flow of the contrast medium is followed by fluoroscopy or images. When the contrast medium reaches the upper lumbar level, the infusion of contrast medium is discontinued. X-ray images are taken of the chest, abdomen, and pelvis to determine the extent of filling of the lymphatic vessels. To examine the lymphatic nodes and to monitor the progress of delayed flow, 24-hr delayed images are taken.

▶ Monitor the patient for complications related to the contrast medium (e.g., allergic reaction, anaphylaxis, bronchospasm).

▶ Remove the needle or catheter and apply a pressure dressing over the puncture site.

▶ Observe/assess the needle/catheter insertion site for bleeding, inflammation, or hematoma formation.

• When the cannula is removed the incision is sutured and bandaged.

POST-TEST:

• A report of the examination will be sent to the requesting HCP, who will discuss the results with the patient.
• Monitor vital signs and neurological status every 15 min for 30 min. Take temperature every 4 hr for 24 hr. Monitor intake and output at least every 8 hr. Compare with baseline values. Notify the HCP if temperature is elevated. Protocols may vary among facilities.
• Observe/assess the cannula insertion site for bleeding, inflammation, or hematoma formation.
• Observe for a delayed allergic reaction to contrast medium or pulmonary embolus, which may include shortness of breath, increased heart rate, pleuritic pain, hypotension, low-grade fever, and cyanosis.
• Instruct the patient to immediately report symptoms such as fast heart rate, difficulty breathing, skin rash, itching, chest pain, persistent right shoulder pain, or abdominal pain. Immediately report symptoms to the appropriate HCP.
• Instruct the patient in the care and assessment of the site.
• Instruct the patient to apply cold compresses to the puncture site as needed to reduce discomfort or edema.
• Instruct the patient to maintain bedrest up to 24 hr to reduce extremity swelling after the procedure, or as ordered.

• Instruct the patient to resume usual medications, as directed by the HCP.
• Recognize anxiety related to test results, and be supportive of perceived loss of independent function. Discuss the implications of abnormal test results on the patient's lifestyle. Provide teaching and information regarding the clinical implications of the test results, as appropriate.
• Reinforce information given by the patient's HCP regarding further testing, treatment, or referral to another HCP. Answer any questions or address any concerns voiced by the patient or family.
• Depending on the results of this procedure, additional testing may be needed to evaluate or monitor progression of the disease process and determine the need for a change in therapy. Evaluate test results in relation to the patient's symptoms and other tests performed.

RELATED MONOGRAPHS:

• Related tests include biopsy bone marrow, biopsy lymph nodes, CBC, CBC WBC count and differential, CT abdomen, CT pelvis, CT thoracic, gallium scan, laparoscopy abdominal, liver and spleen scan, MRI abdomen, mediastinoscopy, and US lymph nodes.
• Refer to the Endocrine and Immune systems tables at the end of the book for tests by related body system.

L

Magnesium, Blood

SYNONYM/ACRONYM: Mg^{2+}.

COMMON USE: To assess electrolyte balance related to magnesium levels to assist in diagnosis, monitoring diseases, and therapeutic interventions such as hemodialysis.

SPECIMEN: Serum (1 mL) collected in a red- or tiger-top tube.

REFERENCE VALUE: (Method: Spectrophotometry)

Age	Conventional Units	Alternative Units (Conventional Units × 0.8229)	SI Units (Conventional Units × 0.4114)
Newborn	1.5–2.2 mg/dL	1.23–1.81 mEq/L	0.62–0.91 mmol/L
Child	1.7–2.1 mg/dL	1.40–1.73 mEq/L	0.70–0.86 mmol/L
Adult	1.6–2.6 mg/dL	1.32–2.14 mEq/L	0.66–1.07 mmol/L

DESCRIPTION: Magnesium is required as a cofactor in numerous crucial enzymatic processes, such as protein synthesis, nucleic acid synthesis, and muscle contraction. Magnesium is also required for the use of adenosine diphosphate as a source of energy. It is the fourth most abundant cation and the second most abundant intracellular ion. Magnesium is needed for the transmission of nerve impulses and muscle relaxation. It controls absorption of sodium, potassium, calcium, and phosphorus; utilization of carbohydrate, lipid, and protein; and activation of enzyme systems that enable the B vitamins to function. Magnesium is also essential for oxidative phosphorylation, nucleic acid synthesis, and blood clotting. Urine magnesium levels reflect magnesium deficiency before serum levels. Magnesium deficiency severe enough to cause hypocalcemia and cardiac arrhythmias can exist despite normal serum magnesium levels.

INDICATIONS
- Determine electrolyte balance in renal failure and chronic alcoholism
- Evaluate cardiac arrhythmias (decreased magnesium levels can lead to excessive ventricular irritability)
- Evaluate known or suspected disorders associated with altered magnesium levels
- Monitor the effects of various drugs on magnesium levels

POTENTIAL DIAGNOSIS

Increased in
- Addison's disease *(related to insufficient production of aldosterone; decreased renal excretion)*
- Adrenocortical insufficiency *(related to decreased renal excretion)*
- Dehydration *(related to hemoconcentration)*
- Diabetic acidosis (severe) *(related to acid-base imbalance)*
- Hypothyroidism *(pathophysiology is unclear)*
- Massive hemolysis *(related to release of intracellular magnesium; intracellular concentration*

is three times higher than normal plasma levels)
- Overuse of antacids *(related to excessive intake of magnesium-containing antacids)*
- Renal insufficiency *(related to decreased urinary excretion)*
- Tissue trauma

Decreased in
- Alcoholism *(related to increased renal excretion and possible insufficient dietary intake)*
- Diabetic acidosis *(insulin treatment lowers blood glucose and appears to increase intracellular transport of magnesium)*
- Glomerulonephritis (chronic) *(related to diminished renal function; magnesium is reabsorbed in the renal tubules)*
- Hemodialysis *(related to loss of magnesium due to dialysis treatment)*
- Hyperaldosteronism *(related to increased excretion)*
- Hypocalcemia *(decreased magnesium is associated with decreased calcium and vitamin D levels)*
- Hypoparathyroidism *(related to decreased calcium)*
- Inadequate intake
- Inappropriate secretion of antidiuretic hormone *(related to fluid overload)*
- Long-term hyperalimentation
- Malabsorption *(related to impaired absorption of calcium and vitamin D)*
- Pancreatitis *(secondary to alcoholism)*
- Pregnancy
- Severe loss of body fluids *(diarrhea, lactation, sweating, laxative abuse)*

CRITICAL FINDINGS
- Less than 1.2 mg/dL
- Greater than 4.9 mg/dL

Note and immediately report to the health-care provider (HCP) any critically increased or decreased values and related symptoms.

Symptoms such as tetany, weakness, dizziness, tremors, hyperactivity, nausea, vomiting, and convulsions occur at decreased (less than 1.2 mg/dL) concentrations. Electrocardiographic (ECG) changes (prolonged P-R and Q-T intervals; broad, flat T waves; and ventricular tachycardia) may also occur. Treatment may include IV or oral administration of magnesium salts, monitoring for respiratory depression and areflexia (IV administration of magnesium salts), and monitoring for diarrhea and metabolic alkalosis (oral administration to replace magnesium).

Respiratory paralysis, decreased reflexes, and cardiac arrest occur at grossly elevated (greater than 15 mg/dL) levels. ECG changes, such as prolonged P-R and Q-T intervals, and bradycardia may be seen. Toxic levels of magnesium may be reversed with the administration of calcium, dialysis treatments, and removal of the source of excessive intake.

INTERFERING FACTORS
- Drugs that may increase magnesium levels include acetylsalicylic acid and progesterone.
- Drugs that may decrease magnesium levels include albuterol, aminoglycosides, amphotericin B, bendroflumethiazide, chlorthalidone, cisplatin, citrates, cyclosporine, digoxin, gentamicin, glucagon, and oral contraceptives.
- Hemolysis results in a false elevation in values; such specimens should be rejected for analysis.
- Specimens should never be collected above an IV line because of the potential for dilution when the

specimen and the IV solution combine in the collection container, falsely decreasing the result. There is also the potential of contaminating the sample with the substance of interest, if it is present in the IV solution, falsely increasing the result.

NURSING IMPLICATIONS AND PROCEDURE

PRETEST:

▶ Positively identify the patient using at least two unique identifiers before providing care, treatment, or services.
▶ *Patient Teaching:* Inform the patient this test can assist in the evaluation of electrolyte balance.
▶ Obtain a history of the patient's complaints, including a list of known allergens, especially allergies or sensitivities to latex.
▶ Obtain a history of the patient's cardiovascular, endocrine, gastrointestinal, genitourinary, and reproductive systems; symptoms; and results of previously performed laboratory tests and diagnostic and surgical procedures.
▶ Obtain a list of the patient's current medications, including herbs, nutritional supplements, and nutraceuticals (see Appendix F).
▶ Review the procedure with the patient. Inform the patient that specimen collection takes approximately 5 to 10 min. Address concerns about pain and explain that there may be some discomfort during the venipuncture.
▶ *Sensitivity to social and cultural issues,* as well as concern for modesty, is important in providing psychological support before, during, and after the procedure.
▶ There are no food, fluid, or medication restrictions unless by medical direction.

INTRATEST:

▶ If the patient has a history of allergic reaction to latex, avoid the use of equipment containing latex.

▶ Instruct the patient to cooperate fully and to follow directions. Direct the patient to breathe normally and to avoid unnecessary movement.
▶ Observe standard precautions, and follow the general guidelines in Appendix A. Positively identify the patient, and label the appropriate tubes with the corresponding patient demographics, date, and time of collection. Perform a venipuncture.
▶ Remove the needle and apply direct pressure with dry gauze to stop bleeding. Observe/assess venipuncture site for bleeding or hematoma formation and secure gauze with adhesive bandage.
▶ Promptly transport the specimen to the laboratory for processing and analysis.

POST-TEST:

▶ A report of the results will be sent to the requesting HCP, who will discuss the results with the patient.
▶ *Nutritional Considerations:* Educate the magnesium-deficient patient regarding good dietary sources of magnesium, such as green vegetables, seeds, legumes, shrimp, and some bran cereals. Advise the patient that high intake of substances such as phosphorus, calcium, fat, and protein interferes with the absorption of magnesium.
▶ Instruct the patient to report any signs or symptoms of electrolyte imbalance, such as dehydration, diarrhea, vomiting, or prolonged anorexia.
▶ Reinforce information given by the patient's HCP regarding further testing, treatment, or referral to another HCP. Answer any questions or address any concerns voiced by the patient or family.
▶ Depending on the results of this procedure, additional testing may be performed to evaluate or monitor progression of the disease process and determine the need for a change in therapy. Evaluate test results in relation to the patient's symptoms and other tests performed.

RELATED MONOGRAPHS:

▶ Related tests include ACTH, aldosterone, anion gap, antiarrhythmic drugs, AST, BUN, calcium, calculus kidney stone panel, CBC WBC count and differential, cortisol, CRP, CK and isoenzymes, creatinine, glucose, homocysteine, LDH and isoenzymes, magnesium urine, myoglobin, osmolality, PTH, phosphorus, potassium, renin, sodium, troponin, and vitamin D.

▶ Refer to the Cardiovascular, Endocrine, Gastrointestinal, Genitourinary, and Reproductive systems tables at the end of the book for related tests by body system.

Magnesium, Urine

SYNONYM/ACRONYM: Urine Mg^{2+}.

COMMON USE: To assess magnesium levels related to renal function.

SPECIMEN: Urine (5 mL) from a random or timed specimen collected in a clean plastic collection container with 6N hydrochloride as a preservative.

REFERENCE VALUE: (Method: Spectrophotometry)

Conventional Units	SI Units (Conventional Units × 0.4114)
6.0–10.0 mEq/24 hr	3.0–5.0 mmol/24 hr

M

DESCRIPTION: Magnesium is required as a cofactor in numerous crucial enzymatic processes, such as protein synthesis, nucleic acid synthesis, and muscle contraction. Magnesium is also required for the use of adenosine diphosphate as a source of energy. It is the fourth most abundant cation and the second most abundant intracellular ion. Magnesium is needed for the transmission of nerve impulses and muscle relaxation. It controls absorption of sodium, potassium, calcium, and phosphorus; utilization of carbohydrate, lipid, and protein; and activation of enzyme systems that enable the B vitamins to function. Magnesium is also essential for oxidative phosphorylation, nucleic acid synthesis, and blood clotting. Urine magnesium levels reflect magnesium deficiency before serum levels. Magnesium deficiency severe enough to cause hypocalcemia and cardiac arrhythmias can exist despite normal serum magnesium levels.

Regulating electrolyte balance is one of the major functions of the kidneys. In normally functioning kidneys, urine levels increase when serum levels are high and decrease when serum levels are low to maintain homeostasis. Analyzing these urinary levels can provide important clues as to the functioning of the kidneys and other major organs. Tests for electrolytes, such as magnesium, in urine usually involve timed urine collections over a 12- or 24-hr period. Measurement of random specimens may also be requested.

INDICATIONS

• Determine the potential cause of renal calculi
• Evaluate known or suspected endocrine disorder
• Evaluate known or suspected renal disease
• Evaluate magnesium imbalance
• Evaluate a malabsorption problem

POTENTIAL DIAGNOSIS

Increased in

• Alcoholism *(related to impaired absorption and increased urinary excretion)*
• Bartter's syndrome *(inherited defect in renal tubules that results in urinary wasting of potassium and magnesium)*
• Transplant recipients on cyclosporine and prednisone *(related to increased excretion by the kidney)*
• Use of corticosteroids *(related to increased excretion by the kidney)*
• Use of diuretics *(related to increased urinary excretion)*

Decreased in

• Abnormal renal function *(related to diminished ability of renal tubules to reabsorb magnesium)*
• Crohn's disease *(related to inadequate intestinal absorption)*
• Inappropriate secretion of antidiuretic hormone *(related to diminished renal absorption)*

• Salt-losing conditions *(related to diminished renal absorption)*

CRITICAL FINDINGS: N/A

INTERFERING FACTORS

• Drugs that may increase urine magnesium levels include cisplatin, cyclosporine, ethacrynic acid, furosemide, mercaptomerin, mercurial diuretics, thiazides, torsemide, and triamterene.
• Drugs that may decrease urine magnesium levels include amiloride, angiotensin, oral contraceptives, parathyroid extract, and phosphates.
• Magnesium levels follow a circadian rhythm, and for this reason 24-hr collections are recommended.
• All urine voided for the timed collection period must be included in the collection, or else falsely decreased values may be obtained. Compare output records with volume collected to verify that all voids were included in the collection.

NURSING IMPLICATIONS AND PROCEDURE

PRETEST:

▶ Positively identify the patient using at least two unique identifiers before providing care, treatment, or services.
▶ *Patient Teaching:* Inform the patient this test can assist in evaluating magnesium balance.
▶ Obtain a history of the patient's complaints, including a list of known allergens, especially allergies or sensitivities to latex.
▶ Obtain a history of the patient's endocrine, gastrointestinal, and genitourinary systems; symptoms; and results of previously performed laboratory tests and diagnostic and surgical procedures.
▶ Obtain a list of the patient's current medications, including herbs, nutritional

M

supplements, and nutraceuticals (see Appendix F).

▸ Review the procedure with the patient. Provide a nonmetallic urinal, bedpan, or toilet-mounted collection device. Address concerns about pain related to the procedure. Explain to the patient that there should be no discomfort during the procedure.

▸ Usually a 24-hr time frame for urine collection is ordered. Inform the patient that all urine must be saved during that 24-hr period. Instruct the patient not to void directly into the laboratory collection container. Instruct the patient to avoid defecating in the collection device and to keep toilet tissue out of the collection device to prevent contamination of the specimen. Place a sign in the bathroom to remind the patient to save all urine.

▸ Instruct the patient to void all urine into the collection device and then to pour the urine into the laboratory collection container. Alternatively, the specimen can be left in the collection device for a health-care staff member to add to the laboratory collection container.

▸ *Sensitivity to social and cultural issues,* as well as concern for modesty, is important in providing psychological support before, during, and after the procedure.

▸ Instruct the patient to avoid excessive exercise and stress during the 24-hr collection of urine.

▸ There are no food, fluid, or medication restrictions unless by medical direction.

INTRATEST:

▸ Ensure that the patient has complied with activity restrictions during the procedure.

▸ If the patient has a history of allergic reaction to latex, avoid the use of equipment containing latex.

▸ Instruct the patient to cooperate fully and to follow directions.

▸ Observe standard precautions, and follow the general guidelines in Appendix A. Positively identify the patient, and label the appropriate tubes with the corresponding patient demographics, date, and time of collection.

Random Specimen (Collect in Early Morning)
Clean-Catch Specimen

▸ Instruct the male patient to (1) thoroughly wash his hands, (2) cleanse the meatus, (3) void a small amount into the toilet, and (4) void directly into the specimen container.

▸ Instruct the female patient to (1) thoroughly wash her hands; (2) cleanse the labia from front to back; (3) while keeping the labia separated, void a small amount into the toilet; and (4) without interrupting the urine stream, void directly into the specimen container.

Indwelling Catheter

▸ Put on gloves. Empty drainage tube of urine. It may be necessary to clamp off the catheter for 15 to 30 min before specimen collection. Cleanse specimen port with antiseptic swab, and then aspirate 5 mL of urine with a 21- to 25-gauge needle and syringe. Transfer urine to a sterile container.

Timed Specimen

▸ Obtain a clean 3-L urine specimen container, toilet-mounted collection device, and plastic bag (for transport of the specimen container). The specimen must be refrigerated or kept on ice throughout the entire collection period. If an indwelling urinary catheter is in place, the drainage bag must be kept on ice.

▸ Begin the test between 6 and 8 a.m. if possible. Collect first voiding and discard. Record the time the specimen was discarded as the beginning of the timed collection period. The next morning, ask the patient to void at the same time the collection was started and add this last voiding to the container. Urinary output should be recorded throughout the collection time.

▸ If an indwelling catheter is in place, replace the tubing and container system at the start of the collection time. Keep the container system on ice during the collection period, or empty the urine into a larger container periodically during the collection period; monitor to ensure continued drainage, and conclude the test the next morning at the same hour the collection was begun.

M

- At the conclusion of the test, compare the quantity of urine with the urinary output record for the collection; if the specimen contains less than what was recorded as output, some urine may have been discarded, invalidating the test.
- Include on the collection container's label the amount of urine, test start and stop times, and ingestion of any foods or medications that can affect test results.
- Promptly transport the specimen to the laboratory for processing and analysis.

POST-TEST:

- A report of the results will be sent to the requesting health-care provider (HCP), who will discuss the results with the patient.
- *Nutritional Considerations:* Educate the magnesium-deficient patient regarding good dietary sources of magnesium, such as green vegetables, seeds, legumes, shrimp, and some bran cereals. Advise the patient that high intake of substances such as phosphorus, calcium, fat, and protein interferes with the absorption of magnesium.
- Instruct the patient to report any signs or symptoms of electrolyte imbalance, such as dehydration, diarrhea, vomiting, or prolonged anorexia.

- Recognize anxiety related to test results. Discuss the implications of abnormal test results on the patient's lifestyle. Provide teaching and information regarding the clinical implications of the test results, as appropriate.
- Reinforce information given by the patient's HCP regarding further testing, treatment, or referral to another HCP. Answer any questions or address any concerns voiced by the patient or family.
- Depending on the results of this procedure, additional testing may be performed to evaluate or monitor progression of the disease process and determine the need for a change in therapy. Evaluate test results in relation to the patient's symptoms and other tests performed.

RELATED MONOGRAPHS:

- Related tests include ACTH, aldosterone, angiography renal, anion gap, BUN, calcium, calculus kidney stone panel, CT renal, cortisol, creatinine, glucose, IVP, magnesium, osmolality, PTH, phosphorus, potassium, renin, renogram, sodium, troponin, UA, US kidney, and vitamin D.
- Refer to the Endocrine, Gastrointestinal, and Genitourinary systems tables at the end of the book for related tests by body system.

M

Magnetic Resonance Angiography

SYNONYM/ACRONYM: MRA.

COMMON USE: To visualize and assess blood flow in diseased and normal vessels to assist with diagnosis of vascular disease and to monitor and evaluate therapeutic interventions.

AREA OF APPLICATION: Vascular.

CONTRAST: Can be done with or without IV contrast (gadolinium).

DESCRIPTION: Magnetic resonance imaging (MRI) uses a magnet and radio waves to produce an energy field that can be displayed as an image. The magnetic field causes the hydrogen atoms in tissue to line up, and when radio waves are directed toward the magnetic field, the atoms absorb the radio waves and change their position. When the radio waves are turned off, the atoms go back to their original position; this change in the energy field is sensed by the equipment, and an image is generated by the attached computer system. MRI produces cross-sectional images of the vessels in multiple planes without the use of ionizing radiation or the interference of bone or surrounding tissue.

Magnetic resonance angiography (MRA) is an application of MRI that provides images of blood flow and diseased and normal blood vessels. In patients who are allergic to iodinated contrast medium, MRA is used in place of angiography. MRA is particularly useful for visualizing vascular abnormalities, dissections, and other pathology. Special imaging sequences allow the visualization of moving blood within the vascular system. Two common techniques to obtain images of flowing blood are time-of-flight and phase-contrast MRA. In time-of-flight imaging, incoming blood makes the vessels appear bright and surrounding tissue is suppressed. Phase-contrast images are produced by subtracting the stationary tissue surrounding the vessels where the blood is moving through vessels during the imaging, producing high-contrast images. MRA is the most accurate technique for imaging blood flowing in

veins and small arteries (*laminar flow*), but it does not accurately depict blood flow in tortuous sections of vessels and distal to bifurcations and stenosis. Swirling blood may cause a signal loss and result in inadequate images, and the degree of vessel stenosis may be overestimated. Images can be obtained in two-dimensional (series of slices) or three-dimensional sequences.

INDICATIONS
- Detect pericardial abnormalities
- Detect peripheral vascular disease
- Detect thoracic and abdominal vascular diseases
- Determine renal artery stenosis
- Differentiate aortic aneurysms from tumors near the aorta
- Evaluate cardiac chambers and pulmonary vessels
- Evaluate postoperative angioplasty sites and bypass grafts
- Identify congenital vascular diseases
- Monitor and evaluate the effectiveness of medical or surgical treatment

POTENTIAL DIAGNOSIS

Normal findings in
- Normal blood flow in the area being examined, including blood flow rate

Abnormal findings in
- Coarctations
- Dissections
- Thrombosis within a vessel
- Tumor invasion of a vessel
- Vascular abnormalities
- Vessel occlusion
- Vessel stenosis

CRITICAL FINDINGS
- Aortic aneurysm
- Aortic dissection
- Occlusion

M

• Tumor with significant mass effect
• Vertebral artery dissection

It is essential that critical diagnoses be communicated immediately to the appropriate health-care provider (HCP). A listing of these diagnoses varies among facilities. Note and immediately report to the HCP abnormal results and related symptoms.

INTERFERING FACTORS

This procedure is contraindicated for

• Patients with certain ferrous metal prosthetics, valves, aneurysm clips, inner ear prostheses, or other metallic objects.
• Patients with metal in their body, such as shrapnel or ferrous metal in the eye.
• ❈ Patients with cardiac pacemakers, because the pacemaker can be deactivated by MRI.
• ❈ Use of gadolinium-based contrast agents (GBCAs) is contraindicated in patients with acute or chronic severe renal insufficiency (glomerular filtration rate less than 30 mL/min/1.73 m^2). Patients should be screened for renal dysfunction prior to administration. The use of GBCAs should be avoided in these patients unless the benefits of the studies outweigh the risks and if essential diagnostic information is not available using non-contrast-enhanced diagnostic studies.
• Patients who are claustrophobic.
• Patients who are pregnant or suspected of being pregnant, unless the potential benefits of the procedure far outweigh the risks to the fetus and mother.

Factors that may impair clear imaging

• Metallic objects (e.g., jewelry, body rings, dental amalgams) within the examination field, which may inhibit organ visualization and cause unclear images.
• Inability of the patient to cooperate or remain still during the procedure because of age, significant pain, or mental status.
• Patients with extreme cases of claustrophobia, unless sedation is given before the study.

Other considerations

• If contrast medium is allowed to seep deep into the muscle tissue, vascular visualization will be impossible.

NURSING IMPLICATIONS AND PROCEDURE

PRETEST:

▶ Positively identify the patient using at least two unique identifiers before providing care, treatment, or services.
▶ *Patient Teaching:* Inform the patient this procedure can assist in assessing the vascular system.
▶ Obtain a history of the patient's complaints, including a list of known allergens, especially allergies or sensitivities to latex, iodine, seafood, contrast medium, anesthetics, or dyes.
▶ Obtain a history of the patient's cardiovascular system, symptoms, and results of previously performed laboratory tests and diagnostic and surgical procedures. Obtain a history of renal dysfunction if the use of GBCA is anticipated.
▶ Ensure the results of BUN, creatinine, and eGFR (estimated glomerular filtration rate) are obtained if GBCA is to be used.
▶ Determine if the patient has ever had any device implanted into his or her body, including copper intrauterine devices, pacemakers, ear implants, and heart valves.
▶ Obtain occupational history to determine the presence of metal in the body, such as shrapnel or flecks of ferrous metal in the eye (which can cause retinal hemorrhage).
▶ Note any recent procedures that can interfere with test results.

M

- Record the date of the last menstrual period and determine the possibility of pregnancy in perimenopausal women.
- Obtain a list of the patient's current medications, including herbs, nutritional supplements, and nutraceuticals (see Appendix F).
- Review the procedure with the patient. Address concerns about pain related to the procedure and explain that no pain will be experienced during the test, but there may be moments of discomfort. Reassure the patient that if contrast is used, it poses no radioactive hazard and rarely produces side effects. Inform the patient the procedure is performed in an MRI department by an HCP who specializes in this procedure, with support staff, and takes approximately 30 to 60 min.
- Inform the patient that the technologist will place him or her in a supine position on a flat table in a large cylindrical scanner.
- Tell the patient to expect to hear loud banging from the scanner and possibly to see magnetophosphenes (flickering lights in the visual field); these will stop when the procedure is over.
- Explain that an IV line may be inserted to allow infusion of IV fluids, contrast medium, or sedatives.
- *Sensitivity to social and cultural issues,* as well as concern for modesty, is important in providing psychological support before, during, and after the procedure.
- Instruct the patient to remove external metallic objects from the area to be examined prior to the procedure.
- There are no food, fluid, or medication restrictions unless by medical direction.

INTRATEST:

- Ensure that the patient has removed external metallic objects from the area to be examined prior to the procedure.
- If the patient has a history of allergic reactions to any substance or drug, administer ordered prophylactic steroids or antihistamines before the procedure.
- Have emergency equipment readily available.
- Instruct the patient to void prior to the procedure and to change into the gown, robe, and foot coverings provided.

- Instruct the patient to cooperate fully and to follow directions. Instruct the patient to remain still throughout the procedure because movement produces unreliable results.
- Observe standard precautions, and follow the general guidelines in Appendix A.
- Supply earplugs to the patient to block out the loud, banging sounds that occur during the test. Instruct the patient to communicate with the technologist during the examination via a microphone within the scanner.
- If an electrocardiogram or respiratory gating is to be performed in conjunction with the scan, apply MRI-safe electrodes to the appropriate sites.
- Establish IV fluid line for the injection of emergency drugs and sedatives.
- Administer an antianxiety agent, as ordered, if the patient has claustrophobia. Administer a sedative to a child or to an uncooperative adult, as ordered.
- Place the patient in the supine position on an examination table.
- If contrast is used, imaging can begin shortly after the injection.
- Ask the patient to inhale deeply and hold his or her breath while the images are taken, and then to exhale after the images are taken.
- Instruct the patient to take slow, deep breaths if nausea occurs during the procedure.
- Monitor the patient for complications related to the procedure (e.g., allergic reaction, anaphylaxis, bronchospasm).
- Remove the needle or catheter and apply a pressure dressing over the puncture site.
- Observe/assess the needle/catheter insertion site for bleeding, inflammation, or hematoma formation.

POST-TEST:

- A report of the results will be sent to the requesting HCP, who will discuss the results with the patient.
- Observe for delayed allergic reactions, such as rash, urticaria, tachycardia, hyperpnea, hypertension, palpitations, nausea, or vomiting.

M

▶ Instruct the patient to immediately report symptoms such as fast heart rate, difficulty breathing, skin rash, itching, chest pain, persistent right shoulder pain, or abdominal pain. Immediately report symptoms to the appropriate HCP.

▶ Instruct the patient in the care and assessment of the injection site.

▶ Instruct the patient to apply cold compresses to the puncture site as needed to reduce discomfort or edema.

▶ Recognize anxiety related to test results. Discuss the implications of abnormal test results on the patient's lifestyle. Provide teaching and information regarding the clinical implications of the test results, as appropriate.

▶ Reinforce information given by the patient's HCP regarding further testing, treatment, or referral to another HCP.

Answer any questions or address any concerns voiced by the patient or family.

▶ Depending on the results of this procedure, additional testing may be performed to evaluate or monitor progression of the disease process and determine the need for a change in therapy. Evaluate test results in relation to the patient's symptoms and other tests performed.

RELATED MONOGRAPHS:

▶ Related tests include angiography of the body area of interest, BUN, CT angiography, creatinine, US arterial Doppler carotid, and US venous Doppler.

▶ Refer to the Cardiovascular System table at the end of the book for related tests by body system.

Magnetic Resonance Imaging, Abdomen

SYNONYM/ACRONYM: Abdominal MRI.

COMMON USE: To visualize and assess abdominal and hepatic structures to assist in diagnosis of tumors, metastasis, aneurysm, and abscess. Also used to monitor medical and surgical therapeutic interventions.

AREA OF APPLICATION: Liver and abdominal area.

CONTRAST: Can be done with or without IV contrast medium (gadolinium).

DESCRIPTION: Magnetic resonance imaging (MRI) uses a magnet and radio waves to produce an energy field that can be displayed as an image. Use of magnetic fields with the aid of radiofrequency energy produces images primarily based on water content of tissue. The magnetic field causes the hydrogen atoms in tissue to line up, and when radio waves are directed toward the magnetic field, the atoms absorb the radio waves and change their position. When the radio waves are turned off, the atoms go back to their original position; this change in the energy field is sensed by the equipment, and an image is generated by the attached computer system. MRI produces cross-sectional images of the abdomen in multiple planes without the use of ionizing radiation or the interference of bone.

Abdominal MRI is performed to assist in diagnosing abnormalities of abdominal and hepatic structures. Contrast-enhanced imaging is effective for distinguishing peritoneal metastases from primary tumors of the gastrointestinal (GI) tract. Primary tumors of the stomach, pancreas, colon, and appendix often spread by intraperitoneal tumor shedding and subsequent peritoneal carcinomatosis. MRI uses the noniodinated contrast medium gadopentetate dimeglumine (Magnevist), which is administered IV to enhance contrast differences between normal and abnormal tissues.

Magnetic resonance angiography (MRA) is an application of MRI that provides images of blood flow and diseased and normal blood vessels. In patients who are allergic to iodinated contrast medium, MRA is used in place of angiography (see monograph titled "Magnetic Resonance Angiography").

INDICATIONS

- Detect abdominal aortic diseases
- Detect and stage cancer (primary or metastatic tumors of liver, pancreas, prostate, uterus, and bladder)
- Detect chronic pancreatitis
- Detect renal vein thrombosis
- Detect soft tissue abnormalities
- Determine and monitor tissue damage in renal transplant patients
- Determine the presence of blood clots, cysts, fluid or fat accumulation in tissues, hemorrhage, and infarctions
- Determine vascular complications of pancreatitis, venous thrombosis, or pseudoaneurysm
- Differentiate aortic aneurysms from tumors near the aorta
- Differentiate liver tumors from liver abnormalities, such as cysts,

cavernous hemangiomas, and hepatic amebic abscesses
- Evaluate postoperative angioplasty sites and bypass grafts
- Monitor and evaluate the effectiveness of medical or surgical interventions and the course of the disease

POTENTIAL DIAGNOSIS

Normal findings in
- Normal anatomic structures, soft tissue density, and biochemical constituents of body tissues, including blood flow

Abnormal findings in
- Acute tubular necrosis
- Aneurysm
- Cholangitis
- Glomerulonephritis
- Hydronephrosis
- Internal bleeding
- Masses, lesions, infections, or inflammations
- Renal vein thrombosis
- Vena cava obstruction

CRITICAL FINDINGS
- Acute GI bleed
- Aortic aneurysm
- Infection
- Tumor with significant mass effect

It is essential that critical diagnoses be communicated immediately to the appropriate health-care provider (HCP). A listing of these diagnoses varies among facilities. Note and immediately report to the HCP abnormal results and related symptoms.

INTERFERING FACTORS

This procedure is contraindicated for
- Patients with certain ferrous metal prostheses, valves, aneurysm clips, inner ear prostheses, or other metallic objects.

M

- ◈ Patients with metal in their body, such as shrapnel or ferrous metal in the eye.
- ◈ Patients with cardiac pacemakers, because the pacemaker can be deactivated by MRI.
- ◈ Use of gadolinium-based contrast agents (GBCAs) is contraindicated in patients with acute or chronic severe renal insufficiency (glomerular filtration rate less than 30 mL/min/1.73 m²). Patients should be screened for renal dysfunction prior to administration. The use of GBCAs should be avoided in these patients unless the benefits of the studies outweigh the risks and if essential diagnostic information is not available using non-contrast-enhanced diagnostic studies.
- Patients with intrauterine devices.
- Patients with iron pigments in tattoos.
- Patients who are claustrophobic.
- Patients who are pregnant or suspected of being pregnant, unless the potential benefits of the procedure far outweigh the risks to the fetus and mother.

Factors that may impair clear imaging

- Metallic objects (e.g., jewelry, body rings, dental amalgams) within the examination field, which may inhibit organ visualization and cause unclear images.
- Inability of the patient to cooperate or remain still during the procedure because of age, significant pain, or mental status.
- Patients with extreme cases of claustrophobia, unless sedation is given before the study or an open MRI is utilized.

Other considerations

- If contrast medium is allowed to seep deep into the muscle tissue, vascular visualization will be impossible.

NURSING IMPLICATIONS AND PROCEDURE

PRETEST:
- Positively identify the patient using at least two unique identifiers before providing care, treatment, or services.
- *Patient Teaching:* Inform the patient this procedure can assist in assessing the abdominal organs and structures.
- Obtain a history of the patient's complaints, including a list of known allergens, especially allergies or sensitivities to latex, iodine, seafood, contrast medium, anesthetics, or dyes.
- Obtain a history of the patient's gastrointestinal, genitourinary, and hepatobiliary systems; symptoms; and results of previously performed laboratory tests and diagnostic and surgical procedures. Obtain a history of renal dysfunction if the use of GBCA is anticipated.
- Ensure the results of BUN, creatinine, and eGFR (estimated glomerular filtration rate) are obtained if GBCA is to be used.
- Determine if the patient has ever had any device implanted into his or her body, including copper intrauterine devices, pacemakers, ear implants, and heart valves.
- Obtain occupational history to determine the presence of metal in the body, such as shrapnel or flecks of ferrous metal in the eye (which can cause retinal hemorrhage).
- Note any recent procedures that can interfere with test results, including examinations using barium- or iodine-based contrast medium.
- Record the date of the last menstrual period and determine the possibility of pregnancy in perimenopausal women.
- Obtain a list of the patient's current medications including herbs, nutritional supplements, and nutraceuticals (see Appendix F).
- Review the procedure with the patient. Address concerns about pain related to the procedure and explain that no pain will be experienced during the test, but there may be moments of discomfort. Reassure the patient that if contrast is used, it poses no radioactive hazard

M

and rarely produces side effects. Inform the patient the procedure is performed in an MRI department by an HCP specializing in this procedure, with support staff, and takes approximately 30 to 60 min.

‣ Inform the patient that the technologist will place him or her in a supine position on a flat table in a large cylindrical scanner.

‣ Tell the patient to expect to hear loud banging from the scanner and possibly to see magnetophosphenes (flickering lights in the visual field); these will stop when the procedure is over.

‣ *Sensitivity to social and cultural issues,* as well as concern for modesty, is important in providing psychological support before, during, and after the procedure.

‣ Explain that an IV line may be inserted to allow infusion of IV fluids, contrast medium, or sedatives.

‣ Instruct the patient to remove jewelry and all other metallic objects from the area to be examined prior to the procedure.

‣ There are no food, fluid, or medication restrictions unless by medical direction.

INTRATEST:

‣ Ensure that the patient has removed all external metallic objects from the area to be examined prior to the procedure.

‣ If the patient has a history of allergic reactions to any substance or drug, administer ordered prophylactic steroids or antihistamines before the procedure.

‣ Have emergency equipment readily available.

‣ Instruct the patient to void prior to the procedure and to change into the gown, robe, and foot coverings provided.

‣ Instruct the patient to cooperate fully and to follow directions. Instruct the patient to remain still throughout the procedure because movement produces unreliable results.

‣ Observe standard precautions, and follow the general guidelines in Appendix A.

‣ Supply earplugs to the patient to block out the loud, banging sounds that

occur during the test. Instruct the patient to communicate with the technologist during the examination via a microphone within the scanner.

‣ Establish an IV fluid line for the injection of emergency drugs and of sedatives.

‣ Administer an antianxiety agent, as ordered, if the patient has claustrophobia. Administer a sedative to a child or to an uncooperative adult, as ordered.

‣ Place the patient in the supine position on an examination table.

‣ If contrast is used, imaging can begin shortly after the injection.

‣ Ask the patient to inhale deeply and hold his or her breath while the images are taken and then to exhale after the images are taken.

‣ Instruct the patient to take slow, deep breaths if nausea occurs during the procedure.

‣ Monitor the patient for complications related to the procedure (e.g., allergic reaction, anaphylaxis, bronchospasm).

‣ Remove the needle or catheter and apply a pressure dressing over the puncture site.

‣ Observe/assess the needle/catheter insertion site for bleeding, inflammation, or hematoma formation.

POST-TEST:

‣ A report of the results will be sent to the requesting HCP, who will discuss the results with the patient.

‣ Observe for delayed allergic reactions, such as rash, urticaria, tachycardia, hyperpnea, hypertension, palpitations, nausea, or vomiting

‣ Instruct the patient to immediately report symptoms such as fast heart rate, difficulty breathing, skin rash, itching, chest pain, persistent right shoulder pain, or abdominal pain. Immediately report symptoms to the appropriate HCP.

‣ Instruct the patient in the care and assessment of the injection site.

‣ Instruct the patient to apply cold compresses to the puncture site as needed to reduce discomfort or edema.

‣ Recognize anxiety related to test results. Discuss the implications of abnormal test results on the patient's

lifestyle. Provide teaching and information regarding the clinical implications of the test results, as appropriate.
▶ Reinforce information given by the patient's HCP regarding further testing, treatment, or referral to another HCP. Answer any questions or address any concerns voiced by the patient or family.
▶ Depending on the results of this procedure, additional testing may be performed to evaluate or monitor progression of the disease process and determine the need for a change in

therapy. Evaluate test results in relation to the patient's symptoms and other tests performed.

RELATED MONOGRAPHS:
▶ Related tests include angiography abdomen, BUN, CT abdomen, creatinine, GI blood loss scan, KUB study, and US liver and biliary system.
▶ Refer to the Gastrointestinal, Genitourinary, and Hepatobiliary systems tables at the end of the book for related tests by body system.

Magnetic Resonance Imaging, Brain

SYNONYM/ACRONYM: Brain MRI.

COMMON USE: To visualize and assess intracranial abnormalities related to tumor, bleeding, lesions, and infarct such as stroke.

AREA OF APPLICATION: Brain area.

CONTRAST: Can be done with or without IV contrast medium (gadolinium).

M

DESCRIPTION: Magnetic resonance imaging (MRI) uses a magnet and radio waves to produce an energy field that can be displayed as an image. Use of magnetic fields with the aid of radiofrequency energy produces images primarily based on water content of tissue. The magnetic field causes the hydrogen atoms in tissue to line up, and when radio waves are directed toward the magnetic field, the atoms absorb the radio waves and change their position. When the radio waves are turned off, the atoms go back to their original position; this change in the energy field is sensed by the equipment, and an image is generated by the attached computer

system. MRI produces cross-sectional images of pathological lesions of the brain in multiple planes without the use of ionizing radiation or the interference of bone or surrounding tissue.

Brain MRI can distinguish solid, cystic, and hemorrhagic components of lesions. This procedure is done to aid in the diagnosis of intracranial abnormalities, including tumors, ischemia, infection, and multiple sclerosis, and in assessment of brain maturation in pediatric patients. Rapidly flowing blood on spin-echo MRI appears as an absence of signal or a void in the vessel's lumen. Blood flow can be evaluated in the cavernous and carotid arteries. Aneurysms may be diagnosed without traditional iodine-based contrast angiography, and old clotted blood in the walls of the aneurysms appears white. MRI uses the noniodinated contrast medium gadopentetate dimeglumine (Magnevist), which is administered IV to enhance contrast differences between normal and abnormal tissues.

Magnetic resonance angiography (MRA) is an application of MRI that provides images of blood flow and diseased and normal blood vessels. In patients who are allergic to iodinated contrast medium, MRA is used in place of angiography (see monograph titled "Magnetic Resonance Angiography").

INDICATIONS
- Detect and locate brain tumors
- Detect cause of cerebrovascular accident, cerebral infarct, or hemorrhage
- Detect cranial bone, face, throat, and neck soft tissue lesions
- Evaluate the cause of seizures, such as intracranial infection, edema, or increased intracranial pressure
- Evaluate cerebral changes associated with dementia
- Evaluate demyelinating disorders
- Evaluate intracranial infections
- Evaluate optic and auditory nerves
- Evaluate the potential causes of headache, visual loss, and vomiting
- Evaluate shunt placement and function in patients with hydrocephalus
- Evaluate the solid, cystic, and hemorrhagic components of lesions
- Evaluate vascularity of the brain and vascular integrity
- Monitor and evaluate the effectiveness of medical or surgical interventions, chemotherapy, radiation therapy, and the course of disease

POTENTIAL DIAGNOSIS

Normal findings in
- Normal anatomic structures, soft tissue density, blood flow rate, face, nasopharynx, neck, tongue, and brain

Abnormal findings in
- Abscess
- Acoustic neuroma
- Alzheimer's disease
- Aneurysm
- Arteriovenous malformation
- Benign meningioma
- Cerebral aneurysm
- Cerebral infarction
- Craniopharyngioma or meningioma
- Granuloma
- Intraparenchymal hematoma or hemorrhage
- Lipoma
- Metastasis
- Multiple sclerosis
- Optic nerve tumor
- Parkinson's disease
- Pituitary microadenoma
- Subdural empyema
- Ventriculitis

CRITICAL FINDINGS
- Abscess
- Cerebral aneurysm
- Cerebral infarct
- Hydrocephalus
- Skull fracture or contusion
- Tumor with significant mass effect

It is essential that critical diagnoses be communicated immediately to the appropriate health-care provider (HCP). A listing of these diagnoses varies among facilities. Note and immediately report to the HCP abnormal results and related symptoms.

INTERFERING FACTORS

This procedure is contraindicated for
- Patients with certain ferrous metal prostheses, valves, aneurysm

M

clips, inner ear prostheses, or other metallic objects.

- ❖ Patients with metal in their body, such as shrapnel or ferrous metal in the eye.
- ❖ Patients with cardiac pacemakers, because the pacemaker can be deactivated by MRI.
- ❖ Use of gadolinium-based contrast agents (GBCAs) is contraindicated in patients with acute or chronic severe renal insufficiency (glomerular filtration rate less than 30 mL/min/1.73 m^2). Patients should be screened for renal dysfunction prior to administration. The use of GBCAs should be avoided in these patients unless the benefits of the studies outweigh the risks and if essential diagnostic information is not available using non-contrast-enhanced diagnostic studies.
- Patients with intrauterine devices.
- Patients with iron pigments in tattoos.
- Patients who are claustrophobic.
- Patients who are pregnant or suspected of being pregnant, unless the potential benefits of the procedure far outweigh the risks to the fetus and mother.

Factors that may impair clear imaging

- Metallic objects (e.g., jewelry, body rings, dental amalgams) within the examination field, which may inhibit organ visualization and cause unclear images.
- Inability of the patient to cooperate or remain still during the procedure because of age, significant pain, or mental status.
- Patients with extreme cases of claustrophobia, unless sedation is given before the study or an open MRI is utilized.

Other considerations

- If contrast medium is allowed to seep deep into the muscle tissue, vascular visualization will be impossible.

M

NURSING IMPLICATIONS AND PROCEDURE

PRETEST:

▸ Positively identify the patient using at least two unique identifiers before providing care, treatment, or services.

▸ *Patient Teaching:* Inform the patient this procedure can assist in assessing the brain.

▸ Obtain a history of the patient's complaints, including a list of known allergens, especially allergies or sensitivities to latex, iodine, seafood, contrast medium, anesthetics, or dyes.

▸ Obtain a history of the patient's cardiovascular and neuromuscular systems, symptoms, and results of previously performed laboratory tests and diagnostic and surgical procedures. Obtain a history of renal dysfunction if the use of GBCA is anticipated.

▸ Ensure the results of BUN, creatinine, and eGFR (estimated glomerular filtration rate) are obtained if GBCA is to be used.

▸ Determine if the patient has ever had any device implanted into his or her body, including copper intrauterine devices, pacemakers, ear implants, and heart valves.

▸ Obtain occupational history to determine the presence of metal in the body, such as shrapnel or flecks of ferrous metal in the eye (which can cause retinal hemorrhage).

▸ Note any recent procedures that can interfere with test results, including examinations using barium- or iodine-based contrast medium.

▸ Record the date of the last menstrual period and determine the possibility of pregnancy in perimenopausal women.

▸ Obtain a list of the patient's current medications, including herbs, nutritional supplements, and nutraceuticals (see Appendix F).

▸ Review the procedure with the patient. Address concerns about pain related to the procedure and explain that no pain will be experienced during the test, but there may be moments of discomfort. Reassure the patient that if contrast is used, it poses no radioactive hazard and rarely produces side effects. Inform the patient the procedure is performed in an MRI department, usually by an HCP who specializes in this procedure, with support staff, and takes approximately 30 to 60 min.

- Inform the patient that the technologist will place him or her in a supine position on a flat table in a large cylindrical scanner.
- Tell the patient to expect to hear loud banging from the scanner and possibly to see magnetophosphenes (flickering lights in the visual field); these will stop when the procedure is over.
- *Sensitivity to social and cultural issues,* as well as concern for modesty, is important in providing psychological support before, during, and after the procedure.
- Explain that an IV line may be inserted to allow infusion of IV fluids, contrast medium, or sedatives.
- Instruct the patient to remove jewelry and all other metallic objects from the area to be examined prior to the procedure.
- There are no food, fluid, or medication restrictions unless by medical direction.

INTRATEST:

- Ensure that the patient has removed all external metallic objects from the area to be examined prior to the procedure.
- If the patient has a history of allergic reactions to any substance or drug, administer ordered prophylactic steroids or antihistamines before the procedure.
- Have emergency equipment readily available.
- Instruct the patient to void prior to the procedure and to change into the gown, robe, and foot coverings provided.
- Instruct the patient to cooperate fully and to follow directions. Instruct the patient to remain still throughout the procedure because movement produces unreliable results.
- Observe standard precautions, and follow the general guidelines in Appendix A.
- Supply earplugs to the patient to block out the loud, banging sounds that occur during the test. Instruct the

patient to communicate with the technologist during the examination via a microphone within the scanner.
- If an electrocardiogram or respiratory gating is to be performed in conjunction with the scan, apply MRI-safe electrodes to the appropriate sites.
- Establish an IV fluid line for the injection of emergency drugs and of sedatives.
- Administer an antianxiety agent, as ordered, if the patient has claustrophobia. Administer a sedative to a child or to an uncooperative adult, as ordered.
- Place the patient in the supine position on an examination table.
- If contrast is used, imaging can begin shortly after the injection.
- Ask the patient to inhale deeply and hold his or her breath while the images are taken and then to exhale after the images are taken.
- Instruct the patient to take slow, deep breaths if nausea occurs during the procedure.
- Monitor the patient for complications related to the procedure (e.g., allergic reaction, anaphylaxis, bronchospasm).
- Remove the needle or catheter and apply a pressure dressing over the puncture site.
- Observe/assess the needle/catheter insertion site for bleeding, inflammation, or hematoma formation.

POST-TEST:

- A report of the results will be sent to the requesting HCP, who will discuss the results with the patient.
- Observe for delayed allergic reactions, such as rash, urticaria, tachycardia, hyperpnea, hypertension, palpitations, nausea, or vomiting, if contrast medium was used.
- Instruct the patient to immediately report symptoms such as fast heart rate, difficulty breathing, skin rash, itching, chest pain, persistent right shoulder pain, or abdominal pain. Immediately report symptoms to the appropriate HCP.
- Instruct the patient to apply cold compresses to the puncture site as needed to reduce discomfort or edema.
- Recognize anxiety related to test results. Discuss the implications of

M

abnormal test results on the patient's lifestyle. Provide teaching and information regarding the clinical implications of the test results, as appropriate.

▶ Reinforce information given by the patient's HCP regarding further testing, treatment, or referral to another HCP. Answer any questions or address any concerns voiced by the patient or family.

▶ Depending on the results of this procedure, additional testing may be performed to evaluate or monitor progression of the disease process and determine the need for a change in therapy. Evaluate test results in relation to the patient's symptoms and other tests performed.

RELATED MONOGRAPHS:

▶ Related tests include Alzheimer's disease markers, angiography of the carotids, BUN, CSF analysis, CT brain, creatinine, EMG, evoked brain potentials, and PET brain.

▶ Refer to the Cardiovascular and Musculoskeletal systems tables at the end of the book for related tests by body system.

Magnetic Resonance Imaging, Breast

SYNONYM/ACRONYM: Breast MRI.

COMMON USE: To visualize and assess abnormalities in breast tissue to assist in evaluating structural abnormalities related to diagnoses such as cancer, abscess, and cysts.

AREA OF APPLICATION: Breast area.

CONTRAST: Can be done with or without IV contrast medium (gadolinium).

DESCRIPTION: Magnetic resonance imaging (MRI) uses a magnet and radio waves to produce an energy field that can be displayed as an image. Use of magnetic fields with the aid of radiofrequency energy produces images primarily based on water content of tissue. The magnetic field causes the hydrogen atoms in tissue to line up, and when radio waves are directed toward the magnetic field, the atoms absorb the radio waves and change their position. When the radio waves are turned off, the atoms go back to their original position; this change in the energy field is sensed by the equipment, and an image is generated by the attached computer system. MRI produces cross-sectional images of the pathological lesions in multiple planes without the use of ionizing radiation or the interference of surrounding tissue, breast implants, or surgically implanted clips.

MRI imaging of the breast is not a replacement for traditional mammography, ultrasound, or biopsy. This examination is extremely helpful in evaluating mammogram abnormalities and identifying early breast cancer in women at high risk. High-risk women include those who have had breast cancer, have an abnormal mutated breast cancer gene (BRCA1 or BRCA2), or have a mother or sister who has been diagnosed with breast cancer. Breast MRI is used most commonly in high-risk women when findings of a mammogram or ultrasound are inconclusive because of dense breast tissue or there is a suspected abnormality that requires further evaluation. MRI is also an excellent examination in the augmented breast, including both the breast implant and the breast tissue surrounding the implant. This same examination is also useful for staging breast cancer and determining the most appropriate treatment. MRI uses the noniodinated contrast medium gadopentetate dimeglumine (Magnevist), which is administered IV to enhance contrast differences between normal and abnormal tissues.

INDICATIONS
- Evaluate breast implants
- Evaluate dense breasts
- Evaluate for residual cancer after lumpectomy
- Evaluate inverted nipples
- Evaluate small abnormalities
- Evaluate tissue after lumpectomy or mastectomy
- Evaluate women at high risk for breast cancer

POTENTIAL DIAGNOSIS

Normal findings in
- Normal anatomic structures, soft tissue density, and blood flow rate

Abnormal findings in
- Breast abscess or cyst
- Breast cancer
- Breast implant rupture
- Hematoma
- Soft tissue masses
- Vascular abnormalities

CRITICAL FINDINGS: N/A

INTERFERING FACTORS

This procedure is contraindicated for
- Patients with certain ferrous metal prostheses, valves, aneurysm clips, inner ear prostheses, or other metallic objects.
- Patients with metal in their body, such as shrapnel or ferrous metal in the eye.
- Patients with cardiac pacemakers, because the pacemaker can be deactivated by MRI.
- Use of gadolinium-based contrast agents (GBCAs) is contraindicated in patients with acute or chronic severe renal insufficiency (glomerular filtration rate less than 30 mL/min/1.73 m^2). Patients should be screened for renal dysfunction prior to administration. The use of GBCAs should be avoided in these patients unless the benefits of the studies outweigh the risks and if essential diagnostic information is not available using non-contrast-enhanced diagnostic studies.
- Patients with intrauterine devices.
- Patients with iron pigments in tattoos.
- Patients who are claustrophobic.
- Patients who are pregnant or suspected of being pregnant, unless the potential benefits of the procedure far outweigh the risks to the fetus and mother.

Factors that may impair clear imaging
- Metallic objects (e.g., jewelry, body rings) within the examination field, which may inhibit organ visualization and cause unclear images.
- Inability of the patient to cooperate or remain still during the procedure because of age, significant pain, or mental status.

M

• Patients with extreme cases of claustrophobia, unless sedation is given before the study or an open MRI is utilized.

Other considerations

• If contrast medium is allowed to seep deep into the muscle tissue, vascular visualization will be impossible.

• The procedure can be nonspecific; the examination is unable to image calcifications that can indicate breast cancer, and there may be difficulty distinguishing between cancerous and noncancerous tumors.

NURSING IMPLICATIONS AND PROCEDURE

PRETEST:

▶ Positively identify the patient using at least two unique identifiers before providing care, treatment, or services.

▶ *Patient Teaching:* Inform the patient this procedure can assist in assessing the breast.

▶ Obtain a history of the patient's complaints, including a list of known allergens, especially allergies or sensitivities to latex, iodine, seafood, contrast medium, anesthetics, or dyes.

▶ Obtain a history of the patient's reproductive system, symptoms, and results of previously performed laboratory tests and diagnostic and surgical procedures. Obtain a history of renal dysfunction if the use of GBCA is anticipated.

▶ Ensure the results of BUN, creatinine, and eGFR (estimated glomerular filtration rate) are obtained if GBCA is to be used.

▶ Determine if the patient has ever had any device implanted into his or her body, including copper intrauterine devices, pacemakers, ear implants, and heart valves.

▶ Obtain occupational history to determine the presence of metal in the body, such as shrapnel or flecks of ferrous metal in the eye (which can cause retinal hemorrhage).

▶ Note any recent procedures that can interfere with test results, including examinations using barium- or iodine-based contrast medium.

▶ Record the date of the last menstrual period and determine the possibility of pregnancy in perimenopausal women.

▶ Obtain a list of the patient's current medications, including herbs, nutritional supplements, and nutraceuticals (see Appendix F).

▶ Review the procedure with the patient. Address concerns about pain related to the procedure and explain that no pain will be experienced during the test, but there may be moments of discomfort. Reassure the patient that if contrast is used, it poses no radioactive hazard and rarely produces side effects. Inform the patient that the procedure is performed in an MRI department by a health-care provider (HCP) who specializes in this procedure, with support staff, and takes approximately 30 to 60 min.

▶ Inform the patient that the technologist will place him or her in a prone position on a special imaging table in a large cylindrical scanner.

▶ Tell the patient to expect to hear loud banging from the scanner and possibly to see magnetophosphenes (flickering lights in the visual field); these will stop when the procedure is over.

▶ *Sensitivity to social and cultural issues,* as well as concern for modesty, is important in providing psychological support before, during, and after the procedure.

▶ Explain that an IV line may be inserted to allow infusion of IV fluids, contrast medium, or sedatives.

▶ Instruct the patient to remove jewelry and all other metallic objects from the area to be examined prior to the procedure.

▶ There are no food, fluid, or medication restrictions unless by medical direction.

INTRATEST:

▶ Ensure that the patient has removed all external metallic objects from the area to be examined prior to the procedure.

▶ If the patient has a history of allergic reactions to any substance or drug, administer ordered prophylactic steroids or antihistamines before the procedure.

▶ Have emergency equipment readily available.

▶ Instruct the patient to void prior to the procedure and to change into the gown, robe, and foot coverings provided.

▶ Instruct the patient to cooperate fully and to follow directions. Instruct the patient to remain still throughout the procedure because movement produces unreliable results.

▶ Observe standard precautions, and follow the general guidelines in Appendix A.

▶ Supply earplugs to the patient to block out the loud, banging sounds that occur during the test. Instruct the patient to communicate with the technologist during the examination via a microphone within the scanner.

▶ Establish an IV fluid line for the injection of emergency drugs and of sedatives.

▶ Administer an antianxiety agent, as ordered, if the patient has claustrophobia. Administer a sedative to a child or to an uncooperative adult, as ordered.

▶ Place the patient in the prone position on a special examination table designed for breast imaging.

▶ If contrast is used, imaging can begin shortly after the injection.

▶ Ask the patient to inhale deeply and hold his or her breath while the images are taken and then to exhale after the images are taken.

▶ Instruct the patient to take slow, deep breaths if nausea occurs during the procedure.

▶ Monitor the patient for complications related to the procedure (e.g., allergic reaction, anaphylaxis, bronchospasm).

▶ Remove the needle or catheter and apply a pressure dressing over the puncture site.

▶ Observe/assess the needle/catheter insertion site for bleeding, inflammation, or hematoma formation.

POST-TEST:

▶ A report of the results will be sent to the requesting HCP, who will discuss the results with the patient.

▶ Observe for delayed allergic reactions, such as rash, urticaria, tachycardia, hyperpnea, hypertension, palpitations, nausea, or vomiting.

▶ Instruct the patient to immediately report symptoms such as fast heart rate, difficulty breathing, skin rash, itching, chest pain, persistent right shoulder pain, or abdominal pain. Immediately report symptoms to the appropriate HCP.

▶ Instruct the patient in the care and assessment of the injection site.

▶ Instruct the patient to apply cold compresses to the puncture site as needed to reduce discomfort or edema.

▶ Recognize anxiety related to test results. Discuss the implications of abnormal test results on the patient's lifestyle. Provide teaching and information regarding the clinical implications of the test results, as appropriate. Educate the patient regarding access to counseling services.

▶ Reinforce information given by the patient's HCP regarding further testing, treatment, or referral to another HCP. Decisions regarding the need for and frequency of breast self-examination, mammography, MRI breast, or other cancer screening procedures should be made after consultation between the patient and HCP. The most current guidelines for breast cancer screening of the general population as well as for individuals with increased risk are available from the American Cancer Society (www.cancer.org), the American College of Obstetricians and Gynecologists (ACOG) (www.acog.org), and the American College of Radiology (www.acr.org). Answer any questions or address any concerns voiced by the patient or family.

▶ Depending on the results of this procedure, additional testing may be performed to evaluate or monitor progression of the disease process and determine the need for a change in therapy. Evaluate test results in relation to the patient's symptoms and other tests performed.

RELATED MONOGRAPHS:

▶ Related tests include biopsy breast, bone scan, BUN, cancer antigens, CT thorax, creatinine, ductography, mammogram, stereotactic biopsy breast, and US breast.

▶ Refer to the Reproductive System table at the end of the book for related tests by body system.

M

Magnetic Resonance Imaging, Chest

SYNONYM/ACRONYM: Chest MRI.

COMMON USE: To visualize and assess pulmonary and cardiovascular structures to assist in diagnosing tumor, masses, aneurysm, infarct, air, fluid, and evaluate the effectiveness of medical, and surgical interventions.

AREA OF APPLICATION: Chest/thorax.

CONTRAST: Can be done with or without IV contrast medium (gadolinium).

DESCRIPTION: Magnetic resonance imaging (MRI) uses a magnet and radio waves to produce an energy field that can be displayed as an image. Use of magnetic fields with the aid of radiofrequency energy produces images primarily based on water content of tissue. The magnetic field causes the hydrogen atoms in tissue to line up, and when radio waves are directed toward the magnetic field, the atoms absorb the radio waves and change their position. When the radio waves are turned off, the atoms go back to their original position; this change in the energy field is sensed by the equipment, and an image is generated by the attached computer system. MRI produces cross-sectional images of pathological lesions in multiple planes without the use of ionizing radiation or the interference of bone or surrounding tissue.

Chest MRI scanning is performed to assist in diagnosing abnormalities of cardiovascular and pulmonary structures. Two special techniques are available for evaluation of cardiovascular structures. One is the electrocardiograph (ECG)–gated multislice spin-echo sequence, used to diagnose anatomic abnormalities of the heart and aorta, and the other is the ECG-referenced gradient refocused sequence, used to diagnose heart function and analyze blood flow patterns.

Magnetic resonance angiography (MRA) is an application of MRI that provides images of blood flow and diseased and normal blood vessels. In patients who are allergic to iodinated contrast medium, MRA is used in place of angiography (see monograph titled "Magnetic Resonance Angiography").

INDICATIONS
- Confirm diagnosis of cardiac and pericardiac masses
- Detect aortic aneurysms
- Detect myocardial infarction and cardiac muscle ischemia
- Detect pericardial abnormalities
- Detect pleural effusion
- Detect thoracic aortic diseases
- Determine blood, fluid, or fat accumulation in tissues, pleuritic space, or vessels
- Determine cardiac ventricular function

M

- Differentiate aortic aneurysms from tumors near the aorta
- Evaluate cardiac chambers and pulmonary vessels
- Evaluate postoperative angioplasty sites and bypass grafts
- Identify congenital heart diseases
- Monitor and evaluate the effectiveness of medical or surgical therapeutic regimen

POTENTIAL DIAGNOSIS

Normal findings in
- Normal heart and lung structures, soft tissue, and function, including blood flow rate

Abnormal findings in
- Aortic dissection
- Congenital heart diseases, including pulmonary atresia, aortic coarctation, agenesis of the pulmonary artery, and transposition of the great vessels
- Constrictive pericarditis
- Intramural and periaortic hematoma
- Myocardial infarction
- Pericardial hematoma or effusion
- Pleural effusion

CRITICAL FINDINGS

- Aortic aneurysm
- Aortic dissection
- Tumor with significant mass effect

It is essential that critical diagnoses be communicated immediately to the appropriate health-care provider (HCP). A listing of these diagnoses varies among facilities. Note and immediately report to the HCP abnormal results and related symptoms.

INTERFERING FACTORS

This procedure is contraindicated for
- Patients with certain ferrous metal prostheses, valves, aneurysm clips, inner ear prostheses, or other metallic objects.

- ◈ Patients with metal in their body, such as shrapnel or ferrous metal in the eye.
- ◈ Patients with cardiac pacemakers, because the pacemaker can be deactivated by MRI.
- ◈ Use of gadolinium-based contrast agents (GBCAs) is contraindicated in patients with acute or chronic severe renal insufficiency (glomerular filtration rate less than 30 mL/min/1.73 m^2). Patients should be screened for renal dysfunction prior to administration. The use of GBCAs should be avoided in these patients unless the benefits of the studies outweigh the risks and if essential diagnostic information is not available using non-contrast-enhanced diagnostic studies.
- Patients with intrauterine devices.
- Patients with iron pigments in tattoos.
- Patients who are claustrophobic.
- Patients who are pregnant or suspected of being pregnant, unless the potential benefits of the procedure far outweigh the risks to the fetus and mother.

Factors that may impair clear imaging
- Metallic objects (e.g., jewelry, body rings, dental amalgams) within the examination field, which may inhibit organ visualization and cause unclear images.
- Inability of the patient to cooperate or remain still during the procedure because of age, significant pain, or mental status.
- Patients with extreme cases of claustrophobia, unless sedation is given before the study or an open MRI is utilized.

Other considerations
- If contrast medium is allowed to seep deep into the muscle tissue, vascular visualization will be impossible.

NURSING IMPLICATIONS AND PROCEDURE

PRETEST:

▶ Positively identify the patient using at least two unique identifiers before providing care, treatment, or services.

▶ *Patient Teaching:* Inform the patient this procedure can assist in assessing organs and structures inside the chest.

▶ Obtain a history of the patient's complaints, including a list of known allergens, especially allergies or sensitivities to latex, iodine, seafood, contrast medium, anesthetics, or dyes.

▶ Obtain a history of the patient's cardiovascular and respiratory systems, symptoms, and results of previously performed laboratory tests and diagnostic and surgical procedures. Obtain a history of renal dysfunction if the use of GBCA is anticipated.

▶ Ensure the results of BUN, creatinine, and eGFR (estimated glomerular filtration rate) are obtained if GBCA is to be used.

▶ Determine if the patient has ever had any device implanted into his or her body, including copper intrauterine devices, pacemakers, ear implants, and heart valves.

▶ Obtain occupational history to determine the presence of metal in the body, such as shrapnel or flecks of ferrous metal in the eye (which can cause retinal hemorrhage).

▶ Note any recent procedures that can interfere with test results, including examinations using barium- or iodine-based contrast medium.

▶ Record the date of the last menstrual period and determine possibility of pregnancy in perimenopausal women.

▶ Obtain a list of the patient's current medications, including herbs, nutritional supplements, and nutraceuticals (see Appendix F).

▶ Review the procedure with the patient. Address concerns about pain related to the procedure and explain that no pain will be experienced during the test, but there may be moments of discomfort. Reassure the patient that if contrast is used, it poses no radioactive hazard and rarely produces side effects. Inform the patient the procedure is performed in an MRI department, usually by an HCP who specializes in these procedures, with support staff, and takes approximately 30 to 60 min.

▶ Inform the patient that the technologist will place him or her in a supine position on a flat table in a large cylindrical scanner.

▶ Tell the patient to expect to hear loud banging from the scanner and possibly to see magnetophosphenes (flickering lights in the visual field); these will stop when the procedure is over.

▶ *Sensitivity to social and cultural issues,* as well as concern for modesty, is important in providing psychological support before, during, and after the procedure.

▶ Explain that an IV line may be inserted to allow infusion of IV fluids, contrast medium, or sedatives.

▶ Instruct the patient to remove jewelry and all other metallic objects from the area to be examined prior to the procedure.

▶ There are no food, fluid, or medication restrictions unless by medical direction.

INTRATEST:

▶ Ensure that the patient has removed all external metallic objects from the area to be examined prior to the procedure.

▶ If the patient has a history of allergic reactions to any substance or drug, administer ordered prophylactic steroids or antihistamines before the procedure.

▶ Have emergency equipment readily available.

▶ Instruct the patient to void prior to the procedure and to change into the gown, robe, and foot coverings provided.

▶ Instruct the patient to cooperate fully and to follow directions. Instruct the patient to remain still throughout the procedure because movement produces unreliable results.

▶ Observe standard precautions, and follow the general guidelines in Appendix A.

▶ Supply earplugs to the patient to block out the loud, banging sounds that occur during the test. Instruct the patient to communicate with the technologist during the examination via a microphone within the scanner.

▶ If an electrocardiogram or respiratory gating is to be performed in conjunction with the scan, apply MRI-safe electrodes to the appropriate sites.

- Establish an IV fluid line for the injection of emergency drugs and of sedatives.
- Administer an antianxiety agent, as ordered, if the patient has claustrophobia. Administer a sedative to a child or to an uncooperative adult, as ordered.
- Place the patient in the supine position on an examination table.
- If contrast is used, imaging can begin shortly after the injection.
- Ask the patient to inhale deeply and hold his or her breath while the images are taken and then to exhale after the images are taken.
- Instruct the patient to take slow, deep breaths if nausea occurs during the procedure.
- Monitor the patient for complications related to the procedure (e.g., allergic reaction, anaphylaxis, bronchospasm).
- Remove the needle or catheter and apply a pressure dressing over the puncture site.
- Observe/assess the needle/catheter insertion site for bleeding, inflammation, or hematoma formation.

POST-TEST:

- A report of the results will be sent to the requesting HCP, who will discuss the results with the patient.
- Observe for delayed allergic reactions, such as rash, urticaria, tachycardia, hyperpnea, hypertension, palpitations, nausea, or vomiting.
- Instruct the patient to immediately report symptoms such as fast heart rate, difficulty breathing, skin rash, itching, chest

pain, persistent right shoulder pain, or abdominal pain. Immediately report symptoms to the appropriate HCP.

- Instruct the patient in the care and assessment of the injection site.
- Instruct the patient to apply cold compresses to the puncture site as needed to reduce discomfort or edema.
- Recognize anxiety related to test results. Discuss the implications of abnormal test results on the patient's lifestyle. Provide teaching and information regarding the clinical implications of the test results, as appropriate.
- Reinforce information given by the patient's HCP regarding further testing, treatment, or referral to another HCP. Answer any questions or address any concerns voiced by the patient or family.
- Depending on the results of this procedure, additional testing may be performed to evaluate or monitor progression of the disease process and determine the need for a change in therapy. Evaluate test results in relation to the patient's symptoms and other tests performed.

RELATED MONOGRAPHS:

- Related tests include AST, BNP, blood gases, blood pool imaging, BUN, chest x-ray, CT cardiac scoring, CT thorax, CRP, CK and isoenzymes, creatinine, echocardiography, exercise stress test, Holter monitor, myocardial infarct scan, myocardial perfusion heart scan, myoglobin, pleural fluid analysis, PET scan of the heart, and troponins.
- Refer to the Cardiovascular and Respiratory systems tables at the end of the book for related tests by body system.

M

Magnetic Resonance Imaging, Musculoskeletal

SYNONYM/ACRONYM: Musculoskeletal (knee, shoulder, hand, wrist, foot, elbow, hip, spine) MRI.

COMMON USE: To visualize and assess bones, joints, and surrounding structures to assist in diagnosing defects, cysts, tumors, and fracture.

AREA OF APPLICATION: Bones, joints, soft tissues.

CONTRAST: Can be done with or without IV contrast medium (gadolinium).

DESCRIPTION: Magnetic resonance imaging (MRI) uses a magnet and radio waves to produce an energy field that can be displayed as an image. Use of magnetic fields with the aid of radiofrequency energy produces images primarily based on water content of tissue. The magnetic field causes the hydrogen atoms in tissue to line up, and when radio waves are directed toward the magnetic field, the atoms absorb the radio waves and change their position. When the radio waves are turned off, the atoms go back to their original position; this change in the energy field is sensed by the equipment, and an image is generated by the attached computer system. MRI produces cross-sectional images of bones and joints in multiple planes without the use of ionizing radiation or the interference of bone or surrounding tissue.

Musculoskeletal MRI is performed to assist in diagnosing abnormalities of bones and joints and surrounding soft tissue structures, including cartilage, synovium, ligaments, and tendons. MRI eliminates the risks associated with exposure to x-rays and causes no harm to cells. Contrast-enhanced imaging is effective for evaluating scarring from previous surgery, vascular abnormalities, and differentiation of metastases from primary tumors. MRI uses the noniodinated contrast medium gadopentetate dimeglumine (Magnevist), which is administered IV to enhance contrast differences between normal and abnormal tissues.

Magnetic resonance angiography (MRA) is an application of MRI that provides images of blood flow and diseased and normal blood vessels. In patients who are allergic to iodinated contrast medium, MRA is used in place of angiography (see monograph titled "Magnetic Resonance Angiography").

INDICATIONS
- Confirm diagnosis of osteomyelitis
- Detect avascular necrosis of the femoral head or knee
- Detect benign and cancerous tumors and cysts of the bone or soft tissue
- Detect bone infarcts in the epiphyseal or diaphyseal sites
- Detect changes in bone marrow
- Detect tears or degeneration of ligaments, tendons, and menisci resulting from trauma or pathology
- Determine cause of low back pain, including herniated disk and spinal degenerative disease
- Differentiate between primary and secondary malignant processes of the bone marrow
- Differentiate between a stress fracture and a tumor
- Evaluate meniscal detachment of the temporomandibular joint

POTENTIAL DIAGNOSIS

Normal findings in
- Normal bones, joints, and surrounding tissue structures; no articular disease, bone marrow disorders, tumors, infections, or trauma to the bones, joints, or muscles

Abnormal findings in

- Avascular necrosis of femoral head or knee, as found in Legg-Calvé-Perthes disease
- Bone marrow disease, such as Gaucher's disease, aplastic anemia, sickle cell disease, or polycythemia
- Degenerative spinal disease, such as spondylosis or arthritis
- Fibrosarcoma
- Hemangioma (muscular or osseous)
- Herniated disk
- Infection
- Meniscal tears or degeneration
- Osteochondroma
- Osteogenic sarcoma
- Osteomyelitis
- Rotator cuff tears
- Spinal stenosis
- Stress fracture
- Synovitis
- Tumor

CRITICAL FINDINGS: N/A

INTERFERING FACTORS

This procedure is contraindicated for

- Patients with certain ferrous metal prostheses, valves, aneurysm clips, inner ear prostheses, or other metallic objects.
- Patients with cardiac pacemakers, because the pacemaker can be deactivated by MRI.
- Use of gadolinium-based contrast agents (GBCAs) is contraindicated in patients with acute or chronic severe renal insufficiency (glomerular filtration rate less than 30 mL/min/1.73 m^2). Patients should be screened for renal dysfunction prior to administration. The use of GBCAs should be avoided in these patients unless the benefits of the studies outweigh the risks and if essential diagnostic information is not available using non-contrast-enhanced diagnostic studies.

- Patients with metal in their body, such as shrapnel or ferrous metal in the eye.
- Patients with intrauterine devices.
- Patients with iron pigments in tattoos.
- Patients who are claustrophobic.
- Patients who are pregnant or suspected of being pregnant, unless the potential benefits of the procedure far outweigh the risks to the fetus and mother.

Factors that may impair clear imaging

- Metallic objects (e.g., jewelry, body rings, dental amalgams) within the examination field, which may inhibit organ visualization and cause unclear images.
- Inability of the patient to cooperate or remain still during the procedure because of age, significant pain, or mental status.
- Patients with extreme cases of claustrophobia, unless sedation is given before the study or an open MRI is utilized.

Other considerations

- If contrast medium is allowed to seep deep into the muscle tissue, vascular visualization will be impossible.

M

NURSING IMPLICATIONS AND PROCEDURE

PRETEST:

- Positively identify the patient using at least two unique identifiers before providing care, treatment, or services.
- *Patient Teaching:* Inform the patient this procedure can assist in assessing bones, muscles, and joints.
- Obtain a history of the patient's complaints, including a list of known allergens, especially allergies or sensitivities to latex, iodine, seafood, contrast medium, anesthetics, or dyes.

▸ Obtain a history of the patient's musculoskeletal system, symptoms, and results of previously performed laboratory tests and diagnostic and surgical procedures. Obtain a history of renal dysfunction if the use of GBCA is anticipated.

▸ Ensure the results of BUN, creatinine, and eGFR (estimated glomerular filtration rate) are obtained if GBCA is to be used.

▸ Determine if the patient has ever had any device implanted into his or her body, including copper intrauterine devices, pacemakers, ear implants, and heart valves.

▸ Obtain occupational history to determine the presence of metal in the body, such as shrapnel or flecks of ferrous metal in the eye (which can cause retinal hemorrhage).

▸ Note any recent procedures that can interfere with test results, including examinations using barium- or iodine-based contrast medium.

▸ Record the date of the last menstrual period and determine the possibility of pregnancy in perimenopausal women.

▸ Obtain a list of the patient's current medications, including herbs, nutritional supplements, and nutraceuticals (see Appendix F).

▸ Review the procedure with the patient. Address concerns about pain related to the procedure and explain that no pain will be experienced during the test, but there may be moments of discomfort. Reassure the patient that if contrast is used, it poses no radioactive hazard and rarely produces side effects. Inform the patient the procedure is performed in an MRI department, usually by a health-care provider (HCP) specializing in this procedure, with support staff, and takes approximately 30 to 60 min.

▸ Inform the patient that the technologist will place him or her in a supine position on a flat table in a large cylindrical scanner.

▸ Tell the patient to expect to hear loud banging from the scanner and possibly to see magnetophosphenes (flickering lights in the visual field); these will stop when the procedure is over.

▸ *Sensitivity to social and cultural issues,* as well as concern for modesty, is important in providing psychological support before, during, and after the procedure.

▸ Explain that an IV line may be inserted to allow infusion of IV fluids, contrast medium, or sedatives.

▸ Instruct the patient to remove jewelry and all other metallic objects from the area to be examined prior to the procedure.

▸ There are no food, fluid, or medication restrictions unless by medical direction.

INTRATEST:

▸ Ensure that the patient has removed all external metallic objects from the area to be examined prior to the procedure.

▸ If the patient has a history of allergic reactions to any substance or drug, administer ordered prophylactic steroids or antihistamines before the procedure.

▸ Have emergency equipment readily available.

▸ Instruct the patient to void prior to the procedure and to change into the gown, robe, and foot coverings provided.

▸ Instruct the patient to cooperate fully and to follow directions. Instruct the patient to remain still throughout the procedure because movement produces unreliable results.

▸ Observe standard precautions, and follow the general guidelines in Appendix A.

▸ Supply earplugs to the patient to block out the loud, banging sounds that occur during the test. Instruct the patient to communicate with the technologist during the examination via a microphone within the scanner.

▸ Establish an IV fluid line for the injection of emergency drugs and of sedatives.

▸ Administer an antianxiety agent, as ordered, if the patient has claustrophobia. Administer a sedative to a child or to an uncooperative adult, as ordered.

▸ Place the patient in the supine position on an examination table.

▸ If contrast is used, imaging can begin shortly after the injection.

▸ Ask the patient to inhale deeply and hold his or her breath while the images are taken and then to exhale after the images are taken.

▸ Instruct the patient to take slow, deep breaths if nausea occurs during the procedure.

- Monitor the patient for complications related to the procedure (e.g., allergic reaction, anaphylaxis, bronchospasm).
- Remove the needle or catheter and apply a pressure dressing over the puncture site.
- Observe/assess the needle/catheter insertion site for bleeding, inflammation, or hematoma formation.

POST-TEST:

- A report of the results will be sent to the requesting HCP, who will discuss the results with the patient.
- Observe for delayed allergic reactions, such as rash, urticaria, tachycardia, hyperpnea, hypertension, palpitations, nausea, or vomiting, if contrast medium was used.
- Instruct the patient to immediately report symptoms such as fast heart rate, difficulty breathing, skin rash, itching, chest pain, persistent right shoulder pain, or abdominal pain. Immediately report symptoms to the appropriate HCP.
- Instruct the patient in the care and assessment of the injection site.
- Instruct the patient to apply cold compresses to the puncture site as needed, to reduce discomfort or edema.

- Recognize anxiety related to test results. Discuss the implications of abnormal test results on the patient's lifestyle. Provide teaching and information regarding the clinical implications of the test results, as appropriate.
- Reinforce information given by the patient's HCP regarding further testing, treatment, or referral to another HCP. Answer any questions or address any concerns voiced by the patient or family.
- Depending on the results of this procedure, additional testing may be performed to evaluate or monitor progression of the disease process and determine the need for a change in therapy. Evaluate test results in relation to the patient's symptoms and other tests performed.

RELATED MONOGRAPHS:

- Related tests include anticyclic citrullinated antibodies, ANA, arthrogram, arthroscopy, bone mineral densitometry, bone scan, BUN, CRP, CT spine, creatinine, ESR, radiography of the bone, synovial fluid analysis, RF, and vertebroplasty.
- Refer to the Musculoskeletal System table at the end of the book for related tests by body system.

M

Magnetic Resonance Imaging, Pancreas

SYNONYM/ACRONYM: Pancreatic MRI.

COMMON USE: To visualize and assess the pancreas for structural defects, tumor, masses, staging cancer, and evaluating the effectiveness of medical and surgical interventions.

AREA OF APPLICATION: Pancreatic/upper abdominal area.

CONTRAST: Can be done with or without IV contrast medium (gadolinium).

DESCRIPTION: Magnetic resonance imaging (MRI) uses a magnet and radio waves to produce an energy field that can be displayed as an image. Use of magnetic fields with the aid of radiofrequency energy produces images primarily based on water content of tissue. The magnetic field causes the hydrogen atoms in tissue to line up, and when radio waves are directed toward the magnetic field, the atoms absorb the radio waves and change their position. When the radio waves are turned off, the atoms go back to their original position; this change in the energy field is sensed by the equipment, and an image is generated by the attached computer system. MRI produces cross-sectional images of the abdominal area in multiple planes without the use of ionizing radiation or the interference of bone or surrounding tissue.

MRI of the pancreas is employed to evaluate small pancreatic adenocarcinomas, islet cell tumors, ductal abnormalities and calculi, or parenchymal abnormalities. A T1-weighted, fat-saturation series of images is probably best for evaluating the pancreatic parenchyma. This sequence is ideal for showing fat planes between the pancreas and peripancreatic structures and for identifying abnormalities such as fatty infiltration of the pancreas, hemorrhage, adenopathy, and carcinomas. T2-weighted images are most useful for depicting intrapancreatic or peripancreatic fluid collections, pancreatic neoplasms, and calculi. Imaging sequences can be adjusted to display fluid in the biliary tree and pancreatic ducts. MRI uses the nonioinated contrast medium gadopentetate dimeglumine (Magnevist), which is administered IV to enhance contrast differences between normal and abnormal tissues.

Magnetic resonance angiography (MRA) is an application of MRI that provides images of blood flow and diseased and normal blood vessels. In patients who are allergic to iodinated contrast medium, MRA is used in place of angiography (see monograph titled "Magnetic Resonance Angiography").

INDICATIONS

- Detect pancreatic fatty infiltration, hemorrhage, and adenopathy
- Detect a pancreatic mass
- Detect pancreatitis
- Detect primary or metastatic tumors of the pancreas and provide cancer staging
- Detect soft tissue abnormalities
- Determine vascular complications of pancreatitis, venous thrombosis, or pseudoaneurysm
- Differentiate tumors from other abnormalities, such as cysts, cavernous hemangiomas, and pancreatic abscesses
- Monitor and evaluate the effectiveness of medical or surgical interventions and course of disease

POTENTIAL DIAGNOSIS

Normal findings in

- Normal anatomic structures and soft tissue density and biochemical constituents of the pancreatic parenchyma, including blood flow

Abnormal findings in

- Islet cell tumor
- Metastasis
- Pancreatic duct obstruction or calculi
- Pancreatic fatty infiltration, hemorrhage, and adenopathy
- Pancreatic mass
- Pancreatitis

CRITICAL FINDINGS: N/A

INTERFERING FACTORS

This procedure is contraindicated for
- Patients with certain ferrous metal prostheses, valves, aneurysm clips, inner ear prostheses, or other metallic objects.
- ✦ Patients with metal in their body, such as shrapnel or ferrous metal in the eye.
- ✦ Patients with cardiac pacemakers, because the pacemaker can be deactivated by MRI.
- ✦ Use of gadolinium-based contrast agents (GBCAs) is contraindicated in patients with acute or chronic severe renal insufficiency (glomerular filtration rate less than 30 mL/min/1.73 m^2). Patients should be screened for renal dysfunction prior to administration. The use of GBCAs should be avoided in these patients unless the benefits of the studies outweigh the risks and if essential diagnostic information is not available using non-contrast-enhanced diagnostic studies.
- Patients with intrauterine devices.
- Patients with iron pigments in tattoos.
- Patients who are claustrophobic.
- Patients who are pregnant or suspected of being pregnant, unless the potential benefits of the procedure far outweigh the risks to the fetus and mother.

Factors that may impair clear imaging
- Metallic objects (e.g., jewelry, body rings, dental amalgams) within the examination field, which may inhibit organ visualization and cause unclear images.
- Inability of the patient to cooperate or remain still during the procedure because of age, significant pain, or mental status.

- Patients with extreme cases of claustrophobia, unless sedation is given before the study or an open MRI is utilized.

Other considerations
- If contrast medium is allowed to seep deep into the muscle tissue, vascular visualization will be impossible.

NURSING IMPLICATIONS AND PROCEDURE

PRETEST:
- Positively identify the patient using at least two unique identifiers before providing care, treatment, or services.
- *Patient Teaching:* Inform the patient this procedure can assist in assessing the pancreas, organs, and structures inside the abdomen.
- Obtain a history of the patient's complaints, including a list of known allergens, especially allergies or sensitivities to latex, iodine, seafood, contrast medium, anesthetics, or dyes.
- Obtain a history of the patient's endocrine and hepatobiliary systems, symptoms, and results of previously performed laboratory tests and diagnostic and surgical procedures. Obtain a history of renal dysfunction if the use of GBCA is anticipated.
- Ensure the results of BUN, creatinine, and eGFR (estimated glomerular filtration rate) are obtained if GBCA is to be used.
- Determine if the patient has ever had any device implanted into his or her body, including copper intrauterine devices, pacemakers, ear implants, and heart valves.
- Obtain occupational history to determine the presence of metal in the body, such as shrapnel or flecks of ferrous metal in the eye (which can cause retinal hemorrhage).
- Note any recent procedures that can interfere with test results, including examinations using barium- or iodine-based contrast medium.

M

- Record the date of the last menstrual period and determine the possibility of pregnancy in perimenopausal women.
- Obtain a list of the patient's current medications, including herbs, nutritional supplements, and nutraceuticals (see Appendix F).
- Review the procedure with the patient. Address concerns about pain related to the procedure and explain that no pain will be experienced during the test, but there may be moments of discomfort. Reassure the patient that if contrast is used, it poses no radioactive hazard and rarely produces side effects. Inform the patient that the procedure is performed in an MRI department by a health-care provider (HCP) specializing in this procedure, with support staff, and takes approximately 30 to 60 min.
- Inform the patient that the technologist will place him or her in a supine position on a flat table in a large cylindrical scanner.
- Tell the patient to expect to hear loud banging from the scanner and possibly to see magnetophosphenes (flickering lights in the visual field); these will stop when the procedure is over.
- *Sensitivity to social and cultural issues,* as well as concern for modesty, is important in providing psychological support before, during, and after the procedure.
- Explain that an IV line may be inserted to allow infusion of IV fluids, contrast medium, or sedatives.
- Instruct the patient to remove jewelry and all other metallic objects from the area to be examined prior to the procedure.
- There are no food, fluid, or medication restrictions unless by medical direction.

INTRATEST:

- Ensure that the patient has removed all external metallic objects from the area to be examined prior to the procedure.
- If the patient has a history of allergic reactions to any substance or drug, administer ordered prophylactic steroids or antihistamines before the procedure.
- Have emergency equipment readily available.

- Instruct the patient to void prior to the procedure and to change into the gown, robe, and foot coverings provided.
- Instruct the patient to cooperate fully and to follow directions. Instruct the patient to remain still throughout the procedure because movement produces unreliable results.
- Observe standard precautions, and follow the general guidelines in Appendix A.
- Supply earplugs to the patient to block out the loud, banging sounds that occur during the test. Instruct the patient to communicate with the technologist during the examination via a microphone within the scanner.
- Establish an IV fluid line for the injection of emergency drugs and of sedatives.
- Administer an antianxiety agent, as ordered, if the patient has claustrophobia. Administer a sedative to a child or to an uncooperative adult, as ordered.
- Place the patient in the supine position on an examination table.
- If contrast is used, imaging can begin shortly after the injection.
- Ask the patient to inhale deeply and hold his or her breath while the images are taken and then to exhale after the images are taken.
- Instruct the patient to take slow, deep breaths if nausea occurs during the procedure.
- Monitor the patient for complications related to the procedure (e.g., allergic reaction, anaphylaxis, bronchospasm).
- Remove the needle or catheter and apply a pressure dressing over the puncture site.
- Observe/assess the needle/catheter insertion site for bleeding, inflammation, or hematoma formation.

POST-TEST:

- A report of the results will be sent to the requesting HCP, who will discuss the results with the patient.
- Observe for delayed allergic reactions, such as rash, urticaria, tachycardia, hyperpnea, hypertension, palpitations, nausea, or vomiting.
- Instruct the patient to immediately report symptoms such as fast heart rate, difficulty breathing, skin

rash, itching, chest pain, persistent right shoulder pain, or abdominal pain. Immediately report symptoms to the appropriate HCP.
- Instruct the patient in the care and assessment of the injection site.
- Instruct the patient to apply cold compresses to the puncture site as needed, to reduce discomfort or edema.
- Recognize anxiety related to test results Discuss the implications of abnormal test results on the patient's lifestyle. Provide teaching and information regarding the clinical implications of the test results, as appropriate.
- Reinforce information given by the patient's HCP regarding further testing, treatment, or referral to another HCP. Answer any questions or address any concerns voiced by the patient or family.

- Depending on the results of this procedure, additional testing may be performed to evaluate or monitor progression of the disease process and determine the need for a change in therapy. Evaluate test results in relation to the patient's symptoms and other tests performed.

RELATED MONOGRAPHS:

- Related tests include amylase, angiography of the abdomen, BUN, calcitonin, cholangiopancreatography endoscopic retrograde, CT abdomen, creatinine, hepatobiliary scan, 5-hydroxyindoleacetic acid, lipase, peritoneal fluid analysis, US liver and biliary system, and US pancreas.
- Refer to the Endocrine and Hepatobiliary systems tables at the end of the book for related tests by body system.

Magnetic Resonance Imaging, Pelvis

SYNONYM/ACRONYM: Pelvis MRI.

COMMON USE: To visualize and assess the pelvis and surrounding structure for tumor, masses, staging cancer, and inflammation and to evaluate the effectiveness of medical and surgical interventions.

AREA OF APPLICATION: Pelvic area.

CONTRAST: Can be done with or without IV contrast medium (gadolinium).

DESCRIPTION: Magnetic resonance imaging (MRI) uses a magnet and radio waves to produce an energy field that can be displayed as an image. Use of magnetic fields with the aid of radiofrequency energy produces images primarily based on water content of tissue. The magnetic field causes the hydrogen atoms in tissue to line up, and when radio waves are directed toward the magnetic field, the atoms absorb the radio waves and change their position. When the radio waves are turned off, the atoms go back to their original position; this change in the energy field is sensed by the equipment, and an image is generated by the attached computer system. MRI produces cross-sectional images of the pelvic area in multiple planes without the use of ionizing radiation or the interference of bone or surrounding tissue.

Pelvic MRI is performed to assist in diagnosing abnormalities of the pelvis and associated structures. Contrast-enhanced MRI is effective for evaluating metastases from primary tumors. MRI is highly effective for depicting small-volume peritoneal tumors, carcinomatosis, and peritonitis and for determining the response to surgical and chemical therapies. MRI uses the noniodinated contrast medium gadopentetate dimeglumine (Magnevist), which is administered IV to enhance contrast differences between normal and abnormal tissues. Oral and rectal contrast administration may be used to isolate the bowel from adjacent pelvic organs and improve organ visualization.

Magnetic resonance angiography (MRA) is an application of MRI that provides images of blood flow and diseased and normal blood vessels. In patients who are allergic to iodinated contrast medium, MRA is used in place of angiography (see monograph titled "Magnetic Resonance Angiography").

INDICATIONS

• Detect cancer (primary or metastatic tumors of ovary, prostate, uterus, and bladder) and provide cancer staging
• Detect pelvic vascular diseases
• Detect peritonitis
• Detect soft tissue abnormalities
• Determine blood clots, cysts, fluid or fat accumulation in tissues, hemorrhage, and infarctions
• Differentiate tumors from tissue abnormalities, such as cysts, cavernous hemangiomas, and abscesses

• Monitor and evaluate the effectiveness of medical or surgical interventions and course of the disease

POTENTIAL DIAGNOSIS

Normal findings in
• Normal pelvic structures and soft tissue density and biochemical constituents of pelvic tissues, including blood flow

Abnormal findings in
• Adenomyosis
• Ascites
• Fibroids
• Masses, lesions, infections, or inflammations
• Peritoneal tumor or carcinomatosis
• Peritonitis
• Pseudomyxoma peritonei

CRITICAL FINDINGS: N/A

INTERFERING FACTORS

This procedure is contraindicated for
• Patients with certain ferrous metal prostheses, valves, aneurysm clips, inner ear prostheses, or other metallic objects.
• ❁ Patients with metal in their body, such as shrapnel or ferrous metal in the eye.
• ❁ Patients with cardiac pacemakers, because the pacemaker can be deactivated by MRI.
• ❁ Use of gadolinium-based contrast agents (GBCAs) is contraindicated in patients with acute or chronic severe renal insufficiency (glomerular filtration rate less than 30 mL/min/1.73 m^2). Patients should be screened for renal dysfunction prior to administration. The use of GBCAs should be avoided in these patients unless the benefits of the studies outweigh the risks and if essential diagnostic information is not available using

non-contrast-enhanced diagnostic studies.
* Patients with intrauterine devices.
* Patients with iron pigments in tattoos.
* Patients who are claustrophobic.
* Patients who are pregnant or suspected of being pregnant, unless the potential benefits of the procedure far outweigh the risks to the fetus and mother.

Factors that may impair clear imaging
* Metallic objects (e.g., jewelry, body rings, dental amalgams) within the examination field, which may inhibit organ visualization and cause unclear images.
* Inability of the patient to cooperate or remain still during the procedure because of age, significant pain, or mental status.
* Patients with extreme cases of claustrophobia, unless sedation is given before the study or an open MRI is utilized.

Other considerations
* If contrast medium is allowed to seep deep into the muscle tissue, vascular visualization will be impossible.

NURSING IMPLICATIONS AND PROCEDURE

PRETEST:

▶ Positively identify the patient using at least two unique identifiers before providing care, treatment, or services.
▶ *Patient Teaching:* Inform the patient this procedure can assist in assessing the pelvis and surrounding structures.
▶ Obtain a history of the patient's complaints, including a list of known allergens, especially allergies or sensitivities to latex, iodine, seafood, contrast medium, anesthetics, or dyes.
▶ Obtain a history of the patient's genitourinary system, symptoms, and results

of previously performed laboratory tests and diagnostic and surgical procedures. Obtain a history of renal dysfunction if the use of GBCA is anticipated.
▶ Ensure the results of BUN, creatinine, and eGFR (estimated glomerular filtration rate) are obtained if GBCA is to be used.
▶ Determine if the patient has ever had any device implanted into his or her body, including copper intrauterine devices, pacemakers, ear implants, and heart valves.
▶ Obtain occupational history to determine the presence of metal in the body, such as shrapnel or flecks of ferrous metal in the eye (which can cause retinal hemorrhage).
▶ Note any recent procedures that can interfere with test results, including examinations using barium- or iodine-based contrast medium.
▶ Record the date of the last menstrual period and determine the possibility of pregnancy in perimenopausal women.
▶ Obtain a list of the patient's current medications, including herbs, nutritional supplements, and nutraceuticals (see Appendix F).
▶ Review the procedure with the patient. Address concerns about pain related to the procedure and explain that no pain will be experienced during the test, but there may be moments of discomfort. Reassure the patient that if contrast is used, it poses no radioactive hazard and rarely produces side effects. Inform the patient the procedure is performed in an MRI department by a health-care provider (HCP) specializing in this procedure, with support staff, and takes approximately 30 to 60 min.
▶ Inform the patient that the technologist will place him or her in a supine position on a flat table in a large cylindrical scanner.
▶ Tell the patient to expect to hear loud banging from the scanner and possibly to see magnetophosphenes (flickering lights in the visual field); these will stop when the procedure is over.
▶ *Sensitivity to social and cultural issues,* as well as concern for modesty, is important in providing psychological support before, during, and after the procedure.

M

- Explain that an IV line may be inserted to allow infusion of IV fluids, contrast medium, or sedatives.
- Instruct the patient to remove jewelry and all other metallic objects from the area to be examined prior to the procedure.
- There are no food, fluid, or medication restrictions unless by medical direction.

INTRATEST:

- Ensure that the patient has removed all external metallic objects from the area to be examined prior to the procedure.
- If the patient has a history of allergic reactions to any substance or drug, administer ordered prophylactic steroids or antihistamines before the procedure.
- Have emergency equipment readily available.
- Instruct the patient to void prior to the procedure and to change into the gown, robe, and foot coverings provided.
- Instruct the patient to cooperate fully and to follow directions. Instruct the patient to remain still throughout the procedure because movement produces unreliable results.
- Observe standard precautions, and follow the general guidelines in Appendix A.
- Supply earplugs to the patient to block out the loud, banging sounds that occur during the test. Instruct the patient to communicate with the technologist during the examination via a microphone within the scanner.
- Establish an IV fluid line for the injection of emergency drugs and of sedatives.
- Administer an antianxiety agent, as ordered, if the patient has claustrophobia. Administer a sedative to a child or to an uncooperative adult, as ordered.
- Place the patient in the supine position on an examination table.
- If contrast is used, imaging can begin shortly after the injection.
- Ask the patient to inhale deeply and hold his or her breath while the images are taken and then to exhale after the images are taken.
- Instruct the patient to take slow, deep breaths if nausea occurs during the procedure.
- Monitor the patient for complications related to the procedure (e.g., allergic reaction, anaphylaxis, bronchospasm).

- Remove the needle or catheter and apply a pressure dressing over the puncture site.
- Observe/assess the needle/catheter insertion site for bleeding, inflammation, or hematoma formation.

POST-TEST:

- A report of the results will be sent to the requesting HCP, who will discuss the results with the patient.
- Observe for delayed allergic reactions, such as rash, urticaria, tachycardia, hyperpnea, hypertension, palpitations, nausea, or vomiting.
- Instruct the patient to immediately report symptoms such as fast heart rate, difficulty breathing, skin rash, itching, chest pain, persistent right shoulder pain, or abdominal pain. Immediately report symptoms to the appropriate HCP.
- Instruct the patient in the care and assessment of the injection site.
- Instruct the patient to apply cold compresses to the puncture site as needed, to reduce discomfort or edema.
- Recognize anxiety related to test results. Discuss the implications of abnormal test results on the patient's lifestyle. Provide teaching and information regarding the clinical implications of the test results, as appropriate.
- Reinforce information given by the patient's HCP regarding further testing, treatment, or referral to another HCP. Answer any questions or address any concerns voiced by the patient or family.
- Depending on the results of this procedure, additional testing may be performed to evaluate or monitor progression of the disease process and determine the need for a change in therapy. Evaluate test results in relation to the patient's symptoms and other tests performed.

RELATED MONOGRAPHS:

- Related tests include BUN, CT pelvis, creatinine, cystourethrography voiding, IVP, KUB study, renogram, and US pelvis.
- Refer to the Genitourinary System table at the end of the book for related tests by body system.

M

Magnetic Resonance Imaging, Pituitary

SYNONYM/ACRONYM: Pituitary MRI, MRI of the parasellar region.

COMMON USE: To visualize and assess the pituitary and surrounding structures of the brain for lesions, hemorrhage, cysts, abscess, tumors, cancer, and infection.

AREA OF APPLICATION: Brain/pituitary area.

CONTRAST: Can be done with or without IV contrast medium (gadolinium).

DESCRIPTION: Magnetic resonance imaging (MRI) uses a magnet and radio waves to produce an energy field that can be displayed as an image. Use of magnetic fields with the aid of radiofrequency energy produces images primarily based on water content of tissue. The magnetic field causes the hydrogen atoms in tissue to line up, and when radio waves are directed toward the magnetic field, the atoms absorb the radio waves and change their position. When the radio waves are turned off, the atoms go back to their original position; this change in the energy field is sensed by the equipment, and an image is generated by the attached computer system. MRI produces cross-sectional images of the pituitary and parasellar region in multiple planes without the use of ionizing radiation or the interference of bone or surrounding tissue.

Pituitary MRI shows the relationship of pituitary lesions to the optic chiasm and cavernous sinuses. MRI has the capability of distinguishing the solid, cystic, and hemorrhagic components of lesions. Rapidly flowing blood on spin-echo MRI appears as an absence of signal or a void in the vessel's lumen. Blood flow can be evaluated in the cavernous and carotid arteries. Suprasellar aneurysms may be diagnosed without angiography, and old clotted blood in the walls of the aneurysms appears white. MRI uses the noniodinated contrast medium gadopentetate dimeglumine (Magnevist), which is administered IV to enhance contrast differences between normal and abnormal tissues.

Magnetic resonance angiography (MRA) is an application of MRI that provides images of blood flow and diseased and normal blood vessels. In patients who are allergic to iodinated contrast medium, MRA is used in place of angiography (see monograph titled "Magnetic Resonance Angiography").

INDICATIONS
- Detect microadenoma or macroadenoma of the pituitary
- Detect parasellar abnormalities
- Detect tumors of the pituitary
- Evaluate potential cause of headache, visual loss, and vomiting
- Evaluate the solid, cystic, and hemorrhagic components of lesions

- Evaluate vascularity of the pituitary
- Monitor and evaluate the effectiveness of medical or surgical interventions and course of disease

POTENTIAL DIAGNOSIS

Normal findings in
- Normal anatomic structures, density, and biochemical constituents of the pituitary, including blood flow

Abnormal findings in
- Abscess
- Aneurysm
- Choristoma
- Craniopharyngioma or meningioma
- Empty sella
- Granuloma
- Infarct or hemorrhage
- Macroadenoma or microadenoma
- Metastasis
- Parasitic infection

CRITICAL FINDINGS: N/A

INTERFERING FACTORS

This procedure is contraindicated for
- Patients with certain ferrous metal prostheses, valves, aneurysm clips, inner ear prostheses, or other metallic objects.
- ❖ Patients with metal in their body, such as shrapnel or ferrous metal in the eye.
- ❖ Patients with cardiac pacemakers, because the pacemaker can be deactivated by MRI.
- ❖ Use of gadolinium-based contrast agents (GBCAs) is contraindicated in patients with acute or chronic severe renal insufficiency (glomerular filtration rate less than 30 mL/min/1.73 m^2). Patients should be screened for renal dysfunction prior to administration. The use of GBCAs should be avoided in these patients unless the benefits of the studies outweigh the risks and if essential diagnostic information is

not available using non-contrast-enhanced diagnostic studies.
- Patients with intrauterine devices.
- Patients with iron pigments in tattoos.
- Patients who are claustrophobic.
- Patients who are pregnant or suspected of being pregnant, unless the potential benefits of the procedure far outweigh the risks to the fetus and mother.

Factors that may impair clear imaging
- Metallic objects (e.g., jewelry, body rings, dental amalgams) within the examination field, which may inhibit organ visualization and cause unclear images.
- Inability of the patient to cooperate or remain still during the procedure because of age, significant pain, or mental status.
- Patients with extreme cases of claustrophobia, unless sedation is given before the study or an open MRI is utilized.

Other considerations
- If contrast medium is allowed to seep deep into the muscle tissue, vascular visualization will be impossible.

NURSING IMPLICATIONS AND PROCEDURE

PRETEST:
- Positively identify the patient using at least two unique identifiers before providing care, treatment, or services.
- *Patient Teaching:* Inform the patient this procedure can assist in assessing the pituitary gland and surrounding brain tissue.
- Obtain a history of the patient's complaints, including a list of known allergens, especially allergies or sensitivities to latex, iodine, seafood, contrast medium, anesthetics, or dyes.
- Obtain a history of the patient's cardiovascular and endocrine systems,

symptoms, and results of previously performed laboratory tests and diagnostic and surgical procedures. Obtain a history of renal dysfunction if the use of GBCA is anticipated.

- Ensure the results of BUN, creatinine, and eGFR (estimated glomerular filtration rate) are obtained if GBCA is to be used.
- Determine if the patient has ever had any device implanted into his or her body, including copper intrauterine devices, pacemakers, ear implants, and heart valves.
- Obtain occupational history to determine the presence of metal in the body, such as shrapnel or flecks of ferrous metal in the eye (which can cause retinal hemorrhage).
- Note any recent procedures that can interfere with test results, including examinations using barium- or iodine-based contrast medium.
- Record the date of the last menstrual period and determine the possibility of pregnancy in perimenopausal women.
- Obtain a list of the patient's current medications, including herbs, nutritional supplements, and nutraceuticals (see Appendix F).
- Review the procedure with the patient. Address concerns about pain related to the procedure and explain that no pain will be experienced during the test, but there may be moments of discomfort. Inform the patient the procedure is performed in an MRI department by a health-care provider (HCP) specializing in this procedure, with support staff, and takes approximately 30 to 60 min.
- Inform the patient that the technologist will place him or her in a supine position on a flat table in a large cylindrical scanner.
- Tell the patient to expect to hear loud banging from the scanner and possibly to see magnetophosphenes (flickering lights in the visual field); these will stop when the procedure is over.
- *Sensitivity to social and cultural issues,* as well as concern for modesty, is important in providing psychological support before, during, and after the procedure.

- Explain that an IV line may be inserted to allow infusion of IV fluids, contrast medium, or sedatives.
- Instruct the patient to remove jewelry and all other metallic objects from the area to be examined prior to the procedure.
- There are no food, fluid, or medication restrictions unless by medical direction.

INTRATEST:

- Ensure that the patient has removed all external metallic objects from the area to be examined prior to the procedure.
- If the patient has a history of allergic reactions to any substance or drug, administer ordered prophylactic steroids or antihistamines before the procedure.
- Have emergency equipment readily available.
- Instruct the patient to void prior to the procedure and to change into the gown, robe, and foot coverings provided.
- Instruct the patient to cooperate fully and to follow directions. Instruct the patient to remain still throughout the procedure because movement produces unreliable results.
- Observe standard precautions, and follow the general guidelines in Appendix A.
- Supply earplugs to the patient to block out the loud, banging sounds that occur during the test. Instruct the patient to communicate with the technologist during the examination via a microphone within the scanner.
- Establish an IV fluid line for the injection of emergency drugs and of sedatives.
- Administer an antianxiety agent, as ordered, if the patient has claustrophobia. Administer a sedative to a child or to an uncooperative adult, as ordered.
- Place the patient in the supine position on an examination table.
- If contrast is used, imaging can begin shortly after the injection.
- Ask the patient to inhale deeply and hold his or her breath while the images are taken and then to exhale after the images are taken.
- Instruct the patient to take slow, deep breaths if nausea occurs during the procedure.

M

▶ Monitor the patient for complications related to the procedure (e.g., allergic reaction, anaphylaxis, bronchospasm).
▶ Remove the needle or catheter and apply a pressure dressing over the puncture site.
▶ Observe/assess the needle/catheter insertion site for bleeding, inflammation, or hematoma formation.

POST-TEST:

▶ A report of the results will be sent to the requesting HCP, who will discuss the results with the patient.
▶ Observe for delayed allergic reactions, such as rash, urticaria, tachycardia, hyperpnea, hypertension, palpitations, nausea, or vomiting.
▶ Instruct the patient to immediately report symptoms such as fast heart rate, difficulty breathing, skin rash, itching, chest pain, persistent right shoulder pain, or abdominal pain. Immediately report symptoms to the appropriate HCP.
▶ Instruct the patient in the care and assessment of the injection site.
▶ Instruct the patient to apply cold compresses to the puncture site as needed to reduce discomfort or edema.

▶ Recognize anxiety related to test results. Discuss the implications of abnormal test results on the patient's lifestyle. Provide teaching and information regarding the clinical implications of the test results, as appropriate.
▶ Reinforce information given by the patient's HCP regarding further testing, treatment, or referral to another HCP. Answer any questions or address any concerns voiced by the patient or family.
▶ Depending on the results of this procedure, additional testing may be performed to evaluate or monitor progression of the disease process and determine the need for a change in therapy. Evaluate test results in relation to the patient's symptoms and other tests performed.

RELATED MONOGRAPHS:

▶ Related tests include ACTH and challenge tests, angiography brain, BUN, cortisol and challenge tests, CT brain, creatinine, EEG, MRI brain, and PET brain.
▶ Refer to the Cardiovascular and Endocrine systems tables at the end of the book for related tests by body system.

M

Mammography

SYNONYM/ACRONYM: Breast x-ray, mammogram.

COMMON USE: To visualize and assess breast tissue and surrounding lymph nodes for cancer, inflammation, abscess, tumor, and cysts.

AREA OF APPLICATION: Breast.

CONTRAST: None.

DESCRIPTION: Mammography, an x-ray examination of the breast, is most commonly used to detect breast cancer; however, it can also be used to detect and evaluate symptomatic changes associated with other breast diseases, including mastitis, abscess, cystic changes, cysts, benign tumors, masses, and lymph nodes.

Mammography is usually performed with traditional x-ray film, but totally electronic image recording is becoming commonplace. Mammography can be used to locate a nonpalpable lesion for biopsy. Mammography cannot detect breast cancer with 100% accuracy. In approximately 15% of breast cancer cases, the cancer is not detected with mammography. To assist in early detection of nonpalpable breast lesions, computer-assisted diagnosis is currently being used. With this technique, a computer performs automated scanning of the mammogram before the health-care provider (HCP) interprets the findings.

When a mass is detected, additional studies are performed to help differentiate the nature of the mass, as follows:

- Magnification views of the area in question
- Focal or "spot" views of the area in question, done with a specialized paddle-style compression device
- Ultrasound images of the area in question, which help differentiate between a fluid-filled cystic lesion and a solid lesion indicative of cancer or fibroadenomas

INDICATIONS

- Differentiate between benign and neoplastic breast disease
- Evaluate breast pain, skin retraction, nipple erosion, or nipple discharge
- Evaluate known or suspected breast cancer
- Evaluate nonpalpable breast masses
- Evaluate opposite breast after mastectomy
- Monitor postoperative and post–radiation treatment status of the breast
- Evaluate size, shape, and position of breast masses

POTENTIAL DIAGNOSIS

Normal findings in
- Normal breast tissue, with no cysts, tumors, or calcifications

Abnormal findings in
- Breast calcifications
- Breast cysts or abscesses
- Breast tumors
- Hematoma resulting from trauma
- Mastitis
- Soft tissue masses
- Vascular calcification

CRITICAL FINDINGS: N/A

INTERFERING FACTORS

This procedure is contraindicated for
- Patients who are pregnant or suspected of being pregnant, unless the potential benefits of the procedure far outweigh the risks to the fetus and mother.
- Patients younger than age 25, because the density of the breast tissue is such that diagnostic x-rays are of limited value.

Factors that may impair clear imaging
- Inability of the patient to cooperate or remain still during the procedure because of age, significant pain, or mental status.
- Metallic objects (e.g., jewelry, body rings) within the examination field, which may inhibit organ visualization and cause unclear images.
- Application of substances such as talcum powder, deodorant, or creams to the skin of breasts or underarms, which may alter test results.
- Previous breast surgery, breast augmentation, or the presence of breast implants, which may

M

decrease the readability of the examination.

Other considerations
- Consultation with an HCP should occur before the procedure for radiation safety concerns regarding infants of patients who are lactating.
- Risks associated with radiation overexposure can result from frequent x-ray procedures. Personnel in the room with the patient should wear a protective lead apron, stand behind a shield, or leave the area while the examination is being done. Personnel working in the examination area should wear badges to record their level of radiation exposure.

NURSING IMPLICATIONS AND PROCEDURE

PRETEST:
- Positively identify the patient using at least two unique identifiers before providing care, treatment, or services.
- *Patient Teaching:* Inform the patient this procedure can assist in assessing breast status.
- Obtain a history of the patient's complaints, including a list of known allergens, especially allergies or sensitivities to latex.
- Obtain a history of the patient's reproductive system, known or suspected breast disease, and family history of breast disease; symptoms; and results of previously performed laboratory tests and diagnostic and surgical procedures.
- Record the date of the last menstrual period and determine the possibility of pregnancy in perimenopausal women.
- Obtain a list of the patient's current medications, including herbs, nutritional supplements, and nutraceuticals (see Appendix F).
- Review the procedure with the patient. Address concerns about pain related to the procedure. Inform the patient

there may be discomfort associated with the study while the breast is being compressed, but the compression allows for better visualization of the breast tissue. Explain to the patient that the radiation dose will be kept to an absolute minimum. Inform the patient that the procedure is performed in the mammography department by a registered mammographer and takes approximately 15 to 30 min to complete.
- Inform the patient that the best time to schedule the examination is 1 week after menses, when breast tenderness is decreased.
- *Sensitivity to social and cultural issues,* as well as concern for modesty, is important in providing psychological support before, during, and after the procedure.
- Inform the patient not to apply deodorant, body creams, or powders on the day of the procedure.
- Instruct the patient to remove jewelry and other metallic objects from the area of examination.
- There are no food, fluid, or medication restrictions unless by medical direction.

INTRATEST:
- Ensure that the patient has removed all jewelry and other metallic objects from the chest area.
- Instruct the patient to void prior to the procedure and to change into the gown and robe provided.
- Instruct the patient to cooperate fully and to follow directions. Instruct the patient to remain still throughout the procedure because movement produces unreliable results.
- Observe standard precautions and follow the general guidelines in Appendix A.
- Assist the patient to a standing or sitting position in front of the x-ray machine, which is adjusted to the level of the breasts. Position the patient's arms out of the range of the area to be imaged.
- Place breasts, one at a time, between the compression apparatus. Two images or exposures are taken of each breast. Ask the patient to hold her

breath during each exposure. Additional images may be taken as requested by the radiologist before the patient leaves the mammography room.

POST-TEST:

▸ A report of the examination will be sent to the requesting HCP, who will discuss the results with the patient.
▸ Determine if the patient has any further questions or concerns.
▸ Recognize anxiety related to test results, and be supportive of fear of shortened life expectancy. Discuss the implications of abnormal test results on the patient's lifestyle. Provide teaching and information regarding the clinical implications of the test results, as appropriate. Educate the patient regarding access to counseling services. Provide contact information, if desired, for the American Cancer Society (www.cancer.org).
▸ Reinforce information given by the patient's HCP regarding further testing, treatment, or referral to another HCP. Decisions regarding the need for and frequency of breast self-examination, mammography, MRI breast, or other cancer screening procedures should be made after consultation between the patient and HCP. The most current guidelines for breast cancer screening of the general population as well as of individuals with increased risk are available from the American Cancer Society, the American College of Obstetricians and Gynecologists (ACOG) (www.acog.org), and the American College of Radiology (www.acr.org). Answer any questions or address any concerns voiced by the patient or family.
▸ Depending on the results of this procedure, additional testing may be performed to evaluate or monitor progression of the disease process and determine the need for a change in therapy. Evaluate test results in relation to the patient's symptoms and other tests performed.

RELATED MONOGRAPHS:

▸ Related tests include biopsy breast, cancer antigens, ductography, MRI breast, stereotactic biopsy breast, and US breast.
▸ Refer to the Reproductive System table at the end of the book for related tests by body system.

M

Meckel's Diverticulum Scan

SYNONYM/ACRONYM: Ectopic gastric mucosa scan, Meckel's scan, Meckel's scintigraphy.

COMMON USE: To assess, evaluate, and diagnose the cause of abdominal pain and gastrointestinal bleeding.

AREA OF APPLICATION: Abdomen.

CONTRAST: IV radioactive technetium-99m pertechnetate.

DESCRIPTION: Meckel's diverticulum scan is a nuclear medicine study performed to assist in diagnosing the cause of abdominal pain or occult gastrointestinal (GI) bleeding and to assess the presence and size of a congenital anomaly of the GI tract. After IV injection of technetium-99m pertechnetate, immediate and delayed imaging is performed, with various views of the abdomen obtained. The radionuclide is taken up and concentrated by parietal cells of the gastric mucosa, whether located in the stomach or in a Meckel's diverticulum. Up to 25% of Meckel's diverticulum is lined internally with ectopic gastric mucosal tissue. This tissue is usually located in the ileum and right lower quadrant of the abdomen; it secretes acid that causes ulceration of intestinal tissue, which results in abdominal pain and occult blood in stools.

INDICATIONS

- Aid in the diagnosis of unexplained abdominal pain and GI bleeding caused by hydrochloric acid and pepsin secreted by ectopic gastric mucosa, which ulcerates nearby mucosa
- Detect sites of ectopic gastric mucosa

POTENTIAL DIAGNOSIS

Normal findings in
- Normal distribution of radionuclide by gastric mucosa at normal sites

Abnormal findings in
- Meckel's diverticulum, as evidenced by focally increased radioactive uptake in areas other than normal structures

CRITICAL FINDINGS: N/A

INTERFERING FACTORS

This procedure is contraindicated for
- Patients who are pregnant or suspected of being pregnant, unless the potential benefits of the procedure far outweigh the risks to the fetus and mother.

Factors that may impair clear imaging
- Inability of the patient to cooperate or remain still during the procedure because of age, significant pain, or mental status.
- Metallic objects (e.g., jewelry, body rings) within the examination field, which may inhibit organ visualization and cause unclear images.
- Retained barium from a previous radiological procedure.
- Other nuclear scans done within the preceding 24 hr.

Other considerations
- Improper injection of the radionuclide may allow the tracer to seep deep into the muscle tissue, producing erroneous hot spots.
- Consultation with a health-care provider (HCP) should occur before the procedure for radiation safety concerns regarding younger patients or patients who are lactating.
- False-positive results may occur from nondiverticular bleeding, intussusception, duplication cysts, inflammatory bowel disease, hemangioma of the bowel, and other organ infections.
- Inadequate amount of gastric mucosa within Meckel's diverticulum can affect the ability to visualize abnormalities.
- Inaccurate timing for imaging after the radionuclide injection can affect the results.
- Failure to follow dietary restrictions before the procedure may cause the procedure to be canceled or repeated.

- Risks associated with radiation overexposure can result from frequent x-ray or radionuclide procedures. Personnel working in the examination area should wear badges to record their level of radiation exposure.

NURSING IMPLICATIONS AND PROCEDURE

PRETEST:

- Positively identify the patient using at least two unique identifiers before providing care, treatment, or services.
- Inform the patient this procedure can assist in assessing gastrointestinal bleeding.
- Obtain a history of the patient's complaints, including a list of known allergens, especially allergies or sensitivities to latex, iodine, seafood, contrast medium, anesthetics, or dyes.
- Obtain a history of the patient's gastrointestinal system, symptoms, and results of previously performed laboratory tests and diagnostic and surgical procedures.
- Note any recent procedures that can interfere with test results.
- Record the date of the last menstrual period and determine the possibility of pregnancy in perimenopausal women.
- Obtain a list of the patient's current medications, including anticoagulants, aspirin and other salicylates, herbs, nutritional supplements, and nutraceuticals, especially those known to affect coagulation (see Appendix F). Such products should be discontinued by medical direction for the appropriate number of days prior to a surgical procedure. Note the last time and dose of medication taken.
- Review the procedure with the patient. Address concerns about pain and explain that some pain may be experienced during the test, but there may be moments of discomfort. Reassure the patient that the radionuclide poses no radioactive hazard and rarely produces side effects. Inform the patient that the procedure is performed in a nuclear medicine department by an HCP specializing in this procedure, with support staff, and takes approximately 60 min.
- *Sensitivity to social and cultural issues,* as well as concern for modesty, is important in providing psychological support before, during, and after the procedure.
- Explain that an IV line may be inserted to allow infusion of IV fluids, contrast medium, dye, or sedatives. Usually normal saline is infused.
- Instruct the patient to remove jewelry and other metallic objects from the area to be examined.
- Instruct the patient to take a histamine blocker, as ordered, 2 days before the study to block GI secretion.
- The patient should fast and refrain from fluids for 8 hr prior to the procedure. Protocols may vary among facilities.

INTRATEST:

- Ensure that the patient has complied with dietary, fluid, and medication restrictions for 8 hr prior to the procedure.
- Ensure that the patient has removed all external metallic objects from the area to be examined prior to the procedure.
- Have emergency equipment readily available.
- Instruct the patient to void prior to the procedure and to change into the gown, robe, and foot coverings provided.
- Record baseline vital signs and assess neurological status. Protocols may vary among facilities.
- Instruct the patient to cooperate fully and to follow directions. Instruct the patient to remain still throughout the procedure because movement produces unreliable results.
- Observe standard precautions, and follow the general guidelines in Appendix A.
- Place the patient in a supine position on a flat table with foam wedges, which help maintain position and immobilization.
- IV radionuclide is administered, and the abdomen is scanned immediately to

M

screen for vascular lesions. Images are taken in various positions every 5 min for the next hour.

- Monitor the patient for complications related to the procedure (e.g., allergic reaction, anaphylaxis, bronchospasm).
- Remove the needle or catheter and apply a pressure dressing over the puncture site.
- Observe/assess the needle/catheter insertion site for bleeding, inflammation, or hematoma formation.

POST-TEST:

- A report of the results will be sent to the requesting HCP, who will discuss the results with the patient.
- Unless contraindicated, advise patient to drink increased amounts of fluids for 24 to 48 hr to eliminate the radionuclide from the body. Inform the patient that radionuclide is eliminated from the body within 6 to 24 hr.
- No other radionuclide tests should be scheduled for 24 to 48 hr after this procedure.
- Instruct the patient to resume usual diet, fluids, and medications, as directed by the HCP.
- Monitor vital signs and neurological status every 15 min for 1 hr, then every 2 hr for 4 hr, and then as ordered by the HCP. Take temperature every 4 hr for 24 hr. Monitor intake and output at least every 8 hr. Compare with baseline values. Notify the HCP if temperature is elevated. Protocols may vary among facilities.
- Observe for delayed allergic reactions, such as rash, urticaria, tachycardia, hyperpnea, hypertension, palpitations, nausea, or vomiting.
- Instruct the patient to immediately report symptoms such as fast heart rate, difficulty breathing, skin rash, itching, chest pain, persistent right shoulder pain, or abdominal pain. Immediately report symptoms to the appropriate HCP.
- Instruct the patient in the care and assessment of the injection site.
- If a woman who is breastfeeding must have a nuclear scan, she should not breastfeed the infant until the radionuclide has been eliminated. This

could take as long as 3 days. She should be instructed to express the milk and discard it during the 3-day period to prevent cessation of milk production.

- Instruct the patient to immediately flush the toilet and to meticulously wash hands with soap and water after each voiding for 24 hr after the procedure.
- Instruct all caregivers to wear gloves when discarding urine for 24 hr after the procedure. Wash gloved hands with soap and water before removing gloves. Then wash hands after the gloves are removed.
- *Nutritional Considerations:* A low-fat, low-cholesterol, and low-sodium diet should be consumed to reduce current disease processes. High fat consumption increases the amount of bile acids in the colon and should be avoided.
- Recognize anxiety related to test results, and be supportive of perceived loss of independent function. Discuss the implications of abnormal test results on the patient's lifestyle. Provide teaching and information regarding the clinical implications of the test results, as appropriate.
- Reinforce information given by the patient's HCP regarding further testing, treatment, or referral to another HCP. Answer any questions or address any concerns voiced by the patient or family.
- Depending on the results of this procedure, additional testing may be needed to evaluate or monitor progression of the disease process and determine the need for a change in therapy. Evaluate test results in relation to the patient's symptoms and other tests performed.

RELATED MONOGRAPHS:

- Related tests include barium swallow, colonoscopy, CT abdomen, CT pelvis, esophageal manometry, EGD, fecal analysis, gastric acid stimulation, gastric emptying scan, gastrin stimulation, GI blood loss, MRI abdomen, MRI pelvis, and upper GI series.
- Refer to the Gastrointestinal System table at the end of the book for related tests by body system.

Mediastinoscopy

SYNONYM/ACRONYM: N/A.

COMMON USE: To visualize and assess structures under the mediastinum to assist in obtaining biopsies for diagnosing and staging cancer and to evaluate the effectiveness of therapeutic interventions.

AREA OF APPLICATION: Mediastinum.

CONTRAST: None.

DESCRIPTION: Mediastinoscopy provides direct visualization of the structures that lie beneath the mediastinum, which is the area behind the sternum and between the lungs. The test is performed under general anesthesia by means of a mediastinoscope inserted through a surgical incision at the suprasternal notch. Structures that can be viewed include the trachea, the esophagus, the heart and its major vessels, the thymus gland, and the lymph nodes that receive drainage from the lungs. The procedure is performed primarily to visualize and obtain biopsy specimens of the mediastinal lymph nodes and to determine the extent of metastasis into the mediastinum for the determination of treatment planning in cancer patients.

INDICATIONS

- Confirm radiological evidence of a thoracic infectious process of an indeterminate nature, coccidioidomycosis, or histoplasmosis
- Confirm radiological or cytological evidence of carcinoma or sarcoidosis
- Detect Hodgkin's disease
- Detect metastasis into the anterior mediastinum or extrapleurally into the chest
- Determine stage of known bronchogenic carcinoma, as indicated by the extent of mediastinal lymph node involvement
- Evaluate a patient with signs and symptoms of obstruction of mediastinal lymph flow and a history of head or neck cancer to determine recurrence or spread

POTENTIAL DIAGNOSIS

Normal findings in
- Normal appearance of mediastinal structures
- No abnormal lymph node tissue

Abnormal findings in
- Bronchogenic carcinoma
- Coccidioidomycosis
- Granulomatous infections
- Histoplasmosis
- Hodgkin's disease
- *Pneumocystis jiroveci* (formerly *P. carinii*)
- Sarcoidosis
- Tuberculosis

CRITICAL FINDINGS: N/A

M

INTERFERING FACTORS

This procedure is contraindicated for

- Patients who have had a previous mediastinoscopy, because scarring can make insertion of the scope and biopsy of lymph nodes difficult.
- Patients who have superior vena cava obstruction, because this condition causes increased venous collateral circulation in the mediastinum.
- Patients who are pregnant or suspected of being pregnant, unless the potential benefits of the procedure far outweigh the risks to the fetus and mother.

Other considerations

- Failure to follow dietary restrictions before the procedure may cause the procedure to be canceled or repeated.

NURSING IMPLICATIONS AND PROCEDURE

PRETEST:

- Positively identify the patient using at least two unique identifiers before providing care, treatment, or services.
- *Patient Teaching:* Inform the patient this procedure can assist in assessing structure in the middle of the chest.
- Obtain a history of the patient's complaints or symptoms, including a list of known allergens, especially allergies or sensitivities to latex, iodine, seafood, contrast medium, and anesthetics.
- Obtain a history of the patient's immune and respiratory systems, symptoms, and results of previously performed laboratory tests and diagnostic and surgical procedures.
- Ensure that the results of blood typing and crossmatching are obtained and recorded before the procedure in the event that an emergency thoracotomy is required.
- Note any recent procedures that can interfere with test results. Ensure that this procedure is performed before an upper gastrointestinal study or barium swallow.
- Record the date of the last menstrual period and determine the possibility of pregnancy in perimenopausal women.
- Obtain a list of the patient's current medications, including herbs, nutritional supplements, and nutraceuticals (see Appendix F).
- Review the procedure with the patient. Inform the patient that prophylactic antibiotics may be administered prior to the procedure. Address concerns about pain related to the procedure and explain that a general anesthesia will be administered to promote relaxation and reduce discomfort prior to the mediastinoscopy. Explain that some pain may be experienced after the test. Meperidine (Demerol) or morphine may be given as a sedative. Inform the patient that the procedure is performed in the operating room by a health-care provider (HCP) specializing in this procedure, with support staff, and usually takes 30 to 60 min to complete.
- *Sensitivity to social and cultural issues,* as well as concern for modesty, is important in providing psychological support before, during, and after the procedure.
- Explain that an IV line will be inserted to allow infusion of IV fluids, antibiotics, anesthetics, and analgesics.
- Instruct the patient to remove jewelry and external metallic objects from the area to be examined prior to the procedure.
- The patient should fast and restrict fluids for 8 hr prior to the procedure. Protocols may vary among facilities. Instruct the patient to avoid taking anticoagulant medication or to reduce dosage as ordered prior to the procedure. Number of days to withhold medication is dependent on the type of anticoagulant.
- *Make sure a written and informed consent has been signed prior to the procedure and before administering any medications.*

INTRATEST:

- Ensure that the patient has complied with food, fluids, and medication restrictions for 8 hr prior to the procedure.

M

- Ensure that the patient has removed jewelry and external metallic objects from the area to be examined prior to the procedure.
- Have emergency equipment readily available.
- Instruct the patient to void prior to the procedure and change into the gown, robe, and foot coverings provided.
- Record baseline vital signs and assess neurological status. Protocols may vary among facilities.
- Observe standard precautions, and follow the general guidelines in Appendix A.
- Establish IV fluid line for the injection of emergency drugs and of sedatives.
- Place electrocardiographic electrodes on the patient for cardiac monitoring. Establish baseline rhythm; determine if the patient has ventricular arrhythmias.
- Avoid using morphine sulfate in patients with asthma or other pulmonary disease. This drug can further exacerbate bronchospasms and respiratory impairment.
- Place the patient in the supine position. General anesthesia is administered via an endotracheal tube.
- An incision is made at the suprasternal notch, and a path for the mediastinoscope is made using finger dissection. The lymph nodes can be palpated at this time. The lymph nodes on the right side of the mediastinum are most accessible and safest to biopsy by medastinoscopy; the lymph nodes on the left side are more difficult to explore and biopsy because of their proximity to the aorta. Biopsy specimens of nodes on the left side of the mediastinum may need to be obtained by mediastinotomy, which involves performing a left anterior thoracotomy.
- Place tissue samples in properly labeled specimen containers, and promptly transport the specimen to the laboratory for processing and analysis.
- The scope is removed, and the incision is closed.
- Observe/assess the incision site for bleeding, inflammation, or hematoma formation.
- If the patient is stable and if no further surgery is immediately indicated, the patient is extubated.

POST-TEST:

- A report of the results will be sent to the requesting HCP, who will discuss the results with the patient.
- Do not allow the patient to eat or drink for 12 to 24 hr.
- Instruct the patient to resume normal activity, medication, and diet in 24 hr or as tolerated after the examination, unless otherwise indicated.
- The patient should remain in a semi-Fowler's position on either side until vital signs revert to preprocedure levels.
- Monitor vital signs and neurological status every 15 min for 1 hr, then every 2 hr for 4 hr, and then as ordered by the HCP. Take temperature every 4 hr for 24 hr. Monitor intake and output, at least every 8 hr. Compare with baseline values. Notify the HCP if temperature changes. Protocols may vary from facility to facility.
- Observe for delayed allergic reactions, such as rash, urticaria, tachycardia, hyperpnea, hypertension, palpitations, nausea, or vomiting.
- Instruct the patient to immediately report symptoms such as fast heart rate, difficulty breathing, skin rash, itching, chest pain, persistent right shoulder pain, or abdominal pain. Immediately report symptoms to the appropriate HCP.
- Instruct the patient in the care and assessment of the site.
- Emphasize that any excessive bleeding; difficulty breathing; excessive coughing after biopsy; fever; or redness, swelling, or pain of the incisional area must be reported to the HCP immediately.
- Recognize anxiety related to test results, and be supportive of perceived loss of independent function. Discuss the implications of abnormal test results on the patient's lifestyle. Provide teaching and information regarding the clinical implications of the test results, as appropriate.
- Reinforce information given by the patient's HCP regarding further testing, treatment, or referral to another HCP. Answer any questions or address any concerns voiced by the patient or family.
- Depending on the results of this procedure, additional testing may be needed to evaluate or monitor progression of

M

the disease process and determine the need for a change in therapy. Evaluate test results in relation to the patient's symptoms and other tests performed.

RELATED MONOGRAPHS:

» Related tests include ACE, β_2-microglobulin, biopsy liver, biopsy lung, biopsy lymph node, blood gases, bronchoscopy, carbon dioxide, chest x-ray, CBC, CBC WBC count and differential, CT thoracic, culture and smear mycobacteria, gallium scan, Gram stain, laparoscopy abdominal, LAP, liver and spleen scan, lung perfusion scan, lung ventilation scan, lymphangiogram, MRI chest, platelet count, pleural fluid analysis, PFT, and TB skin tests.

» Refer to the Immune and Respiratory systems tables at the end of the book for related tests by body system.

Metanephrines

SYNONYM/ACRONYM: N/A.

COMMON USE: To assist in the diagnosis of cancer of the adrenal medulla or to assess for the cause of hypertension.

SPECIMEN: Urine (25 mL) from a timed specimen collected in a clean amber plastic collection container with 6N hydrochloride as a preservative.

REFERENCE VALUE: (Method: High-pressure liquid chromatography)

Age	Conventional Units	SI Units
Normetanephrines (Conventional Units × 5.07)		
3 mo–4 yr	54–249 mcg/24 hr	274–1,262 micromol/day
5–9 yr	31–398 mcg/24 hr	157–2,018 micromol/day
10–17 yr	67–531 mcg/24 hr	340–2,692 micromol/day
18–39 yr	35–482 mcg/24 hr	177–2,444 micromol/day
Greater than 40 yr	88–676 mcg/24 hr	446–3,427 micromol/day
Metanephrines, Total (Conventional Units × 5.07)		
3 mo–4 yr	79–345 mcg/24 hr	401–1,749 micromol/day
5–9 yr	49–409 mcg/24 hr	248–2,074 micromol/day
10–17 yr	107–741 mcg/24 hr	543–3,757 micromol/day
18–39 yr	94–695 mcg/24 hr	477–3,524 micromol/day
40–49 yr	182–739 mcg/24 hr	923–3,747 micromol/day
Greater than 50 yr	224–832 mcg/24 hr	1,136–4,218 micromol/day

M

DESCRIPTION: Metanephrines are the inactive metabolites of epinephrine and norepinephrine. Metanephrines are either excreted or further metabolized into vanillylmandelic acid. Release of metanephrines in the urine is indicative of disorders associated with excessive catecholamine production, particularly pheochromocytoma. Vanillylmandelic acid and catecholamines are normally measured with urinary metanephrines. Creatinine is usually measured simultaneously to ensure adequate collection and to calculate an excretion ratio of metabolite to creatinine.

INDICATIONS

• Assist in the diagnosis of suspected pheochromocytoma
• Assist in identifying the cause of hypertension
• Verify suspected tumors associated with excessive catecholamine secretion

POTENTIAL DIAGNOSIS

Increased in
• Ganglioneuroma
• Neuroblastoma
• Pheochromocytoma
• Severe stress

Decreased in: N/A

CRITICAL FINDINGS: N/A

INTERFERING FACTORS

• Drugs that may increase metanephrine levels include monoamine oxidase inhibitors and prochlorperazine.
• Methylglucamine in x-ray contrast medium may cause false-negative results.
• All urine voided for the timed collection period must be included in the collection or else falsely decreased values may be obtained. Compare output records with volume collected to verify that all voids were included in the collection.

NURSING IMPLICATIONS AND PROCEDURE

PRETEST:

▶ Positively identify the patient using at least two unique identifiers before providing care, treatment, or services.
▶ *Patient Teaching:* Inform the patient this test can assist in diagnosing adrenal gland health and hypertension.
▶ Obtain a history of the patient's complaints, including a list of known allergens, especially allergies or sensitivities to latex.
▶ Obtain a history of the patient's endocrine system, symptoms, and results of previously performed laboratory tests and diagnostic and surgical procedures.
▶ Note any recent procedures that can interfere with test results.
▶ Obtain a list of the patient's current medications, including herbs, nutritional supplements, and nutraceuticals (see Appendix F).
▶ Review the procedure with the patient. Provide a nonmetallic urinal, bedpan, or toilet-mounted collection device. Address concerns about pain and explain that there should be no discomfort during the procedure.
▶ Usually a 24-hr time frame for urine collection is ordered. Inform the patient that all urine must be saved during that 24-hr period. Instruct the patient not to void directly into the laboratory collection container. Instruct the patient to avoid defecating in the collection device and to keep toilet tissue out of the collection device to prevent contamination of the specimen. Place a sign in the bathroom to remind the patient to save all urine.
▶ Instruct the patient to void all urine into the collection device and then to pour the urine into the laboratory collection container. Alternatively, the specimen can be left in the collection device for a health-care staff member to add to the laboratory collection container.

M

▸ At the conclusion of the test, compare the quantity of urine with the urinary output record for the collection; if the specimen contains less than what was recorded as output, some urine may have been discarded, thus invalidating the test.

▸ *Sensitivity to social and cultural issues,* as well as concern for modesty, is important in providing psychological support before, during, and after the procedure.

▸ Instruct the patient to avoid excessive exercise and stress during the 24-hr collection of urine.

▸ There are no food, fluid, or medication restrictions unless by medical direction.

INTRATEST:

▸ Ensure that the patient has complied with activity restrictions during the procedure.

▸ If the patient has a history of allergic reaction to latex, avoid the use of equipment containing latex.

▸ Instruct the patient to cooperate fully and to follow directions.

▸ Observe standard precautions, and follow the general guidelines in Appendix A. Positively identify the patient, and label the appropriate collection container with the corresponding patient demographics, date, and time of collection.

Timed Specimen

▸ Obtain a clean 3-L urine specimen container, toilet-mounted collection device, and plastic bag (for transport of the specimen container). The specimen must be refrigerated or kept on ice throughout the entire collection period. If an indwelling urinary catheter is in place, the drainage bag must be kept on ice.

▸ Begin the test between 6 and 8 a.m. if possible. Collect first voiding and discard. Record the time the specimen was discarded as the beginning of the timed collection period. The next morning, ask the patient to void at the same time the collection was started and add this last voiding to the container. Urinary output should be recorded throughout the collection time.

▸ If an indwelling catheter is in place, replace the tubing and container system at the start of the collection time. Keep the container system on ice

during the collection period, or empty the urine into a larger container periodically during the collection period; monitor to ensure continued drainage, and conclude the test the next morning at the same hour the collection was begun.

▸ At the conclusion of the test, compare the quantity of urine with the urinary output record for the collection; if the specimen contains less than what was recorded as output, some urine may have been discarded, invalidating the test.

▸ Include on the collection container's label the amount of urine and test start and stop times.

▸ Promptly transport the specimen to the laboratory for processing and analysis.

POST-TEST:

▸ A report of the results will be sent to the requesting health-care provider (HCP), who will discuss the results with the patient.

▸ Instruct the patient to resume usual activity, as directed by the HCP.

▸ Recognize anxiety related to test results, and be supportive of fear of shortened life expectancy. Discuss the implications of abnormal test results on the patient's lifestyle. Provide teaching and information regarding the clinical implications of the test results, as appropriate. Educate the patient regarding access to counseling services.

▸ Reinforce information given by the patient's HCP regarding further testing, treatment, or referral to another HCP. Answer any questions or address any concerns voiced by the patient or family.

▸ Depending on the results of this procedure, additional testing may be performed to evaluate or monitor progression of the disease process and determine the need for a change in therapy. Evaluate test results in relation to the patient's symptoms and other tests performed.

RELATED MONOGRAPHS:

▸ Related tests include angiography adrenal, cancer antigens, catecholamines, CT renal, HVA, renin, and VMA.

▸ Refer to the Endocrine System table at the end of the book for related tests by body system.

Methemoglobin

SYNONYM/ACRONYM: Hemoglobin, hemoglobin M, MetHb, Hgb M.

COMMON USE: To assess for cyanosis and hypoxemia associated with polycythemia, pathologies affecting hemoglobin, and potential inhaled drug toxicity.

SPECIMEN: Whole blood (1 mL) collected in green-top (heparin) tube. Specimen should be transported tightly capped and in an ice slurry.

REFERENCE VALUE: (Method: Spectrophotometry)

Conventional Units	SI Units (Conventional Units × 155)
0.06–0.24 g/dL*	9.3–37.2 micromol/L*

*Percentage of total hemoglobin = 0.41 – 1.15%.
Note: The conversion factor of ×155 is based on the molecular weight of hemoglobin of 64,500 daltons (d), or 64.5 kd.

DESCRIPTION: Methemoglobin is a structural hemoglobin variant formed when the heme portion of the deoxygenated hemoglobin is oxidized to a ferric state rather than to the normal ferrous state, rendering it incapable of combining with and transporting oxygen to tissues. Visible cyanosis can result as levels approach 10% to 15% of total hemoglobin.

INDICATIONS

- Assist in the detection of acquired methemoglobinemia caused by the toxic effects of chemicals and drugs
- Assist in the detection of congenital methemoglobinemia, indicated by deficiency of red blood cell nicotinamide adenine dinucleotide (NADH)-methemoglobin reductase or presence of methemoglobin

- Evaluate cyanosis in the presence of normal blood gases

POTENTIAL DIAGNOSIS

Increased in
- Acquired methemoglobinemia (drugs, tobacco smoking, or ionizing radiation)
- Carbon monoxide poisoning *(carbon monoxide is a form of deoxygenated hemoglobin)*
- Hereditary methemoglobinemia *(evidenced by a deficiency of NADH-methemoglobin reductase or related to the presence of a hemoglobinopathy)*

Decreased in: N/A

CRITICAL FINDINGS ✦

Cyanosis can occur at levels greater than 10%.

Dizziness, fatigue, headache, and tachycardia can occur at levels greater than 30%.

M

Signs of central nervous system depression can occur at levels greater than 45%.

Death may occur at levels greater than 70%.

Note and immediately report to the health-care provider (HCP) any critically increased or decreased values and related symptoms.

Possible interventions include airway protection, administration of oxygen, monitoring neurological status every hour, continuous pulse oximetry, hyperbaric oxygen therapy, and exchange transfusion. Administration of activated charcoal or gastric lavage may be effective if performed soon after the toxic agent is ingested. Emesis should never be induced in patients with no gag reflex because of the risk of aspiration. Methylene blue may be used to reverse the process of methemoglobin formation, but it should be used cautiously when methemoglobin levels are greater than 30%. Use of methylene blue is contraindicated in the presence of glucose-6-phosphate dehydrogenase deficiency.

INTERFERING FACTORS

- Drugs that may increase methemoglobin levels include acetanilid, amyl nitrate, aniline derivatives, benzocaine, dapsone, glucosulfone, isoniazid, phenytoin, silver nitrate, sulfonamides, and thiazolsulfone.
- Well water containing nitrate is the most common cause of methemoglobinemia in infants.
- Breastfeeding infants are capable of converting inorganic nitrate from common topical anesthetic applications containing nitrate to the nitrite ion, causing nitrite toxicity and increased methemoglobin.
- Prompt and proper specimen processing, storage, and analysis are important to achieve accurate results. Methemoglobin is unstable and should be transported on ice within a few hours of collection, or else the specimen should be rejected.

NURSING IMPLICATIONS AND PROCEDURE

PRETEST:

- Positively identify the patient using at least two unique identifiers before providing care, treatment, or services.
- *Patient Teaching:* Inform the patient this test can assist in identifying the cause of poor oxygenation.
- Obtain a history of the patient's complaints, including a list of known allergens, especially allergies or sensitivities to latex.
- Obtain a history of the patient's hematopoietic and respiratory systems, symptoms, and results of previously performed laboratory tests and diagnostic and surgical procedures.
- Note any recent procedures that can interfere with test results.
- Obtain a list of the patient's current medications, including herbs, nutritional supplements, and nutraceuticals (see Appendix F).
- Review the procedure with the patient. Inform the patient that specimen collection takes approximately 5 to 10 min. Address concerns about pain and explain that there may be some discomfort during the venipuncture.
- *Sensitivity to social and cultural issues,* as well as concern for modesty, is important in providing psychological support before, during, and after the procedure.
- There are no food, fluid, or medication restrictions unless by medical direction.
- Prepare an ice slurry in a cup or plastic bag to have on hand for immediate transport of the specimen to the laboratory.

INTRATEST:

- If the patient has a history of allergic reaction to latex, avoid the use of equipment containing latex.

M

- Instruct the patient to cooperate fully and to follow directions. Direct the patient to breathe normally and to avoid unnecessary movement.
- Observe standard precautions, and follow the general guidelines in Appendix A. Positively identify the patient, and label the appropriate tubes with the corresponding patient demographics, date, and time of collection. Perform a venipuncture.
- Remove the needle and apply direct pressure with dry gauze to stop bleeding. Observe/assess venipuncture site for bleeding or hematoma formation and secure gauze with adhesive bandage.
- Promptly transport the specimen to the laboratory for processing and analysis. The specimen should be placed in an ice slurry immediately after collection. Information on the specimen label should be protected from water in the ice slurry by first placing the specimen in a protective plastic bag.

POST-TEST:

- A report of the results will be sent to the requesting HCP, who will discuss the results with the patient.

- Instruct the patient to avoid carbon monoxide from firsthand or second-hand smoking, to have home gas furnace checked yearly for leaks, and to use gas appliances such as gas grills in a well-ventilated area.
- Reinforce information given by the patient's HCP regarding further testing, treatment, or referral to another HCP. Answer any questions or address any concerns voiced by the patient or family.
- Depending on the results of this procedure, additional testing may be performed to evaluate or monitor progression of the disease process and determine the need for a change in therapy. Evaluate test results in relation to the patient's symptoms and other tests performed.

RELATED MONOGRAPHS:

- Related tests include alveolar/arterial gradient, blood gases, carboxyhemoglobin, hemoglobin electrophoresis, and pulse oximetry.
- Refer to the Hematopoietic and Respiratory systems tables at the end of the book for related tests by body system.

M

Microalbumin

SYNONYM/ACRONYM: Albumin, urine.

COMMON USE: To assist in the identification and management of early diabetes in order to avoid or delay onset of diabetic associated renal disease.

SPECIMEN: Urine (10 mL) from a random or timed specimen collected in a clean plastic collection container.

REFERENCE VALUE: (Method: Nephelometry immunoassay)

Test	Conventional Units
Random microalbumin	Less than 0.03 mg albumin/mg creatinine

Test	Conventional Units
24-hr microalbumin	
Normal	Less than 30 mg/24 hr
Microalbuminuria	30–299 mg/24 hr
Clinical albuminuria	300 mg or greater/24 hr

Simultaneous measurement of urine creatinine or creatinine clearance may be requested. Normal ratio of microalbumin to creatinine is less than 30:1.

DESCRIPTION: The term *micro-albumin* describes concentrations of albumin in urine that are greater than normal but undetectable by dipstick or traditional spectrophotometry methods. Microalbuminuria precedes the nephropathy associated with diabetes and is often elevated years before creatinine clearance shows abnormal values. Studies have shown that the median duration from onset of microalbuminuria to development of nephropathy is 5 to 7 yr.

INDICATIONS
• Evaluate renal disease
• Screen diabetic patients for early signs of nephropathy

POTENTIAL DIAGNOSIS

Increased in
Conditions resulting in increased renal excretion or loss of protein.
• Cardiomyopathy
• Diabetic nephropathy
• Exercise
• Hypertension (uncontrolled)
• Pre-eclampsia
• Renal disease
• Urinary tract infections

Decreased in: N/A

CRITICAL FINDINGS: N/A

INTERFERING FACTORS
• Drugs that may decrease microalbumin levels include captopril, dipyridamole, enalapril, furosemide, indapamide, perindopril, quinapril, ramipril, tolrestat, and triflusal.
• All urine voided for the timed collection period must be included in the collection, or else falsely decreased values may be obtained. Compare output records with volume collected to verify that all voids were included in the collection.

NURSING IMPLICATIONS AND PROCEDURE

PRETEST:
▸ Positively identify the patient using at least two unique identifiers before providing care, treatment, or services.
▸ *Patient Teaching:* Inform the patient this test can assist in evaluating for early kidney disease.
▸ Obtain a history of the patient's complaints, including a list of known allergens, especially allergies or sensitivities to latex.
▸ Obtain a history of the patient's endocrine and genitourinary systems, symptoms, and results of previously performed laboratory tests and diagnostic and surgical procedures.
▸ Obtain a list of the patient's current medications, including herbs, nutritional supplements, and nutraceuticals (see Appendix F).
▸ Review the procedure with the patient. Provide a nonmetallic urinal, bedpan, or toilet-mounted collection device.

Address concerns about pain and explain that there should be no discomfort during the procedure.

▶ Usually a 24-hr time frame for urine collection is ordered. Inform the patient that all urine must be saved during that 24-hr period. Instruct the patient not to void directly into the laboratory collection container. Instruct the patient to avoid defecating in the collection device and to keep toilet tissue out of the collection device to prevent contamination of the specimen. Place a sign in the bathroom to remind the patient to save all urine.

▶ Instruct the patient to void all urine into the collection device and then to pour the urine into the laboratory collection container. Alternatively, the specimen can be left in the collection device for a health-care staff member to add to the laboratory collection container.

▶ *Sensitivity to social and cultural issues,* as well as concern for modesty, is important in providing psychological support before, during, and after the procedure.

▶ Instruct the patient to avoid excessive exercise and stress during the 24-hr collection of urine.

▶ There are no food, fluid, or medication restrictions unless by medical direction.

INTRATEST:

▶ Ensure that the patient has complied with activity restrictions during the procedure.

▶ If the patient has a history of allergic reaction to latex, avoid the use of equipment containing latex.

▶ Instruct the patient to cooperate fully and to follow directions.

▶ Observe standard precautions, and follow the general guidelines in Appendix A. Positively identify the patient, and label the appropriate collection container with the corresponding patient demographics, date, and time of collection.

Random Specimen (Collect in Early Morning)

Clean-Catch Specimen

▶ Instruct the male patient to (1) thoroughly wash his hands, (2) cleanse the meatus, (3) void a small amount into the toilet, and (4) void directly into the specimen container.

▶ Instruct the female patient to (1) thoroughly wash her hands; (2) cleanse the labia from front to back; (3) while keeping the labia separated, void a small amount into the toilet; and (4) without interrupting the urine stream, void directly into the specimen container.

Indwelling Catheter

▶ Put on gloves. Empty drainage tube of urine. It may be necessary to clamp off the catheter for 15 to 30 min before specimen collection. Cleanse specimen port with antiseptic swab, and then aspirate 5 mL of urine with a 21- to 25-gauge needle and syringe. Transfer urine to a sterile container.

Timed Specimen

▶ Obtain a clean 3-L urine specimen container, toilet-mounted collection device, and plastic bag (for transport of the specimen container). The specimen must be refrigerated or kept on ice throughout the entire collection period. If an indwelling urinary catheter is in place, the drainage bag must be kept on ice.

▶ Begin the test between 6 and 8 a.m. if possible. Collect first voiding and discard. Record the time the specimen was discarded as the beginning of the timed collection period. The next morning, ask the patient to void at the same time the collection was started and add this last voiding to the container. Urinary output should be recorded throughout the collection time.

▶ If an indwelling catheter is in place, replace the tubing and container system at the start of the collection time. Keep the container system on ice during the collection period, or empty the urine into a larger container periodically during the collection period; monitor to ensure continued drainage, and conclude the test the next morning at the same hour the collection was begun.

▶ At the conclusion of the test, compare the quantity of urine with the urinary output record for the collection; if the specimen contains less than what was recorded as output, some urine may have been discarded, invalidating the test.

M

▶ Include on the collection container's label the amount of urine and test start and stop times.

General
▶ Promptly transport the specimen to the laboratory for processing and analysis.

POST-TEST:

▶ A report of the results will be sent to the requesting health-care provider (HCP), who will discuss the results with the patient.
▶ Instruct the patient to resume usual activity, as directed by the HCP.
▶ Instruct the patient and caregiver to report signs and symptoms of hypoglycemia or hyperglycemia.
▶ *Nutritional Considerations:* Increased levels of microalbumin may be associated with diabetes. There is no "diabetic diet"; however, many meal-planning approaches with nutritional goals are endorsed by the American Dietetic Association. Patients who adhere to dietary recommendations report a better general feeling of health, better weight management, greater control of glucose and lipid values, and improved use of insulin. Instruct the patient, as appropriate, in nutritional management of diabetes. In June 2006, the American Heart Association developed a Therapeutic Lifestyle Changes (TLC) diet with goals directed at people with specific risk factors and/or existing medical conditions (e.g., elevated LDL cholesterol levels, other lipid disorders, coronary artery disease [CAD], insulin-dependent diabetes, insulin resistance, or metabolic syndrome). The TLC approach also includes the use of plant stanols or sterols and increased dissolved fiber as an option for lowering LDL cholesterol levels; nutritional recommendations for daily total caloric intake; recommendations for allowable percentage of calories derived from fat (saturated and unsaturated), carbohydrates, protein, and cholesterol; as well as recommendations for daily expenditure of energy. The nutritional needs of each diabetic patient need to be determined individually (especially during

pregnancy) with the appropriate health-care professionals, particularly professionals trained in nutrition.
▶ Recognize anxiety related to test results, and be supportive of perceived loss of independence and fear of shortened life expectancy. Discuss the implications of abnormal test results on the patient's lifestyle. Provide teaching and information regarding the clinical implications of the test results, as appropriate. Emphasize, if indicated, that good glycemic control delays the onset and slows the progression of diabetic retinopathy, nephropathy, and neuropathy. Educate the patient regarding access to counseling services, as appropriate. Provide contact information, if desired, for the American Diabetes Association (www.diabetes.org) or the American Heart Association (www.americanheart.org).
▶ Reinforce information given by the patient's HCP regarding further testing, treatment, or referral to another HCP. Answer any questions or address any concerns voiced by the patient or family.
▶ Depending on the results of this procedure, additional testing may be performed to evaluate or monitor progression of the disease process and determine the need for a change in therapy. Evaluate test results in relation to the patient's symptoms and other tests performed.

RELATED MONOGRAPHS:

▶ Related tests include A/G ratio, angiography renal, blood pool imaging, BUN, CBC, cortisol, creatinine, creatinine clearance, culture urine, cystometry, cystoscopy, cytology urine, echocardiography, echocardiography transesophageal, EPO, fluorescein angiography, fundus photography, glucose, GTT, glycated hemoglobin, gonioscopy, Holter monitor, insulin, insulin antibodies, magnesium, protein total and fractions, renogram, UA, visual fields test, and voiding cystourethrography.
▶ Refer to the Endocrine and Genitourinary systems tables at the end of the book for related tests by body system.

Mumps Serology

SYNONYM/ACRONYM: N/A.

COMMON USE: To assist in diagnosing a present or past mumps infection.

SPECIMEN: Serum (1 mL) collected in a red-top tube.

REFERENCE VALUE: (Method: Indirect immunofluorescence) Negative or less than a fourfold increase in titer.

DESCRIPTION: Mumps serology is done to determine the presence of mumps antibody, indicating exposure to or active presence of mumps. Mumps, also known as *parotitis,* is an infectious viral disease of the parotid glands caused by a myxovirus that is transmitted by direct contact with or droplets spread from the saliva of an infected person. The incubation period averages 3 wk. Virus can be shed in saliva for 2 wk after infection and in urine for 2 wk after the onset of symptoms. Complications of infection include aseptic meningitis; encephalitis; and inflammation of the testes, ovaries, and pancreas. The presence of immunoglobulin M (IgM) antibodies indicates acute infection. The presence of immunoglobulin G (IgG) antibodies indicates current or past infection.

INDICATIONS
- Determine resistance to or protection against the mumps virus by a positive reaction or susceptibility to mumps by a negative reaction
- Document immunity
- Evaluate mumps-like diseases and differentiate between these and actual mumps

POTENTIAL DIAGNOSIS
Past or current mumps infection.

CRITICAL FINDINGS: N/A

INTERFERING FACTORS: N/A

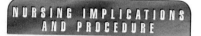

NURSING IMPLICATIONS AND PROCEDURE

PRETEST:
- Positively identify the patient using at least two unique identifiers before providing care, treatment, or services.
- *Patient Teaching:* Inform the patient this test can assist in diagnosing a mumps infection.
- Obtain a history of the patient's complaints, including a list of known allergens, especially allergies or sensitivities to latex. Obtain a history of exposure.
- Obtain a history of the patient's immune system, symptoms, and results of previously performed laboratory tests and diagnostic and surgical procedures.
- Obtain a list of the patient's current medications, including herbs, nutritional supplements, and nutraceuticals (see Appendix F).
- Review the procedure with the patient. Inform the patient that several tests may be necessary to confirm diagnosis. Any individual positive result should be repeated in 7 to 14 days to monitor a change in titer. Inform the

M

patient that specimen collection takes approximately 5 to 10 min. Address concerns about pain and explain that there may be some discomfort during the venipuncture.

▶ *Sensitivity to social and cultural issues,* as well as concern for modesty, is important in providing psychological support before, during, and after the procedure.

▶ There are no food, fluid, or medication restrictions unless by medical direction.

INTRATEST:

▶ If the patient has a history of allergic reaction to latex, avoid the use of equipment containing latex.

▶ Instruct the patient to cooperate fully and to follow directions. Direct the patient to breathe normally and to avoid unnecessary movement.

▶ Observe standard precautions, and follow the general guidelines in Appendix A. Positively identify the patient, and label the appropriate tubes with the corresponding patient demographics, date, and time of collection. Perform a venipuncture.

▶ Remove the needle and apply direct pressure with dry gauze to stop bleeding. Observe/assess venipuncture site for bleeding or hematoma formation and secure gauze with adhesive bandage.

▶ Promptly transport the specimen to the laboratory for processing and analysis.

POST-TEST:

▶ A report of the results will be sent to the requesting health-care provider (HCP), who will discuss the results with the patient.

▶ Instruct the patient in isolation precautions during the time of communicability or contagion.

▶ Emphasize that the patient must return to have a convalescent blood sample taken in 7 to 14 days.

▶ Inform the patient that the presence of mumps antibodies ensures lifelong immunity.

▶ Reinforce information given by the patient's HCP regarding further testing, treatment, or referral to another HCP. Provide information regarding vaccine-preventable diseases where indicated (e.g., encephalitis, hepatitis A and B, human papillomavirus, influenza, measles, mumps, polio, rubella, smallpox, varicella, yellow fever). Answer any questions or address any concerns voiced by the patient or family.

▶ Depending on the results of this procedure, additional testing may be performed to evaluate or monitor progression of the disease process and determine the need for a change in therapy. Evaluate test results in relation to the patient's symptoms and other tests performed.

RELATED MONOGRAPHS:

▶ Refer to the Immune System table at the end of the book for related tests by body system.

Myocardial Infarct Scan

SYNONYM/ACRONYM: PYP cardiac scan, infarct scan, pyrophosphate cardiac scan, acute myocardial infarction scan.

COMMON USE: To differentiate between new and old myocardial infarcts and evaluate myocardial perfusion.

AREA OF APPLICATION: Heart, chest/thorax.

CONTRAST: IV radioactive material, usually technetium-99m stannous pyrophosphate (PYP).

DESCRIPTION: Technetium-99m stannous pyrophosphate (PYP) scanning, also known as *myocardial infarct imaging*, reveals the presence of myocardial perfusion and the extent of myocardial infarction (MI). This procedure can distinguish new from old infarcts when a patient has had abnormal electrocardiograms (ECGs) and cardiac enzymes have returned to normal. PYP uptake by acutely infarcted tissue may be related to the influx of calcium through damaged cell membranes, which accompanies myocardial necrosis; that is, the radionuclide may be binding to calcium phosphates or to hydroxyapatite. The PYP in these damaged cells can be viewed as spots of increased radionuclide uptake that appear in 12 hr at the earliest.

PYP uptake usually takes place 24 to 72 hr after MI, and the radionuclide remains detectable for approximately 10 to 14 days after the MI. PYP uptake is proportional to the blood flow to the affected area; with large areas of necrosis, PYP uptake may be maximal around the periphery of a necrotic area, with little uptake being detectable in the poorly perfused center. Most of the PYP is concentrated in regions that have 20% to 40% of the normal blood flow.

Single-photon emission computed tomography (SPECT) can be used to visualize the heart from multiple angles and planes, enabling areas of MI to be viewed with greater accuracy and resolution. This technique removes overlying structures that may confuse interpretation of the results. With the availability of assays of troponins, myocardial infarct imaging has become less important in the diagnosis of acute MI.

INDICATIONS

- Aid in the diagnosis of (or confirm and locate) acute MI when ECG and enzyme testing do not provide a diagnosis
- Aid in the diagnosis of perioperative MI
- Differentiate between a new and old infarction
- Evaluate possible reinfarction or extension of the infarct
- Obtain baseline information about infarction before cardiac surgery

POTENTIAL DIAGNOSIS

Normal findings in
- Normal coronary blood flow and tissue perfusion, with no PYP localization in the myocardium
- No uptake above background activity in the myocardium (*Note:* when PYP uptake is present, it is graded in relation to adjacent rib activity)

Abnormal findings in
- MI, indicated by increased PYP uptake in the myocardium

CRITICAL FINDINGS: N/A

INTERFERING FACTORS

This procedure is contraindicated for
- Patients who are pregnant or suspected of being pregnant, unless the potential benefits of the procedure far outweigh the risk of radiation exposure to the fetus.
- Patients with hypersensitivity to the radionuclide.

M

Factors that may impair clear imaging

- Inability of the patient to cooperate or remain still during the procedure because of age, significant pain, or mental status.
- Metallic objects (e.g., jewelry, body rings) within the examination field, which may inhibit organ visualization and cause unclear images.
- Other nuclear scans done within the previous 24 to 48 hr.
- Conditions such as chest wall trauma, cardiac trauma, or recent cardioversion procedure.
- Myocarditis.
- Pericarditis.
- Left ventricular aneurysm.
- Metastasis.
- Valvular and coronary artery calcifications.
- Cardiac neoplasms.
- Aneurysms.

Other considerations

- Improper injection of the radionuclide may allow the tracer to seep deep into the muscle tissue, producing erroneous hot spots.
- Consultation with a health-care provider (HCP) should occur before the procedure for radiation safety concerns regarding younger patients or patients who are lactating.
- Risks associated with radiation overexposure can result from frequent x-ray or radionuclide procedures. Personnel working in the examination area should wear badges to record their level of radiation.

NURSING IMPLICATIONS AND PROCEDURE

PRETEST:

- Positively identify the patient using at least two unique identifiers before providing care, treatment, or services.
- *Patient Teaching:* Inform the patient this procedure can assess blood flow to the heart.
- Obtain a history of the patient's complaints, including a list of known allergens, especially allergies or sensitivities to latex, iodine, seafood, contrast medium, anesthetics, or dyes.
- Obtain a history of the patient's cardiovascular system, symptoms, and results of previously performed laboratory tests and diagnostic and surgical procedures.
- Note any recent procedures that can interfere with test results, including examinations using iodine-based contrast medium.
- Record the date of the last menstrual period and determine the possibility of pregnancy in perimenopausal women.
- Obtain a list of the patient's current medications, including herbs, nutritional supplements, and nutraceuticals (see Appendix F).
- Review the procedure with the patient. Address concerns about pain related to the procedure and explain that some pain may be experienced during the test, and there may be moments of discomfort. Reassure the patient that the radionuclide poses no radioactive hazard and rarely produces side effects. Inform the patient that the procedure is performed in a nuclear medicine department by an HCP specializing in this procedure, with support staff, and will take approximately 30 to 60 min. Inform the patient that the technologist will administer an IV injection of the radionuclide and that he or she will need to return 2 to 3 hr later for the scan.
- *Sensitivity to social and cultural issues,* as well as concern for modesty, is important in providing psychological support before, during, and after the procedure.
- The patient should fast, restrict fluids, and refrain from smoking for 4 hr prior to the procedure. Instruct the patient to withhold medications for 24 hr before the procedure. Protocols may vary among facilities.
- Instruct the patient to remove jewelry and other metallic objects from the area to be examined.

INTRATEST:

▶ Ensure that the patient has complied with dietary and medication restrictions and other pretesting preparations.

▶ Ensure that the patient has removed all external metallic objects prior to the procedure.

▶ Have emergency equipment readily available.

▶ Instruct the patient to void prior to the procedure and to change into the gown, robe, and foot coverings provided.

▶ Instruct the patient to cooperate fully and to follow directions. Instruct the patient to lie very still during the procedure because movement will produce unclear images.

▶ Observe standard precautions, and follow the general guidelines in Appendix A.

▶ Place the patient in a supine position on a flat table with foam wedges to help maintain position and immobilization.

▶ IV radionuclide is administered. The heart is scanned 2 to 4 hr after injection in various positions. In most circumstances, however, SPECT is done so that the heart can be viewed from multiple angles and planes.

▶ Monitor the patient for complications related to the procedure (e.g., allergic reaction, anaphylaxis, bronchospasm).

▶ Remove the needle or catheter and apply a pressure dressing over the puncture site.

▶ Observe/assess the needle/catheter insertion site for bleeding, inflammation, or hematoma formation.

POST-TEST:

▶ A report of the results will be sent to the requesting HCP, who will discuss the results with the patient.

▶ Instruct the patient to resume normal activity and diet as directed by the HCP.

▶ Unless contraindicated, advise the patient to drink increased amounts of fluids for 24 to 48 hr to eliminate the radionuclide from the body. Inform the patient that radionuclide is eliminated from the body within 6 to 24 hr.

▶ No other radionuclide tests should be scheduled for 24 to 48 hr after this procedure.

▶ Evaluate the patient's vital signs. Monitor vital signs and neurological status every 15 min for 1 hr, then every 2 hr for 4 hr, and then as ordered by HCP. Take temperature every 4 hr for 24 hr. Monitor intake and output at least every 8 hr. Compare with baseline values. Notify the HCP if temperature is elevated. Protocols may vary among facilities.

▶ Observe for delayed allergic reactions, such as rash, urticaria, tachycardia, hyperpnea, hypertension, palpitations, nausea, or vomiting.

▶ Instruct the patient to immediately report symptoms such as fast heart rate, difficulty breathing, skin rash, itching, chest pain, persistent right shoulder pain, or abdominal pain. Immediately report symptoms to the appropriate HCP.

▶ Instruct the patient in the care and assessment of the injection site.

▶ If the patient must return for additional imaging, advise the patient to rest in the interim and restrict diet to liquids before redistribution studies.

▶ If a woman who is breastfeeding must have a nuclear scan, she should not breastfeed the infant until the radionuclide has been eliminated. This could take as long as 3 days. She should be instructed to express the milk and discard it during the 3-day period to prevent cessation of milk production.

▶ Instruct the patient to flush the toilet immediately after each voiding following the procedure and to meticulously wash hands with soap and water after each voiding for 24 hr after the procedure.

▶ Instruct all caregivers to wear gloves when discarding urine for 24 hr after the procedure. Wash gloved hands with soap and water before removing gloves. Then wash hands after the gloves are removed.

▶ *Nutritional Considerations:* Abnormal findings may be associated with cardiovascular disease. The American Heart Association and National Heart, Lung, and Blood Institute (NHBLI)

M

recommend nutritional therapy for individuals identified to be at high risk for developing coronary artery disease (CAD) or individuals who have specific risk factors and/or existing medical conditions (e.g., elevated LDL cholesterol levels, other lipid disorders, insulin-dependent diabetes, insulin resistance, or metabolic syndrome). If overweight, the patient should be encouraged to achieve a normal weight. The NHLBI's National Cholesterol Education Program (NCEP) revised its dietary guidelines for reducing CAD in 2001. Guidelines for the Therapeutic Lifestyle Changes (TLC) diet are outlined in the Third Report of the Expert Panel on Detection, Evaluation, and Treatment of High Blood Cholesterol in Adults (Adult Treatment Panel III [ATP III]). The TLC diet emphasizes a reduction in foods high in saturated fats and cholesterol. Red meats, eggs, and dairy products are the major sources of saturated fats and cholesterol. If triglycerides also are elevated, the patient should be advised to eliminate or reduce alcohol and simple carbohydrates from the diet. The TLC approach also includes the use of plant stanols or sterols and increased dissolved fiber as an option for lowering LDL cholesterol levels; nutritional recommendations for daily total caloric intake; recommendations for allowable percentage of calories derived from fat (saturated and unsaturated), carbohydrates, protein, and cholesterol; as well as recommendations for daily expenditure of energy.

▶ *Nutritional Considerations:* Overweight patients with high blood pressure should be encouraged to achieve a normal weight. Other changeable risk factors warranting patient education include strategies to safely decrease sodium intake, increase physical activity, decrease alcohol consumption, eliminate tobacco use, and decrease cholesterol levels.

▶ *Social and Cultural Considerations:* Numerous studies point to the prevalence of excess body weight in American children and adolescents. Experts estimate that obesity is present in 25% of the population ages 6 to 11 yr. The medical, social, and emotional consequences of excess body weight are significant. Special attention should be given to instructing the child and caregiver regarding health risks and weight-control education.

▶ Recognize anxiety related to test results, and be supportive of fear of shortened life expectancy. Discuss the implications of abnormal test results on the patient's lifestyle. Provide teaching and information regarding the clinical implications of the test results, as appropriate. Educate the patient regarding access to counseling services. Provide contact information, if desired, for the American Heart Association (www.americanheart.org) or the NHLBI (www.nhlbi.nih.gov).

▶ Reinforce information given by the patient's HCP regarding further testing, treatment, or referral to another HCP. Answer any questions or address any concerns voiced by the patient or family.

▶ Depending on the results of this procedure, additional testing may be needed to evaluate or monitor progression of the disease process and determine the need for a change in therapy. Evaluate test results in relation to the patient's symptoms and other tests performed.

RELATED MONOGRAPHS:

▶ Related tests include angiography abdominal, AST, BNP, blood pool imaging, chest x-ray, CT abdominal, CT thoracic, CK and isoenzymes, culture viral, echocardiography, echocardiography transesophageal, ECG, MRA, MRI chest, myocardial perfusion scan, pericardial fluid analysis, and PET heart.

▶ Refer to the Cardiovascular System table at the end of the book for related tests by body system.

Myocardial Perfusion Heart Scan

SYNONYM/ACRONYM: Sestamibi scan, stress thallium, thallium scan.

COMMON USE: To assess cardiac blood flow to evaluate for and assist in diagnosing coronary artery disease and myocardial infarction.

AREA OF APPLICATION: Heart, chest/thorax.

CONTRAST: IV contrast medium.

DESCRIPTION: Cardiac scanning is a nuclear medicine study that reveals clinical information about coronary blood flow, ventricular size, and cardiac function. Thallium-201 chloride rest or stress studies are used to evaluate myocardial blood flow to assist in diagnosing or determining the risk for ischemic cardiac disease, coronary artery disease (CAD), and myocardial infarction (MI). This procedure is an alternative to angiography or cardiac catheterization in cases in which these procedures may pose a risk to the patient. Thallium-201 is a potassium analogue and is taken up by myocardial cells proportional to blood flow to the cell and cell viability. During stress studies, the radionuclide is injected at peak exercise, after which the patient continues to exercise for several minutes. During exercise, areas of heart muscle supplied by normal arteries increase their blood supply, as well as the supply of thallium-201 delivery to the heart muscle, to a greater extent than regions of the heart muscle supplied by stenosed coronary arteries. This discrepancy in blood flow becomes apparent and quantifiable in subsequent imaging. Comparison of early stress images with images taken after 3 to 4 hr

redistribution (delayed images) enables differentiation between normally perfused, healthy myocardium (which is normal at rest but ischemic on stress) and infarcted myocardium.

Technetium-99m agents such as sestamibi (2-methoxyisobutylisonitrile) are delivered similarly to thallium-201 during myocardial perfusion imaging, but they are extracted to a lesser degree on the first pass through the heart and are taken up by the mitochondria. Over a short period, the radionuclide concentrates in the heart to the same degree as thallium-201. The advantage to technetium-99m agents is that immediate imaging is unnecessary because the radionuclide remains fixed to the heart muscle for several hours. The examination requires two separate injections, one for the rest portion and one for the stress portion of the procedure. These injections can take place on the same day or preferably over a 2-day period. Examination quality is improved if the patient is given a light, fatty meal after the radionuclide is injected to facilitate hepatobiliary clearance of the radioactivity.

If stress testing cannot be performed by exercising, dipyridamole

M

(Persantine) or adenosine, a vasodilator, can be administered orally or IV. A coronary vasodilator is administered before the thallium-201 or other radionuclide, and the scanning procedure is then performed. Vasodilators increase blood flow in normal coronary arteries twofold to threefold without exercise, and they reveal perfusion defects when blood flow is compromised by vessel pathology. Vasodilator-mediated myocardial perfusion scanning is reserved for patients who are unable to participate in treadmill, bicycle, or handgrip exercises for stress testing because of lung disease, neurological disorders (e.g., multiple sclerosis, spinal cord injury), morbid obesity, and orthopedic disorders (e.g., arthritis, limb amputation).

Single-photon emission computed tomography can be used to visualize the heart from multiple angles and planes, enabling areas of MI to be viewed with greater accuracy and resolution. This technique removes overlying structures that may confuse interpretation of the results.

INDICATIONS

- Aid in the diagnosis of CAD or risk for CAD
- Determine rest defects and reperfusion with delayed imaging in unstable angina
- Evaluate the extent of CAD and determine cardiac function
- Assess the function of collateral coronary arteries
- Evaluate bypass graft patency and general cardiac status after surgery
- Evaluate the site of an old MI to determine obstruction to cardiac muscle perfusion
- Evaluate the effectiveness of medication regimen and balloon angioplasty procedure on narrow coronary arteries

POTENTIAL DIAGNOSIS

Normal findings in
- Normal wall motion, coronary blood flow, tissue perfusion, and ventricular size and function

Abnormal findings in
- Abnormal stress and resting images, indicating previous MI
- Abnormal stress images with normal resting images, indicating transient ischemia
- Cardiac hypertrophy, indicated by increased radionuclide uptake in the myocardium
- Enlarged left ventricle
- Heart chamber disorder
- Ventricular septal defects

CRITICAL FINDINGS: N/A

INTERFERING FACTORS

This procedure is contraindicated for
- ❖ Patients who have taken sildenafil (Viagra) within the previous 48 hr, because this test may require the use of nitrates (nitroglycerin) that can precipitate life-threatening low blood pressure.
- Patients with bleeding disorders.
- Patients who are pregnant or suspected of being pregnant, unless the potential benefits of the procedure far outweigh the risk of radiation exposure to the fetus.
- Patients with hypersensitivity to the radionuclide.
- Patients with left ventricular hypertrophy, right and left bundle branch block, hypokalemia, and patients receiving cardiotonic therapy.
- Patients with anginal pain at rest or patients with severe atherosclerotic coronary vessels in whom dipyridamole testing cannot be performed.

- Patients with asthma, because chemical stress with vasodilators can cause bronchospasms.

Factors that may impair clear imaging

- Inability of the patient to cooperate or remain still during the procedure because of age, significant pain, or mental status.
- Medications such as digitalis and quinidine, which can alter cardiac contractility, and nitrates, which can affect cardiac performance.
- Single-vessel disease, which can produce false-negative thallium-201 scanning results.
- Conditions such as chest wall or cardiac trauma, angina that is difficult to control, significant cardiac arrhythmias, and recent cardioversion procedure.
- Suboptimal cardiac stress or patient exhaustion preventing maximum heart rate testing.
- Excessive eating or exercising between initial and redistribution imaging 4 hr later, which produces false-positive results.
- Improper adjustment of the radiological equipment to accommodate obese or thin patients, which can cause overexposure or underexposure and a poor-quality study.
- Patients who are very obese or who may exceed the weight limit for the equipment.
- Incorrect positioning of the patient, which may produce poor visualization of the area to be examined.
- Metallic objects (e.g., jewelry, body rings) within the examination field, which may inhibit organ visualization and cause unclear images.

Other considerations

- Failure to follow dietary restrictions before the procedure may cause the procedure to be canceled or repeated.
- Improper injection of the radionuclide that allows the tracer to seep deep into the muscle tissue produces erroneous hot spots.
- Inaccurate timing for imaging after radionuclide injection can affect the results.
- Consultation with a health-care provider (HCP) should occur before the procedure for radiation safety concerns regarding younger patients or patients who are lactating.
- Risks associated with radiation overexposure can result from frequent x-ray or radionuclide procedures. Personnel working in the examination area should wear badges to reveal their level of exposure to radiation.

NURSING IMPLICATIONS AND PROCEDURE

PRETEST:

- Positively identify the patient using at least two unique identifiers before providing care, treatment, or services.
- *Patient Teaching:* Inform the patient this procedure can assist in assessing blood flow to the heart.
- Obtain a history of the patient's complaints and symptoms, including a list of known allergens, especially allergies or sensitivities to latex.
- Obtain a history of the patient's cardiovascular system, symptoms, and results of previously performed laboratory tests and diagnostic and surgical procedures.
- Record the date of the last menstrual period and determine the possibility of pregnancy in perimenopausal women.
- Obtain a list of the patient's current medications, including herbs, nutritional supplements, and nutraceuticals (see Appendix F).
- Review the procedure with the patient. Address concerns about pain and explain that some pain may be experienced during the test, or there may be moments of discomfort. Inform the patient that the procedure is performed in a special department, usually in a radiology or vascular suite, by an HCP specializing in this procedure, with support staff, and takes approximately 30 to 60 min.

Sensitivity to social and cultural issues, as well as concern for modesty, is important in providing psychological support before, during, and after the procedure.

- Explain that an IV line may be inserted to allow infusion of IV fluids, contrast medium, dye, or sedatives. Usually normal saline is infused.
- Instruct the patient to wear walking shoes (if treadmill exercise testing is to be performed), and emphasize the importance of reporting fatigue, pain, or shortness of breath.
- Instruct the patient to remove dentures, jewelry, and other metallic objects from the area to be examined prior to the procedure.
- Instruct the patient to fast for 4 hr, refrain from smoking for 4 to 6 hr, and withhold medications for 24 hr before the test. Instruct the patient to avoid taking anticoagulant medication or to reduce dosage as ordered prior to the procedure. Protocols may vary among facilities.
- *Make sure a written and informed consent has been signed prior to the procedure and before administering any medications.*
- This procedure may be terminated if chest pain, severe cardiac arrhythmias, or signs of a cerebrovascular accident occur.

INTRATEST:

- Ensure that the patient has complied with dietary, tobacco, and medication restrictions and other pretesting preparations for 4 to 6 hr prior to the procedure.
- Ensure that the patient has removed external metallic objects from the area to be examined prior to the procedure.
- Have emergency equipment readily available.
- If the patient has a history of allergic reactions to any substance or drug, administer ordered prophylactic steroids or antihistamines before the procedure. Use nonionic contrast medium for the procedure.
- Instruct the patient to void prior to the procedure and change into the gown, robe, and foot coverings provided.

- Record baseline vital signs and assess neurological status. Protocols may vary among facilities.
- Instruct the patient to cooperate fully and to follow directions.
- Observe standard precautions, and follow the general guidelines in Appendix A.
- Establish IV fluid line for the injection of emergency drugs and of sedatives.
- Place electrocardiographic (ECG) electrodes on the patient for cardiac monitoring. Establish baseline rhythm; determine if the patient has ventricular arrhythmias. Monitor the patient's blood pressure throughout the procedure by using an automated blood pressure machine.
- Assist the patient onto the treadmill or bicycle ergometer and ask the patient to exercise to a calculated 80% to 85% of the maximum heart rate, as determined by the protocol selected.
- Wear gloves during the radionuclide injection and while handling the patient's urine.
- Thallium-201 is injected 60 to 90 sec before exercise is terminated, and imaging is done immediately in the supine position and repeated in 4 hr.
- Patients who cannot exercise are given dipyridamole 4 min before thallium-201 is injected.
- Inform the patient that movement during the resting procedure affects the results and makes interpretation difficult.
- Monitor the patient for complications related to the procedure (e.g., allergic reaction, anaphylaxis, or brochospasm).
- Remove the needle or catheter and apply a pressure dressing over the puncture site.
- Observe/assess the needle/catheter insertion site for bleeding, inflammation, or hematoma formation.
- The results are recorded on film or in a computerized system for recall and postprocedure interpretation by the appropriate HCP.

POST-TEST:

- A report of the results will be sent to the requesting HCP, who will discuss the results with the patient.
- Instruct the patient to resume normal diet and activity, as directed by the HCP.

- Unless contraindicated, advise patient to drink increased amounts of fluids for 24 to 48 hr to eliminate the radionuclide from the body. Inform the patient that radionuclide is eliminated from the body within 6 to 24 hr.
- No other radionuclide tests should be scheduled for 24 to 48 hr after this procedure.
- Evaluate the patient's vital signs. Monitor vital signs and neurological status every 15 min for 1 hr, then every 2 hr for 4 hr, and then as ordered by HCP. Take temperature every 4 hr for 24 hr. Monitor intake and output at least every 8 hr. Compare with baseline values. Notify the HCP if temperature is elevated. Protocols may vary among facilities.
- Observe for delayed allergic reactions, such as rash, urticaria, tachycardia, hyperpnea, hypertension, palpitations, nausea, or vomiting.
- Instruct the patient to immediately report symptoms such as fast heart rate, difficulty breathing, skin rash, itching, chest pain, persistent right shoulder pain, or abdominal pain. Immediately report symptoms to the appropriate HCP.
- Instruct the patient in the care and assessment of the injection site.
- If the patient must return for additional imaging, advise the patient to rest in the interim and restrict diet to liquids before redistribution studies.
- If a woman who is breastfeeding must have a nuclear scan, she should not breastfeed the infant until the radionuclide has been eliminated. This could take as long as 3 days. She should be instructed to express the milk and discard it during the 3-day period to prevent cessation of milk production.
- Instruct the patient to flush the toilet immediately after each voiding following the procedure and to meticulously wash hands with soap and water after each voiding for 24 hr after the procedure.
- Instruct all caregivers to wear gloves when discarding urine for 24 hr after the procedure. Wash gloved hands with soap and water before removing gloves. Then wash hands after the gloves are removed.

- **Nutritional Considerations:** Abnormal findings may be associated with cardiovascular disease. The American Heart Association and National Heart, Lung, and Blood Institute (NHBLI) recommend nutritional therapy for individuals identified to be at high risk for developing CAD or individuals who have specific risk factors and/or existing medical conditions (e.g., elevated LDL cholesterol levels, other lipid disorders, insulin-dependent diabetes, insulin resistance, or metabolic syndrome). If overweight, the patient should be encouraged to achieve a normal weight. The NHLBI's National Cholesterol Education Program (NCEP) revised its dietary guidelines for reducing CAD in 2001. Guidelines for the Therapeutic Lifestyle Changes (TLC) diet are outlined in the Third Report of the Expert Panel on Detection, Evaluation, and Treatment of High Blood Cholesterol in Adults (Adult Treatment Panel III [ATP III]). The TLC diet emphasizes a reduction in foods high in saturated fats and cholesterol. Red meats, eggs, and dairy products are the major sources of saturated fats and cholesterol. If triglycerides also are elevated, the patient should be advised to eliminate or reduce alcohol and simple carbohydrates from the diet. The TLC approach also includes the use of plant stanols or sterols and increased dissolved fiber as an option for lowering LDL cholesterol levels; nutritional recommendations for daily total caloric intake; recommendations for allowable percentage of calories derived from fat (saturated and unsaturated), carbohydrates, protein, and cholesterol; as well as recommendations for daily expenditure of energy.
- **Nutritional Considerations:** Overweight patients with high blood pressure should be encouraged to achieve a normal weight. Other changeable risk factors warranting patient education include strategies to safely decrease sodium intake, increase physical activity, decrease alcohol consumption, eliminate tobacco use, and decrease cholesterol levels.
- **Social and Cultural Considerations:** Numerous studies point to the prevalence of excess body weight in

M

American children and adolescents. Experts estimate that obesity is present in 25% of the population ages 6 to 11 yr. The medical, social, and emotional consequences of excess body weight are significant. Special attention should be given to instructing the child and caregiver regarding health risks and weight-control education.

▶ Recognize anxiety related to test results, and be supportive of fear of shortened life expectancy. Discuss the implications of abnormal test results on the patient's lifestyle. Provide teaching and information regarding the clinical implications of the test results, as appropriate. Educate the patient regarding access to counseling services. Provide contact information, if desired, for the American Heart Association (www.americanheart.org) or the NHLBI (www.nhlbi.nih.gov).

▶ Reinforce information given by the patient's HCP regarding further testing, treatment, or referral to another HCP. Answer any questions or address any concerns voiced by the patient or family.

▶ Depending on the results of this procedure, additional testing may be needed to evaluate or monitor progression of the disease process and determine the need for a change in therapy. Evaluate test results in relation to the patient's symptoms and other tests performed.

RELATED MONOGRAPHS:

▶ Related tests include antiarrhythmic drugs, apolipoprotein A and B, AST, atrial natriuretic peptide, BNP, calcium, cholesterol (total, HDL, LDL), CT cardiac scoring, CRP, CK and isoenzymes, echocardiography, echocardiography transesophageal, ECG, exercise stress test, glucose, glycated hemoglobin, Holter monitor, homocysteine, ketones, LDH and isos, lipoprotein electrophoresis, magnesium, MRI chest, MI infarct scan, myoglobin, PET heart, potassium, triglycerides, and troponin.

▶ Refer to the Cardiovascular System table at the end of the book for related tests by body system.

Myoglobin

SYNONYM/ACRONYM: MB.

COMMON USE: A general assessment of damage to skeletal or cardiac muscle from trauma or inflammation.

SPECIMEN: Serum (1 mL) collected in a red- or tiger-top tube.

REFERENCE VALUE: (Method: Nephelometry)

Conventional & SI Units
5–70 mcg/L

Values are higher in males.

DESCRIPTION: Myoglobin is an oxygen-binding muscle protein normally found in skeletal and cardiac muscle. It is released into the bloodstream after muscle damage from ischemia, trauma, or inflammation. Although myoglobin testing is more sensitive than creatinine kinase and isoenzymes, it does not indicate the specific site involved.

Timing for Appearance and Resolution of Serum/Plasma Cardiac Markers in Acute Myocardial Infarction

Cardiac Marker	Appearance (Hours)	Peak (Hours)	Resolution (Days)
AST	6–8	24–48	3–4
CK (total)	4–6	24	2–3
CK-MB	4–6	15–20	2–3
LDH	12	24–48	10–14
Myoglobin	1–3	4–12	1
Troponin I	2–6	15–20	5–7

INDICATIONS

- Assist in predicting a flare-up of polymyositis
- Estimate damage from skeletal muscle injury or myocardial infarction (MI)

POTENTIAL DIAGNOSIS

Increased in
Conditions that cause muscle damage; damaged muscle cells release myoglobin into circulation.

- Cardiac surgery
- Cocaine use *(rhabdomyolysis is a complication of cocaine use or overdose)*
- Exercise
- Malignant hyperthermia
- MI
- Progressive muscular dystrophy
- Renal failure
- Rhabdomyolysis
- Shock
- Thrombolytic therapy

Decreased in
- Myasthenia gravis
- Presence of antibodies to myoglobin, as seen in patients with polymyositis
- Rheumatoid arthritis

CRITICAL FINDINGS: N/A

INTERFERING FACTORS: N/A

NURSING IMPLICATIONS AND PROCEDURE

PRETEST:

- Positively identify the patient using at least two unique identifiers before providing care, treatment, or services.
- *Patient Teaching:* Inform the patient this test can assist in diagnosing cardiac or skeletal muscle damage.
- Obtain a history of the patient's complaints, including a list of known allergens, especially allergies or sensitivities to latex.
- Obtain a history of the patient's cardiovascular and musculoskeletal systems, symptoms, and results of previously performed laboratory tests and diagnostic and surgical procedures.
- Obtain a list of the patient's current medications, including herbs, nutritional supplements, and nutraceuticals (see Appendix F).
- Review the procedure with the patient. Inform the patient that specimen

M

collection takes approximately 5 to 10 min. Address concerns about pain and explain that there may be some discomfort during the venipuncture.

- *Sensitivity to social and cultural issues,* as well as concern for modesty, is important in providing psychological support before, during, and after the procedure.
- There are no food, fluid, or medication restrictions unless by medical direction.

INTRATEST:

- If the patient has a history of allergic reaction to latex, avoid the use of equipment containing latex.
- Instruct the patient to cooperate fully and to follow directions. Direct the patient to breathe normally and to avoid unnecessary movement.
- Observe standard precautions, and follow the general guidelines in Appendix A. Positively identify the patient, and label the appropriate tubes with the corresponding patient demographics, date, and time of collection. Perform a venipuncture.
- Remove the needle and apply direct pressure with dry gauze to stop bleeding. Observe/assess venipuncture site for bleeding or hematoma formation and secure gauze with adhesive bandage.
- Promptly transport the specimen to the laboratory for processing and analysis.

POST-TEST:

- A report of the results will be sent to the requesting health-care provider (HCP), who will discuss the results with the patient.
- *Nutritional Considerations:* Abnormal myoglobin levels may be associated with cardiovascular disease. The American Heart Association and National Heart, Lung, and Blood Institute (NHBLI) recommend nutritional therapy for individuals identified to be at high risk for developing coronary artery disease (CAD) or individuals who have specific risk factors and/or existing medical conditions (e.g., elevated

LDL cholesterol levels, other lipid disorders, insulin-dependent diabetes, insulin resistance, or metabolic syndrome). If overweight, the patient should be encouraged to achieve a normal weight. The NHLBI's National Cholesterol Education Program (NCEP) revised its dietary guidelines for reducing CAD in 2001. Guidelines for the Therapeutic Lifestyle Changes (TLC) diet are outlined in the Third Report of the Expert Panel on Detection, Evaluation, and Treatment of High Blood Cholesterol in Adults (Adult Treatment Panel III [ATP III]). The TLC diet emphasizes a reduction in foods high in saturated fats and cholesterol. Red meats, eggs, and dairy products are the major sources of saturated fats and cholesterol. If triglycerides also are elevated, the patient should be advised to eliminate or reduce alcohol and simple carbohydrates from the diet. The TLC approach also includes the use of plant stanols or sterols and increased dissolved fiber as an option for lowering LDL cholesterol levels; nutritional recommendations for daily total caloric intake; recommendations for allowable percentage of calories derived from fat (saturated and unsaturated), carbohydrates, protein, and cholesterol; as well as recommendations for daily expenditure of energy.

- *Nutritional Considerations:* Overweight patients with high blood pressure should be encouraged to achieve a normal weight. Other changeable risk factors warranting patient education include strategies to safely decrease sodium intake, increase physical activity, decrease alcohol consumption, eliminate tobacco use, and decrease cholesterol levels.
- Recognize anxiety related to test results, and be supportive of fear of shortened life expectancy. Discuss the implications of abnormal test results on the patient's lifestyle. Provide teaching and information regarding the clinical implications of the test results, as appropriate. Educate the patient regarding access

to counseling services. Provide contact information, if desired, for the American Heart Association (www.americanheart.org) or the NHLBI (www.nhlbi.nih.gov).

▶ Reinforce information given by the patient's HCP regarding further testing, treatment, or referral to another HCP. Answer any questions or address any concerns voiced by the patient or family.

▶ Depending on the results of this procedure, additional testing may be performed to evaluate or monitor progression of the disease process and determine the need for a change in therapy. Evaluate test results in relation to the patient's symptoms and other tests performed.

RELATED MONOGRAPHS:

▶ Related tests include antiarrhythmic drugs, apolipoprotein A and B, AST, ANP, blood gases, BNP, calcium, cholesterol (total, HDL, and LDL), CRP, CK and isoenzymes, CT cardiac scoring, echocardiography, echocardiography transesophageal, ECG, exercise stress test, glucose, glycated hemoglobin, Holter monitor, homocysteine, ketones, LDH and isoenzymes, lipoprotein electrophoresis, magnesium, MRI chest, MI infarct scan, myoglobin, pericardial fluid analysis, PET heart, potassium, triglycerides, and troponin.

▶ Refer to the Cardiovascular and Musculoskeletal systems tables at the end of the book for related tests by body system.

M

Nerve Fiber Analysis

SYNONYM/ACRONYM: NFA.

COMMON USE: To assist in measuring the thickness of the retinal nerve fiber layer, to assist in diagnosing diseases of the eye such as glaucoma.

AREA OF APPLICATION: Eyes.

CONTRAST: N/A.

DESCRIPTION: There are over 1 million ganglion nerve cells in the retina of each eye. Each nerve cell has a long fiber that travels through the nerve fiber layer of the retina and exits the eye through the optic nerve. The optic nerve is made up of all the ganglion nerve fibers and connects the eye to the brain for vision to occur. As the ganglion cells die, the nerve fiber layer becomes thinner and an empty space in the optic nerve, called the cup, becomes larger. The thinning of the nerve fiber layer and the enlargement of the nerve fiber cup are measurements used to gauge the extent of damage to the retina. Significant damage to the nerve fiber layer occurs before loss of vision is noticed by the patient. Damage can be caused by glaucoma or by aging or occlusion of the vessels in the retina. Ganglion cell loss due to glaucoma begins in the periphery of the retina, thereby first affecting peripheral vision. This change in vision can also be detected by visual field testing. There are several different techniques for measuring nerve fiber layer thickness. One of the most common employs a laser that emits polarizing light waves. The laser's computer measures the change in direction of alignment of the light beam after it passes through the nerve fiber layer tissue. The amount of change in polarization correlates to the thickness of the retinal nerve fiber layer.

INDICATIONS
- Assist in the diagnosis of eye diseases
- Determine retinal nerve fiber layer thickness
- Monitor the effects of various therapies or the progression of conditions resulting in loss of vision

POTENTIAL DIAGNOSIS

Normal findings in
- Normal nerve fiber layer thickness

Abnormal findings in
- Glaucoma or suspicion of glaucoma
- Ocular hypertension

CRITICAL FINDINGS: N/A

INTERFERING FACTORS

Factors that may impair the results of the examination
- Inability of the patient to fixate on focal point.
- Corneal disorder that prevents proper alignment of the retinal nerve fibers.
- Dense cataract that prevents visualization of a clear nerve fiber image.
- Inability of the patient to cooperate or remain still during the test because of age, significant pain, or mental status.

NURSING IMPLICATIONS AND PROCEDURE

PRETEST:

- Positively identify the patient using at least two unique identifiers before providing care, treatment, or services.
- *Patient Teaching:* Inform the patient this procedure can assist in diagnosing eye disease.
- Obtain a history of the patient's complaints, including a list of known allergens.
- Obtain a history of narrow-angle glaucoma. Obtain a history of known or suspected visual impairment, changes in visual acuity, and use of glasses or contact lenses.
- Obtain a history of the patient's known or suspected vision loss, including type and cause; eye conditions with treatment regimens; eye surgery; and other tests and procedures to assess and diagnose visual deficit.
- Obtain a history of symptoms and results of previously performed laboratory tests and diagnostic and surgical procedures.
- Obtain a list of the patient's current medications, including herbs, nutritional supplements, and nutraceuticals (see Appendix F).
- Instruct the patient to remove contact lenses or glasses, as appropriate. Instruct the patient regarding the importance of keeping the eyes open for the test.
- Review the procedure with the patient. Explain that the patient will be requested to fixate the eyes during the procedure. Address concerns about pain and explain that no pain will be experienced during the test, but there may be moments of discomfort. Explain to the patient that some discomfort may be experienced after the test when the numbness wears off from anesthetic drops administered prior to the test. Inform the patient that a health-care provider (HCP) performs the test and that to evaluate both eyes, the test can take 10 to 15 min.

- *Sensitivity to social and cultural issues,* as well as concern for modesty, is important in providing psychological support before, during, and after the procedure.
- There are no food, fluid, or medication restrictions unless by medical direction.

INTRATEST:

- Instruct the patient to cooperate fully and to follow directions. Ask the patient to remain still during the procedure because movement produces unreliable results.
- Seat the patient comfortably. Instruct the patient to look straight ahead, keeping the eyes open and unblinking.
- Instill topical anesthetic in each eye, as ordered, and allow time for it to work. Topical anesthetic drops are placed in the eye with the patient looking up and the solution directed at the six o'clock position of the sclera (white of the eye) near the limbus (gray, semitransparent area of the eyeball where the cornea and sclera meet). Neither the dropper nor the bottle should touch the eyelashes.
- The equipment used to perform the test determines whether dilation of the pupils is required (OCT) or avoided (GDX).
- Request that the patient look straight ahead at a fixation light with the chin in the chin rest and forehead against the support bar. The patient should be reminded not to move the eyes or blink the eyelids as the measurement is taken. The person performing the test can store baseline data or retrieve previous images from the equipment. The equipment can create the mean image from current and previous data, and its computer can make a comparison against previous images.

POST-TEST:

- A report of the results will be sent to the requesting HCP, who will discuss the results with the patient.
- Recognize anxiety related to test results, and be supportive of impaired activity related to vision loss or anticipated loss of driving privileges. Discuss

N

the implications of abnormal test results on the patient's lifestyle. Provide teaching and information regarding the clinical implications of the test results, as appropriate. Provide contact information, if desired, for the Glaucoma Research Foundation (www .glaucoma.org).

▶ Reinforce information given by the patient's HCP regarding further testing, treatment, or referral to another HCP. Instruct the patient in the use of any ordered medications, usually eye drops. Explain the importance of adhering to the therapy regimen, especially because glaucoma does not present symptoms. Instruct the patient in both the ocular side effects and systemic reactions associated with the pre-scribed medication. Encourage him or her to review corresponding literature provided by a pharmacist. Answer any questions or address any concerns voiced by the patient or family.

▶ Depending on the results of this proce-dure, additional testing may be per-formed to evaluate or monitor progres-sion of the disease process and deter-mine the need for a change in therapy. Evaluate test results in relation to the patient's symptoms and other tests performed.

RELATED MONOGRAPHS:

▶ Related tests include fundus photogra-phy, gonioscopy, pachymetry, slit-lamp biomicroscopy, and visual field testing.
▶ Refer to the Ocular System table at the end of the book for related tests by body system.

N

Osmolality, Blood and Urine

SYNONYM/ACRONYM: Osmo.

COMMON USE: To assess fluid and electrolyte balance related to hydration, acid-base balance, and toxic screening, to assist in diagnosing diseases such as diabetes

SPECIMEN: Serum (1 mL) collected in a red- or tiger-top tube; urine (5 mL) from an unpreserved random specimen collected in a clean plastic collection container.

REFERENCE VALUE: (Method: Freezing point depression)

	Conventional Units	SI Units (Conventional Units × 1)
Serum	275–295 mOsm/kg	275–295 mmol/kg
Urine		
Newborn	75–300 mOsm/kg	75–300 mmol/kg
Children and adults	250–900 mOsm/kg	250–900 mmol/kg

DESCRIPTION: Osmolality is the number of particles in a solution; it is independent of particle size, shape, and charge. Measurement of osmotic concentration in serum provides clinically useful information about water and dissolved-particle transport across fluid compartment membranes. Osmolality is used to assist in the diagnosis of metabolic, renal, and endocrine disorders. The simultaneous determination of serum and urine osmolality provides the opportunity to compare values between the two fluids. A normal urine-to-serum ratio is approximately 0.2 to 4.7 for random samples and greater than 3.0 for first-morning samples (dehydration normally occurs overnight). The major dissolved particles that contribute to osmolality are sodium, chloride, bicarbonate, urea, and glucose. Some of these substances are used in the following calculated estimate:

$$\text{Serum osmolality} = (2 \times Na^+) + (\text{glucose}/18) + (BUN/2.8)$$

Measured osmolality is higher than the estimated value. The osmolal gap is the difference between the measured and calculated values and is normally 5 to 10 mOsm/kg. If the difference is greater than 15 mOsm/kg, consider ethylene glycol, isopropanol, methanol, or ethanol toxicity. These substances behave like antifreeze, lowering the freezing point in the blood, and provide misleadingly high results.

INDICATIONS

Serum
- Assist in the evaluation of antidiuretic hormone (ADH) function
- Assist in rapid screening for toxic substances, such as ethylene glycol, ethanol, isopropanol, and methanol
- Evaluate electrolyte and acid-base balance
- Evaluate state of hydration

0

Urine

- Evaluate concentrating ability of the kidneys
- Evaluate diabetes insipidus
- Evaluate neonatal patients with protein or glucose in the urine
- Perform work-up for renal disease

POTENTIAL DIAGNOSIS

Increased in

- Serum

  Azotemia *(related to accumulation of nitrogen-containing waste products that contribute to osmolality)*

  Dehydration *(related to hemoconcentration)*

  Diabetes insipidus *(related to excessive loss of water through urination that results in hemoconcentration)*

  Diabetic ketoacidosis *(related to excessive loss of water through urination that results in hemoconcentration)*

  Hypercalcemia *(related to electrolyte imbalance that results in water loss and hemoconcentration)*

  Hypernatremia *(related to insufficient intake of water or excessive loss of water; sodium is a major cation in the determination of osmolality)*

- Urine

  Amyloidosis

  Azotemia *(related to decrease in renal blood flow; decrease in water excreted by the kidneys results in a more concentrated urine)*

  Congestive heart failure *(decrease in renal blood flow related to diminished cardiac output; decrease in water excreted by the kidneys results in a more concentrated urine)*

  Dehydration *(related to decrease in water excreted by the kidneys that results in a more concentrated urine)*

  Hyponatremia

  Syndrome of inappropriate antidiuretic hormone production (SIADH) *(related to decrease in water excreted by the kidneys that results in a more concentrated urine)*

Decreased in

- Serum

  Adrenocorticoid insufficiency

  Hyponatremia *(sodium is a major influence on osmolality; decreased sodium contributes to decreased osmolality)*

  SIADH *(related to increase in water reabsorbed by the kidneys that results in a more dilute serum)*

  Water intoxication *(related to excessive water intake, which has a dilutional effect)*

- Urine

  Diabetes insipidus *(related to decreased ability of the kidneys to concentrate urine)*

  Hypernatremia *(related to increased water excreted by the kidneys that results in a more dilute urine)*

  Hypokalemia *(related to increased water excreted by the kidneys that results in a more dilute urine)*

  Primary polydipsia *(related to increase in water intake that results in dilute urine)*

CRITICAL FINDINGS ✦

Serum

- Less than 265 mOsm/kg
- Greater than 320 mOsm/kg

Note and immediately report to the health-care provider (HCP) any critically increased or decreased values and related symptoms.

Serious clinical conditions may be associated with elevated or decreased serum osmolality. The following conditions are associated with elevated serum osmolality:

- *Respiratory arrest*: 360 mOsm/kg
- *Stupor of hyperglycemia:* 385 mOsm/kg
- *Grand mal seizures*: 420 mOsm/kg
- *Death*: greater than 420 mOsm/kg

Symptoms of critically high levels include poor skin turgor, listlessness, acidosis (decreased pH), shock, seizures, coma, and cardiopulmonary arrest.

Intervention may include close monitoring of electrolytes, administering intravenous fluids with the appropriate composition to shift water either into or out of the intravascular space as needed, monitoring cardiac signs, continuing neurological checks, and taking seizure precautions.

INTERFERING FACTORS

- Drugs that may increase serum osmolality include corticosteroids, glycerin, inulin, ioxitalamic acid, mannitol, and methoxyflurane.
- Drugs that may decrease serum osmolality include bendroflumethiazide, carbamazepine, chlorpromazine, chlorthalidone, cyclophosphamide, cyclothiazide, doxepin, hydrochlorothiazide, lorcainide, methyclothiazide, and polythiazide.
- Drugs that may increase urine osmolality include anesthetic agents, chlorpropamide, cyclophosphamide, furosemide, mannitol, metolazone, octreotide, phloridzin, and vincristine.
- Drugs that may decrease urine osmolality include captopril, demeclocycline, glyburide, lithium, methoxyflurane, octreotide, tolazamide, and verapamil.

NURSING IMPLICATIONS AND PROCEDURE

PRETEST:

- Positively identify the patient using at least two unique identifiers before providing care, treatment, or services.
- *Patient Teaching:* Inform the patient that the test is used to evaluate electrolyte and water balance.
- Obtain a history of the patient's complaints, including a list of known allergens, especially allergies or sensitivities to latex.
- Obtain a history of the patient's endocrine and genitourinary systems, symptoms, and results of previously performed laboratory tests and diagnostic and surgical procedures.
- Obtain a list of the patient's current medications, including herbs, nutritional supplements, and nutraceuticals (see Appendix F).
- Review the procedure with the patient. Inform the patient that blood specimen collection takes approximately 5 to 10 min; random urine collection takes approximately 5 min and depends on the cooperation of the patient. Urine specimen collection may also be timed. Address concerns about pain and explain that there may be some discomfort during the venipuncture; there will be no discomfort during urine collection.
- *Sensitivity to social and cultural issues,* as well as concern for modesty, is important in providing psychological support before, during, and after the procedure.
- There are no food, fluid, or medication restrictions unless by medical direction.

INTRATEST:

- Direct the patient to breathe normally and to avoid unnecessary movement during the venipuncture.
- Observe standard precautions, and follow the general guidelines in Appendix A. Positively identify the patient, and label the appropriate tubes or collection containers with the corresponding patient demographics, date, and time of collection.

Blood

- If the patient has a history of allergic reaction to latex, avoid the use of equipment containing latex.
- Perform a venipuncture.
- Remove the needle and apply direct pressure with dry gauze to stop bleeding. Observe/assess venipuncture site for bleeding or hematoma formation and secure gauze with adhesive bandage.

Urine

- Provide a nonmetallic urinal, bedpan, or toilet-mounted collection device.
- Either a random specimen or a timed collection may be requested. For timed specimens, a 12- or 24-hr time frame for urine collection may be ordered. Inform the patient that all urine must be

saved during that 12- or 24-hr period. Instruct the patient not to void directly into the laboratory collection container. Instruct the patient to avoid defecating in the collection device and to keep toilet tissue out of the collection device to prevent contamination of the specimen. Place a sign in the bathroom to remind the patient to save all urine.

▶ Instruct the patient to void all urine into the collection device and then to pour the urine into the laboratory collection container. Alternatively, the specimen can be left in the collection device for a health-care staff member to add to the laboratory collection container.

Clean-Catch Specimen
▶ Instruct the male patient to (1) thoroughly wash his hands, (2) cleanse the meatus, (3) void a small amount into the toilet, and (4) void directly into the specimen container.
▶ Instruct the female patient to (1) thoroughly wash her hands; (2) cleanse the labia from front to back; (3) while keeping the labia separated, void a small amount into the toilet; and (4) without interrupting the urine stream, void directly into the specimen container.

Indwelling Catheter
▶ Put on gloves. Empty drainage tube of urine. It may be necessary to clamp off the catheter for 15 to 30 min before specimen collection. Cleanse specimen port with antiseptic swab, and then aspirate 5 mL of urine with a 21- to 25-gauge needle and syringe. Transfer urine to a sterile container.

Blood or Urine
▶ Promptly transport the specimen to the laboratory for processing and analysis.

▶ A report of the results will be sent to the requesting HCP, who will discuss the results with the patient.
▶ *Nutritional Considerations:* Decreased osmolality may be associated with overhydration. Observe the patient for signs and symptoms of fluid-volume

excess related to excess electrolyte intake, fluid-volume deficit related to active body fluid loss, or risk of injury related to an alteration in body chemistry. (For electrolyte-specific dietary references, see monographs titled "Chloride," "Potassium," and "Sodium.")
▶ Increased osmolality may be associated with dehydration. Evaluate the patient for signs and symptoms of dehydration. Dehydration is a significant and common finding in geriatric and other patients in whom renal function has deteriorated.
▶ Recognize anxiety related to test results. Discuss the implications of abnormal test results on the patient's lifestyle. Provide teaching and information regarding the clinical implications of the test results, as appropriate. Educate the patient regarding access to counseling services. Provide contact information, if desired, for the National Kidney Foundation (www.kidney.org).
▶ Reinforce information given by the patient's HCP regarding further testing, treatment, or referral to another HCP. Answer any questions or address any concerns voiced by the patient or family.
▶ Depending on the results of this procedure, additional testing may be performed to evaluate or monitor progression of the disease process and determine the need for a change in therapy. Evaluate test results in relation to the patient's symptoms and other tests performed.

▶ Related tests include ACTH, anion gap, ammonia, ADH, ANP, BNP, BUN, calcium, carbon dioxide, chloride, CBC hematocrit, CBC hemoglobin, cortisol, creatinine, echocardiography, echocardiography transesophageal, ethanol, glucose, ketones, lung perfusion scan, magnesium, phosphorus, potassium, sodium, and UA.
▶ Refer to the Endocrine and Genitourinary systems tables at the end of the book for related tests by body system.

Osmotic Fragility

SYNONYM/ACRONYM: Red blood cell osmotic fragility, OF.

COMMON USE: To assess the fragility of erythrocytes related to red blood cell lysis to assist in diagnosing diseases such as hemolytic anemia.

SPECIMEN: Whole blood (1 mL) collected in a green-top (heparin) tube and two peripheral blood smears.

REFERENCE VALUE: (Method: Spectrophotometry) Hemolysis (unincubated) begins at 0.5 w/v sodium chloride (NaCl) solution and is complete at 0.3 w/v NaCl solution. Results are compared to a normal curve.

POTENTIAL DIAGNOSIS

Increased in
Conditions that produce RBCs with a small surface-to-volume ratio or RBCs that are rounder than normal will have increased osmotic fragility.
- Acquired immune hemolytic anemias *(abnormal RBCs in size and shape; spherocytes)*
- Hemolytic disease of the newborn *(abnormal RBCs in size and shape; spherocytes)*
- Hereditary spherocytosis *(abnormal RBCs in size and shape; spherocytes)*
- Malaria *(related to effect of parasite on RBC membrane integrity)*
- Pyruvate kinase deficiency *(abnormal RBCs in size and shape; spherocytes)*

Decreased in
Conditions that produce RBCs with a large surface-to-volume ratio or RBCs that are flatter than normal will have decreased osmotic fragility.
- Asplenia *(abnormal cells are not removed from circulation due to absence of spleen; target cells)*
- Hemoglobinopathies *(abnormal RBCs in size and shape; target cells, drepanocytes)*
- Iron-deficiency anemia *(abnormal RBCs in size and shape; target cells)*
- Liver disease *(abnormal RBCs in size and shape; target cells)*
- Thalassemias *(abnormal RBCs in size and shape; target cells)*

CRITICAL FINDINGS: N/A

O

Find and print out the full monograph at DavisPlus (http://davisplus.fadavis.com, keyword Van Leeuwen).

Osteocalcin

SYNONYM/ACRONYM: Bone GLA protein, BGP.

COMMON USE: To assist in assessment of risk for osteoporosis and to evaluate effectiveness of therapeutic interventions.

SPECIMEN: Serum (1 mL) collected in a red-top tube.

REFERENCE VALUE: (Method: Radioimmunoassay)

Age and Sex	Conventional Units	SI Units (Conventional Units × 1)
Newborn	20–40 ng/mL	20–40 mcg/L
1–17 yr	2.8–41 ng/mL	2.8–41 mcg/L
Adult		
Male	3–13 ng/mL	3–13 mcg/L
Female		
Premenopausal	0.4–8.2 ng/mL	0.4–8.2 mcg/L
Postmenopausal	1.5–11 ng/mL	1.5–11 mcg/L

DESCRIPTION: Osteocalcin is an important bone cell matrix protein and a sensitive marker in bone metabolism. It is produced by osteoblasts during the matrix mineralization phase of bone formation and is the most abundant noncollagenous bone cell protein. Synthesis of osteocalcin is dependent on vitamin K. Osteocalcin levels parallel alkaline phosphatase levels. Osteocalcin levels are affected by a number of factors, including the hormone estrogen. Assessment of osteocalcin levels permits indirect measurement of osteoblast activity and bone formation. Because it is released into the bloodstream during bone resorption, there is some question as to whether osteocalcin might also be considered a marker for bone matrix degradation and turnover.

INDICATIONS
- Assist in the diagnosis of bone cancer
- Evaluate bone disease
- Evaluate bone metabolism
- Monitor effectiveness of estrogen replacement therapy

POTENTIAL DIAGNOSIS

Increased in
- Adolescents undergoing a growth spurt *(levels in the blood increase as the rate of bone formation increases)*

• Chronic renal failure *(related to accumulation in circulation due to decreased renal excretion)*
• Hyperthyroidism (primary and secondary) *(related to increased bone turnover)*
• Metastatic skeletal disease *(levels in the blood increase as bone destruction releases it into circulation)*
• Paget's disease *(levels in the blood increase as bone destruction releases it into circulation)*
• Renal osteodystrophy *(related to bone degeneration secondary to hyperparathyroidism of chronic renal failure)*
• Some patients with osteoporosis *(levels in the blood increase as bone destruction releases it into circulation)*

Decreased in
• Growth hormone deficiency *(bone mineralization is stimulated by growth hormone)*
• Pregnancy *(increased demand by developing fetus results in an increase in maternal bone resorption)*
• Primary biliary cirrhosis *(related to increased bone loss)*

CRITICAL FINDINGS: N/A

INTERFERING FACTORS
• Drugs that may increase osteocalcin levels include anabolic steroids, calcitonin, calcitriol, danazol, nafarelin, pamidronate, parathyroid hormone, and stanozolol.
• Drugs that may decrease osteocalcin levels include alendronate, antithyroid therapy, corticosteroids, cyproterone, estradiol valerate, estrogen/progesterone therapy, glucocorticoids, hormone replacement therapy, methylprednisolone, oral contraceptives, pamidronate, parathyroid hormone, prednisolone, prednisone, raloxifene, tamoxifen, and vitamin D.

• Recent radioactive scans or radiation within 1 wk before the serum osteocalcin test can interfere with test results when radioimmunoassay is the test method.

NURSING IMPLICATIONS AND PROCEDURE

PRETEST:
▶ Positively identify the patient using at least two unique identifiers before providing care, treatment, or services.
▶ *Patient Teaching:* Inform the patient this test can assist in evaluating for bone disease.
▶ Obtain a history of the patient's complaints, including a list of known allergens, especially allergies or sensitivities to latex.
▶ Obtain a history of the patient's musculoskeletal system, symptoms, and results of previously performed laboratory tests and diagnostic and surgical procedures.
▶ Note any recent procedures that can interfere with test results.
▶ Obtain a list of the patient's current medications, including herbs, nutritional supplements, and nutraceuticals (see Appendix F).
▶ Review the procedure with the patient. Inform the patient that specimen collection takes approximately 5 to 10 min. Address concerns about pain and explain that there may be some discomfort during the venipuncture.
▶ *Sensitivity to social and cultural issues,* as well as concern for modesty, is important in providing psychological support before, during, and after the procedure
▶ There are no food, fluid, or medication restrictions unless by medical direction.

INTRATEST:
▶ If the patient has a history of allergic reaction to latex, avoid the use of equipment containing latex.
▶ Instruct the patient to cooperate fully and to follow directions. Direct the

O

patient to breathe normally and to avoid unnecessary movement.

▶ Observe standard precautions, and follow the general guidelines in Appendix A. Positively identify the patient, and label the appropriate tubes with the corresponding patient demographics, date, and time of collection. Perform a venipuncture.

▶ Remove the needle and apply direct pressure with dry gauze to stop bleeding. Observe/assess venipuncture site for bleeding or hematoma formation and secure gauze with adhesive bandage.

▶ Promptly transport the specimen to the laboratory for processing and analysis.

POST-TEST:

▶ A report of the results will be sent to the requesting health-care provider (HCP), who will discuss the results with the patient.

▶ *Nutritional Considerations:* Increased osteocalcin levels may be associated with skeletal disease. Nutritional therapy is indicated for individuals identified as being at high risk for developing osteoporosis. Educate the patient regarding the National Osteoporosis Foundation's guidelines, which include a regular regimen of weight-bearing exercises, limited alcohol intake, avoidance of tobacco products, and adequate dietary intake of vitamin D (400 to 800 IU/day) and calcium (120 mg/day). Dietary calcium can be obtained from animal or plant sources. Milk and milk products, sardines, clams, oysters, salmon, rhubarb, spinach, beet greens, broccoli, kale, tofu, legumes, and fortified orange juice are high in calcium. Milk and

milk products also contain vitamin D and lactose, which assist calcium absorption. Cooked vegetables yield more absorbable calcium than raw vegetables. Patients should be informed of the substances that can inhibit calcium absorption by irreversibly binding to some of the calcium, making it unavailable for absorption, such as oxalates, which naturally occur in some vegetables; phytic acid, found in some cereals; and insoluble dietary fiber (in excessive amounts). Excessive protein intake can also negatively affect calcium absorption, especially if it is combined with foods high in phosphorus. Vitamin D is synthesized by the skin and is also available in fortified dairy foods and cod liver oil.

▶ Reinforce information given by the patient's HCP regarding further testing, treatment, or referral to another HCP. Answer any questions or address any concerns voiced by the patient or family.

▶ Depending on the results of this procedure, additional testing may be performed to evaluate or monitor progression of the disease process and determine the need for a change in therapy. Evaluate test results in relation to the patient's symptoms and other tests performed.

RELATED MONOGRAPHS:

▶ Related tests include ALP, biopsy bone, BMD, bone scan, calcium, collagen cross-linked N-telopeptide, MRI musculoskeletal, PTH, phosphorus, radiography bone, and vitamin D.

▶ Refer to the Musculoskeletal System table at the end of the book for related tests by body system.

Otoscopy

SYNONYM/ACRONYM: N/A.

COMMON USE: To visualize and assess internal and external structures of the ear to evaluate for pain or hearing loss.

AREA OF APPLICATION: Ears.

CONTRAST: N/A.

DESCRIPTION: This noninvasive procedure is used to inspect the external ear, auditory canal, and tympanic membrane. Otoscopy is an essential part of any general physical examination but is also done before any other audiological studies when symptoms of ear pain or hearing loss are present.

INDICATIONS

- Detect causes of deafness, obstruction, stenosis, or swelling of the pinna or canal causing a narrowing or closure that prevents sound from entering
- Detect ear abnormalities during routine physical examination
- Diagnose cause of ear pain
- Remove impacted cerumen (with a dull ring curette) or foreign bodies (with a forceps) that are obstructing the entrance of sound waves into the ear
- Evaluate acute or chronic otitis media and effectiveness of therapy in controlling infections

POTENTIAL DIAGNOSIS

Normal findings in
- Normal structure and appearance of the external ear, auditory canal, and tympanic membrane.
  Pinna: Funnel-shaped cartilaginous structure; no evidence of infection, pain, dermatitis with swelling, redness, or itching
- *External auditory canal:* S-shaped canal lined with fine hairs, sebaceous and ceruminous glands; no evidence of redness, lesions, edema, scaliness, pain, accumulation of cerumen, drainage, or presence of foreign bodies
  Tympanic membrane: Shallow, circular cone that is shiny and pearl gray in color, semitransparent whitish cord crossing from front to back just under the upper edge, cone of light on the right side at the 4 o'clock position; no evidence of bulging, retraction, lusterless membrane, or obliteration of the cone of light

Abnormal findings in
- Cerumen accumulation
- Ear trauma
- Foreign bodies
- Otitis externa
- Otitis media
- Tympanic membrane perforation or rupture

CRITICAL FINDINGS: N/A

INTERFERING FACTORS

Factors that may impair the results of the examination
- Obstruction of the auditory canal with cerumen, dried drainage, or foreign bodies that prevent introduction of the otoscope.

O

NURSING IMPLICATIONS AND PROCEDURE

PRETEST:

▶ Positively identify the patient using at least two unique identifiers before providing care, treatment, or services.

▶ *Patient Teaching:* Inform the patient this procedure can assist in investigating suspected ear disorders.

▶ Obtain a history of the patient's complaints, including a list of known allergens, especially allergies or sensitivities to latex.

▶ Obtain a history of the patient's known or suspected hearing loss, including type and cause; ear conditions with treatment regimens; ear surgery; and other tests and procedures to assess and diagnose auditory deficit. Obtain a history of the patient's complaints of pain, itching, drainage, deafness, or presence of tympanotomy tube.

▶ Obtain a history of symptoms and results of previously performed laboratory tests, diagnostic and surgical procedures.

▶ Obtain a list of the patient's current medications, especially antibiotic regimen, as well as herbs, nutritional supplements, and nutraceuticals (see Appendix F).

▶ Review the procedure with the patient. Inform the caregiver that he or she may need to restrain a child in order to prevent damage to the ear if the child cannot remain still. Address concerns about pain and explain that no discomfort will be experienced during the test. Inform the patient that a health-care provider (HCP) performs the test and that to evaluate both ears, the test can take 5 to 10 min.

▶ *Sensitivity to social and cultural issues,* as well as concern for modesty, is important in providing psychological support before, during, and after the procedure.

▶ There are no food, fluid, or medication restrictions unless by medical direction.

▶ Ensure that the external auditory canal is clear of impacted cerumen.

INTRATEST:

▶ Instruct the patient to cooperate fully and to follow directions. Ask the patient to remain still during the procedure because movement produces unreliable results.

▶ Administer ear drops or irrigation to prepare for cerumen removal, if ordered.

▶ Place adult patient in a sitting position; place a child in a supine position on the caregiver's lap. Request that the patient remain very still during the examination; a child can be restrained by the caregiver if necessary.

▶ Assemble the otoscope with the correct-size speculum to fit the size of the patient's ear, and check the light source. For the adult, tilt the head slightly away and, with the nondominant hand, pull the pinna upward and backward. For a child, hold the head steady or have the caregiver hold the child's head steady, depending on the age, and pull the pinna downward. Gently and slowly insert the speculum into the ear canal downward and forward with the handle of the otoscope held downward. For the child, hold the handle upward while placing the edge of the hand holding the otoscope on the head to steady it during insertion. If the speculum resists insertion, withdraw and attach a smaller one.

▶ Place an eye to the lens of the otoscope, turn on the light source, and advance the speculum into the ear canal until the tympanic membrane is visible. Examine the posterior and anterior membrane, cone of light, outer rim (annulus), umbo, handle of the malleus, folds, and pars tensa.

▶ Culture any effusion with a sterile swab and culture tube (see "Culture, Bacterial, Ear," monograph); alternatively, an HCP will perform a needle aspiration from the middle ear through the tympanic membrane during the examination. Other procedures such as cerumen and foreign body removal can also be performed.

▶ Pneumatic otoscopy can be done to determine tympanic membrane flexibility. This test permits the introduction of air into the canal that reveals a reduction in movement of the membrane in otitis media and absence of movement in chronic otitis media.

POST-TEST:

▶ A report of the results will be sent to the requesting HCP, who will discuss the results with the patient.

▶ Administer ear drops of a soothing oil, as ordered, if the canal is irritated by removal of cerumen or foreign bodies.

▶ Recognize anxiety related to test results, and be supportive of impaired activity related to hearing loss. Discuss the implications of abnormal test results on the patient's lifestyle. Provide teaching and information regarding the clinical implications of the test results, as appropriate.

▶ Reinforce information given by the patient's HCP regarding further testing, treatment, or referral to another HCP. Answer any questions or address any concerns voiced by the patient or family.

▶ Depending on the results of this procedure, additional testing may be performed to evaluate or monitor progression of the disease process and determine the need for a change in therapy. Evaluate test results in relation to the patient's symptoms and other tests performed.

RELATED MONOGRAPHS:

▶ Related tests include antibiotic drugs, audiometry hearing loss, culture bacterial (ear), and Gram stain.

▶ Refer to the Auditory System table at the end of the book for related tests by body system.

Ova and Parasites, Stool

SYNONYM/ACRONYM: O & P.

COMMON USE: To assess for the presence of parasites, larvae, or eggs in stool to assist in diagnosing a parasitic infection.

SPECIMEN: Stool collected in a clean plastic, tightly capped container.

REFERENCE VALUE: (Method: Macroscopic and microscopic examination) No presence of parasites, ova, or larvae.

DESCRIPTION: This test evaluates stool for the presence of intestinal parasites and their eggs. Some parasites are nonpathogenic; others, such as protozoa and worms, can cause serious illness.

INDICATIONS
• Assist in the diagnosis of parasitic infestation.

POTENTIAL DIAGNOSIS

Positive findings in
• Amebiasis—*Entamoeba histolytica* infection

• Ascariasis—*Ascaris lumbricoides* infection
• Blastocystis—*Blastocystis hominis* infection
• Cryptosporidiosis—*Cryptosporidium parvum* infection
• Enterobiasis—*Enterobius vermicularis* (pinworm) infection
• Giardiasis—*Giardia lamblia* infection
• Hookworm disease—*Ancylostoma duodenale, Necator americanus* infection
• Isospora—*Isospora belli* infection
• Schistosomiasis—*Schistosoma haematobium, S. japonicum, S. mansoni* infection

O

- Strongyloidiasis—*Strongyloides stercoralis* infection
- Tapeworm disease—*Diphyllobothrium, Hymenolepiasis, Taenia saginata, T. solium* infection
- Trematode disease—*Clonorchis sinensis, Fasciola hepatica, Fasciolopsis buski* infection
- Trichuriasis—*Trichuris trichiura* infection

CRITICAL FINDINGS: N/A

INTERFERING FACTORS
- Failure to test a fresh specimen may yield a false-negative result.
- Antimicrobial or antiamebic therapy within 10 days of test may yield a false-negative result.
- Failure to wait 1 wk after a gastrointestinal study using barium or after laxative use can affect test results.
- Medications such as antacids, antibiotics, antidiarrheal compounds, bismuth, castor oil, iron, magnesia, or psyllium fiber (Metamucil) may interfere with analysis.

NURSING IMPLICATIONS AND PROCEDURE

PRETEST:
- Positively identify the patient using at least two unique identifiers before providing care, treatment, or services.
- *Patient Teaching:* Inform the patient this test can assist in diagnosing a parasitic infection.
- Obtain a history of the patient's complaints, including a list of known allergens. Document any travel to foreign countries.
- Obtain a history of the patient's gastrointestinal and immune systems, symptoms, and results of previously performed laboratory tests and diagnostic and surgical procedures.
- Note any recent therapies that can interfere with test results.

- Obtain a list of the patient's current medications, including herbs, nutritional supplements, and nutraceuticals (see Appendix F).
- Review the procedure with the patient. Instruct the patient on hand-washing procedures, and inform the patient that the infection may be contagious. Warn the patient not to contaminate the specimen with urine, toilet paper, or toilet water. Address concerns about pain and explain to the patient that there should be no discomfort during the procedure.
- *Sensitivity to social and cultural issues,* as well as concern for modesty, is important in providing psychological support before, during, and after the procedure.
- Instruct the patient to avoid medications that interfere with test results.
- There are no food or fluid restrictions unless by medical direction.

INTRATEST:
- Instruct the patient to cooperate fully and to follow directions.
- Observe standard precautions, and follow the general guidelines in Appendix A. Positively identify the patient, and label the appropriate collection container with the corresponding patient demographics, date, and time of collection.
- Collect a stool specimen directly into the container. If the patient is bedridden, use a clean bedpan and transfer the specimen into the container using a tongue depressor.
- Specimens to be examined for the presence of pinworms are collected by the "Scotch tape" method in the morning before bathing or defecation. A small paddle with a piece of cellophane tape (sticky side facing out) is pressed against the perianal area. The tape is placed in a collection container and submitted to determine if ova are present. Sometimes adult worms are observed protruding from the rectum.
- Promptly transport the specimen to the laboratory for processing and analysis.

POST-TEST:
- A report of the results will be sent to the requesting health-care provider

(HCP), who will discuss the results with the patient.

» Recognize anxiety related to test results. Discuss the implications of abnormal test results on the patient's lifestyle. Provide teaching and information regarding the clinical implications of the test results, as appropriate.

» Reinforce information given by the patient's HCP regarding further testing, treatment, or referral to another HCP. Educate the patient with positive findings on the transmission of the parasite, as indicated. Warn the patient that one negative result does not rule out parasitic infestation and that additional specimens may be required. Answer

any questions or address any concerns voiced by the patient or family.

» Depending on the results of this procedure, additional testing may be performed to evaluate or monitor progression of the disease process and determine the need for a change in therapy. Evaluate test results in relation to the patient's symptoms and other tests performed.

RELATED MONOGRAPHS:

» Related tests include biopsy intestinal, biopsy liver, biopsy muscle, culture stool, fecal analysis, and IgE.
» Refer to the Gastrointestinal and Immune systems tables at the end of the book for related tests by body system.

Oxalate, Urine

SYNONYM/ACRONYM: N/A.

COMMON USE: To identify patients who are at risk for renal calculus formation or hyperoxaluria related to malabsorption.

SPECIMEN: Urine (25 mL) from a timed specimen collected in a clean plastic collection container with hydrogen chloride (HCl) as a preservative.

REFERENCE VALUE: (Method: Spectrophotometry)

Conventional Units	SI Units (Conventional Units × 11.4)
0–40 mg/24 hr	0–456 micromol/24 hr

DESCRIPTION: Oxalate is derived from the metabolism of oxalic acid, glycine, and ascorbic acid. Some individuals with malabsorption disorders absorb and excrete abnormally high amounts of oxalate, resulting in *hyperoxaluria*. Hyperoxaluria may be seen in patients who consume large amounts of animal protein, certain fruits and vegetables, or

megadoses of vitamin C (ascorbic acid). Hyperoxaluria is also associated with ethylene glycol poisoning (oxalic acid is used in cleaning and bleaching agents). Patients who absorb and excrete large amounts of oxalate may form calcium oxalate kidney stones. Simultaneous measurement of serum and urine calcium is often requested.

INDICATIONS

- Assist in the evaluation of patients with ethylene glycol poisoning
- Assist in the evaluation of patients with a history of kidney stones
- Assist in the evaluation of patients with malabsorption syndromes or patients who have had jejunoileal bypass surgery

POTENTIAL DIAGNOSIS

Increased in
Conditions that result in malabsorption for any reason can lead to increased levels. Chronic diarrhea results in excessive loss of calcium to bind oxalate. Increased oxalate is absorbed by the intestine and excreted by the kidneys.

- Bacterial overgrowth
- Biliary tract disease
- Bowel disease
- Celiac disease
- Cirrhosis
- Crohn's disease
- Diabetes
- Ethylene glycol poisoning *(ethylene glycol is metabolized to oxalate and excreted by the kidneys; crystals are present in urine)*
- Ileal resection
- Jejunal shunt
- Pancreatic disease
- Primary hereditary hyperoxaluria (rare)
- Pyridoxine (vitamin B_6) deficiency *(pyridoxine is a cofactor in an enzyme reaction that converts glyoxylic acid to glycine; deficiency results in an increase in oxalate)*
- Sarcoidosis

Decreased in
- Hypercalciuria *(related to formation of calcium oxalate crystals)*
- Renal failure *(related to oxalate kidney stone disease)*

CRITICAL FINDINGS: N/A

INTERFERING FACTORS

- Drugs and vitamins that may increase oxalate levels include ascorbic acid, calcium, and methoxyflurane.
- Drugs that may decrease oxalate levels include nifedipine and pyridoxine.
- Failure to follow dietary restrictions before the procedure may cause the procedure to be canceled or repeated.
- Failure to collect sample in proper preservative may cause the procedure to be repeated. HCl helps keep oxalate dissolved in the urine. If the pH rises above 3.0, oxalate may precipitate from the sample, causing falsely decreased values. The acid also prevents oxidation of vitamin C to oxalate in the sample, causing falsely increased values.

NURSING IMPLICATIONS AND PROCEDURE

PRETEST:

- Positively identify the patient using at least two unique identifiers before providing care, treatment, or services.
- *Patient Teaching:* Inform the patient this test can assist in evaluating risk for kidney stones.
- Obtain a history of the patient's complaints, including a list of known allergens, especially allergies or sensitivities to latex.
- Obtain a history of the patient's gastrointestinal and genitourinary systems, symptoms, and results of previously performed laboratory tests and diagnostic and surgical procedures.
- Obtain a list of the patient's current medications, including herbs, nutritional supplements, and nutraceuticals (see Appendix F).
- Review the procedure with the patient. Provide a nonmetallic urinal, bedpan, or toilet-mounted collection device.

Address concerns about pain and explain that there should be no discomfort during the procedure.

▶ *Sensitivity to social and cultural issues*, as well as concern for modesty, is important in providing psychological support before, during, and after the procedure.

▶ Usually a 24-hr time frame for urine collection is ordered. Inform the patient that all urine must be saved during that 24-hr period. Instruct the patient not to void directly into the laboratory collection container. Instruct the patient to avoid defecating in the collection device and to keep toilet tissue out of the collection device to prevent contamination of the specimen. Place a sign in the bathroom to remind the patient to save all urine.

▶ Instruct the patient to void all urine into the collection device and then to pour the urine into the laboratory collection container. Alternatively, the specimen can be left in the collection device for a health-care staff member to add to the laboratory collection container.

▶ There are no fluid or medication restrictions unless by medical direction.

▶ Calcium supplements, gelatin, rhubarb, spinach, strawberries, tomatoes, and vitamin C should be restricted for at least 24 hr before the test. High-protein meals should also be avoided 24 hr before specimen collection. Protocols may vary among facilities.

INTRATEST:

▶ Ensure that the patient has complied with dietary restrictions; assure that restricted foods have been avoided for at least 24 hr prior to the procedure.

▶ If the patient has a history of allergic reaction to latex, avoid the use of equipment containing latex.

▶ Instruct the patient to cooperate fully and to follow directions.

▶ Observe standard precautions, and follow the general guidelines in Appendix A. Positively identify the patient, and label the appropriate tubes with the corresponding patient demographics, date, and time of collection.

Random Specimen (Collect in Early Morning)
Clean-Catch Specimen

▶ Instruct the male patient to (1) thoroughly wash his hands, (2) cleanse the meatus, (3) void a small amount into the toilet, and (4) void directly into the specimen container.

▶ Instruct the female patient to (1) thoroughly wash her hands; (2) cleanse the labia from front to back; (3) while keeping the labia separated, void a small amount into the toilet; and (4) without interrupting the urine stream, void directly into the specimen container.

Indwelling Catheter

▶ Put on gloves. Empty drainage tube of urine. It may be necessary to clamp off the catheter for 15 to 30 min before specimen collection. Cleanse specimen port with antiseptic swab, and then aspirate 5 mL of urine with a 21- to 25-gauge needle and syringe. Transfer urine to a sterile container.

Timed Specimen

▶ Obtain a clean 3-L urine specimen container, toilet-mounted collection device, and plastic bag (for transport of the specimen container). The specimen must be refrigerated or kept on ice throughout the entire collection period. If an indwelling urinary catheter is in place, the drainage bag must be kept on ice.

▶ Begin the test between 6 and 8 a.m. if possible. Collect first voiding and discard. Record the time the specimen was discarded as the beginning of the timed collection period. The next morning, ask the patient to void at the same time the collection was started and add this last voiding to the container. Urinary output should be recorded throughout the collection time.

▶ If an indwelling catheter is in place, replace the tubing and container system at the start of the collection system. Keep the container system on ice during the collection period, or empty the urine into a larger container periodically during the collection period; monitor to ensure continued drainage, and conclude the test the next morning at the same hour the collection was begun.

O

▶ At the conclusion of the test, compare the quantity of urine with the urinary output record for the collection; if the specimen contains less than what was recorded as output, some urine may have been discarded, invalidating the test.

▶ Include on the collection container's label the amount of urine, test start and stop times, and ingestion of any foods or medications that can affect test results.

General

▶ Promptly transport the specimen to the laboratory for processing and analysis.

POST-TEST:

▶ A report of the results will be sent to the requesting health-care provider (HCP), who will discuss the results with the patient.

▶ Instruct the patient to resume usual diet, as directed by the HCP.

▶ *Nutritional Considerations:* Consideration may be given to lessening dietary intake of oxalate if urine levels are increased. Encourage patients with abnormal results to seek advice regarding dietary modifications from a trained nutritionist. Magnesium supplementation may be recommended for patients with GI disease to prevent the development of calcium oxalate kidney stones.

▶ Recognize anxiety related to test results, and be supportive of fear of shortened life expectancy. Discuss the implications of abnormal test results on the patient's lifestyle. Provide teaching and information regarding the clinical implications of the test results, as appropriate. Educate the patient regarding access to counseling services.

▶ Reinforce information given by the patient's HCP regarding further testing, treatment, or referral to another HCP. Answer any questions or address any concerns voiced by the patient or family.

▶ Depending on the results of this procedure, additional testing may be performed to evaluate or monitor progression of the disease process and determine the need for a change in therapy. Evaluate test results in relation to the patient's symptoms and other tests performed.

RELATED MONOGRAPHS:

▶ Related tests include calcium, calculus kidney stone panel, UA, urine uric acid, and vitamin C.

▶ Refer to the Gastrointestinal and Genitourinary systems tables at the end of the book for related tests by body system.

Pachymetry

SYNONYM/ACRONYM: N/A.

COMMON USE: To assess the thickness of the cornea prior to LASIK surgery and evaluate glaucoma risk.

AREA OF APPLICATION: Eyes.

CONTRAST: N/A.

DESCRIPTION: Pachymetry is the measurement of the thickness of the cornea using an ultrasound device called a pachymeter. Refractive surgery procedures such as LASIK (laser-assisted in-situ keratomileusis) remove tissue from the cornea. Pachymetry is used to ensure that enough central corneal tissue remains after surgery to prevent ectasia, or abnormal bowing, of thin corneas. Also, studies point to a correlation between increased risk of glaucoma and decreased corneal thickness. This correlation has influenced some health-care providers (HCPs) to include pachymetry as a part of a regular eye health examination for patients who have a family history of glaucoma or who are part of a high-risk population. African Americans have a higher incidence of glaucoma than any other ethnic group.

INDICATIONS

- Assist in the diagnosis of glaucoma (*Note:* the intraocular pressure in glaucoma patients with a thin cornea, 530 micron or less, may be higher than in patients whose corneal thickness is within normal limits)
- Determine corneal thickness in potential refractive surgery candidates
- Monitor the effects of various therapies using eye drops, laser, or filtering surgery

POTENTIAL DIAGNOSIS

Normal findings in
- Normal corneal thickness of 535 to 555 micron

Abnormal findings in
- Bullous keratopathy
- Corneal rejection after penetrating keratoplasty
- Fuchs' endothelial dystrophy
- Glaucoma

CRITICAL FINDINGS: N/A

INTERFERING FACTORS

Factors that may impair the results of the examination:
- Inability of the patient to cooperate or remain still during the test because of age, significant pain, or mental status.
- Improper technique during application of the probe tip to the cornea.

NURSING IMPLICATIONS AND PROCEDURE

PRETEST:
- Positively identify the patient using at least two unique identifiers before providing care, treatment, or services.
- *Patient Teaching:* Inform the patient this procedure can assist in measuring the thickness of the cornea in the eye.
- Obtain a history of the patient's complaints, including a list of known allergens, especially allergies or sensitivities to latex.
- Obtain a history of narrow-angle glaucoma. Obtain a history of known or suspected visual impairment, changes

in visual acuity, and use of glasses or contact lenses.

▶ Obtain a history of the patient's known or suspected vision loss, including type and cause; eye conditions with treatment regimens; eye surgery; and other tests and procedures to assess and diagnose visual deficit.

▶ Obtain a history of symptoms and results of previously performed laboratory tests, diagnostic and surgical procedures.

▶ Obtain a list of the patient's current medications, including herbs, nutritional supplements, and nutraceuticals (see Appendix F).

▶ Instruct the patient to remove contact lenses or glasses, as appropriate. Instruct the patient regarding the importance of keeping the eyes open for the test.

▶ Review the procedure with the patient. Explain that the patient will be requested to fixate the eyes during the procedure. Address concerns about pain and explain that no pain will be experienced during the test, but there may be moments of discomfort. Explain that some discomfort may be experienced after the test when the numbness wears off from anesthetic drops administered prior to the test, or discomfort may occur if too much pressure is used during the test. Inform the patient that an HCP performs the test and that to evaluate both eyes, the test can take 3 to 5 min.

▶ *Sensitivity to social and cultural issues,* as well as concern for modesty, is important in providing psychological support before, during, and after the procedure.

▶ There are no food, fluid, or medication restrictions unless by medical direction.

INTRATEST:

▶ Instruct the patient to cooperate fully and to follow directions. Ask the patient to remain still during the procedure because movement produces unreliable results.

▶ Seat the patient comfortably. Instruct the patient to look straight ahead, keeping the eyes open and unblinking.

▶ Instill topical anesthetic in each eye, as ordered, and allow time for it to work. Topical anesthetic drops are placed in the eye with the patient looking up and

the solution directed at the six o'clock position of the sclera (white of the eye) near the limbus (gray, semitransparent area of the eyeball where the cornea and sclera meet). Neither the dropper nor the bottle should touch the eyelashes.

▶ Request that the patient look straight ahead while the probe of the pachymeter is applied directly on the cornea of the eye. Take an average of three readings for each eye. Individual readings should be within 10 microns. Results on both eyes should be similar.

POST-TEST:

▶ A report of the results will be sent to the requesting HCP, who will discuss the results with the patient.

▶ Recognize anxiety related to test results. Encourage the family to recognize and be supportive of impaired activity related to vision loss, anticipated loss of driving privileges, or the possibility of requiring corrective lenses (self-image). Discuss the implications of test results on the patient's lifestyle. Reassure the patient regarding concerns related to impending cataract surgery. Provide teaching and information regarding the clinical implications of the test results, as appropriate. Provide contact information, if desired, for the Glaucoma Research Foundation (www.glaucoma.org).

▶ Reinforce information given by the patient's HCP regarding further testing, treatment, or referral to another HCP. Answer any questions or address any concerns voiced by the patient or family.

▶ Depending on the results of this procedure, additional testing may be performed to evaluate or monitor progression of the disease process and determine the need for a change in therapy. Evaluate test results in relation to the patient's symptoms and other tests performed.

RELATED MONOGRAPHS:

▶ Related tests include fundus photography, gonioscopy, intraocular pressure, and visual field testing.

▶ Refer to the Ocular System table at the end of the book for related tests by body system.

Papanicolaou Smear

SYNONYM/ACRONYM: Pap smear, cervical smear.

COMMON USE: To establish a histological diagnosis of cervical and vaginal disease and identify the presence of genital infections, such as cancer, herpes, and cytomegalovirus.

SPECIMEN: Cervical and endocervical cells.

REFERENCE VALUE: (Method: Microscopic examination of fixed and stained smear) Reporting of Pap smear findings may follow one of several formats and may vary by laboratory. Simplified content of the two most common formats for interpretation are listed in the table.

Bethesda System	Description
Specimen type	Conventional, liquid-based, or other
Specimen adequacy	*Satisfactory* for evaluation—endocervical transformation zone component is described as present or absent, along with other quality indicators (e.g., partially obscuring blood, inflammation)
	Unsatisfactory for evaluation—either the specimen is rejected and the reason given or the specimen is processed and examined but not evaluated for epithelial abnormalities and the reason is given
General categorization	*Negative* for intraepithelial lesion or malignancy. Epithelial cell abnormality (abnormality is specified in the interpretation section of the report).
	Other comments
Automated review	Indicates the case was examined by an automated device and the results are listed along with the name of the device
Ancillary testing	Describes the test method and result
Interpretation/result	Organisms—*Trichomonas vaginalis,* fungal organisms consistent with *Candida* spp., shift in flora suggestive of bacterial vaginosis, bacteria morphologically consistent with *Actinomyces* spp., cellular changes consistent with herpes simplex virus

P

Bethesda System	Description
	Other nonneoplastic findings—reactive cellular changes associated with inflammation, radiation, intrauterine device; glandular cell status post-hysterectomy; atrophy; endometrial cells (in a woman of 40 yr or greater)
Epithelial cell abnormalities Squamous cell	ASC • of undetermined significance (ASC-US) • cannot exclude HSIL (ASC-H) LSIL • encompassing HPV, mild dysplasia, CIN 1 HSIL • encompassing moderate and severe dysplasia CIS/CIN 2 and CIN 3 • with features suspicious for invasion (if invasion is suspected) Squamous cell carcinoma
Glandular cell	Atypical • endocervical cells (not otherwise specified [NOS] or specify otherwise) • endometrial cells (NOS or specify otherwise) • glandular cells (NOS or specify otherwise) Atypical • endocervical cells, favor neoplastic • glandular cells, favor neoplastic Endocervical carcinoma in situ Adenocarcinoma • endocervical • endometrial • extrauterine • NOS
Other malignant neoplasms	Specify
Educational notes and suggestions	Should be consistent with clinical follow-up guidelines published by professional organizations with references included

ASC = atypical squamous cells; ASC-H = high-grade atypical squamous cells; ASC-US = atypical squamous cells undetermined significance; CIN = cervical intraepithelial neoplasia = CIN; CIS = carcinoma in situ; HSIL = high-grade squamous intraepithelial lesion; LSIL = low-grade squamous intraepithelial lesion.

DESCRIPTION: The Papanicolaou (Pap) smear is primarily used for the early detection of cervical cancer. The interpretation of Pap smears is as heavily dependent on the collection and fixation technique as it is on the completeness and accuracy of the clinical information provided with the specimen. The patient's age, date of last menstrual period, parity, surgical status, postmenopausal status, use of hormone therapy (including use of oral contraceptives), history of radiation or chemotherapy, history of abnormal vaginal bleeding, and history of previous Pap smears are essential for proper interpretation. Human papillomavirus (HPV) is the most common sexually transmitted virus and primary causal factor in the development of cervical cancer. Therefore, specimens for HPV are often collected simultaneously with the PAP smear. The laboratory should be consulted about the availability of this option prior to specimen collection because specific test kits are required to allow for simultaneous sample collection. HPV infection can be successfully treated once it has been identified. Gardasil, the first vaccine developed against HPV, is given at 2 and 6 mo respectively after the initial injection. The Centers for Disease Control and Prevention recommends vaccination for females age 11 and 12 yr. Vaccination is also recommended for females age 13 to 26 yr who have not been previously vaccinated.

A wet prep can be prepared simultaneously from a cervical or vaginal sample. The swab is touched to a microscope slide, and a small amount of saline is dropped on the slide. The slide is examined by microscope to determine the presence of harmful bacteria or *Trichomonas*.

A Schiller's test entails applying an iodine solution to the cervix. Normal cells pick up the iodine and stain brown. Abnormal cells do not pick up any color.

Improvements in specimen preparation have added to the increased quality of screening procedures. The Cytyc ThinPrep Pap test (www.cytyc.com), approved by the U.S. Food and Drug Administration in 1996, is a technique that provides a uniform monolayer of cells free of debris such as blood and mucus. Computerized scanning systems are also being used to reduce the number of smears that require manual review by a cytotechnologist or pathologist.

There are now some alternatives to cone biopsy and cryosurgery for the treatment of cervical dysplasia. Patients with abnormal Pap smear results may have a cervical loop electrosurgical excision procedure (LEEP) performed to remove or destroy abnormal cervical tissue. In the LEEP procedure, a speculum is inserted into the vagina, the cervix is numbed, and a special electrically charged wire loop is used to painlessly remove the suspicious area. Postprocedure cramping and bleeding can occur. Laser ablation is another technique that can be employed for the precise removal of abnormal cervical tissue.

P

INDICATIONS
- Assist in the diagnosis of cervical dysplasia
- Assist in the diagnosis of endometriosis, condyloma, and vaginal adenosis
- Assist in the diagnosis of genital infections (herpes, *Candida* spp., *Trichomonas vaginalis,* Cytomegalovirus, *Chlamydia*, lymphogranuloma venereum, HPV, and *Actinomyces* spp.)

• Assist in the diagnosis of primary and metastatic neoplasms
• Evaluate hormonal function

POTENTIAL DIAGNOSIS

Positive findings in
(See table [Bethesda system])

Decreased in: N/A

CRITICAL FINDINGS: N/A

INTERFERING FACTORS

• The smear should not be allowed to air dry before fixation.
• Lubricating jelly should not be used on the speculum.
• Improper collection site may result in specimen rejection. Samples for cancer screening are obtained from the posterior vaginal fornix and from the cervix. Samples for hormonal evaluation are obtained from the vagina.
• Douching, sexual intercourse, using tampons, or using vaginal medication within 24 hr prior to specimen collection can interfere with the specimen's results.
• Collection of other specimens prior to the collection of the Pap smear may be cause for specimen rejection.
• Contamination with blood from samples collected during the patient's menstrual period may be cause for specimen rejection.

NURSING IMPLICATIONS AND PROCEDURE

PRETEST:

▶ Positively identify the patient using at least two unique identifiers before providing care, treatment, or services.
▶ *Patient Teaching:* Inform the patient this procedure can assist in diagnosing disease of the reproductive system.
▶ Obtain a history of the patient's complaints, including a list of known allergens, especially allergies or sensitivities to latex.

▶ Obtain a history of the patient's immune and reproductive systems, symptoms, and results of previously performed laboratory tests and diagnostic and surgical procedures.
▶ Record the date of the last menstrual period and determine the possibility of pregnancy in perimenopausal women.
▶ Note any recent procedures that can interfere with test results.
▶ Obtain a list of the patient's current medications, including herbs, nutritional supplements, and nutraceuticals (see Appendix F).
▶ Review the procedure with the patient. Instruct the patient to avoid douching or sexual intercourse for 24 hr before specimen collection. Verify that the patient is not menstruating. Address concerns about pain and explain that there may be some discomfort during the procedure. Inform the patient that specimen collection is performed by a health-care provider (HCP) specializing in this procedure and takes approximately 5 to 10 min.
▶ *Sensitivity to social and cultural issues,* as well as concern for modesty, is important in providing psychological support before, during, and after the procedure.
▶ There are no food, fluid, or medication restrictions unless by medical direction.
▶ If the patient is taking vaginal antibiotic medication, testing should be delayed for 1 mo after the treatment has been completed.
▶ *Make sure a written and informed consent has been signed prior to the procedure and before administering any medications.*

INTRATEST:

▶ Have the patient void before the procedure.
▶ Have the patient remove clothes below the waist.
▶ Instruct the patient to cooperate fully and to follow directions. Ask the patient to breathe normally and to avoid unnecessary movement during the procedure.
▶ Observe standard precautions, and follow the general guidelines in Appendix A. Positively identify the patient, and label the appropriate collection containers with the corresponding patient demographics, date and time of collection, and site location.

P

- Assist the patient into a lithotomy position on a gynecological examination table (with feet in stirrups). Drape the patient's legs.
- A plastic or metal speculum is inserted into the vagina and is opened to gently spread apart the vagina for inspection of the cervix. The speculum may be dipped in warm water to aid in comfortable insertion.
- After the speculum is properly positioned, the cervical and vaginal specimens are obtained. A synthetic fiber brush is inserted deep enough into the cervix to reach the endocervical canal. The brush is then rotated one turn and removed. A plastic or wooden spatula is used to lightly scrape the cervix and vaginal wall.

Conventional Collection

- Specimens from both the brush and the spatula are plated on the glass slide. The brush specimen is plated using a gentle rolling motion, whereas the spatula specimen is plated using a light gliding motion across the slide. The specimens are immediately fixed to the slide with a liquid or spray containing 95% ethanol. The speculum is removed from the vagina. A pelvic and/or rectal examination is usually performed after specimen collection is completed.

ThinPrep Collection

- The ThinPrep bottle lid is opened and removed, exposing the solution. The brush and spatula specimens are then gently swished in the ThinPrep solution to remove the adhering cells. The brush and spatula are then removed from the ThinPrep solution, and the bottle lid is replaced and secured.

General

- Place samples in properly labeled specimen container and promptly transport the specimen to the laboratory for processing and analysis.

POST-TEST:

- A report of the results will be sent to the requesting HCP, who will discuss the results with the patient.
- Cleanse or allow the patient to cleanse secretions or excess lubricant (if a pelvic and/or rectal examination is also performed) from the perineal area. Provide a sanitary pad if cervical bleeding occurs.
- Recognize anxiety related to test results, and offer support. Discuss the implications of abnormal test results on the patient's lifestyle. Provide teaching and information regarding the clinical implications of the test results, as appropriate. Educate the patient regarding access to counseling services.
- Decisions regarding the need for and frequency of conventional or liquid-based Pap tests or other cancer screening procedures should be made after consultation between the patient and HCP. The most current guidelines for cervical cancer screening of the general population as well as of individuals with increased risk are available from the American Cancer Society (www.cancer.org) and the American College of Obstetricians and Gynecologists (ACOG) (www.acog.org).
- Reinforce information given by the patient's HCP regarding further testing, treatment, or referral to another HCP. Inform the patient, as appropriate, that repeat testing may be requested in the event of specimen rejection or abnormal findings. Answer any questions or address any concerns voiced by the patient or family.
- Depending on the results of this procedure, additional testing may be performed to evaluate or monitor progression of the disease process and determine the need for a change in therapy. Evaluate test results in relation to the patient's symptoms and other tests performed.

RELATED MONOGRAPHS:

- Related tests include biopsy cervical, cancer antigens, *Chlamydia* group antibody, colposcopy, culture anal/genital, culture throat, culture urine, culture viral, CMV, cytology urine, laparoscopy gynecologic, US pelvis, and UA.
- Refer to the Immune and Reproductive systems tables at the end of the book for related tests by body system.

P

Parathyroid Hormone

SYNONYM/ACRONYM: Parathormone, PTH, intact PTH, whole molecule PTH.

COMMON USE: To assist in the diagnosis of parathyroid disease and disorders of calcium balance. Also used to monitor patients receiving renal dialysis.

SPECIMEN: Serum (1 mL) collected in a red- or tiger-top tube. Specimen should be transported tightly capped and in an ice slurry.

REFERENCE VALUE: (Method: Immunoassay)

Age	Conventional Units	SI Units (Conventional Units × 1)
Cord blood	Less than 3 pg/mL	Less than 3 ng/L
2–20 yr	9–52 pg/mL	9–52 ng/L
Adult	10–65 pg/mL	10–65 ng/L

DESCRIPTION: Parathyroid hormone (PTH) is secreted by the parathyroid glands in response to decreased levels of circulating calcium. PTH assists in the mobilization of calcium from bone into the bloodstream, promoting renal tubular reabsorption of calcium and depression of phosphate reabsorption, thereby reducing calcium excretion and increasing phosphate excretion by the kidneys. PTH also decreases the renal secretion of hydrogen ions, which leads to increased renal excretion of bicarbonate and chloride. PTH enhances renal production of active vitamin D metabolites, causing increased calcium absorption in the small intestine. The net result of PTH action is maintenance of adequate serum calcium levels. C-terminal and N-terminal assays were used prior to the development of reliable intact or whole molecule PTH assays. A rapid PTH assay has been developed specifically for intraoperative monitoring of PTH in the surgical treatment of primary hyperparathyroidism. Rapid PTH assays have proved valuable because the decision of whether the hyperparathyroidism involves one or multiple glands depends on measurement of circulating PTH levels. Surgical outcomes indicate that a 50% decrease or more in intraoperative PTH from baseline measurements can predict successful treatment with up to 97% accuracy. An intraoperative decrease of less than 50% indicates the need to identify and remove additional malfunctioning parathyroid tissue. In healthy individuals, intact PTH has a circulating half-life of about 5 min. N-terminal PTH has a circulating half-life of about 2 min and is found in very small quantities. Intact and N-terminal PTH are the only biologically active forms of the hormone.

Ninety percent of circulating PTH is composed of inactive C-terminal and midregion fragments. PTH is cleared from the body by the kidneys.

INDICATIONS

- Assist in the diagnosis of hyperparathyroidism
- Assist in the diagnosis of suspected secondary hyperparathyroidism due to chronic renal failure, malignant tumors that produce ectopic PTH, and malabsorption syndromes
- Detect incidental damage or inadvertent removal of the parathyroid glands during thyroid or neck surgery
- Differentiate parathyroid and nonparathyroid causes of hypercalcemia
- Evaluate autoimmune destruction of the parathyroid glands
- Evaluate parathyroid response to altered serum calcium levels, especially those that result from malignant processes, leading to decreased PTH production
- Evaluate source of altered calcium metabolism

POTENTIAL DIAGNOSIS

Increased in

- Fluorosis *(skeletal fluorosis can cause a condition resembling secondary hyperparathyroidism, disruption in calcium homeostasis, and excessive PTH production)*
- Primary, secondary, or tertiary hyperparathyroidism *(all result in excess PTH production)*
- Pseudogout *(calcium is lost due to deposits in the joint; decrease in calcium stimulates PTH production)*
- Pseudohypoparathyroidism
- Zollinger-Ellison syndrome *(related to poor intestinal absorption of calcium and vitamin D; decreased calcium stimulates PTH production)*

Decreased in

- Autoimmune destruction of the parathyroids *(related to decreased parathyroid function)*
- DiGeorge's syndrome *(related to hypoparathyroidism)*
- Hyperthyroidism *(related to increased calcium from bone loss; increased calcium levels inhibit PTH production)*
- Hypomagnesemia *(magnesium is a calcium channel blocker; low magnesium levels allow for increased calcium, which inhibits PTH production)*
- Nonparathyroid hypercalcemia (in the absence of renal failure) *(increased calcium levels inhibit PTH production)*
- Sarcoidosis *(related to increased calcium levels)*
- Secondary hypoparathyroidism due to surgery

CRITICAL FINDINGS: N/A

INTERFERING FACTORS

- Drugs that may increase PTH levels include clodronate, estrogen/progestin therapy, foscarnet, furosemide, hydrocortisone, isoniazid, lithium, nifedipine, octreotide, pamidronate, phosphates, prednisone, tamoxifen, and verapamil.
- Drugs and vitamins that may decrease PTH levels include alfacalcidol, aluminum hydroxide, calcitriol, diltiazem, magnesium sulfate, parathyroid hormone, pindolol, prednisone, and vitamin D.
- PTH levels are subject to diurnal variation, with highest levels occurring in the morning.
- PTH levels should always be measured in conjunction with calcium for proper interpretation.

P

• Failure to follow dietary restrictions before the procedure may cause the procedure to be canceled or repeated.

NURSING IMPLICATIONS AND PROCEDURE

PRETEST:

▶ Positively identify the patient using at least two unique identifiers before providing care, treatment, or services.

▶ *Patient Teaching:* Inform the patient this test can assist in diagnosing parathyroid disease.

▶ Obtain a history of the patient's complaints, including a list of known allergens, especially allergies or sensitivities to latex.

▶ Obtain a history of the patient's endocrine system, symptoms, and results of previously performed laboratory tests and diagnostic and surgical procedures.

▶ Obtain a list of the patient's current medications, including herbs, nutritional supplements, and nutraceuticals (see Appendix F).

▶ Review the procedure with the patient. Early-morning specimen collection is recommended because of the diurnal variation in PTH levels. Inform the patient that specimen collection takes approximately 5 to 10 min. Address concerns about pain and explain that there may be some discomfort during the venipuncture.

▶ *Sensitivity to social and cultural issues,* as well as concern for modesty, is important in providing psychological support before, during, and after the procedure.

▶ The patient should fast for 12 hr before specimen collection. Protocols may vary among facilities.

▶ There are no fluid or medication restrictions unless by medical direction.

▶ Prepare an ice slurry in a cup or plastic bag to have on hand for immediate transport of the specimen to the laboratory.

INTRATEST:

▶ Ensure that the patient has complied with dietary restrictions; ensure that food has been restricted for at least 12 hr prior to the procedure.

▶ If the patient has a history of allergic reaction to latex, avoid the use of equipment containing latex.

▶ Instruct the patient to cooperate fully and to follow directions. Direct the patient to breathe normally and to avoid unnecessary movement.

▶ Observe standard precautions, and follow the general guidelines in Appendix A. Positively identify the patient, and label the appropriate tubes with the corresponding patient demographics, date, and time of collection. Perform a venipuncture.

▶ Remove the needle and apply direct pressure with dry gauze to stop bleeding. Observe/assess venipuncture site for bleeding or hematoma formation and secure gauze with adhesive bandage.

▶ Promptly transport the specimen to the laboratory for processing and analysis. The sample should be placed in an ice slurry immediately after collection. Information on the specimen label should be protected from water in the ice slurry by first placing the specimen in a protective plastic bag.

POST-TEST:

▶ A report of the results will be sent to the requesting health-care provider (HCP), who will discuss the results with the patient.

▶ Instruct the patient to resume usual diet, as directed by the HCP.

▶ *Nutritional Considerations:* Patients with abnormal parathyroid levels are also likely to experience the effects of calcium-level imbalances. Instruct the patient to report signs and symptoms of hypocalcemia and hypercalcemia to the HCP. (For critical values, signs, and symptoms of calcium imbalance and for nutritional information, see monographs titled "Calcium, Blood"; "Calcium, Ionized"; and "Calcium, Urine.")

▶ Reinforce information given by the patient's HCP regarding further testing, treatment, or referral to another HCP. Answer any questions or address any concerns voiced by the patient or family.

▶ Depending on the results of this procedure, additional testing may be

performed to evaluate or monitor progression of the disease process and determine the need for a change in therapy. Evaluate test results in relation to the patient's symptoms and other tests performed.

RELATED MONOGRAPHS:

▶ Related tests include ALP, arthroscopy, calcitonin, calcium, collagen cross-linked telopeptides, evoked brain potentials, fecal fat, gastric emptying scan, gastric acid stimulation, gastrin stimulation test, parathyroid scan, phosphorus, RAIU, synovial fluid analysis, TSH, thyroxine, US thyroid and parathyroid, uric acid, UA, and vitamin D.

▶ Refer to the Endocrine System table at the end of the book for related tests by body system.

Parathyroid Scan

SYNONYM/ACRONYM: Parathyroid scintiscan.

COMMON USE: To assess the parathyroid gland to assist in diagnosing cancer and perform postoperative evaluation of the parathyroid gland.

AREA OF APPLICATION: Parathyroid.

CONTRAST: IV technetium-99m (Tc-99m) pertechnetate, Tc-99m sestamibi, oral iodine-123, and thallium.

DESCRIPTION: Parathyroid scanning is performed to assist in the preoperative localization of parathyroid adenomas in clinically proven primary hyperparathyroidism; it is useful for distinguishing between intrinsic and extrinsic parathyroid adenomas. It is also performed after surgery to verify the presence of the parathyroid gland in children, and it is done after thyroidectomy as well.

The radionuclide is administered 10 to 20 min before the imaging is performed. The thyroid and surrounding tissues should be carefully palpated.

Fine-needle aspiration biopsy guided by ultrasound is occasionally necessary to differentiate thyroid pathology, as well as pathology of other tissues, from parathyroid neoplasia.

INDICATIONS

- Aid in the diagnosis of hyperparathyroidism
- Differentiate between extrinsic and intrinsic parathyroid adenoma but not between benign and malignant conditions
- Evaluate the parathyroid in patients with severe hypercalcemia or in patients before parathyroidectomy

POTENTIAL DIAGNOSIS

Normal findings in
- No areas of increased perfusion or uptake in the thyroid or parathyroid

Abnormal findings in
- Intrinsic and extrinsic parathyroid adenomas

P

CRITICAL FINDINGS: N/A

INTERFERING FACTORS

This procedure is contraindicated for

- Patients who are pregnant or suspected of being pregnant, unless the potential benefits of the procedure far outweigh the risks to the fetus and mother.

Factors that may impair clear imaging

- Inability of the patient to cooperate or remain still during the procedure because of age, significant pain, or mental status.
- Ingestion of foods containing iodine (e.g., iodized salt) and medications containing iodine (e.g., cough syrup, potassium iodide, vitamins, Lugol's solution, thyroid replacement medications), which can decrease uptake of the radionuclide.
- Other nuclear scans or iodinated contrast medium radiographic studies done within the previous 24 to 48 hr.
- Metallic objects (e.g., jewelry, body rings) within the examination field, which may inhibit organ visualization and cause unclear images.

Other considerations

- Improper injection of the radionuclide that allows the tracer to seep deep into the muscle tissue produces erroneous hot spots.
- Consultation with a health-care provider (HCP) should occur before the procedure for radiation safety concerns regarding younger patients or patients who are lactating.
- Risks associated with radiation overexposure can result from frequent x-ray or radionuclide procedures. Personnel working in the examination area should wear badges to record their level of radiation exposure.

NURSING IMPLICATIONS AND PROCEDURE

PRETEST:

- Positively identify the patient using at least two unique identifiers before providing care, treatment, or services.
- *Patient Teaching:* Inform the patient this procedure can assist in diagnosing parathyroid disease.
- Obtain a history of the patient's complaints, including a list of known allergens, especially allergies or sensitivities to latex, iodine, seafood, contrast medium, or anesthetics.
- Note any recent procedures that can interfere with test results, including examinations using iodinated contrast medium or radioactive nuclides.
- Obtain a history of the patient's endocrine system, symptoms, and results of previously performed laboratory tests and diagnostic and surgical procedures.
- Record the date of the last menstrual period and determine the possibility of pregnancy in perimenopausal women.
- Obtain a list of the patient's current medications, including herbs, nutritional supplements, and nutraceuticals (see Appendix F).
- Review the procedure with the patient. Address concerns about pain related to the procedure and explain that some pain may be experienced during the test. Inform the patient that the procedure is performed in a nuclear medicine department, usually by an HCP specializing in this procedure, with support staff, and takes approximately 30 to 60 min.
- *Sensitivity to social and cultural issues,* as well as concern for modesty, is important in providing psychological support before, during, and after the procedure.
- Instruct the patient to remove jewelry and other metallic objects from the area to be examined.
- There are no food, fluid, or medication restrictions unless by medical direction.
- *Make sure a written and informed consent has been signed prior to the procedure and before administering any medications.*

INTRATEST:

▶ Ensure that the patient has removed all external metallic objects from the area to be examined prior to the procedure.

▶ Instruct the patient to void prior to the procedure and to change into the gown, robe, and foot coverings provided.

▶ Instruct the patient to cooperate fully and to follow directions. Instruct the patient to remain still throughout the procedure because movement produces unreliable results.

▶ Observe standard precautions, and follow the general guidelines in Appendix A.

▶ Technetium-99m (Tc-99m) pertechnetate is injected IV before scanning.

▶ Place the patient in a supine position under a radionuclide gamma camera. Images are preformed 15 min after the injection.

▶ With the patient in the same position, Tc-99m sestamibi is injected, and a second image is obtained after 10 min.

▶ Iodine-123 may be administered orally in place of Tc-99m pertechnetate; the imaging sequence, as described previously, is performed 24 hr later.

▶ Remove the needle or catheter and apply a pressure dressing over the puncture site.

▶ Observe/assess the needle/catheter insertion site for bleeding, inflammation, or hematoma formation.

POST-TEST:

▶ A report of the results will be sent to the requesting HCP, who will discuss the results with the patient.

▶ Observe/assess the needle/catheter insertion site for bleeding, inflammation, or hematoma formation.

▶ Instruct the patient in the care and assessment of the injection site.

▶ Advise the patient to drink increased amounts of fluids for 24 to 48 hr to eliminate the radionuclide from the body, unless contraindicated. Tell the patient that radionuclide is eliminated from the body within 6 to 24 hr.

▶ If a woman who is breastfeeding must have a nuclear scan, she should not breastfeed the infant until the radionuclide has been eliminated. This could take as long as 3 days. She should be instructed to express the milk and discard it during the 3-day period to prevent cessation of milk production.

▶ Instruct the patient to flush the toilet immediately and to meticulously wash hands with soap and water after each voiding for 24 hr after the procedure.

▶ Instruct all caregivers to wear gloves when discarding urine for 24 hr after the procedure. Wash gloved hands with soap and water before removing gloves. Then wash hands after the gloves are removed.

▶ Recognize anxiety related to test results, and be supportive of perceived loss of independent function. Discuss the implications of abnormal test results on the patient's lifestyle. Provide teaching and information regarding the clinical implications of the test results, as appropriate.

▶ Reinforce information given by the patient's HCP regarding further testing, treatment, or referral to another HCP. Answer any questions or address any concerns voiced by the patient or family.

▶ Depending on the results of this procedure, additional testing may be needed to evaluate or monitor progression of the disease process and determine the need for a change in therapy. Evaluate test results in relation to the patient's symptoms and other tests performed.

RELATED MONOGRAPHS:

▶ Related tests include calcitonin, calcium, CT thoracic and MRI chest, PTH, phosphorus, US thyroid and parathyroid, and vitamin D.

▶ Refer to the Endocrine System table at the end of the book for related tests by body system.

Partial Thromboplastin Time, Activated

SYNONYM/ACRONYM: aPTT, APTT.

COMMON USE: To assist in assessing coagulation disorders and monitor the effectiveness of therapeutic interventions.

SPECIMEN: Plasma (1 mL) collected in a completely filled blue-top (3.2% sodium citrate) tube. If the patient's hematocrit exceeds 55%, the volume of citrate in the collection tube must be adjusted.

REFERENCE VALUE: (Method: Clot detection) 25 to 39 sec. Reference ranges vary with respect to the equipment and reagents used to perform the assay.

DESCRIPTION: The activated partial thromboplastin time (aPTT) coagulation test evaluates the function of the intrinsic (factors XII, XI, IX, and VIII) and common (factors V, X, II, and I) pathways of the coagulation sequence, specifically the intrinsic thromboplastin system. It represents the time required for a firm fibrin clot to form after tissue thromboplastin or phospholipid reagents similar to thromboplastin and calcium are added to the specimen. The aPTT is abnormal in 90% of patients with coagulation disorders and is useful in monitoring the inactivation of factor II effect of heparin therapy. The test is prolonged when there is a 30% to 40% deficiency in one of the factors required or when factor inhibitors (e.g., antithrombin III, protein C, or protein S) are present. The aPTT has additional activators, such as kaolin, celite, or elegiac acid, that more rapidly activate factor XII, making this test faster and more reliably reproducible than the partial thromboplastin time (PTT). The aPTT and prothrombin time (PT)

tests assist in identifying the cause of bleeding or as preoperative tests to identify coagulation defects. A comparison between the results of aPTT and PT tests can allow some inferences to be made that a factor deficiency exists. A normal aPTT with a prolonged PT can occur only with factor VII deficiency. A prolonged aPTT with a normal PT could indicate a deficiency in factors XII, XI, IX, VIII, and VIII:C (von Willebrand factor). Factor deficiencies can also be identified by correction or substitution studies using normal serum. These studies are easy to perform and are accomplished by adding plasma from a healthy patient to a sample from a patient suspected to be factor deficient. When the aPTT is repeated and is corrected, or is within the reference range, it can be assumed that the prolonged aPTT is caused by a factor deficiency. If the result remains uncorrected, the prolonged aPTT is most likely due to a circulating anticoagulant. The administration of prophylactic low-dose heparin does not require serial monitoring of aPTT. (For more information on factor deficiencies, see monograph titled "Fibrinogen.")

INDICATIONS

- Detect congenital deficiencies in clotting factors, as seen in diseases such as hemophilia A (factor VIII) and hemophilia B (factor IX)
- Evaluate response to anticoagulant therapy with heparin or coumarin derivatives
- Identify individuals who may be prone to bleeding during surgical, obstetric, dental, or invasive diagnostic procedures
- Identify the possible cause of abnormal bleeding, such as epistaxis, hematoma, gingival bleeding, hematuria, and menorrhagia
- Monitor the hemostatic effects of conditions such as liver disease, protein deficiency, and fat malabsorption

POTENTIAL DIAGNOSIS

Prolonged in

- Afibrinogenemia *(related to insufficient levels of fibrinogen, which is required for clotting)*
- Circulating anticoagulants *(related to the presence of coagulation factor inhibitors, e.g., developed from long-term factor VIII therapy, or circulating anticoagulants associated with conditions like tuberculosis, systemic lupus erythematosus, rheumatoid arthritis, and chronic glomerulonephritis)*
- Circulating products of fibrin and fibrinogen degradation *(related to the presence of circulating breakdown products of fibrin)*
- Disseminated intravascular coagulation *(related to increased consumption of clotting factors)*
- Factor deficiencies *(related to insufficient levels of coagulation factors)*
- Hemodialysis patients *(related to the anticoagulant effect of heparin)*
- Severe liver disease *(insufficient production of clotting factors related to liver damage)*
- Vitamin K deficiency *(related to insufficient vitamin K levels required for clotting)*
- Von Willebrand's disease *(related to a congenital deficiency of clotting factors)*

CRITICAL FINDINGS

- Greater than 60 sec

Note and immediately report to the health-care provider (HCP) any critically increased values and related symptoms.

Important signs to note are prolonged bleeding from cuts or gums, hematoma at a puncture site, hemorrhage, blood in the stool, persistent epistaxis, heavy or prolonged menstrual flow, and shock. Monitor vital signs, unusual ecchymosis, occult blood, severe headache, unusual dizziness, and neurological changes until aPTT is within normal range.

INTERFERING FACTORS

- Drugs and vitamins such as anistreplase, antihistamines, chlorpromazine, salicylates, and ascorbic acid may cause prolonged aPTT.
- Anticoagulant therapy with heparin will prolong the aPTT.
- Copper is a component of factor V, and severe copper deficiencies may result in prolonged aPTT values.
- Traumatic venipunctures can activate the coagulation sequence by contamination of the sample with tissue thromboplastin and can produce falsely shortened results.

P

- Failure to fill the tube sufficiently to yield a proper blood-to-anticoagulant ratio invalidates the results and is reason for specimen rejection.
- Excessive agitation that causes sample hemolysis can falsely shorten the aPTT because the hemolyzed cells activate plasma-clotting factors.
- Inadequate mixing of the tube can produce erroneous results.
- Specimens left unprocessed for longer than 24 hr should be rejected for analysis.
- High platelet count or inadequate centrifugation will result in decreased values.
- Hematocrit greater than 55% may cause falsely prolonged results because of anticoagulant excess relative to plasma volume.
- Incompletely filled collection tubes, specimens contaminated with heparin, clotted specimens, or unprocessed specimens not delivered to the laboratory within 1 to 2 hr of collection should be rejected.

NURSING IMPLICATIONS AND PROCEDURE

PRETEST:

- Positively identify the patient using at least two unique identifiers before providing care, treatment, or services.
- *Patient Teaching:* Inform the patient this test can assist in evaluating the effectiveness of blood clotting.
- Obtain a history of the patient's complaints, including a list of known allergens, especially allergies or sensitivities to latex.
- Obtain a history of the patient's hematopoietic and hepatobiliary systems, especially any bleeding disorders and other symptoms, as well as results of previously performed laboratory tests and diagnostic and surgical procedures.
- Obtain a list of the patient's current medications, including anticoagulants, aspirin and other salicylates, herbs, nutritional supplements, and nutraceuticals (see Appendix F). Such products should be discontinued by medical direction for the appropriate number of days prior to a surgical procedure. If the patient is receiving anticoagulant therapy, note the time and amount of the last dose.
- Review the procedure with the patient. Inform the patient that specimen collection takes approximately 5 to 10 min. Address concerns about pain and explain there may be some discomfort during the venipuncture.
- *Sensitivity to social and cultural issues,* as well as concern for modesty, is important in providing psychological support before, during, and after the procedure.
- There are no food, fluid, or medication restrictions unless by medical direction.

INTRATEST:

- If the patient has a history of allergic reaction to latex, avoid the use of equipment containing latex.
- Instruct the patient to cooperate fully and to follow directions. Direct the patient to breathe normally and to avoid unnecessary movement.
- Observe standard precautions, and follow the general guidelines in Appendix A. Positively identify the patient, and label the appropriate tubes with the corresponding patient demographics, date, and time of collection. Perform a venipuncture. Fill tube completely. *Important note:* Two different concentrations of sodium citrate preservative are currently added to blue-top tubes for coagulation studies: 3.2% and 3.8%. The Clinical and Laboratory Standards Institute (CLSI; formerly the National Committee for Clinical Laboratory Standards [NCCLS]) guideline for sodium citrate is 3.2%. Laboratories establish reference ranges for coagulation testing based on numerous factors, including sodium citrate concentration, test equipment, and test reagents. It is important to ask the laboratory which concentration

it recommends, because each concentration will have its own specific reference range. When multiple specimens are drawn, the blue-top tube should be collected after sterile (i.e., blood culture) tubes. Otherwise, when using a standard vacutainer system, the blue-top tube is the first tube collected. When a butterfly is used and due to the added tubing, an extra red-top tube should be collected before the blue-top tube to ensure complete filling of the blue-top tube.

- Remove the needle and apply direct pressure with dry gauze to stop bleeding. Observe/assess venipuncture site for bleeding or hematoma formation and secure gauze with adhesive bandage.
- Promptly transport the specimen to the laboratory for processing and analysis. If delays in specimen transport and processing occur, it is important to consult with the testing laboratory. Whole blood specimens are stable at room temperature for up to 24 hr. Specimen stability requirements may also vary if the patient is receiving heparin therapy. Some laboratories require frozen plasma if testing will not be performed within 1 hr of collection. Criteria for rejection of specimens based on collection time may vary among facilities.
- If the patient has a known hematocrit above 55%, adjust the amount of anticoagulant in the collection tube before drawing the blood according to the CLSI guidelines:

Anticoagulant vol. [x] = (100 − hematocrit)/(595 − hematocrit) × total vol. of anticoagulated blood required

Example:

Patient hematocrit = 60% = [(100 − 60)/(595 − 60) × 5.0] = 0.37 mL

sodium citrate for a 5-mL standard drawing tube

POST-TEST:

- A report of the results will be sent to the requesting HCP, who will discuss the results with the patient.
- Instruct the patient to report severe bruising or bleeding from any areas of the skin or mucous membranes.
- Inform the patient with prolonged aPTT values of the importance of taking precautions against bruising and bleeding, including the use of a soft bristle toothbrush, use of an electric razor, avoidance of constipation, avoidance of acetylsalicylic acid and similar products, and avoidance of intramuscular injections.
- Inform the patient of the importance of periodic laboratory testing while taking an anticoagulant.
- Reinforce information given by the patient's HCP regarding further testing, treatment, or referral to another HCP. Answer any questions or address any concerns voiced by the patient or family.
- Depending on the results of this procedure, additional testing may be performed to evaluate or monitor progression of the disease process and determine the need for a change in therapy. Evaluate test results in relation to the patient's symptoms and other tests performed.

RELATED MONOGRAPHS:

- Related tests include antithrombin III, bleeding time, coagulation factors, CBC, CBC platelet count, copper, D-dimer, FDP, plasminogen, protein C, protein S, PT/INR, and vitamin K.
- Refer to the Hematopoietic and Hepatobiliary systems tables at the end of the book for related tests by body system.

P

Parvovirus B19 Immunoglobulin G and Immunoglobulin M Antibodies

SYNONYM/ACRONYM: N/A.

COMMON USE: To assist in confirming a diagnosis of a present or past parvovirus infection.

SPECIMEN: Serum (2 mL) collected in a red- or tiger-top tube.

REFERENCE VALUE: (Method: Immunoassay)

Negative	Less than 0.8
Equivocal	0.8–1.2

hybridization using a polymerase chain reaction.

DESCRIPTION: Parvovirus B19, a single-stranded DNA virus transmitted by respiratory secretions, is the only parvovirus known to infect humans. Its primary site of replication is in red blood cell precursors in the bone marrow. It is capable of causing disease along a wide spectrum ranging from a self-limited erythema (fifth disease) to bone marrow failure or aplastic crisis in patients with sickle cell anemia, spherocytosis, or thalassemia. Fetal hydrops and spontaneous abortion may also occur as a result of infection during pregnancy. The incubation period is approximately 1 wk after exposure. B19-specific antibodies appear in the serum approximately 3 days after the onset of symptoms. The presence of immunoglobulin M (IgM) antibodies indicates acute infection. The presence of immunoglobin G (IgG) antibodies indicates past infection and is believed to confer lifelong immunity. Parvovirus B19 can also be detected by DNA

INDICATIONS
• Assist in establishing a diagnosis of parvovirus B19 infection

POTENTIAL DIAGNOSIS

Positive findings in Parvovirus infection can be evidenced in a variety of conditions.
• Arthritis
• Erythema infectiosum (fifth disease)
• Erythrocyte aplasia
• Hydrops fetalis

Negative findings in: N/A

CRITICAL FINDINGS: N/A

INTERFERING FACTORS
• Immunocompromised patients may not develop sufficient antibody to be detected.

NURSING IMPLICATIONS AND PROCEDURE

PRETEST:
▶ Positively identify the patient using at least two unique identifiers before providing care, treatment, or services.

P

- *Patient Teaching:* Inform the patient this test can assist in diagnosing a viral infection.
- Obtain a history of the patient's complaints, including a list of known allergens, especially allergies or sensitivities to latex.
- Obtain a history of the patient's immune system, symptoms, and results of previously performed laboratory tests and diagnostic and surgical procedures.
- Obtain a list of the patient's current medications, including herbs, nutritional supplements, and nutraceuticals (see Appendix F).
- Review the procedure with the patient. Inform the patient that specimen collection takes approximately 5 to 10 min. Inform the patient that a subsequent sample will be required in 7 to 14 days. Address concerns about pain and explain that there may be some discomfort during the venipuncture.
- *Sensitivity to social and cultural issues,* as well as concern for modesty, is important in providing psychological support before, during, and after the procedure.
- There are no food, fluid, or medication restrictions unless by medical direction.

INTRATEST:

- If the patient has a history of allergic reaction to latex, avoid the use of equipment containing latex.
- Instruct the patient to cooperate fully and to follow directions. Direct the patient to breathe normally and to avoid unnecessary movement.
- Observe standard precautions, and follow the general guidelines in Appendix A. Positively identify the patient, and label the appropriate tubes with the corresponding patient demographics, date, and time of collection. Perform a venipuncture.
- Remove the needle and apply direct pressure with dry gauze to stop

bleeding. Observe/assess venipuncture site for bleeding or hematoma formation and secure gauze with adhesive bandage.
- Promptly transport the specimen to the laboratory for processing and analysis.

POST-TEST:

- A report of the results will be sent to the requesting health-care provider (HCP), who will discuss the results with the patient.
- Recognize anxiety related to test results, and be supportive of impaired activity related to lack of neuromuscular control, perceived loss of independence, and fear of shortened life expectancy. Discuss the implications of abnormal test results on the patient's lifestyle. Provide teaching and information regarding the clinical implications of the test results, as appropriate. Educate the patient regarding access to counseling services.
- Reinforce information given by the patient's HCP regarding further testing, treatment, or referral to another HCP. Emphasize the need for the patient to return to have a convalescent blood sample taken in 7 to 14 days. Answer any questions or address any concerns voiced by the patient or family.
- Depending on the results of this procedure, additional testing may be performed to evaluate or monitor progression of the disease process and determine the need for a change in therapy. Evaluate test results in relation to the patient's symptoms and other tests performed.

RELATED MONOGRAPHS:

- Related tests include CBC, CBC RBC morphology, and CBC WBC count and differential.
- Refer to the Immune System table at the end of the book for related tests by body system.

P

Pericardial Fluid Analysis

SYNONYM/ACRONYM: None.

COMMON USE: To evaluate and classifying the type of fluid between the pericardium membranes to assist with diagnosis of infection or fluid balance disorder.

SPECIMEN: Pericardial fluid (5 mL) collected in a red- or green-top (heparin) tube for glucose, a lavender-top (EDTA) tube for cell count, and sterile containers for microbiology specimens; 200 to 500 mL of fluid in a clear container for cytology. Ensure that there is an equal amount of fixative and fluid in the container for cytology.

REFERENCE VALUE: (Method: Spectrophotometry for glucose; automated or manual cell count, macroscopic examination of cultured organisms, and microscopic examination of specimen for microbiology and cytology; microscopic examination of cultured microorganisms)

Pericardial Fluid	Reference Value
Appearance	Clear
Color	Pale yellow
Glucose	Parallels serum values
Red blood cell count	None seen
White blood cell count	Less than 300/mm^3
Culture	No growth
Gram stain	No organisms seen
Cytology	No abnormal cells seen

DESCRIPTION: The heart is located within a protective membrane called the *pericardium*. The fluid between the pericardial membranes is called *serous fluid*. Normally only a small amount of fluid is present because the rates of fluid production and absorption are about the same. Many abnormal conditions can result in the buildup of fluid within the pericardium. Specific tests are usually ordered in addition to a common battery of tests used to distinguish a transudate from an exudate. *Transudates* are effusions that form as a result of a systemic disorder that disrupts the regulation of fluid balance, such as a suspected perforation. *Exudates* are caused by conditions involving the tissue of the membrane itself, such as an infection or malignancy. Fluid is withdrawn from the pericardium by needle aspiration and tested as listed in the previous and following tables.

Characteristic	Transudate	Exudate
Appearance	Clear	Cloudy or turbid
Specific gravity	Less than 1.015	Greater than 1.015
Total protein	Less than 2.5 g/dL	Greater than 3.0 g/dL
Fluid-to-serum protein ratio	Less than 0.5	Greater than 0.5
LDH	Parallels serum value	Less than 200 units/L
Fluid-to-serum LDH ratio	Less than 0.6	Greater than 0.6
Fluid cholesterol	Less than 55 mg/dL	Greater than 55 mg/dL
White blood cell count	Less than 100/mm^3	Greater than 1,000/mm^3

LDH = lactate dehydrogenase.

INDICATIONS

- Evaluate effusion of unknown etiology
- Investigate suspected hemorrhage, immune disease, malignancy, or infection

POTENTIAL DIAGNOSIS

Increased in

Condition/Test Showing Increased Result

- Bacterial pericarditis (red blood cell [RBC] count, white blood cell [WBC] count with a predominance of neutrophils)
- Hemorrhagic pericarditis (RBC count, WBC count)
- Malignancy (RBC count, abnormal cytology)
- Post–myocardial infarction syndrome, also called Dressler's syndrome (RBC count, WBC count with a predominance of neutrophils)
- Rheumatoid disease or systemic lupus erythematosus (SLE) (RBC count, WBC count)
- Tuberculous or fungal pericarditis (RBC count, WBC count with a predominance of lymphocytes)
- Viral pericarditis (RBC count, WBC count with a predominance of neutrophils)

Decreased in

Condition/Test Showing Decreased Result

- Bacterial pericarditis (glucose)
- Malignancy (glucose)
- Rheumatoid disease or SLE (glucose)

CRITICAL FINDINGS ✣

Positive culture findings in any sterile body fluid.

Note and immediately report to the health-care provider (HCP) positive culture results, if ordered, and related symptoms.

INTERFERING FACTORS

- Bloody fluid may be the result of a traumatic tap.
- Unknown hyperglycemia or hypoglycemia may be misleading in the comparison of fluid and serum glucose levels. Therefore, it is advisable to collect comparative serum samples a few hours before performing pericardiocentesis.
- Failure to follow dietary restrictions before the procedure may cause the procedure to be canceled or repeated.

P

NURSING IMPLICATIONS AND PROCEDURE

PRETEST:

▸ Positively identify the patient using at least two unique identifiers before providing care, treatment, or services.

- *Patient Teaching:* Inform the patient this procedure can assist with evaluating fluid around the heart.
- Obtain a history of the patient's complaints, including a list of known allergens, especially allergies or sensitivities to latex.
- Obtain a history of the patient's cardiovascular and immune system, especially any bleeding disorders and other symptoms, as well as results of previously performed laboratory tests and diagnostic and surgical procedures.
- Note any recent procedures that can interfere with test results.
- Record the date of the last menstrual period and determine the possibility of pregnancy in perimenopausal women.
- Obtain a list of the patient's current medications, including anticoagulants, aspirin and other salicylates, herbs, nutritional supplements, and nutraceuticals (see Appendix F). Such products should be discontinued by medical direction for the appropriate number of days prior to the surgical procedure.
- Review the procedure with the patient. Inform the patient that it may be necessary to remove hair from the site before the procedure. Address concerns about pain and explain that a sedative and/or analgesia will be administered to promote relaxation and reduce discomfort prior to needle insertion through the chest wall. Explain that any discomfort with the needle insertion will be minimized with local anesthetics and systemic analgesics. Explain that the anesthetic injection may cause a stinging sensation. Explain that after the skin has been anesthetized, a large needle will be inserted through the chest to obtain the fluid. Inform the patient that specimen collection is performed by an HCP specializing in this procedure and usually takes approximately 30 min to complete.
- Explain that an IV line will be inserted to allow infusion of IV fluids, antibiotics, anesthetics, and analgesics.
- *Sensitivity to social and cultural issues,* as well as concern for modesty, is important in providing psychological support before, during, and after the procedure.
- Food and fluids should be restricted for 6 to 8 hr before the procedure, as directed

by the HCP, unless the procedure is performed in an emergency situation to correct pericarditis. The requesting HCP may request that anticoagulants and aspirin be withheld. The number of days to withhold medication is dependent on the type of anticoagulant. Protocols may vary among facilities.
- *Make sure a written and informed consent has been signed prior to the procedure and before administering any medications.*

INTRATEST:

- Ensure that the patient has complied with dietary and fluids restrictions; assure that food has been restricted for at least 6 to 8 hr prior to the procedure.
- Ensure that anticoagulant therapy has been withheld for the appropriate number of days prior to the procedure. Notify the HCP if patient anticoagulant therapy has not been withheld.
- Have emergency equipment readily available.
- Have the patient void before the procedure.
- Have the patient remove clothes above the waist and put on a gown.
- If the patient has a history of allergic reaction to latex, avoid the use of equipment containing latex.
- Instruct the patient to cooperate fully and to follow directions. Direct the patient to breathe normally and to avoid unnecessary movement during the local anesthetic and the procedure.
- Record baseline vital signs, and continue to monitor throughout the procedure. Protocols may vary among facilities.
- Observe standard precautions, and follow the general guidelines in Appendix A. Positively identify the patient, and label the appropriate collection containers with the corresponding patient demographics, date and time of collection, and site location.
- Establish an IV line to allow infusion of IV fluids, anesthetics, analgesics, or IV sedation.
- Assist the patient into a comfortable supine position with the head elevated 45° to 60°.
- Prior to the administration of local anesthesia, cleanse the site with an

antiseptic solution, and drape the area with sterile towels. The skin at the injection site is then anesthetized.

- The precordial (V) cardiac lead wire is attached to the cardiac needle with an alligator clip. The cardiac needle is inserted just below and to the left of the breastbone, and fluid is removed.
- Monitor vital signs every 15 min for signs of hypovolemia or shock. Monitor electrocardiogram for needle-tip positioning to indicate accidental puncture of the right atrium.
- The needle is withdrawn, and slight pressure is applied to the site. Apply a sterile dressing to the site.
- Monitor the patient for complications related to the procedure (e.g., allergic reaction, anaphylaxis).
- Place samples in properly labeled specimen containers, and promptly transport the specimens to the laboratory for processing and analysis.

POST-TEST:

- A report of the results will be sent to the requesting HCP, who will discuss the results with the patient.
- Instruct the patient to resume usual diet and medications, as directed by the HCP.
- Monitor vital signs and cardiac status every 15 min for the first hour, every 30 min for the next 2 hr, every hr for the next 4 hr, and every 4 hr for the next 24 hr. Take the patient's temperature every 4 hr for 24 hr. Monitor intake and output for 24 hr. Notify the HCP if temperature is elevated. Protocols may vary among facilities.
- Observe/assess the patient for signs of respiratory and cardiac distress, such as shortness of breath, cyanosis, or rapid pulse.
- Continue IV fluids until vital signs are stable and the patient can resume fluid intake independently.
- Inform the patient that 1 hr or more of bed rest is required after the procedure.
- Observe/assess the puncture site for bleeding or drainage and signs of

inflammation each time vital signs are taken and daily thereafter for several days. Report to HCP if bleeding is present.

- Observe/assess for nausea and pain. Administer antiemetic and analgesic medications as needed and as directed by the HCP.
- Administer antibiotics, as ordered, and instruct the patient in the importance of completing the entire course of antibiotic therapy even if no symptoms are present.
- Recognize anxiety related to test results, and offer support. Discuss the implications of abnormal test results on the patient's lifestyle. Provide teaching and information regarding the clinical implications of the test results, as appropriate. Educate the patient regarding access to counseling services, if appropriate.
- Reinforce information given by the patient's HCP regarding further testing, treatment, or referral to another HCP. Answer any questions or address any concerns voiced by the patient or family.
- Depending on the results of this procedure, additional testing may be performed to evaluate or monitor progression of the disease process and determine the need for a change in therapy. Evaluate test results in relation to the patient's symptoms and other tests performed.

RELATED MONOGRAPHS:

- Related tests include AST, atrial natriuretic peptide, blood gases, B-type natriuretic peptide, cancer antigens, chest x-ray, CBC WBC count and differential, CK and isoenzymes, culture and smear mycobacteria, culture blood, culture fungal, culture viral, ECG, echocardiography, α_1-fetoprotein, homocysteine, LDH and isoenzymes, magnesium, MRI chest, MI scan, myoglobin, and troponin.
- Refer to the Cardiovascular and Immune systems tables at the end of the book for related tests by body system.

P

Peritoneal Fluid Analysis

SYNONYM/ACRONYM: Ascites fluid analysis.

COMMON USE: To evaluate and classify the type of fluid within the peritoneal cavity to assist with diagnosis of cancer, infection, necrosis, and perforation.

SPECIMEN: Peritoneal fluid (5 mL) collected in a red- or green-top (heparin) tube for amylase, glucose, and alkaline phosphatase; lavender-top (EDTA) tube for cell count; sterile containers for microbiology specimens; 200 to 500 mL of fluid in a clear container with anticoagulant for cytology. Ensure that there is an equal amount of fixative and fluid in the container for cytology.

REFERENCE VALUE: (Method: Spectrophotometry for glucose, amylase, and alkaline phosphatase; automated or manual cell count, macroscopic examination of cultured organisms, and microscopic examination of specimen for microbiology and cytology; microscopic examination of cultured microorganisms)

Peritoneal Fluid	Reference Value
Appearance	Clear
Color	Pale yellow
Amylase	Parallels serum values
Alkaline phosphatase	Parallels serum values
Glucose	Parallels serum values
Red blood cell count	Less than $100,000/mm^3$
White blood cell count	Less than $300/mm^3$
Culture	No growth
Acid-fast stain	No organisms seen
Gram stain	No organisms seen
Cytology	No abnormal cells seen

DESCRIPTION: The peritoneal cavity and organs within it are lined with a protective membrane. The fluid between the membranes is called *serous fluid*. Normally only a small amount of fluid is present because the rates of fluid production and absorption are about the same. Many abnormal conditions can result in the buildup of fluid within the peritoneal cavity. Specific tests are usually ordered in addition to a common battery of tests used to distinguish a transudate from an exudate. *Transudates* are effusions that form as a result of a systemic disorder that disrupts the regulation of fluid balance, such as a suspected perforation. *Exudates* are caused by conditions involving the tissue of the membrane itself, such as an infection or malignancy. Fluid is withdrawn from the peritoneal cavity by needle aspiration and tested as listed in the previous and following tables.

P

INDICATIONS

- Evaluate ascites of unknown cause
- Investigate suspected peritoneal rupture, perforation, malignancy, or infection.

Characteristic	Transudate	Exudate
Appearance	Clear	Cloudy or turbid
Specific gravity	Less than 1.015	Greater than 1.015
Total protein	Less than 2.5 g/dL	Greater than 3.0 g/dL
Fluid-to-serum protein ratio	Less than 0.5	Greater than 0.5
LDH	Parallels serum value	Less than 200 units/L
Fluid-to-serum LDH ratio	Less than 0.6	Greater than 0.6
Fluid cholesterol	Less than 55 mg/dL	Greater than 55 mg/dL
White blood cell count	Less than 100/mm^3	Greater than 1,000/mm^3

LDH = lactate dehydrogenase.

POTENTIAL DIAGNOSIS

Increased in

Condition/Test Showing Increased Result

- Abdominal malignancy (red blood cell [RBC] count, carcinoembryonic antigen, abnormal cytology)
- Abdominal trauma (RBC count greater than 100,000/mm^3)
- Ascites caused by cirrhosis (white blood cell [WBC] count, neutrophils greater than 25% but less than 50%, absolute granulocyte count greater than 250/mm^3)
- Bacterial peritonitis (WBC count, neutrophils greater than 50%, absolute granulocyte count greater than 250/mm^3)
- Peritoneal effusion due to gastric strangulation, perforation, or necrosis (amylase, ammonia, alkaline phosphatase)
- Peritoneal effusion due to pancreatitis, pancreatic trauma, or pancreatic pseudocyst (amylase)
- Rupture or perforation of urinary bladder (ammonia, creatinine, urea)
- Tuberculous effusion (elevated lymphocyte count, positive acid-fast bacillus smear and culture [25% to 50% of cases])

Decreased in

Condition/Test Showing Decreased Result

- Abdominal malignancy (glucose)
- Tuberculous effusion (glucose)

CRITICAL FINDINGS ◈

Positive culture findings in any sterile body fluid.

Note and immediately report to the health-care provider (HCP) positive culture results, if ordered, and related symptoms.

INTERFERING FACTORS

- Bloody fluids may result from a traumatic tap.
- Unknown hyperglycemia or hypoglycemia may be misleading in the comparison of fluid and serum glucose levels. Therefore, it is advisable to collect comparative serum samples a few hours before performing paracentesis.

NURSING IMPLICATIONS AND PROCEDURE

PRETEST:

▶ Positively identify the patient using at least two unique identifiers before providing care, treatment, or services.

▶ *Patient Teaching:* Inform the patient this procedure can assist with evaluation of fluid surrounding the abdominal organs.

▶ Obtain a history of the patient's complaints, including a list of known allergens, especially allergies or sensitivities to latex.

▶ Obtain a history of the patient's gastrointestinal and immune system, especially any bleeding disorders and other symptoms, as well as results of previously performed laboratory tests and diagnostic and surgical procedures.

▶ Note any recent procedures that can interfere with test results.

▶ Record the date of the last menstrual period and determine the possibility of pregnancy in perimenopausal women.

▶ Obtain a list of the patient's current medications, including anticoagulants, aspirin and other salicylates, herbs, nutritional supplements, and nutraceuticals (see Appendix F). Such products should be discontinued by medical direction for the appropriate number of days prior to a surgical procedure.

▶ Review the procedure with the patient. If patient has ascites, obtain weight and measure abdominal girth. Inform the patient that it may be necessary to remove hair from the site before the procedure. Address concerns about pain and explain that a sedative and/or analgesia will be administered to promote relaxation and reduce discomfort prior to needle insertion through the abdomen wall. Explain that any discomfort with the needle insertion will be minimized with local anesthetics and systemic analgesics. Explain that the anesthetic injection may cause an initial stinging sensation. Explain that after the skin has been anesthetized, a large needle will be inserted through the abdominal wall and a "popping" sensation may be experienced as the needle penetrates the peritoneum. Inform the patient that specimen collection is performed under sterile conditions by an HCP specializing in this procedure and usually takes approximately 30 min to complete.

▶ Explain that an IV line will be inserted to allow infusion of IV fluids, antibiotics, anesthetics, and analgesics.

▶ *Sensitivity to social and cultural issues,* as well as concern for modesty, is important in providing psychological support before, during, and after the procedure.

▶ There are no food or fluid restrictions unless by medical direction. The requesting HCP may request that anticoagulants and aspirin be withheld. The number of days to withhold medication is dependent on the type of anticoagulant.

▶ *Make sure a written and informed consent has been signed prior to the procedure and before administering any medications.*

INTRATEST:

▶ Ensure that anticoagulant therapy has been withheld for the appropriate number of days prior to the procedure. Notify the HCP if patient anticoagulant therapy has not been withheld.

▶ Have emergency equipment readily available.

▶ Have the patient void, or catheterize the patient to avoid accidental puncture of the bladder if he or she is unable to void.

▶ Have the patient remove clothing and change into a gown for the procedure.

▶ If the patient has a history of allergic reaction to latex, avoid the use of equipment containing latex.

▶ Instruct the patient to cooperate fully and to follow directions. Direct the patient to breathe normally and to avoid unnecessary movement during the local anesthetic and the procedure.

▶ Observe standard precautions, and follow the general guidelines in Appendix A. Positively identify the patient, and label the appropriate collection containers with the corresponding patient demographics, date and time of collection, and site location.

▶ Record baseline vital signs and continue to monitor throughout the procedure. Protocols may vary among facilities.

▶ Establish an IV line to allow infusion of IV fluids, anesthetics, analgesics, or IV sedation.

▶ Assist the patient to a comfortable seated position with feet and back supported or in high Fowler's position.

- Prior to the administration of local anesthesia, shave and cleanse the site with an antiseptic solution, and drape the area with sterile towels. The skin at the injection site is then anesthetized.
- The paracentesis needle is inserted 1 to 2 in. below the umbilicus, and fluid is removed. If lavage fluid is required (helpful if malignancy is suspected), saline or Ringer's lactate can be infused via the needle over a 15- to 20-min period before the lavage fluid is removed. Monitor vital signs every 15 min for signs of hypovolemia or shock.
- No more than 1,500 to 2,000 mL of fluid should be removed at a time, even in the case of a therapeutic paracentesis, because of the risk of hypovolemia and shock.
- The needle is withdrawn, and slight pressure is applied to the site. Apply a sterile dressing to the site.
- Monitor the patient for complications related to the procedure (e.g., allergic reaction, anaphylaxis).
- Place samples in properly labeled specimen containers, and promptly transport the specimens to the laboratory for processing and analysis.

POST-TEST:

- A report of the results will be sent to the requesting HCP, who will discuss the results with the patient.
- Instruct the patient to resume usual medications, as directed by the HCP.
- Monitor vital signs every 15 min for the first hr, every 30 min for the next 2 hr, every hour for the next 4 hr, and every 4 hr for the next 24 hr. Take the patient's temperature every 4 hr for 24 hr. Monitor intake and output for 24 hr. Notify the HCP if temperature is elevated. Protocols may vary among facilities.
- Observe/assess the puncture site for bleeding or drainage and signs of inflammation each time vital signs are taken and daily thereafter for several days. Report to the HCP if bleeding is present.
- If a large amount of fluid was removed, obtain weight and measure abdominal girth.

- Inform the patient that 1 hr or more of bed rest is required after the procedure.
- Instruct the patient to immediately report severe abdominal pain. (Note: Rigidity of abdominal muscles indicates developing peritonitis.) Report to HCP if abdominal rigidity or pain is present.
- Observe/assess for nausea and pain. Administer antiemetic and analgesic medications as needed and as directed by the HCP.
- Administer antibiotics, as ordered, and instruct the patient in the importance of completing the entire course of antibiotic therapy even if no symptoms are present.
- Recognize anxiety related to test results, and offer support. Discuss the implications of abnormal test results on the patient's lifestyle. Provide teaching and information regarding the clinical implications of the test results, as appropriate. Educate the patient regarding access to counseling services, if appropriate.
- Reinforce information given by the patient's HCP regarding further testing, treatment, or referral to another HCP. Answer any questions or address any concerns voiced by the patient or family.
- Depending on the results of this procedure, additional testing may be performed to evaluate or monitor progression of the disease process and determine the need for a change in therapy. Evaluate test results in relation to the patient's symptoms and other tests performed.

RELATED MONOGRAPHS:

- Related tests include cancer antigens, CBC, CBC WBC count and differential, CT abdomen, CT biliary tract and liver, culture and smear mycobacteria, culture blood, culture fungal, culture viral, KUB studies, laparoscopy abdominal, liver and spleen scan, MRI abdomen, and US spleen.
- Refer to the Gastrointestinal and Immune systems tables at the end of the book for related tests by body system.

P

Phosphorus, Blood

SYNONYM/ACRONYM: Inorganic phosphorus, phosphate, PO_4.

COMMON USE: To assist in evaluating multiple body system functions by monitoring phosphorus levels in relation to other electrolytes. Used specifically to evaluate renal function in at-risk patients.

SPECIMEN: Serum (1 mL) collected in a red- or tiger-top tube. Plasma (1 mL) collected in green-top (heparin) tube is also acceptable.

REFERENCE VALUE: (Method: Spectrophotometry)

Age	Conventional Units	SI Units (Conventional Units × 0.323)
0–5 day	4.6–8.0 mg/dL	1.5–2.6 mmol/L
1–3 yr	3.9–6.5 mg/dL	1.3–2.1 mmol/L
4–6 yr	4.0–5.4 mg/dL	1.3–1.7 mmol/L
7–11 yr	3.7–5.6 mg/dL	1.2–1.8 mmol/L
12–13 yr	3.3–5.4 mg/dL	1.1–1.7 mmol/L
14–15 yr	2.9–5.4 mg/dL	0.9–1.7 mmol/L
16–19 yr	2.8–4.6 mg/dL	0.9–1.5 mmol/L
Adult	2.5–4.5 mg/dL	0.8–1.4 mmol/L

Values may be slightly decreased in older adults due to dietary insufficiency or the effects of medications and the presence of multiple chronic or acute diseases with or without muted symptoms.

DESCRIPTION: Phosphorus, in the form of phosphate, is distributed throughout the body. Approximately 85% of the body's phosphorus is stored in bones; the remainder is found in cells and body fluids. It is the major intracellular anion and plays a crucial role in cellular metabolism, maintenance of cellular membranes, and formation of bones and teeth. Phosphorus also indirectly affects the release of oxygen from hemoglobin by affecting the formation of 2,3-bisphosphoglycerate. Levels of phosphorus are dependent on dietary intake.

Phosphorus excretion is regulated by the kidneys. Calcium and phosphorus are interrelated with respect to absorption and metabolic function. They have an inverse relationship with respect to concentration: Serum phosphorus is increased when serum calcium is decreased. Hyperphosphatemia can result in an infant fed only cow's milk during the first few weeks of life because of the combination of a high phosphorus content in cow's milk and the inability of infants' kidneys to clear the excess phosphorus.

INDICATIONS
• Assist in establishing a diagnosis of hyperparathyroidism
• Assist in the evaluation of renal failure

POTENTIAL DIAGNOSIS

Increased in

- Acromegaly *(related to increased renal absorption)*
- Bone metastases *(related to release from bone stores)*
- Diabetic ketoacidosis *(acid-base imbalance causes intracellular phosphorus to move into the extracellular fluid)*
- Excessive levels of vitamin D *(vitamin D promotes intestinal absorption of phosphorus; excessive levels promote phosphorus release from bone stores)*
- Hyperthermia *(tissue damage causes intracellular phosphorus to be released into circulation)*
- Hypocalcemia *(calcium and phosphorus have an inverse relationship)*
- Hypoparathyroidism *(related to increased renal absorption)*
- Lactic acidosis *(acid-base imbalance causes intracellular phosphorus to move into the extracellular fluid)*
- Milk alkali syndrome *(increased dietary intake)*
- Pseudohypoparathyroidism *(related to increased renal absorption)*
- Pulmonary embolism *(related to respiratory acid-base imbalance and compensatory mechanisms)*
- Renal failure *(related to decreased renal excretion)*
- Respiratory acidosis *(acid-base imbalance causes intracellular phosphorus to move into the extracellular fluid)*

Decreased in

- Acute gout *(related to decreased circulating calcium in calcium crystal–induced gout; calcium and phosphorus have an inverse relationship)*
- Alcohol withdrawal *(related to malnutrition)*
- Gram-negative bacterial septicemia

- Growth hormone deficiency
- Hyperalimentation therapy
- Hypercalcemia *(calcium and phosphorus have an inverse relationship)*
- Hyperinsulinism *(insulin increases intracellular movement of phosphorus)*
- Hyperparathyroidism *(parathyroid hormone [PTH] increases renal excretion)*
- Hypokalemia
- Impaired renal absorption *(decreases return of phosphorus to general circulation)*
- Malabsorption syndromes *(related to insufficient intestinal absorption of phosphorus)*
- Malnutrition *(related to deficient intake)*
- Osteomalacia *(evidenced by hypophosphatemia)*
- PTH-producing tumors *(PTH increases renal excretion)*
- Primary hyperparathyroidism *(PTH increases renal excretion)*
- Renal tubular acidosis
- Renal tubular defects *(related to decreased renal absorption)*
- Respiratory alkalosis
- Respiratory infections
- Rickets *(related to vitamin D deficiency)*
- Salicylate poisoning
- Severe burns
- Severe vomiting and diarrhea *(related to excessive loss)*
- Vitamin D deficiency *(related to vitamin D deficiency, which reduces intestinal and renal tubular absorption of phosphorus)*

CRITICAL FINDINGS ✦

Values less than 1.0 mg/dL may have significant effects on the neuromuscular, gastrointestinal (GI), cardiopulmonary, and skeletal systems.

Note and immediately report to the health-care provider (HCP) any critically increased or decreased

P

values and related symptoms. Interventions including IV replacement therapy with sodium or potassium phosphate may be necessary. Close monitoring of both phosphorus and calcium is important during replacement therapy.

INTERFERING FACTORS

- Drugs that may increase phosphorus levels include anabolic steroids, β-adrenergic blockers, ergocalciferol, furosemide, hydrochlorothiazide, methicillin (occurs with nephrotoxicity), oral contraceptives, parathyroid extract, phosphates, sodium etidronate, tetracycline (occurs with nephrotoxicity), and vitamin D.
- Drugs that may decrease phosphorus levels include acetazolamide, albuterol, aluminum salts, amino acids (via IV hyperalimentation), anesthetic agents, anticonvulsants, calcitonin, epinephrine, fibrin hydrolysate, fructose, glucocorticoids, glucose, insulin, mannitol, oral contraceptives, pamidronate, phenothiazine, phytate, and plicamycin.
- Serum phosphorus levels are subject to diurnal variation: They are highest in late morning and lowest in the evening; therefore, serial samples should be collected at the same time of day for consistency in interpretation.
- Hemolysis will falsely increase phosphorus values.
- Specimens should never be collected above an IV line because of the potential for dilution when the specimen and the IV solution combine in the collection container, thereby falsely decreasing the result. There is also the potential of contaminating the sample with the substance of interest if it is present in the IV solution, thereby falsely increasing the result.

NURSING IMPLICATIONS AND PROCEDURE

PRETEST:

- Positively identify the patient using at least two unique identifiers before providing care, treatment, or services.
- *Patient Teaching:* Inform the patient this test can assist in a general evaluation of body systems.
- Obtain a history of the patient's complaints, including a list of known allergens, especially allergies or sensitivities to latex.
- Obtain a history of the patient's endocrine, gastrointestinal, genitourinary, and musculoskeletal systems; symptoms; and results of previously performed laboratory tests and diagnostic and surgical procedures.
- Obtain a list of the patient's current medications, including herbs, nutritional supplements, and nutraceuticals (see Appendix F).
- Review the procedure with the patient. Inform the patient that specimen collection takes approximately 5 to 10 min. Address concerns about pain and explain that there may be some discomfort during the venipuncture.
- *Sensitivity to social and cultural issues,* as well as concern for modesty, is important in providing psychological support before, during, and after the procedure.
- There are no food, fluid, or medication restrictions unless by medical direction.

INTRATEST:

- If the patient has a history of allergic reaction to latex, avoid the use of equipment containing latex.
- Instruct the patient to cooperate fully and to follow directions. Direct the patient to breathe normally and to avoid unnecessary movement.
- Observe standard precautions, and follow the general guidelines in Appendix A. Positively identify the patient, and label the appropriate tubes with the corresponding patient demographics, date, and time of collection. Perform a venipuncture.
- Remove the needle and apply direct pressure with dry gauze to stop

bleeding. Observe/assess venipuncture site for bleeding or hematoma formation and secure gauze with adhesive bandage.

- Promptly transport the specimen to the laboratory for processing and analysis.

POST-TEST:

- A report of the results will be sent to the requesting HCP, who will discuss the results with the patient.
- *Nutritional Considerations:* Severe hypophosphatemia is common in elderly patients or patients who have been hospitalized for long periods of time. Good dietary sources of phosphorus include meat, dairy products, nuts, and legumes.
- *Nutritional Considerations:* To decrease phosphorus levels to normal in the patient with hyperphosphatemia, dietary restriction may be recommended. Other interventions may include the administration of phosphate binders or calcitriol (the activated form of vitamin D).
- Reinforce information given by the patient's HCP regarding further testing, treatment, or referral to another HCP.

- Answer any questions or address any concerns voiced by the patient or family.
- Depending on the results of this procedure, additional testing may be performed to evaluate or monitor progression of the disease process and determine the need for a change in therapy. Evaluate test results in relation to the patient's symptoms and other tests performed.

RELATED MONOGRAPHS:

- Related tests include biopsy bone, blood gases, BUN, calcitonin, calcium, calculus kidney stone panel, carbon dioxide, chloride, collagen cross-linked N-telopeptides, CBC WBC count and differential, creatinine, fecal analysis, fecal fat, FDP, glucagon, glucose, GH, insulin, lactic acid, lung perfusion scan, lung ventilation scan, osmolality, osteocalcin, PTH, parathyroid scan, phosphorus urine, potassium, and vitamin D.
- Refer to the Endocrine, Gastrointestinal, Genitourinary, and Musculoskeletal systems tables at the end of the book for related tests by body system.

Phosphorus, Urine

SYNONYM/ACRONYM: Urine phosphate.

COMMON USE: To assist in evaluating calcium and phosphorus levels related to use of diuretics in progression of renal disease.

SPECIMEN: Urine (5 mL) from an unpreserved random or timed specimen collected in a clean plastic collection container.

REFERENCE VALUE: (Method: Spectrophotometry) Reference values are dependent on phosphorus and calcium intake. Phosphate excretion exhibits diurnal variation and is significantly higher at night.

Conventional Units	SI Units (Conventional Units × 32.3)
0.4–1.3 g/24 hr	12.9–42.0 g/24 hr

DESCRIPTION: Phosphorus, in the form of phosphate, is distributed throughout the body. Approximately 85% of the body's phosphorus is stored in bones; the remainder is found in cells and body fluids. It is the major intracellular anion and plays a crucial role in cellular metabolism, maintenance of cellular membranes, and formation of bones and teeth. Phosphorus also indirectly affects the release of oxygen from hemoglobin by affecting the formation of 2,3-bisphosphoglycerate. Levels of phosphorus are dependent on dietary intake.

Analyzing urinary phosphorus levels can provide important clues to the functioning of the kidneys and other major organs. Tests for phosphorus in urine usually involve timed urine collections over a 12- or 24-hr period. Measurement of random specimens may also be requested. Children with thalassemia may have normal phosphorus absorption but increased excretion, which may result in a phosphorus deficiency.

INDICATIONS

- Assist in the diagnosis of hyperparathyroidism
- Assist in the evaluation of calcium and phosphorus balance
- Assist in the evaluation of nephrolithiasis
- Assist in the evaluation of renal tubular disease

POTENTIAL DIAGNOSIS

Increased in
- Abuse of diuretics *(related to increased renal excretion)*
- Primary hyperparathyroidism *(parathyroid hormone [PTH] increases renal excretion)*
- Renal tubular acidosis
- Vitamin D deficiency *(related to decreased renal reabsorption)*

Decreased in
- Hypoparathyroidism *(PTH enhances renal excretion; therefore, a lack of PTH will decrease urine phosphorus levels)*
- Pseudohypoparathyroidism *(PTH enhances renal reabsorption; therefore, a lack of response to PTH, as in pseudohypoparathyroidism, will decrease urine phosphorus levels)*
- Vitamin D intoxication *(vitamin D promotes renal excretion of phosphorus)*

CRITICAL FINDINGS: N/A

INTERFERING FACTORS

- Drugs and vitamins that can cause an increase in urine phosphorus levels include acetazolamide, acetylsalicylic acid, bismuth salts, calcitonin, corticosteroids, dihydrotachysterol, glucocorticoids, hydrochlorothiazide, mestranol, metolazone, parathyroid extract, and parathyroid hormone.
- Drugs that can cause a decrease in urine phosphorus levels include aluminum-containing antacids and diltiazem.
- Urine phosphorus levels are subject to diurnal variation: Output is highest in the afternoon, which is why 24-hr urine collections are recommended.
- All urine voided for the timed collection period must be included in the collection or else falsely decreased values may be obtained. Compare output records with volume collected to verify that all voids were included in the collection.

NURSING IMPLICATIONS AND PROCEDURE

PRETEST:

▸ Positively identify the patient using at least two unique identifiers before providing care, treatment, or services.

- **Patient Teaching:** Inform the patient this test can assist in evaluating calcium and phosphorus balance.
- Obtain a history of the patient's complaints, including a list of known allergens, especially allergies or sensitivities to latex.
- Obtain a history of the patient's endocrine and genitourinary systems, symptoms, and results of previously performed laboratory tests and diagnostic and surgical procedures.
- Obtain a list of the patient's current medications, including herbs, nutritional supplements, and nutraceuticals (see Appendix F).
- Review the procedure with the patient. Provide a nonmetallic urinal, bedpan, or toilet-mounted collection device. Address concerns about pain and explain that there should be no discomfort during the procedure.
- **Sensitivity to social and cultural issues,** as well as concern for modesty, is important in providing psychological support before, during, and after the procedure.
- Usually a 24-hr time frame for urine collection is ordered. Inform the patient that all urine must be saved during that 24-hr period. Instruct the patient not to void directly into the laboratory collection container. Instruct the patient to avoid defecating in the collection device and to keep toilet tissue out of the collection device to prevent contamination of the specimen. Place a sign in the bathroom to remind the patient to save all urine.
- Instruct the patient to void all urine into the collection device and then to pour the urine into the laboratory collection container. Alternatively, the specimen can be left in the collection device for a health-care staff member to add to the laboratory collection container.
- **Sensitivity to social and cultural issues,** as well as concern for modesty, is important in providing psychological support before, during, and after the procedure.
- Instruct the patient to avoid excessive exercise and stress during the 24-hr collection of urine.
- There are no food, fluid, or medication restrictions unless by medical direction.

INTRATEST:

- Ensure that the patient has complied with activity restrictions and pretesting preparations; assure that excessive exercise and stress have been restricted during the 24-hr procedure.
- If the patient has a history of allergic reaction to latex, avoid the use of equipment containing latex.
- Instruct the patient to cooperate fully and to follow directions.
- Observe standard precautions, and follow the general guidelines in Appendix A. Positively identify the patient, and label the appropriate tubes with the corresponding patient demographics, date, and time of collection.

Random Specimen (Collect in Early Morning)
Clean-Catch Specimen
- Instruct the male patient to (1) thoroughly wash his hands, (2) cleanse the meatus, (3) void a small amount into the toilet, and (4) void directly into the specimen container.
- Instruct the female patient to (1) thoroughly wash her hands; (2) cleanse the labia from front to back; (3) while keeping the labia separated, void a small amount into the toilet; and (4) without interrupting the urine stream, void directly into the specimen container.

Indwelling Catheter
- Put on gloves. Empty drainage tube of urine. It may be necessary to clamp off the catheter for 15 to 30 min before specimen collection. Cleanse specimen port with antiseptic swab, and then aspirate 5 mL of urine with a 21- to 25-gauge needle and syringe. Transfer urine to a sterile container.

Timed Specimen
- Obtain a clean 3-L urine specimen container, toilet-mounted collection device, and plastic bag (for transport of the specimen container). The specimen must be refrigerated or kept on ice throughout the entire collection period. If an indwelling urinary catheter is in place, the drainage bag must be kept on ice.
- Begin the test between 6 and 8 a.m. if possible. Collect first voiding and discard. Record the time the specimen

P

was discarded as the beginning of the timed collection period. The next morning, ask the patient to void at the same time the collection was started and add this last voiding to the container. Urinary output should be recorded throughout the collection time.

▶ If an indwelling catheter is in place, replace the tubing and container system at the start of the collection time. Keep the container system on ice during the collection period, or empty the urine into a larger container periodically during the collection period; monitor to ensure continued drainage, and conclude the test the next morning at the same hour the collection was begun.

▶ At the conclusion of the test, compare the quantity of urine with the urinary output record for the collection; if the specimen contains less than what was recorded as output, some urine may have been discarded, invalidating the test.

▶ Include on the collection container's label the amount of urine, test start and stop times, and ingestion of any foods or medications that can affect test results.

General

▶ Promptly transport the specimen to the laboratory for processing and analysis.

POST-TEST:

▶ A report of the results will be sent to the requesting health-care provider (HCP), who will discuss the results with the patient.

▶ *Nutritional Considerations:* Vitamin D is necessary for the body to absorb phosphorus. Vitamin D is added to food products such as milk, cheese, and orange juice.

The recommended daily intake of vitamin D is 200 IU per day for men and women under 50 and 400 IU per day for men and women over age 50.

▶ Increased urine phosphorus levels may be associated with the formation of kidney stones. Educate the patient, if appropriate, on the importance of drinking a sufficient amount of water when kidney stones are suspected.

▶ Recognize anxiety related to test results. Discuss the implications of abnormal test results on the patient's lifestyle. Provide teaching and information regarding the clinical implications of the test results, as appropriate.

▶ Reinforce information given by the patient's HCP regarding further testing, treatment, or referral to another HCP. Answer any questions or address any concerns voiced by the patient or family.

▶ Depending on the results of this procedure, additional testing may be performed to evaluate or monitor progression of the disease process and determine the need for a change in therapy. Evaluate test results in relation to the patient's symptoms and other tests performed.

RELATED MONOGRAPHS:

▶ Related tests include ALP, calcitonin, calcium, calculus kidney stone panel, chloride, CT abdomen, cystoscopy, IVP, KUB studies, PTH, parathyroid scan, phosphorus blood, potassium, renogram, retrograde ureteropyelography, uric acid, and UA.

▶ Refer to the Endocrine and Genitourinary systems tables at the end of the book for related tests by body system.

Plasminogen

SYNONYM/ACRONYM: Profibrinolysin, PMG.

COMMON USE: To assess thrombolytic disorders such as disseminated intravascular coagulation (DIC) and monitor thrombolytic therapy.

SPECIMEN: Plasma (1 mL) collected in a completely filled blue-top (3.2% sodium citrate) tube. If the patient's hematocrit exceeds 55%, the volume of citrate in the collection tube must be adjusted.

REFERENCE VALUE: (Method: Chromogenic substrate) 80% to 120% of normal for plasma.

DESCRIPTION: Plasminogen is a plasma glycoprotein produced by the liver. It is the circulating, inactive precursor to plasmin. Damaged tissues release a substance called *plasminogen activator* that initiates the conversion of plasminogen to plasmin. Plasmin participates in fibrinolysis and is capable of degrading fibrin, factor I (fibrinogen), factor V, and factor VIII. (For more information on fibrin degradation, see monograph titled "Fibrinogen.")

INDICATIONS

Evaluate the level of circulating plasminogen in patients with thrombosis or disseminated intravascular coagulation (DIC).

POTENTIAL DIAGNOSIS

Increased in
- Pregnancy (late) *(pathophysiology is unclear)*

Decreased in
- DIC *(related to increased consumption during the hyperfibrinolytic state by conversion to plasmin)*
- Fibrinolytic therapy with tissue plasminogen activators such as streptokinase or urokinase *(related to increased consumption by conversion to plasmin)*
- Hereditary deficiency
- Liver disease *(related to decreased production by damaged liver cells)*
- Neonatal hyaline membrane disease *(possibly related to deficiency of plasminogen)*

- Postsurgical period *(possibly related to trauma of surgery)*

CRITICAL FINDINGS: N/A

INTERFERING FACTORS
- Drugs that may decrease plasminogen levels include streptokinase and urokinase.
- Hematocrit greater than 55% may cause falsely prolonged results because of anticoagulant excess relative to plasma volume.
- Incompletely filled collection tubes, specimens contaminated with heparin, clotted specimens, or unprocessed specimens not delivered to the laboratory within 1 to 2 hr of collection should be rejected.

NURSING IMPLICATIONS AND PROCEDURE

PRETEST:
- Positively identify the patient using at least two unique identifiers before providing care, treatment, or services.
- *Patient Teaching:* Inform the patient that this test can assist in evaluating the effectiveness of blood clotting.
- Obtain a history of the patient's complaints, including a list of known allergens, especially allergies or sensitivities to latex.
- Obtain a history of the patient's hematopoietic system, symptoms, and results of previously performed laboratory tests and diagnostic and surgical procedures.
- Obtain a list of the patient's current medications, including herbs, nutritional supplements, and nutraceuticals (see Appendix F).

P

- Review the procedure with the patient. Inform the patient that specimen collection takes approximately 5 to 10 min. Address concerns about pain and explain that there may be some discomfort during the venipuncture.
- *Sensitivity to social and cultural issues,* as well as concern for modesty, is important in providing psychological support before, during, and after the procedure.
- There are no food, fluid, or medication restrictions unless by medical direction.

INTRATEST:

- If the patient has a history of allergic reaction to latex, avoid the use of equipment containing latex.
- Instruct the patient to cooperate fully and to follow directions. Direct the patient to breathe normally and to avoid unnecessary movement.
- Observe standard precautions, and follow the general guidelines in Appendix A. Positively identify the patient, and label the appropriate tubes with the corresponding patient demographics, date, and time of collection. Perform a venipuncture. Fill tube completely. *Important note*: Two different concentrations of sodium citrate preservative are currently added to blue-top tubes for coagulation studies: 3.2% and 3.8%. The Clinical and Laboratory Standards Institute (CLSI; formerly the National Committee for Clinical Laboratory Standards [NCCLS]) guideline for sodium citrate is 3.2%. Laboratories establish reference ranges for coagulation testing based on numerous factors, including sodium citrate concentration, test equipment, and test reagents. It is important to ask the laboratory which concentration it recommends, because each concentration will have its own specific reference range. When multiple specimens are drawn, the blue-top tube should be collected after sterile (i.e., blood culture) tubes. Otherwise, when using a standard vacutainer system, the blue-top tube is the first tube collected. When a butterfly is used and due to the added tubing, an extra red-top tube should be collected before the blue-top tube to ensure complete filling of the blue-top tube.

- Remove the needle and apply direct pressure with dry gauze to stop bleeding. Observe/assess venipuncture site for bleeding or hematoma formation and secure gauze with adhesive bandage.
- Promptly transport the specimen to the laboratory for processing and analysis. The CLSI recommendation for processed and unprocessed samples stored in unopened tubes is that testing should be completed within 1 to 4 hr of collection. If the patient has a known hematocrit above 55%, adjust the amount of anticoagulant in the collection tube before drawing the blood according to the CLSI guidelines:

$$\text{Anticoagulant vol. [x]} = (100 - \text{hematocrit})/(595 - \text{hematocrit}) \times \text{total vol. of anticoagulated blood required}$$

Example:

$$\text{Patient hematocrit} = 60\%$$
$$= [(100 - 60)/(595 - 60) \times 5.0] = 0.37$$
mL sodium citrate for a 5-mL standard drawing tube

POST-TEST:

- A report of the results will be sent to the requesting health-care provider (HCP), who will discuss the results with the patient.
- Reinforce information given by the patient's HCP regarding further testing, treatment, or referral to another HCP. Answer any questions or address any concerns voiced by the patient or family.
- Depending on the results of this procedure, additional testing may be performed to evaluate or monitor progression of the disease process and determine the need for a change in therapy. Evaluate test results in relation to the patient's symptoms and other tests performed.

RELATED MONOGRAPHS:

- Related tests include AT-III, CBC platelet count, coagulation factors, FDP, fibrinogen, aPTT, protein S, and PT/INR.
- Refer to the Hematopoietic System table at the end of the book for related tests by body system.

Platelet Antibodies

SYNONYM/ACRONYM: Antiplatelet antibody; platelet-bound IgG/IgM, direct and indirect.

COMMON USE: To assess for the presence of platelet antibodies to assist in diagnosing thrombocytopenia related to autoimmune conditions and platelet transfusion compatibility issues.

SPECIMEN: Serum (1 mL) collected in a red-top tube for indirect immunoglobulin G (IgG) antibody. Whole blood (7 mL) collected in a lavender-top (EDTA) tube for direct antibody.

REFERENCE VALUE: (Method: Solid-phase enzyme-linked immunoassay) Negative.

DESCRIPTION: Platelet antibodies can be formed by autoimmune response, or they can be acquired in reaction to transfusion products or medications. Platelet autoantibodies are immunoglobulins of autoimmune origin (i.e., immunoglobulin G [IgG]), and they are present in various autoimmune disorders, including thrombocytopenias. Platelet alloantibodies develop in patients who become sensitized to platelet antigens of transfused blood. As a result, destruction of both donor and native platelets occurs along with a shortened survival time of platelets in the transfusion recipient. The platelet antibody detection test is also used for platelet typing, which allows compatible platelets to be transfused to patients with disorders such as aplastic anemia and cancer. Platelet typing decreases the alloimmunization risk resulting from repeated transfusions from random donors. Platelet typing may also provide additional support for a diagnosis of post-transfusional purpura.

INDICATIONS
- Assist in the detection of platelet alloimmune disorders
- Determine platelet type for refractory patients

POTENTIAL DIAGNOSIS

Increased in

Development of platelet antibodies is associated with autoimmune conditions and medications.

- AIDS *(related to medications used therapeutically)*
- Acute myeloid leukemia *(related to medications used therapeutically)*
- Idiopathic thrombocytopenic purpura *(related to development of platelet-associated IgG antibodies)*
- Immune complex diseases
- Multiple blood transfusions *(related in most cases to sensitization to PLA1 antigens on donor red blood cells that will stimulate formation of antiplatelet antibodies)*
- Multiple myeloma *(related to medications used therapeutically)*
- Neonatal immune thrombocytopenia *(related to maternal platelet-sociated antibodies directed against fetal platelets)*
- Paroxysmal hemoglobinuria

P

- Rheumatoid arthritis *(related to medications used therapeutically)*
- Systemic lupus erythematosus *(related to medications used therapeutically)*
- Thrombocytopenias provoked by drugs (see monograph titled Complete Blood Count, Platelet Count)

Decreased in: N/A

CRITICAL FINDINGS: N/A

INTERFERING FACTORS

- There are many drugs that may induce immune thrombocytopenia (production of antibodies that destroy platelets in response to the drugs). The most common include acetaminophen, gold salts, heparin (Type II HIT), oral diabetic medications, penicillin, quinidine, quinine, salicylates, sulfonamides, and sulfonylurea.
- There are many drugs that may induce nonimmune thrombocytopenia (effect of the drug includes bone marrow suppression or non-immune platelet destruction). The most common include anticancer medications (e.g. bleomycin), ethanol, heparin (Type I HIT), procarbazine, protamine, ristocetin, thiazide, and valproic acid.
- Hemolyzed or clotted specimens will affect results.

P

NURSING IMPLICATIONS AND PROCEDURE

PRETEST:

- Positively identify the patient using at least two unique identifiers before providing care, treatment, or services.
- *Patient Teaching:* Inform the patient this test can assist in evaluating for issues related to platelet compatibility.
- Obtain a history of the patient's complaints, including a list of known allergens, especially allergies or sensitivities to latex.

- Obtain a history of the patient's hematopoietic and immune systems, especially any bleeding disorders and other symptoms, as well as results of previously performed laboratory tests and diagnostic and surgical procedures.
- Obtain a list of the patient's current medications, including anticoagulants, aspirin and other salicylates, herbs, nutritional supplements, and nutraceuticals (see Appendix F). Note the last time and dose of medication taken.
- Review the procedure with the patient. Inform the patient that specimen collection takes approximately 5 to 10 min. Address concerns about pain and explain that there may be some discomfort during the venipuncture.
- *Sensitivity to social and cultural issues,* as well as concern for modesty, is important in providing psychological support before, during, and after the procedure.
- There are no food, fluid, or medication restrictions unless by medical direction.

INTRATEST:

- If the patient has a history of allergic reaction to latex, avoid the use of equipment containing latex.
- Instruct the patient to cooperate fully and to follow directions. Direct the patient to breathe normally and to avoid unnecessary movement.
- Observe standard precautions, and follow the general guidelines in Appendix A. Positively identify the patient, and label the appropriate tubes with the corresponding patient demographics, date, and time of collection. Perform a venipuncture.
- Remove the needle and apply direct pressure with dry gauze to stop bleeding. Observe/assess venipuncture site for bleeding or hematoma formation and secure gauze with adhesive bandage.
- Promptly transport the specimen to the laboratory for processing and analysis.

POST-TEST:

- A report of the results will be sent to the requesting health-care provider (HCP), who will discuss the results with the patient.

- Note the patient's response to platelet transfusions.
- Instruct the patient to report severe bruising or bleeding from any areas of the skin or mucous membranes.
- Inform the patient who has developed platelet antibodies of the importance of taking precautions against bruising and bleeding, including the use of a soft bristle toothbrush, use of an electric razor, avoidance of constipation, avoidance of acetylsalicylic acid and similar products, and avoidance of intramuscular injections.
- Reinforce information given by the patient's HCP regarding further testing, treatment, or referral to another HCP. Answer any questions or address any concerns voiced by the patient or family.

- Depending on the results of this procedure, additional testing may be performed to evaluate or monitor progression of the disease process and determine the need for a change in therapy. Evaluate test results in relation to the patient's symptoms and other tests performed.

RELATED MONOGRAPHS:

- Related tests include angiography abdominal, biopsy bone marrow, bleeding time, clot retraction, CBC platelet count, CT brain, Ham's test, hemosiderin, and LAP.
- Refer to the Hematopoietic and Immune systems tables at the end of the book for related tests by body system.

Plethysmography

SYNONYM/ACRONYM: Impedance plethysmography, PVR.

COMMON USE: To measure changes in blood vessel size or changes in gas volume in the lungs to assist in diagnosis of diseases such as deep vein thrombosis (DVT), chronic obstructive pulmonary disease (COPD), and some peripheral vascular disorders.

AREA OF APPLICATION: Veins, arteries, and lungs.

CONTRAST: None.

DESCRIPTION: Plethysmography is a noninvasive diagnostic manometric study used to measure changes in the size of blood vessels by determining volume changes in the blood vessels of the eye, extremities, and neck or to measure gas volume changes in the lungs.

Arterial plethysmography assesses arterial circulation in an upper or lower limb; it is used to diagnose extremity arteriosclerotic disease and to rule out occlusive disease. The test requires a normal extremity for comparison of results. The test is performed by applying a series of three blood pressure cuffs to the extremity. The amplitude of each pulse wave is then recorded.

Venous plethysmography, done with a series of cuffs, measures changes in venous capacity and outflow (volume and rate of outflow); it is used to diagnose a thrombotic condition that causes obstruction of the major veins of the extremity. When the cuffs are applied to an extremity in patients with venous obstruction, no initial increase in leg volume is recorded because the venous volume of the leg cannot dissipate quickly.

Body plethysmography measures the total amount (volume) of air within the thorax, whether or not the air is in ventilatory communication with the lung; the elasticity (compliance) of the lungs; and the resistance to airflow in the respiratory tree. It is used in conjunction with pulmonary stress testing and pulmonary function testing.

Impedance plethysmography is widely used to detect acute deep vein thrombosis (DVT) of the leg, but it can also be used in the arm, abdomen, neck, or thorax. Doppler flow studies now are used to identify DVT, but ultrasound studies are less accurate in examinations below the knee.

INDICATIONS

Arterial Plethysmography
- Confirm suspected acute arterial embolization
- Detect vascular changes associated with Raynaud's phenomenon and disease
- Determine changes in toe or finger pressures when ankle pressures are elevated as a result of arterial calcifications
- Determine the effect of trauma on the arteries in an extremity
- Determine peripheral small-artery changes (ischemia) caused by diabetes, and differentiate these changes from neuropathy

- Evaluate suspected arterial occlusive disease
- Locate and determine the degree of arterial atherosclerotic obstruction and vessel patency in peripheral atherosclerotic disease, as well as inflammatory changes causing obliteration in the vessels in thromboangiitis obliterans

Venous Plethysmography
- Detect partial or total venous thrombotic obstruction
- Determine valve competency in conjunction with Doppler ultrasonography in the diagnosis of varicose veins

Body Plethysmography
- Detect acute pulmonary disorders, such as atelectasis
- Detect or determine the status of chronic obstructive pulmonary disease (COPD), such as emphysema, asthma, or chronic bronchitis
- Detect or determine the status of restrictive pulmonary disease, such as fibrosis
- Detect infectious pulmonary diseases, such as pneumonia
- Determine baseline pulmonary status before pulmonary rehabilitation to determine potential therapeutic benefit
- Differentiate between obstructive and restrictive pulmonary pathology

Impedance Plethysmography
- Act as a diagnostic screen for patients at risk for DVT
- Detect and evaluate DVT
- Evaluate degree of resolution of DVT after treatment
- Evaluate patients with suspected pulmonary embolism (most pulmonary emboli are complications of DVT in the leg)

POTENTIAL DIAGNOSIS

Normal findings in
- Arterial plethysmography:

Normal arterial pulse waves: Steep upslope, more gradual downslope with narrow pointed peaks

Normal pressure: Less than 20 mm Hg systolic difference between the lower and upper extremities; toe pressure greater than or equal to 80% of ankle pressure and finger pressure greater than or equal to 80% of wrist pressure

- Venous plethysmography:
  Normal venous blood flow in the extremities
  Venous filling times greater than 20 sec
- Body plethysmography:
  Thoracic gas volume: 2,400 mL
  Compliance: 0.2 L/cm H_2O
  Airway resistance: 0.6 to 2.5 cm H_2O/L per sec
- Impedance plethysmography:
  Sharp rise in volume with temporary occlusion
  Rapid venous outflow with release of the occlusion

Abnormal findings in

- COPD, restrictive lung disease, lung infection, or atelectasis (body plethysmography)
- DVT (arterial, venous, or impedance plethysmography)
- Incompetent valves, thrombosis, or thrombotic obstruction in a major vein in an extremity
- Small-vessel diabetic changes
- Vascular disease (Raynaud's phenomenon)
- Vascular trauma

CRITICAL FINDINGS

- DVT

It is essential that critical diagnoses be communicated immediately to the appropriate health-care provider (HCP). A listing of these diagnoses varies among facilities. Note and immediately report to the HCP abnormal results and related symptoms.

INTERFERING FACTORS

Arterial Plethysmography

Factors that may impair the results of the examination
- Cigarette smoking 2 hr before the study, which causes inaccurate results because the nicotine constricts the arteries.
- Alcohol consumption.
- Low cardiac output.
- Shock.
- Compression of pelvic veins (tumors or external compression by dressings).
- Environmental temperatures (hot or cold).
- Arterial occlusion proximal to the extremity to be examined, which can prevent blood flow to the limb.

Venous Plethysmography

Factors that may impair the results of the examination
- Low environmental temperature or cold extremity, which constricts the vessels.
- High anxiety level or muscle tenseness.
- Venous thrombotic occlusion proximal to the extremity to be examined, which can affect blood flow to the limb.

Body Plethysmography

Factors that may impair the results of the examination
- Inability of the patient to follow breathing instructions during the procedure.

Impedance Plethysmography

Factors that may impair the results of the examination
- Movement of the extremity during electrical impedance recording, poor electrode contact, or nonlinear

P

electrical output, which can cause false-positive results.
• Constricting clothing or bandages.

NURSING IMPLICATIONS AND PROCEDURE

PRETEST:

▶ Positively identify the patient using at least two unique identifiers before providing care, treatment, or services.
▶ *Patient Teaching:* Inform the patient this procedure can assist in evaluating blood vessel size and lung ventilation.
▶ Obtain a history of the patient's complaints including a list of known allergens, especially allergies or sensitivities to latex, iodine, seafood, contrast medium, or anesthetics.
▶ Obtain a history of the patient's cardiovascular and pulmonary systems, symptoms, and results of laboratory tests and diagnostic and surgical procedures.
▶ Record the date of the last menstrual period and determine the possibility of pregnancy in perimenopausal women.
▶ Obtain a list of the patient's current medications, including herbs, nutritional supplements, and nutraceuticals (see Appendix F).
▶ Review the procedure with the patient. Address concerns about pain related to the procedure and explain to the patient that no discomfort will be experienced during the test. Explain that there may be some discomfort during insertion of the nasoesophageal catheter if compliance testing is done. Inform the patient that the procedure is generally performed in a specialized area or at the bedside by an HCP who specializes in this procedure, with support staff, and usually takes 30 to 60 min.
▶ Assess the patient's ability to comply with directions given for rest, positioning, and activity before and during the procedure.

▶ For body plethysmography, record the patient's weight, height, and gender. Determine whether the patient is claustrophobic.
▶ *Sensitivity to social and cultural issues,* as well as concern for modesty, is important in providing psychological support before, during, and after the procedure.
▶ Instruct the patient to refrain from smoking for 2 hr prior to the procedure.
▶ There are no food, fluid, or medication restrictions unless by medical direction.

INTRATEST:

▶ Ensure the patient has refrained from smoking for 2 hr before the procedure.
▶ Instruct the patient to void prior to the procedure and to change into the gown, robe, and foot coverings provided.
▶ Obtain and record baseline vital signs.
▶ Instruct the patient to report any unexpected symptoms that occur during the test.
▶ Observe standard precautions, and follow the general guidelines in Appendix A.

Arterial Plethysmography
▶ Explain to the patient that cuffs are applied to the extremity to measure and compare blood flow.
▶ Place the patient in a semi-Fowler's position on an examination table or in bed.
▶ Ask the patient to notify medical personnel if he or she has unexpected symptoms during the test.
▶ Instruct the patient to remain still during the procedure.
▶ Apply three blood pressure cuffs to the extremity and attach a pulse volume recorder (plethysmograph), which records the amplitude of each pulse wave.
▶ Inflate the cuffs to 65 mm Hg to measure the pulse waves of each cuff. When compared with a normal limb, these measurements determine the presence of arterial occlusive disease.

Venous Plethysmography
▶ Explain to the patient that cuffs are applied to the extremity to measure and compare blood flow.

- Place the patient in a semi-Fowler position on an examination table or in bed.
- Instruct the patient to remain still during the procedure.
- Apply two blood pressure cuffs to the extremity, one on the proximal part of the extremity (occlusion cuff) and the other on the distal part of the extremity (recorder cuff). Attach a third cuff to the pulse volume recorder.
- Inflate the recorder cuff to 10 mm Hg, and evaluate the effects of respiration on venous volume: Absence of changes during respirations indicates venous thrombotic occlusion.
- Inflate the occlusion cuff to 50 mm Hg, and record venous volume on the pulse monitor. Deflate the occlusion cuff after the highest volume is recorded in the recorder cuff. A delay in the return to preocclusion volume indicates venous thrombotic occlusion.

Body Plethysmography

- Place the patient in a sitting position on a chair in the body box. Explain to the patient that the cuffs are applied to the extremities to measure and compare blood flow.
- Position a nose clip to prevent breathing through the nose, and connect a mouthpiece to a measuring instrument.
- Ask the patient to breathe through the mouthpiece.
- Close the door to the box, and record the start time of the procedure. At the beginning of the study, instruct the patient to pant rapidly and shallowly, without allowing the glottis to close.
- For compliance testing, a double-lumen nasoesophageal catheter is inserted, and the bag is inflated with air. Intraesophageal pressure is recorded during normal breathing.

Impedance Plethysmography

- Explain to the patient that cuffs are applied to the extremity to measure and compare blood flow.
- Place the patient on his or her back with the leg being tested above the heart level.
- Flex the patient's knee slightly, and rotate the hips by shifting weight to the same side as the leg being tested.

- Apply conductive gel and electrodes to the legs, near the cuffs.
- Apply a blood pressure cuff to the thigh.
- Inflate the pressure cuff attached to the thigh temporarily to occlude venous return without interfering with arterial blood flow. Expect the blood volume in the other calf to increase.
- A tracing of changes in electrical impedance occurring during inflation and for 15 sec after cuff deflation is recorded.
- With DVT, blood volume increases less than expected because the veins are already at capacity.

POST-TEST:

- A report of the examination will be sent to the requesting HCP, who will discuss the results with the patient.
- Remove conductive gel and electrodes, as applied.
- Instruct the patient to resume usual activity and diet, as directed by the HCP.
- Monitor for severe ischemia, ulcers, and pain of the extremity after arterial, venous, or impedance plethysmography, and handle the extremity gently.
- Monitor respiratory pattern after body plethysmography, and allow the patient time to resume a normal breathing pattern.
- Monitor vital signs every 15 min until they return to baseline levels.
- Recognize anxiety related to test results, and be supportive of perceived loss of independent function. Discuss the implications of abnormal test results on the patient's lifestyle. Provide teaching and information regarding the clinical implications of the test results, as appropriate.
- Reinforce information given by the patient's HCP regarding further testing, treatment, or referral to another HCP. Answer any questions or address any concerns voiced by the patient or family.
- Depending on the results of this procedure, additional testing may be needed to evaluate or monitor progression of the disease process and determine the need for a change in therapy. Evaluate

P

test results in relation to the patient's symptoms and other tests performed.

RELATED MONOGRAPHS:

▶ Related tests include α₁-AT, angiography pulmonary, anion gap, arterial/alveolar oxygen ratio, AT-III, biopsy lung, blood gases, bronchoscopy, carboxyhemoglobin, cardiolipin antibodies, chest x-ray, chloride sweat, cold agglutinin, CBC, CBC hemoglobin, CBC WBC count and differential, CT angiography, CT thoracic, culture and smear for mycobacteria, culture bacterial sputum, culture viral, cytology sputum, D-dimer, echocardiography, ECG, EMG, ENG, fibrinogen, gram stain, IgE, lactic acid, lung perfusion scan, lung ventilation scan, lupus anticoagulant antibodies, MR angiography, MRI chest, osmolality, phosphorus, plasminogen, pleural fluid analysis, potassium, PET chest, PFT, pulse oximetry, sodium, TB skin test, and US arterial and venous Doppler of the extremities.

▶ Refer to the Cardiovascular and Pulmonary systems tables at the end of the book for related tests by body system.

Pleural Fluid Analysis

SYNONYM/ACRONYM: Thoracentesis fluid analysis.

COMMON USE: To assess and categorize fluid obtained from within the pleural space for infection, cancer, and blood as well as identify the cause of its accumulation.

SPECIMEN: Pleural fluid (5 mL) collected in a green-top (heparin) tube for amylase, cholesterol, glucose, lactate dehydrogenase (LDH), pH, protein, and triglycerides; lavender-top (EDTA) tube for cell count; sterile containers for microbiology specimens; 200 to 500 mL of fluid in a clear container with anticoagulant for cytology. Ensure that there is an equal amount of fixative and fluid in the container for cytology.

REFERENCE VALUE: (Method: Spectrophotometry for amylase, cholesterol, glucose, LDH, protein, and triglycerides; ion-selective electrode for pH; automated or manual cell count; macroscopic and microscopic examination of cultured microorganisms; microscopic examination of specimen for microbiology and cytology)

Appearance	Clear
Color	Pale yellow
Amylase	Parallels serum values
Cholesterol	Parallels serum values
Glucose	Parallels serum values
LDH	Less than 200 units/L

Appearance	Clear
Fluid LDH–to–serum LDH ratio	0.6 or less
Protein	3.0 g/dL
Fluid protein–to–serum protein ratio	0.5 or less
Triglycerides	Parallel serum values
pH	7.37–7.43
RBC count	Less than 1,000/mm³
WBC count	Less than 1,000/mm³
Culture	No growth
Gram stain	No organisms seen
Cytology	No abnormal cells seen

LDH = lactate dehydrogenase; RBC = red blood cell; WBC = white blood cell.

DESCRIPTION: The pleural cavity and organs within it are lined with a protective membrane. The fluid between the membranes is called *serous fluid*. Normally, only a small amount of fluid is present because the rates of fluid production and absorption are about the same. Many abnormal conditions can result in the buildup of fluid within the pleural cavity. Specific tests are usually ordered in addition to a common battery of tests used to distinguish a transudate from an exudate. *Transudates* are effusions that form as a result of a systemic disorder that disrupts the regulation of fluid balance, such as a suspected perforation. *Exudates* are caused by conditions involving the tissue of the membrane itself, such as an infection or malignancy. Fluid is withdrawn from the pleural cavity by needle aspiration and tested as listed in the previous and following tables.

Characteristic	Transudate	Exudate
Appearance	Clear	Cloudy or turbid
Specific gravity	Less than 1.015	Greater than 1.015
Total protein	Less than 2.5 g/dL	Greater than 3.0 g/dL
Fluid protein–to–serum protein ratio	Less than 0.5	Greater than 0.5
LDH	Parallels serum value	Less than 200 units/L
Fluid LDH–to–serum LDH ratio	Less than 0.6	Greater than 0.6
Fluid cholesterol	Less than 55 mg/dL	Greater than 55 mg/dL
WBC count	Less than 100/mm³	Greater than 1,000/mm³

LDH = lactate dehydrogenase; WBC = white blood cell.

INDICATIONS

- Differentiate transudates from exudates
- Evaluate effusion of unknown cause
- Investigate suspected rupture, immune disease, malignancy, or infection

POTENTIAL DIAGNOSIS

- *Bacterial or tuberculous empyema:* Red blood cell (RBC) count less

P

than 5,000/mm³, white blood cell (WBC) count 25,000 to 100,000/mm³ with a predominance of neutrophils, increased fluid protein-to-serum protein ratio, increased fluid LDH-to-serum LDH ratio, decreased glucose, pH less than 7.3

- *Chylous pleural effusion:* Marked increase in both triglycerides (two to three times serum level) and chylomicrons
- *Effusion caused by pneumonia:* RBC count less than 5,000/mm³, WBC count 5,000 to 25,000/mm³ with a predominance of neutrophils and some eosinophils, increased fluid protein-to-serum protein ratio, increased fluid LDH-to-serum LDH ratio, pH less than 7.4 (and decreased glucose if bacterial pneumonia)
- *Esophageal rupture:* Significantly decreased pH (6.0) and elevated amylase
- *Hemothorax:* Bloody appearance, increased RBC count, elevated hematocrit
- *Malignancy:* RBC count 1,000 to 100,000/mm³, WBC count 5,000 to 10,000/mm³ with a predominance of lymphocytes, abnormal cytology, increased fluid protein-to-serum protein ratio, increased fluid LDH-to-serum LDH ratio, decreased glucose, pH less than 7.3
- *Pancreatitis:* RBC count 1,000 to 10,000/mm³, WBC count 5,000 to 20,000/mm³ with a predominance of neutrophils, pH greater than 7.3, increased fluid protein-to-serum protein ratio, increased fluid LDH-to-serum LDH ratio, increased amylase
- *Pulmonary infarction:* RBC count 10,000 to 100,000/mm³, WBC count 5,000 to 15,000/mm³ with a predominance of neutrophils, pH greater than 7.3, normal glucose, increased fluid protein-to-serum

protein ratio, and increased fluid LDH-to-serum LDH ratio.

- *Pulmonary tuberculosis:* RBC count 10,000/mm³, WBC count 5,000 to 10,000/mm³ with a predominance of lymphocytes, positive acid-fast bacillus stain and culture, increased protein, decreased glucose, pH less than 7.3
- *Rheumatoid disease:* Normal RBC count, WBC count 1,000 to 20,000/mm³ with a predominance of either lymphocytes or neutrophils, pH less than 7.3, decreased glucose, increased fluid protein-to-serum protein ratio, increased fluid LDH-to-serum LDH ratio, increased immunoglobulins
- *Systemic lupus erythematosus:* Similar findings as with rheumatoid disease, except that glucose is usually not decreased

CRITICAL FINDINGS ✦

Positive culture findings in any sterile body fluid.

Note and immediately report to the health-care provider (HCP) positive culture results, if ordered, and related symptoms. pH 7.1 to 7.2 indicates need for immediate drainage.

INTERFERING FACTORS

- Bloody fluids may be the result of a traumatic tap.
- Unknown hyperglycemia or hypoglycemia may be misleading in the comparison of fluid and serum glucose levels. Therefore, it is advisable to collect comparative serum samples a few hours before performing thoracentesis.

NURSING IMPLICATIONS AND PROCEDURE

PRETEST:

▶ Positively identify the patient using at least two unique identifiers before providing care, treatment, or services.

• *Patient Teaching:* Inform the patient this test can assist in identifying the type of fluid being produced within the body cavity.

• Obtain a history of the patient's complaints, including a list of known allergens, especially allergies or sensitivities to latex.

• Obtain a history of the patient's immune and respiratory systems, especially any bleeding disorders and other symptoms, as well as results of previously performed laboratory tests and diagnostic and surgical procedures.

• Note any recent procedures that can interfere with test results.

• Record the date of the last menstrual period and determine the possibility of pregnancy in perimenopausal women.

• Obtain a list of the patient's current medications, including anticoagulants, aspirin and other salicylates, herbs, nutritional supplements, and nutraceuticals (see Appendix F). Such products should be discontinued by medical direction for the appropriate number of days prior to a surgical procedure.

• Review the procedure with the patient. Inform the patient that it may be necessary to remove hair from the site before the procedure. Discuss with the patient that the requesting HCP may request that a cough suppressant be given before the thoracentesis. Address concerns about pain and explain that a sedative and/or analgesia will be administered to promote relaxation and reduce discomfort prior to needle insertion through the chest wall into the pleural space. Explain that any discomfort with the needle insertion will be minimized with local anesthetics and systemic analgesics. Explain that the local anesthetic injection may cause an initial stinging sensation. Meperidine (Demerol) or morphine may be given as a sedative. Inform the patient that the needle insertion is performed under sterile conditions by

an HCP specializing in this procedure. The procedure usually takes about 20 min to complete.

• Explain that an IV line will be inserted to allow infusion of IV fluids, antibiotics, anesthetics, and analgesics.

• *Sensitivity to social and cultural issues,* as well as concern for modesty, is important in providing psychological support before, during, and after the procedure.

• There are no food or fluid restrictions unless by medical direction. The requesting HCP may request that anticoagulants and aspirin be withheld. The number of days to withhold medication is dependent on the type of anticoagulant.

• *Make sure a written and informed consent has been signed prior to the procedure and before administering any medications.*

INTRATEST:

• Ensure that anticoagulant therapy has been withheld for the appropriate number of days prior to the procedure. Notify the HCP if patient anticoagulant therapy has not been withheld.

• Have emergency equipment readily available. Keep resuscitation equipment on hand in the case of respiratory impairment or laryngospasm after the procedure.

• Avoid using morphine sulfate in those with asthma or other pulmonary disease. This drug can further exacerbate bronchospasms and respiratory impairment.

• Have the patient remove clothing and change into a gown for the procedure.

• Instruct the patient to cooperate fully and to follow directions. Direct the patient to breathe normally and to avoid unnecessary movement during the local anesthetic and the procedure.

• Observe standard precautions, and follow the general guidelines in Appendix A. Positively identify the patient, and label the appropriate collection containers with the corresponding patient demographics, date and time of collection, and site location.

- Record baseline vital signs and continue to monitor throughout the procedure. Protocols may vary among facilities.
- Establish an IV line to allow infusion of IV fluids, anesthetics, analgesics, or IV sedation.
- Assist the patient into a comfortable sitting or side-lying position.
- Prior to the administration of local anesthesia, shave and cleanse the site with an antiseptic solution and drape the area with sterile towels. The skin at the injection site is then anesthetized.
- The thoracentesis needle is inserted, and fluid is removed.
- The needle is withdrawn, and pressure is applied to the site with a petroleum jelly gauze. A pressure dressing is applied over the petroleum jelly gauze.
- Monitor the patient for complications related to the procedure (e.g., allergic reaction, anaphylaxis).
- Place samples in properly labeled specimen container, and promptly transport the specimen to the laboratory for processing and analysis.

POST-TEST:

- A report of the examination will be sent to the requesting HCP, who will discuss the results with the patient.
- Instruct the patient to resume usual medications, as directed by the HCP.
- Monitor vital signs every 15 min for the first hr, every 30 min for the next 2 hr, every hour for the next 4 hr, and every 4 hr for the next 24 hr. Take the patient's temperature every 4 hr for 24 hr. Monitor intake and output for 24 hr. Notify the HCP if temperature is elevated. Protocols may vary among facilities.
- Observe/assess the patient for signs of respiratory distress or skin color changes.
- Observe/assess the thoracentesis site for bleeding, inflammation, or hematoma formation each time vital signs are taken and daily thereafter for several days.

- Observe/assess the patient for hemoptysis, difficulty breathing, cough, air hunger, pain, or absent breathing sounds over the affected area. Report to HCP.
- Inform the patient that 1 hr or more of bed rest (lying on the unaffected side) is required after the procedure. Elevate the patient's head for comfort.
- Evaluate the patient for symptoms indicating the development of pneumothorax, such as dyspnea, tachypnea, anxiety, decreased breathing sounds, or restlessness. Prepare the patient for a chest x-ray, if ordered, to ensure that a pneumothorax has not occurred as a result of the procedure.
- Observe/assess for nausea and pain. Administer antiemetic and analgesic medications as needed and as directed by the HCP.
- Administer antibiotics, as ordered, and instruct the patient in the importance of completing the entire course of antibiotic therapy even if no symptoms are present.
- Recognize anxiety related to test results, and offer support. Discuss the implications of abnormal test results on the patient's lifestyle. Provide teaching and information regarding the clinical implications of the test results, as appropriate. Educate the patient regarding access to counseling services, if appropriate.
- Reinforce information given by the patient's HCP regarding further testing, treatment, or referral to another HCP. Answer any questions or address any concerns voiced by the patient or family.
- Depending on the results of this procedure, additional testing may be performed to evaluate or monitor progression of the disease process and determine the need for a change in therapy. Evaluate test results in relation to the patient's symptoms and other tests performed.

RELATED MONOGRAPHS:

- Related tests include antibodies anti-cyclic citrullinated peptide, ANA, biopsy lung, blood gases, cancer antigens, chest x-ray, CBC WBC count and differential, CT thoracic, CRP, culture and smear mycobacteria, culture blood, culture fungal, culture viral, ECG, ESR, MRI chest, and RF.

◗ Refer to the Immune and Respiratory systems tables at the end of the book for related tests by body system.

Porphyrins, Urine

SYNONYM/ACRONYM: Coproporphyrin, porphobilinogen, urobilinogen, and other porphyrins.

COMMON USE: To assess for porphyrias in the urine to assist with diagnosis of genetic disorders associated with porphyrin synthesis as well as heavy metal toxicity.

SPECIMEN: Urine (10 mL) from a random or timed specimen collected in a clean, amber-colored plastic collection container with sodium carbonate as a preservative.

REFERENCE VALUE: (Method: Chromatography for uroporphyrins; spectrophotometry for δ-aminolevulinic acid, urobilinogen, and porphobilinogen)

Test	Conventional Units	SI Units
Total porphyrins	Less than 105 mcg/24 hr	
Coproporphyrin		(Conventional Units × 1.53)
Male	Less than 96 mcg/24 hr	Less than 147 nmol/24 hr
Female	Less than 60 mcg/24 hr	Less than 92 nmol/24 hr
Uroporphyrins	Less than 4 mcg/24 hr	(Conventional Units × 1.43) Less than 6 nmol/24 hr
Hexacarboxylporphyrin	Less than 1 mcg/24 hr	(Conventional Units × 1.34) Less than 1.34 nmol/24 hr
Heptacarboxylporphyrin	Less than 4 mcg/24 hr	(Conventional Units × 1.27) Less than 5.1 nmol/24 hr
Porphobilinogen	Less than 2.0 mg/24 hr	(Conventional Units × 4.42) Less than 8.8 micromol/ 24 hr
Urobilinogen	0.5–4.0 Ehrlich units/24 hr	(Conventional Units × 1) 0.5–4.0 Ehrlich units/24 hr
δ-Aminolevulinic acid	1.5–7.5 mg/24 hr	(Conventional Units × 7.626) 11.4–57.2 micromol/24 hr

P

DESCRIPTION: Porphyrins are produced during the synthesis of heme. If heme synthesis is disturbed, these precursors accumulate and are excreted in the urine in excessive amounts. Conditions producing increased levels of heme precursors are called *porphyrias*. The two main categories of genetically determined porphyrias are erythropoietic porphyrias, in which major abnormalities occur in red blood cell chemistry, and hepatic porphyrias, in which heme precursors are found in urine and feces. Erythropoietic and hepatic porphyrias are rare. Acquired porphyrias are characterized by greater accumulation of precursors in urine and feces than in red blood cells. Lead poisoning is the most common cause of acquired porphyrias. Porphyrins are reddish fluorescent compounds. Depending on the type of porphyrin present, the urine may be reddish, resembling port wine. Porphobilinogen is excreted as a colorless compound. A color change may occur in an acidic sample containing porphobilinogen if the sample is exposed to air for several hours.

INDICATIONS
- Assist in the diagnosis of congenital or acquired porphyrias characterized by abdominal pain, tachycardia, emesis, fever, leukocytosis, and neurological abnormalities
- Detect suspected lead poisoning, as indicated by elevated porphyrins

POTENTIAL DIAGNOSIS

Increased in
- Acute hepatic porphyrias
- Congenital or acquired porphyrias

- Heavy metal, benzene, or carbon tetrachloride toxicity
- Variegated porphyrias

Decreased in: N/A

CRITICAL FINDINGS: N/A

INTERFERING FACTORS
- Drugs that may increase urine porphyrin levels include acriflavine, aminopyrine, ethoxazene, griseofulvin, hexachlorobenzene, oxytetracycline, and sulfonmethane.
- Numerous drugs are suspected as potential initiators of acute attacks, but drugs classified as unsafe for high-risk individuals include aminopyrine, aminoglutethimide, antipyrine, barbiturates, *N*-butylscopolammonium bromide, carbamazepine, carbromal, chlorpropamide, danazol, dapsone, diclofenac, diphenylhydantoin, ergot preparations, ethchlorvynol, ethinamate, glutethimide, griseofulvin, *N*-isopropyl meprobamate, mephenytoin, meprobamate, methyprylon, novobiocin, phenylbutazone, primidone, pyrazolone preparations, succinimides, sulfonamide antibiotics, sulfonethylmethane, sulfonmethane, synthetic estrogens and progestins, tolazamide, tolbutamide, trimethadione, and valproic acid.
- Exposure of the specimen to light can falsely decrease values.
- Screening methods are not well standardized and can produce false-negative results.
- Failure to collect all urine and store specimen properly during the 24-hour test period will interfere with results.

NURSING IMPLICATIONS AND PROCEDURE

PRETEST:

- Positively identify the patient using at least two unique identifiers before providing care, treatment, or services.
- *Patient Teaching:* Inform the patient this test can assist in evaluating for conditions producing increased levels of heme precursors called porphyrias.
- Obtain a history of the patient's complaints, including a list of known allergens, especially allergies or sensitivities to latex.
- Obtain a history of the patient's hematopoietic system, symptoms, and results of previously performed laboratory tests and diagnostic and surgical procedures.
- Obtain a list of the patient's current medications, including herbs, nutritional supplements, and nutraceuticals (see Appendix F).
- Review the procedure with the patient. Provide a nonmetallic urinal, bedpan, or toilet-mounted collection device. Address concerns about pain and explain that there should be no discomfort during the procedure.
- Usually a 24-hr time frame for urine collection is ordered. Inform the patient that all urine must be saved during that 24-hr period. Instruct the patient not to void directly into the laboratory collection container. Instruct the patient to avoid defecating in the collection device and to keep toilet tissue out of the collection device to prevent contamination of the specimen. Place a sign in the bathroom to remind the patient to save all urine.
- Instruct the patient to void all urine into the collection device and then to pour the urine into the laboratory collection container. Alternatively, the specimen can be left in the collection device for a health-care staff member to add to the laboratory collection container.

- *Sensitivity to social and cultural issues,* as well as concern for modesty, is important in providing psychological support before, during, and after the procedure.
- There are no food, fluid, or medication restrictions unless by medical direction.

INTRATEST:

- If the patient has a history of allergic reaction to latex, avoid the use of equipment containing latex.
- Instruct the patient to cooperate fully and to follow directions.
- Observe standard precautions, and follow the general guidelines in Appendix A. Positively identify the patient, and label the appropriate tubes with the corresponding patient demographics, date, and time of collection.

Random Specimen (Collect in Early Morning)

Clean-Catch Specimen
- Instruct the male patient to (1) thoroughly wash his hands, (2) cleanse the meatus, (3) void a small amount into the toilet, and (4) void directly into the specimen container.
- Instruct the female patient to (1) thoroughly wash her hands; (2) cleanse the labia from front to back; (3) while keeping the labia separated, void a small amount into the toilet; and (4) without interrupting the urine stream, void directly into the specimen container.

Indwelling Catheter
- Put on gloves. Empty drainage tube of urine. It may be necessary to clamp off the catheter for 15 to 30 minutes before specimen collection. Cleanse specimen port with antiseptic swab, and then aspirate 5 mL of urine with a 21- to 25-gauge needle and syringe. Transfer urine to a sterile container.

Timed Specimen
- Obtain a clean 3-L urine specimen container, toilet-mounted collection

P

device, and plastic bag (for transport of the specimen container). The specimen must be refrigerated or kept on ice throughout the entire collection period. If an indwelling urinary catheter is in place, the drainage bag must be kept on ice.

▶ Begin the test between 6 and 8 a.m. if possible. Collect first voiding and discard. Record the time the specimen was discarded as the beginning of the timed collection period. The next morning, ask the patient to void at the same time the collection was started and add this last voiding to the container. Urinary output should be recorded throughout the collection time.

▶ If an indwelling catheter is in place, replace the tubing and container system at the start of the collection time. Keep the container system on ice during the collection period, or empty the urine into a larger container periodically during the collection period; monitor to ensure continued drainage, and conclude the test the next morning at the same hour the collection was begun.

▶ At the conclusion of the test, compare the quantity of urine with the urinary output record for the collection; if the specimen contains less than what was recorded as output, some urine may have been discarded, invalidating the test.

▶ Include on the collection container's label the amount of urine, test start and stop times, and ingestion of any foods or medications that can affect test results.

General

▶ Promptly transport the specimen to the laboratory for processing and analysis.

POST-TEST:

▶ A report of the results will be sent to the requesting health-care provider (HCP), who will discuss the results with the patient.

▶ Recognize anxiety related to test results. Discuss the implications of abnormal test results on the patient's lifestyle. Provide teaching and information regarding the clinical implications of the test results, as appropriate. Educate the patient regarding access to counseling services. Provide contact information, if desired, for the American Porphyria Foundation at www.porphyriafoundation.com.

▶ Reinforce information given by the patient's HCP regarding further testing, treatment, or referral to another HCP. Answer any questions or address any concerns voiced by the patient or family.

▶ Depending on the results of this procedure, additional testing may be performed to evaluate or monitor progression of the disease process and determine the need for a change in therapy. Evaluate test results in relation to the patient s symptoms and other tests performed.

RELATED MONOGRAPHS:

▶ Related tests include δ-aminolevulinic acid, erythrocyte protoporphyrin, and lead.

▶ Refer to the Hematopoietic System table at the end of the book for related tests by body system.

P

Positron Emission Tomography, Brain

SYNONYM/ACRONYM: PET scan of the brain.

COMMON USE: To assess blood flow and metabolic processes of the brain to assist in diagnosis of disorders such as ischemic or hemorrhagic stroke or cancer and to evaluate head trauma.

AREA OF APPLICATION: Brain.

CONTRAST: IV radioactive material (fluorodeoxyglucose [FDG]).

DESCRIPTION: Positron emission tomography (PET) combines the biochemical properties of nuclear medicine with the accuracy of computed tomography (CT). PET uses positron emissions from specific radionuclides (oxygen, nitrogen, carbon, and fluorine) to produce detailed functional images within the body. After the radionuclide becomes concentrated in the brain, PET images of blood flow or metabolic processes at the cellular level can be obtained. Fluorine-18, in the form of fluorodeoxyglucose (FDG), is one of the more commonly used radionuclides. FDG is a glucose analogue, and because every cell uses glucose, the metabolic activity occurring in neurological conditions can be measured. There is little localization of FDG in normal tissue, allowing rapid detection of abnormal disease states. The brain uses oxygen and glucose almost exclusively to meet its energy needs, and therefore the brain's metabolism has been studied widely with PET.

The positron radiopharmaceuticals generally have short half-lives, ranging from a few seconds to a few hours, and therefore they must be produced in a cyclotron located near where the test is being done. The PET scanner translates the emissions from the radioactivity as the positron combines with the negative electrons from the tissues and forms gamma rays that can be detected by the scanner. This information is transmitted to the computer, which determines the location and its distribution and translates the emissions as color-coded images for viewing, quantitative measurements, activity changes in relation to time, and three-dimensional computer-aided analysis. Each radionuclide tracer is designed to measure a specific body process, such as glucose metabolism, blood flow, or brain tissue perfusion. The radionuclide can be administered IV or inhaled as a gas. PET has had the greatest clinical impact in patients with epilepsy, dementia, neurodegenerative diseases, inflammation, cerebrovascular disease (indirectly), and brain tumors.

The expense of the study and the limited availability of radiopharmaceuticals limit the use of PET even though it is more sensitive than traditional nuclear scanning

P

and single-photon emission computed tomography. Changes in reimbursement and the advent of mobile technology have increased the availability of this procedure in the community setting.

INDICATIONS

- Detect Parkinson's disease and Huntington's disease, as evidenced by decreased metabolism
- Determine the effectiveness of therapy, as evidenced by biochemical activity of normal and abnormal tissues
- Determine physiological changes in psychosis and schizophrenia
- Differentiate between tumor recurrence and radiation necrosis
- Evaluate Alzheimer's disease and differentiate it from other causes of dementia, as evidenced by decreased cerebral flow and metabolism
- Evaluate cranial tumors pre- and postoperatively and determine stage and appropriate treatment or procedure
- Identify cerebrovascular accident or aneurysm, as evidenced by decreased blood flow and oxygen use
- Identify focal seizures, as evidenced by decreased metabolism between seizures

POTENTIAL DIAGNOSIS

Normal findings in
- Normal patterns of tissue metabolism, blood flow, and radionuclide distribution

Abnormal findings in
- Alzheimer's disease
- Aneurysm
- Cerebral metastases
- Cerebrovascular accident
- Creutzfeldt-Jakob disease
- Dementia
- Head trauma
- Huntington's disease
- Migraine
- Parkinson's disease
- Schizophrenia
- Seizure disorders
- Tumors

CRITICAL FINDINGS

- Aneurysm
- Cerebrovascular accident
- Tumor with significant mass effect

It is essential that critical diagnoses be communicated immediately to the appropriate health-care provider (HCP). A listing of these diagnoses varies among facilities. Note and immediately report to the HCP abnormal results and related symptoms.

INTERFERING FACTORS

This procedure is contraindicated for
- Patients who are pregnant or suspected of being pregnant, unless the potential benefits of the procedure far outweigh the risks to the fetus and mother.

Factors that may impair clear imaging
- Inability of the patient to cooperate or remain still during the procedure because of age, significant pain, or mental status.
- Drugs that alter glucose metabolism, such as tranquilizers or insulin, because hypoglycemia can alter PET results.
- The use of alcohol, tobacco, or caffeine-containing drinks at least 24 hr before the study, because the effects of these substances would make it difficult to evaluate the patient's true physiological state (e.g., alcohol is a vasconstrictor and would decrease blood flow to the target organ).
- Metallic objects (e.g., jewelry, body rings) within the examination field, which may inhibit organ visualization and cause unclear images.

Other considerations

- Failure to follow dietary restrictions before the procedure may cause the procedure to be canceled or repeated.
- Improper injection of the radionuclide that allows the tracer to seep deep into the muscle tissue produces erroneous hot spots.
- False-positive findings may occur as a result of normal gastrointestinal tract uptake and uptake in areas of infection or inflammation.
- Consultation with a HCP should occur before the procedure for radiation safety concerns regarding younger patients or patients who are lactating.
- Risks associated with radiation overexposure can result from frequent x-ray or radionuclide procedures. Personnel working in the examination area should wear badges to record their level of radiation exposure.

NURSING IMPLICATIONS AND PROCEDURE

PRETEST:

- Positively identify the patient using at least two unique identifiers before providing care, treatment, or services.
- *Patient Teaching:* Inform the patient that this procedure can assist in assessing blood flow to the brain and brain tissue metabolism.
- Obtain a history of the patient's complaints, including a list of known allergens, especially allergies or sensitivities to latex, iodine, seafood, contrast medium, or anesthetics.
- Obtain a history of the patient's musculoskeletal system, symptoms, and results of previously performed laboratory tests and diagnostic and surgical procedures.
- Note any recent procedures that can interfere with test results, including examinations using barium- or iodine-based contrast medium.

- Record the date of the last menstrual period and determine the possibility of pregnancy in perimenopausal women.
- Obtain a list of the patient's current medications, including herbs, nutritional supplements, and nutraceuticals (see Appendix F).
- Review the procedure with the patient. Address concerns about pain related to the procedure and explain that some pain may be experienced during the test, or there may be moments of discomfort. Reassure the patient that radioactive material poses minimal radioactive hazard because of its short half-life and rarely produces side effects. Inform the patient that the procedure is performed in a special department, usually in a radiology suite, by an HCP specializing in this procedure, with support staff, and takes approximately 60 to 120 min.
- *Sensitivity to social and cultural issues,* as well as concern for modesty, is important in providing psychological support before, during, and after the procedure.
- Sometimes FDG examinations are done after blood has been drawn to determine circulating blood glucose levels. If blood glucose levels are high, insulin may be given.
- Instruct the patient to remove jewelry and other metallic objects from the area to be examined prior to the procedure.
- Instruct the patient to avoid taking anticoagulant medication or to reduce dosage as ordered prior to the procedure.
- Instruct the patient to restrict food for 4 hr; restrict alcohol, nicotine, or caffeine-containing drinks for 24 hr; and withhold medications for 24 hr before the test. Protocols may vary among facilities.
- *Make sure a written and informed consent has been signed prior to the procedure and before administering any medications.*

INTRATEST:

- Ensure that the patient has complied with dietary, fluid, and medication restrictions and pretesting preparations.

P

• Ensure the patient has removed all jewelry and external metallic objects from the area to be examined prior to the procedure.

• Have emergency equipment readily available.

• Instruct the patient to void prior to the procedure and to change into the gown, robe, and foot coverings provided.

• Instruct the patient to cooperate fully and to follow directions. Ask the patient to remain still throughout the procedure because movement produces unreliable results.

• Observe standard precautions, and follow the general guidelines in Appendix A.

• Record baseline vital signs and assess neurological status. Protocols may vary among facilities.

• Place the patient in the supine position on an examination table.

• The radionuclide is injected, and imaging is started after a 30-min delay. If comparative studies are indicated, additional injections may be needed.

• The patient may be asked to perform different cognitive activities (e.g., reading) to measure changes in brain activity during reasoning or remembering.

• The patient may be blindfolded or asked to use earplugs to decrease auditory and visual stimuli.

• Monitor the patient for complications related to the procedure (e.g., allergic reaction, anaphylaxis, bronchospasm).

• Remove the needle or catheter and apply a pressure dressing over the puncture site.

• Observe/assess the needle/catheter insertion site for bleeding, inflammation, or hematoma formation.

POST-TEST:

• A report of the results will be sent to the requesting HCP, who will discuss the results with the patient.

• Instruct the patient to resume pretest diet, fluids, medications, or activity.

• Observe for delayed allergic reactions, such as rash, urticaria, tachycardia, hyperpnea, hypertension, palpitations, nausea, or vomiting.

• Instruct the patient to immediately report symptoms such as fast heart rate, difficulty breathing, skin rash, itching, chest pain, persistent right shoulder pain, or abdominal pain. Immediately report symptoms to the appropriate HCP.

• Observe/assess the needle/catheter insertion site for bleeding, inflammation, or hematoma formation.

• Instruct the patient in the care and assessment of the injection site.

• Instruct the patient to apply cold compresses to the puncture site as needed to reduce discomfort or edema.

• Instruct the patient to drink increased amounts of fluids for 24 to 48 hr to eliminate the radionuclide from the body, unless contraindicated. Educate the patient that radionuclide is eliminated from the body within 6 to 24 hr.

• Instruct the patient to flush the toilet immediately after each voiding and to meticulously wash hands with soap and water for 24 hr after the procedure.

• Instruct all caregivers to wear gloves when discarding urine for 24 hr after the procedure. Wash gloved hands with soap and water before removing gloves. Then wash hands after the gloves are removed.

• If a woman who is breastfeeding must have a nuclear scan, she should not breastfeed the infant until the radionuclide has been eliminated, about 3 days. Instruct her to express the milk and discard it during the 3-day period to prevent cessation of milk production.

• No other radionuclide tests should be scheduled for 24 to 48 hr after this procedure.

• Recognize anxiety related to test results, and be supportive of perceived loss of independent function. Discuss the implications of abnormal test results on the patient's lifestyle. Provide teaching and information regarding the clinical implications of the test results, as appropriate.

• Reinforce information given by the patient's HCP regarding further testing, treatment, or referral to another HCP. Answer any questions or address any concerns voiced by the patient or family.

▶ Depending on the results of this procedure, additional testing may be needed to evaluate or monitor progression of the disease process and determine the need for a change in therapy. Evaluate test results in relation to the patient's symptoms and other tests performed.

RELATED MONOGRAPHS:
▶ Related tests include Alzheimer's disease markers, CT brain, EEG, MRI brain, and US arterial Doppler of the carotids.
▶ Refer to the Musculoskeletal System table at the end of the book for related tests by body system.

Positron Emission Tomography, FDG

SYNONYM/ACRONYM: Fluorodeoxyglucose (FDG)-positron emission tomography (PET).

COMMON USE: To assist in assessment, staging, and monitoring of metabolically active malignant lesions in the breast, abdomen, brain, and heart, such as breast cancer, Parkinson's disease, and Alzheimer's disease.

AREA OF APPLICATION: Abdomen, brain, breast, heart, pelvis.

CONTRAST: IV radioactive material fluorodeoxyglucose (FDG).

DESCRIPTION: Fluorine-18, in the form of fluorodeoxyglucose (FDG), is one of the more commonly used radionuclides. FDG is a glucose analogue, and because every cell uses glucose, the metabolic activity occurring in neurological conditions can be measured. There is little localization of FDG in normal tissue, allowing rapid detection of abnormal disease states. The brain uses oxygen and glucose almost exclusively to meet its energy needs, and therefore the brain's metabolism has been studied widely with positron emission tomography (PET). The role of this procedure is to detect metabolically active malignant lesions. FDG-PET scan may also be used to stage and monitor the response to the malignant disease.

PET combines the biochemical properties of nuclear medicine with the accuracy of computed tomography (CT). PET uses positron emissions from specific radionuclides (oxygen, nitrogen, carbon, and fluorine) to produce detailed functional images within the body. The positron radiopharmaceuticals generally have short half-lives, ranging from a few seconds to a few hours, and therefore they must be produced in a cyclotron located near where the test is being done. The PET scanner translates the emissions from the radioactivity as the positron combines with the negative electrons from the tissues and forms gamma rays that can be detected by the scanner. This information is transmitted to the computer, which determines the location and its distribution and translates the emissions as color-coded images

P

for viewing, quantitative measurements, activity changes in relation to time, and three-dimensional computer-aided analysis.

The expense of the study and the limited availability of radiopharmaceuticals limit the use of PET, even though it is more sensitive than traditional nuclear scanning and single-photon emission computed tomography. Changes in reimbursement and the advent of mobile technology have increased the availability of this procedure in the community setting.

INDICATIONS

- Detect Parkinson's disease and Huntington's disease, as evidenced by decreased metabolism
- Determine physiological changes in psychosis and schizophrenia
- Evaluate Alzheimer's disease and differentiate it from other causes of dementia, as evidenced by decreased cerebral flow and metabolism
- Evaluate coronary artery disease (CAD), as evidenced by decreased myocardial blood flow and myocardial perfusion
- Evaluate myocardial viability, as evidenced by low glucose metabolism
- Evaluate tumors preoperatively and postoperatively and determine grade, stage, and appropriate treatment or procedure
- Identify cerebrovascular accident or aneurysm, as evidenced by decreased blood flow and oxygen use
- Identify focal seizures, as evidenced by decreased metabolism between seizures

POTENTIAL DIAGNOSIS

Normal findings in
- Normal patterns of tissue metabolism, blood flow, and radionuclide distribution

Abnormal findings in
- Alzheimer's disease
- Brain trauma
- Breast cancer
- Colorectal cancer
- CAD
- Epilepsy
- Heart muscle dysfunction
- Huntington's disease
- Infections
- Lung cancer
- Lymphoma
- Melanoma
- Metastatic disease
- Myeloma
- Ovarian cancer
- Pancreatic cancer
- Parkinson's disease

CRITICAL FINDINGS: N/A

INTERFERING FACTORS

This procedure is contraindicated for
- Patients who are pregnant or suspected of being pregnant, unless the potential benefits of the procedure far outweigh the risks to the fetus and mother.

Factors that may impair clear imaging
- Inability of the patient to cooperate or remain still during the procedure because of age, significant pain, or mental status.
- Drugs that alter glucose metabolism, such as tranquilizers, sedatives, or insulin, because hypoglycemia can alter PET results.
- The use of alcohol, tobacco, or caffeine-containing drinks at least 24 hr before the study, because the effects of these substances, make it difficult to evaluate the patient's true physiological state (e.g., alcohol is a vasoconstrictor and would decrease blood flow to the target organ).
- Excessive exercise in the preceding 3 days, which can cause factitious

uptake of the contrast material in the musculature.

- Excessive anxiety may affect valuation of brain function.
- Metallic objects (e.g., jewelry, body rings) within the examination field, which may inhibit organ visualization and cause unclear images.

Other considerations

- Failure to follow dietary restrictions before the procedure may cause the procedure to be canceled or repeated.
- Consultation with a health-care provider (HCP) should occur before the procedure for radiation safety concerns regarding younger patients or patients who are lactating.
- Risks associated with radiation overexposure can result from frequent x-ray or radionuclide procedures. Personnel working in the examination area should wear badges to record their level of radiation exposure.

NURSING IMPLICATIONS AND PROCEDURE

PRETEST:

- Positively identify the patient using at least two unique identifiers before providing care, treatment, or services.
- *Patient Teaching:* Inform the patient this test can assist in assessing blood flow and tissue metabolism.
- Obtain a history of the patient's complaints, including a list of known allergens, especially allergies or sensitivities to latex, iodine, seafood, anesthetics, or contrast medium.
- Obtain a history of the patient's cardiovascular, hematopoietic, neuromuscular, and reproductive systems; symptoms; and results of previously performed laboratory tests and diagnostic and surgical procedures.
- Note any recent procedures that can interfere with test results, including

examinations using barium- or iodine-based contrast medium.

- Record the date of last menstrual period and determine the possibility of pregnancy in perimenopausal women.
- Obtain a list of the patient's current medications, including herbs, nutritional supplements, and nutraceuticals (see Appendix F).
- Review the procedure with the patient. Address concerns about pain related to the procedure and explain that no pain will be experienced during the test, but there may be moments of discomfort. Reassure the patient the radionuclide poses no radioactive hazard and rarely produces side effects. Inform the patient that the procedure is performed in a nuclear medicine department, by an HCP specializing in this procedure, with support staff, and takes approximately 1 to 3 hr.
- *Sensitivity to social and cultural issues,* as well as concern for modesty, is important in providing psychological support before, during, and after the procedure.
- Instruct patients with diabetes to take their pretest dose of insulin at a meal 4 hr before the test.
- Sometimes FDG examinations are done after blood has been drawn to determine circulating blood glucose levels. If blood glucose levels are high, insulin may be given.
- Instruct the patient to remove jewelry and other metallic objects from the area to be examined prior to the procedure.
- Instruct the patient to restrict food for 4 to 6 hr; restrict alcohol, nicotine, or caffeine-containing drinks for 24 hr; and withhold medications for 24 hr before the test. The exception is that there are no dietary restrictions for patients undergoing cardiac imaging. Protocols may vary among facilities.
- *Make sure a written and informed consent has been signed prior to the procedure and before administering any medications.*

INTRATEST:

- Ensure that the patient has complied with dietary, fluid, and medication

P

restrictions and pretesting preparations prior to the procedure.

- Ensure that the patient has removed external metallic objects from the area to be examined prior to the procedure.
- Have emergency equipment readily available.
- Instruct the patient to void prior to the procedure and to change into the gown, robe, and foot coverings provided.
- Instruct the patient to cooperate fully and to follow directions. Instruct the patient to remain still throughout the procedure because movement produces unreliable results.
- Observe standard precautions, and follow the general guidelines in Appendix A.
- Record baseline vital signs and assess neurological status. Protocols may vary among facilities.
- Cardiac imaging patients may be asked to drink glucose prior to the radionuclide injection.
- Place the patient in the supine position on an examination table.
- The radionuclide is injected, and imaging is started after a 30-min delay. Images may be recorded for up to 3 hr postinjection.
- Monitor the patient for complications related to the procedure (e.g., allergic reaction, anaphylaxis, bronchospasm).
- Remove the needle or catheter and apply a pressure dressing over the puncture site.
- Observe/assess the needle/catheter insertion site for bleeding, inflammation, or hematoma formation.

POST-TEST:

- A report of the results will be sent to the requesting HCP, who will discuss the results with the patient.
- Instruct the patient to resume pretest diet, fluids, medications, and activity.
- Observe for delayed allergic reactions, such as rash, urticaria, tachycardia, hyperpnea, hypertension, palpitations, nausea, or vomiting.
- Instruct the patient to immediately report symptoms such as fast heart rate, difficulty breathing, skin rash, itching, chest pain, persistent right shoulder pain, or abdominal pain.

Immediately report symptoms to the appropriate HCP.

- Observe/assess the needle/catheter insertion site for bleeding, inflammation, or hematoma formation.
- Instruct the patient in the care and assessment of the injection site.
- Instruct the patient to apply cold compresses to the puncture site as needed, to reduce discomfort or edema.
- Instruct the patient to drink increased amounts of fluids for 24 to 48 hr to eliminate the radionuclide from the body, unless contraindicated. Educate the patient that radionuclide is eliminated from the body within 6 to 24 hr.
- Instruct the patient to flush the toilet immediately after each voiding and to meticulously wash hands with soap and water for 24 hr after the procedure.
- Instruct all caregivers to wear gloves when discarding urine for 24 hr after the procedure. Wash gloved hands with soap and water before removing gloves. Then wash hands after the gloves are removed.
- If a woman who is breastfeeding must have a nuclear scan, she should not breastfeed the infant until the radionuclide has been eliminated, about 3 days. Instruct her to express the milk and discard it during the 3-day period to prevent cessation of milk production.
- *Nutritional Considerations:* Abnormal findings may be associated with cardiovascular disease. The American Heart Association and National Heart, Lung, and Blood Institute (NHBLI) recommend nutritional therapy for individuals identified to be at high risk for developing CAD or individuals who have specific risk factors or existing medical conditions (e.g., elevated LDL cholesterol levels, other lipid disorders, insulin-dependent diabetes, insulin resistance, or metabolic syndrome). If overweight, the patient should be encouraged to achieve a normal weight. The NHLBI's National Cholesterol Education Program (NCEP) revised its dietary guidelines for reducing CAD in 2001. Guidelines for the Therapeutic Lifestyle Changes (TLC) diet are outlined in the Third Report of the Expert Panel on Detection, Evaluation, and Treatment of High

Blood Cholesterol in Adults (Adult Treatment Panel III [ATP III]). The TLC diet emphasizes a reduction in foods high in saturated fats and cholesterol. Red meats, eggs, and dairy products are the major sources of saturated fats and cholesterol. If triglycerides also are elevated, the patient should be advised to eliminate or reduce alcohol and simple carbohydrates from the diet. The TLC approach also includes the use of plant stanols or sterols and increased dissolved fiber as an option for lowering LDL cholesterol levels; nutritional recommendations for daily total caloric intake; recommendations for allowable percentage of calories derived from fat (saturated and unsaturated), carbohydrates, protein, and cholesterol; as well as recommendations for daily expenditure of energy.

▶ *Nutritional Considerations:* Overweight patients with high blood pressure should be encouraged to achieve a normal weight. Other changeable risk factors warranting patient education include strategies to safely decrease sodium intake, increase physical activity, decrease alcohol consumption, eliminate tobacco use, and decrease cholesterol levels.

▶ No other radionuclide tests should be scheduled for 24 to 48 hr after this procedure.

▶ Recognize anxiety related to test results. Discuss the implications of abnormal test results on the patient's lifestyle. Provide teaching and information regarding the clinical implications of the test results, as appropriate.

▶ Reinforce information given by the patient's HCP regarding further testing, treatment, or referral to another HCP. Decisions regarding the need for and frequency of breast self-examination, mammography, magnetic resonance imaging (MRI) of the breast, or other cancer screening procedures should be made after consultation between the patient and HCP. The most current guidelines for breast cancer screening of the general population as well as of individuals with increased risk are available from the American Cancer Society (www.cancer.org), the American College of Obstetricians and Gynecologists (ACOG) (www.acog.org), and the American College of Radiology (www.acr.org). Answer any questions or address any concerns voiced by the patient or family.

▶ Depending on the results of this procedure, additional testing may be needed to evaluate or monitor progression of the disease process and determine the need for a change in therapy. Evaluate test results in relation to the patient's symptoms and other tests performed.

RELATED MONOGRAPHS:

▶ Related tests include AFP, Alzheimer's disease markers, amino acid screen, amylase, barium enema, biopsy breast, biopsy lung, bronchoscopy, calcitonin, cancer antigens, CBC WBC count and differential, CSF analysis, colonoscopy, CT abdomen, CT brain, CT pancreas, CT pelvis, cytology sputum, evoked brain potentials, exercise stress test, fecal analysis, gallium scan, laparoscopy abdominal, laparoscopy gyn, lymphangiogram, mammography, MRI abdomen, MRI brain, MRI breast, MRI pelvis, myocardial perfusion heart scan, peritoneal fluid analysis, PET brain, PET heart, PET pelvis, proctosigmoidoscopy, stereotactic breast biopsy, US breast, US pancreas, US pelvis gyn, and WBC scan.

▶ Refer to the Cardiovascular, Musculoskeletal, and Reproductive systems tables at the end of the book for related tests by body system.

P

Positron Emission Tomography, Heart

SYNONYM/ACRONYM: PET scan of the heart.

COMMON USE: To assess blood flow and metabolic process of the heart to assist in diagnosis of disorders such as coronary artery disease, infarct, and aneurysm.

AREA OF APPLICATION: Heart, chest/thorax, vascular system.

CONTRAST: IV radioactive material (fluorodeoxyglucose [FDG]).

DESCRIPTION: Positron emission tomography (PET) combines the biochemical properties of nuclear medicine with the accuracy of computed tomography (CT). PET uses positron emissions from specific radionuclides (oxygen, nitrogen, carbon, and fluorine) to produce detailed functional images within the body. After the radionuclide becomes concentrated in the heart, PET images of blood flow or metabolic processes at the cellular level can be obtained. Fluorine-18, in the form of fluorodeoxyglucose (FDG), is one of the more commonly used radionuclides. FDG is a glucose analogue, and because every cell uses glucose, the metabolic activity occurring in heart conditions such as myocardial viability can be measured. There is little localization of FDG in normal tissue, allowing rapid detection of abnormal disease states.

The positron radiopharmaceuticals generally have short half-lives, ranging from a few seconds to a few hours, and therefore they must be produced in a cyclotron located near where the test is being done. The PET scanner translates the emissions from the radioactivity as the positron combines with the negative electrons from the tissues and forms gamma rays that can be detected by the scanner. This information is transmitted to the computer, which determines the location and its distribution and translates the emissions as color-coded images for viewing, quantitative measurements, activity changes in relation to time, and three-dimensional computer-aided analysis. Each radionuclide tracer is designed to measure a specific body process, such as glucose metabolism, blood flow, or tissue perfusion. The radionuclide can be administered IV or inhaled as a gas.

The expense of the study and the limited availability of radiopharmaceuticals limit the use of PET, even though it is more sensitive than traditional nuclear scanning and single-photon emission computed tomography. Changes in reimbursement and the advent of mobile technology have increased the availability of this procedure in the community setting.

INDICATIONS
- Assess tissue permeability
- Determine the effects of therapeutic drugs on malfunctioning or diseased tissue

- Determine localization of areas of heart metabolism
- Determine the presence of coronary artery disease (CAD), as evidenced by metabolic state during ischemia and after angina
- Determine the size of heart infarcts
- Identify cerebrovascular accident or aneurysm, as evidenced by decreasing blood flow and oxygen use

POTENTIAL DIAGNOSIS

Normal findings in
- Normal patterns of tissue metabolism, blood flow, and radionuclide distribution

Abnormal findings in
- Chronic obstructive pulmonary disease
- Decreased blood flow and decreased glucose concentration **(indicating necrotic, scarred tissue)**
- Enlarged left ventricle
- Heart chamber disorder
- Myocardial infarction **(indicating increased radionuclide uptake in the myocardium)**
- Pulmonary edema
- Reduced blood flow but increased glucose concentration **(indicating ischemia)**

CRITICAL FINDINGS: N/A

INTERFERING FACTORS

This procedure is contraindicated for
- Patients who are pregnant or suspected of being pregnant, unless the potential benefits of the procedure far outweigh the risks to the fetus and mother.

Factors that may impair clear imaging
- Inability of the patient to cooperate or remain still during the procedure because of age, significant pain, or mental status.

- Drugs that alter glucose metabolism, such as tranquilizers or insulin, because hypoglycemia can alter PET results.
- The use of alcohol, tobacco, or caffeine-containing drinks at least 24 hr before the study, because the effects of these substances would make it difficult to evaluate the patient's true physiological state (e.g., alcohol is a vasoconstrictor and would decrease blood flow to the target organ).
- Metallic objects (e.g., jewelry, body rings) within the examination field, which may inhibit organ visualization and cause unclear images.

Other considerations
- Failure to follow dietary restrictions before the procedure may cause the procedure to be canceled or repeated.
- Improper injection of the radionuclide that allows the tracer to seep deep into the muscle tissue produces erroneous hot spots.
- False-positive findings may occur as a result of normal gastrointestinal tract uptake and uptake in areas of infection or inflammation.
- Consultation with a health-care provider (HCP) should occur before the procedure for radiation safety concerns regarding younger patients or patients who are lactating.
- Risks associated with radiation overexposure can result from frequent x-ray or radionuclide procedures. Personnel working in the examination area should wear badges to record their level of radiation exposure.

NURSING IMPLICATIONS AND PROCEDURE

PRETEST:
▶ Positively identify the patient using at least two unique identifiers before providing care, treatment, or services.

P

▶ *Patient Teaching:* Inform the patient this procedure can assist in assessing blood flow to the heart.

▶ Obtain a history of the patient's complaints, including a list of known allergens, especially allergies or sensitivities to latex, iodine, seafood, contrast medium, or anesthetics.

▶ Obtain a history of the patient's cardiovascular and respiratory systems, symptoms, and results of previously performed laboratory tests and diagnostic and surgical procedures.

▶ Note any recent procedures that can interfere with test results, including examinations using barium- or iodine-based contrast medium.

▶ Record the date of the last menstrual period and determine the possibility of pregnancy in perimenopausal women.

▶ Obtain a list of the patient's current medications, including herbs, nutritional supplements, and nutraceuticals (see Appendix F).

▶ Review the procedure with the patient. Address concerns about pain related to the procedure and explain that some pain may be experienced during the test, or there may be moments of discomfort. Reassure the patient that radioactive material poses minimal radioactive hazard because of its short half-life and rarely produces side effects. Inform the patient that the procedure is performed in a special department, usually in a radiology suite, by an HCP specializing in this procedure, with support staff, and takes approximately 60 to 120 min.

▶ *Sensitivity to social and cultural issues,* as well as concern for modesty, is important in providing psychological support before, during, and after the procedure.

▶ Sometimes FDG examinations are done after blood has been drawn to determine circulating blood glucose levels. If blood glucose levels are high, insulin may be given.

▶ Instruct the patient to remove jewelry and other metallic objects from the area to be examined prior to the procedure.

▶ Instruct the patient to avoid taking anticoagulant medication or to reduce dosage as ordered prior to the procedure.

▶ Instruct the patient to restrict food for 4 hr; restrict alcohol, nicotine, or caffeine-containing drinks for 24 hr; and withhold medications for 24 hr before the test. Protocols may vary among facilities.

▶ *Make sure a written and informed consent has been signed prior to the procedure and before administering any medications.*

INTRATEST:

▶ Ensure that the patient has complied with dietary, fluid, and medication restrictions and pretesting preparations.

▶ Ensure the patient has removed all jewelry and external metallic objects from the area to be examined prior to the procedure.

▶ Have emergency equipment readily available.

▶ Instruct the patient to void prior to the procedure and to change into the gown, robe, and foot coverings provided.

▶ Instruct the patient to cooperate fully and to follow directions. Ask the patient to remain still throughout the procedure because movement produces unreliable results.

▶ Observe standard precautions, and follow the general guidelines in Appendix A.

▶ Record baseline vital signs and assess neurological status. Protocols may vary among facilities.

▶ Place the patient in the supine position on an examination table.

▶ The radionuclide is injected and imaging is done at periodic intervals, with continuous scanning done for 1 hr. If comparative studies are indicated, additional injections may be needed.

▶ Monitor the patient for complications related to the procedure (e.g., allergic reaction, anaphylaxis, bronchospasm).

▶ Remove the needle or catheter and apply a pressure dressing over the puncture site.

▶ Observe/assess the needle site for bleeding, inflammation, or hematoma formation.

POST-TEST:

▶ A report of the results will be sent to the requesting HCP, who will discuss the results with the patient.

- Instruct the patient to resume pretest diet, fluids, medications, and activity.
- Observe for delayed allergic reactions, such as rash, urticaria, tachycardia, hyperpnea, hypertension, palpitations, nausea, or vomiting.
- Instruct the patient to immediately report symptoms such as fast heart rate, difficulty breathing, skin rash, itching, chest pain, persistent right shoulder pain, or abdominal pain. Immediately report symptoms to the appropriate HCP.
- Observe/assess the needle/catheter insertion site for bleeding, inflammation, or hematoma formation.
- Instruct the patient to apply cold compresses to the puncture site as needed, to reduce discomfort or edema.
- Instruct the patient to drink increased amounts of fluids for 24 to 48 hr to eliminate the radionuclide from the body, unless contraindicated. Educate the patient that radionuclide is eliminated from the body within 6 to 24 hr.
- Instruct the patient to flush the toilet immediately after each voiding and to meticulously wash hands with soap and water for 24 hr after the procedure.
- Instruct all caregivers to wear gloves when discarding urine for 24 hr after the procedure. Wash gloved hands with soap and water before removing gloves. Then wash hands after the gloves are removed.
- If a woman who is breastfeeding must have a nuclear scan, she should not breastfeed the infant until the radionuclide has been eliminated, about 3 days. Instruct her to express the milk and discard it during the 3-day period to prevent cessation of milk production.
- No other radionuclide tests should be scheduled for 24 to 48 hr after this procedure.
- **Nutritional Considerations:** Abnormal findings may be associated with cardiovascular disease. The American Heart Association and National Heart, Lung, and Blood Institute (NHBLI) recommend nutritional therapy for individuals identified to be at high risk for developing CAD or individuals who have specific risk factors and/or existing medical conditions (e.g., elevated LDL

cholesterol levels, other lipid disorders, insulin-dependent diabetes, insulin resistance, or metabolic syndrome). If overweight, the patient should be encouraged to achieve a normal weight. The NHLBI's National Cholesterol Education Program (NCEP) revised its dietary guidelines for reducing CAD in 2001. Guidelines for the Therapeutic Lifestyle Changes (TLC) diet are outlined in the Third Report of the Expert Panel on Detection, Evaluation, and Treatment of High Blood Cholesterol in Adults (Adult Treatment Panel III [ATP III]). The TLC diet emphasizes a reduction in foods high in saturated fats and cholesterol. Red meats, eggs, and dairy products are the major sources of saturated fats and cholesterol. If triglycerides also are elevated, the patient should be advised to eliminate or reduce alcohol and simple carbohydrates from the diet. The TLC approach also includes the use of plant stanols or sterols and increased dissolved fiber as an option for lowering LDL cholesterol levels; nutritional recommendations for daily total caloric intake; recommendations for allowable percentage of calories derived from fat (saturated and unsaturated), carbohydrates, protein, and cholesterol; as well as recommendations for daily expenditure of energy.
- **Nutritional Considerations:** Overweight patients with high blood pressure should be encouraged to achieve a normal weight. Other changeable risk factors warranting patient education include strategies to safely decrease sodium intake, increase physical activity, decrease alcohol consumption, eliminate tobacco use, and decrease cholesterol levels.
- Recognize anxiety related to test results, and be supportive of perceived loss of independent function. Discuss the implications of abnormal test results on the patient's lifestyle. Provide teaching and information regarding the clinical implications of the test results, as appropriate.
- Reinforce information given by the patient's HCP regarding further testing, treatment, or referral to another HCP. Answer any questions or address any concerns voiced by the patient or family.

P

▶ Depending on the results of this procedure, additional testing may be needed to evaluate or monitor progression of the disease process and determine the need for a change in therapy. Evaluate test results in relation to the patient's symptoms and other tests performed.

RELATED MONOGRAPHS:

▶ Related tests for cardiac indications include anion gap, antiarrhythmic drugs, apolipoprotein A and B, arterial/alveolar oxygen ratio, AST, ANP, α_1-AT, biopsy lung, blood gases, blood pool imaging, BNP, bronchoscopy, calcium, ionized calcium, carboxyhemoglobin, chest x-ray, chloride sweat, cholesterol (total, HDL, and LDL), CRP, CBC, CT cardiac scoring, CT thoracic, CK and isoenzymes, culture and smear for mycobacteria, culture bacterial sputum, culture viral, cytology sputum, echocardiography, echocardiography transesophageal, ECG, electrolytes, exercise stress test, glucose, glycated hemoglobin, gram stain, Hgb, Holter monitor, homocysteine, ketones, LDH and isoenzymes, lipoprotein electrophoresis, magnesium, MRI chest, MI infarct scan, IgE, lactic acid, lung perfusion scan, lung ventilation scan, myocardial perfusion heart scan, myoglobin, osmolality, pericardial fluid analysis, phosphorus, plethysmography, pleural fluid analysis, PET heart, PFT, potassium, pulse oximetry, TB skin test, and triglycerides. Related tests for pulmonary indications include α_1-AT, anion gap, arterial/alveolar oxygen ratio, biopsy lung, bronchoscopy, carboxyhemoglobin, chest x-ray, chloride sweat, CBC, CBC hemoglobin, CBC WBC count and differential, culture and smear for mycobacteria, culture bacterial sputum, culture viral, cytology sputum, electrolytes, gram stain, IgE, lactic acid, lung perfusion scan, lung ventilation scan, osmolality, phosphorus, plethysmography, pleural fluid analysis, and pulse oximetry.

▶ Refer to the Cardiovascular and Respiratory systems tables at the end of the book for related tests by body system.

Positron Emission Tomography, Pelvis

SYNONYM/ACRONYM: PET scan of the pelvis.

COMMON USE: To assess blood flow and metabolism to the pelvis to assist in diagnosis of disorders such as colorectal tumor, assist in tumor staging, and monitor the effectiveness of therapeutic interventions.

AREA OF APPLICATION: Pelvis.

CONTRAST: IV radioactive material (fluorodeoxyglucose [FDG]).

DESCRIPTION: Positron emission tomography (PET) combines the biochemical properties of nuclear medicine with the accuracy of computed tomography (CT). PET uses positron emissions from specific radionuclides (oxygen, nitrogen, carbon, and fluorine) to produce detailed functional images within the body. After the radionuclide becomes concentrated in the pelvis, PET images of blood flow or metabolic processes at the cellular level can be obtained. Colorectal tumor detection, tumor staging, evaluation of the effects of therapy, detection of recurrent disease, and detection of metastases are the main reasons to do a pelvic PET scan. Fluorine-18, in the form of fluorodeoxyglucose (FDG), is one of the more commonly used radionuclides. FDG is a glucose analogue, and because every cell uses glucose, the metabolic activity occurring in pelvic conditions such as colorectal cancer can be measured. There is little localization of FDG in normal tissue, allowing rapid detection of abnormal disease states.

The positron radiopharmaceuticals generally have short half-lives, ranging from a few seconds to a few hours, and therefore they must be produced in a cyclotron located near where the test is being done. The PET scanner translates the emissions from the radioactivity as the positron combines with the negative electrons from the tissues and forms gamma rays that can be detected by the scanner. This information is transmitted to the computer, which determines the location and its distribution and translates the emissions as color-coded images for viewing, quantitative measurements, activity changes in relation to time, and three-dimensional computer-aided analysis. Each radionuclide tracer is designed to measure a specific body process, such as glucose metabolism, blood flow, or tissue perfusion.

The expense of the study and the limited availability of radiopharmaceuticals limit the use of PET, even though it is more sensitive than traditional nuclear scanning and single-photon emission computed tomography. Changes in reimbursement and the advent of mobile technology have increased the availability of this procedure in the community setting.

INDICATIONS
- Determine the effects of therapy
- Determine the presence of colorectal cancer
- Determine the presence of metastases of a cancerous tumor
- Determine the recurrence of tumor or cancer
- Identify the site for biopsy

POTENTIAL DIAGNOSIS

Normal findings in
- Normal patterns of tissue metabolism, blood flow, and radionuclide distribution
- No focal uptake of radionuclide

Abnormal findings in
- Focal uptake of the radionuclide in pelvis
- Focal uptake in abnormal lymph nodes
- Focal uptake in tumor
- Focal uptake in metastases

CRITICAL FINDINGS: N/A

INTERFERING FACTORS

This procedure is contraindicated for
- Patients who are pregnant or suspected of being pregnant, unless the potential benefits of the procedure far outweigh the risks to the fetus and mother.

Factors that may impair clear imaging

- Inability of the patient to cooperate or remain still during the procedure because of age, significant pain, or mental status.
- Drugs that alter glucose metabolism, such as tranquilizers or insulin, because hypoglycemia can alter PET results.
- The use of alcohol, tobacco, or caffeine-containing drinks at least 24 hr before the study, because the effects of these substances would make it difficult to evaluate the patient's true physiological state (e.g., alcohol is a vasconstrictor and would decrease blood flow to the target organ).
- Metallic objects within the examination field (e.g., jewelry, body rings), which may inhibit organ visualization and can produce unclear images.

Other considerations

- Failure to follow dietary restrictions before the procedure may cause the procedure to be canceled or repeated.
- Improper injection of the radionuclide that allows the tracer to seep deep into the muscle tissue produces erroneous hot spots.
- False-positive findings may occur as a result of normal gastrointestinal (GI) tract uptake and uptake in areas of infection or inflammation.
- Consultation with a health-care provider (HCP) should occur before the procedure for radiation safety concerns regarding younger patients or patients who are lactating.
- Risks associated with radiation overexposure can result from frequent x-ray or radionuclide procedures. Personnel working in the examination area should wear badges to record their level of radiation exposure.

NURSING IMPLICATIONS AND PROCEDURE

PRETEST:

- Positively identify the patient using at least two unique identifiers before providing care, treatment, or services.
- *Patient Teaching:* Inform the patient this procedure can assist in assessing the pelvis related to abnormal organ function.
- Obtain a history of the patient's complaints, including a list of known allergens, especially allergies or sensitivities to latex, iodine, seafood, contrast medium, or anesthetics.
- Obtain a history of the patient's gastrointestinal system, symptoms, and results of previously performed laboratory tests and diagnostic and surgical procedures.
- Note any recent procedures that can interfere with test results, including examinations using barium- or iodine-based contrast medium.
- Record the date of the last menstrual period and determine the possibility of pregnancy in perimenopausal women.
- Obtain a list of the patient's current medications, including herbs, nutritional supplements, and nutraceuticals (see Appendix F).
- Review the procedure with the patient. Address concerns about pain related to the procedure and explain that some pain may be experienced during the test, and there may be moments of discomfort. Reassure the patient that radioactive material poses minimal radioactive hazard because of its short half-life and rarely produces side effects. Inform the patient that the procedure is performed in a special department, usually in a radiology suite, by an HCP specializing in this procedure, with support staff, and takes approximately 30 to 60 min.
- *Sensitivity to social and cultural issues,* as well as concern for modesty, is important in providing psychological support before, during, and after the procedure.
- Sometimes FDG examinations are done after blood has been drawn to determine circulating blood glucose levels. If blood glucose levels are high, insulin may be given.

P

- Instruct the patient to remove jewelry and other metallic objects in the area to be examined.
- Instruct the patient to avoid taking anticoagulant medication or to reduce dosage as ordered prior to the procedure.
- Instruct the patient to restrict food for 4 hr; restrict alcohol, nicotine, or caffeine-containing drinks for 24 hr; and withhold medications for 24 hr before the test. Protocols may vary among facilities.
- *Make sure a written and informed consent has been signed prior to the procedure and before administering any medications.*

INTRATEST:

- Ensure that the patient has complied with dietary, fluid, and medication restrictions and pretesting preparations.
- Ensure the patient has removed all jewelry and external metallic objects from the area to be examined prior to the procedure.
- Have emergency equipment readily available.
- Instruct the patient to void prior to the procedure and to change into the gown, robe, and foot coverings provided.
- Instruct the patient to cooperate fully and to follow directions. Ask the patient to remain still throughout the procedure because movement produces unreliable results.
- Observe standard precautions, and follow the general guidelines in Appendix A.
- Record baseline vital signs and assess neurological status. Protocols may vary among facilities.
- Place the patient in the supine position on an examination table.
- The radionuclide is injected, and imaging is started after a 45-min delay. Continuous scanning may be done for 1 hr. If comparative studies are indicated, additional injections of radionuclide may be needed.
- If required, the bladder may need to be lavaged via a urinary catheter with 2 L of 0.9% saline solution to remove concentrated radionuclide.
- Monitor the patient for complications related to the procedure (e.g., allergic reaction, anaphylaxis, bronchospasm).

- Remove the needle or catheter and apply a pressure dressing over the puncture site.
- Observe/assess the needle/catheter insertion site for bleeding, inflammation, or hematoma formation.

POST-TEST:

- A report of the results will be sent to the requesting HCP, who will discuss the results with the patient.
- Instruct the patient to resume pretest diet, fluids, medications, and activity.
- Observe for delayed allergic reactions, such as rash, urticaria, tachycardia, hyperpnea, hypertension, palpitations, nausea, or vomiting.
- Instruct the patient to immediately report symptoms such as fast heart rate, difficulty breathing, skin rash, itching, chest pain, persistent right shoulder pain, or abdominal pain. Immediately report symptoms to the appropriate HCP.
- Observe/assess the needle/catheter insertion site for bleeding, inflammation, or hematoma formation.
- Instruct the patient to apply cold compresses to the puncture site as needed, to reduce discomfort or edema.
- Instruct the patient to drink increased amounts of fluids for 24 to 48 hr to eliminate the radionuclide from the body, unless contraindicated. Tell the patient that radionuclide is eliminated from the body within 6 to 24 hr.
- Instruct the patient to flush the toilet immediately after each voiding and to meticulously wash hands with soap and water for 24 hr after the procedure.
- Tell all caregivers to wear gloves when discarding urine for 24 hr after the procedure. Wash gloved hands with soap and water before removing gloves. Then wash hands after the gloves are removed.
- If a woman who is breastfeeding must have a nuclear scan, she should not breastfeed the infant until the radionuclide has been eliminated, about 3 days. Instruct her to express the milk and discard it during the 3-day period to prevent cessation of milk production.

P

No other radionuclide tests should be scheduled for 24 to 48 hr after this procedure.

Recognize anxiety related to test results, and be supportive of perceived loss of independent function. Discuss the implications of abnormal test results on the patient's lifestyle. Provide teaching and information regarding the clinical implications of the test results, as appropriate.

Reinforce information given by the patient's HCP regarding further testing, treatment, or referral to another HCP. Decisions regarding the need for and frequency of occult blood testing, colonoscopy, or other cancer screening procedures should be made after consultation between the patient and HCP. The most current guidelines for colon cancer screening of the general population as well as of individuals with increased risk are available from the American Cancer Society (www.cancer.org) and the American College of Gastroenterology (www.gi.org). Answer any questions or address any concerns voiced by the patient or family.

Depending on the results of this procedure, additional testing may be needed to evaluate or monitor progression of the disease process and determine the need for a change in therapy. Evaluate test results in relation to the patient's symptoms and other tests performed.

RELATED MONOGRAPHS:

Related tests include barium enema, biopsy intestinal, capsule endoscopy, cancer antigens, CT abdomen, fecal analysis, KUB, CT colonoscopy, MRI abdomen, and proctosigmoidoscopy.

Refer to the Gastrointestinal System table at the end of the book for related tests by body system.

Potassium, Blood

SYNONYM/ACRONYM: Serum K^+.

COMMON USE: To evaluate fluid and electrolyte balance related to potassium levels to assist in diagnosing disorders such as acidosis, renal failure, dehydration, and monitor the effectiveness of therapeutic interventions.

SPECIMEN: Serum (1 mL) collected in a red- or tiger-top tube. Plasma (1 mL) collected in green-top (heparin) tube is also acceptable.

REFERENCE VALUE: (Method: Ion-selective electrode)

Serum	Conventional Units	SI Units (Conventional Units × 1)
Newborn	3.7–5.9 mEq/L	3.7–5.9 mmol/L
Infant	4.1–5.3 mEq/L	4.1–5.3 mmol/L
Child	3.4–4.7 mEq/L	3.4–4.7 mmol/L
Adult–older adult	3.5–5.0 mEq/L	3.5–5.0 mmol/L

Note: Serum values are 0.1 mmol/L higher than plasma values, and reference ranges should be adjusted accordingly. It is important that serial measurements be collected using the same type of collection container to reduce variability of results from collection to collection.

DESCRIPTION: Electrolytes dissociate into electrically charged ions when dissolved. Cations, including potassium, carry a positive charge. Body fluids contain approximately equal numbers of anions and cations, although the nature of the ions and their mobility differs between the intracellular and extracellular compartments. Both types of ions affect the electrical and osmolar functions of the body. Electrolyte quantities and the balance among them are controlled by oxygen and carbon dioxide exchange in the lungs; absorption, secretion, and excretion of many substances by the kidneys; and secretion of regulatory hormones by the endocrine glands. Potassium is the most abundant intracellular cation. It is essential for the transmission of electrical impulses in cardiac and skeletal muscle. It also functions in enzyme reactions that transform glucose into energy and amino acids into proteins. Potassium helps maintain acid-base equilibrium, and it has a significant and inverse relationship to pH: A decrease in pH of 0.1 increases the potassium level by 0.6 mEq/L.

Abnormal potassium levels can be caused by a number of contributing factors, which can be categorized as follows:

Altered renal excretion: Normally, 80% to 90% of the body's potassium is filtered out through the kidneys each day (the remainder is excreted in sweat and stool); renal disease can result in abnormally high potassium levels.

Altered dietary intake: A severe potassium deficiency can be caused by an inadequate intake of dietary potassium.

Altered cellular metabolism: Damaged red blood cells (RBCs) release potassium into the circulating fluid, resulting in increased potassium levels.

INDICATIONS
- Assess a known or suspected disorder associated with renal disease, glucose metabolism, trauma, or burns
- Assist in the evaluation of electrolyte imbalances; this test is especially indicated in elderly patients, patients receiving hyperalimentation supplements, patients on hemodialysis, and patients with hypertension
- Evaluate cardiac arrhythmia to determine whether altered potassium levels are contributing to the problem, especially during digitalis therapy, which leads to ventricular irritability
- Evaluate the effects of drug therapy, especially diuretics
- Evaluate the response to treatment for abnormal potassium levels
- Monitor known or suspected acidosis, because potassium moves from RBCs into the extracellular fluid in acidotic states
- Routine screen of electrolytes in acute and chronic illness

POTENTIAL DIAGNOSIS

Increased in
- Acidosis *(intracellular potassium ions are expelled in exchange for hydrogen ions in order to achieve electrical neutrality)*
- Acute renal failure *(potassium excretion is diminished, and it accumulates in the blood)*
- Addison's disease *(due to lack of aldosterone, potassium excretion is diminished, and it accumulates in the blood)*

- Asthma *(related to chronic inflammation and damage to lung tissue)*
- Burns *(related to tissue damage and release by damaged cells)*
- Chronic interstitial nephritis *(potassium excretion is diminished, and it accumulates in the blood)*
- Dehydration *(related to hemoconcentration)*
- Dialysis *(dialysis treatments simulate kidney function, but potassium builds up between treatments)*
- Diet *(related to excessive intake of salt substitutes or of potassium salts in medications)*
- Exercise *(related to tissue damage and release by damaged cells)*
- Hemolysis (massive) *(potassium is the major intracellular cation)*
- Hyperventilation *(in response to respiratory alkalosis, blood levels of potassium are increased in order to achieve electrical neutrality)*
- Hypoaldosteronism *(due to lack of aldosterone, potassium excretion is diminished, and it accumulates in the blood)*
- Insulin deficiency *(insulin deficiency results in movement of potassium from the cell into the extracellular fluid)*
- Ketoacidosis *(insulin deficiency results in movement of potassium from the cell into the extracellular fluid)*
- Leukocytosis
- Muscle necrosis *(related to tissue damage and release by damaged cells)*
- Near drowning
- Pregnancy
- Prolonged periods of standing
- Tissue trauma *(related to release by damaged cells)*
- Transfusion of old banked blood *(aged cells hemolyze and release intracellular potassium)*
- Tubular unresponsiveness to aldosterone
- Uremia

Decreased in
- Alcoholism *(related to insufficient dietary intake)*
- Alkalosis *(potassium uptake by cells is increased in response to release of hydrogen ions from cells)*
- Anorexia nervosa *(related to significant changes in renal function that result in hypokalemia)*
- Bradycardia *(hypokalemia can cause bradycardia)*
- Chronic, excessive licorice ingestion (from licorice root)
- Congestive heart failure *(related to fluid retention and hemodilution)*
- Crohn's disease *(insufficient intestinal absorption)*
- Cushing's syndrome *(aldosterone facilitates the excretion of potassium by the kidneys)*
- Diet deficient in meat and vegetables *(insufficient dietary intake)*
- Excess insulin *(insulin causes glucose and potassium to move into cells)*
- Familial periodic paralysis *(related to fluid retention)*
- Gastrointestinal (GI) loss due to vomiting, diarrhea, nasogastric suction, or intestinal fistula
- Hyperaldosteronism *(aldosterone facilitates the excretion of potassium by the kidneys)*
- Hypertension *(medications used to treat hypertension may result in loss of potassium; hypertension is often related to diabetes and renal disease, which affect cellular retention and renal excretion of potassium respectively)*
- Hypomagnesemia *(magnesium levels tend to parallel potassium levels)*
- IV therapy with inadequate potassium supplementation
- Laxative abuse *(related to medications that cause potassium wasting)*
- Malabsorption *(related to insufficient intestinal absorption)*

- Pica (eating substances of no nutritional value, e.g., clay)
- Renal tubular acidosis *(condition results in excessive loss of potassium)*
- Sweating *(related to increased loss)*
- Theophylline administration, excessive *(theophylline drives potassium into cells, reducing circulating levels)*
- Thyrotoxicosis *(related to changes in renal function)*

CRITICAL FINDINGS ✦

- Less than 2.5 mEq/L
- Greater than 6.5 mEq/L

Note and immediately report to the health-care provider (HCP) any critically increased or decreased values and related symptoms, especially symptoms of fluid imbalance.

Symptoms of hyperkalemia include irritability, diarrhea, cramps, oliguria, difficulty speaking, and cardiac arrhythmias (peaked T waves and ventricular fibrillation). Continuous cardiac monitoring is indicated. Administration of sodium bicarbonate or calcium chloride may be requested. If the patient is receiving an IV supplement, verify that the patient is voiding.

Symptoms of hypokalemia include malaise, thirst, polyuria, anorexia, weak pulse, low blood pressure, vomiting, decreased reflexes, and electrocardiographic changes (depressed T waves and ventricular ectopy). Replacement therapy is indicated.

INTERFERING FACTORS

- Drugs that can cause an increase in potassium levels include dexamethasone, enalapril, mannitol, methicillin, metoprolol, NSAIDs, some drugs with potassium salts, propranolol, spironolactone, and succinylcholine.
- Drugs that can cause a decrease in potassium levels include acetazolamide, acetylsalicylic acid, alanine, albuterol, aldosterone, ammonium chloride, amphotericin B, bicarbonate, bisacodyl, captopril, carbenicillin, cathartics, cisplatin, clorexolone, desoxycorticosterone, dexamethasone, digoxin, diuretics, enalapril, furosemide, hydrocortisone, hydroflumethiazide, laxatives, moxalactam (common when coadministered with amikacin), large doses of any IV penicillin, phenolphthalein (with chronic laxative abuse), phosphates, IV theophylline, thiazides, and triamterene. A number of these medications initially increase the serum potassium level, but they also have a diuretic effect, which promotes potassium loss in the urine except in cases of renal insufficiency.
- Leukocytosis, as seen in leukemia, causes elevated potassium levels.
- False elevations can occur with vigorous pumping of the hand during venipuncture. Hemolysis of the sample and high platelet counts also increase potassium levels, as follows: (1) Because potassium is an intracellular ion and concentrations are approximately 150 times extracellular concentrations, even a slight amount of hemolysis can cause a significant increase in levels. (2) Platelets release potassium during the clotting process, and therefore serum samples collected from patients with elevated platelet counts may produce spuriously high potassium levels. Plasma is the specimen of choice in patients known to have elevated platelet counts.
- False increases are seen in unprocessed samples left at room temperature because a significant amount of potassium leaks out of the cells within a few hours. Plasma or serum should be separated from cells within 4 hr of collection.
- Storage of unprocessed blood causes potassium levels to increase because a significant amount of potassium leaks out of the cells

within a few hours. Plasma or serum should be separated from cells within 4 hr of collection.

• Specimens should never be collected above an IV line because of the potential for dilution when the specimen and the IV solution combine in the collection container, falsely decreasing the result. There is also the potential of contaminating the sample with the substance of interest, if it is present in the IV solution, falsely increasing the result.

NURSING IMPLICATIONS AND PROCEDURE

PRETEST:

▶ Positively identify the patient using at least two unique identifiers before providing care, treatment, or services.

▶ *Patient Teaching:* Inform the patient this test can assist in evaluating electrolyte balance.

▶ Obtain a history of the patient's complaints, including a list of known allergens, especially allergies or sensitivities to latex. Especially note complaints of weakness and confusion.

▶ Obtain a history of the patient's cardiovascular, endocrine, gastrointestinal, genitourinary, immune, and respiratory systems; symptoms; and results of previously performed laboratory tests and diagnostic and surgical procedures.

▶ Obtain a list of the patient's current medications, including herbs, nutritional supplements, and nutraceuticals (see Appendix F).

▶ Review the procedure with the patient. Inform the patient that specimen collection takes approximately 5 to 10 min. Address concerns about pain and explain that there may be some discomfort during the venipuncture.

▶ *Sensitivity to social and cultural issues,* as well as concern for modesty, is important in providing psychological support before, during, and after the procedure.

▶ There are no food, fluid, or medication restrictions unless by medical direction.

INTRATEST:

▶ If the patient has a history of allergic reaction to latex, avoid the use of equipment containing latex.

▶ Instruct the patient to cooperate fully and to follow directions. Direct the patient to breathe normally and to avoid unnecessary movement. Instruct the patient not to clench and unclench the fist immediately before or during specimen collection.

▶ Observe standard precautions, and follow the general guidelines in Appendix A. Positively identify the patient, and label the appropriate tubes with the corresponding patient demographics, date, and time of collection. Perform a venipuncture.

▶ Remove the needle and apply direct pressure with dry gauze to stop bleeding. Observe/assess venipuncture site for bleeding or hematoma formation and secure gauze with adhesive bandage.

▶ Promptly transport the specimen to the laboratory for processing and analysis.

POST-TEST:

▶ A report of the results will be sent to the requesting HCP, who will discuss the results with the patient.

▶ *Nutritional Considerations:* In 2004, the Institute of Medicine's Food and Nutrition Board established 4.7 g/day as the recommended maximum daily intake of dietary potassium for adults and 3.8 g/day for children. Potassium is present in all plant and animal cells, making dietary replacement simple to achieve in the potassium-deficient patient.

▶ Observe the patient for signs and symptoms of fluid volume excess related to excess potassium intake (hyperkalemia), fluid volume deficit related to active loss (hypokalemia), or risk of injury related to an alteration in body chemistry. Symptoms of hypokalemia and hyperkalemia include dehydration, diarrhea, vomiting, or prolonged anorexia.

▶ Increased potassium levels may be associated with dehydration. Evaluate the patient for signs and symptoms of dehydration. Dehydration is a significant and common finding in geriatric patients and other patients in whom renal function has deteriorated.

P

▸ Decreased potassium levels may occur in patients receiving digoxin or potassium-wasting diuretics. Potassium levels should be monitored carefully because cardiac arrhythmias can occur. Instruct the patient in electrolyte replacement therapy and changes in dietary intake that affect electrolyte levels, as ordered.

▸ Reinforce information given by the patient's HCP regarding further testing, treatment, or referral to another HCP. Answer any questions or address any concerns voiced by the patient or family.

▸ Depending on the results of this procedure, additional testing may be performed to evaluate or monitor progression of the disease process and determine the need for a change in therapy. Evaluate test results in relation to the patient's symptoms and other tests performed.

RELATED MONOGRAPHS:

▸ Related tests include ACTH, aldosterone, anion gap, antiarrhythmic drugs, alveolar/arterial gradient, ANP, BNP, blood gases, BUN, calcium, carbon dioxide, chloride, complement, CBC hematocrit, CBC hemoglobin, CBC WBC count and differential, Coomb's antiglobulin (direct and indirect), cortisol, CK and isoenzymes, creatinine, DHEAS, echocardiography, echocardiography transesophageal, fecal fat, glucose, G6PD, Ham's test, haptoglobin, hemosiderin, insulin, ketones, lactic acid, lung perfusion scan, magnesium, osmolality, osmotic fragility, plethysmography, urine potassium, PFT, PK, renin, sickle cell screen, and sodium.

▸ Refer to the Cardiovascular, Endocrine, Gastrointestinal, Genitourinary, Immune, and Respiratory systems tables at the end of the book for related tests by body system.

Potassium, Urine

SYNONYM/ACRONYM: Urine K⁺.

COMMON USE: To evaluate electrolyte balance, acid-base balance, and hypokalemia.

SPECIMEN: Urine (5 mL) from an unpreserved random or timed specimen collected in a clean plastic collection container.

REFERENCE VALUE: (Method: Ion-selective electrode)

Age	Conventional Units	SI Units (Conventional Units × 1)
6–10 yr		
Male	17–54 mEq/24 hr	17–54 mmol/24 hr
Female	8–37 mEq/24 hr	8–37 mmol/24 hr
10–14 yr		
Male	22–57 mEq/24 hr	22–57 mmol/24 hr
Female	18–58 mEq/24 hr	18–58 mmol/24 hr
Adult–older adult	26–123 mEq/24 hr	26–123 mmol/24 hr

Note: Reference values depend on potassium intake and diurnal variation. Excretion is significantly higher at night.

DESCRIPTION: Electrolytes dissociate into electrically charged ions when dissolved. Cations, including potassium, carry a positive charge. Body fluids contain approximately equal numbers of anions and cations, although the nature of the ions and their mobility differs between the intracellular and extracellular compartments. Both types of ions affect the electrical and osmolar functions of the body. Electrolyte quantities and the balance among them are controlled by oxygen and carbon dioxide exchange in the lungs; absorption, secretion, and excretion of many substances by the kidneys; and secretion of regulatory hormones by the endocrine glands. Potassium is the most abundant intracellular cation. It is essential for the transmission of electrical impulses in cardiac and skeletal muscle. It also functions in enzyme reactions that transform glucose into energy and amino acids into proteins. Potassium helps maintain acid-base equilibrium, and it has a significant and inverse relationship to pH: A decrease in pH of 0.1 increases the potassium level by 0.6 mEq/L.

Abnormal potassium levels can be caused by a number of contributing factors, which can be categorized as follows:

Altered renal excretion: Normally, 80% to 90% of the body's potassium is filtered out through the kidneys each day (the remainder is excreted in sweat and stool); renal disease can result in abnormally high potassium levels.

Altered dietary intake: A severe potassium deficiency can be caused by an inadequate intake of dietary potassium.

Altered cellular metabolism: Damaged red blood cells (RBCs) release potassium into the circulating fluid, resulting in increased potassium levels.

Regulating electrolyte balance is one of the major functions of the kidneys. In normally functioning kidneys, urine potassium levels increase when serum levels are high and decrease when serum levels are low to maintain homeostasis. The kidneys respond to alkalosis by excreting potassium to retain hydrogen ions and increase acidity. In acidosis, the body excretes hydrogen ions and retains potassium. Analyzing these urinary levels can provide important clues to the functioning of the kidneys and other major organs. Urine potassium tests usually involve timed urine collections over a 12- or 24-hr period. Measurement of random specimens also may be requested.

INDICATIONS
- Determine the potential cause of renal calculi
- Evaluate known or suspected endocrine disorder
- Evaluate known or suspected renal disease
- Evaluate malabsorption disorders

POTENTIAL DIAGNOSIS

Increased in
- Albright-type renal disease *(related to excessive production of cortisol)*
- Cushing's syndrome *(excessive corticosteroids, especially aldosterone levels, will increase urinary excretion of potassium)*
- Diabetic ketoacidosis *(insulin deficiency forces potassium into the extracellular fluid; excess potassium is excreted in the urine)*

- Diuretic therapy *(related to potassium-wasting effects of the medications)*
- Hyperaldosteronism *(excessive aldosterone levels will increase urinary excretion of potassium)*
- Starvation (onset) *(cells involved in providing energy through tissue breakdown release potassium into circulation)*
- Vomiting *(elevated urine potassium is a hallmark of bulimia)*

Decreased in
- Addison's disease *(reduced aldosterone levels will diminish excretion of potassium by the kidneys)*
- Potassium deficiency (chronic)
- Renal failure with decreased urine flow

CRITICAL FINDINGS: N/A

INTERFERING FACTORS

- Drugs and substances that can cause an increase in urine potassium levels include acetazolamide, acetylsalicylic acid, ammonium chloride, bendroflumethiazide, carbenoxolone, chlorthalidone, clopamide, corticosteroids, cortisone, desoxycorticosterone, dexamethasone, diuretics, ethacrynic acid, intra-amniotic saline, mefruside, niacinamide, some oral contraceptives, thiazides, triflocin, and viomycin.
- Drugs that can cause a decrease in urine potassium levels include amiloride, anesthetic agents, felodipine, and levarterenol.
- A dietary deficiency or excess of potassium can lead to spurious results.
- Diuretic therapy with excessive loss of electrolytes into the urine may falsely elevate results.
- All urine voided for the timed collection period must be included in the collection, or else falsely decreased values may be obtained.

Compare output records with volume collected to verify that all voids were included in the collection.
- Potassium levels are subject to diurnal variation (output being highest at night), which is why 24-hr collections are recommended.

NURSING IMPLICATIONS AND PROCEDURE

PRETEST:

- Positively identify the patient using at least two unique identifiers before providing care, treatment, or services.
- *Patient Teaching:* Inform the patient this test can assist in evaluating electrolyte balance.
- Obtain a history of the patient's complaints, including a list of known allergens, especially allergies or sensitivities to latex.
- Obtain a history of the patient's endocrine, gastrointestinal, and genitourinary systems; symptoms; and results of previously performed laboratory tests and diagnostic and surgical procedures.
- Obtain a list of the patient's current medications, including herbs, nutritional supplements, and nutraceuticals (see Appendix F).
- Review the procedure with the patient. Provide a nonmetallic urinal, bedpan, or toilet-mounted collection device. Address concerns about pain and explain that there should be no discomfort during the procedure.
- *Sensitivity to social and cultural issues,* as well as concern for modesty, is important in providing psychological support before, during, and after the procedure.
- Usually a 24-hr time frame for urine collection is ordered. Inform the patient that all urine must be saved during that 24-hr period. Instruct the patient not to void directly into the laboratory collection container. Instruct the patient to avoid defecating in the collection device and to keep toilet tissue out of the collection device to prevent contamination of the specimen. Place a

P

sign in the bathroom to remind the patient to save all urine.

▶ Instruct the patient to void all urine into the collection device and then to pour the urine into the laboratory collection container. Alternatively, the specimen can be left in the collection device for a health-care staff member to add to the laboratory collection container.

▶ There are no food, fluid, or medication restrictions unless by medical direction.

▶ If the patient has a history of allergic reaction to latex, avoid the use of equipment containing latex.

▶ Instruct the patient to cooperate fully and to follow directions.

▶ Observe standard precautions, and follow the general guidelines in Appendix A. Positively identify the patient, and label the appropriate collection container with the corresponding patient demographics, date, and time of collection.

Random Specimen (Collect in Early Morning)

Clean-Catch Specimen

▶ Instruct the male patient to (1) thoroughly wash his hands, (2) cleanse the meatus, (3) void a small amount into the toilet, and (4) void directly into the specimen container.

▶ Instruct the female patient to (1) thoroughly wash her hands; (2) cleanse the labia from front to back; (3) while keeping the labia separated, void a small amount into the toilet; and (4) without interrupting the urine stream, void directly into the specimen container.

Indwelling Catheter

▶ Put on gloves. Empty drainage tube of urine. It may be necessary to clamp off the catheter for 15 to 30 min before specimen collection. Cleanse specimen port with antiseptic swab, and then aspirate 5 mL of urine with a 21- to 25-gauge needle and syringe. Transfer urine to a sterile container.

Timed Specimen

▶ Obtain a clean 3-L urine specimen container, toilet-mounted collection device, and plastic bag (for transport of the specimen container). The specimen must be refrigerated or kept on ice throughout the entire collection period. If an indwelling urinary catheter is in place, the drainage bag must be kept on ice.

▶ Begin the test between 6 and 8 a.m. if possible. Collect first voiding and discard. Record the time the specimen was discarded as the beginning of the timed collection period. The next morning, ask the patient to void at the same time the collection was started and add this last voiding to the container. Urinary output should be recorded throughout the collection time.

▶ If an indwelling catheter is in place, replace the tubing and container system at the start of the collection time. Keep the container system on ice during the collection period, or empty the urine into a larger container periodically during the collection period; monitor to ensure continued drainage, and conclude the test next morning at the same hour the collection was begun.

▶ At the conclusion of the test, compare the quantity of urine with the urinary output record for the collection; if the specimen contains less than what was recorded as output, some urine may have been discarded, invalidating the test.

▶ Include on the collection container's label the amount of urine, test start and stop times, and ingestion of any foods or medications that can affect test results.

General

▶ Promptly transport the specimen to the laboratory for processing and analysis.

▶ A report of the results will be sent to the requesting health-care provider (HCP), who will discuss the results with the patient.

▶ *Nutritional Considerations:* In 2004, the Institute of Medicine's Food and Nutrition Board established 4.7 g/day as the recommended maximum daily intake of dietary potassium for adults and 3.8 g/day for children. Potassium is present in all plant and animal cells,

P

making dietary replacement simple to achieve in the potassium-deficient patient.

▶ Observe the patient for signs and symptoms of fluid volume excess related to excess potassium intake, fluid volume deficit related to active loss, or risk of injury related to an alteration in body chemistry. Symptoms include dehydration, diarrhea, vomiting, or prolonged anorexia. Instruct the patient in electrolyte replacement therapy and changes in dietary intake that affect electrolyte levels, as ordered.

▶ Increased potassium levels may be associated with dehydration. Evaluate the patient for signs and symptoms of dehydration. Dehydration is a significant and common finding in geriatric patients and other patients in whom renal function has deteriorated.

▶ Patients receiving digoxin or diuretics should have potassium levels monitored carefully because cardiac arrhythmias can occur.

▶ Increased urine potassium levels may be associated with the formation of kidney stones. Educate the patient, if appropriate, on the importance of drinking a sufficient amount of water when kidney stones are suspected. Water consumption should include six to eight 8-oz glasses of water per day, or water consumption equivalent to half of the body's weight in fluid ounces (32 fl oz = 1 qt; 34 fl oz = 1 L).

▶ Recognize anxiety related to test results. Discuss the implications of abnormal test results on the patient's lifestyle. Provide teaching and information regarding the clinical implications of the test results, as appropriate.

▶ Reinforce information given by the patient's HCP regarding further testing, treatment, or referral to another HCP. Answer any questions or address any concerns voiced by the patient or family.

▶ Depending on the results of this procedure, additional testing may be performed to evaluate or monitor progression of the disease process and determine the need for a change in therapy. Evaluate test results in relation to the patient's symptoms and other tests performed.

RELATED MONOGRAPHS:

▶ Related tests include ACTH, aldosterone, anion gap, BUN, calcium, calculus kidney stone panel, carbon dioxide, chloride, cortisol, creatinine, DHEAS, glucose, insulin, ketones, lactic acid, magnesium, osmolality, phosphorus, potassium, renin, sodium, and UA.

▶ Refer to the Endocrine, Gastrointestinal, and Genitourinary systems tables at the end of the book for related tests by body system.

P

Prealbumin

SYNONYM/ACRONYM: Transthyretin.

COMMON USE: To assess nutritional status and evaluate liver function to assist in diagnosing disorders such as malnutrition and chronic renal failure.

SPECIMEN: Serum (1 mL) collected in a red- or tiger-top tube.

REFERENCE VALUE: (Method: Nephelometry)

Age	Conventional Units	SI Units (Conventional Units × 10)
Newborn–1 mo	7.0–39.0 mg/dL	70–390 mg/L
1–6 mo	8.3–34.0 mg/dL	83–340 mg/L
6 mo–4 yr	2.0–36.0 mg/dL	20–360 mg/L
5–6 yr	12.0–30.0 mg/dL	120–300 mg/L
7 yr–adult/older adult	12.0–42.0 mg/dL	120–420 mg/L

DESCRIPTION: Prealbumin is a protein primarily produced by the liver. It is the major transport protein for triiodothyronine and thyroxine. It is also important in the metabolism of retinol-binding protein, which is needed for transporting vitamin A (retinol). Prealbumin has a short biological half-life of 2 days. This makes it a good indicator of protein status and an excellent marker for malnutrition. Prealbumin is often measured simultaneously with transferrin and albumin.

INDICATIONS

Evaluate nutritional status

POTENTIAL DIAGNOSIS

Increased in
- Alcoholism *(related to leakage of prealbumin from damaged hepatocytes and/or poor nutrition)*
- Chronic renal failure *(related to rapid turnover of prealbumin, which reflects a perceived elevation in the presence of overall loss of other proteins that take longer to produce)*
- Patients receiving steroids *(these drugs stimulate production of prealbumin)*

Decreased in
- Acute-phase inflammatory response *(prealbumin is a negative acute-phase reactant protein; levels decrease in the presence of inflammation)*
- Diseases of the liver *(related to decreased ability of the damaged liver to synthesize protein)*
- Hepatic damage *(related to decreased ability of the damaged liver to synthesize protein)*
- Malnutrition *(synthesis is decreased due to lack of proper diet)*
- Tissue necrosis *(prealbumin is a negative acute-phase reactant protein; levels decrease in the presence of inflammation)*

CRITICAL FINDINGS: N/A

INTERFERING FACTORS
- Drugs that may increase prealbumin levels include anabolic steroids, anticonvulsants, danazol, oral contraceptives, prednisolone, prednisone, and propranolol.
- Drugs that may decrease prealbumin levels include amiodarone and diethylstilbestrol.
- Fasting 4 hr before specimen collection is highly recommended. Reference ranges are often based on fasting populations to provide some level of standardization for comparison. The presence of lipids in the blood may also interfere with the test method; fasting eliminates this potential source of error, especially if the patient has elevated lipid levels.

P

NURSING IMPLICATIONS AND PROCEDURE

PRETEST:

▶ Positively identify the patient using at least two unique identifiers before providing care, treatment, or services.

▶ *Patient Teaching:* Inform the patient this test can assist in assessing nutritional status.

▶ Obtain a history of the patient's complaints, including a list of known allergens, especially allergies or sensitivities to latex.

▶ Obtain a history of the patient's endocrine, gastrointestinal, and hepatobiliary systems; symptoms; and results of previously performed laboratory tests and diagnostic and surgical procedures.

▶ Obtain a list of the patient's current medications, including herbs, nutritional supplements, and nutraceuticals (see Appendix F).

▶ Review the procedure with the patient. Inform the patient that specimen collection takes approximately 5 to 10 min. Address concerns about pain and explain that there may be some discomfort during the venipuncture.

▶ *Sensitivity to social and cultural issues,* as well as concern for modesty, is important in providing psychological support before, during, and after the procedure.

▶ Instruct the patient to fast for 4 hr before specimen collection.

▶ There are no fluid or medication restrictions, unless by medical direction.

INTRATEST:

▶ Ensure that the patient has complied with dietary restrictions; ensure that food has been restricted for at least 4 hr prior to the procedure.

▶ If the patient has a history of allergic reaction to latex, avoid the use of equipment containing latex.

▶ Instruct the patient to cooperate fully and to follow directions. Direct the patient to breathe normally and to avoid unnecessary movement.

▶ Observe standard precautions, and follow the general guidelines in Appendix A. Positively identify the patient, and label the appropriate tubes with the corresponding patient demographics, date, and time of collection. Perform a venipuncture.

▶ Remove the needle and apply direct pressure with dry gauze to stop bleeding. Observe/assess venipuncture site for bleeding or hematoma formation and secure gauze with adhesive bandage.

▶ Promptly transport the specimen to the laboratory for processing and analysis.

POST-TEST:

▶ A report of the results will be sent to the requesting health-care provider (HCP), who will discuss the results with the patient.

▶ Instruct the patient to resume usual diet, as directed by the HCP.

▶ *Nutritional Considerations:* Nutritional therapy may be indicated for patients with decreased prealbumin levels. Educate the patient, as appropriate, that good dietary sources of complete protein (containing all eight essential amino acids) include meat, fish, eggs, and dairy products and that good sources of incomplete protein (lacking one or more of the eight essential amino acids) include grains, nuts, legumes, vegetables, and seeds.

▶ Reinforce information given by the patient's HCP regarding further testing, treatment, or referral to another HCP. Answer any questions or address any concerns voiced by the patient or family.

▶ Depending on the results of this procedure, additional testing may be performed to evaluate or monitor progression of the disease process and determine the need for a change in therapy. Evaluate test results in relation to the patient's symptoms and other tests performed.

RELATED MONOGRAPHS:

▶ Related tests include albumin, chloride, ferritin, iron/TIBC, potassium, protein, sodium, T_4, T_3, transferrin, and vitamin A.

▶ Refer to the Endocrine, Gastrointestinal, and Hepatobiliary systems tables at the end of the book for related tests by body system.

Proctosigmoidoscopy

SYNONYM/ACRONYM: Anoscopy (anal canal), proctoscopy (rectum), flexible fiberoptic sigmoidoscopy, flexible proctosigmoidoscopy, sigmoidoscopy (sigmoid colon).

COMMON USE: To visualize and assess the colon, rectum, and anus to assist in diagnosing disorders such as cancer, inflammation, prolapse, and evaluate the effectiveness of medical and surgical therapeutic interventions.

AREA OF APPLICATION: Anus, rectum, colon.

CONTRAST: Air.

DESCRIPTION: Proctosigmoidoscopy allows direct visualization of the mucosa of the anal canal (anoscopy), rectum (proctoscopy), and distal sigmoid colon (sigmoidoscopy). The procedure can be performed using a rigid or flexible fiberoptic endoscope, but the flexible instrument is generally preferred. The endoscope is a multichannel device allowing visualization of the mucosal lining of the colon, instillation of air, removal of fluid and foreign objects, obtainment of tissue biopsy specimens, and use of a laser for the destruction of tissue and control of bleeding. The endoscope is advanced approximately 60 cm into the colon. This procedure is commonly used in patients with lower abdominal and perineal pain; changes in bowel habits; rectal prolapse during defecation; or passage of blood, mucus, or pus in the stool. Proctosigmoidoscopy can also be a therapeutic procedure, allowing removal of polyps or hemorrhoids or reduction of a volvulus. Biopsy specimens of suspicious sites may be obtained during the procedure.

INDICATIONS

- Confirm the diagnosis of diverticular disease
- Confirm the diagnosis of Hirschsprung's disease and colitis in children
- Determine the cause of pain and rectal prolapse during defecation
- Determine the cause of rectal itching, pain, or burning
- Evaluate the cause of blood, pus, or mucus in the stool
- Evaluate postoperative anastomosis of the colon
- Examine the distal colon before barium enema (BE) x-ray to obtain improved visualization of the area, and after a BE when x-ray findings are inconclusive
- Reduce volvulus of the sigmoid colon
- Remove hemorrhoids by laser therapy
- Screen for and excise polyps
- Screen for colon cancer

POTENTIAL DIAGNOSIS

Normal findings in
- Normal mucosa of the anal canal, rectum, and sigmoid colon

Abnormal findings in
- Anal fissure or fistula
- Anorectal abscess

- Benign lesions
- Bleeding sites
- Bowel infection or inflammation
- Crohn's disease
- Diverticula
- Hypertrophic anal papillae
- Internal and external hemorrhoids
- Polyps
- Rectal prolapse
- Tumors
- Ulcerative colitis
- Vascular abnormalities

CRITICAL FINDINGS: N/A

INTERFERING FACTORS

This procedure is contraindicated for

- Patients with bleeding disorders, especially disorders associated with uremia and cytotoxic chemotherapy.
- Patients with cardiac conditions or arrhythmias.
- Patients with bowel perforation, acute peritonitis, ischemic bowel necrosis, toxic megacolon, diverticulitis, recent bowel surgery, advanced pregnancy, severe cardiac or pulmonary disease, recent myocardial infarction, known or suspected pulmonary embolus, large abdominal aortic or iliac aneurysm, or coagulation abnormality.

Factors that may impair clear imaging

- Inability of the patient to cooperate or remain still during the procedure because of age, significant pain, or mental status.
- Strictures or other abnormalities preventing passage of the scope.
- Barium swallow or upper gastrointestinal (GI) series within the preceding 48 hr.
- Severe lower GI bleeding or the presence of feces, barium, blood, or blood clots.

Other considerations

- Failure to follow dietary restrictions before the procedure may cause

the procedure to be canceled or repeated.
- Use of bowel preparations that include laxatives or enemas should be avoided in pregnant patients or patients with inflammatory bowel disease unless specifically directed by a health-care provider (HCP).

NURSING IMPLICATIONS AND PROCEDURE

PRETEST:

- Positively identify the patient using at least two unique identifiers before providing care, treatment, or services.
- *Patient Teaching:* Inform the patient this procedure can assist in evaluating the rectum and lower colon for disease.
- Obtain a history of the patient's complaints, including a list of known allergens, especially allergies or sensitivities to latex, iodine, seafood, contrast medium, and anesthetics.
- Obtain a history of the patient's gastrointestinal system, symptoms, and results of previously performed laboratory tests and diagnostic and surgical procedures.
- Note any recent procedures that can interfere with test results. Ensure that this procedure is performed before an upper GI study or barium swallow.
- Record the date of the last menstrual period and determine the possibility of pregnancy in perimenopausal women.
- Obtain a list of the patient's current medications, including anticoagulants, aspirin and other salicylates, herbs, nutritional supplements, and nutraceuticals (see Appendix F). Such products should be discontinued by medical direction for the appropriate number of days prior to a surgical procedure. Note time and date of last dose.
- Note intake of oral iron preparations within 1 wk before the procedure because these cause black, sticky feces that are difficult to remove with bowel preparation.
- Review the procedure with the patient. Address concerns about pain related to the procedure and explain that some pain may be experienced during

P

the test, and there may be moments of discomfort. Explain that a sedative and/or analgesia will be administered to promote relaxation and reduce discomfort prior to insertion of the anoscope. Inform the patient that the procedure is performed in a GI lab by an HCP specializing in this procedure, with support staff, and takes approximately 30 to 60 min.

▶ *Sensitivity to social and cultural issues,* as well as concern for modesty, is important in providing psychological support before, during, and after the procedure.

▶ Instruct the patient that a laxative may be needed the day before the procedure, with cleansing enemas on the morning of the procedure, depending on the institution's policy.

▶ Inform the patient that the urge to defecate may be experienced when the scope is passed. Encourage slow, deep breathing through the mouth to help alleviate the feeling.

▶ Inform the patient that flatus may be expelled during and after the procedure owing to air that is injected into the scope to improve visualization.

▶ Instruct the patient to eat a low-residue diet for 3 days prior to the procedure. Consume clear liquids only the evening before, and restrict food and fluids for 8 hr prior to the procedure. Protocols may vary among facilities.

▶ *Make sure a written and informed consent has been signed prior to the procedure and before administering any medications.*

P

INTRATEST:

▶ Ensure that the patient has complied with food, fluid, and medication restrictions and pretesting preparations.

▶ Administer two small-volume enemas 1 hr before the procedure.

▶ Have emergency equipment readily available.

▶ Instruct the patient to void prior to the procedure and change into the gown, robe, and foot coverings provided.

▶ Observe standard precautions, and follow the general guidelines in Appendix A. Wear gloves and gown throughout the procedure.

▶ Record baseline vital signs and continue to monitor throughout the procedure. Protocols may vary among facilities.

▶ Place the patient on an examination table in the left lateral decubitus position or the knee-chest position and drape with the buttocks exposed. The buttocks are placed at or extending slightly beyond the edge of the examination table or bed, preferably on a special examining table that tilts the patient into the desired position.

▶ The HCP visually inspects the perianal area and then performs a digital rectal examination with a well-lubricated, gloved finger. A fecal specimen may be obtained from the glove when the finger is removed from the rectum.

▶ A lubricated anoscope (7 cm in length) is inserted, and the anal canal is inspected (anoscopy). The anoscope is removed, and a lubricated proctoscope (27 cm in length) or flexible sigmoidoscope (35 to 60 cm in length) is inserted.

▶ The scope is manipulated gently to facilitate passage, and air may be insufflated through the scope to improve visualization. Suction and cotton swabs also are used to remove materials that hinder visualization.

▶ The patient is instructed to take deep breaths to aid in movement of the scope downward through the ascending colon to the cecum and into the terminal portion of the ileum.

▶ Examination is done as the scope is gradually withdrawn. Photographs are obtained for future reference.

▶ At the end of the procedure, the scope is completely withdrawn, and residual lubricant is cleansed from the anal area.

▶ Place fecal or tissue samples and polyps in properly labeled specimen containers, and promptly transport the specimen to the laboratory for processing and analysis.

POST-TEST:

▶ A report of the results will be sent to the requesting HCP, who will discuss the results with the patient.

▶ Monitor vital signs and neurological status every 15 min for 1 hr, then every 2 hr for 4 hr, and then as ordered by the HCP. Monitor temperature every 4 hr for

24 hr. Monitor intake and output at least every 8 hr. Compare with baseline values. Notify the HCP if temperature changes. Protocols may vary among facilities.

- Monitor for any rectal bleeding.
- Instruct the patient to resume diet, medication, and activity, as directed by the HCP.
- Instruct the patient to expect slight rectal bleeding for 2 days after removal of polyps or biopsy specimens, but heavy rectal bleeding must be immediately reported to the HCP.
- Instruct the patient that any abdominal pain, tenderness, or distention; pain on defecation; or fever must be reported to the HCP immediately.
- Inform the patient that any bloating or flatulence is the result of air insufflation.
- Encourage the patient to drink several glasses of water to help replace fluid lost during test preparation.
- Recognize anxiety related to test results, and be supportive of perceived loss of independence and fear of shortened life expectancy. Discuss the implications of abnormal test results on the patient's lifestyle. Provide teaching and information regarding the clinical implications of the test results, as appropriate. Educate the patient regarding access to counseling services.

- Reinforce information given by the patient's HCP regarding further testing, treatment, or referral to another HCP. Decisions regarding the need for and frequency of occult blood testing, colonoscopy, or other cancer screening procedures should be made after consultation between the patient and HCP. The most current guidelines for colon cancer screening of the general population as well as of individuals with increased risk are available from the American Cancer Society (www.cancer.org) and the American College of Gastroenterology (www.gi.org). Answer any questions or address any concerns voiced by the patient or family.
- Depending on the results of this procedure, additional testing may be needed to evaluate or monitor progression of the disease process and determine the need for a change in therapy. Evaluate test results in relation to the patient's symptoms and other tests performed.

RELATED MONOGRAPHS:

- Related tests include barium enema, capsule endoscopy, colonoscopy, CBC, CT abdomen, fecal analysis, fecal fat, GI blood loss scan, MRI abdomen, and US prostate transrectal.
- Refer to the Gastrointestinal System table at the end of the book for related tests by body system.

P

Progesterone

SYNONYM/ACRONYM: N/A.

COMMON USE: To assess ovarian function, assist in fertility work-ups, and monitor placental function during pregnancy related to disorders such as tumor, cysts, and threatened abortion.

SPECIMEN: Serum (1 mL) collected in a red- or tiger-top tube.

REFERENCE VALUE: (Method: Immunochemiluminometric assay [ICMA])

Hormonal State	Conventional Units	SI Units (Conventional Units × 3.18)
Prepubertal	7–52 ng/dL	0.2–1.7 nmol/L
Adult male	13–97 ng/dL	0.4–3.1 nmol/L
Adult female		
Follicular phase	15–70 ng/dL	0.5–2.2 nmol/L
Luteal phase	200–2,500 ng/dL	6.4–79.5 nmol/L
Pregnancy, first trimester	725–4,400 ng/dL	23.0–140.0 nmol/L
Pregnancy, second trimester	1,950–8,250 ng/dL	62.0–262.4 nmol/L
Pregnancy, third trimester	6,500–22,900 ng/dL	206.7–728.2 nmol/L
Postmenopausal period	Less than 40 ng/dL	Less than 127.2 nmol/L

DESCRIPTION: Progesterone is a female sex hormone. Its function is to prepare the uterus for pregnancy and the breasts for lactation. Progesterone testing can be used to confirm that ovulation has occurred and to assess the functioning of the corpus luteum. Serial measurements can be performed to help determine the day of ovulation.

INDICATIONS

- Assist in the diagnosis of luteal-phase defects (performed in conjunction with endometrial biopsy)
- Evaluate patients at risk for early or spontaneous abortion
- Identify patients at risk for ectopic pregnancy and assessment of corpus luteum function
- Monitor patients ovulating during the induction of human chorionic gonadotropin (HCG), human menopausal gonadotropin, follicle-stimulating hormone/luteinizing hormone–releasing hormone, or clomiphene (serial measurements can assist in pinpointing the day of ovulation)
- Monitor patients receiving progesterone replacement therapy

POTENTIAL DIAGNOSIS

Increased in

- Chorioepithelioma of the ovary *(related to progesterone-secreting tumor)*
- Congenital adrenal hyperplasia *(related to excessive production of progesterone precursors)*
- Hydatidiform mole *(related to progesterone-secreting tumor)*
- Lipoid ovarian tumor *(related to progesterone-secreting tumor)*
- Ovulation *(related to normal production of progesterone)*
- Pregnancy *(related to normal production of progesterone)*
- Theca lutein cyst *(related to progesterone-secreting cyst)*

Decreased in

- Galactorrhea-amenorrhea syndrome *(progesterone is not produced in the absence of ovulation)*

- Primary or secondary hypogonadism *(related to diminished production of progesterone)*
- Short luteal phase syndrome *(related to diminished time frame for production and secretion)*
- Threatened abortion, fetal demise, toxemia of pregnancy, preeclampsia, placental failure *(related to decreased production by threatened placenta)*

CRITICAL FINDINGS: N/A

INTERFERING FACTORS

- Drugs that may increase progesterone levels include clomiphene, corticotropin, hydroxyprogesterone, ketoconazole, mifepristone, progesterone, tamoxifen, and valproic acid.
- Drugs that may decrease progesterone levels include ampicillin, danazol, epostane, goserelin, and leuprolide.

NURSING IMPLICATIONS AND PROCEDURE

PRETEST:

- Positively identify the patient using at least two unique identifiers before providing care, treatment, or services.
- *Patient Teaching:* Inform the patient this test can assist in evaluating hormone level during pregnancy.
- Obtain a history of the patient's complaints, including a list of known allergens, especially allergies or sensitivities to latex.
- Obtain a history of the patient's endocrine and reproductive systems, symptoms, and results of previously performed laboratory tests and diagnostic and surgical procedures.
- Record the date of the last menstrual period and determine the possibility of pregnancy in perimenopausal women.
- Obtain a list of the patient's current medications, including herbs, nutritional supplements, and nutraceuticals (see Appendix F).
- Review the procedure with the patient. Inform the patient that specimen collection takes approximately 5 to 10 min. Address concerns about pain and explain that there may be some discomfort during the venipuncture.
- *Sensitivity to social and cultural issues,* as well as concern for modesty, is important in providing psychological support before, during, and after the procedure.
- There are no food, fluid, or medication restrictions unless by medical direction.

INTRATEST:

- If the patient has a history of allergic reaction to latex, avoid the use of equipment containing latex.
- Instruct the patient to cooperate fully and to follow directions. Direct the patient to breathe normally and to avoid unnecessary movement.
- Observe standard precautions, and follow the general guidelines in Appendix A. Positively identify the patient, and label the appropriate tubes with the corresponding patient demographics, date, and time of collection. Perform a venipuncture.
- Remove the needle and apply direct pressure with dry gauze to stop bleeding. Observe/assess venipuncture site for bleeding or hematoma formation and secure gauze with adhesive bandage.
- Promptly transport the specimen to the laboratory for processing and analysis.

POST-TEST:

- A report of the results will be sent to the requesting health-care provider (HCP), who will discuss the results with the patient.
- Recognize anxiety related to test results, and provide support. Provide teaching and information regarding the clinical implications of the test results, as appropriate. Provide a nonjudgmental, nonthreatening atmosphere for exploring other options (e.g., adoption). Educate the patient regarding access to counseling services, as appropriate.
- Reinforce information given by the patient's HCP regarding further testing, treatment, or referral to another HCP. Instruct the patient in the use of home pregnancy test kits approved by the U.S. Food and Drug Administration. Answer

P

any questions or address any concerns voiced by the patient or family.

▶ Depending on the results of this procedure, additional testing may be performed to evaluate or monitor progression of the disease process and determine the need for a change in therapy. Evaluate test results in relation to the patient's symptoms and other tests performed.

RELATED MONOGRAPHS:

▶ Related tests include ACTH, AFP, amniotic fluid analysis, antibodies cardiolipin, biopsy chorionic villus, estradiol, fetal fibronectin, FSH, HCG, LH, prolactin, testosterone, and US BPP obstetric.

▶ Refer to the Endocrine and Reproductive systems tables at the end of the book for related tests by body system.

Prolactin

SYNONYM/ACRONYM: Luteotropic hormone, lactogenic hormone, lactogen, HPRL, PRL.

COMMON USE: To assess for lactation disorders and identify the presence of prolactin-secreting tumors to assist in diagnosing disorders such as lactation failure.

SPECIMEN: Serum (1 mL) collected in a red- or tiger-top tube. Specimen should be transported tightly capped and in an ice slurry.

REFERENCE VALUE: (Method: Immunoassay)

Age	Conventional Units	SI Units (Conventional Units × 1)
Prepubertal males and females	3.2–20.0 ng/mL	3.2–20.0 mcg/L
Adult males	4.0–23.0 ng/mL	4.0–23.0 mcg/L
Adult females	4.0–30.0 ng/mL	4.0–30.0 mcg/L
Pregnant	5.3–215.3 ng/mL	5.3–215.3 mcg/L
Postmenopausal	2.4–24.0 ng/mL	2.4–24.0 mcg/L

DESCRIPTION: Prolactin is secreted by the pituitary gland. It is unique among hormones in that it responds to inhibition by the hypothalamus rather than to stimulation. The only known function of prolactin is to induce milk production in female breasts that are already stimulated by high estrogen levels. When milk production is established, lactation can continue without elevated prolactin levels. Prolactin levels rise late in pregnancy, peak with the initiation of lactation, and surge each time a woman breastfeeds. The function of prolactin in males is unknown.

INDICATIONS

- Assist in the diagnosis of primary hypothyroidism, as indicated by elevated levels
- Assist in the diagnosis of suspected tumor involving the lungs or kidneys (elevated levels indicating ectopic prolactin production)
- Evaluate failure of lactation in the postpartum period
- Evaluate sexual dysfunction of unknown cause in men and women
- Evaluate suspected postpartum hypophyseal infarction (Sheehan's syndrome), as indicated by decreased levels

POTENTIAL DIAGNOSIS

Increased in

- Adrenal insufficiency *(secondary to hypopituitarism)*
- Amenorrhea *(pathophysiology is unclear)*
- Anorexia nervosa *(pathophysiology is unclear)*
- Breastfeeding *(stimulates secretion of prolactin)*
- Chiari-Frommel and Argonz–Del Castillo syndromes *(endocrine disorders in which pituitary or hypothalamic tumors secrete excessive amounts of prolactin)*
- Chest wall injury *(trauma in this location can stimulate production of prolactin)*
- Chronic renal failure *(related to decreased renal excretion)*
- Ectopic prolactin-secreting tumors (e.g., lung, kidney)
- Galactorrhea *(production of breast milk related to prolactin-secreting tumor)*
- Hypothalamic and pituitary disorders
- Hypothyroidism (primary) *(related to pituitary gland dysfunction)*
- Pituitary tumor
- Polycystic ovary (Stein-Leventhal) syndrome
- Pregnancy

- Stress *(stimulates secretion of prolactin)*
- Surgery (pituitary stalk section)

Decreased in

- Sheehan's syndrome *(severe hemorrhage after obstetric delivery that causes pituitary infarct; secretion of all pituitary hormones is diminished)*

CRITICAL FINDINGS: N/A

INTERFERING FACTORS

- Drugs and hormones that may increase prolactin levels include amitriptyline, amoxapine, azosemide, benserazide, butaperazine, butorphanol, carbidopa, chlorophenylpiperazine, chlorpromazine, cimetidine, clomipramine, desipramine, diethylstilbestrol, enalapril, β-endorphin, enflurane, fenfluramine, fenoldopam, flunarizine, fluphenazine, fluvoxamine, furosemide, growth hormone–releasing hormone, haloperidol, hexarelin, imipramine, insulin, interferon-b, labetalol, loxapine, megestrol, mestranol, methyldopa, metoclopramide, molindone, morphine, nitrous oxide, oral contraceptives, oxcarbazepine, parathyroid hormone, pentagastrin, perphenazine, phenytoin, pimozide, prochlorperazine, promazine, ranitidine, remoxipride, reserpine, sulpiride, sultopride, thiethylperazine, thioridazine, thiothixene, thyrotropin-releasing hormone, trifluoperazine, trimipramine, tumor necrosis factor, veralipride, verapamil, and zometapine.
- Drugs and hormones that may decrease prolactin levels include anticonvulsants, apomorphine, bromocriptine, cabergoline, calcitonin, cyclosporine, dexamethasone, D-Trp-6-LHRH, levodopa, metoclopramide, morphine, nifedipine, octreotide, pergolide, ranitidine, rifampin, ritanserin, ropinirole, secretin, and tamoxifen.

- Episodic elevations can occur in response to sleep, stress, exercise, hypoglycemia, and breastfeeding.
- Venipuncture can cause falsely elevated levels.
- Prolactin secretion is subject to diurnal variation with highest levels occurring in the morning.
- Failure to follow dietary restrictions before the procedure may cause the procedure to be canceled or repeated.

NURSING IMPLICATIONS AND PROCEDURE

PRETEST:

- Positively identify the patient using at least two unique identifiers before providing care, treatment, or services.
- *Patient Teaching:* Inform the patient that test can assist in evaluating breast feeding hormone level.
- Obtain a history of the patient's complaints, including a list of known allergens, especially allergies or sensitivities to latex.
- Obtain a history of the patient's endocrine and reproductive systems, symptoms, and results of previously performed laboratory tests and diagnostic and surgical procedures.
- Obtain a list of the patient's current medications, including herbs, nutritional supplements, and nutraceuticals (see Appendix F).
- Review the procedure with the patient. Specimen collection should occur between 8 and 10 a.m. Inform the patient that specimen collection takes approximately 5 to 10 min. Address concerns about pain and explain there may be some discomfort during the venipuncture.
- *Sensitivity to social and cultural issues,* as well as concern for modesty, is important in providing psychological support before, during, and after the procedure.
- The patient should fast for 12 hr before specimen collection.
- There are no fluid or medication restrictions unless by medical direction.

- Prepare an ice slurry in a cup or plastic bag to have on hand for immediate transport of the specimen to the laboratory.

INTRATEST:

- Ensure that the patient has complied with dietary restrictions; ensure that food has been restricted for at least 12 hr prior to the procedure.
- If the patient has a history of allergic reaction to latex, avoid the use of equipment containing latex.
- Instruct the patient to cooperate fully and to follow directions. Direct the patient to breathe normally and to avoid unnecessary movement.
- Observe standard precautions, and follow the general guidelines in Appendix A. Positively identify the patient, and label the appropriate tubes with the corresponding patient demographics, date, and time of collection. Perform a venipuncture.
- Remove the needle and apply direct pressure with dry gauze to stop bleeding. Observe/assess venipuncture site for bleeding or hematoma formation and secure gauze with adhesive bandage.
- Promptly transport the specimen to the laboratory for processing and analysis. The specimen should be placed in an ice slurry immediately after collection. Information on the specimen label should be protected from water in the ice slurry by first placing the specimen in a protective plastic bag.

POST-TEST:

- A report of the results will be sent to the requesting health-care provider (HCP), who will discuss the results with the patient.
- Instruct the patient to resume usual diet, as directed by the HCP.
- Reinforce information given by the patient's HCP regarding further testing, treatment, or referral to another HCP. Answer any questions or address any concerns voiced by the patient or family.
- Depending on the results of this procedure, additional testing may be performed to evaluate or monitor progression of the disease process and determine the need for a change

in therapy. Evaluate test results in relation to the patient's symptoms and other tests performed.

RELATED MONOGRAPHS:
- Related tests include ACE, BMD, CT pituitary, DHEAS, estradiol, FSH,
GH, HCG, insulin, laparoscopy gynecologic, LH, MRI pituitary, progesterone, RAIU, TSH, and thyroxine.
- Refer to the Endocrine and Reproductive systems tables at the end of the book for related tests by body system.

Prostate-Specific Antigen

SYNONYM/ACRONYM: PSA.

COMMON USE: To assess prostate health and assist in diagnosis of disorders such as prostate cancer, inflammation, and benign tumor and to evaluate effectiveness of medical and surgical therapeutic interventions.

SPECIMEN: Serum (1 mL) collected in a red- or tiger-top tube.

REFERENCE VALUE: (Method: Immunoassay)

Gender	Conventional Units	SI Units (Conventional Units × 1)
Male	Less than 4 ng/mL	Less than 4 mcg/L
Female	Less than 0.5 ng/mL	Less than 0.5 mcg/L

DESCRIPTION: Prostate-specific antigen (PSA) is produced exclusively by the epithelial cells of the prostate, periurethral, and perirectal glands. Used in conjunction with the digital rectal examination (DRE), PSA is a useful test for identifying and monitoring cancer of the prostate. Risk of diagnosis is higher in African American men, who are 61% more likely than Caucasian men to develop prostate cancer. Family history and age at diagnosis are other strong correlating factors. PSA circulates in both free and bound (complexed) forms. A low ratio of free to complexed PSA (i.e., less than 10%) is suggestive of prostate cancer; a ratio of greater than 30% is rarely associated with prostate cancer. New technology makes it possible to combine data such as analysis of molecular biomarkers and cellular structure specific to the individual's biopsy tissue, standard tissue biopsy results, Gleason score, number of positive tumor cores, tumor stage, presurgical and postsurgical PSA levels, and postsurgical margin status with computerized mathematical programs to create a personalized report that predicts the likelihood of post-prostatectomy disease progression. Serial measurements of PSA in the blood

P

are often performed before and after surgery. PSA velocity, the rate of PSA increase over time, is being used to identify the potential aggressiveness of the cancer. Approximately 15% to 40% of patients who have had their prostate removed will encounter an increase in PSA. Patients treated for prostate cancer and who have had a PSA recurrence can still develop a metastasis for as long as 8 years after the postsurgical PSA level increased. The majority of prostate tumors develop slowly and require minimal intervention, but patients with an increase in PSA greater than 2.0 ng/mL in a year are more likely to have an aggressive form of prostate cancer with a greater risk of death. Personalized medicine provides a technology to predict the progression of prostate cancer, likelihood of recurrence, or development of related metastatic disease. PSA is also produced in females, most notably in breast tissue. There is some evidence that elevated PSA levels in breast cancer patients are associated with positive estrogen and progesterone status. *Important note:* When following patients using serial testing, the same method of measurement should be consistently used.

INDICATIONS

- Evaluate the effectiveness of treatment for prostate cancer (prostatectomy): Levels decrease if treatment is effective; rising levels are associated with recurrence and a poor prognosis
- Investigate or evaluate an enlarged prostate gland, especially if prostate cancer is suspected
- Stage prostate cancer

POTENTIAL DIAGNOSIS

Increased in

A breach in the protective barrier between the prostatic lumen and the bloodstream due to significant disease will allow measurable levels of circulating PSA.

- Benign prostatic hypertrophy
- Prostate cancer
- Prostatic infarct
- Prostatitis
- Urinary retention

Decreased in: N/A

CRITICAL FINDINGS: N/A

INTERFERING FACTORS

- Drugs that decrease PSA levels include buserelin, dutasteride, finasteride, and flutamide.
- Increases may occur if ejaculation occurs within 24 hr prior to specimen collection. Increases can occur due to prostatic needle biopsy, cystoscopy, or prostatic infarction either by undergoing catheterization or the presence of an indwelling catheter; therefore, specimens should be collected prior to or 6 wk after the procedure. There is conflicting information regarding the effect of DRE on PSA values, and some health-care providers (HCPs) may specifically request specimen collection prior to DRE.

NURSING IMPLICATIONS AND PROCEDURE

PRETEST:

- Positively identify the patient using at least two unique identifiers before providing care, treatment, or services.
- *Patient Teaching:* Inform the patient this test can assist in assessing prostate health.
- Obtain a history of the patient's complaints, including a list of known allergens, especially allergies or sensitivities to latex.

- Obtain a history of the patient's genitourinary system, symptoms, and results of previously performed laboratory tests and diagnostic and surgical procedures.
- Note any recent procedures that can interfere with test results.
- Obtain a list of the patient's current medications, including herbs, nutritional supplements, and nutraceuticals (see Appendix F).
- Review the procedure with the patient. Inform the patient that specimen collection takes approximately 5 to 10 min. Address concerns about pain and explain that there may be some discomfort during the venipuncture.
- *Sensitivity to social and cultural issues,* as well as concern for modesty, is important in providing psychological support before, during, and after the procedure.
- There are no food, fluid, or medication restrictions unless by medical direction.

INTRATEST:

- If the patient has a history of allergic reaction to latex, avoid the use of equipment containing latex.
- Instruct the patient to cooperate fully and to follow directions. Direct the patient to breathe normally and to avoid unnecessary movement.
- Observe standard precautions, and follow the general guidelines in Appendix A. Positively identify the patient, and label the appropriate tubes with the corresponding patient demographics, date, and time of collection. Perform a venipuncture.
- Remove the needle and apply direct pressure with dry gauze to stop bleeding. Observe/assess venipuncture site for bleeding or hematoma formation and secure gauze with adhesive bandage.
- Promptly transport the specimen to the laboratory for processing and analysis.

POST-TEST:

- A report of the results will be sent to the requesting HCP, who will discuss the results with the patient.
- *Nutritional Considerations:* There is growing evidence that inflammation and oxidation play key roles in the development of numerous diseases, including prostate cancer. Research also indicates that diets containing dried beans, fresh fruits and vegetables, nuts, spices, whole grains, and smaller amounts of red meats can increase the amount of protective antioxidants. Regular exercise, especially in combination with a healthy diet, can bring about changes in the body's metabolism that decrease inflammation and oxidation.
- Recognize anxiety related to test results, and offer support. Counsel the patient, as appropriate, that sexual dysfunction related to altered body function, drugs, or radiation may occur. Discuss the implications of abnormal test results on the patient's lifestyle. Provide teaching and information regarding the clinical implications of the test results, as appropriate. Educate the patient regarding access to counseling services. Provide contact information, if desired, for the Prostate Cancer Foundation (www.prostatecancerfoundation.org).
- Reinforce information given by the patient's HCP regarding further testing, treatment, or referral to another HCP. Answer any questions or address any concerns voiced by the patient or family. Decisions regarding the need for and frequency of routine PSA testing or other cancer screening procedures should be made after consultation between the patient and HCP. The most current guidelines for prostate cancer screening of the general population as well as of individuals with increased risk are available from the American Cancer Society (www.cancer.org) and the American Urological Association (www.aua.org).
- Depending on the results of this procedure, additional testing may be performed to evaluate or monitor progression of the disease process and determine the need for a change in therapy. Evaluate test results in relation to the patient's symptoms and other tests performed.

RELATED MONOGRAPHS:

- Related tests include biopsy prostate (including Gleason score), cystoscopy, cystourethrography voiding, PAP, retrograde ureteropyelography, semen analysis, and US prostate.
- Refer to the Genitourinary System table at the end of the book for related tests by body system.

P

Protein, Blood, Total and Fractions

SYNONYM/ACRONYM: TP, SPEP (fractions include albumin, α_1-globulin, α_2-globulin, β-globulin, and γ-globulin).

COMMON USE: To assess nutritional status related to various disease and conditions such as dehydration, burns, and malabsorption.

SPECIMEN: Serum (1 mL) collected in a red- or tiger-top tube.

REFERENCE VALUE: (Method: Spectrophotometry for total protein, electrophoresis for protein fractions)

Total Protein

Age	Conventional Units	SI Units (Conventional units × 10)
Newborn–5 days	3.8–6.2 g/dL	38–62 g/L
1–3 yr	5.9–7.0 g/dL	59–70 g/L
4–6 yr	5.9–7.8 g/dL	59–78 g/L
7–9 yr	6.2–8.1 g/dL	62–81 g/L
10–19 yr	6.3–8.6 g/dL	63–86 g/L
Adult	6.0–8.0 g/dL	60–80 g/L

Values may be slightly decreased in older adults due to insufficient intake or the effects of medications and the presence of multiple chronic or acute diseases with or without muted symptoms.

Protein Fractions

	Conventional Units	SI Units (Conventional Units × 10)
Albumin	3.4–4.8 g/dL	34–48 g/L
α_1-Globulin	0.2–0.4 g/dL	2–4 g/L
α_2-Globulin	0.4–0.8 g/dL	4–8 g/L
β-Globulin	0.5–1.0 g/dL	5–10 g/L
γ-Globulin	0.6–1.2 g/dL	6–12 g/L

Values may be slightly decreased in older adults due to insufficient intake or the effects of medications and the presence of multiple chronic or acute diseases with or without muted symptoms.

DESCRIPTION: Protein is essential to all physiological functions. Proteins consist of amino acids, the building blocks of blood and body tissues. Protein is also required for the regulation of metabolic processes, immunity, and proper water balance. Total protein includes albumin and globulins. Albumin, the protein present in the highest concentrations, is the main transport protein in the body. Albumin also significantly affects plasma oncotic pressure, which regulates the distribution of body fluid between blood vessels, tissues, and cells. α_1-Globulin includes α_1-antitrypsin, α_1-fetoprotein, α_1-acid glycoprotein, α_1-antichymotrypsin, inter-α_1-trypsin inhibitor, high-density lipoproteins, and group-specific component (vitamin D–binding protein). α_2-Globulin includes haptoglobin, ceruloplasmin, and α_2-macroglobulin. β-Globulin includes transferrin, hemopexin, very-low-density lipoproteins, low-density lipoproteins, β_2-microglobulin, fibrinogen, complement, and C-reactive protein. γ-Globulin includes immunoglobulin (Ig) G, IgA, IgM, IgD, and IgE. After an acute infection or trauma, levels of many of the liver-derived proteins increase, whereas albumin level decreases; these conditions may not reflect an abnormal total protein determination.

INDICATIONS

- Evaluation of edema, as seen in patients with low total protein and low albumin levels
- Evaluation of nutritional status

POTENTIAL DIAGNOSIS

Increased in

- α_1-Globulin proteins in acute and chronic inflammatory diseases
- α_2-Globulin proteins occasionally in diabetes, pancreatitis, and hemolysis
- β-Globulin proteins in hyperlipoproteinemias and monoclonal gammopathies
- γ-Globulin proteins in chronic liver diseases, chronic infections, autoimmune disorders, hepatitis, cirrhosis, and lymphoproliferative disorders

- Total protein:
  Dehydration *(related to hemoconcentration)*
  Monoclonal and polyclonal gammopathies *(related to excessive γ-globulin protein synthesis)*
  Myeloma *(related to excessive γ-globulin protein synthesis)*
  Sarcoidosis *(related to excessive γ-globulin protein synthesis)*
  Some types of chronic liver disease
  Tropical diseases (e.g., leprosy) *(related to inflammatory reaction)*
  Waldenström's macroglobulinemia *(related to excessive γ-globulin protein synthesis)*

Decreased in

- α_1-Globulin proteins in hereditary deficiency
- α_2-Globulin proteins in nephrotic syndrome, malignancies, numerous subacute and chronic inflammatory disorders, and recovery stage of severe burns
- β-Globulin proteins in hypo-β-lipoproteinemias and IgA deficiency
- γ-Globulin proteins in immune deficiency or suppression
- Total protein:
  Administration of IV fluids *(related to hemodilution)*
  Burns *(related to fluid retention, loss of albumin from chronic open burns)*
  Chronic alcoholism *(related to insufficient dietary intake; diminished protein synthesis by damaged liver)*
  Chronic ulcerative colitis *(related to poor intestinal absorption)*
  Cirrhosis *(related to damaged liver, which cannot synthesize adequate amount of protein)*
  Crohn's disease *(related to poor intestinal absorption)*
  Glomerulonephritis *(related to alteration in permeability that results in excessive loss by kidneys)*
  Heart failure *(related to fluid retention)*
  Hyperthyroidism *(possibly related to increased metabolism and corresponding protein synthesis)*
  Malabsorption *(related to insufficient intestinal absorption)*

P

Malnutrition *(related to insufficient intake)*

Neoplasms

Nephrotic syndrome *(related to alteration in permeability that results in excessive loss by kidneys)*

Pregnancy *(related to fluid retention, dietary insufficiency, increased demands of growing fetus)*

Prolonged immobilization *(related to fluid retention)*

Protein-losing enteropathies *(related to excessive loss)*

Severe skin disease

Starvation *(related to insufficient intake)*

CRITICAL FINDINGS: N/A

INTERFERING FACTORS

• Drugs that may increase protein levels include amino acids (if given IV), anabolic steroids, angiotensin, anticonvulsants, corticosteroids, corticotropin, furosemide, insulin, isotretinoin, levonorgestrel, oral contraceptives, progesterone, radiographic agents, and thyroid agents.

• Drugs and substances that may decrease protein levels include acetylsalicylic acid, arginine, benzene, carvedilol, citrates, floxuridine, laxatives, mercury compounds, oral contraceptives, pentastarch, phosgene, pyrazinamide, rifampin, trimethadione, and valproic acid.

• Values are significantly lower (5% to 10%) in recumbent patients.

• Hemolysis can falsely elevate results.

• Venous stasis can falsely elevate results; the tourniquet should not be left on the arm for longer than 60 sec.

NURSING IMPLICATIONS AND PROCEDURE

PRETEST:

▶ Positively identify the patient using at least two unique identifiers before providing care, treatment, or services.

▶ *Patient Teaching:* Inform the patient this test can assist in assessing nutritional status related to disease process.

▶ Obtain a history of the patient's complaints, including a list of known allergens especially allergies or sensitivities to latex.

▶ Obtain a history of the patient's gastrointestinal, hepatobiliary, and immune systems; symptoms; and results of previously performed laboratory tests and diagnostic and surgical procedures.

▶ Obtain a list of the patient's current medications, including herbs, nutritional supplements, and nutraceuticals (see Appendix F).

▶ Review the procedure with the patient. Inform the patient that specimen collection takes approximately 5 to 10 min. Address concerns about pain and explain that there may be some discomfort during the venipuncture.

▶ *Sensitivity to social and cultural issues,* as well as concern for modesty, is important in providing psychological support before, during, and after the procedure.

▶ There are no food, fluid, or medication restrictions unless by medical direction.

INTRATEST:

▶ If the patient has a history of allergic reaction to latex, avoid the use of equipment containing latex.

▶ Instruct the patient to cooperate fully and to follow directions. Direct the patient to breathe normally and to avoid unnecessary movement.

▶ Observe standard precautions, and follow the general guidelines in Appendix A. Positively identify the patient, and label the appropriate tubes with the corresponding patient demographics, date, and time of collection. Perform a venipuncture.

▶ Remove the needle and apply direct pressure with dry gauze to stop bleeding. Observe venipuncture site for bleeding or hematoma formation and secure gauze with adhesive bandage.

▶ Promptly transport the specimen to the laboratory for processing and analysis.

POST-TEST:

▶ A report of the results will be sent to the requesting health-care provider (HCP), who will discuss the results with the patient.

Nutritional Considerations: Educate the patient, as appropriate, that good dietary sources of complete protein (containing all eight essential amino acids) include meat, fish, eggs, and dairy products and that good sources of incomplete protein (lacking one or more of the eight essential amino acids) include grains, nuts, legumes, vegetables, and seeds.

Reinforce information given by the patient's HCP regarding further testing, treatment, or referral to another HCP. Answer any questions or address any concerns voiced by the patient or family.

Depending on the results of this procedure, additional testing may be performed to evaluate or monitor progression of the disease process and determine the need for a change in therapy.

Evaluate test results in relation to the patient's symptoms and other tests performed.

RELATED MONOGRAPHS:

Related tests include albumin, ALP, ACE, anion gap, AST, biopsy liver, biopsy lung, calcium, carbon dioxide, chloride, CBC WBC count and differential, cryoglobulin, fecal analysis, fecal fat, gallium scan, GGT, IgA, IgG, IgM, IFE, liver and spleen scan, magnesium, mediastinoscopy, β_2-microglobulin, osmolality, protein urine total and fractions, PFT, radiography bone, RF, sodium, TSH, thyroxine, and UA.

Refer to the Gastrointestinal, Hepatobiliary, and Immune systems tables at the end of the book for related tests by body system.

Protein C

SYNONYM/ACRONYM: Protein C antigen, protein C functional.

COMMON USE: To assess coagulation function and assist in diagnosis of disorders such as thrombosis and protein C deficiency.

SPECIMEN: Plasma (1 mL) collected in a completely filled blue-top (3.2% sodium citrate) tube. If the patient's hematocrit exceeds 55%, the volume of citrate in the collection tube must be adjusted.

REFERENCE VALUE: (Method: Chromogenic) 70% to 140% activity. Values are significantly reduced in children because of liver immaturity. Levels rise to approximately 50% of adult levels by age 5 yr and reach adult levels by age 16 yr.

DESCRIPTION: Protein C is a vitamin K–dependent protein that originates in the liver and circulates in plasma. Protein C activation occurs on thrombomodulin receptors on the endothelial cell surface. Thrombin bound to thrombomodulin receptors preferentially activates protein C. Freely circulating thrombin mainly converts fibrinogen to fibrin. Other steps in the activation process require calcium and protein S cofactor binding (see monographs titled "Protein S" and "Fibrinogen"). Activated protein C exhibits potent anticoagulant effects by degrading activated factors V and VIII. Factor V Leiden is a genetic variant of factor V and is resistant to inactivation by protein C. Factor V Leiden is the most common inherited hypercoagulability disorder identified among individuals of Eurasian descent. There are two types of protein C deficiency:

Type I: Decreased antigen and function, detected by functional and antigenic assays

Type II: Normal antigen but decreased function, detected only by a functional assay

Functional assays are recommended for initial evaluation because of their greater sensitivity.

INDICATIONS
- Differentiate inherited deficiency from acquired deficiency
- Investigate the mechanism of idiopathic venous thrombosis

POTENTIAL DIAGNOSIS

Increased in: N/A

Decreased in
- Congenital deficiency
- Disseminated intravascular coagulation (DIC) *(related to increased consumption)*
- Liver disease *(related to decreased synthesis by the liver)*
- Oral anticoagulant therapy *(patients deficient in protein C may be at risk of developing Coumadin-induced skin necrosis unless an immediate-acting anticoagulant like heparin is administered until therapeutic Coumadin levels are achieved)*
- Vitamin K deficiency *(related to production of dysfunctional protein in the absence of vitamin K)*

CRITICAL FINDINGS: N/A

INTERFERING FACTORS
- Drugs that may increase protein C levels include desmopressin and oral contraceptives.
- Drugs that may decrease protein C levels include coumarin and warfarin (Coumadin).
- Placement of tourniquet for longer than 60 sec can result in venous stasis and changes in the concentration of plasma proteins to be measured. Platelet activation may also occur under these conditions, causing erroneous results.
- Vascular injury during phlebotomy can activate platelets and coagulation factors, causing erroneous results.
- Hemolyzed specimens must be rejected because hemolysis is an indication of platelet and coagulation factor activation.
- Icteric or lipemic specimens interfere with optical testing methods, producing erroneous results.
- Hematocrit greater than 55% may cause falsely prolonged results because of anticoagulant excess relative to plasma volume.
- Incompletely filled collection tubes, specimens contaminated with heparin, clotted specimens, or unprocessed specimens not delivered to the laboratory within 1 to 2 hr of collection should be rejected.

NURSING IMPLICATIONS AND PROCEDURE

PRETEST:
- Positively identify the patient using at least two unique identifiers before providing care, treatment, or services.
- *Patient Teaching:* Inform the patient this test can assist in assessing anticoagulant function.
- Obtain a history of the patient's complaints, including a list of known allergens, especially allergies or sensitivities to latex.
- Obtain a history of the patient's hematopoietic and hepatobiliary systems, symptoms, and results of previously performed laboratory tests and diagnostic and surgical procedures.
- Obtain a list of the patient's current medications, including herbs, nutritional

supplements, and nutraceuticals (see Appendix F).

▶ Review the procedure with the patient. Inform the patient that specimen collection takes approximately 5 to 10 min. Address concerns about pain and explain that there may be some discomfort during the venipuncture.

▶ *Sensitivity to social and cultural issues,* as well as concern for modesty, is important in providing psychological support before, during, and after the procedure.

▶ There are no food, fluid, or medication restrictions unless by medical direction.

INTRATEST:

▶ If the patient has a history of allergic reaction to latex, avoid the use of equipment containing latex.

▶ Instruct the patient to cooperate fully and to follow directions. Direct the patient to breathe normally and to avoid unnecessary movement.

▶ Observe standard precautions, and follow the general guidelines in Appendix A. Positively identify the patient, and label the appropriate tubes with the corresponding patient demographics, date, and time of collection. Perform a venipuncture. Fill tube completely. *Important note:* Two different concentrations of sodium citrate preservative are currently added to blue-top tubes for coagulation studies: 3.2% and 3.8%. The Clinical and Laboratory Standards Institute (CLSI; formerly the National Committee for Clinical Laboratory Standards [NCCLS]) guideline for sodium citrate is 3.2%. Laboratories establish reference ranges for coagulation testing based on numerous factors, including sodium citrate concentration, test equipment, and test reagents. It is important to ask the laboratory which concentration it recommends, because each concentration will have its own specific reference range. When multiple specimens are drawn, the blue-top tube should be collected after sterile (i.e., blood culture) tubes. Otherwise, when using a standard vacutainer system, the blue-top tube is the first tube collected. When a butterfly is used and due to the added tubing, an extra red-top tube should be collected before the blue-top tube to ensure complete filling of the blue-top tube.

▶ Remove the needle and apply direct pressure with dry gauze to stop bleeding. Observe/assess venipuncture site for bleeding or hematoma formation and secure gauze with adhesive bandage.

▶ Promptly transport the specimen to the laboratory for processing and analysis. The CLSI recommendation for processed and unprocessed samples stored in unopened tubes is that testing should be completed within 1 to 4 hr of collection. If the patient has a known hematocrit above 55%, adjust the amount of anticoagulant in the collection tube before drawing the blood according to the CLSI guidelines:

Anticoagulant vol. [x] = (100 − hematocrit)/(595 − hematocrit) × total vol. of anticoagulated blood required

Example:

Patient hematocrit = 60%
= [(100 − 60)/(595 − 60) × 5.0] = 0.37 mL sodium citrate for a 5-mL standard drawing tube

POST-TEST:

▶ A report of the results will be sent to the requesting health-care provider (HCP), who will discuss the results with the patient.

▶ Reinforce information given by the patient's HCP regarding further testing, treatment, or referral to another HCP. Answer any questions or address any concerns voiced by the patient or family.

▶ Depending on the results of this procedure, additional testing may be performed to evaluate or monitor progression of the disease process and determine the need for a change in therapy. Evaluate test results in relation to the patient's symptoms and other tests performed.

RELATED MONOGRAPHS:

▶ Related tests include antibody anticardiolipin, antithrombin III, calcium, CBC, coagulation factors (factor V), FDP, fibrinogen, lupus anticoagulant, aPTT, protein S, PT/INR, and vitamin K.

▶ Refer to the Hematopoietic and Hepatobiliary systems tables at the end of the book for related tests by body system.

Protein S

SYNONYM/ACRONYM: Protein S antigen, protein S functional.

COMMON USE: To assess coagulation function, assist in the diagnosis of disorders such as disseminated intravascular coagulation (DIC), and evaluate oral anticoagulation therapy.

SPECIMEN: Plasma (1 mL) collected in a completely filled blue-top (3.2% sodium citrate) tube. If the patient's hematocrit exceeds 55%, the volume of citrate in the collection tube must be adjusted.

REFERENCE VALUE: (Method: Clot detection)

	Conventional Units
Adult	70%–140% activity
Pediatric	12%–60% activity

Note: The low end of "normal" is lower in children younger than age 16 because of the immaturity of the liver.

DESCRIPTION: Protein S is a vitamin K–dependent protein that originates in the liver and circulates in plasma. It is a cofactor required for the activation of protein C (see monographs titled "Protein C" and "Fibrinogen"). Protein S exists in two forms: free (biologically active) and bound. Approximately 40% of protein S circulates in the free form; the remainder is bound and is functionally inactive. There are two types of protein S deficiency:

Type I: Decreased antigen and function, detected by functional and antigenic assays
Type II: Normal antigen but decreased function, detected only by a functional assay

Functional assays are recommended for initial evaluation because of their greater sensitivity.

INDICATIONS
Investigate the cause of hypercoagulable states.

POTENTIAL DIAGNOSIS

Increased in: N/A

Decreased in
- Acute phase reactions *(related to increased levels of C4b-binding protein in response to inflammation, which decrease levels of available functional protein)*
- Congenital deficiency
- Disseminated intravascular coagulation (DIC) *(related to increased consumption)*
- Estrogen (replacement therapy, oral contraceptives, and pregnancy) *(elevated estrogen levels are associated with decreased protein levels; estrogen does not stimulate hypercoagulable states)*
- Liver disease *(related to decreased synthesis by the liver)*
- Oral anticoagulant therapy
- Vitamin K deficiency *(related to production of dysfunctional protein in the absence of vitamin K)*

CRITICAL FINDINGS: N/A

INTERFERING FACTORS

- Drugs that may decrease protein S levels include coumarin, estrogen, and warfarin (Coumadin).
- Placement of tourniquet for longer than 60 sec can result in venous stasis and changes in the concentration of plasma proteins to be measured. Platelet activation may also occur under these conditions, causing erroneous results.
- Vascular injury during phlebotomy can activate platelets and coagulation factors, causing erroneous results.
- Hemolyzed specimens must be rejected because hemolysis is an indication of platelet and coagulation factor activation.
- Icteric or lipemic specimens interfere with optical testing methods, producing erroneous results.
- Hematocrit greater than 55% may cause falsely prolonged results because of anticoagulant excess relative to plasma volume.
- Incompletely filled collection tubes, specimens contaminated with heparin, clotted specimens, or unprocessed specimens not delivered to the laboratory within 1 to 2 hr of collection should be rejected.

NURSING IMPLICATIONS AND PROCEDURE

PRETEST:

- Positively identify the patient using at least two unique identifiers before providing care, treatment, or services.
- *Patient Teaching:* Inform the patient this test can assist in assessing anticoagulant function.
- Obtain a history of the patient's complaints, including a list of known allergens, especially allergies or sensitivities to latex.
- Obtain a history of the patient's hematopoietic and hepatobiliary systems, symptoms, and results of previously performed laboratory tests and diagnostic and surgical procedures.

- Obtain a list of the patient's current medications, including herbs, nutritional supplements, and nutraceuticals (see Appendix F).
- Review the procedure with the patient. Inform the patient that specimen collection takes approximately 5 to 10 min. Address concerns about pain and explain that there may be some discomfort during the venipuncture.
- *Sensitivity to social and cultural issues,* as well as concern for modesty, is important in providing psychological support before, during, and after the procedure.
- There are no food, fluid, or medication restrictions unless by medical direction.

INTRATEST:

- If the patient has a history of allergic reaction to latex, avoid the use of equipment containing latex.
- Instruct the patient to cooperate fully and to follow directions. Direct the patient to breathe normally and to avoid unnecessary movement.
- Observe standard precautions, and follow the general guidelines in Appendix A. Positively identify the patient, and label the appropriate tubes with the corresponding patient demographics, date, and time of collection. Perform a venipuncture. Fill tube completely. *Important note:* Two different concentrations of sodium citrate preservative are currently added to blue-top tubes for coagulation studies: 3.2% and 3.8%. The Clinical and Laboratory Standards Institute (CLSI; formerly the National Committee for Clinical Laboratory Standards [NCCLS]) guideline for sodium citrate is 3.2%. Laboratories establish reference ranges for coagulation testing based on numerous factors, including sodium citrate concentration, test equipment, and test reagents. It is important to ask the laboratory which concentration it recommends, because each concentration will have its own specific reference range. When multiple specimens are drawn, the blue-top tube should be collected after sterile (i.e., blood culture) tubes. Otherwise, when using a standard vacutainer system, the blue-top tube is the first tube collected.

P

When a butterfly is used and due to the added tubing, an extra red-top tube should be collected before the blue-top tube to ensure complete filling of the blue-top tube.

▸ Remove the needle and apply direct pressure with dry gauze to stop bleeding. Observe/assess venipuncture site for bleeding or hematoma formation and secure gauze with adhesive bandage.

▸ Promptly transport the specimen to the laboratory for processing and analysis. The CLSI recommendation for processed and unprocessed samples stored in unopened tubes is that testing should be completed within 1 to 4 hr of collection. If the patient has a known hematocrit above 55%, adjust the amount of anticoagulant in the collection tube before drawing the blood according to the CLSI guidelines:

Anticoagulant vol. [x] = (100 − hematocrit)/(595 − hematocrit) × total vol. of anticoagulated blood required

Example:

Patient hematocrit = 60% = [(100 − 60)/(595 − 60) × 5.0] = 0.37 mL sodium citrate for a 5-mL standard drawing tube

POST-TEST:

▸ A report of the results will be sent to the requesting health-care provider (HCP), who will discuss the results with the patient.

▸ Reinforce information given by the patient's HCP regarding further testing, treatment, or referral to another HCP. Answer any questions or address any concerns voiced by the patient or family.

▸ Depending on the results of this procedure, additional testing may be performed to evaluate or monitor progression of the disease process and determine the need for a change in therapy. Evaluate test results in relation to the patient's symptoms and other tests performed.

RELATED MONOGRAPHS:

▸ Related tests include, anticardiolipin antibody, AT-III, calcium, CBC, coagulation factors (factor V), FDP, fibrinogen, lupus anticoagulant, aPTT, protein C, PT/INR, and vitamin K.

▸ Refer to the Hematopoietic and Hepatobiliary systems tables at the end of the book for related test by body system.

Protein, Urine: Total Quantitative and Fractions

P

SYNONYM/ACRONYM: None.

COMMON USE: To assess for the presence of protein in the urine to assist in diagnosing disorders affecting the kidneys and urinary tract, such as cancer, infection, and preeclampsia.

SPECIMEN: Urine (5 mL) from an unpreserved random or timed specimen collected in a clean plastic collection container.

REFERENCE VALUE: (Method: Spectrophotometry for total protein, electrophoresis for protein fractions)

	Conventional Units	SI Units (Conventional Units × 0.001)
Total protein	30–150 mg/24 hr	0.03–0.15 g/24 hr

Electrophoresis for fractionation is qualitative: No monoclonal gammopathy detected. (Urine protein electrophoresis should be ordered along with serum protein electrophoresis.)

DESCRIPTION: Most proteins, with the exception of the immuno-globulins, are synthesized and catabolized in the liver, where they are broken down into amino acids. The amino acids are converted to ammonia and ketoacids. Ammonia is converted to urea via the urea cycle. Urea is excreted in the urine.

INDICATIONS

- Assist in the detection of Bence Jones proteins (light chains)
- Assist in the diagnosis of myeloma, Waldenström's macroglobulinemia, lymphoma, and amyloidosis
- Evaluate kidney function

POTENTIAL DIAGNOSIS

Increased in

- Diabetic nephropathy *(related to disease involving renal glomeruli, which increases permeability of protein)*
- Fanconi's syndrome *(related to abnormal protein deposits in the kidney, which can cause Fanconi's syndrome)*
- Heavy metal poisoning *(related to disease involving renal glomeruli, which increases permeability of protein)*
- Malignancies of the urinary tract *(tumors secrete protein into the urine)*
- Monoclonal gammopathies *(evidenced by large amounts of Bence Jones protein light chains excreted in the urine)*
- Multiple myeloma *(evidenced by large amounts of Bence Jones*

protein light chains excreted in the urine)
- Nephrotic syndrome *(related to disease involving renal glomeruli, which increases permeability of protein)*
- Postexercise period *(related to muscle exertion)*
- Preeclampsia *(numerous factors contribute to increased permeability of the kidneys to protein)*
- Sickle cell disease *(related to increased destruction of red blood cells and excretion of hemoglobin protein)*
- Urinary tract infections *(related to disease involving renal glomeruli, which increases permeability of protein)*

Decreased in: N/A

CRITICAL FINDINGS: N/A

INTERFERING FACTORS

- Drugs and substances that may increase urine protein levels include acetaminophen, aminosalicylic acid, amphotericin B, ampicillin, antimony compounds, antipyrine, arsenicals, ascorbic acid, bacitracin, bismuth subsalicylate, bromate, capreomycin, captopril, carbamazepine, carbarsone, carbenoxolone, carbutamide, cephaloglycin, cephaloridine, chlorpromazine, chlorpropamide, chlorthalidone, chrysarobin, colistimethate, colistin, corticosteroids, cyclosporine, demeclocycline, 1,2-diaminopropane, diatrizoic acid, dihydrotachysterol, doxycycline, enalapril, gentamicin, gold, hydrogen sulfide, iodoalphionic acid, iodopyracet, iopanoic acid, iophenoxic acid,

P

ipodate, kanamycin, corn oil (Lipomul), lithium, mefenamic acid, melarsonyl, melarsoprol, mercury compounds, methicillin, methylbromide, mezlocillin, mitomycin, nafcillin, naphthalene, neomycin, NSAIDs, oxacillin, paraldehyde, penicillamine, penicillin, phenolphthalein, phenols, phensuximide, phosphorus, picric acid, piperacillin, plicamycin, polymyxin, probenecid, promazine, pyrazolones, quaternary ammonium compounds, radiographic agents, rifampin, sodium bicarbonate, streptokinase, sulfisoxazole, suramin, tetracyclines, thallium, thiosemicarbazones, tolbutamide, tolmetin, triethylenemelamine, and vitamin D.

- Drugs that may decrease urine protein levels include benazepril, captopril, cyclosporine, diltiazem, enalapril, fosinopril, interferon, lisinopril, losartan, lovastatin, prednisolone, prednisone, and quinapril.

- All urine voided for the timed collection period must be included in the collection, or else falsely decreased values may be obtained. Compare output records with volume collected to verify that all voids were included in the collection.

NURSING IMPLICATIONS AND PROCEDURE

PRETEST:

- Positively identify the patient using at least two unique identifiers before providing care, treatment, or services.
- *Patient Teaching:* Inform the patient this test can assist in assessing the cause of protein in the urine.
- Obtain a history of the patient's complaints, including a list of known allergens, especially allergies or sensitivities to latex.
- Obtain a history of the patient's genitourinary and immune systems, symptoms, and results of previously performed laboratory tests and diagnostic and surgical procedures.

- Obtain a list of the patient's current medications, including herbs, nutritional supplements, and nutraceuticals (see Appendix F).
- Review the procedure with the patient. Provide a nonmetallic urinal, bedpan, or toilet-mounted collection device. Address concerns about pain and explain that there should be no discomfort during the procedure.
- Usually a 24-hr time frame for urine collection is ordered. Inform the patient that all urine must be saved during that 24-hr period. Instruct the patient not to void directly into the laboratory collection container. Instruct the patient to avoid defecating in the collection device and to keep toilet tissue out of the collection device to prevent contamination of the specimen. Place a sign in the bathroom to remind the patient to save all urine.
- Instruct the patient to void all urine into the collection device and then to pour the urine into the laboratory collection container. Alternatively, the specimen can be left in the collection device for a health-care staff member to add to the laboratory collection container.
- *Sensitivity to social and cultural issues,* as well as concern for modesty, is important in providing psychological support before, during, and after the procedure.
- There are no food, fluid, or medication restrictions unless by medical direction.

INTRATEST:

- If the patient has a history of allergic reaction to latex, avoid the use of equipment containing latex.
- Instruct the patient to cooperate fully and to follow directions.
- Observe standard precautions, and follow the general guidelines in Appendix A. Positively identify the patient, and label the appropriate collection container with the corresponding patient demographics, date, and time of collection.

Random Specimen (Collect in Early Morning)

Clean-Catch Specimen
- Instruct the male patient to (1) thoroughly wash his hands, (2) cleanse the meatus, (3) void a small amount into

the toilet, and (4) void directly into the specimen container.

▸ Instruct the female patient to (1) thoroughly wash her hands; (2) cleanse the labia from front to back; (3) while keeping the labia separated, void a small amount into the toilet; and (4) without interrupting the urine stream, void directly into the specimen container.

Indwelling Catheter

▸ Put on gloves. Empty drainage tube of urine. It may be necessary to clamp off the catheter for 15 to 30 min before specimen collection. Cleanse specimen port with antiseptic swab, and then aspirate 5 mL of urine with a 21- to 25-gauge needle and syringe. Transfer urine to a sterile container.

Timed Specimen

▸ Obtain a clean 3-L urine specimen container, toilet-mounted collection device, and plastic bag (for transport of the specimen container). The specimen must be refrigerated or kept on ice throughout the entire collection period. If an indwelling urinary catheter is in place, the drainage bag must be kept on ice.

▸ Begin the test between 6 and 8 a.m. if possible. Collect first voiding and discard. Record the time the specimen was discarded as the beginning of the timed collection period. The next morning, ask the patient to void at the same time the collection was started and add this last voiding to the container. Urinary output should be recorded throughout the collection time.

▸ If an indwelling catheter is in place, replace the tubing and container system at the start of the collection time. Keep the container system on ice during the collection period, or empty the urine into a larger container periodically during the collection period; monitor to ensure continued drainage, and conclude the test the next morning at the same hour the collection was begun.

▸ At the conclusion of the test, compare the quantity of urine with the urinary output record for the collection; if the specimen contains less than the

recorded output, some urine may have been discarded, invalidating the test.

▸ Include on the collection container's label the amount of urine collected and test start and stop times.

General

▸ Promptly transport the specimen to the laboratory for processing and analysis.

POST-TEST:

▸ A report of the results will be sent to the requesting health-care provider (HCP), who will discuss the results with the patient.

▸ Recognize anxiety related to test results. Discuss the implications of abnormal test results on the patient's lifestyle. Provide teaching and information regarding the clinical implications of the test results, as appropriate.

▸ Reinforce information given by the patient's HCP regarding further testing, treatment, or referral to another HCP. Answer any questions or address any concerns voiced by the patient or family.

▸ Depending on the results of this procedure, additional testing may be performed to evaluate or monitor progression of the disease process and determine the need for a change in therapy. Evaluate test results in relation to the patient's symptoms and other tests performed.

RELATED MONOGRAPHS:

▸ Related tests include amino acid screen, ACE, β_2-microglobulin, biopsy bladder, biopsy bone marrow, bladder cancer markers, BUN, calcium, CBC, CT pelvis, CT renal, creatinine, cryoglobulin, culture urine, cytology urine, cystometry, cystoscopy, glucose, glycated hemoglobin, Hgb electrophoresis, IgA, IgG, IgM, IFE, IVP, lead, LAP, MRI musculoskeletal, microalbumin, osmolality, porphyrins, protein blood total and fractions, renogram, sickle cell screen, US bladder, US spleen, UA, and voiding cystourethrography.

▸ Refer to the Genitourinary and Immune systems tables at the end of the book for related tests by body system.

P

Prothrombin Time and International Normalized Ratio

SYNONYM/ACRONYM: Protime, PT.

COMMON USE: To assess and monitor coagulation status related to therapeutic interventions and disorders such as vitamin K deficiency.

SPECIMEN: Plasma (1 mL) collected in a completely filled blue-top (sodium citrate) tube.

REFERENCE VALUE: (Method: Clot detection) 10 to 13 sec.

- International normalized ratio (INR) = Less than 2.0 for patients not receiving anticoagulation therapy, 2.0 to 3.0 for patients receiving treatment for venous thrombosis, pulmonary embolism, and valvular heart disease.
- INR = 2.5 to 3.5 for patients with mechanical heart valves and/or receiving treatment for recurrent systemic embolism.

DESCRIPTION: Prothrombin time (PT) is a coagulation test performed to measure the time it takes for a firm fibrin clot to form after tissue thromboplastin (factor III) and calcium are added to the sample. It is used to evaluate the extrinsic pathway of the coagulation sequence in patients receiving oral warfarin or coumarin-type anticoagulants. Prothrombin is a vitamin K–dependent protein produced by the liver; measurement is reported as time in seconds or percentage of normal activity.

The goal of long-term anticoagulation therapy is to achieve a balance between in vivo thrombus formation and hemorrhage. It is a delicate clinical balance, and because of differences in instruments and reagents, there is a wide variation in PT results among laboratories. Worldwide concern for the need to provide more consistency in monitoring patients receiving anticoagulant therapy led to the development of an international committee. In the early 1980s, manufacturers of instruments and reagents began comparing their measurement systems with a single reference material provided by the World Health Organization (WHO). The international effort successfully developed an algorithm to provide comparable PT values regardless of differences in laboratory methodology. Reagent and instrument manufacturers compare their results to the WHO reference and derive a factor called an international sensitivity index (ISI) that is applied to a mathematical formula to standardize the results. Laboratories convert their PT values into an international normalized ratio (INR) by using the following formula:

$$INR = (patient\ PT\ result / normal\ patient\ average)^{(ISI)}$$

PT evaluation can now be based on an INR using a standardized thromboplastin reagent to assist in making decisions regarding oral anticoagulation therapy. Interest is also growing in the area of pharma-cogenetic testing to manage dosing and decrease the number of adverse drug reactions with numerous medications, including the anticoagulant warfarin (Coumadin). Cytochrome (CY) P450 is a large and very diverse group of enzymes found in plants and mammals. In humans, this enzyme system is responsible for metabolizing up to 30% of all prescribed drugs. The CYP450 genes are distributed differently and in predictable frequency among various ethnic groups. CYP450 testing is available and should be used in conjunction with other factors, including all prescription and over-the-counter medications being used; mode of drug administration; use of tobacco products, foods, and supplements; age, weight, environment, activity level, and diseases with which the patient may be dealing.

Some inferences of factor deficiency can be made by comparison of results obtained from the activated partial thromboplastin time (aPTT) and PT tests. A normal aPTT with a prolonged PT can occur only with factor VII deficiency. A prolonged aPTT with a normal PT could indicate a deficiency in factors XII, XI, IX, and VIII as well as VIII:C (von Willebrand factor). Factor deficiencies can also be identified by correction or substitution studies using normal serum. These studies are easy to perform and are accomplished by adding plasma from a healthy patient to a sample from a suspected factor-deficient patient. When the PT is repeated and corrected, or within the reference range, it can be assumed that the prolonged PT is due to a factor deficiency (see monograph titled "Coagulation Factors"). If the result remains uncorrected, the prolonged PT is most likely due to a circulating anticoagulant.

INDICATIONS

- Differentiate between deficiencies of clotting factors II, V, VII, and X, which prolong the PT, and congenital coagulation disorders such as hemophilia A (factor VIII) and hemophilia B (factor IX), which do not alter the PT
- Evaluate the response to anticoagulant therapy with coumarin derivatives and determine dosage required to achieve therapeutic results
- Identify individuals who may be prone to bleeding during surgical, obstetric, dental, or invasive diagnostic procedures
- Identify the possible cause of abnormal bleeding, such as epistaxis, hematoma, gingival bleeding, hematuria, and menorrhagia
- Monitor the effects of conditions such as liver disease, protein deficiency, and fat malabsorption on hemostasis
- Screen for prothrombin deficiency
- Screen for vitamin K deficiency

POTENTIAL DIAGNOSIS

Increased in

- Afibrinogenemia, dysfibrinogenemia, or hypofibrinogenemia *(related to insufficient levels of fibrinogen, which is required for clotting; its absence prolongs PT)*
- Biliary obstruction *(related to poor absorption of fat-soluble vitamin K; vitamin K is required for clotting and its absence prolongs PT)*
- Disseminated intravascular coagulation *(related to increased consumption of clotting factors; PT is increased)*

P

- Hereditary deficiencies of factors II, V, VII, and X *(related to deficiency of factors required for clotting; their absence prolongs PT)*
- Liver disease (cirrhosis) *(related to decreased liver function, which results in decreased production of clotting factors and prolonged PT)*
- Massive transfusion of packed red blood cells (RBCs) *(related to dilutional effect of replacing a significant fraction of the total blood volume; there are insufficient clotting factors in plasma-poor, packed RBC products. Blood products contain anticoagulants, which compound the lack of adequate clotting factors in the case of massive transfusion)*
- Poor fat absorption *(tropical sprue, celiac disease, and chronic diarrhea are conditions that prevent absorption of fat-soluble vitamins, including vitamin K, which is required for clotting; its absence prolongs PT)*
- Presence of circulating anticoagulant *(related to the production of inhibitors of specific factors, e.g., developed from long-term factor VIII therapy or circulating anticoagulants associated with conditions like tuberculosis, systemic lupus erythematosus, rheumatoid arthritis, and chronic glomerulonephritis)*
- Salicylate intoxication *(related to decreased liver function)*
- Vitamin K deficiency *(vitamin K is required for clotting; its absence prolongs PT)*

Decreased in
- Ovarian hyperfunction
- Regional enteritis or ileitis

CRITICAL FINDINGS ✸

INR
- Greater than 5

Prothrombin Time
- Greater than 27 sec

Note and immediately report to the health-care provider (HCP) any critically increased values and related symptoms.

Important signs to note are prolonged bleeding from cuts or gums, hematoma at a puncture site, hemorrhage, blood in the stool, persistent epistaxis, heavy or prolonged menstrual flow, and shock. Monitor vital signs, unusual ecchymosis, occult blood, severe headache, unusual dizziness, and neurological changes until PT is within normal range. Intramuscular administration of vitamin K, an anticoagulant reversal agent, may be requested by the HCP.

INTERFERING FACTORS
- Drugs that may increase the PT in patients receiving anticoagulation therapy include acetaminophen, acetylsalicylic acid, amiodarone, anabolic steroids, anisindione, anistreplase, antibiotics, antipyrine, carbenicillin, cathartics, chloral hydrate, chlorthalidone, cholestyramine, clofibrate, corticotropin, demeclocycline, dextrothyroxine, diazoxide, diflunisal, disulfiram, diuretics, doxycycline, erythromycin, ethyl alcohol, hydroxyzine, laxatives, mercaptopurine, miconazole, nalidixic acid, neomycin, niacin, oxyphenbutazone, phenytoin, quinidine, quinine, sulfachlorpyridazine, thyroxine, and tosylate bretylium.
- Drugs that may decrease the PT in patients receiving anticoagulation therapy include aminoglutethimide, amobarbital, anabolic steroids, antacids, antihistamines, barbiturates, carbamazepine, chloral hydrate, chlordane, chlordiazepoxide, cholestyramine, clofibrate,

colchicine, corticosteroids, dichloralphenazone, diuretics, oral contraceptives, penicillin, primidone, raloxifene, rifabutin, rifampin, simethicone, spironolactone, tacrolimus, tolbutamide, and vitamin K.

- Traumatic venipunctures can activate the coagulation sequence by contaminating the sample with tissue thromboplastin and producing falsely shortened PT.
- Hematocrit greater than 55% may cause falsely prolonged results because of anticoagulant excess relative to plasma volume.
- Incompletely filled collection tubes, specimens contaminated with heparin, clotted or hemolyzed specimens, or unprocessed specimens not delivered to the laboratory within 24 hr of collection should be rejected.
- Excessive agitation causing sample hemolysis can falsely shorten the PT because the hemolyzed cells activate plasma-clotting factors.

NURSING IMPLICATIONS AND PROCEDURE

PRETEST:

- Positively identify the patient using at least two unique identifiers before providing care, treatment, or services.
- *Patient Teaching:* Inform the patient this test can assist in evaluating coagulation and monitor therapy.
- Obtain a history of the patient's complaints, including a list of known allergens, especially allergies or sensitivities to latex.
- Obtain a history of the patient's cardiovascular, hematopoietic, and hepatobiliary systems, especially any bleeding disorders and other symptoms, as well as results of previously performed laboratory tests and diagnostic and surgical procedures.
- Obtain a list of the patient's current medications, including anticoagulants, aspirin and other salicylates, herbs,

nutritional supplements, and nutraceuticals (see Appendix F). Such products should be discontinued by medical direction for the appropriate number of days prior to a surgical procedure. Note the last time and dose of medication taken.

- Review the procedure with the patient. Inform the patient that specimen collection takes approximately 5 to 10 min. Address concerns about pain and explain that there may be some discomfort during the venipuncture.
- *Sensitivity to social and cultural issues,* as well as concern for modesty, is important in providing psychological support before, during, and after the procedure.
- There are no food, fluid, or medication restrictions unless by medical direction.

INTRATEST:

- If the patient has a history of allergic reaction to latex, avoid the use of equipment containing latex.
- Instruct the patient to cooperate fully and to follow directions. Direct the patient to breathe normally and to avoid unnecessary movement.
- Observe standard precautions, and follow the general guidelines in Appendix A. Positively identify the patient, and label the appropriate tubes with the corresponding patient demographics, date, and time of collection. Perform a venipuncture. Fill tube completely. *Important note:* Two different concentrations of sodium citrate preservative are currently added to blue-top tubes for coagulation studies: 3.2% and 3.8%. The Clinical and Laboratory Standards Institute (CLSI; formerly the National Committee for Clinical Laboratory Standards [NCCLS]) guideline for sodium citrate is 3.2%. Laboratories establish reference ranges for coagulation testing based on numerous factors, including sodium citrate concentration, test equipment, and test reagents. It is important to ask the laboratory which concentration it recommends, because each concentration will have its own specific reference range. When multiple specimens are drawn, the blue-top tube should be collected after sterile (i.e., blood

P

culture) tubes. Otherwise, when using a standard vacutainer system, the blue-top tube is the first tube collected. When a butterfly is used and due to the added tubing, an extra red-top tube should be collected before the blue-top tube to ensure complete filling of the blue-top tube.

▸ Remove the needle and apply direct pressure with dry gauze to stop bleeding. Observe/assess venipuncture site for bleeding or hematoma formation and secure gauze with adhesive bandage.

▸ Promptly transport the specimen to the laboratory for processing and analysis. If delays in specimen transport and processing occur, it is important to consult with the testing laboratory. Whole blood specimens are stable at room temperature for up to 24 hr. Some laboratories will accept refrigerated whole blood samples up to 48 hr from the time of collection. Criteria for rejection of specimens based on collection time may vary among facilities.

▸ If the patient has a known hematocrit above 55%, adjust the amount of anticoagulant in the collection tube before drawing the blood according to the CLSI guidelines:

Anticoagulant vol. [x] = $(100 - \text{hematocrit})/(595 - \text{hematocrit}) \times$ total vol. of anticoagulated blood required

Example:

Patient hematocrit = 60% = $[(100 - 60)/(595 - 60) \times 5.0] = 0.37$ mL sodium citrate for a 5-mL standard drawing tube

POST-TEST:

▸ A report of the results will be sent to the requesting HCP, who will discuss the results with the patient.

▸ Instruct the patient to report bleeding from any areas of the skin or mucous membranes.

▸ Inform the patient with prolonged PT/INR of the importance of taking precautions against bruising and bleeding, including the use of a soft bristle toothbrush, use of an electric razor, avoidance of constipation, avoidance of aspirin products, and avoidance of intramuscular injections.

▸ Inform the patient of the importance of periodic laboratory testing while taking an anticoagulant.

▸ *Nutritional Considerations:* Foods high in vitamin K should be avoided by the patient on anticoagulant therapy. Foods that contain vitamin K include cabbage, cauliflower, chickpeas, egg yolks, green tea, liver, milk, soybean products, tomatoes, and green leafy vegetables such as Brussels sprouts, kale, spinach, and turnip greens.

▸ *Nutritional Considerations:* Avoid alcohol and alcohol products while taking warfarin because the combination of the two increases the risk of gastrointestinal bleeding.

▸ Reinforce information given by the patient's HCP regarding further testing, treatment, or referral to another HCP. Answer any questions or address any concerns voiced by the patient or family.

▸ Depending on the results of this procedure, additional testing may be performed to evaluate or monitor progression of the disease process and determine the need for a change in therapy. Evaluate test results in relation to the patient's symptoms and other tests performed.

RELATED MONOGRAPHS:

▸ Related tests include, ALP, ALT, ANA, AT-III, AST, bilirubin, biopsy liver, bleeding time, calcium, coagulation factors, CBC, CBC platelet count, CT liver and biliary tract, cryoglobulin, D-dimer, fecal analysis, fecal fat, FDP, fibrinogen, GGT, gastric acid emptying scan, hepatitis antibodies (A, B, C, D), liver and spleen scan, lupus anticoagulant, aPTT, plasminogen, protein C, protein S, US liver, and vitamin K.

▸ Refer to the Cardiovascular, Hematopoietic, and Hepatobiliary systems tables at the end of the book for related tests by body system.

P

Pseudocholinesterase and Dibucaine Number

SYNONYM/ACRONYM: CHS, PCHE, AcCHS.

COMMON USE: To assess for pseudocholinesterase deficiency to assist in diagnosing disorders such as congenital deficiency and cancer. Special attention must be given to results for preoperative patients because positive results indicate risk for apnea with use of succinylcholine as an anesthetic agent.

SPECIMEN: Plasma (1 mL) collected in a lavender-top (EDTA) tube. Serum (1 mL) collected in a red-top tube is also acceptable.

REFERENCE VALUE: (Method: Spectrophotometry, kinetic)

Test	Conventional Units
Pseudocholinesterase	
Males	3,334–7,031 IU/L
Females	2,504–6,297 IU/L

Dibucaine Number	Fraction (%) of Activity Inhibited
Normal homozygote	79%–84%
Heterozygote	55%–70%
Abnormal homozygote	16%–28%

POTENTIAL DIAGNOSIS

Increased in
Increased levels are observed in a number of conditions without specific cause.
- Diabetes
- Hyperthyroidism
- Nephrotic syndrome
- Obesity

Decreased in
The enzyme is produced in the liver, and any condition affecting liver function may result in decreased production of circulating enzyme.
- Acute infection
- Anemia (severe)
- Carcinomatosis
- Cirrhosis
- Congenital deficiency
- Hepatic carcinoma
- Hepatocellular disease
- Infectious hepatitis
- Insecticide exposure *(organic phosphate exposure decreases enzyme activity)*
- Malnutrition *(possibly related to decreased availability of transport proteins; condition associated with decreased enzyme activity)*
- Muscular dystrophy
- Myocardial infarction
- Plasmapheresis *(iatragenic cause)*

P

- Succinylcholine hypersensitivity *(this chemical is a trigger in susceptible individuals)*
- Tuberculosis *(chronic infection is known to decrease enzyme activity)*
- Uremia *(pathological condition known to decrease enzyme activity)*

CRITICAL FINDINGS:

A positive result indicates that the patient is at risk for prolonged or unrecoverable apnea related to the inability to metabolize succinylcholine.

Notify the anesthesiologist if the test result is positive and surgery is scheduled.

Find and print out the full monograph at DavisPlus (http://davisplus.fadavis .com, keyword Van Leeuwen).

Pulmonary Function Studies

SYNONYM/ACRONYM: Pulmonary function tests (PFTs).

COMMON USE: To assess respiratory function to assist in evaluating obstructive versus restrictive lung disease and to monitor and assess the effectiveness of therapeutic interventions.

AREA OF APPLICATION: Lungs, respiratory system.

CONTRAST: None.

DESCRIPTION: Pulmonary function studies provide information about the volume, pattern, and rates of airflow involved in respiratory function. These studies may also include tests involving the diffusing capabilities of the lungs (i.e., volume of gases diffusing across a membrane). A complete pulmonary function study includes the determination of all lung volumes, spirometry, diffusing capacity, maximum voluntary ventilation, flow-volume loop (see figure), and maximum expiratory and inspiratory pressures. Other studies include small airway volumes.

Pulmonary function studies are classified according to lung volumes and capacities, rates of flow, and gas exchange. The exception is the diffusion test, which records the movement of a gas during inspiration and expiration. Lung volumes and capacities constitute the amount of air inhaled or exhaled from the lungs; this value is compared to normal reference values specific for the patient's age, height, and gender. The following are volumes and capacities measured by spirometry that do not require timed testing.

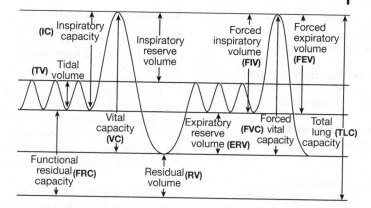

Tidal volume
Total amount of air inhaled and exhaled with one breath.

Residual volume
Amount of air remaining in the lungs after a maximum expiration effort (not measured by spirometry, but can be calculated from the functional residual capacity [FRC] minus the expiratory reserve volume [ERV]); this indirect type of measurement can be done by body plethysmography (see monograph titled "Plethysmography")

Inspiratory reserve volume
Maximum amount of air inhaled after normal inspirations

Expiratory reserve volume
Maximum amount of air exhaled after a resting expiration (can be calculated by the vital capacity [VC] minus the inspiratory capacity [IC])

Vital capacity
Maximum amount of air exhaled after a maximum inspiration (can be calculated by adding the IC and the ERV)

Total lung capacity
Total amount of air that the lungs can hold after maximal inspiration (can be calculated by adding the VC and the residual volume [RV])

Inspiratory capacity
Maximum amount of air inspired after normal expiration (can be calculated by adding the inspiratory RV and tidal volume)

Functional residual capacity
Volume of air that remains in the lungs after normal expiration (can be calculated by adding the RV and ERV)

The volumes, capacities, and rates of flow measured by spirometry that do require timed testing include the following:

Forced vital capacity in 1 sec
Maximum amount of air that can be forcefully exhaled after a full inspiration

Forced expiratory volume
Amount of air exhaled in the first second (can also be determined at 2 or 3 sec) of forced vital capacity (FVC, which is the amount of air exhaled in seconds, expressed as a percentage)

Maximal midexpiratory flow
Also known as forced expiratory flow rate (FEF_{25-75}), or the maximal rate of airflow during a forced expiration

Forced inspiratory flow rate
Volume inspired from the RV at a point of measurement (can be

P

expressed as a percentage to identify the corresponding volume pressure and inspired volume)

Peak inspiratory flow rate
Maximum airflow during a forced maximal inspiration

Peak expiratory flow rate
Maximum airflow expired during FVC

Flow-volume loops
Flows and volumes recorded during forced expiratory volume and forced inspiratory VC procedures (see figure)

Maximal inspiratory-expiratory pressures
Measures the strength of the respiratory muscles in neuromuscular disorders

Maximal voluntary ventilation
Maximal volume of air inspired and expired in 1 min (may be done for shorter periods and multiplied to equal 1 min)

Other studies for gas-exchange capacity, small airway abnormalities, and allergic responses in hyperactive airway disorders can be performed during the conventional pulmonary function study. These include the following:

Diffusing capacity of the lungs
Rate of transfer of carbon monoxide through the alveolar and capillary membrane in 1 min

Closing volume
Measures the closure of small airways in the lower alveoli by monitoring volume and percentage of alveolar nitrogen after inhalation of 100% oxygen

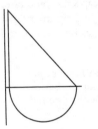

Normal

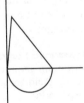

Restrictive

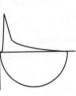

Obstructive

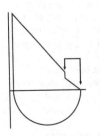

Small airway disease

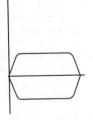

Fixed upper airway obstruction

Variable upper airway obstruction

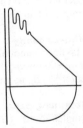

Sleep apnea disorder

Isoflow volume

Flow-volume loop test followed by inhalation of a mixture of helium and oxygen to determine small airway disease

Body plethysmography

Measures thoracic gas volume and airway resistance

Bronchial provocation

Quantifies airway response after inhalation of methacholine

Arterial blood gases

Measure oxygen, pH, and carbon dioxide in arterial blood

Values are expressed in units of mL, %, L, L/sec, and L/min, depending on the test performed.

INDICATIONS

- Detect chronic obstructive pulmonary disease (COPD) and/or restrictive pulmonary diseases that affect the chest wall (e.g., neuromuscular disorders, kyphosis, scoliosis) and lungs, as evidenced by abnormal airflows and volumes
- Determine airway response to inhalants in patients with an airway-reactive disorder
- Determine the diffusing capacity of the lungs (DCOL)
- Determine the effectiveness of therapy regimens, such as bronchodilators, for pulmonary disorders
- Determine the presence of lung disease when other studies, such as x-rays, do not provide a definitive diagnosis, or determine the progression and severity of known COPD and restrictive pulmonary disease
- Evaluate the cause of dyspnea occurring with or without exercise
- Evaluate lung compliance to determine changes in elasticity, as evidenced by changes in lung volumes (decreased in restrictive pulmonary disease, increased in COPD and in elderly patients)
- Evaluate pulmonary disability for legal or insurance claims
- Evaluate pulmonary function after surgical pneumonectomy, lobectomy, or segmental lobectomy
- Evaluate the respiratory system to determine the patient's ability to tolerate procedures such as surgery or diagnostic studies
- Screen high-risk populations for early detection of pulmonary conditions (e.g., patients with exposure to occupational or environmental hazards, smokers, patients with a hereditary predisposition)

POTENTIAL DIAGNOSIS

Normal findings in

- Normal respiratory volume and capacities, gas diffusion, and distribution
- No evidence of COPD or restrictive pulmonary disease

Normal adult lung volumes, capacities, and flow rates are as follows:

TV	500 mL at rest
RV	1,200 mL (approximate)
IRV	3,000 mL (approximate)
ERV	1,100 mL (approximate)
VC	4,600 mL (approximate)
TLC	5,800 mL (approximate)

(table continues on page 1118)

IC	3,500 mL (approximate)
FRC	2,300 mL (approximate)
FVC	3,000–5,000 mL (approximate)
FEV_1/FVC	81%–83%
MMEF	25%–75%
FIF	25%–75%
MVV	25%–35% or 170 L/min
PIFR	300 L/min
PEFR	450 L/min
F-V loop	Normal curve
DCOL	25 mL/min per mm Hg (approximate)
CV	10%–20% of VC
V_{iso}	Based on age formula
Bronchial provocation	No change, or less than 20% reduction in FEV_1

Note: Normal values listed are estimated values for adults. Actual pediatric and adult values are based on age, height, and gender. These normal values are included on the patient's pulmonary function laboratory report.

CV = closing volume; DCOL = diffusing capacity of the lungs; ERV = expiratory reserve volume; FEV_1 = forced expiratory volume in 1 sec; FIF = forced inspiratory flow rate; FRC = functional residual capacity; FVC = forced vital capacity; IC = inspiratory capacity; IRV = inspiratory reserve volume; MMEF = maximal midexpiratory flow (also known as FEF_{25-75}); MVV = maximal voluntary ventilation; PEFR = peak expiratory flow rate; PIFR = peak inspiratory flow rate; RV = residual volume; TLC = total lung capacity; TV = tidal volume; VC = vital capacity; V_{iso} = isoflow volume.

Abnormal findings in
- Allergy
- Asbestosis
- Asthma
- Bronchiectasis
- Chest trauma
- Chronic bronchitis
- Curvature of the spine
- Emphysema
- Myasthenia gravis
- Obesity
- Pulmonary fibrosis
- Pulmonary tumors
- Respiratory infections
- Sarcoidosis

CRITICAL FINDINGS: N/A

INTERFERING FACTORS
- The aging process can cause decreased values (FVC, DCOL) depending on the study done.
- Inability of the patient to put forth the necessary breathing effort affects the results.
- Medications such as bronchodilators can affect results.
- Improper placement of the nose clamp or mouthpiece that allows for leakage can affect volume results.
- Confusion or inability to understand instructions or cooperate during the study can cause inaccurate results.
- Testing is contraindicated in patients with cardiac insufficiency, recent myocardial infarction, and presence of chest pain that affects inspiration or expiration ability.
- Exercise caution with patients who have upper respiratory infections, such as a cold or acute bronchitis.

NURSING IMPLICATIONS AND PROCEDURE

PRETEST:

▸ Positively identify the patient using at least two unique identifiers before providing care, treatment, or services.

▸ *Patient Teaching:* Inform the patient this procedure can assist in assessing lung function.

▸ Obtain a history of the patient's complaints or symptoms, including a list of known allergens, especially allergies or sensitivities to latex, iodine, seafood, anesthetics, or contrast mediums.

▸ Obtain a history of the patient's cardiovascular and respiratory systems, symptoms, and results of previously performed laboratory tests and diagnostic and surgical procedures.

▸ Obtain a list of the patient's current medications, including herbs, nutritional supplements, and nutraceuticals (see Appendix F).

▸ Review the procedure with the patient. Address concerns about pain related to the procedure and explain that no discomfort will be experienced during the test. Explain that the procedure is generally performed in a specially equipped room or in a health-care provider's (HCP's) office by an HCP specializing in this procedure and usually lasts 1 hr.

▸ *Sensitivity to social and cultural issues,* as well as concern for modesty, is important in providing psychological support before, during, and after the procedure.

▸ Record the patient's height and weight.

▸ The patient should avoid bronchodilators (oral or inhalant) for at least 4 hr before the study, as directed by the HCP.

▸ Instruct the patient to refrain from smoking tobacco or eating a heavy meal for 4 to 6 hr prior to the study. Protocols may vary among facilities.

INTRATEST:

▸ Ensure the patient has complied with dietary and medication restrictions and pretesting preparations.

▸ Obtain an inhalant bronchodilator to treat any bronchospasms that may occur with testing.

▸ Instruct the patient to void and to loosen any restrictive clothing.

▸ Instruct the patient to cooperate fully and to follow directions.

▸ Observe standard precautions, and follow the general guidelines in Appendix A.

▸ Place the patient in a sitting position on a chair near the spirometry equipment.

▸ Place a soft clip on the patient's nose to restrict nose breathing, and instruct the patient to breathe through the mouth.

▸ Place a mouthpiece in the mouth and instruct the patient to close his or her lips around it to form a seal.

▸ Tubing from the mouthpiece attaches to a cylinder that is connected to a computer that measures, records, and calculates the values for the tests done.

▸ Instruct the patient to inhale deeply and then to quickly exhale as much air as possible into the mouthpiece.

▸ Additional breathing maneuvers are performed on inspiration and expiration (normal, forced, and breath-holding).

POST-TEST:

▸ A report of the examination will be sent to the requesting HCP, who will discuss the results with the patient.

▸ Assess the patient for dizziness or weakness after the testing.

▸ Allow the patient to rest as long as needed to recover.

▸ Instruct the patient to resume usual diet and medications, as directed by the HCP.

▸ Recognize anxiety related to test results, and be supportive of perceived loss of independent function. Discuss the implications of abnormal test results on the patient's lifestyle. Provide teaching and information regarding the clinical implications of the test results, as appropriate.

▸ Reinforce information given by the patient's HCP regarding further testing, treatment, or referral to another HCP.

P

Answer any questions or address any concerns voiced by the patient or family.

▶ Depending on the results of this procedure, additional testing may be performed to evaluate or monitor progression of the disease process and determine the need for a change in therapy. Evaluate test results in relation to the patient's symptoms and other tests performed.

RELATED MONOGRAPHS:

▶ Related tests include α_1-AT, anion gap, arterial/alveolar oxygen ratio, biopsy lung, blood gases, bronchoscopy, carboxyhemoglobin, chest x-ray, chloride sweat, CBC, CBC hemoglobin, CBC WBC count and differential, CT angiography, CT thoracic, culture and smear for mycobacteria, culture bacterial sputum, culture viral, cytology sputum, echocardiography, ECG, Gram stain, IgE, lactic acid, lung perfusion scan, lung ventilation scan, MR angiography, MRI chest, osmolality, phosphorus, plethysmography, pleural fluid analysis, potassium, PET chest, pulse oximetry, sodium, and TB skin test.

▶ Refer to the Cardiovascular and Respiratory systems tables at the end of the book for related tests by body system.

Pulse Oximetry

SYNONYM/ACRONYM: Oximetry, pulse ox.

COMMON USE: To assess arterial blood oxygenation to assist in evaluating respiratory status during ventilation, acute illness, activity, and sleep and to evaluate the effectiveness of therapeutic interventions.

AREA OF APPLICATION: Earlobe, fingertip; for infants, use the large toe, top or bottom of the foot, or sides of the ankle.

CONTRAST: None.

P

DESCRIPTION: Pulse oximetry is a noninvasive study that provides continuous readings of arterial blood oxygen saturation (SpO_2) using a sensor site (earlobe or fingertip). The SpO_2 equals the ratio of the amount of O_2 contained in the hemoglobin to the maximum amount of O_2 contained, with hemoglobin expressed as a percentage. The results obtained may compare favorably with O_2 saturation levels obtained by arterial blood gas analysis without the need to perform successive arterial punctures. The device used is a clip or probe that produces a light beam with two different wavelengths on one side. A sensor on the opposite side measures the absorption of each of the wavelengths of light to determine the O_2 saturation reading. The displayed result is a ratio, expressed as a percentage, between the actual O_2 content of the hemoglobin and the potential maximum O_2-carrying capacity of the hemoglobin.

INDICATIONS

- Determine the effectiveness of pulmonary gas exchange function
- Evaluate suspected nocturnal hypoxemia in chronic obstructive pulmonary disease
- Monitor oxygenation during testing for sleep apnea
- Monitor oxygenation perioperatively and during acute illnesses
- Monitor oxygenation status in patients on a ventilator, during surgery, and during bronchoscopy
- Monitor O_2 saturation during activities such as pulmonary exercise stress testing or pulmonary rehabilitation exercises to determine optimal tolerance
- Monitor response to pulmonary drug regimens, especially flow and O_2 content

POTENTIAL DIAGNOSIS

Normal findings in
- Greater than or equal to 95%

Abnormal findings in
- Abnormal gas exchange
- Hypoxemia with levels less than 95%
- Impaired cardiopulmonary function

CRITICAL FINDINGS: N/A

INTERFERING FACTORS

This procedure is contraindicated for
- Patients who smoke or have suffered carbon monoxide inhalation, because O_2 levels may be falsely elevated.

Factors that may result in incorrect values
- Patients with anemic conditions reflecting a reduction in hemoglobin, the O_2-carrying component in the blood.
- Excessive light surrounding the patient, such as from surgical lights.
- Impaired cardiopulmonary function.
- Lipid emulsion therapy and presence of certain dyes.
- Movement of the finger or ear or improper placement of probe or clip.
- Nail polish, artificial fingernails, and skin pigmentation when a finger probe is used.
- Vasoconstriction from cool skin temperature, drugs, hypotension, or vessel obstruction causing a decrease in blood flow.

Other considerations
- Accuracy for most units is plus or minus 4% with a standard deviation of 1%.

NURSING IMPLICATIONS AND PROCEDURE

PRETEST:
- Positively identify the patient using at least two unique identifiers before providing care, treatment, or services.
- *Patient Teaching:* Inform the patient this procedure can assist in monitoring oxygen in the blood.
- Obtain a history of the patient's complaints, including a list of known allergens, especially allergies or sensitivities to latex, iodine, seafood, contrast medium, or anesthetics.
- Obtain a history of the patient's cardiovascular and respiratory systems, symptoms, and results of previously performed laboratory tests and diagnostic and surgical procedures.
- Obtain a list of the patient's current medications, including herbs, nutritional

P

supplements, and nutraceuticals (see Appendix F).

- Review the procedure with the patient. Address concerns about pain related to the procedure and explain that no pain is associated with the procedure. Inform the patient that the procedure is generally performed at the bedside, in the operating room during a surgical procedure, or in the office of a health-care provider (HCP). Explain that the procedure lasts as long as the monitoring is needed and could be continuous.
- *Sensitivity to social and cultural issues,* as well as concern for modesty, is important in providing psychological support before, during, and after the procedure.
- If a finger probe is used, instruct the patient to remove artificial fingernails and nail polish.
- When used in the presence of flammable gases, the equipment must be approved for that specific use.
- Instruct the patient not to smoke for 24 hr before the procedure.
- There are no food, fluid, or medication restrictions unless by medical direction.

INTRATEST:

- Ensure that the patient has complied with pretesting instructions.
- If a finger probe is used, instruct the patient not to grip treadmill rail or bed rail tightly; doing so restricts blood flow.
- Instruct the patient to cooperate fully and to follow directions.
- Observe standard precautions, and follow the general guidelines in Appendix A.
- Massage or apply a warm towel to the upper earlobe or finger to increase the blood flow.
- The index finger is normally used, but if the patient's finger is too large for the probe, a smaller finger can be used.
- If the earlobe is used, make sure good contact is achieved.
- The big toe, top or bottom of the foot, or sides of the heel may be used in infants.
- Place the photodetector probe over the finger in such a way that the light beams and sensors are opposite each other. Turn the power switch to the oximeter monitor, which will display information about heart rate and peripheral capillary saturation (SaO_2).
- Remove the clip used for monitoring when the procedure is complete.

POST-TEST:

- A report of the examination will be sent to the requesting HCP, who will discuss the results with the patient.
- Closely observe SpO_2, and report to the HCP if it decreases to 90%.
- Recognize anxiety related to test results, and be supportive of perceived loss of independent function. Discuss the implications of abnormal test results on the patient's lifestyle. Provide teaching and information regarding the clinical implications of the test results, as appropriate.
- Reinforce information given by the patient's HCP regarding further testing, treatment, or referral to another HCP. Answer any questions or address any concerns voiced by the patient or family.
- Depending on the results of this procedure, additional testing may be performed to evaluate or monitor progression of the disease process and determine the need for a change in therapy. Evaluate test results in relation to the patient's symptoms and other tests performed.

RELATED MONOGRAPHS:

- Related tests include α_1-AT, anion gap, arterial/alveolar oxygen ratio, biopsy lung, blood gases, bronchoscopy, carboxyhemoglobin, chest x-ray, chloride sweat, CBC, CBC hemoglobin, CBC WBC count and differential, CT angiography, culture and smear for mycobacteria, culture bacterial sputum, culture viral, cytology sputum, ECG, Gram stain, IgE, lactic acid, lung perfusion scan, lung ventilation scan, MR angiography, MR chest, osmolality, phosphorus, plethysmography, pleural fluid analysis, potassium, pulmonary function tests, sodium, and TB skin test.
- Refer to the Cardiovascular and Respiratory systems tables at the end of the book for related tests by body system.

Pyruvate Kinase

SYNONYM/ACRONYM: PK.

COMMON USE: To assess for an enzyme deficiency to assist in diagnosis of hemolytic anemia.

SPECIMEN: Whole blood collected in yellow-top (acid-citrate-dextrose [ACD]) tube. Specimens collected in a lavender-top (EDTA) or green-top (heparin) tube also may be acceptable in some laboratories.

REFERENCE VALUE: (Method: Spectrophotometry) 6 to 19 micromol $NAD(H)_2$/min/g hemoglobin (37°C).

POTENTIAL DIAGNOSIS

Increased in
Related to release of skeletal and cardiac specific isoenzymes of PK from damaged tissue cells.
- Carriers of Duchenne's muscular dystrophy
- Muscle disease
- Myocardial infarction

Decreased in
- Hereditary pyruvate kinase deficiency (evidenced by autosomal recessive trait for PK enzyme deficiency):
Congenital nonspherocytic hemolytic anemia
- Acquired pyruvate kinase deficiency (related to interaction of medications used for therapy; related to release of leukocyte specific isoenzymes from damaged leukocytes):
Acute leukemia
Aplasias
Other anemias

CRITICAL FINDINGS: N/A

Find and print out the full monograph at DavisPlus (http://davisplus.fadavis.com, keyword Van Leeuwen).

Radioactive Iodine Uptake

SYNONYM/ACRONYM: RAIU, thyroid uptake.

COMMON USE: To assess thyroid function to assist in diagnosing disorders such as hyperthyroidism and goiter.

AREA OF APPLICATION: Thyroid.

CONTRAST: Oral radioactive iodine.

DESCRIPTION: Radioactive iodine uptake (RAIU) is a nuclear medicine study used for evaluating thyroid function. It directly measures the ability of the thyroid gland to concentrate and retain circulating iodide for the synthesis of thyroid hormone. RAIU assists in the diagnosis of both hyperthyroidism and hypothyroidism, but it is more useful in the diagnosis of hyperthyroidism.

A very small dose of radioactive iodine-123 (I-123) or I-131 is administered orally, and images are taken at specified intervals after the initial dose is administered. The radionuclide emits gamma radiation, which allows external measurement. The uptake of radionuclide in the thyroid gland is measured as the percentage of radionuclide absorbed in a specific amount of time. The iodide not used is excreted in the urine. The thyroid gland does not distinguish between radioactive and nonradioactive iodine. Uptake values are used in conjunction with measurements of circulating thyroid hormone levels to differentiate primary and secondary thyroid disease, and serial measurements are helpful in long-term management of thyroid disease and its treatment.

INDICATIONS
- Evaluate hyperthyroidism and/or hypothyroidism
- Evaluate neck pain
- Evaluate the patient as part of a complete thyroid evaluation for symptomatic patients (e.g., swollen neck, neck pain, extreme sensitivity to heat or cold, jitters, sluggishness)
- Evaluate thyroiditis, goiter, or pituitary failure
- Monitor response to therapy for thyroid disease

POTENTIAL DIAGNOSIS

Normal findings in
- Variations in normal ranges of iodine uptake can occur with differences in dietary intake, geographic location, and protocols among laboratories:

Iodine Uptake	Percentage of Radionuclide
2-hr absorption	1%–13%
6-hr absorption	2%–25%
24-hr absorption	15%–45%

R

Abnormal findings in

- Decreased iodine intake or increased iodine excretion
- Graves' disease
- Iodine-deficient goiter
- Hashimoto's thyroiditis (early)
- Hyperthyroidism, increased uptake of radionuclide:
  Rebound thyroid hormone withdrawal
  Drugs and hormones such as barbiturates, diuretics, estrogens, lithium carbonate, phenothiazines, and thyroid-stimulating hormone
- Hypothyroidism, decreased uptake of 0% to 10% radionuclide over 24-hr period:
  Hypoalbuminemia
  Malabsorption
  Renal failure
  Subacute thyroiditis
  Thyrotoxicosis as a result of ectopic thyroid metastasis

CRITICAL FINDINGS: N/A

INTERFERING FACTORS

This procedure is contraindicated for

- Patients who are pregnant or suspected of being pregnant, unless the potential benefits of the procedure far outweigh the risks to the fetus and mother.

Factors that may impair clear imaging

- Inability of the patient to cooperate or remain still during the procedure because of age, significant pain, or mental status.
- Recent use of iodinated contrast medium for radiographic studies (within the last 4 wk) or nuclear medicine procedures done within the previous 24 to 48 hr.
- Iodine deficiency (e.g., patients with inadequate dietary intake,

patients on phenothiazine therapy), which can increase radionuclide uptake.

- Certain drugs and other external sources of excess iodine, which can decrease radionuclide uptake, as follows:
  Foods containing iodine (e.g., iodized salt)
  Drugs such as aminosalicylic acid, antihistamines, antithyroid medications (e.g., propylthiouracil, iodothiouracil), corticosteroids, cough syrup, isoniazid, levothyroxine sodium/T_4, L-triiodothyronine, Lugol's solution, nitrates, penicillins, potassium iodide, propylthiouracil, saturated solution of potassium iodide, sulfonamides, thiocyanate, thyroid extract, tolbutamide, and warfarin
  Multivitamins containing minerals
- Vomiting, severe diarrhea, and gastroenteritis, which can affect absorption of the oral radionuclide dose.
- Metallic objects (e.g., jewelry, body rings) within the examination field, which may inhibit organ visualization and cause unclear images.

Other considerations

- Failure to follow dietary restrictions before the procedure may cause the procedure to be canceled or repeated.
- Consultation with a health-care provider (HCP) should occur before the procedure for radiation safety concerns regarding younger patients or patients who are lactating.
- Risks associated with radiation overexposure can result from frequent x-ray or radionuclide procedures. Personnel working in the examination area should wear badges to record their level of radiation exposure.

R

NURSING IMPLICATIONS AND PROCEDURE

PRETEST:

▶ Positively identify the patient using at least two unique identifiers before providing care, treatment, or services.

▶ *Patient Teaching:* Inform the patient this test can assist in assessing thyroid function.

▶ Obtain a history of the patient's complaints, including a list of known allergens, especially allergies or sensitivities to latex, iodine, seafood, contrast medium, anesthetics, or dyes.

▶ Obtain a history of the patient's endocrine system, symptoms, and results of previously performed laboratory tests and diagnostic and surgical procedures.

▶ Note any recent procedures that can interfere with test results, including examinations using iodine-based contrast medium.

▶ Ensure that this procedure is performed before all radiographic procedures using iodinated contrast medium.

▶ Record the date of the last menstrual period and determine the possibility of pregnancy in perimenopausal women.

▶ Obtain a list of the patient's current medications, including herbs, nutritional supplements, and nutraceuticals (see Appendix F).

▶ Review the procedure with the patient. Address concerns about pain related to the procedure and explain that some pain may be experienced during the test, and there may be moments of discomfort. Inform the patient that the procedure is performed in a nuclear medicine department by an HCP who specializes in this procedure, with support staff, and takes approximately 15 to 30 min. Delayed images or data collection is needed 24 hr later.

▶ *Sensitivity to social and cultural issues,* as well as concern for modesty, is important in providing psychological support before, during, and after the procedure.

▶ Instruct the patient to remove jewelry and other metallic objects from the area to be examined.

▶ Instruct the patient to fast and restrict fluids for 8 to 12 hr before the procedure. The patient may eat 4 hr after the injection unless otherwise indicated. Protocols may vary among facilities.

INTRATEST:

▶ Ensure the patient has complied with dietary, fluid, and medication restrictions for 8 to 12 hr before the procedure.

▶ Ensure that the patient has removed all external metallic objects from the area to be examined prior to the procedure.

▶ Instruct the patient to cooperate fully and to follow directions. Instruct the patient to remain still throughout the procedure because movement produces unreliable results.

▶ Observe standard precautions, and follow the general guidelines in Appendix A.

▶ Administer the I-123 orally (pill form).

▶ Place the patient in a sitting or supine position in front of a radionuclide detector at 2, 6, and 24 hr after ingestion for uptake images.

POST-TEST:

▶ A report of the results will be sent to the requesting HCP, who will discuss the results with the patient.

▶ Instruct the patient to resume usual diet, as directed by the HCP.

▶ Advise patient to drink increased amounts of fluids for 24 hr to eliminate the radionuclide from the body, unless contraindicated. Tell the patient that radionuclide is eliminated from the body within 24 to 48 hr.

▶ If a woman who is breastfeeding must have a nuclear scan, she should not breastfeed the infant until the radionuclide has been eliminated. This could take as long as 3 days. She should be instructed to express the milk and discard it during the 3-day period to prevent cessation of milk production.

▶ Instruct the patient to immediately flush the toilet and to meticulously wash hands with soap and water after each voiding for 24 hr after the procedure.

▶ Instruct all caregivers to wear gloves when discarding urine for 24 hr after the procedure. Wash gloved hands with soap and water before removing gloves. Then wash hands after the gloves are removed.

▸ Recognize anxiety related to test results, and be supportive of perceived loss of independent function. Discuss the implications of abnormal test results on the patient's lifestyle. Provide teaching and information regarding the clinical implications of the test results, as appropriate.

▸ Reinforce information given by the patient's HCP regarding further testing, treatment, or referral to another HCP. Answer any questions or address any concerns voiced by the patient or family.

▸ Depending on the results of this procedure, additional testing may be needed to evaluate or monitor progression of the disease process and determine the need for a change in therapy. Evaluate test results in relation to the patient's symptoms and other tests performed.

RELATED MONOGRAPHS:

▸ Related tests include ACTH, albumin, ACE, antibodies antithyroglobulin, biopsy thyroid, BUN, CT spine, copper, creatinine, cystoscopy, fecal analysis, fecal fat, FSH, gastric emptying scan, GH, LH, PTH, protein, thyroglobulin, thyroid binding inhibitory immunoglobulins, thyroid scan, TSH, TSI, thyroxine, free T_4, triiodothyronine, free T_3, US thyroid, upper GI series, and UA.

▸ Refer to the Endocrine System table at the end of the book for tests by related body system.

Radiofrequency Ablation, Liver

SYNONYM/ACRONYM: RFA, RF ablation.

COMMON USE: To assist in treating tumors of the liver that are too small for surgery or have poor response to chemotherapy.

AREA OF APPLICATION: Liver.

CONTRAST: Done without contrast.

DESCRIPTION: One minimally invasive therapy to eliminate tumors in organs such as the liver is called radiofrequency ablation (RFA). This technique works by passing electrical current in the range of radiofrequency waves between the needle electrode and the grounding pads placed on the patient's skin. A special needle electrode is placed in the tumor under the guidance of an imaging method such as ultrasound (US), computed tomography (CT) scanning, or magnetic resonance imaging (MRI). A radiofrequency current is then passed through the electrode to heat the tumor tissue near the needle tip and to ablate, or eliminate, it. The current creates heat around the electrode inside the tumor, and this heat spreads out to destroy the entire tumor but little of the surrounding normal liver tissue. The heat from radiofrequency energy also closes

R

up small blood vessels, thereby minimizing the risk of bleeding. Because healthy liver tissue withstands more heat than a tumor, RFA is able to destroy a tumor and a small rim of normal tissue about its edges without affecting most of the normal liver. The dead tumor cells are gradually replaced by scar tissue that shrinks over time. Some liver tumors may have failed to respond to chemotherapy or have recurred after initial surgery, and they may be treated by RFA. If there are multiple tumor nodules, they may be treated in one or more sessions. In general, RFA causes only minimal discomfort and may be done as an outpatient procedure without general anesthesia. RFA is most effective if the tumor is less than 2 in. in diameter; results are not as good when RFA is used to treat larger tumors. Similar therapy is being used to treat tumors in the kidney, pancreas, bone, thyroid, breast, adrenal gland, and lung.

INDICATIONS

- Ablation of metastases to the liver
- Ablation of primary liver tumors, with hepatocellular carcinoma
- Therapy for multiple small liver tumors that are too spread out to remove surgically
- Therapy for recurrent liver tumors
- Therapy for tumors that are less than 2 in. in diameter
- Therapy for tumors that have failed to respond to chemotherapy
- Therapy for tumors that have recurred after initial surgery

Risks

- May cause brief or long-lasting shoulder pain
- May cause inflammation of the gallbladder

- May cause damage to the bile ducts with resulting biliary obstruction
- May cause thermal damage to the bowel
- The patient may experience flu-like symptoms that appear 3 to 5 days after the procedure and last for approximately 5 days
- The patient may experience bleeding; if bleeding is severe, surgery may be needed

POTENTIAL DIAGNOSIS

Normal findings in

- Decrease in tumor size
- Normal size, position, contour, and texture of the liver

Abnormal findings in: N/A

CRITICAL FINDINGS: N/A

INTERFERING FACTORS

This procedure is contraindicated for

- Patients with bleeding disorders.
- Patients who are pregnant or suspected of being pregnant, unless the potential benefits of the procedure far outweigh the risks to the fetus and mother.

Factors that may impair clear imaging

- Metallic objects (e.g., jewelry, rings, surgery clips) within the examination field, which may inhibit organ visualization and cause unclear images.
- Inability of the patient to cooperate or remain still during the procedure because of age, significant pain, or mental status.

Other considerations

- Failure to follow dietary restrictions and other pretesting preparations before the procedure may cause the procedure to be canceled or repeated.

R

- Consultation with a health-care provider (HCP) should occur before the procedure for radiation safety concerns regarding younger patients or patients who are lactating.
- Risks associated with radiation overexposure can result from frequent x-ray procedures. Personnel in the room with the patient should wear a protective lead apron, stand behind a shield, or leave the area while the examination is being done. Personnel working in the examination area should wear badges to record their level of radiation exposure.

NURSING IMPLICATIONS AND PROCEDURE

PRETEST:

- Positively identify the patient using at least two unique identifiers before providing care, treatment, or services.
- *Patient Teaching:* Inform the patient this procedure can assist in assessing liver function.
- Obtain a history of the patient's complaints, including a list of known allergens, especially allergies or sensitivities to latex, iodine, seafood, contrast medium, and anesthetics.
- Obtain a history of the patient's hepatobiliary system, symptoms, and results of previously performed laboratory tests and diagnostic and surgical procedures.
- Note any recent procedures that can interfere with test results, including barium examinations.
- Record the date of the last menstrual period and determine the possibility of pregnancy in perimenopausal women.
- Obtain a list of the patient's current medications, including anticoagulant therapy, aspirin and other salicylates, herbs, nutritional supplements, and nutraceuticals, especially those known to affect coagulation (see Appendix F). Such products should be discontinued by medical direction for the appropriate

number of days prior to a surgical procedure. Note the last time and dose of medication taken.

- Review the procedure with the patient. Address concerns about pain related to the procedure and explain that a sedative and/or analgesia will be administered to promote relaxation and reduce discomfort prior to the needle electrode insertion. Explain that any discomfort with the needle electrode will be minimized with local anesthetics and systemic analgesics. Inform the patient that the procedure is performed in the radiology department by an HCP, with support staff, and takes approximately 30 to 90 min.
- Explain that an IV line may be inserted to allow infusion of IV fluids or sedatives. Usually normal saline is infused.
- *Sensitivity to social and cultural issues,* as well as concern for modesty, is important in providing psychological support before, during, and after the procedure.
- Instruct the patient to remove jewelry and other metallic objects from the area to be examined prior to the procedure.
- This procedure may be terminated if chest pain or severe cardiac arrhythmias occur.
- Instruct the patient to fast and restrict fluids for 8 hr prior to the procedure. Instruct the patient to avoid taking anticoagulant medication or to reduce dosage as ordered prior to the procedure. Protocols may vary among facilities.
- *Make sure a written and informed consent has been signed prior to the procedure and before administering any medications.*

INTRATEST:

- Ensure that the patient has complied with dietary, fluid, and medication restrictions and pretesting preparations.
- Ensure that the patient has removed all external metallic objects from the area to be examined prior to the procedure.
- Have emergency equipment readily available.
- If the patient has a history of allergic reactions to any substance or drug,

R

administer ordered prophylactic steroids or antihistamines before the procedure.

▶ Instruct the patient to void and change into the gown, robe, and foot coverings provided.

▶ Instruct the patient to cooperate fully and to follow directions. Instruct the patient to remain still throughout the procedure because movement produces unreliable results.

▶ Record baseline vital signs and assess neurological status. Protocols may vary among facilities.

▶ Observe standard precautions, and follow the general guidelines in Appendix A.

▶ Establish an IV fluid line for the injection of emergency drugs and of sedatives.

▶ Administer an antianxiety agent, as ordered, if the patient has claustrophobia. Administer a sedative to a child or to an uncooperative adult, as ordered.

▶ Place electrocardiographic electrodes on the patient for cardiac monitoring. Establish baseline rhythm; determine if the patient has ventricular arrhythmias.

▶ Place the patient in the supine position on an examination table. Cleanse the selected area, and cover with a sterile drape.

▶ A local anesthetic is injected at the site, and a needle electrode is inserted under ultrasound, CT, or MRI guidance.

▶ A radiofrequency current is passed through the needle electrode, and the tumor is ablated.

▶ Instruct the patient to take slow, deep breaths if nausea occurs during the procedure. Monitor and administer an antiemetic agent if ordered. Ready an emesis basin for use.

▶ The needle electrode is removed, and a pressure dressing is applied over the puncture site.

▶ Observe/assess the needle electrode insertion site for bleeding, inflammation, or hematoma formation.

▶ Monitor the patient for complications related to the procedure (e.g., allergic reaction, anaphylaxis, bronchospasm).

POST-TEST:

▶ A report of the results will be sent to the requesting HCP, who will discuss the results with the patient.

▶ Instruct the patient to resume usual diet, fluids, medications, and activity, as directed by the HCP.

▶ Monitor vital signs and neurological status every 15 min for 1 hr, then every 2 hr for 4 hr, and as ordered. Take temperature every 6 hr for 24 hr. Compare with baseline values. Notify the HCP if temperature is elevated. Protocols may vary among facilities.

▶ Observe for delayed allergic reactions, such as rash, urticaria, tachycardia, hyperpnea, hypertension, palpitations, nausea, or vomiting.

▶ Instruct the patient to immediately report symptoms such as fast heart rate, difficulty breathing, skin rash, itching, chest pain, persistent right shoulder pain, or abdominal pain. Immediately report symptoms to the appropriate HCP.

▶ Instruct the patient to immediately report bile leakage, inflammation, any pleuritic pain, persistent right shoulder pain, or abdominal pain.

▶ Observe/assess the needle electrode insertion site for bleeding, inflammation, or hematoma formation.

▶ Instruct the patient in the care and assessment of the site.

▶ Instruct the patient to apply cold compresses to the puncture site as needed to reduce discomfort or edema.

▶ Instruct the patient to maintain bed rest for 4 to 6 hr after the procedure or as ordered.

▶ Recognize anxiety related to test results, and be supportive of impaired activity related to physical activity. Discuss the implications of abnormal test results on the patient's lifestyle. Provide teaching and information regarding the clinical implications of the test results, as appropriate.

▶ Reinforce information given by the patient's HCP regarding further testing, treatment, or referral to another HCP. Answer any questions or address any concerns voiced by the patient or family.

R

▶ Depending on the results of this procedure, additional testing may be performed to evaluate or monitor progression of the disease process and determine the need for a change in therapy. Evaluate test results in relation to the patient's symptoms and other tests performed.

RELATED MONOGRAPHS:

▶ Related tests include angiography abdomen, AST, biopsy liver, CT liver, MRI abdomen, and US liver and biliary system.
▶ Refer to the Hepatobiliary System table at the end of the book for related tests by body system.

Radiography, Bone

SYNONYM/ACRONYM: Arm x-rays, bone x-rays, leg x-rays, rib x-rays, spine x-rays.

COMMON USE: To assist in evaluating bone pain, trauma, and abnormalities related to disorders or events such as dislocation, fracture, abuse, and degenerative disease.

AREA OF APPLICATION: Skeleton.

CONTRAST: None.

DESCRIPTION: Skeletal x-rays are used to evaluate extremity pain or discomfort due to trauma, bone and spine abnormalities, or fluid within a joint. Serial skeletal x-rays are used to evaluate growth pattern. Radiation emitted from the x-ray machine passes through the patient onto a photographic plate or x-ray film. X-rays pass through air freely and are mostly absorbed by the photographic media. Bones and tissues absorb the x-rays in varying degrees, thereby causing white and shades of gray on the x-ray recording media: Bones are very dense and therefore absorb most of the x-ray and appear white; organs are denser than air but not as dense as bone, so they appear in shades of gray. All metals absorb x-rays. Because the x-ray is absorbed or blocked, metal appears totally white on the film and thus facilitates the search for foreign bodies in the patient.

INDICATIONS
- Assist in detecting bone fracture, dislocation, deformity, and degeneration
- Evaluate for child abuse
- Evaluate growth pattern
- Identify abnormalities of bones, joints, and surrounding tissues
- Monitor fracture healing process

POTENTIAL DIAGNOSIS

Normal findings in
- *Infants and children:* Thin plate of cartilage, known as growth plate or

R

epiphyseal plate, between the shaft and both ends
• *Adolescents and adults:* By age 17, calcification of cartilage plate; no evidence of fracture, congenital abnormalities, tumors, or infection

Abnormal findings in
• Arthritis
• Bone degeneration
• Bone spurs
• Foreign bodies
• Fracture
• Genetic disturbance (achondroplasia, dysplasia, dyostosis)
• Hormonal disturbance
• Infection, including osteomyelitis
• Injury
• Joint dislocation or effusion
• Nutritional or metabolic disturbances
• Osteoporosis or osteopenia
• Soft tissue abnormalities
• Tumor or neoplastic disease (osteogenic sarcoma, Paget's disease, myeloma)

CRITICAL FINDINGS: N/A

INTERFERING FACTORS

This procedure is contraindicated for
• Patients who are pregnant or suspected of being pregnant, unless the potential benefits of the procedure far outweigh the risks to the fetus and mother.

Factors that may impair clear imaging
• Retained barium from a previous radiological procedure.
• Metallic objects (e.g., jewelry, body rings) within the examination field, which may inhibit organ visualization and can produce unclear images.
• Inability of the patient to cooperate or remain still during the procedure because of age, significant pain, or mental status.

Other considerations
• Consultation with a health-care provider (HCP) should occur before the procedure for radiation safety concerns regarding younger patients or patients who are lactating.
• Risks associated with radiation overexposure can result from frequent x-ray procedures. Personnel in the room with the patient should wear a protective lead apron, stand behind a shield, or leave the area while the examination is being done. Personnel working in the examination area should wear badges to record their level of radiation exposure.

NURSING IMPLICATIONS AND PROCEDURE

PRETEST:

▶ Positively identify the patient using at least two unique identifiers before providing care, treatment, or services.
▶ *Patient Teaching:* Inform the patient this procedure can assist in examining bone structure.
▶ Obtain a history of the patient's complaints, including a list of known allergens, especially allergies or sensitivities to latex, iodine, seafood, anesthetics, or contrast medium.
▶ Obtain a history of the patient's musculoskeletal system, symptoms, and results of previously performed laboratory tests and diagnostic and surgical procedures.
▶ Record the date of the last menstrual period and determine the possibility of pregnancy in perimenopausal women.
▶ Obtain a list of the patient's current medications, including herbs, nutritional supplements, and nutraceuticals (see Appendix F).
▶ Review the procedure with the patient. Explain that numerous x-rays may be taken depending on the bones or joint affected. Address concerns about pain and explain that some pain may be experienced during the test, or there

may be moments of discomfort. Inform the patient that the procedure is performed in the radiology department by an HCP, with support staff, and takes approximately 10 to 30 min.

▶ *Sensitivity to social and cultural issues,* as well as concern for modesty, is important in providing psychological support before, during, and after the procedure.

▶ Instruct the patient to inhale deeply and hold his or her breath while the image is taken. Warn the patient that the extremity's position during the procedure may be uncomfortable, but ask the patient to hold very still during the procedure because movement will produce unclear images.

▶ Instruct the patient to remove jewelry and other metallic objects from the area to be examined prior to the procedure.

▶ There are no food, fluid, or medication restrictions unless by medical direction.

INTRATEST:

▶ Ensure that the patient has removed all external metallic objects from the area to be examined prior to the procedure.

▶ Have emergency equipment readily available.

▶ Instruct the patient to void prior to the procedure and to change into the gown, robe, and foot coverings provided.

▶ Observe standard precautions, and follow the general guidelines in Appendix A.

▶ Place patient in a standing, sitting, or recumbent position in front of the image receptor.

▶ Ask the patient to inhale deeply and hold his or her breath while the x-ray images are taken.

▶ Instruct the patient to cooperate fully and to follow directions. Ask the patient

to remain still throughout the procedure because movement produces unreliable results.

POST-TEST:

▶ A report of the examination will be sent to the requesting HCP, who will discuss the results with the patient.

▶ Recognize anxiety related to test results, and be supportive of impaired activity related to the perceived loss of daily function. Discuss the implications of abnormal test results on the patient's lifestyle. Provide teaching and information regarding the clinical implications of the test results, as appropriate.

▶ Reinforce information given by the patient's HCP regarding further testing, treatment, or referral to another HCP. Explain the importance of adhering to the therapy regimen. Answer any questions or address any concerns voiced by the patient or family.

▶ Depending on the results of this procedure, additional testing may be performed to evaluate or monitor progression of the disease process and determine the need for a change in therapy. Evaluate test results in relation to the patient's symptoms and other tests performed.

RELATED MONOGRAPHS:

▶ Related tests include antibodies anti-cyclic citrullinated peptide, ANA, arthrogram, arthroscopy, biopsy bone, BMD, bone scan, calcium, CBC, CRP, collagen cross-linked telopeptides, CT spine, ESR, MRI musculoskeletal, osteocalcin, phosphorus, synovial fluid analysis, RF, vitamin D, and WBC scan.

▶ Refer to the Musculoskeletal System table at the end of the book for related tests by body system.

R

Red Blood Cell Cholinesterase

SYNONYM/ACRONYM: Acetylcholinesterase (AChE), erythrocyte cholinesterase, true cholinesterase.

COMMON USE: To assess for pesticide toxicity and screen for cholinesterase deficiency, which may contribute to unrecoverable apnea after surgical induction with succinylcholine.

SPECIMEN: Whole blood (1 mL) collected in a lavender-top (EDTA) tube.

REFERENCE VALUE: (Method: Spectrophotometry, kinetic)

Test	Conventional Units
RBC cholinesterase	5,300–10,000 international units/L

DESCRIPTION: There are two types of cholinesterase enzyme: *acetylcholinesterase (AChE)*, which is found in red blood cells (RBCs), lung, and brain (nerve) tissue, and cholinesterase, which is mainly found in the plasma, liver, and heart. RBC AChE is highly specific for acetylcholine. Cholinesterase has broader esterolytic activity and is referred to as "pseudocholinesterase." Pseudocholinesterase is the test used to indicate succinylcholine sensitivity (see monograph titled "Pseudocholinesterase and Dibucaine Number"). RBC cholinesterase is used to assist in the diagnosis of chronic carbamate or organophosphate insecticide (e.g., parathion, malathion) toxicity. Organophosphate pesticides bind irreversibly with cholinesterase, inhibiting normal enzyme activity. Carbamate insecticides bind reversibly. Serum or plasma pseudocholinesterase is used more frequently to measure acute pesticide toxicity.

Patients with inherited cholinesterase deficiency are at risk during anesthesia if succinylcholine is administered as an anesthetic. Succinylcholine, a short-acting muscle relaxant, is a reversible inhibitor of acetylcholinesterase and is hydrolyzed by cholinesterase. Succinylcholine-sensitive patients may be unable to metabolize the anesthetic quickly, resulting in prolonged or unrecoverable apnea. This test, along with the pseudocholinesterase test, is also used to identify individuals with atypical forms of the enzyme cholinesterase. The prevalence of succinylcholine sensitivity is 1 in 1,500 patients. Widespread preoperative screening is not routinely performed.

INDICATIONS
- Monitor cumulative exposure to organic phosphate insecticides
- Verify suspected exposure to organic phosphate insecticides

POTENTIAL DIAGNOSIS

Increased in
- Hemolytic anemias (e.g., sickle cell anemia, thalassemias, spherocytosis, and acquired hemolytic anemias) *(increased in hemolytic anemias as AChE is released from the hemolyzed RBCs)*

Decreased in
- Insecticide exposure *(organic phosphate insecticides inhibit AChE activity)*
- Late pregnancy *(related to anemia of pregnancy)*
- Paroxysmal nocturnal hemoglobinuria *(related to lack of RBC production by bone marrow)*
- Relapse of megaloblastic anemia *(related to underproduction of normal RBCs containing AChE)*

CRITICAL FINDINGS: N/A

INTERFERING FACTORS

- Drugs and substances that may increase RBC cholinesterase levels include echothiophate, parathion, and antiepileptic drugs such as carbamazepine, phenobarbital, phenytoin, and valproic acid.
- Improper anticoagulant; fluoride interferes with the measurement and causes a falsely decreased value.

NURSING IMPLICATIONS AND PROCEDURE

PRETEST:

- Positively identify the patient using at least two unique identifiers before providing care, treatment, or services.
- *Patient Teaching:* Inform the patient this test can assist in identification of pesticide poisoning.
- Obtain a history of the patient's complaints, including a list of known allergens, especially allergies or sensitivities to latex. Particularly important to report is exposure to pesticides causing symptoms including blurred vision, muscle weakness, nausea, vomiting, headaches, pulmonary edema, salivation, sweating, or convulsions.
- Obtain a history of exposure to occupational hazards and medication regimen.
- Obtain a history of the patient's hematopoietic system, symptoms, and results of previously performed laboratory tests and diagnostic and surgical procedures.
- Obtain a list of the patient's current medications, including herbs, nutritional supplements, and nutraceuticals (see Appendix F).
- Review the procedure with the patient. Inform the patient that specimen collection takes approximately 5 to 10 min. Address concerns about pain and explain that there may be some discomfort during the venipuncture.
- *Sensitivity to social and cultural issues,* as well as concern for modesty, is important in providing psychological support before, during, and after the procedure.
- There are no food, fluid, or medication restrictions, unless by medical direction.

INTRATEST:

- If the patient has a history of allergic reaction to latex, avoid the use of equipment containing latex.
- Instruct the patient to cooperate fully and to follow directions. Direct the patient to breathe normally and to avoid unnecessary movement.
- Observe standard precautions, and follow the general guidelines in Appendix A. Positively identify the patient, and label the appropriate tubes with the corresponding patient demographics, date, and time of collection. Perform a venipuncture.
- Remove the needle and apply direct pressure with dry gauze to stop bleeding. Observe/assess venipuncture site for bleeding or hematoma formation and secure gauze with adhesive bandage.
- Promptly transport the specimen to the laboratory for processing and analysis.

- A report of the results will be sent to the requesting health-care provider (HCP), who will discuss the results with the patient.
- Reinforce information given by the patient's HCP regarding further testing, treatment, or referral to another HCP. Answer any questions or address any concerns voiced by the patient or family.
- Depending on the results of this procedure, additional testing may be performed to evaluate or monitor progression of the disease process and determine the need for a change in therapy. Evaluate test results in relation to the patient's symptoms and other tests performed.

RELATED MONOGRAPHS:

- Related tests include biopsy bone marrow, CBC, CBC RBC indices, CBC RBC morphology, Ham's test, pseudocholinesterase, sickle cell screen, and vitamin B_{12}.
- Refer to the Hematopoietic System table at the end of the book for related tests by body system.

Refraction

SYNONYM/ACRONYM: N/A.

COMMON USE: To assess the visual acuity of the eyes to assist in evaluating the eyes prior to therapeutic interventions such as LASIK surgery.

AREA OF APPLICATION: Eyes.

CONTRAST: N/A.

DESCRIPTION: This noninvasive procedure tests the visual acuity (VA) of the eyes and determines abnormalities or refractive errors that need correction. Refractions are performed using a combination of different pieces of equipment. Refractive error can be quickly and accurately measured using computerized automatic refractors or manually with a viewing system consisting of an entire set of trial lenses mounted on a circular wheel (phoropter). A projector may also be used to display test letters and characters for use in assessing VA. If the VA is worse than 20/20, the pinhole test may be used to quickly assess the best corrected vision. Refractive errors of the peripheral cornea and lens can be reduced or eliminated by having the patient look through a pinhole at the vision test. Patients with cataracts or visual field defects will not show improved results using the pinhole test. The retinoscope is probably the most valuable instrument that can be used to objectively assess VA. It is also the only objective means of assessing refractive error in pediatric patients and patients who are unable to cooperate with other techniques of assessing refractive error due to illiteracy, senility, or inability to speak the same language as the examiner. Visual defects identified through refraction, such as hyperopia (farsightedness), in which the point of focus lies behind the

R

retina; myopia (nearsightedness), in which the point of focus lies in front of the retina; and astigmatism, in which the refraction is unequal in different curvatures of the eyeball, can be corrected by glasses, contact lenses, or refractive surgery.

INDICATIONS

• Determine if an optical defect is present and if light rays entering the eye focus correctly on the retina
• Determine the refractive error prior to refractive surgery such as radial keratotomy (RK), photorefractive keratotomy (PRK), laser assisted in situ keratomileusis (LASIK), intracorneal rings (Intacs), limbal relaxing incisions (LRI), implantable contact lens (phakic IOL), clear lens replacement
• Determine the type of corrective lenses (e.g., biconvex or plus lenses for hyperopia, biconcave or minus lenses for myopia, compensatory lenses for astigmatism) needed for refractive errors
• Diagnose refractive errors in vision

POTENTIAL DIAGNOSIS

Visual Acuity Scale

Foot	Meter	Decimal
20/200	6/60	0.1
20/160	6/48	0.13
20/120	6/36	0.17
20/100	6/30	0.2
20/80	6/24	0.25
20/60	6/18	0.33
20/50	6/15	0.4
20/40	6/12	0.5
20/30	6/9	0.67
20/25	6/7.5	0.8
20/20	6/6	1
20/16	6/4.8	1.25
20/12	6/3.6	1.67
20/10	6/3	2

VA can be expressed fractionally in feet, fractionally in meters, or as a decimal where perfect vision of 20/20 feet or 6/6 meters is equal to 1. A patient who cannot achieve best corrected VA of 20/200 or above in his or her better eye is considered legally blind in the United States. Comparing the fraction in feet or meters to the decimal helps demonstrate that "less than" 20/20 is "worse" vision, while acuity "greater than" 20/20 is "better."

Normal findings in
• Normal visual acuity; 20/20 (with corrective lenses if appropriate).

Uncorrected Visual Acuity	Foot	Meter	Decimal
Mild vision loss	20/30–20/70	6/9–6/21	0.67–0.29
Moderate vision loss	20/80–20/160	6/24–6/48	0.25–0.13
Severe vision loss	20/200–20/400	6/60–6/120	0.1–0.05
Profound vision loss	20/500–20/1,000	6/150–6/300	0.04–0.02

Abnormal findings in
- Refractive errors such as astigmatism, hyperopia, and myopia.

CRITICAL FINDINGS: N/A

INTERFERING FACTORS

This procedure is contraindicated for
- Patients with narrow-angle glaucoma if pupil dilation is performed because dilation can initiate a severe and sight-threatening open-angle attack.
- Patients with allergies to mydriatics if pupil dilation using mydriatics is performed.

Factors that may impair clear imaging
- Improper pupil dilation may prevent adequate examination for refractive error.
- Inability of the patient to cooperate and remain still during the procedure because of age, significant pain, or mental status may interfere with the test results.
- Failure to follow medication restrictions before the procedure may cause the procedure to be canceled or repeated.

NURSING IMPLICATIONS AND PROCEDURE

PRETEST:
- Positively identify the patient using at least two unique identifiers before providing care, treatment, or services.

- *Patient Teaching:* Inform the patient this procedure can assist in assessing visual acuity.
- Obtain a history of the patient's complaints, including a list of known allergens, especially mydriatics if dilation is to be performed.
- Obtain a history of the patient's known or suspected vision loss; changes in visual acuity, including type and cause; use of glasses or contact lenses; eye conditions with treatment regimens; eye surgery; and other tests and procedures to assess and diagnose visual deficit.
- Obtain a history of symptoms and results of previously performed laboratory tests and diagnostic and surgical procedures.
- Obtain a list of the patient's current medications, including herbs, nutritional supplements, and nutraceuticals (see Appendix F).
- Instruct the patient to remove contact lenses or glasses, as appropriate. Instruct the patient regarding the importance of keeping the eyes open for the test.
- Review the procedure with the patient. Address concerns about pain and explain that mydriatics, if used, may cause blurred vision and sensitivity to light. There may also be a brief stinging sensation when the drop is put in the eye. Inform the patient that a health-care provider (HCP) performs the test, in a quiet, darkened room, and that to evaluate both eyes, the test can take up 30 min (including time for the pupils to dilate before the test is actually performed).
- *Sensitivity to social and cultural issues,* as well as concern for modesty, is important in providing psychological

support before, during, and after the procedure.

▸ There are no food or fluid restrictions unless by medical direction.

▸ The patient should withhold eye medications (particularly mydriatic eyedrops if the patient has glaucoma) for at least 1 day prior to the test.

▸ Ensure that the patient understands that he or she must refrain from driving until the pupils return to normal (about 4 hours) after the test and has made arrangements to have someone else be responsible for transportation after the test.

INTRATEST:

▸ Ensure that the patient has complied with medication restrictions and pre-testing preparations; assure that eye medications, especially mydriatics, have been restricted for at least 1 day prior to the procedure.

▸ Instruct the patient to cooperate fully and to follow directions. Ask the patient to remain still during the procedure because movement produces unreliable results.

▸ If dilation is to be performed, administer the ordered mydriatic to each eye and repeat in 5 to 15 min. Drops are placed in the eye with the patient looking up and the solution directed at the six o'clock position of the sclera (white of the eye) near the limbus (gray, semitransparent area of the eyeball where the cornea and sclera meet). The dropper bottle should not touch the eyelashes.

▸ Ask the patient to place the chin in the chin rest and gently press the forehead against the support bar. The examiner will sit about 2 ft away at eye level with the patient. The retinascope light is held in front of the eyes and directed through the pupil. Each eye is also examined for the characteristics of the red reflex, the reflection of the light from the retinascope, which normally moves in the same direction as the light.

▸ Request that the patient look straight ahead while the eyes are examined with the instrument and while different lenses are tried to provide the best corrective lenses to be prescribed. When optimal VA is obtained with the trial lenses in each eye, a prescription for corrective lenses is written.

POST-TEST:

▸ A report of the results will be sent to the requesting HCP, who will discuss the results with the patient.

▸ Instruct the patient to resume usual medications, as directed by the HCP.

▸ Recognize anxiety related to test results, and be supportive of impaired activity related to vision loss, anticipated loss of driving privileges, or the possibility of requiring corrective lenses (self-image). Discuss the implications of abnormal test results on the patient's lifestyle. Provide teaching and information regarding the clinical implications of the test results, as appropriate. Provide contact information, if desired, for a general patient education Web site on the topic of eye care (e.g., www.allaboutvision.com).

▸ Reinforce information given by the patient's HCP regarding further testing, treatment, or referral to another HCP. Inform the patient that visual acuity and responses to light may change. Suggest that the patient wear dark glasses after the test until the pupils return to normal size. Answer any questions or address any concerns voiced by the patient or family.

▸ Depending on the results of this procedure, additional testing may be performed to evaluate or monitor progression of the disease process and determine the need for a change in therapy. Evaluate test results in relation to the patient's symptoms and other tests performed.

RELATED MONOGRAPHS:

▸ Related tests include color perception test, intraocular muscle function, intraocular pressure, Schirmer tear test, and slit-lamp biomicroscopy.

▸ Refer to the Ocular System table at the end of the book for related tests by body system.

R

Renin

SYNONYM/ACRONYM: Plasma renin activity (PRA).

COMMON USE: To assist in evaluating for a possible cause of hypertension.

SPECIMEN: Plasma (3 mL) collected in a lavender-top (EDTA) tube.

REFERENCE VALUE: (Method: Radioimmunoassay)

Age and Position	Conventional Units	SI Units (Conventional Units × 1)
Newborn–12 mo Supine, normal sodium diet	2.0–35.0 ng/mL/hr	2.0–35.0 mcg/L/hr
1–3 yr	1.7–11.2 ng/mL/hr	1.7–11.2 mcg/L/hr
4–5 yr	1.0–6.5 ng/mL/hr	1.0–6.5 mcg/L/hr
6–10 yr	0.5–5.9 ng/mL/hr	0.5–5.9 mcg/L/hr
11–15 yr	0.5–3.3 ng/mL/hr	0.5–3.3 mcg/L/hr
Adult	0.2–2.3 ng/mL/hr	0.2–2.3 mcg/L/hr
Upright, normal sodium diet Adult–older adult	1.3–4.0 ng/mL/hr	1.3–4.0 mcg/L/hr

Values vary according to the laboratory performing the test, as well as the patient's age, gender, dietary pattern, state of hydration, posture, and physical activity.

DESCRIPTION: Renin is an enzyme that activates the renin-angiotensin system. It is released into the renal veins by the juxtaglomerular cells of the kidney in response to sodium depletion and hypovolemia. Renin converts angiotensinogen to angiotensin I. Angiotensin I is converted to angiotensin II, the biologically active form. Angiotensin II is a powerful vasoconstrictor that stimulates aldosterone production in the adrenal cortex. Angiotensin II and aldosterone increase blood pressure. Excessive amounts of angiotensin II cause renal hypertension. The renin assay screens for essential, renal, or renovascular hypertension.

Plasma renin is expressed as the rate of angiotensin I formation per unit of time. The random collection of specimens without prior dietary preparations does not provide clinically significant information. Values should also be evaluated along with simultaneously collected aldosterone levels (see monographs titled "Aldosterone" and "Angiotensin-Converting Enzyme").

INDICATIONS

• Assist in the identification of primary hyperaldosteronism resulting from aldosterone-secreting adrenal adenoma

- Assist in monitoring patients on mineralocorticoid therapy
- Assist in the screening of the origin of essential, renal, or renovascular hypertension

POTENTIAL DIAGNOSIS

Increased in
- Addison's disease *(related to hyponatremia, which stimulates production of renin)*
- Bartter's syndrome *(related to hereditary defect in loop of Henle that affects sodium resorption; hyponatremia stimulates renin production)*
- Cirrhosis *(related to fluid buildup, which dilutes sodium concentration; hyponatremia is a strong stimulus for production of renin)*
- Congestive heart failure *(related to fluid buildup, which dilutes sodium concentration; hyponatremia is a strong stimulus for production of renin)*
- Gastrointestinal disorders with electrolyte loss *(related to hyponatremia, which stimulates production of renin)*
- Hepatitis *(related to fluid buildup, which dilutes sodium concentration; hyponatremia is a strong stimulus for production of renin)*
- Hypokalemia *(related to decreased potassium levels, which stimulate renin production)*
- Malignant hypertension *(related to secondary hyperaldosteronism that constricts the blood vessels and results in hypertension)*
- Nephritis *(the kidneys can produce renin in response to inflammation or disease)*
- Nephropathies with sodium or potassium wasting *(related to hyponatremia, which stimulates production of renin)*

- Pheochromocytoma *(related to renin production in response to hypertension)*
- Pregnancy *(related to retention of fluid and hyponatremia that stimulates renin production; normal pregnancy is associated with changes in the balance between renin and angiotensin)*
- Renin-producing renal tumors
- Renovascular hypertension *(related to decreased renal blood flow, which stimulates release of renin)*

Decreased in
- Cushing's syndrome *(related to excessive production of glucocorticoids, which increase sodium levels and decrease potassium levels, inhibiting renin production)*
- Primary hyperaldosteronism *(related to aldosterone-secreting adrenal tumor; aldosterone inhibits renin production)*

CRITICAL FINDINGS: N/A

INTERFERING FACTORS

- Drugs that may increase renin levels include albuterol, amiloride, azosemide, benazepril, bendroflumethiazide, captopril, chlorthalidone, cilazapril, cromakalim, desmopressin, diazoxide, dihydralazine, doxazosin, enalapril, endralazine, felodipine, fenoldopam, fosinopril, furosemide, hydralazine, hydrochlorothiazide, laxatives, lisinopril, lithium, methyclothiazide, metolazone, muzolimine, nicardipine, nifedipine, opiates, oral contraceptives, perindopril, ramipril, spironolactone, triamterene, and xipamide.
- Drugs and substances that may decrease renin levels include acetylsalicylic acid, angiotensin, angiotensin II, atenolol, bopindolol,

R

bucindolol, carbenoxolone, carve-dilol, clonidine, cyclosporin A, dexfenfluramine, glycyrrhiza, ibu-profen, indomethacin, levodopa, metoprolol, naproxen, nicardipine, nonsteroidal anti-inflammatory drugs, oral contraceptives, oxpre-nolol, propranolol, sulindax, and vasopressin.

• Upright body posture, stress, and strenuous exercise can increase renin levels.

• Recent radioactive scans or radia-tion can interfere with test results when radioimmunoassay is the test method.

• Diet can significantly affect results (e.g., low-sodium diets stimulate the release of renin).

• Hyperkalemia, acute increase in blood pressure, and increased blood volume may suppress renin secretion.

• Failure to follow dietary restrictions before the procedure may cause the procedure to be canceled or repeated.

NURSING IMPLICATIONS AND PROCEDURE

PRETEST:

▸ Positively identify the patient using at least two unique identifiers before pro-viding care, treatment, or services.

▸ *Patient Teaching:* Inform the patient this test can assist in evaluating for high blood pressure.

▸ Obtain a history of the patient's complaints, including a list of known allergens, especially allergies or sensitivities to latex.

▸ Obtain a history of the patient's endocrine and genitourinary systems, symptoms, and results of previously performed laboratory tests and diagnostic and surgical procedures.

▸ Note any recent procedures that can interfere with test results.

▸ Obtain a list of the patient's current medications, including herbs, nutritional supplements, and nutraceuticals (see Appendix F).

▸ Review the procedure with the patient. Inform the patient or family member that the position required (supine or upright) must be maintained for 2 hr before specimen collection. Inform the patient that multiple specimens may be required. Inform the patient that speci-men collection takes approximately 5 to 10 min. Address concerns about pain and explain that there may be some discomfort during the venipuncture.

▸ *Sensitivity to social and cultural issues,* as well as concern for modesty, is impor-tant in providing psychological support before, during, and after the procedure.

▸ The patient should be on a normal sodium diet (1 to 2 g sodium per day) for 2 to 4 wk before the test. Protocols may vary among facilities.

▸ By medical direction, the patient should avoid diuretics, antihypertensive drugs, herbals, cyclic progestogens, and estrogens for 2 to 4 wk before the test.

▸ Prepare an ice slurry in a cup or plastic bag to have ready for immediate trans-port of the specimen to the laboratory.

INTRATEST:

▸ Ensure that the patient has complied with diet and medication restrictions and pretesting dietary preparations; ensure that specific medications have been restricted for at least 2 to 4 wk prior to the procedure.

▸ If the patient has a history of allergic reaction to latex, avoid the use of equipment containing latex.

▸ Instruct the patient to cooperate fully and to follow directions. Direct the patient to breathe normally and to avoid unnecessary movement.

▸ Observe standard precautions, and follow the general guidelines in Appendix A. Positively identify the patient, and label the appropriate tubes with the corresponding patient demographics, date, and time of collection. Specify patient position (upright or supine) and exact source of specimen (peripheral vs. arterial). Perform a venipuncture after the patient has been in the upright (sitting or standing) position for 2 hr. If a supine specimen is requested on an inpatient, the specimen should be collected early in the morning before the patient rises.

▸ Remove the needle and apply direct pressure with dry gauze to stop bleeding. Observe/assess venipuncture site for bleeding or hematoma formation and secure gauze with adhesive bandage.

▸ The sample should be placed in an ice slurry immediately after collection. Information on the specimen label should be protected from water in the ice slurry by first placing the specimen in a protective plastic bag. Promptly transport the specimen to the laboratory for processing and analysis.

POST-TEST:

▸ A report of the results will be sent to the requesting health-care provider (HCP), who will discuss the results with the patient.

▸ Instruct the patient to resume usual medications, as directed by the HCP.

▸ *Nutritional Considerations:* Instruct the patient to notify the requesting HCP of any signs and symptoms of dehydration or fluid overload related to abnormal renin levels or compromised sodium regulatory mechanisms. Fluid loss or dehydration is signaled by the thirst response. Decreased skin turgor, dry mouth, and multiple longitudinal furrows in the tongue are symptoms of dehydration. Fluid overload may be signaled by a loss of appetite and nausea. Excessive fluid also causes pitting edema: When firm pressure is placed on the skin over a bone (e.g., the ankle), the indentation will remain after 5 sec.

▸ *Nutritional Considerations:* Educate patients of the importance of proper water balance. Adults should consume six to eight 8-oz of water per day or the equivalent of half of the body's weight in fluid ounces (32 oz = 1 qt; 34 fl oz = 1 L); infants need more because their basal metabolic heat production is much higher. In buildings with hard water, untreated tap water contains minerals such as calcium, magnesium, and iron. Water-softening systems replace these minerals with sodium, and therefore patients on a low-sodium diet should avoid drinking treated tap water and drink bottled water instead.

▸ *Nutritional Considerations:* Renin levels affect the regulation of fluid balance and electrolytes. If appropriate, educate patients with low sodium levels that the major source of dietary sodium is found in table salt. Many foods, such as milk and other dairy products, are also good sources of dietary sodium. Most other dietary sodium is available through the consumption of processed foods. Patients on low-sodium diets should be advised to avoid beverages such as colas, ginger ale, sports drinks, lemon-lime sodas, and root beer. Many over-the-counter medications, including antacids, laxatives, analgesics, sedatives, and antitussives, contain significant amounts of sodium. The best advice is to emphasize the importance of reading all food, beverage, and medicine labels. In 2004, the Institute of Medicine's Food and Nutrition Board established 2,300 mg as the recommended maximum daily intake of dietary sodium for adults and 1,900 mg/day for children. The requesting HCP or nutritionist should be consulted before the patient on a low-sodium diet begins using salt substitutes. In 2004, the Institute of Medicine's Food and Nutrition Board established 4.7 g as the recommended maximum daily intake of dietary potassium for adults and 3.8 g/day for children. Potassium is present in all plant and animal cells, making dietary replacement fairly simple to achieve.

▸ Reinforce information given by the patient's HCP regarding further testing, treatment, or referral to another HCP. Answer any questions or address any concerns voiced by the patient or family.

▸ Depending on the results of this procedure, additional testing may be performed to evaluate or monitor progression of the disease process and determine the need for a change in therapy. Evaluate test results in relation to the patient's symptoms and other tests performed.

R

Renogram

SYNONYM/ACRONYM: Radioactive renogram, renocystography, renocystogram, renal scintigraphy.

COMMON USE: To assist in diagnosing renal disorders such as embolism, obstruction, infection, inflammation, trauma, stones, and bleeding.

AREA OF APPLICATION: Kidneys.

CONTRAST: IV radioactive material.

DESCRIPTION: A renogram is a nuclear medicine study performed to assist in diagnosing renal disorders, such as abnormal blood flow, collecting-system defects, and excretion dysfunction. Because renography uses no iodinated contrast medium, it is safe to use in patients who have iodine allergies or compromised renal function.

After IV administration of the radioisotope, information about the structures of the kidneys is obtained. The radioactive material is detected by a gamma camera, which can detect the gamma rays emitted by the radionuclide in the kidney. Renography simultaneously tracks the rate at which the radionuclide flows into *(vascular phase)*, through *(tubular phase)*, and out of *(excretory phase)* the kidneys. The times are plotted on a graph and compared to normal parameters of organ function. Differential estimates of left and right kidney contributions to glomerular filtration rate and effective renal plasma flow can be calculated. With the use of diuretic stimulation during the excretory phase, it is possible to differentiate between anatomic obstruction and non-obstructive residual dilation from previous hydronephrosis. All information obtained is stored in a computer to be used for further interpretation and computations. Renal function can be monitored by serially repeating this test and comparing results.

INDICATIONS

- Aid in the diagnosis of renal artery embolism or renal infarction causing obstruction
- Aid in the diagnosis of renal artery stenosis resulting from renal dysplasia or atherosclerosis and causing arterial hypertension and reduced glomerular filtration rate
- Aid in the diagnosis of renal vein thrombosis resulting from dehydration in infants or obstruction of blood flow in the presence of renal tumors in adults
- Detect renal infectious or inflammatory diseases, such as acute or chronic pyelonephritis, renal abscess, or nephritis
- Determine the presence and effects of renal trauma, such as arterial injury, renal contusion, hematoma, rupture, arteriovenous fistula, or urinary extravasation
- Determine the presence, location, and cause of obstructive uropathy, such as calculi, neoplasm, congenital disorders, scarring, or inflammation
- Evaluate acute and chronic renal failure
- Evaluate chronic urinary tract infections, especially in children
- Evaluate kidney transplant for acute or chronic rejection
- Evaluate obstruction caused by stones or tumor

POTENTIAL DIAGNOSIS

Normal findings in

- Normal shape, size, position, symmetry, vasculature, perfusion, and function of the kidneys
- Radionuclide material circulates bilaterally, symmetrically, and without interruption through the renal parenchyma, ureters, and urinary bladder, with 50% of the radionuclide excreted within the first 10 min

Abnormal findings in

- Acute tubular necrosis
- Congenital anomalies (e.g., absence of a kidney)
- Decreased renal function
- Diminished blood supply
- Infection or inflammation (pyelonephritis, glomerulonephritis)
- Masses
- Obstructive uropathy
- Renal failure, infarction, cyst, or abscess
- Renal vascular disease, including renal artery stenosis or renal vein thrombosis
- Trauma

CRITICAL FINDINGS: N/A

INTERFERING FACTORS

This procedure is contraindicated for

- Patients who are pregnant or suspected of being pregnant, unless the potential benefits of the procedure far outweigh the risks to the fetus and mother.

Factors that may impair clear imaging

- Inability of the patient to cooperate or remain still during the procedure because of age, significant pain, or mental status.
- Serum creatinine levels greater than or equal to 3 mg/dL (depending on the radionuclide used), which can decrease renal perfusion.
- Other nuclear medicine studies done within the previous 24 to 48 hr.
- Medications such as antihypertensives, angiotensin-converting enzyme (ACE) inhibitors, and β-blockers taken within 24 hr of the test.
- Dehydration, which can accentuate abnormalities, or overhydration, which can mask abnormalities.

R

• Metallic objects (e.g., jewelry, body rings) within the examination field, which may inhibit organ visualization.

Other considerations

• Consultation with a health-care provider (HCP) should occur before the procedure for radiation safety concerns regarding younger patients or patients who are lactating.

• Risks associated with radiation overexposure can result from frequent x-ray or radionuclide procedures. Personnel working in the examination area should wear badges to record their level of radiation exposure.

• Inaccurate timing of imaging after the radionuclide injection can affect the results.

NURSING IMPLICATIONS AND PROCEDURE

PRETEST:

▸ Positively identify the patient using at least two unique identifiers before providing care, treatment, or services.

▸ *Patient Teaching:* Inform the patient this procedure can assist in assessing the renal system.

▸ Obtain a history of the patient's complaints, including a list of known allergens, especially allergies or sensitivities to latex, iodine, seafood, anesthetics, or contrast medium.

▸ Obtain a history of the patient's genitourinary system, symptoms, and results of previously performed laboratory tests and diagnostic and surgical procedures.

▸ Record the date of the last menstrual period and determine the possibility of pregnancy in perimenopausal women.

▸ Obtain a list of the patient's current medications, including herbs, nutritional supplements, and nutraceuticals (see Appendix F).

▸ Review the procedure with the patient. Address concerns about pain related to the procedure and explain that some pain may be experienced during the test, and there may be moments of discomfort. Reassure the patient that radioactive material poses minimal radioactive hazard because of its short half-life and rarely produces side effects. Inform the patient that the procedure is performed in a nuclear medicine department by an HCP and usually takes approximately 60 to 90 min, and that delayed images are needed 2 to 24 hr later. The patient may leave the department and return later to undergo delayed imaging.

▸ *Sensitivity to social and cultural issues,* as well as concern for modesty, is important in providing psychological support before, during, and after the procedure.

▸ Instruct the patient to remove jewelry and other metallic objects from the area to be examined prior to the procedure.

▸ Inform the patient that he or she will be asked to drink several glasses of fluid before the study for hydration, unless the patient has a restricted fluid intake for other reasons.

▸ There are no food or medication restrictions unless by medical direction.

INTRATEST:

▸ Ensure that the patient has removed external metallic objects from the area to be examined prior to the procedure.

▸ Instruct the patient to void and change into the gown, robe, and foot coverings provided.

▸ Observe standard precautions, and follow the general guidelines in Appendix A.

▸ Administer sedative to a child or to an uncooperative adult, as ordered.

▸ Place the patient in a supine position on a flat table with foam wedges to help maintain position and immobilization.

▸ The radionuclide is administered IV, and the kidney area is scanned immediately with images taken every minute for 30 min.

- During the flow and static imaging, the diuretic furosemide (Lasix) or ACE inhibitor (captopril) can be administered IV and images obtained.
- Urine and blood laboratory studies are done after the renogram to correlate findings before diagnosis.
- If a study for vesicoureteral reflux is done, the patient is asked to void, and a catheter is inserted into the bladder. The radionuclide is instilled into the bladder, and multiple images are obtained during bladder filling. The patient is then requested to void, with the catheter in place or after catheter removal, depending on department policy. Imaging is continued during and after voiding. Reflux is determined by calculating the urine volume and counts obtained by imaging.
- Gloves should be worn during the radionuclide administration and while handling the patient's urine.
- Remove the needle or catheter and apply a pressure dressing over the puncture site.
- Observe/assess the needle/catheter insertion site for bleeding, inflammation, or hematoma formation.

- A report of the results will be sent to the requesting HCP, who will discuss the results with the patient.
- Unless contraindicated, advise patient to drink increased amounts of fluids for 24 hr to eliminate the radionuclide from the body. Inform the patient that radionuclide is eliminated from the body within 6 to 24 hr.
- Instruct the patient to immediately flush the toilet and to meticulously wash hands with soap and water after each voiding for 24 hr after the procedure.
- Instruct all caregivers to wear gloves when discarding urine for 24 hr after

the procedure. Wash gloved hands with soap and water before removing gloves. Then wash ungloved hands after the gloves are removed.
- Observe/assess the needle/catheter site for bleeding, hematoma formation, and inflammation.
- Instruct the patient in the care and assessment of the site.
- Instruct the patient to apply cold compresses to the puncture site as needed to reduce discomfort or edema.
- Recognize anxiety related to test results. Discuss the implications of abnormal test results on the patient's lifestyle. Provide teaching and information regarding the clinical importance of the test results, as appropriate.
- Reinforce information given by the patient's HCP regarding further testing, treatment, or referral to another HCP. Answer any questions or address any concerns voiced by the patient or family.
- Depending on the results of this procedure, additional testing may be needed to evaluate or monitor progression of the disease process and determine the need for a change in therapy. Evaluate test results in relation to the patient's symptoms and other tests performed.

- Related tests include angiography renal, antibodies anti-glomerular basement membrane, biopsy kidney, bladder cancer markers, BUN, calculus kidney stone panel, C4, CT abdomen, CT pelvis, CT renal, creatinine, creatinine clearance, cystoscopy, IVP, KUB studies, MRA, MRI abdomen, retrograde ureteropyelography, strep group A, US kidney, and UA.
- Refer to the Genitourinary System table at the end of the book for related tests by body system.

R

Reticulocyte Count

SYNONYM/ACRONYM: Retic count.

COMMON USE: To assess reticulocyte count in relation to bone marrow activity to assist in diagnosing anemias such as pernicious, iron deficiency, and hemolytic; to monitor response of therapeutic interventions.

SPECIMEN: Whole blood (1 mL) collected in a lavender-top (EDTA) tube.

REFERENCE VALUE: (Method: Microscopic examination of specially stained peripheral blood smear or automated analyzer)

Age	Total Erythrocyte Count*
Newborn	3%–7%
1–12 mo	0.2%–2.8%
Adult–older adult	1.5%–2.5%

*Values are expressed as percentage of the red blood cell count.

DESCRIPTION: Normally, as it matures, the red blood cell (RBC) loses its nucleus. The remaining ribonucleic acid (RNA) produces a characteristic color when special stains are used, making these cells easy to identify and enumerate. The presence of reticulocytes is an indication of the level of erythropoietic activity in the bone marrow. In abnormal conditions, reticulocytes are prematurely released into circulation. (See monographs titled "Complete Blood Count, RBC Count" and "Complete Blood Count, RBC Morphology and Inclusions.")

production. The calculation corrects the count for anemia and for the premature release of reticulocytes into the peripheral blood during periods of hemolysis or significant bleeding. The RPI also takes into consideration the maturation time of large polychromatophilic cells or nucleated RBCs seen on the peripheral smear:

$$RPI = \% \text{ reticulocytes} \times [\text{patient hematocrit (Hct)/normal Hct}] \times (1/\text{maturation time})$$

As the formula shows, the RPI is inversely proportional to Hct, as follows:

INDICATIONS
- Evaluate erythropoietic activity
- Monitor response to therapy for anemias

POTENTIAL DIAGNOSIS
The reticulocyte production index (RPI) is a good estimate of RBC

Hematocrit (%)	Maturation Time (days)
45	1.0
35	1.5
25	2.0
15	2.5

Increased in

Conditions that result in excessive RBC loss or destruction stimulate a compensatory bone marrow response by increasing production of RBCs.

- Blood loss
- Hemolytic anemias
- Iron-deficiency anemia
- Megaloblastic anemia

Decreased in

- Alcoholism *(decreased production related to nutritional deficit)*
- Anemia of chronic disease
- Aplastic anemia *(related to overall lack of RBC)*
- Bone marrow replacement *(new marrow fails to produce RBCs until it engrafts)*
- Endocrine disease *(hypometabolism related to hypothyroidism is reflected by decreased bone marrow activity)*
- RBC aplasia *(related to overall lack of RBCs)*
- Renal disease *(diseased kidneys cannot produce erythropoietin, which stimulates the bone marrow to produce RBCs)*
- Sideroblastic anemia *(RBCs are produced but are abnormal in that they cannot incorporate iron into hemoglobin, resulting in anemia)*

CRITICAL FINDINGS: N/A

INTERFERING FACTORS

- Drugs that may increase reticulocyte counts include acetanilid, acetylsalicylic acid, amyl nitrate, antimalarials, antipyretics, antipyrine, arsenicals, corticotropin, dimercaprol, etretinate, furaltadone, furazolidone, levodopa, methyldopa, nitrofurans, penicillin, procainamide, and sulfones.

- Drugs that may decrease reticulocyte counts include azathioprine, dactinomycin, hydroxyurea, methotrexate, and zidovudine.
- Reticulocyte count may be falsely increased by the presence of RBC inclusions (Howell-Jolly bodies, Heinz bodies, and Pappenheimer bodies) that stain with methylene blue.
- Reticulocyte count may be falsely decreased as a result of the dilutional effect after a recent blood transfusion.
- Specimens that are clotted or hemolyzed should be rejected for analysis.

NURSING IMPLICATIONS AND PROCEDURE

PRETEST:

- Positively identify the patient using at least two unique identifiers before providing care, treatment, or services.
- *Patient Teaching:* Inform the patient this test can assist in assessing for anemia.
- Obtain a history of the patient's complaints, including a list of known allergens, especially allergies or sensitivities to latex.
- Obtain a history of the patient's hematopoietic system, symptoms, and results of previously performed laboratory tests and diagnostic and surgical procedures.
- Note any recent procedures that can interfere with test results.
- Obtain a list of the patient's current medications, including herbs, nutritional supplements, and nutraceuticals (see Appendix F).
- Review the procedure with the patient. Inform the patient that specimen collection takes approximately 5 to 10 min. Address concerns about pain and explain that there may be some discomfort during the venipuncture.
- *Sensitivity to social and cultural issues,* as well as concern for modesty, is important in providing psychological

R

support before, during, and after the procedure.

▶ There are no food, fluid, or medication restrictions unless by medical direction.

INTRATEST:

▶ If the patient has a history of allergic reaction to latex, avoid the use of equipment containing latex.

▶ Instruct the patient to cooperate fully and to follow directions. Direct the patient to breathe normally and to avoid unnecessary movement.

▶ Observe standard precautions, and follow the general guidelines in Appendix A. Positively identify the patient, and label the appropriate tubes with the corresponding patient demographics, date, and time of collection. Perform a venipuncture.

▶ Remove the needle and apply direct pressure with dry gauze to stop bleeding. Observe/asses venipuncture site for bleeding or hematoma formation and secure gauze with adhesive bandage.

▶ Promptly transport the specimen to the laboratory for processing and analysis.

POST-TEST:

▶ A report of the results will be sent to the requesting health-care provider

(HCP), who will discuss the results with the patient.

▶ Reinforce information given by the patient's HCP regarding further testing, treatment, or referral to another HCP. Answer any questions or address any concerns voiced by the patient or family.

▶ Depending on the results of this procedure, additional testing may be performed to evaluate or monitor progression of the disease process and determine the need for a change in therapy. Evaluate test results in relation to the patient's symptoms and other tests performed.

RELATED MONOGRAPHS:

▶ Related tests include biopsy bone marrow, complement, CBC, CBC hematocrit, CBC hemoglobin, CBC RBC count, CBC RBC indices, CBC RBC morphology, Coomb's antiglobulin direct and indirect, erythropoietin, iron/TIBC, ferritin, folate, G6PD, Ham's test, Hgb electrophoresis, lead, osmotic fragility, PK, sickle cell screen, and vitamin B_{12}.

▶ Refer to the Hematopoietic System table at the end of the book for related tests by body system.

Retrograde Ureteropyelography

SYNONYM/ACRONYM: Retrograde.

COMMON USE: To assess the urinary tract for trauma, obstruction, stones, infection, and abscess that can interfere with function.

AREA OF APPLICATION: Renal calyces, ureter.

CONTRAST: Radiopaque iodine-based contrast medium.

DESCRIPTION: Retrograde ureteropyelography uses a contrast medium introduced through a ureteral catheter during cystography and radiographic visualization to view the renal collecting system (calyces, renal pelvis, and urethra). During a cystoscopic examination, a catheter is advanced through the ureters and into the kidney; contrast medium is injected through the catheter into the kidney. This procedure is primarily used in patients who are known to be hypersensitive to IV injected iodine-based contrast medium and when excretory ureterography does not adequately reveal the renal collecting system. The incidence of allergic reaction to the contrast medium is reduced because there is less systemic absorption of the contrast medium when injected into the kidney than when injected IV. Retrograde ureteropyelography sometimes provides more information about the anatomy of the different parts of the collecting system than can be obtained by excretory ureteropyelography. The procedure is not hampered by impaired renal function, but it carries the risk of urinary tract infection and sepsis.

INDICATIONS

- Evaluate the effects of urinary system trauma
- Evaluate known or suspected ureteral obstruction
- Evaluate placement of a ureteral stent or catheter
- Evaluate the presence of calculi in the kidneys, ureters, or bladder
- Evaluate the renal collecting system when excretory urography is unsuccessful
- Evaluate space-occupying lesions or congenital anomalies of the urinary system
- Evaluate the structure and integrity of the renal collecting system

POTENTIAL DIAGNOSIS

Normal findings in
- Normal outline and opacification of renal pelvis and calyces
- Normal size and uniform filling of the ureters
- Symmetrical and bilateral outline of structures

Abnormal findings in
- Congenital renal or urinary tract abnormalities
- Hydronephrosis
- Neoplasms
- Obstruction as a result of tumor, blood clot, stricture, or calculi
- Obstruction of ureteropelvic junction
- Perinephric abscess
- Perinephric inflammation or suppuration
- Polycystic kidney disease
- Prostatic enlargement
- Tumor of the kidneys or the collecting system

CRITICAL FINDINGS: N/A

INTERFERING FACTORS

This procedure is contraindicated for
- Patients with allergies to shellfish or iodinated dye. The contrast medium used may cause a life-threatening allergic reaction. Patients with a known hypersensitivity to the contrast medium may benefit from premedication with corticosteroids or the use of nonionic contrast medium.
- Patients who are pregnant or suspected of being pregnant, unless the potential benefits of the procedure far outweigh the risks to the fetus and mother.
- Elderly and other patients who are chronically dehydrated before the test, because of their risk of contrast-induced renal failure.
- Patients who are in renal failure.

R

- Patients with renal insufficiency, indicated by a blood urea nitrogen value greater than 40 mg/dL, because contrast medium can complicate kidney function.
- Young patients (17 yr and younger), unless the benefits of the x-ray diagnosis outweigh the risks of exposure to high levels of radiation.
- Patients with multiple myeloma, who may experience decreased kidney function subsequent to administration of contrast medium.

Factors that may impair clear imaging

- Gas or feces in the gastrointestinal tract resulting from inadequate cleansing or failure to restrict food intake before the study.
- Retained barium from a previous radiological procedure.
- Metallic objects (e.g., jewelry, body rings) within the examination field, which may inhibit organ visualization and cause unclear images.
- Inability of the patient to cooperate or remain still during the procedure because of age, significant pain, or mental status.

Other considerations

- Consultation with a health-care provider (HCP) should occur before the procedure for radiation safety concerns regarding younger patients or patients who are lactating.
- Risks associated with radiation overexposure can result from frequent x-ray procedures. Personnel in the room with the patient should wear a protective lead apron, stand behind a shield or leave the area while the examination is being done. Personnel working in the examination area should wear badges to record their level of radiation exposure.

- Failure to follow dietary restrictions and other pretesting preparations may cause the procedure to be canceled or repeated.

NURSING IMPLICATIONS AND PROCEDURE

PRETEST:

▶ Positively identify the patient using at least two unique identifiers before providing care, treatment, or services.

▶ *Patient Teaching:* Inform the patient this procedure can assist in assessing the urinary tract.

▶ Obtain a history of the patient's complaints, including a list of known allergens, especially allergies or sensitivities to latex, iodine, seafood, anesthetics, or contrast medium.

▶ Obtain a history of the patient's genitourinary system, symptoms, and results of previously performed laboratory tests and diagnostic and surgical procedures.

▶ Note any recent procedures that can interfere with test results, including examinations using barium.

▶ Record the date of the last menstrual period and determine the possibility of pregnancy in perimenopausal women.

▶ Obtain a list of the patient's current medications, including herbs, nutritional supplements, and nutraceuticals (see Appendix F).

▶ Patients receiving metformin (Glucophage) for non-insulin-dependent (type 2) diabetes should discontinue the drug on the day of the test and continue to withhold it for 48 hr after the test. Failure to do so may result in lactic acidosis.

▶ Review the procedure with the patient. Address concerns about pain related to the procedure and explain that some pain may be experienced during the test, or there may be moments of discomfort. Inform the patient that the procedure is performed in a special department, usually in a radiology or vascular suite, by an HCP, with support staff, and takes approximately 30 to 60 min.

R

▶ *Sensitivity to social and cultural issues,* as well as concern for modesty, is important in providing psychological support before, during, and after the procedure.

▶ Inform the patient that he or she may receive a laxative the night before the test and an enema or a cathartic the morning of the test, as ordered.

▶ Explain that an IV line may be inserted to allow infusion of IV fluids, contrast medium, or sedatives. Usually normal saline is infused.

▶ Inform the patient that if a local anesthetic is used, the patient may feel (1) some pressure in the kidney area as the catheter is introduced and contrast medium injected and (2) the urgency to void.

▶ Instruct the patient to remove jewelry and other metallic objects from the area to be examined prior to the procedure.

▶ Instruct the patient to fast and restrict fluids for 8 hr prior to the procedure. Instruct the patient to avoid taking anticoagulant medication or to reduce dosage as ordered prior to the procedure. Protocols may vary among facilities.

▶ This procedure may be terminated if chest pain, severe cardiac arrhythmias, or signs of a cerebrovascular accident occur.

▶ *Make sure a written and informed consent has been signed prior to the procedure and before administering any medications.*

INTRATEST:

▶ Ensure that the patient has complied with dietary, fluid, and medication restrictions for 8 hr prior to the procedure.

▶ Ensure the patient has removed all external metallic objects from the area to be examined prior to the procedure.

▶ If the patient has a history of allergic reactions to any substance or drug, administer ordered prophylactic steroids or antihistamines before the procedure. Use nonionic contrast medium for the procedure.

▶ Have emergency equipment readily available.

▶ Instruct the patient to void prior to the procedure and to change into the gown, robe, and foot coverings provided.

▶ Instruct the patient to cooperate fully and to follow directions. Instruct the patient to remain still throughout the procedure because movement produces unreliable results.

▶ Record baseline vital signs and assess neurological status. Protocols may vary among facilities.

▶ Observe standard precautions, and follow the general guidelines in Appendix A.

▶ Establish an IV fluid line for the injection of emergency drugs and of sedatives.

▶ Administer an antianxiety agent, as ordered, if the patient has claustrophobia. Administer a sedative to a child or to an uncooperative adult, as ordered.

▶ Place electrocardiographic electrodes on the patient for cardiac monitoring. Establish baseline rhythm; determine if the patient has ventricular arrhythmias.

▶ Place patient supine on the table in the lithotomy position.

▶ A kidney, ureter, and bladder (KUB) or plain image is taken to ensure that no barium or stool will obscure visualization of the urinary system. The patient may be asked to hold his or her breath to facilitate visualization.

▶ The patient is given a local anesthetic, and a cystoscopic examination is performed and the bladder is inspected.

▶ A catheter is inserted, and the renal pelvis is emptied by gravity. Contrast medium is introduced into the catheter. Inform the patient that the contrast medium may cause a temporary flushing of the face, a feeling of warmth, or nausea.

▶ X-ray images are made and the results processed. Inform the patient that additional images may be necessary to visualize the area in question.

▶ Additional contrast medium is injected through the catheter to outline the ureters as the catheter is withdrawn.

▶ The catheter may be kept in place and attached to a gravity drainage unit until urinary flow has returned or is corrected.

R

◗ Additional x-ray images are taken 10 to 15 min after the catheter is removed to evaluate retention of the contrast medium, indicating urinary stasis.

◗ Remove the needle or catheter and apply a pressure dressing over the puncture site.

◗ Observe/assess the needle/catheter insertion site for bleeding, inflammation, or hematoma formation.

POST-TEST:

◗ A report of the examination will be sent to the requesting HCP, who will discuss the results with the patient.

◗ Instruct the patient to resume usual diet, fluids, medications, and activity, as directed by the HCP. Renal function should be assessed before metformin is resumed.

◗ Monitor vital signs and neurological status every 15 min for 1 hr, then every 2 hr for 4 hr, and then as ordered. Take temperature every 4 hr for 24 hr. Monitor intake and output at least every 8 hr. Compare with baseline values. Notify the HCP if temperature is elevated. Protocols may vary among facilities.

◗ Observe for delayed allergic reactions, such as rash, urticaria, tachycardia, hyperpnea, hypertension, palpitations, nausea, or vomiting.

◗ Instruct the patient to immediately report symptoms such as fast heart rate, difficulty breathing, skin rash, itching, chest pain, persistent right shoulder pain, or abdominal pain. Immediately report symptoms to the appropriate HCP.

◗ Observe/assess the needle/catheter insertion site for bleeding, inflammation, or hematoma formation.

◗ Instruct the patient in the care and assessment of the site.

◗ Instruct the patient to apply cold compresses to the puncture site as needed to reduce discomfort or edema.

◗ Monitor for signs of sepsis and severe pain in the kidney area.

◗ Maintain the patient on adequate hydration after the procedure. Encourage the patient to drink lots of fluids to prevent stasis and to prevent the buildup of bacteria.

◗ Recognize anxiety related to test results, and be supportive of perceived loss of independent function. Discuss the implications of abnormal test results on the patient's lifestyle. Provide teaching and information regarding clinical implications of the test results, as appropriate.

◗ Reinforce information given by the patient's HCP regarding further testing, treatment, or referral to another HCP. Answer any questions or address any concerns voiced by the patient or family.

◗ Instruct the patient in the use of any ordered medications. Explain the importance of adhering to the therapy regimen. As appropriate, instruct the patient in significant side effects and systemic reactions associated with the prescribed medication. Encourage him or her to review corresponding literature provided by a pharmacist.

◗ Depending on the results of this procedure, additional testing may be needed to evaluate or monitor progression of the disease process and determine the need for a change in therapy. Evaluate test results in relation to the patient's symptoms and other tests performed.

RELATED MONOGRAPHS:

◗ Related tests include angiography renal, BUN, calculus kidney stone panel, CT abdomen, creatinine, cystoscopy, IVP, KUB, MRI abdomen, PT/INR, PSA, renogram, US kidney, UA, and voiding cystourethrography.

◗ Refer to the Genitourinary System table at the end of the book for related tests by body system.

R

Rheumatoid Factor

SYNONYM/ACRONYM: RF, RA.

COMMON USE: To primarily assist in diagnosing rheumatoid arthritis.

SPECIMEN: Serum (1 mL) collected in a red-top tube.

REFERENCE VALUE: (Method: Immunoturbidometric) Less than 14 international units/mL.

DESCRIPTION: Rheumatoid arthritis (RA) is a chronic, systemic autoimmune disease that damages the joints. Inflammation caused by autoimmune responses can affect other organs and body systems. The current American Academy of Rheumatology criteria state that a patient must have four of seven criteria to be diagnosed with RA: morning stiffness, arthritis of three or more joint areas, arthritis of hand joints, symmetric arthritis, rheumatoid nodules, abnormal amounts of rheumatoid factor, and radiographic changes. The study of RA is complex, and it is believed that multiple genes may be involved in the manifestation of RA. Individuals with RA harbor a macroglobulin-type antibody called *rheumatoid factor (RF)* in their blood. Patients with other diseases (e.g., systemic lupus erythematosus [SLE] and occasionally tuberculosis, chronic hepatitis, infectious mononucleosis, and subacute bacterial endocarditis) may also test positive for RF. RF antibodies are usually immunoglobulin (Ig) M but may also be IgG or IgA. Women are two to three times more likely to develop RA than men. While RA is most likely to affect people aged 35 to 50, it can affect all ages.

INDICATIONS

Assist in the diagnosis of rheumatoid arthritis, especially when clinical diagnosis is difficult

POTENTIAL DIAGNOSIS

Increased in
Pathophysiology is unclear, but RF is present in numerous conditions, including rheumatoid arthritis.
- Chronic hepatitis
- Chronic viral infections
- Cirrhosis
- Dermatomyositis
- Infectious mononucleosis
- Leishmaniasis
- Leprosy
- Malaria
- Rheumatoid arthritis
- Sarcoidosis
- Scleroderma
- Sjögren's syndrome
- SLE
- Syphilis
- Tuberculosis
- Waldenström's macroglobulinemia

Decreased in: N/A

CRITICAL FINDINGS: N/A

INTERFERING FACTORS

- Older patients may have higher values.

R

- Recent blood transfusion, multiple vaccinations or transfusions, or an inadequately activated complement may affect results.
- Serum with cryoglobulin or high lipid levels may cause a false-positive test and may require that the test be repeated after a fat-restriction diet.

NURSING IMPLICATIONS AND PROCEDURE

PRETEST:

▶ Positively identify the patient using at least two unique identifiers before providing care, treatment, or services.

▶ *Patient Teaching:* Inform the patient this test can assist in diagnosing arthritic disorders.

▶ Obtain a history of the patient's complaints, including a list of known allergens, especially allergies or sensitivities to latex.

▶ Obtain a history of the patient's immune and musculoskeletal systems, symptoms, and results of previously performed laboratory tests and diagnostic and surgical procedures.

▶ Obtain a list of the patient's current medications, including herbs, nutritional supplements, and nutraceuticals (see Appendix F).

▶ Review the procedure with the patient. Inform the patient that specimen collection takes approximately 5 to 10 min. Address concerns about pain and explain that there may be some discomfort during the venipuncture.

▶ *Sensitivity to social and cultural issues,* as well as concern for modesty, is important in providing psychological support before, during, and after the procedure.

▶ There are no food, fluid, or medication restrictions unless by medical direction.

INTRATEST:

▶ If the patient has a history of allergic reaction to latex, avoid the use of equipment containing latex.

▶ Instruct the patient to cooperate fully and to follow directions. Direct the patient to breathe normally and to avoid unnecessary movement.

▶ Observe standard precautions, and follow the general guidelines in Appendix A. Positively identify the patient, and label the appropriate tubes with the corresponding patient demographics, date, and time of collection. Perform a venipuncture.

▶ Remove the needle and apply direct pressure with dry gauze to stop bleeding. Observe venipuncture site for bleeding or hematoma formation and secure gauze with adhesive bandage.

▶ Promptly transport the specimen to the laboratory for processing and analysis.

POST-TEST:

▶ A report of the results will be sent to the requesting health-care provider (HCP), who will discuss the results with the patient.

▶ Recognize anxiety related to test results, and be supportive of impaired activity related to anticipated chronic pain resulting from joint inflammation, impairment in mobility, musculoskeletal deformity, and loss of independence. Discuss the implications of abnormal test results on the patient's lifestyle. Provide teaching and information regarding the clinical implications of the test results, as appropriate. Educate the patient regarding access to counseling services, as appropriate. Provide contact information, if desired, for the Arthritis Foundation (www.arthritis.org).

▶ Reinforce information given by the patient's HCP regarding further testing, treatment, or referral to another HCP. Advise the patient, as appropriate, that additional studies may be undertaken to determine treatment regimen or to determine the possible causes of symptoms if the test is negative for RA. Answer any questions or address any concerns voiced by the patient or family.

▶ Depending on the results of this procedure, additional testing may be performed to evaluate or monitor

progression of the disease process and determine the need for a change in therapy. Evaluate test results in relation to the patient's symptoms and other tests performed.

RELATED MONOGRAPHS:

- Related laboratory tests include antibodies anticyclic citrullinated peptide, ANA, arthrogram, arthroscopy, biopsy bone, BMD, bone scan, calcium, collagen cross-linked telopeptides, CBC, CT spine, CRP, ESR, MRI musculoskeletal, osteocalcin, phosphorus, radiography bone, synovial fluid analysis, uric acid, vitamin D, and WBC scan.
- Refer to the Immune and Musculoskeletal systems tables at the end of the book for related tests by body system.

Rubella Antibodies

SYNONYM/ACRONYM: German measles serology.

COMMON USE: To assess for antibodies related to rubella immunity or for presence of rubella infection.

SPECIMEN: Serum (1 mL) collected in a red-top tube.

REFERENCE VALUE: (Method: Indirect immunofluorescence) Immune or less than a fourfold increase in titer.

DESCRIPTION: Rubella, commonly known as German measles, is a communicable viral disease transmitted by contact with respiratory secretions and aerosolized droplets of the secretions. The incubation period is 14 to 21 days. This disease produces a pink, macular rash that disappears in 2 to 3 days. Rubella infection induces immunoglobulin (Ig) G and IgM antibody production. This test can determine current infection or immunity from past infection. Rubella serology is part of the TORCH (*t*oxoplasmosis, *r*ubella, *c*ytomegalovirus, and *h*erpes simplex type 2) panel routinely performed on pregnant women. Fetal infection during the first trimester can cause spontaneous abortion or congenital defects. Ideally, the immune status of women of childbearing age should be ascertained before pregnancy, when vaccination can be administered to provide lifelong immunity. The presence of IgM antibodies indicates acute infection. The presence of IgG antibodies indicates current or past infection. Susceptibility to rubella is indicated by a negative reaction. Many laboratories use a qualitative assay that detects the presence of both IgM and IgG rubella antibodies. IgM- and IgG-specific enzyme immunoassays

R

are also available to help distinguish acute infection from immune status. A rise in titer greater than fourfold in paired specimens is an indication of current infection.

INDICATIONS

• Assist in the diagnosis of rubella infection
• Determine presence of rubella antibodies
• Determine susceptibility to rubella, particularly in pregnant women
• Perform as part of routine prenatal serological testing

POTENTIAL DIAGNOSIS

Positive findings in
• Rubella infection (past or present)

CRITICAL FINDINGS ❖

A nonimmune status in pregnant patients may present significant health consequences for the developing fetus if the mother is exposed to an infected individual.

Note and immediately report to the health-care provider (HCP) patients with rubella nonimmune status.

INTERFERING FACTORS: N/A

NURSING IMPLICATIONS AND PROCEDURE

PRETEST:

▶ Positively identify the patient using at least two unique identifiers before providing care, treatment, or services.
▶ *Patient Teaching:* Inform the patient this test can indicate rubella infection or immunity.
▶ Obtain a history of the patient's complaints, including a list of known

allergens, especially allergies or sensitivities to latex.
▶ Obtain a history of exposure to rubella.
▶ Obtain a history of the patient's immune and reproductive systems, symptoms, and results of previously performed laboratory tests and diagnostic and surgical procedures.
▶ Obtain a list of the patient's current medications, including herbs, nutritional supplements, and nutraceuticals (see Appendix F).
▶ Review the procedure with the patient. Inform the patient that several tests may be necessary to confirm diagnosis. Any individual positive result should be repeated in 7 to 14 days to monitor a change in titer. Inform the patient that specimen collection takes approximately 5 to 10 min. Address concerns about pain and explain that there may be some discomfort during the venipuncture.
▶ *Sensitivity to social and cultural issues,* as well as concern for modesty, is important in providing psychological support before, during, and after the procedure.
▶ There are no food, fluid, or medication restrictions unless by medical direction.

INTRATEST:

▶ If the patient has a history of allergic reaction to latex, avoid the use of equipment containing latex.
▶ Instruct the patient to cooperate fully and to follow directions. Direct the patient to breathe normally and to avoid unnecessary movement.
▶ Observe standard precautions, and follow the general guidelines in Appendix A. Positively identify the patient, and label the appropriate tubes with the corresponding patient demographics, date, and time of collection. Perform a venipuncture.
▶ Remove the needle and apply direct pressure with dry gauze to stop bleeding. Observe/assess venipuncture site for bleeding or hematoma formation and secure gauze with adhesive bandage.
▶ Promptly transport the specimen to the laboratory for processing and analysis.

- A report of the results will be sent to the requesting HCP, who will discuss the results with the patient.
- *Vaccination Considerations:* Record the date of the last menstrual period and determine the possibility of pregnancy prior to administration of rubella vaccine to female rubella-nonimmune patients. Instruct patient not to become pregnant for 1 mo after being vaccinated with the rubella vaccine to protect any fetus from contracting the disease and having serious birth defects. Instruct on birth control methods to prevent pregnancy, if appropriate. Delay rubella vaccination in pregnancy until after childbirth, and give immediately prior to discharge from the hospital.
- Recognize anxiety related to test results, and provide emotional support if results are positive and the patient is pregnant. Encourage the family to seek counseling if concerned with pregnancy termination. Provide teaching and information regarding the clinical implications of the test results, as appropriate. Decisions regarding elective abortion should take place in the presence of both parents. Provide a nonjudgmental, nonthreatening atmosphere for discussing the risks and difficulties of delivering and raising a developmentally challenged infant as well as for exploring other options

(e.g., termination of pregnancy or adoption). Educate the patient regarding access to counseling services, as appropriate.
- Reinforce information given by the patient's HCP regarding further testing, treatment, or referral to another HCP. Instruct the patient in isolation precautions during time of communicability or contagion. Emphasize the need to return to have a convalescent blood sample taken in 7 to 14 days. Provide information regarding vaccine-preventable diseases where indicated (e.g., encephalitis, hepatitis A and B, human papillomavirus, influenza, measles, mumps, polio, rubella, smallpox, varicella, yellow fever). Answer any questions or address any concerns voiced by the patient or family.
- Depending on the results of this procedure, additional testing may be performed to evaluate or monitor progression of the disease process and determine the need for a change in therapy. Evaluate test results in relation to the patient's symptoms and other tests performed.

RELATED MONOGRAPHS:

- Related tests include culture viral, CMV, rubeola, *Toxoplasma,* and varicella antibody.
- Refer to the Immune and Reproductive systems tables at the end of the book for related tests by body system.

Rubeola Antibodies

R

SYNONYM/ACRONYM: Measles serology.

COMMON USE: To assess for a rubeola infection or immunity.

SPECIMEN: Serum (1 mL) collected in a red-top tube.

REFERENCE VALUE: (Method: Indirect immunofluorescence) Negative or less than a fourfold increase in titer.

DESCRIPTION: Measles is caused by a single-stranded ribonucleic acid (RNA) paramyxovirus that invades the respiratory tract and lymphoreticular tissues. It is transmitted by respiratory secretions and aerosolized droplets of the secretions. The incubation period is 10 to 11 days. Symptoms initially include conjunctivitis, cough, and fever. Koplik's spots develop 4 to 5 days later, followed by papular eruptions, body rash, and lymphadenopathy. The presence of immunoglobulin (Ig) M antibodies indicates acute infection. The presence of IgG antibodies indicates current or past infection. Susceptibility to measles is indicated by a negative reaction. Many laboratories use a qualitative assay that detects the presence of both IgM and IgG rubeola antibodies. IgM- and IgG-specific enzyme immunoassays are also available to help distinguish acute infection from immune status. A rise in titer greater than fourfold in paired specimens is an indication of current infection.

INDICATIONS

- Determine resistance to or protection against measles virus
- Differential diagnosis of viral infection, especially in pregnant women with a history of exposure to measles

POTENTIAL DIAGNOSIS

Positive findings in
- Measles infection

CRITICAL FINDINGS: N/A

INTERFERING FACTORS: N/A

NURSING IMPLICATIONS AND PROCEDURE

PRETEST:

- Positively identify the patient using at least two unique identifiers before providing care, treatment, or services.
- *Patient Teaching:* Inform the patient this test is to assess for measles.
- Obtain a history of the patient's complaints, including a list of known allergens, especially allergies or sensitivities to latex.
- Obtain a history of exposure to measles.
- Obtain a history of the patient's immune system, symptoms, and results of previously performed laboratory tests and diagnostic and surgical procedures.
- Obtain a list of the patient's current medications, including herbs, nutritional supplements, and nutraceuticals (see Appendix F).
- Review the procedure with the patient. Inform the patient that several tests may be necessary to confirm the diagnosis. Any individual positive result should be repeated in 7 to 14 days to monitor a change in titer. Inform the patient that specimen collection takes approximately 5 to 10 min. Address concerns about pain and explain that there may be some discomfort during the venipuncture.
- *Sensitivity to social and cultural issues,* as well as concern for modesty, is important in providing psychological support before, during, and after the procedure.
- There are no food, fluid, or medication restrictions, unless by medical direction.

INTRATEST:

- If the patient has a history of allergic reaction to latex, avoid the use of equipment containing latex.
- Instruct the patient to cooperate fully and to follow directions. Direct the patient to breathe normally and to avoid unnecessary movement.
- Observe standard precautions, and follow the general guidelines in Appendix A. Positively identify the

R

patient, and label the appropriate tubes with the corresponding patient demographics, date, and time of collection. Perform a venipuncture.

▶ Remove the needle and apply direct pressure with dry gauze to stop bleeding. Observe/assess venipuncture site for bleeding or hematoma formation and secure gauze with adhesive bandage.

▶ Promptly transport the specimen to the laboratory for processing and analysis.

POST-TEST:

▶ A report of the results will be sent to the requesting health-care provider (HCP), who will discuss the results with the patient.

▶ Reinforce information given by the patient's HCP regarding further testing, treatment, or referral to another HCP. Instruct the patient in isolation precautions during time of communicability or contagion. Emphasize the need to return to have a convalescent blood sample taken in 7 to 14 days. Provide information regarding vaccine-preventable diseases where indicated (e.g., encephalitis, hepatitis A and B, human papillomavirus, influenza, measles, mumps, polio, rubella, smallpox, varicella, yellow fever). Answer any questions or address any concerns voiced by the patient or family.

▶ Depending on the results of this procedure, additional testing may be performed to evaluate or monitor progression of the disease process and determine the need for a change in therapy. Evaluate test results in relation to the patient's symptoms and other tests performed.

RELATED MONOGRAPHS:

▶ Related tests include culture viral, rubella, and varicella.

▶ Refer to the Immune System table at the end of the book for related tests by body system.

R

Schirmer Tear Test

SYNONYM/ACRONYM: N/A.

COMMON USE: To assess tear duct function.

AREA OF APPLICATION: Eyelids.

CONTRAST: N/A.

DESCRIPTION: The tear film, secreted by the lacrimal, Krause, and Wolfring glands, covers the surface of the eye. Blinking spreads tears over the eye and moves them toward an opening in the lower eyelid known as the punctum. Tears drain through the punctum into the nasolacrimal duct and into the nose. The Schirmer tear test simultaneously tests both eyes to assess lacrimal gland function by determining the amount of moisture accumulated on standardized filter paper or strips held against the conjuctival sac of each eye. The Schirmer test measures both reflex and basic secretion of tears. The Schirmer II test measures basic tear secretion and is used to evaluate the accessory glands of Krause and Wolfring. The Schirmer test is performed by instilling a topical anesthetic before insertion of filter paper. The topical anesthetic inhibits reflex tearing of major lacrimal glands by the filter paper, allowing testing of the accessory glands. The Schirmer II test is performed by irritating the nostril with a cotton swab to stimulate tear production.

INDICATIONS

- Assess adequacy of tearing for contact lens comfort
- Assess suspected tearing deficiency

POTENTIAL DIAGNOSIS

Normal findings in
- 10 mm of moisture on test strip after 5 min. It may be slightly less than 10 mm in elderly patients.

Abnormal findings in
- Tearing deficiency related to aging, dry eye syndrome, or Sjögren's syndrome
- Tearing deficiency secondary to leukemia, lymphoma, or rheumatoid arthritis

CRITICAL FINDINGS: N/A

INTERFERING FACTORS

Factors that may impair the results of the examination
- Inability of the patient to remain still and cooperative during the test may interfere with the test results.
- Rubbing or squeezing the eyes may affect results.

NURSING IMPLICATIONS AND PROCEDURE

PRETEST:

- Positively identify the patient using at least two unique identifiers before providing care, treatment, or services.
- *Patient Teaching:* Inform the patient this procedure can assist in evaluating tear duct function.
- Obtain a history of the patient's complaints, including a list of known allergens, especially topical anesthetic eyedrops.
- Obtain a history of the patient's known or suspected vision loss; changes in

visual acuity, including type and cause; use of glasses or contact lenses; eye conditions with treatment regimens; eye surgery; and other tests and procedures to assess and diagnose visual deficit.
- Obtain a history of the patient's symptoms and results of previously performed laboratory tests and diagnostic and surgical procedures.
- Obtain a list of the patient's current medications, including herbs, nutritional supplements, and nutraceuticals (see Appendix F).
- Instruct the patient to remove contact lenses or glasses, as appropriate. Instruct the patient regarding the importance of keeping the eyes open for the test.
- Review the procedure with the patient. Address concerns about pain and explain that no pain will be experienced during the test, but there may be moments of discomfort. Explain to the patient that some discomfort may be experienced after the test when the numbness wears off from anesthetic drops administered prior to the test. Inform the patient that the test is performed by a health-care provider (HCP) and takes about 15 min to complete.
- *Sensitivity to social and cultural issues,* as well as concern for modesty, is important in providing psychological support before, during, and after the procedure.
- There are no food, fluid, or medication restrictions unless by medical direction.

INTRATEST:

- Instruct the patient to cooperate fully and to follow directions. Ask the patient to remain still during the procedure because movement produces unreliable results.
- Observe standard precautions, and follow the general guidelines in Appendix A.
- Seat the patient comfortably. Instruct the patient to look straight ahead, keeping the eyes open and unblinking.
- Instill topical anesthetic in each eye, as ordered, and provide time for it to

work. Topical anesthetic drops are placed in the eye with the patient looking up and the solution directed at the six o'clock position of the sclera (white of the eye) near the limbus (gray, semitransparent area of the eyeball where the cornea and sclera meet). Neither the dropper nor the bottle should touch the eyelashes. Insert a test strip in each eye. The strip should be folded over the midportion of both lower eyelids.

POST-TEST:

- A report of the results will be sent to the requesting HCP, who will discuss the results with the patient.
- Assess for corneal abrasion caused by patient rubbing the eye before topical anesthetic has worn off.
- Instruct the patient to avoid rubbing the eyes for 30 min after the procedure.
- If appropriate, instruct the patient not to reinsert contact lenses for 2 hr.
- Recognize anxiety related to test results, and be supportive of pain related to decreased lacrimation or inflammation. Discuss the implications of abnormal test results on the patient's lifestyle. Provide teaching and information regarding the clinical implications of the test results, as appropriate. Provide contact information, if desired, for a general patient education Web site on the topic of eye care (e.g., www.allaboutvision.com).
- Reinforce information given by the patient's HCP regarding further testing, treatment, or referral to another HCP. Answer any questions or address any concerns voiced by the patient or family.
- Instruct the patient in the use of any ordered medications. Explain the importance of adhering to the therapy regimen. As appropriate, instruct the patient in significant side effects and systemic reactions associated with the prescribed medication. Encourage him or her to review corresponding literature provided by a pharmacist.

S

▶ Depending on the results of this procedure, additional testing may be performed to evaluate or monitor progression of the disease process and determine the need for a change in therapy. Evaluate test results in relation to the patient's symptoms and other tests performed.

RELATED MONOGRAPHS:
▶ Related tests include antibodies ANA, refraction, rheumatoid factor, and slit-lamp biomicroscopy.
▶ Refer to the Ocular System table at the end of the book for related tests by body system.

Semen Analysis

SYNONYM/ACRONYM: N/A.

COMMON USE: To assess for male infertility related to disorders such as obstruction, testicular failure, and atrophy.

SPECIMEN: Semen from ejaculate specimen collected in a clean, dry, glass container known to be free of detergent. The specimen container should be kept at body temperature (37°C) during transportation.

REFERENCE VALUE: (Method: Macroscopic and microscopic examination)

Test	Normal Result
Volume	2–5 mL
Color	White or opaque
Appearance	Viscous (pours in droplets, not clumps or strings)
Clotting and liquefaction	Complete in 20–30 min, rarely over 60 min
pH	7.2–8.0
Sperm count	Greater than 20 million/mL
Total sperm count	Greater than 40 million/ejaculate
Motility	At least 50%
Morphology	At least 70% normal oval-headed forms

DESCRIPTION: Semen analysis is a valid measure of overall male fertility. Semen contains a combination of elements produced by various parts of the male reproductive system. Spermatozoa are produced in the testes and account for only a small volume of seminal fluid.

Fructose and other nutrients are provided by fluid produced in the seminal vesicles. The prostate gland provides acid phosphatase and other enzymes required for coagulation and liquefaction of semen. Sperm motility depends on the presence of a sufficient level of ionized calcium. If the specimen has an abnormal appearance (e.g., bloody, oddly colored, turbid), the patient may have an infection. Specimens can be tested with a leukocyte esterase strip to detect the presence of white blood cells.

INDICATIONS
• Assist in the diagnosis of azoospermia and oligospermia
• Evaluate infertility
• Evaluate effectiveness of vasectomy

• Evaluate the effectiveness of vasectomy reversal
• Support or disprove sterility in paternity suit

POTENTIAL DIAGNOSIS
There is marked intraindividual variation in sperm count. Indications of suboptimal fertility should be investigated by serial analysis of two to three samples collected over several months. If abnormal results are obtained, additional testing may be requested.

Abnormality	Test Ordered	Normal Result
Decreased count	Fructose	Present (greater than 150 mg/dL)
Decreased motility with clumping	Male antisperm antibodies	Absent
Normal semen analysis with infertility	Female antisperm antibodies	Absent

Increased in: N/A

Decreased in
• Hyperpyrexia *(unusual and abnormal elevation in body temperature may result in insufficient sperm production)*
• Infertility *(related to insufficient production of sperm)*
• Obstruction of ejaculatory system
• Orchitis *(insufficient sperm production usually related to viral infection, rarely bacterial infection)*
• Postvasectomy period *(related to obstruction of the vas deferens)*
• Primary and secondary testicular failure *(congenital, as in Kleinfelter's syndrome, or acquired via infection)*
• Testicular atrophy (e.g., recovery from mumps)
• Varicocele *(abnormal enlargement of the blood vessels in the scrotal area eventually damages testicular tissue and affects sperm production)*

CRITICAL FINDINGS: N/A

INTERFERING FACTORS
• Drugs and substances that may decrease sperm count include arsenic, azathioprine, cannabis, cimetidine, cocaine, cyclophosphamide, estrogens, fluoxymesterone, ketoconazole, lead, methotrexate, methyltestosterone, nitrofurantoin, nitrogen mustard, procarbazine, sulfasalazine, and vincristine.
• Testicular radiation may decrease sperm counts.
• Cigarette smoking is associated with decreased production of semen.
• Caffeine consumption is associated with increased sperm density and number of abnormal forms.

• Delays in transporting the specimen and failure to keep the specimen warm during transportation are the most common reasons for specimen rejection.

NURSING IMPLICATIONS AND PROCEDURE

PRETEST:

▶ Positively identify the patient using at least two unique identifiers before providing care, treatment, or services.

▶ *Patient Teaching:* Inform the patient this test can assess for infertility.

▶ Obtain a history of the patient's complaints, including a list of known allergens, especially allergies or sensitivities to latex.

▶ Obtain a history of the patient's immune and reproductive systems, symptoms, and results of previously performed laboratory tests and diagnostic and surgical procedures.

▶ Obtain a list of the patient's current medications, including herbs, nutritional supplements, and nutraceuticals (see Appendix F).

▶ Note any recent procedures that can interfere with test results.

▶ Review the procedure with the patient. Instruct the patient to refrain from any sexual activity for 3 days before specimen collection. Instruct the patient to bring the specimen to the laboratory within 30 to 60 min of collection and to keep the specimen warm (close to body temperature) during transportation. The requesting health-care provider (HCP) usually provides the patient with instructions for specimen collection. Address concerns about pain and explain that there should be no discomfort during the procedure.

▶ *Sensitivity to social and cultural issues,* as well as concern for modesty, is important in providing psychological support before, during, and after the procedure.

▶ There are no food, fluid, or medication restrictions unless by medical direction.

INTRATEST:

▶ Instruct the patient to cooperate fully and to follow directions.

▶ Observe standard precautions, and follow the general guidelines in Appendix A. Positively identify the patient, and label the appropriate collection container with the corresponding patient demographics, date, and time of collection.

Ejaculated Specimen

▶ Ideally, the specimen is obtained by masturbation in a private location close to the laboratory. In cases in which the patient expresses psychological or religious concerns about masturbation, the specimen can be obtained during coitus interruptus, through the use of a condom, or through postcoital collection of samples from the cervical canal and vagina of the patient's sexual partner. The patient should be warned about the possible loss of the sperm-rich portion of the sample if coitus interruptus is the collection approach. If a condom is used, the patient must be carefully instructed to wash and dry the condom completely before use to prevent contamination of the specimen with spermicides.

Cervical Vaginal Specimen

▶ Assist the patient's partner to the lithotomy position on the examination table. A speculum is inserted, and the specimen is obtained by direct smear or aspiration of saline lavage.

Specimens Collected From Skin or Clothing

▶ Dried semen may be collected by sponging the skin with a gauze soaked in saline or by soaking the material in a saline solution.

General

▶ Promptly transport the specimen to the laboratory for processing and analysis.

S

POST-TEST:

- A report of the results will be sent to the requesting HCP, who will discuss the results with the patient.
- Recognize anxiety related to test results. Provide a supportive, nonjudgmental environment when assisting a patient through the process of fertility testing. Discuss the implications of abnormal test results on the patient's lifestyle. Provide teaching and information regarding the clinical implications of the test results, as appropriate. Encourage the patient or family to seek counseling and other support services if concerned with infertility.
- Reinforce information given by the patient's HCP regarding further testing, treatment, or referral to another HCP. Answer any questions or address any concerns voiced by the patient or family.
- Depending on the results of this procedure, additional testing may be performed to evaluate or monitor progression of the disease process and determine the need for a change in therapy. Evaluate test results in relation to the patient's symptoms and other tests performed.

RELATED MONOGRAPHS:

- Related tests include antisperm antibodies, cancer antigens, *Chlamydia* group antibodies, estradiol, FSH, hysterosalpingography, laparoscopy gynecologic, LH, testosterone, and US scrotal.
- Refer to the Immune and Reproductive systems tables at the end of the book for related tests by body system.

Sialography

SYNONYM/ACRONYM: Salivary gland studies.

COMMON USE: To assess parotid, submaxillary, sublingual, and submandibular ducts for structure, tumors, and inflammation related to pain, swelling, and tenderness.

AREA OF APPLICATION: Base of the tongue, mandible, parotid gland, submandibular gland, sublingual gland.

CONTRAST: Water-soluble iodionated contrast medium.

DESCRIPTION: Sialography is the radiographic visualization of the salivary glands and ducts. These glands secrete saliva into the mouth, and there are three pairs of salivary glands: the parotid, the submandibular, and the sublingual. Sialography involves the introduction of a water-soluble contrast agent into the orifices of the salivary gland ducts with a small cannula, followed by a series of radiographic images. The evaluation of the salivary glands is usually done with computed tomography or magnetic resonance imaging; however, sialography is the method of choice when a definite diagnosis is required for pathology such as

S

sialadenitis (inflammation of the salivary glands) or if the oral component of Sjögren's syndrome is a concern.

INDICATIONS

POTENTIAL DIAGNOSIS

Normal findings in
- Normal salivary ducts with no indication of gland abnormalities

Abnormal findings in
- Calculi
- Fistulas
- Mixed parotid tumors
- Sialectasia (dilation of a duct)
- Strictures of the ducts

CRITICAL FINDINGS: N/A

INTERFERING FACTORS

This procedure is contraindicated for
- Patients with allergies to shellfish and iodinated dye. The contrast medium used may cause life-threatening allergic reaction. Patients with a known hypersensitivity to the contrast medium may benefit from premedication with corticosteroids or the use of nonionic contrast medium.

Factors that may impair clear imaging
- Inability of the patient to cooperate or remain still during the test because of age, significant pain, or mental status may interfere with the test results.

Other considerations
- Risks associated with radiation overexposure can result from frequent x-ray procedures. Personnel in the room with the patient should wear a protective lead apron, stand behind a shield,

or leave the area while the examination is being done. Personnel working in the examination area should wear badges to record the level of radiation exposure.

NURSING IMPLICATIONS AND PROCEDURE

PRETEST:

- Positively identify the patient using at least two unique identifiers before providing care, treatment, or services.
- *Patient Teaching:* Inform the patient that this procedure can assist in assessing duct glands in the neck and mouth.
- Obtain a history of the patient's complaints, including a list of known allergens, especially allergies or sensitivities to latex, iodine, seafood, contrast medium, anesthetics, or dyes.
- Obtain a history of the patient's endocrine system, symptoms, and results of previously performed laboratory tests and diagnostic and surgical procedures.
- Record the date of last menstrual period and determine the possibility of pregnancy in perimenopausal women.
- Obtain a list of the patient's current medications, including anticoagulants, aspirin and other salicylates, herbs, nutritional supplements, and nutraceuticals (see Appendix F).
- Instruct the patient to remove dentures or removable bridgework prior to examination.
- Review the procedure with the patient. Inform the patient that the procedure is usually done with the patient awake and laying on a table. Address concerns about pain and explain that the patient may be asked to suck on a lemon slice to dilate the salivary orifice, and a local anesthetic spray or liquid may be applied to the throat to ease with insertion of the cannula. Inform the patient that the procedure is performed in a radiology department

S

by a health-care provider (HCP) specializing in this procedure, with support staff, and takes approximately 15 to 30 min.

▶ *Sensitivity to social and cultural issues,* as well as concern for modesty, is important in providing psychological support before, during, and after the procedure.

▶ There are no food, fluid, or medication restrictions unless by medical direction.

▶ *Make sure a written and informed consent has been signed prior to the procedure and before administering any medications.*

INTRATEST:

▶ Ensure that the patient has removed dentures and removable bridgework prior to the procedure.

▶ If the patient has a history of severe allergic reactions to any substance or drug, administer ordered prophylactic steroids or antihistamines before the procedure. Use nonionic contrast medium for the procedure.

▶ Have emergency equipment readily available.

▶ Instruct the patient to cooperate fully and to follow directions. Instruct the patient to remain still throughout the procedure because movement produces unreliable results.

▶ Observe standard precautions, and follow the general guidelines in Appendix A.

▶ Place the patient in the supine position on an examination table. Instill ordered topical anesthetic in the throat, as ordered, and allow time for it to work.

▶ The salivary duct is located and dilated. Following insertion of the cannula, the contrast medium is injected, and a series of images is taken. Delayed images may be taken to examine the ducts in cases of ductal obstruction.

▶ Ask the patient to inhale deeply and hold his or her breath while the x-ray images are taken, and then to exhale after the images are taken.

▶ Monitor the patient for complications related to the procedure (e.g., allergic reaction, anaphylaxis, bronchospasm).

▶ Remove the needle or cannula.

▶ Observe/assess the needle/cannula insertion site for bleeding or inflammation.

POST-TEST:

▶ A report of the results will be sent to the requesting HCP, who will discuss the results with the patient.

▶ Instruct the patient to wait until the numbness in the throat wears off before attempting to eat or drink following the procedure.

▶ Observe for delayed allergic reactions, such as rash, urticaria, tachycardia, hyperpnea, hypertension, palpitations, nausea, or vomiting.

▶ Instruct the patient to immediately report symptoms such as fast heart rate, difficulty breathing, skin rash, itching, chest pain, persistent right shoulder pain, or abdominal pain. Immediately report symptoms to the appropriate HCP.

▶ Observe/assess the needle/cannula insertion site for bleeding or inflammation.

▶ Instruct the patient in the care and assessment of the site.

▶ Instruct the patient to apply cold compresses to the puncture site as needed to reduce discomfort or edema.

▶ Recognize anxiety related to test results. Discuss the implications of abnormal test results on the patient's lifestyle. Provide teaching and information regarding the clinical implications of the test results, as appropriate.

▶ Reinforce information given by the patient's HCP regarding further testing, treatment, or referral to another HCP. Answer any questions or address any concerns voiced by the patient or family.

▶ Depending on the results of this procedure, additional testing may be needed to evaluate or monitor progression of the disease process and determine the need for a change in therapy. Evaluate test results in relation to the patient's symptoms and other tests performed.

RELATED MONOGRAPHS:

▶ Related tests include CT brain, MRI brain, and radiography bone.

▶ Refer to the Musculoskeletal System table at the end of the book for related tests by body system.

S

Sickle Cell Screen

SYNONYM/ACRONYM: Sickle cell test.

COMMON USE: To assess for hemoglobin S to assist in diagnosing sickle cell anemia.

SPECIMEN: Whole blood (1 mL) collected in a lavender-top (EDTA) tube.

REFERENCE VALUE: (Method: Hemoglobin high-salt solubility) Negative.

DESCRIPTION: The sickle cell screen is one of several screening tests for a group of hereditary hemoglobinopathies. The test is positive in the presence of rare sickling hemoglobin (Hgb) variants such as Hgb S and Hgb C Harlem. Hgb S results from an amino acid substitution during Hgb synthesis whereby valine replaces glutamic acid. Hemoglobin C Harlem results from the substitution of lysine for glutamic acid. Individuals with sickle cell disease have chronic anemia because the abnormal Hgb is unable to carry oxygen. The red blood cells of affected individuals are also abnormal in shape, resembling a crescent or sickle rather than the normal disk shape. This abnormality, combined with cell-wall rigidity, prevents the cells from passing through smaller blood vessels. Blockages in blood vessels result in hypoxia, damage, and pain. Individuals with the sickle cell trait do not have the clinical manifestations of the disease but may pass the disease on to children if the other parent has the trait (or the disease) as well.

INDICATIONS
• Detect sickled red blood cells
• Evaluate hemolytic anemias

POTENTIAL DIAGNOSIS

Positive findings in
Deoxygenated Hgb S is insoluble in the presence of a high-salt solution and will form a cloudy turbid suspension when present.
• Combination of Hgb S with other hemoglobinopathies
• Hgb C Harlem anemia
• Sickle cell anemia
• Sickle cell trait
• Thalassemias

Negative findings in: N/A

CRITICAL FINDINGS: N/A

INTERFERING FACTORS
• Drugs that may increase sickle cells in vitro include prostaglandins.
• A positive test does not distinguish between the sickle trait and sickle cell anemia; to make this determination, follow-up testing by Hgb electrophoresis should be performed.
• False-negative results may occur in children younger than 3 mo of age.
• False-negative results may occur in patients who have received a

recent blood transfusion before specimen collection, as a result of the dilutional effect.

- False-positive results may occur in patients without the trait or disease who have received a blood transfusion from a sickle cell–positive donor; this effect can last for 4 mo after the transfusion.

- Test results are unreliable if the patient has pernicious anemia or polycythemia.

NURSING IMPLICATIONS AND PROCEDURE

PRETEST:

▶ Positively identify the patient using at least two unique identifiers before providing care, treatment, or services.

▶ *Patient Teaching:* Inform the patient this test can assist in diagnosing anemia.

▶ Obtain a history of the patient's complaints, including a list of known allergens, especially allergies or sensitivities to latex.

▶ Obtain a history of the patient's hematopoietic system, symptoms, and results of previously performed laboratory tests and diagnostic and surgical procedures.

▶ Note any recent procedures that can interfere with test results.

▶ Obtain a list of the patient's current medications, including herbs, nutritional supplements, and nutraceuticals (see Appendix F).

▶ Review the procedure with the patient. Inform the patient that specimen collection takes approximately 5 to 10 min. Address concerns about pain and explain that there may be some discomfort during the venipuncture.

▶ *Sensitivity to social and cultural issues,* as well as concern for modesty, is important in providing psychological support before, during, and after the procedure.

▶ There are no food, fluid, or medication restrictions unless by medical direction.

INTRATEST:

▶ If the patient has a history of allergic reaction to latex, avoid the use of equipment containing latex.

▶ Instruct the patient to cooperate fully and to follow directions. Direct the patient to breathe normally and to avoid unnecessary movement.

▶ Observe standard precautions, and follow the general guidelines in Appendix A. Positively identify the patient, and label the appropriate tubes with the corresponding patient demographics, date, and time of collection. Perform a venipuncture.

▶ Remove the needle and apply direct pressure with dry gauze to stop bleeding. Observe/assess venipuncture site for bleeding or hematoma formation and secure gauze with adhesive bandage.

▶ Promptly transport the specimen to the laboratory for processing and analysis.

POST-TEST:

▶ A report of the results will be sent to the requesting health-care provider (HCP), who will discuss the results with the patient.

▶ Advise the patient with sickle cell disease to avoid situations in which hypoxia may occur, such as strenuous exercise, staying at high altitudes, or traveling in an unpressurized aircraft. Obstetric and surgical patients with sickle cell anemia are at risk for hypoxia and therefore require close observation: Obstetric patients are at risk for hypoxia during the stress of labor and delivery, and surgical patients may become hypoxic while under general anesthesia.

▶ Recognize anxiety related to test results, and offer support, as appropriate. Discuss the implications of abnormal test results on the patient's lifestyle. Provide teaching and information regarding the clinical implications of the test results, as appropriate. Educate the patient regarding access to counseling services (www.sicklecelldisease.org).

▶ Reinforce information given by the patient's HCP regarding further testing, treatment, or referral to another HCP. Inform the patient that further testing may be indicated if results are positive.

S

Answer any questions or address any concerns voiced by the patient or family.

▶ Depending on the results of this procedure, additional testing may be performed to evaluate or monitor progression of the disease process and determine the need for a change in therapy. Evaluate test results in relation to the patient's symptoms and other tests performed.

RELATED MONOGRAPHS:

▶ Related tests include biopsy bone marrow, CBC, CBC RBC morphology, CBC RBC indices, ESR, Hgb electrophoresis, hemosiderin, LAP, MRI musculoskeletal, RBC cholinesterase, and US spleen.

▶ Refer to the Hematopoietic System table at the end of the book for related tests by body system.

Slit-Lamp Biomicroscopy

SYNONYM/ACRONYM: Slit-lamp examination.

COMMON USE: To detect abnormalities in the external and anterior eye structures to assist in diagnosing disorders such as corneal injury, hemorrhage, ulcers, and abrasion.

AREA OF APPLICATION: Eyes.

CONTRAST: N/A.

DESCRIPTION: This noninvasive procedure is used to visualize the anterior portion of the eye and its parts, including the eyelids and eyelashes, sclera, conjunctiva, cornea, iris, lens, and anterior chamber, and to detect pathology of any of these areas of the eyes. The slit lamp has a binocular microscope and light source that can be adjusted to examine the fluid, tissues, and structures of the eyes. Special attachments to the slit lamp are used for special studies and more detailed views of specific areas. Dilating drops or mydriatics may be used to enlarge the pupil in order to allow the examiner to see the eye in greater detail. Mydriatics work either by temporarily paralyzing the muscle that makes the pupil smaller or by stimulating the iris dilator muscle. Blue or hazel eyes dilate faster than brown eyes.

INDICATIONS

• Detect conjunctival and corneal injuries by foreign bodies and determine if ocular penetration or anterior chamber hemorrhage is present

• Detect corneal abrasions, ulcers, or abnormal curvatures (keratoconus)

- Detect deficiency in tear formation indicative of lacrimal dysfunction causing dry eye disease that can lead to corneal erosions or infection
- Detect lens opacities indicative of cataract formation
- Determine the presence of blepharitis, conjunctivitis, hordeolum, entropion, ectropion, trachoma, scleritis, and iritis
- Evaluate the fit of contact lenses

POTENTIAL DIAGNOSIS

Normal findings in
- Normal anterior tissues and structures of the eyes

Abnormal findings in
- Blepharitis
- Conjunctivitis
- Corneal abrasions
- Corneal ulcers
- Ectropion
- Entropion
- Hordeolum
- Iritis
- Keratoconus (abnormal curvatures)
- Lens opacities
- Scleritis
- Trachoma

CRITICAL FINDINGS: N/A

INTERFERING FACTORS

- Patients with narrow-angle glaucoma if pupil dilation is performed, because dilation can initiate a severe and sight-threatening open-angle attack.
- Patients with allergies to mydriatics if pupil dilation using mydriatics is performed.
- Inability of the patient to cooperate and remain still during the procedure because of age, significant pain, or mental status may interfere with the test results.

- Failure to follow medication restrictions before the procedure may cause the procedure to be canceled or repeated.

NURSING IMPLICATIONS AND PROCEDURE

PRETEST:

- Positively identify the patient using at least two unique identifiers before providing care, treatment, or services.
- *Patient Teaching:* Inform the patient this procedure can assist in evaluating the structures of the eye.
- Obtain a history of the patient's complaints, including a list of known allergens, especially mydriatics if dilation is to be performed.
- Obtain a history of the patient's known or suspected vision loss, changes in visual acuity, including type and cause; use of glasses or contact lenses; eye conditions with treatment regimens; eye surgery; and other tests and procedures to assess and diagnose visual deficit.
- Obtain a history of the patient's symptoms and results of previously performed laboratory tests and diagnostic and surgical procedures.
- Obtain a list of the patient's current medications, including herbs, nutritional supplements, and nutraceuticals (see Appendix F).
- Instruct the patient to remove contact lenses or glasses, as appropriate, unless the study is being done to check the fit and effectiveness of the contact lenses. Instruct the patient regarding the importance of keeping the eyes open for the test.
- Review the procedure with the patient. Address concerns about pain and explain that mydriatics, if used, may cause blurred vision and sensitivity to light. There may also be a brief stinging sensation when the drop is put in the eye. Inform the patient that a health-care provider (HCP) performs the test in a quiet, darkened room, and that to evaluate both eyes, the test can take up 30 min (including time for the pupils to dilate before the test is actually performed).

S

▶ *Sensitivity to social and cultural issues,* as well as concern for modesty, is important in providing psychological support before, during, and after the procedure.

▶ There are no food or fluid restrictions unless by medical direction.

▶ The patient should withhold eye medications (particularly mydriatic eyedrops if the patient has glaucoma) for at least 1 day prior to the procedure.

▶ Ensure that the patient understands that he or she must refrain from driving until the pupils return to normal (about 4 hr) after the test and has made arrangements to have someone else be responsible for transportation after the test.

INTRATEST:

▶ Ensure that the patient has complied with medication restrictions and pretesting preparations; assure that eye medications, especially mydriatics, have been restricted for at least 1 day prior to the procedure.

▶ Instruct the patient to cooperate fully and to follow directions. Ask the patient to remain still during the procedure because movement produces unreliable results.

▶ Seat the patient comfortably. If dilation is to be performed, administer the ordered mydriatic to each eye and repeat in 5 to 15 min. Drops are placed in the eye with the patient looking up and the solution directed at the six o'clock position of the sclera (white of the eye) near the limbus (gray, semitransparent area of the eyeball where the cornea and sclera meet). Neither dropper nor bottle should touch the eyelashes.

▶ Ask the patient to place the chin in the chin rest and gently press the forehead against the support bar.

▶ The HCP places the slit lamp in front of the patient's eyes in line with the examiner's eyes. The external structures of the eyes are inspected with the special bright light and microscope of the slit lamp. The light is then directed into the patient's eyes to inspect the anterior fluids and structures and is adjusted for shape, intensity, and depth needed to visualize these areas. Magnification of the microscope is also adjusted to optimize visualization of the eye structures.

▶ Special attachments and procedures can also be used to obtain further diagnostic information about the eyes. These may include, for example, a camera to photograph specific parts, gonioscopy to determine anterior chamber closure, and a cobalt-blue filter to detect minute corneal scratches, breaks, and abrasions with corneal staining.

POST-TEST:

▶ A report of the results will be sent to the requesting HCP, who will discuss the results with the patient.

▶ Instruct the patient to resume usual medications, as directed by the HCP.

▶ Recognize anxiety related to test results, and encourage the family to recognize and be supportive of impaired activity related to vision loss, anticipated loss of driving privileges, or the possibility of requiring corrective lenses (self-image). Discuss the implications of the abnormal test results on the patient's lifestyle. Provide contact information, if desired, for a general patient education Web site on the topic of eye care (e.g., www.allaboutvision.com).

▶ Reinforce information given by the patient's HCP regarding further testing, treatment, or referral to another HCP. Inform the patient that visual acuity and responses to light may change. Suggest that the patient wear dark glasses after the test until the pupils return to normal size. Answer any questions or address any concerns voiced by the patient or family.

▶ Depending on the results of this procedure, additional testing may be performed to evaluate or monitor progression of the disease process and determine the need for a change in therapy. Evaluate test results in relation to the patient's symptoms and other tests performed.

S

- Related tests include color perception test, fluorescein angiography, gonioscopy, intraocular muscle function, intraocular pressure, nerve fiber analysis, refraction, Schirmer tear test, and visual field testing.
- Refer to the Ocular System table at the end of the book for related tests by body system.

Sodium, Blood

SYNONYM/ACRONYM: Serum Na+.

COMMON USE: To assess electrolyte balance related to hydration levels and disorders such as diarrhea and vomiting and to monitor the effect of diuretic use.

SPECIMEN: Serum (1 mL) collected in a red- or tiger-top tube. Plasma (1 mL) collected in a green-top (heparin) tube is also acceptable.

REFERENCE VALUE: (Method: Ion-selective electrode)

Age	Conventional Units	SI Units (Conventional Units × 1)
Newborn	133–146 mEq/L	133–146 mmol/L
Infant	133–144 mEq/L	133–144 mmol/L
Child	135–145 mEq/L	135–145 mmol/L
Adult–older adult	135–145 mEq/L	135–145 mmol/L

DESCRIPTION: Sodium is the most abundant cation in the extracellular fluid and, together with the accompanying chloride and bicarbonate anions, accounts for 92% of serum osmolality. Sodium plays a major role in maintaining homeostasis in a variety of ways, including maintaining the osmotic pressure of extracellular fluid, regulating renal retention and excretion of water, maintaining acid-base balance, regulating potassium and chloride levels, stimulating neuromuscular reactions, and maintaining systemic blood pressure. *Hypernatremia* (elevated sodium level) occurs when there is excessive water loss or abnormal retention of sodium. *Hyponatremia* (low

S

sodium level) occurs when there is inadequate sodium retention or inadequate intake.

INDICATIONS
- Determine whole-body stores of sodium, because the ion is predominantly extracellular
- Monitor the effectiveness of drug therapy, especially diuretics, on serum sodium levels

POTENTIAL DIAGNOSIS

Increased in
- Azotemia *(related to increased renal retention)*
- Burns *(hemoconcentration related to excessive loss of free water)*
- Cushing's disease
- Dehydration
- Diabetes *(dehydration related to frequent urination)*
- Diarrhea *(related to water loss in excess of salt loss)*
- Excessive intake
- Excessive saline therapy *(related to administration of IV fluids)*
- Excessive sweating *(related to loss of free water, which can cause hemoconcentration)*
- Fever *(related to loss of free water through sweating)*
- Hyperaldosteronism *(related to excessive production of aldosterone, which increases renal absorption of sodium and increases blood levels)*
- Lactic acidosis *(related to diabetes)*
- Nasogastric feeding with inadequate fluid *(related to dehydration and hemoconcentration)*
- Vomiting *(related to dehydration)*

Decreased in
- Central nervous system disease
- Congestive heart failure *(diminished renal blood flow due to reduced cardiac capacity decreases urinary excretion and increases blood sodium levels)*
- Cystic fibrosis *(related to loss from chronic diarrhea; poor intestinal absorption)*
- Excessive antidiuretic hormone production *(related to excessive loss through renal excretion)*
- Excessive use of diuretics *(related to excessive loss through renal excretion; renal absorption is blocked)*
- Hepatic failure *(hemodilution related to fluid retention)*
- Hypoproteinemia *(related to fluid retention)*
- Insufficient intake
- IV glucose infusion *(hypertonic glucose draws water into extracellular fluid and sodium is diluted)*
- Mineralocorticoid deficiency (Addison's disease) *(related to inadequate production of aldosterone, which results in decreased absorption by the kidneys)*
- Nephrotic syndrome *(related to decreased ability of renal tubules to reabsorb sodium)*

CRITICAL FINDINGS ✦
- *Hyponatremia:* Less than 120 mEq/L
- *Hypernatremia:* Greater than 160 mEq/L

Note and immediately report to the health-care provider (HCP) any critically increased or decreased values and related symptoms especially fluid imbalance.

Signs and symptoms of hyponatremia include confusion, irritability, convulsions, tachycardia, nausea, vomiting, and loss of consciousness. Possible interventions include maintenance of airway, monitoring for convulsions, fluid restriction, and performance of hourly neurological checks. Administration of saline for replacement requires close attention to serum and urine osmolality.

Signs and symptoms of hypernatremia include restlessness, intense thirst, weakness, swollen tongue, seizures, and coma. Possible interventions include treatment of the underlying cause of water loss or sodium excess, which includes sodium restriction and administration of diuretics combined with IV solutions of 5% dextrose in water (D_5W).

INTERFERING FACTORS

- Drugs that may increase serum sodium levels include anabolic steroids, angiotensin, bicarbonate, carbenoxolone, cisplatin, corticotropin, cortisone, gamma globulin, and mannitol.
- Drugs that may decrease serum sodium levels include amphotericin B, bicarbonate, cathartics (excessive use), chlorpropamide, chlorthalidone, diuretics, ethacrynic acid, fluoxetine, furosemide, laxatives (excessive use), methyclothiazide, metolazone, nicardipine, quinethazone, theophylline (IV infusion), thiazides, and triamterene.
- Specimens should never be collected above an IV line because of the potential for dilution when the specimen and the IV solution combine in the collection container, falsely decreasing the result. There is also the potential of contaminating the sample with the substance of interest, if it is present in the IV solution, falsely increasing the result.

NURSING IMPLICATIONS AND PROCEDURE

PRETEST:

- Positively identify the patient using at least two unique identifiers before providing care, treatment, or services.
- *Patient Teaching:* Inform the patient this test can assist in evaluating electrolyte balance.
- Obtain a history of the patient's complaints, including a list of known allergens, especially allergies or sensitivities to latex.
- Obtain a history of the patient's cardiovascular, endocrine, and genitourinary systems; symptoms; and results of previously performed laboratory tests and diagnostic and surgical procedures.
- Obtain a list of the patient's current medications, including herbs, nutritional supplements, and nutraceuticals (see Appendix F).
- Review the procedure with the patient. Inform the patient that specimen collection takes approximately 5 to 10 min. Address concerns about pain and explain that there may be some discomfort during the venipuncture.
- *Sensitivity to social and cultural issues,* as well as concern for modesty, is important in providing psychological support before, during, and after the procedure.
- There are no food, fluid, or medication restrictions unless by medical direction.

INTRATEST:

- If the patient has a history of allergic reaction to latex, avoid the use of equipment containing latex.
- Instruct the patient to cooperate fully and to follow directions. Direct the patient to breathe normally and to avoid unnecessary movement.
- Observe standard precautions, and follow the general guidelines in Appendix A. Positively identify the patient, and label the appropriate tubes with the corresponding patient demographics, date, and time of collection. Perform a venipuncture.

S

▶ Remove the needle and apply direct pressure with dry gauze to stop bleeding. Observe/assess venipuncture site for bleeding or hematoma formation and secure gauze with adhesive bandage.

▶ Promptly transport the specimen to the laboratory for processing and analysis.

POST-TEST:

▶ A report of the results will be sent to the requesting HCP, who will discuss the results with the patient.

▶ *Nutritional Considerations:* Evaluate the patient for signs and symptoms of dehydration. Decreased skin turgor, dry mouth, and multiple longitudinal furrows in the tongue are symptoms of dehydration. Dehydration is a significant and common finding in geriatric and other patients in whom renal function has deteriorated.

▶ *Nutritional Considerations:* If appropriate, educate patients with low sodium levels that the major source of dietary sodium is found in table salt. Many foods, such as milk and other dairy products, are also good sources of dietary sodium. Most other dietary sodium is available through the consumption of processed foods. Patients on low-sodium diets should be advised to avoid beverages such as colas, ginger ale, sports drinks, lemon-lime sodas, and root beer. Many over-the-counter medications, including antacids, laxatives, analgesics, sedatives, and antitussives, contain significant amounts of sodium. The best advice is to emphasize the importance of reading all food, beverage, and medicine labels. In 2004, the Institute of Medicine's Food and Nutrition Board established 2,300 mg as the recommended maximum daily intake of dietary sodium for adults and 1,900 mg/day for children.

▶ Reinforce information given by the patient's HCP regarding further testing, treatment, or referral to another HCP. Answer any questions or address any concerns voiced by the patient or family.

▶ Depending on the results of this procedure, additional testing may be performed to evaluate or monitor progression of the disease process and determine the need for a change in therapy. Evaluate test results in relation to the patient's symptoms and other tests performed.

RELATED MONOGRAPHS:

▶ Related tests include ACTH, aldosterone, anion gap, ANP, BNP, blood gases, BUN, calculus kidney stone panel, BUN, calcium, carbon dioxide, chloride, chloride sweat, cortisol, creatinine, DHEAS, echocardiography, glucose, insulin, ketones, lactic acid, lung perfusion scan, magnesium, osmolality, potassium, renin, urine sodium, and UA.

▶ Refer to the Cardiovascular, Endocrine, and Genitourinary systems tables at the end of the book for related tests by body system.

S

Sodium, Urine

SYNONYM/ACRONYM: Urine Na⁺

COMMON USE: To assist in evaluating for acute renal failure, acute oliguria, and to assist in the differential diagnosis of hyponatremia.

SPECIMEN: Urine (5 mL) from an unpreserved random or timed specimen collected in a clean plastic collection container.

REFERENCE VALUE: (Method: Ion-selective electrode)

Age	Conventional Units	SI Units (Conventional Units × 1)
6–10 yr		
Male	41–115 mEq/24 hr	41–115 mmol/24 hr
Female	20–69 mEq/24 hr	20–69 mmol/24 hr
10–14 yr		
Male	63–177 mEq/24 hr	63–177 mmol/24 hr
Female	48–168 mEq/24 hr	48–168 mmol/24 hr
Adult–older adult	27–287 mEq/24 hr	27–287 mmol/24 hr

Values vary markedly depending on dietary intake and hydration state.

DESCRIPTION: Regulating electrolyte balance is a major function of the kidneys. In normally functioning kidneys, urine sodium levels increase when serum levels are high and decrease when serum levels are low to maintain homeostasis. Analyzing these urinary levels can provide important clues to the functioning of the kidneys and other major organs. There is diurnal variation in excretion of sodium, with values lower at night. Urine sodium tests usually involve timed urine collections over a 12- or 24-hr period. Measurement of random specimens may also be requested.

INDICATIONS

- Determine potential cause of renal calculi
- Evaluate known or suspected endocrine disorder
- Evaluate known or suspected renal disease
- Evaluate malabsorption disorders

POTENTIAL DIAGNOSIS

Increased in

- Adrenal failure *(inadequate production of aldosterone results in decreased renal sodium absorption)*
- Diabetes *(increased glucose levels result in hypertonic extracellular fluid; dehydration from excessive urination can cause hemoconcentration)*

- Diuretic therapy *(medication causes sodium to be lost by the kidneys)*
- Excessive intake
- Renal tubular acidosis *(related to diabetes)*
- Salt-losing nephritis *(related to diminished capacity of the kidneys to reabsorb sodium)*

Decreased in

- Adrenal hyperfunction *(overproduction of aldosterone and other corticosteroids stimulate renal absorption of sodium decreasing urine sodium levels)*
- Congestive heart failure *(decreased renal blood flow related to diminished cardiac output)*
- Diarrhea *(related to decreased intestinal absorption; a decrease in blood levels will cause sodium to be retained by the kidneys and will lower urine sodium levels)*
- Excessive sweating *(excessive loss of sodium through sweat; sodium will be retained by the kidneys)*
- Extrarenal sodium loss with adequate hydration
- Insufficient intake
- Postoperative period (first 24 to 48 hr)
- Prerenal azotemia
- Sodium retention *(premenstrual)*

CRITICAL FINDINGS: N/A

INTERFERING FACTORS

- Drugs that may increase urine sodium levels include acetazolamide, acetylsalicylic acid, amiloride, ammonium chloride, azosemide, benzthiazide, bumetanide, calcitonin, chlorothiazide, clopamide, cyclothiazide, diapamide, dopamine, ethacrynic acid, furosemide, hydrocortisone, hydroflumethiazide, isosorbide, levodopa, mercurial diuretics, methyclothiazide, metolazone, polythiazide, quinethazone, spironolactone, sulfates, tetracycline, thiazides, torasemide, triamterene, trichlormethiazide, triflocin, verapamil, and vincristine.
- Drugs that may decrease urine sodium levels include aldosterone, anesthetics, angiotensin, corticosteroids, cortisone, etodolac, indomethacin, levarterenol, lithium, and propranolol.
- Sodium levels are subject to diurnal variation (output being lowest at night), which is why 24-hr collections are recommended.

NURSING IMPLICATIONS AND PROCEDURE

PRETEST:

- Positively identify the patient using at least two unique identifiers before providing care, treatment, or services.
- *Patient Teaching:* Inform the patient this test can assist in evaluating kidney function.
- Obtain a history of the patient's complaints, including a list of known allergens, especially allergies or sensitivities to latex.
- Obtain a history of the patient's endocrine and genitourinary systems, symptoms, and results of previously performed laboratory tests and diagnostic and surgical procedures.
- Obtain a list of the patient's current medications, including herbs, nutritional supplements, and nutraceuticals (see Appendix F).
- Review the procedure with the patient. Provide a nonmetallic urinal, bedpan, or toilet-mounted collection device. Address concerns about pain and explain that there should be no discomfort during the procedure.
- *Sensitivity to social and cultural issues,* as well as concern for modesty, is important in providing psychological support before, during, and after the procedure.
- Usually a 24-hr time frame for urine collection is ordered. Inform the patient

that all urine must be saved during that 24-hr period. Instruct the patient not to void directly into the laboratory collection container. Instruct the patient to avoid defecating in the collection device and to keep toilet tissue out of the collection device to prevent contamination of the specimen. Place a sign in the bathroom to remind the patient to save all urine.

▶ Instruct the patient to void all urine into the collection device and then to pour the urine into the laboratory collection container. Alternatively, the specimen can be left in the collection device for a health care staff member to add to the laboratory collection container.

▶ There are no food, fluid, or medication restrictions unless by medical direction.

INTRATEST:

▶ If the patient has a history of allergic reaction to latex, avoid the use of equipment containing latex.

▶ Instruct the patient to cooperate fully and to follow directions.

▶ Observe standard precautions, and follow the general guidelines in Appendix A. Positively identify the patient, and label the appropriate collection containers with the corresponding patient demographics, date, and time of collection.

Random Specimen (Collect in Early Morning)

Clean-Catch Specimen

▶ Instruct the male patient to (1) thoroughly wash his hands, (2) cleanse the meatus, (3) void a small amount into the toilet, and (4) void directly into the specimen container.

▶ Instruct the female patient to (1) thoroughly wash her hands; (2) cleanse the labia from front to back; (3) while keeping the labia separated, void a small amount into the toilet; and (4) without interrupting the urine stream, void directly into the specimen container.

Indwelling Catheter

▶ Put on gloves. Empty drainage tube of urine. It may be necessary to clamp off the catheter for 15 to 30 min before specimen collection. Cleanse specimen

port with antiseptic swab, and then aspirate 5 mL of urine with a 21- to 25-gauge needle and syringe. Transfer urine to a sterile container.

Timed Specimen

▶ Obtain a clean 3-L urine specimen container, toilet-mounted collection device, and plastic bag (for transport of the specimen container). The specimen must be refrigerated or kept on ice throughout the entire collection period. If an indwelling urinary catheter is in place, the drainage bag must be kept on ice.

▶ Begin the test between 6 and 8 a.m., if possible. Collect first voiding and discard. Record the time the specimen was discarded as the beginning of the timed collection period. The next morning, ask the patient to void at the same time the collection was started and add this last voiding to the container. Urinary output should be recorded throughout the collection time.

▶ If an indwelling catheter is in place, replace the tubing and container system at the start of the collection time. Keep the container system on ice during the collection period, or empty the urine into a larger container periodically during the collection period; monitor to ensure continued drainage, and conclude the test the next morning at the same hour the collection was begun.

▶ At the conclusion of the test, compare the quantity of urine with the urinary output record for the collection; if the specimen contains less than what was recorded as output, some urine may have been discarded, invalidating the test.

▶ Include on the collection container's label the amount of urine, test start and stop times, and any foods or medications that can affect test results.

General

▶ Promptly transport the specimen to the laboratory for processing and analysis.

POST-TEST:

▶ A report of the results will be sent to the requesting health-care provider (HCP), who will discuss the results with the patient.

▶ Instruct the patient to resume usual diet, fluids, medications, and activity, as directed by the HCP.

▶ *Nutritional Considerations:* If appropriate, educate patients with low sodium levels that the major source of dietary sodium is found in table salt. Many foods, such as milk and other dairy products, are also good sources of dietary sodium. Most other dietary sodium is available through the consumption of processed foods. Patients on low-sodium diets should be advised to avoid beverages such as colas, ginger ale, sports drinks, lemon-lime sodas, and root beer. Many over-the-counter medications, including antacids, laxatives, analgesics, sedatives, and antitussives, contain significant amounts of sodium. The best advice is to emphasize the importance of reading all food, beverage, and medicine labels. In 2004, the Institute of Medicine's Food and Nutrition Board established 2,300 mg as the recommended maximum daily intake of dietary sodium for adults; 1,900 mg/day for children.

▶ Recognize anxiety related to test results. Discuss the implications of abnormal test results on the patient's lifestyle. Provide teaching and information regarding the clinical implications of the test results, as appropriate.

▶ Reinforce information given by the patient's HCP regarding further testing, treatment, or referral to another HCP. Answer any questions or address any concerns voiced by the patient or family.

▶ Depending on the results of this procedure, additional testing may be performed to evaluate or monitor progression of the disease process and determine the need for a change in therapy. Evaluate test results in relation to the patient's symptoms and other tests performed.

RELATED MONOGRAPHS:

▶ Related tests include ACTH, aldosterone, anion gap, ANP, BNP, blood gases, BUN, calcium, calculus kidney stone panel, carbon dioxide, chloride, chloride sweat, cortisol, creatinine, DHEAS, echocardiography, glucose, insulin, ketones, lactic acid, lung perfusion scan, magnesium, osmolality, potassium, renin, sodium, and UA.

▶ Refer to the Endocrine and Genitourinary system tables at the end of the book for related tests by body system.

Spondee Speech Recognition Threshold

SYNONYM/ACRONYM: SRT, speech reception threshold.

COMMON USE: To evaluate for hearing loss related to speech discrepancies.

AREA OF APPLICATION: Ears.

CONTRAST: N/A.

DESCRIPTION: This noninvasive speech audiometric procedure measures the degree of hearing loss for speech. The speech recognition threshold is the lowest hearing level at which speech can barely be recognized or understood. In this test, a number of spondaic words are presented to the patient at different intensities. Spondaic words, or spondees, are words containing two syllables that are equally accented or emphasized when they are spoken to the patient. The SRT is defined as the lowest hearing level at which the patient correctly repeats 50% of a list of spondaic words. Examples are airplane, hot dog, outside, ice cream, and baseball.

INDICATIONS

- Determine appropriate gain during hearing aid selection
- Determine the extent of hearing loss related to speech recognition, as evidenced by the faintest level at which spondee words are correctly repeated
- Differentiate a real hearing loss from pseudohypoacusis
- Verify pure tone results

POTENTIAL DIAGNOSIS

Normal findings in

- Normal spondee threshold of about 6 to 10 dB (decibels) of the normal pure tone threshold with 50% of the words presented being correctly repeated at the appropriate intensity (see monograph titled "Audiometry, Hearing Loss")
- Normal speech recognition with 90% to 100% of the words presented being correctly repeated at an appropriate intensity

Abnormal findings in

- Conductive hearing loss
- Impacted cerumen
- Obstruction of external ear canal *(related to presence of a foreign body)*
- Otitis externa *(related to infection in ear canal)*

- Otitis media *(related to poor eustachian tube function or infection)*
- Otitis media serus *(related to fluid in middle ear due to allergies or a cold)*
- Otosclerosis
- High-frequency hearing loss *(normal hearing range is 20 Hz to 20,000 Hz; high-frequency range begins at 4,000 Hz)*
- Presbyacusis *(related to gradual hearing loss experienced in advancing age, which occurs in the high-frequency range)*
- Noise induced *(related to exposure over long periods of time)*
- Sensorineural hearing loss (acoustic nerve impairment)
- Congenital damage or malformations of the inner ear
- Ménière's disease
- Ototoxic drugs *(aminoglycosides, e.g., gentamicin or tobramycin; salicylates, e.g., aspirin)*
- Presbyacusis *(related to gradual hearing loss experienced in advancing age)*
- Serious infections *(meningitis, measles, mumps, other viral, syphilis)*
- Trauma to the inner ear *(related to exposure to noise in excess of 90 dB or as a result of physical trauma)*
- Tumor *(e.g., acoustic neuroma, cerebellopontine angle tumor, meningioma)*
- Vascular disorders

CRITICAL FINDINGS: N/A

INTERFERING FACTORS

Factors that may impair the results of the examination

- Inability of the patient to cooperate or remain still during the procedure because of age or mental status may interfere with the test results.

S

- Unfamiliarity with the language in which the words are presented or with the words themselves will alter the results.
- Improper placement of the earphones and inconsistency in frequency of word presentation will affect results.

NURSING IMPLICATIONS AND PROCEDURE

PRETEST:

▶ Positively identify the patient using at least two unique identifiers before providing care, treatment, or services.

▶ *Patient Teaching:* Inform the patient this procedure can assist in measuring hearing loss related to speech.

▶ Obtain a history of the patient's complaints, including a list of known allergens.

▶ Obtain a history of the patient's known or suspected hearing loss, including type and cause; ear conditions with treatment regimens; ear surgery; and other tests and procedures to assess and diagnose hearing deficit.

▶ Obtain a history of the patient's symptoms and results of previously performed laboratory tests and diagnostic and surgical procedures.

▶ Obtain a list of the patient's current medications, including herbs, nutritional supplements, and nutraceuticals (see Appendix F).

▶ Review the procedure with the patient. Ensure that the patient understands words and sounds in the language to be used for the test. Inform the patient that a series of words that change from loud to soft tones will be presented using earphones and that he or she will be asked to repeat the word. Explain that each ear is tested separately. Address concerns about pain and explain that no discomfort will be experienced during the test. Inform the patient that a health-care provider (HCP) performs the test, in a quiet, soundproof room, and that the evaluation takes 5 to 10 min.

▶ *Sensitivity to social and cultural issues,* as well as concern for modesty, is important in providing psychological support before, during, and after the procedure.

▶ There are no food, fluid, or medication restrictions unless by medical direction.

INTRATEST:

▶ Instruct the patient to cooperate fully and to follow directions. Ask the patient to remain still during the procedure because movement produces unreliable results.

▶ Seat the patient on a chair in a soundproof booth. Place the earphones on the patient's head and secure them over the ears. The audiometer is set at 20 dB above the known pure tone threshold obtained from audiometry. The test represents hearing levels at speech frequencies of 500, 1,000, and 2,000 Hz.

▶ The spondee words are presented to the ear with the best auditory response using a speech audiometer. The intensity is decreased and then increased to the softest sound at which the patient is able to hear the words and respond correctly to 50% of them. The procedure is then repeated for the other ear.

POST-TEST:

▶ A report of the results will be sent to the requesting HCP, who will discuss the results with the patient.

▶ Recognize anxiety related to test results, and be supportive of activity related to impaired hearing and perceived loss of independence. Discuss the implications of abnormal test results on the patient's lifestyle. Provide teaching and information regarding the clinical implications of the test results, as appropriate. Educate the patient regarding access to counseling services. Provide contact information, if desired, for the American Speech-Language-Hearing Association (www.asha.org).

▶ Reinforce information given by the patient's HCP regarding further testing, treatment, or referral to another HCP. Answer any questions or address any concerns voiced by the patient or family.

S

Depending on the results of this procedure, additional testing may be performed to evaluate or monitor progression of the disease process and determine the need for a change in therapy. Evaluate test results in relation to the patient's symptoms and other tests performed.

RELATED MONOGRAPHS:

Related tests include antibiotic drugs, analgesic and antipyretic drugs, audiometry hearing loss, culture bacterial (ear), and Gram stain.

Refer to the Auditory System table at the end of the book for related tests by body system.

Stereotactic Biopsy, Breast

SYNONYM/ACRONYM: N/A.

COMMON USE: To assess suspicious breast tissue for cancer.

SPECIMEN: Breast tissue or cells.

REFERENCE VALUE: (Method: Macroscopic and microscopic examination of tissue) No abnormal cells or tissue.

DESCRIPTION: A stereotactic breast biopsy is helpful when a mammogram or ultrasound examination shows a mass, a cluster of microcalcifications (tiny calcium deposits that are closely grouped together), or an area of abnormal tissue change, usually with no lump being felt on a careful breast examination. A number of biopsy instruments and methods are utilized with x-ray guidance. They include core biopsy, which uses a large-bore needle to remove a generous sample of breast tissue, and a vacuum-assisted needle biopsy device. As an alternative to an open-core surgical biopsy, which removes an entire breast lump for microscopic analysis, a narrow needle may be passed through the skin into the area under investigation. This is accomplished with the help of special breast x-rays.

Images of the breast are obtained with a mammography machine, and the images are recorded in a computer. An initial x-ray locates the abnormality, and two stereo views are obtained, each angled 15° to either side of the initial image. The computer calculates how much the area of interest has changed with each image and determines the exact site in three-dimensional space. A small sample of breast tissue is obtained and can show whether the breast mass is cancerous. A pathologist examines the tissue that was removed and makes a final diagnosis to allow for effective treatment.

INDICATIONS

• A mammogram showing a suspicious cluster of small calcium deposits

- A mammogram showing a suspicious solid mass that cannot be felt on breast examination
- Evidence of breast lesion by palpation, mammography, or ultrasound
- New mass or area of calcium deposits present at a previous surgery site
- Observable breast changes such as "peau d'orange" skin, scaly skin of the areola, drainage from the nipple, or ulceration of the skin
- Patient preference for a nonsurgical method of lesion assessment
- Structure of the breast tissue is distorted

POTENTIAL DIAGNOSIS
- Positive findings in carcinoma of the breast

CRITICAL FINDINGS: N/A

INTERFERING FACTORS
- This procedure is contraindicated in patients with bleeding disorders.

Factors that may impair clear imaging
- Failure to restrict food intake before the study.
- Metallic objects (e.g., jewelry, body rings, dental amalgams) within the examination field, which may inhibit organ visualization and cause unclear images.
- Inability of the patient to cooperate or remain still during the procedure because of age, significant pain, or mental status.

Other considerations
- Complications of the procedure include hemorrhage, infection at the insertion site, and cardiac arrhythmias.
- Failure to follow dietary restrictions before the procedure may cause the procedure to be canceled or repeated.

- Consultation with a health-care practitioner (HCP) should occur before the procedure for radiation safety concerns regarding younger patients or patients who are lactating.
- Risks associated with radiation overexposure can result from frequent x-ray procedures. Personnel in the room with the patient should wear a protective lead apron, stand behind a shield, or leave the area while the examination is being done. Personnel working in the examination area should wear badges to record their level of radiation exposure.

NURSING IMPLICATIONS AND PROCEDURE

PRETEST:
- Positively identify the patient using at least two unique identifiers before providing care, treatment, or services.
- *Patient Teaching:* Inform the patient this procedure can assist in assessing breast health.
- Obtain a history of the patient's complaints, including a list of known allergens, especially allergies or sensitivities to latex or anesthetics.
- Obtain a history of the patient's reproductive system, symptoms, and results of previously performed laboratory tests and diagnostic and surgical procedures.
- Note any recent procedures that can interfere with test results.
- Record the date of the last menstrual period and determine the possibility of pregnancy in perimenopausal women.
- Obtain a list of the patient's current medications, including anticoagulant therapy, aspirin and other salicylates, herbs, nutritional supplements, and nutraceuticals, especially those known to affect coagulation (see Appendix F). It is recommended that use be discontinued 14 days before surgical procedures. The requesting HCP and laboratory should be advised if the patient regularly uses these products

so that their effects can be taken into consideration when reviewing results.

▶ Review the procedure with the patient. Address concerns about pain related to the procedure and explain that some pain will be experienced during the test, or there may be moments of discomfort. Inform the patient that the procedure is performed in a special room, usually a mammography suite, by an HCP specializing in this procedure, with support staff, and takes approximately 30 to 60 min.

▶ *Sensitivity to social and cultural issues,* as well as concern for modesty, is important in providing psychological support before, during, and after the procedure.

▶ Explain that an IV line may be inserted to allow infusion of IV fluids or sedatives. Usually normal saline is infused.

▶ Instruct the patient to remove jewelry and other metallic objects from the area of the procedure.

▶ Instruct the patient to avoid taking anticoagulant medication or to reduce dosage as ordered prior to the procedure. Number of days to withhold medication is dependent on the type of anticoagulant.

▶ Instruct the patient to fast and restrict fluids for 4 hr prior to the procedure. Protocols may vary among facilities.

▶ *Make sure a written and informed consent has been signed prior to the procedure and before administering any medications.*

▶ The procedure may be terminated if chest pain or severe cardiac arrhythmias occur.

INTRATEST:

▶ Ensure that the patient has complied with dietary and medication restrictions for 4 hr prior to the procedure.

▶ Ensure that anticoagulant therapy has been withheld for the appropriate number of days prior to the procedure. Number of days to withhold medication is dependent on the type of anticoagulant. Notify the HCP if patient anticoagulant therapy has not been withheld.

▶ Ensure the patient has removed all external metallic objects from the area to be examined prior to the procedure.

▶ Have emergency equipment readily available.

▶ If the patient has a history of severe allergic reactions to any substance or drug, administer ordered prophylactic steroids or antihistamines before the procedure.

▶ Instruct the patient to void and change into the gown, robe, and foot coverings provided.

▶ Observe standard precautions, and follow the general guidelines in Appendix A. Positively identify the patient, and label the appropriate specimen containers with the corresponding patient demographics, date and time of collection, and site location (left or right breast).

▶ Instruct the patient to cooperate fully and to follow directions. Instruct the patient to remain still throughout the procedure because movement produces unreliable results.

▶ Record baseline vital signs and assess neurological status. Protocols may vary among facilities.

▶ Establish an IV fluid line for the injection of emergency drugs and of sedatives.

▶ Place the patient in the prone or sitting position on an examination table. Cleanse the selected area, and cover with a sterile drape.

▶ A local anesthetic is injected at the site, and a small incision is made or a needle inserted.

▶ Instruct the patient to inhale deeply and hold his or her breath while the images are taken, and then to exhale after the images are taken.

▶ Instruct the patient to take slow, deep breaths if nausea occurs during the procedure. Monitor and administer an antiemetic agent if ordered. Ready an emesis basin for use.

▶ Monitor the patient for complications related to the procedure (e.g., allergic reaction, anaphylaxis, bronchospasm).

▶ Remove the needle or catheter and apply a pressure dressing over the puncture site.

▶ Observe/assess the needle/catheter insertion site for bleeding, inflammation, or hematoma formation.

▶ Place tissue samples in properly labeled specimen containers, and promptly transport the specimens to the laboratory for processing and analysis.

POST-TEST:

- A report of the results will be sent to the requesting HCP, who will discuss the results with the patient.
- Instruct the patient to resume usual diet and medications, as directed by the HCP.
- Monitor vital signs and neurological status every 15 min for 1 hr, then every 2 hr for 4 hr, and then as ordered by the HCP. Take temperature every 4 hr for 24 hr. Monitor intake and output at least every 8 hr. Compare with baseline values. Notify the HCP if temperature is elevated. Protocols may vary among facilities.
- Observe for delayed allergic reactions, such as rash, urticaria, tachycardia, hyperpnea, hypertension, palpitations, nausea, or vomiting.
- Instruct the patient to immediately report symptoms such as fast heart rate, difficulty breathing, skin rash, itching, chest pain, persistent right shoulder pain, or abdominal pain. Immediately report symptoms to the appropriate HCP.
- Observe/assess the biopsy site for bleeding, inflammation, or hematoma formation.
- Instruct the patient in the care and assessment of the site.
- Recognize anxiety related to test results, and be supportive of the potential perceived loss of body image. Discuss the implications of abnormal test results on the patient's lifestyle. Provide teaching and information regarding the clinical implications of the test results, as appropriate. Educate the patient regarding access to counseling services. Provide contact information, if desired, for the American Cancer Society (www.cancer.org).
- Reinforce information given by the patient's HCP regarding further testing, treatment, or referral to another HCP. Decisions regarding the need for and frequency of breast self-examination, mammography, magnetic resonance imaging (MRI) of the breast, or other cancer screening procedures should be made after consultation between the patient and HCP. The most current guidelines for breast cancer screening of the general population as well as of individuals with increased risk are available from the American Cancer Society (www.cancer.org), the American College of Obstetricians and Gynecologists (ACOG) (www.acog.org), and the American College of Radiology (www.acr.org). Answer any questions or address any concerns voiced by the patient or family.
- Depending on the results of this procedure, additional testing may be performed to evaluate or monitor progression of the disease process and determine the need for a change in therapy. Evaluate test results in relation to the patient's symptoms and other tests performed.

RELATED MONOGRAPHS:

- Related tests include biopsy breast, cancer antigens, ductography, mammography, MRI breast, and US breast.
- Refer to the Reproductive System table at the end of the book for related tests by body system.

S

Synovial Fluid Analysis

SYNONYM/ACRONYM: Arthrocentesis, joint fluid analysis, knee fluid analysis.

COMMON USE: To identify the presence and assist in the management of joint disease related to disorders such as arthritis and gout.

SPECIMEN: Synovial fluid collected in a red-top tube for antinuclear antibodies (ANAs), complement, crystal examination, protein, rheumatoid factor (RF), and uric acid; sterile (red-top) tube for microbiological testing; lavender-top (EDTA) tube for mucin clot/viscosity, complete blood count (CBC) and differential; gray-top (sodium fluoride [NaFl]) tube for glucose; green-top (heparin) tube for lactic acid and pH.

REFERENCE VALUE: (Method: Macroscopic evaluation of appearance; spectrophotometry for glucose, lactic acid, protein, and uric acid; Gram stain, acid-fast stain, and culture for microbiology; microscopic examination of fluid for cell count and evaluation of crystals; ion-selective electrode for pH; nephelometry for RF and C3 complement; indirect fluorescence for ANAs)

Test	Normal Result
Color	Colorless to pale yellow
Clarity	Clear
Viscosity	High
ANA	Parallels serum level
C3	Parallels serum level
Glucose	Less than 10 mg/dL of blood level
Lactic acid	5–20 mg/dL
pH	7.2–7.4
Protein	Less than 3 g/dL
RF	Parallels serum level
Uric acid	Parallels serum level
Crystals	None present
RBC count	None
WBC count	Less than $0.2 \times 10^3/mm^3$ (or $200/mm^3$)
Neutrophils	Less than 25%
WBC morphology	No abnormal cells or inclusions
Gram stain and culture	No organisms present
AFB smear and culture	No AFB present

AFB = acid-fast bacilli; ANA = antinuclear antibodies; C3 = complement; RBC = red blood cell; RF = rheumatoid factor; WBC = white blood cell.

DESCRIPTION: Synovial fluid analysis is performed via arthrocentesis, an invasive procedure involving insertion of a needle into the joint space. Synovial effusions are associated with disorders or injuries involving the joints. The most commonly aspirated joint is the knee, although samples also can be obtained from the shoulder, hip, elbow, wrist, and ankle if clinically indicated. Joint disorders can be classified into five categories: noninflammatory, inflammatory, septic, crystal-induced, and hemorrhagic. The mucin clot test is used to correlate the qualitative assessment of synovial fluid viscosity with the presence of hyaluronic acid. The test is performed by mixing equal amounts of synovial fluid and 5% acetic acid solution on a glass slide and grading the ropiness of the subsequent clot as good, fair, or poor. Long, ropy strands are seen in normal synovial fluid.

INDICATIONS
- Assist in the evaluation of joint effusions
- Differentiate gout from pseudogout

POTENTIAL DIAGNOSIS

Fluid Values Increased In
- Acute bacterial infection: White blood cell (WBC) count greater than $50 \times 10^3/mm^3$, marked predominance of neutrophils (greater than 90% neutrophils), positive Gram stain, positive cultures, possible presence of rice bodies, increased lactic acid (produced by bacteria), and complement levels paralleling those found in serum (may be elevated or decreased)
- *Gout:* WBC count variable: $(0.5 - 200) \times 10^3/mm^3$ with a predominance of neutrophils (90% neutrophils), presence of monosodium urate crystals, increased uric acid, and complement levels paralleling those of serum (may be elevated or decreased)
- *Osteoarthritis, traumatic arthritis degenerative joint disease:* WBC count less than $3 \times 10^3/mm^3$ with less than 25% neutrophils and the presence of cartilage cells
- *Pseudogout:* Presence of calcium pyrophosphate crystals
- *Rheumatoid arthritis:* WBC count $(3 - 50) \times 10^3/mm^3$ with a predominance of neutrophils (greater than 70% neutrophils), presence of ragocyte cells and possibly rice bodies, presence of cholesterol crystals if effusion is chronic, increased

protein, increased lactic acid, and presence of rheumatoid factor
- *Systemic lupus erythematosus (SLE):* $(3 - 50) \times 10^3/mm^3$ with a predominance of neutrophils, presence of SLE cells, and presence of antinuclear antibodies
- *Trauma, joint tumors, or hemophilic arthritis:* Elevated RBC count, increased protein level, and presence of fat droplets (if trauma involved)
- *Tuberculous arthritis:* WBC count $(2 - 100) \times 10^3/mm^3$ with a predominance of neutrophils (up to 90% neutrophils), possible presence of rice bodies, presence of cholesterol crystals if effusion is chronic, in some cases a positive culture and smear for acid-fast bacilli (results frequently negative), and lactic acid

Fluid Values Decreased In (Analytes in Parentheses Are Decreased)
- Acute bacterial arthritis (glucose and pH)
- Gout (glucose)
- Rheumatoid arthritis (glucose, pH, and complement)
- SLE (glucose, pH, and complement)
- Tuberculous arthritis (glucose and pH)

CRITICAL FINDINGS: N/A

INTERFERING FACTORS
- Blood in the sample from traumatic arthrocentesis may falsely elevate the RBC count.
- Undetected hypoglycemia or hyperglycemia may produce misleading glucose values.
- Refrigeration of the sample may result in an increase in monosodium urate crystals secondary to decreased solubility of uric acid; exposure of the sample to room air with a resultant loss of carbon

dioxide and rise in pH encourages the formation of calcium pyrophosphate crystals.

NURSING IMPLICATIONS AND PROCEDURE

PRETEST:

▶ Positively identify the patient using at least two unique identifiers before providing care, treatment, or services.

▶ *Patient Teaching:* Inform the patient this procedure can assist in assessing joint health.

▶ Obtain a history of the patient's complaints, including a list of known allergens, especially allergies or sensitivities to latex.

▶ Obtain a history of the patient's immune and musculoskeletal systems, especially any bleeding disorders and other symptoms, and results of previously performed laboratory tests and diagnostic and surgical procedures.

▶ Note any recent procedures that can interfere with test results.

▶ Record the date of the last menstrual period and determine the possibility of pregnancy in perimenopausal women.

▶ Obtain a list of the patient's current medications, anticoagulants, aspirin and other salicylates, herbs, nutritional supplements, and nutraceuticals (see Appendix F). Such products should be discontinued by medical direction for the appropriate number of days prior to a surgical procedure.

▶ Review the procedure with the patient. Inform the patient that it may be necessary to remove hair from the site before the procedure. Address concerns about pain and explain that a sedative and/or analgesia will be administered to promote relaxation and reduce discomfort prior to needle insertion through the joint space. Explain that any discomfort with the needle insertion will be minimized with local anesthetics and systemic analgesics. Explain that the anesthetic injection may cause an initial stinging sensation. Explain that, after the skin has been anesthetized, a large needle will be inserted through the joint space, and a "popping" sensation may be experienced as the needle penetrates the joint. Inform the patient that the procedure is performed by a health-care provider (HCP) specializing in this procedure. The procedure usually takes approximately 20 min to complete.

▶ *Sensitivity to social and cultural issues,* as well as concern for modesty, is important in providing psychological support before, during, and after the procedure.

▶ There are no fluid restrictions unless by medical direction. Fasting for at least 12 hr before the procedure is recommended if fluid glucose measurements are included in the analysis. Instruct the patient to avoid taking anticoagulant medication or to reduce dosage as ordered prior to the procedure. Protocols may vary among facilities.

▶ *Make sure a written and informed consent has been signed prior to the procedure and before administering any medications.*

INTRATEST:

▶ Ensure that the patient has complied with dietary and medication restrictions and pretesting preparations; assure that food has been restricted for at least 12 hr prior to the procedure. Ensure that anticoagulant medications and aspirin have been withheld, as ordered.

▶ Assemble the necessary equipment, including an arthrocentesis tray with solution for skin preparation, local anesthetic, a 20-mL syringe, needles of various sizes, sterile drapes, and sterile gloves for the tests to be performed.

▶ Instruct the patient to cooperate fully and to follow directions. Direct the patient to breathe normally and to avoid unnecessary movement during the local anesthetic and the procedure.

▶ Observe standard precautions, and follow the general guidelines in Appendix A. Positively identify the patient, and label the appropriate collection containers with the corresponding patient demographics, date and time of collection, and site location, especially left or right.

S

- Assist the patient into a comfortable sitting or supine position, as appropriate.
- Prior to the administration of general or local anesthesia, shave the site and cleanse it with an antiseptic solution, and drape the area with sterile towels.
- After the local anesthetic is administered, the needle is inserted at the collection site, and fluid is removed by syringe. Manual pressure may be applied to facilitate fluid removal.
- If medication is injected into the joint, the syringe containing the sample is detached from the needle and replaced with the one containing the drug. The medication is injected with gentle pressure. The needle is withdrawn, and digital pressure is applied to the site for a few minutes. If there is no evidence of bleeding, a sterile dressing is applied to the site. An elastic bandage can be applied to the joint.
- Monitor the patient for complications related to the procedure (allergic reaction, anaphylaxis).
- Place samples in properly labeled specimen containers and promptly transport the specimens to the laboratory for processing and analysis. If bacterial culture and sensitivity tests are to be performed, record on the specimen containers any antibiotic therapy the patient is receiving.

POST-TEST:

- A report of the results will be sent to the requesting HCP, who will discuss the results with the patient.
- Instruct the patient to resume usual diet and medications, as directed by the HCP.
- After local anesthesia, monitor vital signs and compare with baseline values. Notify the HCP if temperature is elevated. Protocols may vary among facilities.
- Observe/assess puncture site for bleeding, bruising, inflammation, and excessive drainage of synovial fluid approximately every 4 hr for 24 hr and daily thereafter for several days.
- Instruct the patient to report excessive pain, bleeding, or swelling to the requesting HCP immediately. Report to

HCP if severe pain is present or the patient is unable to move the joint.
- Observe/assess for nausea and pain. Administer antiemetic and analgesic medications as needed and as directed by the HCP.
- Instruct the patient to apply an ice pack to the site for 24 to 48 hr.
- Administer antibiotics, as ordered, and instruct the patient in the importance of completing the entire course of antibiotic therapy even if no symptoms are present.
- Recognize anxiety related to test results, and offer support. Discuss the implications of abnormal test results on the patient's lifestyle. Provide teaching and information regarding the clinical implications of the test results, as appropriate.
- Reinforce information given by the patient's HCP regarding further testing, treatment, or referral to another HCP. Instruct the patient or caregiver to handle linen and dispose of dressings cautiously, especially if septic arthritis is suspected. Instruct the patient to avoid excessive use of the joint for several days to prevent pain and swelling. Instruct the patient to return for a follow-up visit as scheduled. Answer any questions or address any concerns voiced by the patient or family.
- Depending on the results of this procedure, additional testing may be performed to evaluate or monitor progression of the disease process and determine the need for a change in therapy. Evaluate test results in relation to the patient's symptoms and other tests performed.

RELATED MONOGRAPHS:

- Related tests include antibodies anticyclic citrullinated, ANA, arthrogram, arthroscopy, BMD, bone scan, CRP, cholesterol, CBC, CBC WBC count and differential, ESR, MRI musculoskeletal, radiography bone, RF, synovial fluid analysis, and uric acid.
- Refer to the Immune and Musculoskeletal systems tables at the end of the book for related tests by body system.

Syphilis Serology

SYNONYM/ACRONYM: Automated reagin testing (ART), fluorescent treponemal antibody testing (FTA-ABS), microhemagglutination–*Treponema pallidum* (MHA-TP), rapid plasma reagin (RPR), treponemal studies, Venereal Disease Research Laboratory (VDRL) testing.

COMMON USE: To indicate past or present syphilis infection.

SPECIMEN: Serum (1 mL) collected in a red- or tiger-top tube.

REFERENCE VALUE: (Method: Dark-field microscopy, rapid plasma reagin, enzyme-linked immunosorbent assay [ELISA], microhemagglutination, fluorescence) Nonreactive or absence of treponemal organisms.

DESCRIPTION: There are numerous methods for detecting *Treponema pallidum*, the organism known to cause syphilis. Syphilis serology is routinely ordered as part of a prenatal work-up and is required for evaluating donated blood units before release for transfusion. Selection of the proper testing method is important. Automated reagin testing (ART), rapid plasma reagin (RPR), and Venereal Disease Research Laboratory (VDRL) testing should be used for screening purposes. Fluorescent treponemal antibody testing (FTA-ABS) and microhemagglutination–*Treponema pallidum* (MHA-TP) are confirmatory methods for samples that screen positive or reactive. Cerebrospinal fluid should be tested only by the FTA-ABS method. Cord blood should not be submitted for testing by any of the aforementioned methods; instead, the mother's serum should be tested to establish whether the infant should be treated.

INDICATIONS
- Monitor effectiveness of treatment for syphilis
- Screen for and confirm the presence of syphilis

POTENTIAL DIAGNOSIS

Positive findings in
- Syphilis

False-Positive or False-Reactive Findings in Screening (RPR, VDRL) Tests
- Infectious:
  Bacterial endocarditis
  Chancroid
  Chickenpox
  HIV
  Infectious mononucleosis
  Leprosy
  Leptospirosis
  Lymphogranuloma venereum
  Malaria
  Measles
  Mumps
  Mycoplasma pneumoniae
  Pneumococcal pneumonia
  Psittacosis
  Relapsing fever
  Rickettsial disease
  Scarlet fever
  Trypanosomiasis

S

Tuberculosis
Vaccinia (live or attenuated)
Viral hepatitis

- **Noninfectious:**
  Advanced cancer
  Advancing age
  Chronic liver disease
  Connective tissue diseases
  IV drug use
  Multiple blood transfusions
  Multiple myeloma and other
    immunological disorders
  Narcotic addiction
  Pregnancy

False-Positive or False-Reactive Findings in Confirmatory (FTA-ABS, MHA-TP) Tests

- **Infectious:**
  Infectious mononucleosis
  Leprosy
  Leptospirosis
  Lyme disease
  Malaria
  Relapsing fever

- **Noninfectious:**
  Systemic lupus erythematosus

Negative findings in: N/A

CRITICAL FINDINGS: N/A

INTERFERING FACTORS: N/A

NURSING IMPLICATIONS AND PROCEDURE

PRETEST:

- Positively identify the patient using at least two unique identifiers before providing care, treatment, or services.
- *Patient Teaching:* Inform the patient this test can assist in diagnosing syphilis.
- Obtain a history of the patient's complaints, including a list of known allergens, especially allergies or sensitivities to latex.
- Obtain a history of exposure.
- Obtain a history of the patient's immune and reproductive systems,

symptoms, and results of previously performed laboratory tests and diagnostic and surgical procedures.

- Obtain a list of the patient's current medications, including herbs, nutritional supplements, and nutraceuticals (see Appendix F).
- Review the procedure with the patient. Inform the patient that specimen collection takes approximately 5 to 10 min. Address concerns about pain and explain that there may be some discomfort during the venipuncture.
- *Sensitivity to social and cultural issues,* as well as concern for modesty, is important in providing psychological support before, during, and after the procedure.
- There are no food, fluid, or medication restrictions unless by medical direction.

INTRATEST:

- If the patient has a history of allergic reaction to latex, avoid the use of equipment containing latex.
- Instruct the patient to cooperate fully and to follow directions. Direct the patient to breathe normally and to avoid unnecessary movement.
- Observe standard precautions, and follow the general guidelines in Appendix A. Positively identify the patient, and label the appropriate tubes with the corresponding patient demographics, date, and time of collection. Perform a venipuncture.
- Remove the needle and apply direct pressure with dry gauze to stop bleeding. Observe/assess venipuncture site for bleeding or hematoma formation and secure gauze with adhesive bandage.
- Promptly transport the specimen to the laboratory for processing and analysis.

POST-TEST:

- A report of the results will be sent to the requesting health-care provider (HCP), who will discuss the results with the patient.
- Recognize anxiety related to test results, and offer support. Counsel the patient, as appropriate, regarding the risk of transmission and proper prophylaxis, and reinforce the

importance of strict adherence to the treatment regimen. Inform the patient that positive findings must be reported to local health department officials, who will question him or her regarding sexual partners. Provide teaching and information regarding the clinical implications of the test results, as appropriate. Educate the patient regarding access to counseling services.

▸ Reinforce information given by the patient's HCP regarding further testing, treatment, or referral to another HCP. Inform the patient that repeat testing may be needed at 3-mo intervals for 1 yr to monitor the effectiveness of treatment. Answer any questions or address any concerns voiced by the patient or family.

▸ Offer support, as appropriate, to patients who may be the victim of rape or sexual assault. Educate the patient regarding access to counseling services. Provide a nonjudgmental, nonthreatening atmosphere for a discussion during which risks of sexually transmitted diseases are explained. It is also important to discuss problems the patient may experience (e.g., guilt, depression, anger).

▸ Depending on the results of this procedure, additional testing may be performed to evaluate or monitor progression of the disease process and determine the need for a change in therapy. Evaluate test results in relation to the patient's symptoms and other tests performed.

RELATED MONOGRAPHS:

▸ Related tests include acid phosphatase, cerebrospinal fluid analysis, *Chlamydia* group antibody, culture bacterial anal, Gram stain, hepatitis B, hepatitis C, HIV, and β_2-microglobulin.

▸ Refer to the Immune and Reproductive systems tables at the end of the book for related tests by body system.

S

Testosterone, Total

SYNONYM/ACRONYM: N/A.

COMMON USE: To evaluate testosterone to assist in identification of disorders related to early puberty, late puberty, and infertility while assessing gonadal and adrenal function.

SPECIMEN: Serum (1 mL) collected in a red- or tiger-top tube. Plasma (1 mL) collected in green-top (heparin) tube is also acceptable.

REFERENCE VALUE: (Method: Immunochemiluminometric assay [ICMA])

Age	Conventional Units	SI Units (Conventional Units × 0.0347)
1–5 mo		
Male	1–177 ng/dL	0.03–6.14 nmol/L
Female	1–5 ng/dL	0.03–0.17 nmol/L
6–11 mo		
Male	2–7 ng/dL	0.07–0.24 nmol/L
Female	2–5 ng/dL	0.07–0.17 nmol/L
1–5 yr		
Male and female	0–10 ng/dL	0.00–0.35 nmol/L
6–7 yr		
Male	0–20 ng/dL	0.00–0.69 nmol/L
Female	0–10 ng/dL	0.00–0.35 nmol/L
8–10 yr		
Male	0–25 ng/dL	0.00–0.87 nmol/L
Female	0–30 ng/dL	0.00–1.0 nmol/L
11–12 yr		
Male	0–350 ng/dL	0.00–12.1 nmol/L
Female	0–50 ng/dL	0.00–1.74 nmol/L
13–15 yr		
Male	15–500 ng/dL	0.52–17.35 nmol/L
Female	0–50 ng/dL	0.00–1.74 nmol/L
Adult–older adult		
Male	241–827 ng/dL	8.36–28.70 nmol/L
Female	15–70 ng/dL	0.52–2.43 nmol/L

Tanner Stage	Male	Female
I	2–23 ng/dL	2–10 ng/dL
II	5–70 ng/dL	5–30 ng/dL
III	15–280 ng/dL	10–30 ng/dL
IV	105–545 ng/dL	15–40 ng/dL
V	265–800 ng/dL	10–40 ng/dL

DESCRIPTION: Testosterone is the major androgen responsible for sexual differentiation. In males, testosterone is made by the Leydig cells in the testicles and is responsible for spermatogenesis and the development of secondary sex characteristics. In females, the ovary and adrenal gland secrete small amounts of this hormone; however, most of the testosterone in females comes from the metabolism of androstenedione. In males, a testicular, adrenal, or pituitary tumor can cause an overabundance of testosterone, triggering precocious puberty. In females, adrenal tumors, hyperplasia, and medications can cause an overabundance of this hormone, resulting in masculinization or hirsutism.

INDICATIONS

- Assist in the diagnosis of hypergonadism
- Assist in the diagnosis of male sexual precocity before age 10
- Distinguish between primary and secondary hypogonadism
- Evaluate hirsutism
- Evaluate male infertility

POTENTIAL DIAGNOSIS

Increased in
- Adrenal hyperplasia (*oversecretion of the androgen precursor DHEA*)
- Adrenocortical tumors (*oversecretion of the androgen precursor DHEA*)
- Hirsutism (*any condition that results in increased production of testosterone or its precursors*)
- Hyperthyroidism (*high thyroxine levels increase the production of sex hormone–binding protein, which increases measured levels of total testosterone*)
- Idiopathic sexual precocity (*related to stimulation of testosterone production by elevated levels of luteinizing hormone [LH]*)
- Polycystic ovaries (*high estrogen levels increase the production of sex hormone–binding protein, which increases measured levels of total testosterone*)
- Syndrome of androgen resistance
- Testicular or extragonadal tumors (*related to excessive secretion of testosterone*)
- Trophoblastic tumors during pregnancy
- Virilizing ovarian tumors

Decreased in
- Anovulation
- Cryptorchidism (*related to dysfunctional testes*)
- Delayed puberty
- Down syndrome (*related to diminished or dysfunctional testes*)
- Excessive alcohol intake (*alcohol inhibits secretion of testosterone*)
- Hepatic insufficiency (*related to decreased binding protein and reflects decreased measured levels of total testosterone*)
- Impotence (*decreased testosterone levels can result in impotence*)
- Klinefelter's syndrome (*chromosome abnormality XXY associated with testicular failure*)
- Malnutrition
- Myotonic dystrophy (*related to testicular atrophy*)
- Orchiectomy (*testosterone production occurs in the testes*)
- Primary and secondary hypogonadism
- Primary and secondary hypopituitarism
- Uremia

CRITICAL FINDINGS: N/A

INTERFERING FACTORS

- Drugs that may increase testosterone levels include barbiturates, bromocriptine, cimetidine, flutamide, gonadotropin, levonorgestrel, mifepristone, moclobemide, nafarelin (males), nilutamide, oral contraceptives, rifampin, and tamoxifen.
- Drugs that may decrease testosterone levels include cyclophosphamide, cyproterone, danazol, dexamethasone, diethylstilbestrol, digoxin, D-Trp-6-LHRH, fenoldopam, goserelin, ketoconazole, leuprolide, magnesium sulfate, medroxyprogesterone, methylprednisone, nandrolone, oral contraceptives, pravastatin, prednisone, pyridoglutethimide, spironolactone, stanozolol, tetracycline, and thioridazine.

NURSING IMPLICATIONS AND PROCEDURE

PRETEST:

- Positively identify the patient using at least two unique identifiers before providing care, treatment, or services.
- *Patient Teaching:* Inform the patient this test can assist with evaluating hormone levels.
- Obtain a history of the patient's complaints, including a list of known allergens, especially allergies or sensitivities to latex.
- Obtain a history of the patient's endocrine and reproductive systems, symptoms, and results of previously performed laboratory tests and diagnostic and surgical procedures.
- Obtain a list of the patient's current medications, including herbs, nutritional supplements, and nutraceuticals (see Appendix F).
- Review the procedure with the patient. Inform the patient that specimen collection takes approximately 5 to 10 min. Address concerns about pain and explain that there may be some discomfort during the venipuncture.

- *Sensitivity to social and cultural issues,* as well as concern for modesty, is important in providing psychological support before, during, and after the procedure.
- There are no food, fluid, or medication restrictions unless by medical direction.

INTRATEST:

- If the patient has a history of allergic reaction to latex, avoid the use of equipment containing latex.
- Instruct the patient to cooperate fully and to follow directions. Direct the patient to breathe normally and to avoid unnecessary movement.
- Observe standard precautions, and follow the general guidelines in Appendix A. Positively identify the patient, and label the appropriate tubes with the corresponding patient demographics, date, and time of collection. Perform a venipuncture.
- Remove the needle and apply direct pressure with dry gauze to stop bleeding. Observe/assess venipuncture site for bleeding or hematoma formation and secure gauze with adhesive bandage.
- Promptly transport the specimen to the laboratory for processing and analysis.

POST-TEST:

- A report of the results will be sent to the requesting health-care provider (HCP), who will discuss the results with the patient.
- Recognize anxiety related to test results, and offer support, as appropriate. Discuss the implications of abnormal test results on the patient's lifestyle. Provide teaching and information regarding the clinical implications of the test results, as appropriate. Educate the patient regarding access to counseling services.
- Reinforce information given by the patient's HCP regarding further testing, treatment, or referral to another HCP. Answer any questions or address any concerns voiced by the patient or family.
- Depending on the results of this procedure, additional testing may be performed to evaluate or monitor progression of the disease process and determine the need for a change in therapy.

Evaluate test results in relation to the patient's symptoms and other tests performed.

RELATED MONOGRAPHS:

▶ Related tests include angiography adrenal gland scan, ACE, antibodies antisperm, biopsy thyroid, chromosome analysis, CT renal, DHEAS, estradiol, FSH, LH, PTH, RAIU, semen analysis, US scrotal, thyroid scan, TSH, and thyroxine.

▶ Refer to the Endocrine and Reproductive systems tables at the end of the book for related test by body system.

Thyroglobulin

SYNONYM/ACRONYM: Tg.

COMMON USE: To evaluate thyroid gland function related to disorders such as tumor, inflammation, structural damage, and cancer.

SPECIMEN: Serum (1 mL) collected in a red- or tiger-top tube.

REFERENCE VALUE: (Method: Chemiluminescent enzyme immunoassay)

Age	Conventional Units	SI Units (Conventional Units × 1)
Premature infant		
1 day	107–395 ng/mL	107–395 mcg/L
3 days	49–163 ng/mL	49–163 mcg/L
Cord blood	5–65 ng/mL	5–65 mcg/L
1 day	6–93 ng/mL	6–93 mcg/L
10 days	9–148 ng/mL	9–148 mcg/L
1 mo	17–63 ng/mL	17–63 mcg/L
7–12 yr	20–50 ng/mL	20–50 mcg/L
12–18 yr	9–27 ng/mL	9–27 mcg/L
Adult–older adult	0–50 ng/mL	0–50 mcg/L

DESCRIPTION: Thyroglobulin is an iodinated glycoprotein secreted by follicular epithelial cells of the thyroid gland. It is the storage form of the thyroid hormones thyroxine (T_4) and triiodothyronine (T_3). When thyroid hormones are released into the bloodstream, they split from thyroglobulin in response to thyroid-stimulating hormone. Values greater than 55 ng/mL are indicative of tumor recurrence in athyrotic patients.

T

INDICATIONS

- Assist in the diagnosis of subacute thyroiditis
- Assist in the diagnosis of suspected disorders of excess thyroid hormone
- Management of differentiated or metastatic cancer of the thyroid
- Monitor response to treatment of goiter
- Monitor T_4 therapy in patients with solitary nodules

POTENTIAL DIAGNOSIS

Increased in

Thyroglobulin is secreted by normal, abnormal, and cancerous thyroid tissue cells.

- Differentiated thyroid cancer
- Graves' disease (untreated) *(autoimmune destruction of thyroid tissue cells)*
- Surgery or irradiation of the thyroid *(elevated levels indicate residual or disseminated carcinoma)*
- T_4-binding globulin deficiency
- Thyroiditis *(related to leakage from inflamed, damaged thyroid tissue cells)*
- Thyrotoxicosis

Decreased in

- Administration of thyroid hormone *(feedback loop suppresses production)*
- Congenital athyrosis (neonates) *(related to insufficient synthesis)*
- Thyrotoxicosis factitia

CRITICAL FINDINGS: N/A

INTERFERING FACTORS

- Drugs that may decrease thyroglobulin levels include neomycin and T_4.
- Autoantibodies to thyroglobulin can cause decreased values.
- Recent thyroid surgery or needle biopsy can interfere with test results.

NURSING IMPLICATIONS AND PROCEDURE

PRETEST:

- Positively identify the patient using at least two unique identifiers before providing care, treatment, or services.
- *Patient Teaching:* Inform the patient this test can assist in assessing the thyroid gland.
- Obtain a history of the patient's complaints, including a list of known allergens, especially allergies or sensitivities to latex.
- Obtain a history of the patient's endocrine system, symptoms, and results of previously performed laboratory tests and diagnostic and surgical procedures.
- Obtain a list of the patient's current medications, including herbs, nutritional supplements, and nutraceuticals (see Appendix F).
- Review the procedure with the patient. Inform the patient that specimen collection takes approximately 5 to 10 min. Address concerns about pain and explain that there may be some discomfort during the venipuncture.
- *Sensitivity to social and cultural issues,* as well as concern for modesty, is important in providing psychological support before, during, and after the procedure.
- There are no food, fluid, or medication restrictions unless by medical direction.

INTRATEST:

- If the patient has a history of allergic reaction to latex, avoid the use of equipment containing latex.
- Instruct the patient to cooperate fully and to follow directions. Direct the patient to breathe normally and to avoid unnecessary movement.
- Observe standard precautions, and follow the general guidelines in Appendix A. Positively identify the patient, and label the appropriate tubes with the corresponding patient demographics, date, and time of collection. Perform a venipuncture.
- Remove the needle and apply direct pressure with dry gauze to stop

T

bleeding. Observe/assess venipuncture site for bleeding or hematoma formation and secure gauze with adhesive bandage.
- Promptly transport the specimen to the laboratory for processing and analysis.

performed to evaluate or monitor progression of the disease process and determine the need for a change in therapy. Evaluate test results in relation to the patient's symptoms and other tests performed.

POST-TEST:

- A report of the results will be sent to the requesting health-care provider (HCP), who will discuss the results with the patient.
- Reinforce information given by the patient's HCP regarding further testing, treatment, or referral to another HCP. Answer any questions or address any concerns voiced by the patient or family.
- Depending on the results of this procedure, additional testing may be

RELATED MONOGRAPHS:

- Related tests include ACTH, albumin, ACE, antibodies thyroglobulin, biopsy thyroid, copper, follicle-stimulating hormone, growth hormone, luteinizing hormone, PTH, protein, RAIU, TBII, thyroid scan, TSH, TSI, T_4, free T_4, T_3, free T_3, and US thyroid.
- Refer to the Endocrine System table at the end of the book for related tests by body system.

Thyroid-Binding Inhibitory Immunoglobulin

SYNONYM/ACRONYM: Thyrotropin receptor antibodies, thyrotropin-binding inhibitory immunoglobulin, TBII.

COMMON USE: To assist in diagnosing Graves' disease related to thyroid function.

SPECIMEN: Serum (1 mL) collected in a red-top tube.

REFERENCE VALUE: (Method: Radioreceptor) Less than 10% inhibition. *Note:* In patients with Graves' disease, inhibition is expected to be 10% to 100%.

POTENTIAL DIAGNOSIS

Increased in
Evidenced by antibodies that block the action of TSH and result in hyperthyroid conditions.
- Graves' disease
- Hyperthyroidism (various forms)

- Maternal thyroid disease
- Neonatal thyroid disease
- Toxic goiter

Decreased in: N/A

CRITICAL FINDINGS: N/A

Find and print out the full monograph at DavisPlus (http://davisplus.fadavis.com, keyword Van Leeuwen).

Thyroid Scan

SYNONYM/ACRONYM: Iodine thyroid scan, technetium thyroid scan, thyroid scintiscan.

COMMON USE: To assess thyroid gland size, structure, function, and shape to assist in diagnosing disorders such as tumor, inflammation, cancer, and bleeding.

AREA OF APPLICATION: Thyroid.

CONTRAST: Oral radioactive iodine or IV technetium-99m pertechnetate.

DESCRIPTION: The thyroid scan is a nuclear medicine study performed to assess thyroid size, shape, position, and function. It is useful for evaluating thyroid nodules, multinodular goiter, and thyroiditis; assisting in the differential diagnosis of masses in the neck, base of the tongue, and mediastinum; and ruling out possible ectopic thyroid tissue in these areas. Thyroid scanning is performed after oral administration of radioactive iodine-123 (I-123) or I-131 or IV injection of technetium-99m (Tc-99m). Increased or decreased uptake by the thyroid gland and surrounding area and tissue is noted: Areas of increased radionuclide uptake ("hot spots") are caused by hyperfunctioning thyroid nodules, which are usually nonmalignant; areas of decreased uptake ("cold spots") are caused by hypofunctioning nodules, which are more likely to be malignant. Ultrasound imaging may be used to determine if the cold spot is a solid, semicystic lesion or a pure cyst (cysts are rarely cancerous). To determine whether the cold spot depicts a malignant neoplasm, however, a biopsy must be performed.

INDICATIONS

- Assess palpable nodules and differentiate between a benign tumor or cyst and a malignant tumor
- Assess the presence of a thyroid nodule or enlarged thyroid gland
- Detect benign or malignant thyroid tumors
- Detect causes of neck or substernal masses
- Detect forms of thyroiditis (e.g., acute, chronic, Hashimoto's)
- Detect thyroid dysfunction
- Differentiate between Graves' disease and Plummer's disease, both of which cause hyperthyroidism
- Evaluate thyroid function in hyperthyroidism and hypothyroidism (analysis combined with interpretation of laboratory tests, thyroid function panel including thyroxine and triiodothyronine, and thyroid uptake tests)

POTENTIAL DIAGNOSIS

Normal findings in
- Normal size, contour, position, and function of the thyroid gland with homogeneous uptake of the radionuclide

Abnormal findings in
- Adenoma
- Cysts
- Fibrosis

- Goiter
- Graves' disease (diffusely enlarged, hyperfunctioning gland)
- Hematoma
- Metastasis
- Plummer's disease (nodular hyper-functioning gland)
- Thyroiditis (Hashimoto's)
- Thyrotoxicosis
- Tumors, benign or malignant

CRITICAL FINDINGS: N/A

INTERFERING FACTORS

This procedure is contraindicated for

- Patients who are pregnant or suspected of being pregnant, unless the potential benefits of the procedure far outweigh the risks to the fetus or mother.

Factors that may impair clear imaging

- Inability of the patient to cooperate or remain still during the procedure because of age, significant pain, or mental status.
- Other nuclear scans or iodinated contrast medium radiographic studies done within the previous 24 to 48 hr.
- Ingestion of foods containing iodine (iodized salt) or medications containing iodine (cough syrup, potassium iodide, vitamins, Lugol's solution, thyroid replacement medications), which can decrease the uptake of the radionuclide.
- Antithyroid medications (propyl-thiouracil), corticosteroids, antihistamines, warfarin, sulfonamides, nitrates, corticosteroids, thyroid hormones, and isoniazid, which can decrease the uptake of the radionuclide.
- Increased uptake of iodine in persons with an iodine-deficient diet or who are on phenothiazine therapy.

- Vomiting and severe diarrhea, which can affect absorption of orally administered radionuclide.
- Gastroenteritis, which can interfere with absorption of orally administered radionuclide.
- Metallic objects (e.g., jewelry, body rings) within the examination field, which may inhibit organ visualization and cause unclear images.

Other considerations

- Improper injection of the radionuclide that allows the tracer to seep deep into the muscle tissue can produce erroneous hot spots.
- Consultation with a health-care provider (HCP) should occur before the procedure for radiation safety concerns regarding younger patients or patients who are lactating.
- Risks associated with radiation overexposure can result from frequent x-ray or radionuclide procedures. Personnel working in the examination area should wear badges to record their level of radiation exposure.

NURSING IMPLICATIONS AND PROCEDURE

PRETEST:

- Positively identify the patient using at least two unique identifiers before providing care, treatment, or services.
- *Patient Teaching:* Inform the patient this procedure can assist in evaluating the thyroid glands structure and function.
- Obtain a history of the patient's complaints, including a list of known allergens, especially allergies or sensitivities to latex, iodine, seafood, contrast medium, anesthetics, or dyes.
- Obtain a history of the patient's endocrine system, symptoms, and results of previously performed laboratory tests and diagnostic and surgical procedures.
- Ensure thyroid blood tests are completed prior to this procedure.

- Note any recent procedures that can interfere with test results, including examinations using iodinated contrast medium or radioactive nuclides.
- Ensure that this procedure is performed before all radiographic procedures using iodinated contrast medium.
- Record the date of the last menstrual period and determine the possibility of pregnancy in perimenopausal women.
- Obtain a list of the patient's current medications, including herbs, nutritional supplements, and nutraceuticals (see Appendix F).
- Review the procedure with the patient. Address concerns about pain related to the procedure and explain that some pain may be experienced during the test. Inform the patient that the procedure is performed in a nuclear medicine department, usually by an HCP specializing in this procedure, with support staff, and takes approximately 30 to 60 min.
- *Sensitivity to social and cultural issues,* as well as concern for modesty, is important in providing psychological support before, during, and after the procedure.
- Instruct the patient to remove jewelry and other metallic objects from the area to be examined.
- The patient should fast for 8 to 12 hr prior to the procedure. Protocols may vary among facilities.
- *Make sure a written and informed consent has been signed prior to the procedure and before administering any medications.*

INTRATEST:

- Ensure that the patient has complied with dietary restrictions for 8 to 12 hr prior to the procedure.
- Ensure that the patient has removed all external metallic objects from the area to be examined prior to the procedure.
- Instruct the patient to void prior to the procedure and to change into the gown, robe, and foot coverings provided.
- Instruct the patient to cooperate fully and to follow directions. Ask the patient to lie still during the procedure because movement produces unclear images.

- Observe standard precautions, and follow the general guidelines in Appendix A.
- Administer sedative to a child or to an uncooperative adult, as ordered.
- Tc-99m pertechnetate is injected IV 20 min before scanning.
- If oral radioactive nuclide is used instead, administer I-123 24 hr before scanning.
- Place the patient in a supine position on a flat table to obtain images of the neck area.
- Remove the needle or catheter and apply a pressure dressing over the puncture site.
- Observe/assess the needle/catheter insertion site for bleeding, inflammation, or hematoma formation.

POST-TEST:

- A report of the results will be sent to the requesting HCP, who will discuss the results with the patient.
- Observe/assess the needle/catheter insertion site for bleeding, inflammation, or hematoma formation.
- Instruct the patient in the care and assessment of the injection site.
- Advise the patient to drink increased amounts of fluids for 24 to 48 hr to eliminate the radionuclide from the body, unless contraindicated. Tell the patient that radionuclide is eliminated from the body within 6 to 24 hr.
- If a woman who is breastfeeding must have a nuclear scan, she should not breastfeed the infant until the radionuclide has been eliminated. This could take as long as 3 days. She should be instructed to express the milk and discard it during the 3-day period to prevent cessation of milk production.
- Instruct the patient to flush the toilet immediately and to meticulously wash hands with soap and water after each voiding for 24 hr after the procedure.
- Instruct all caregivers to wear gloves when discarding urine for 24 hr after the procedure. Wash gloved hands with soap and water before removing gloves. Then wash hands after the gloves are removed.
- Recognize anxiety related to test results, and be supportive of perceived loss of

independent function. Discuss the implications of abnormal test results on the patient's lifestyle. Provide teaching and information regarding the clinical implications of the test results, as appropriate.

▶ Reinforce information given by the patient's HCP regarding further testing, treatment, or referral to another HCP. Answer any questions or address any concerns voiced by the patient or family.

▶ Depending on the results of this procedure, additional testing may be needed to evaluate or monitor progression of the disease process and determine the need for a change in therapy. Evaluate test results in relation to the patient's symptoms and other tests performed.

RELATED MONOGRAPHS:

▶ Related tests include ACTH, angiography adrenal, biopsy thyroid, calcium, CT renal, cortisol, glucose, radioactive iodine uptake, sodium, thyroglobulin, thyroid antibodies, TBII, thyroid scan, TSH, TT_3, T_4, FT_4, and US thyroid.

▶ Refer to the Endocrine System table at the end of the book for related tests by body system.

Thyroid-Stimulating Hormone

SYNONYM/ACRONYM: Thyrotropin, TSH.

COMMON USE: To evaluate thyroid gland function related to the primary cause of hypothyroidism and assess for congenital disorders, tumor, cancer, and inflammation.

SPECIMEN: Serum (1 mL) collected in a red- or tiger-top tube; for a neonate, use filter paper.

REFERENCE VALUE: (Method: Immunoassay)

Age	Conventional Units	SI Units (Conventional Units × 1)
Neonates–3 days	Less than 20 micro-international units/mL	Less than 20 milli-international units/L
2 wk–5 mo	1.7–9.1 micro-international units/mL	1.7–9.1 milli-international units/L
6 mo–20 yr	0.7–6.4 micro-international units/mL	0.7–6.4 milli-international units/L
21–54 yr	0.4–4.2 micro-international units/mL	0.4–4.2 milli-international units/L
55–87 yr	0.5–8.9 micro-international units/mL	0.5–8.9 milli-international units/L

DESCRIPTION: Thyroid-stimulating hormone (TSH) is produced by the pituitary gland in response to stimulation by thyrotropin-releasing hormone (TRH), a hypothalamic-releasing factor. TRH regulates the release and circulating levels of thyroid hormones in response to variables such as cold, stress, and increased metabolic need. Thyroid and pituitary function can be evaluated by TSH measurement. TSH exhibits diurnal variation, peaking between midnight and 4 a.m. and troughing between 5 and 6 p.m. TSH values are high at birth but reach adult levels in the first week of life. Elevated TSH levels combined with decreased thyroxine (T_4) levels indicate hypothyroidism and thyroid gland dysfunction. In general, decreased TSH and T_4 levels indicate secondary congenital hypothyroidism and pituitary hypothalamic dysfunction. A normal TSH level and a depressed T_4 level may indicate (1) hypothyroidism owing to a congenital defect in T_4-binding globulin or (2) transient congenital hypothyroidism owing to hypoxia or prematurity. Early diagnosis and treatment in the neonate are crucial for the prevention of cretinism and mental retardation.

INDICATIONS
- Assist in the diagnosis of congenital hypothyroidism
- Assist in the diagnosis of hypothyroidism or hyperthyroidism or suspected pituitary or hypothalamic dysfunction
- Differentiate functional euthyroidism from true hypothyroidism in debilitated individuals

POTENTIAL DIAGNOSIS

Increased in
A decrease in thyroid hormone levels activates the feedback loop to increase production of TSH.

- Congenital hypothyroidism in the neonate (filter paper test)
- Ectopic TSH-producing tumors (lung, breast)
- Primary hypothyroidism *(related to a dysfunctional thyroid gland)*
- Secondary hyperthyroidism owing to pituitary hyperactivity
- Thyroid hormone resistance
- Thyroiditis (Hashimoto's autoimmune disease)

Decreased in
An increase in thyroid hormone levels activates the feedback loop to decrease production of TSH.

- Excessive thyroid hormone replacement
- Graves' disease
- Primary hyperthyroidism
- Secondary hypothyroidism *(related to pituitary involvement that decreases production of TSH)*
- Tertiary hypothyroidism *(related to hypothalamic involvement that decreases production of TRH)*

CRITICAL FINDINGS: N/A

INTERFERING FACTORS
- Drugs and hormones that may increase TSH levels include amiodarone, benserazide, erythrosine, flunarizine (males), iobenzamic acid, iodides, lithium, methimazole, metoclopramide, morphine, propranolol, radiographic agents, TRH, and valproic acid.
- Drugs and hormones that may decrease TSH levels include acetylsalicylic acid, amiodarone, anabolic steroids, carbamazepine, corticosteroids, glucocorticoids, hydrocortisone, interferon-alfa-2b, iodamide, levodopa (in hypothyroidism), levothyroxine, methergoline, nifedipine, T_4, and triiodothyronine (T_3).
- Failure to let the filter paper sample dry may affect test results.

NURSING IMPLICATIONS AND PROCEDURE

PRETEST:

- Positively identify the patient using at least two unique identifiers before providing care, treatment, or services.
- *Patient Teaching:* Inform the patient this test can assist in evaluating thyroid function.
- Obtain a history of the patient's complaints, including a list of known allergens, especially allergies or sensitivities to latex.
- Obtain a history of the patient's endocrine system, symptoms, and results of previously performed laboratory tests and diagnostic and surgical procedures.
- Obtain a list of the patient's current medications, including herbs, nutritional supplements, and nutraceuticals (see Appendix F).
- Review the procedure with the patient. Inform the patient that specimen collection takes approximately 5 to 10 min. Address concerns about pain and explain that there may be some discomfort during the venipuncture.
- *Sensitivity to social and cultural issues,* as well as concern for modesty, is important in providing psychological support before, during, and after the procedure.
- There are no food, fluid, or medication restrictions unless by medical direction.

INTRATEST:

- If the patient has a history of allergic reaction to latex, avoid the use of equipment containing latex.
- Instruct the patient to cooperate fully and to follow directions. Direct the patient to breathe normally and to avoid unnecessary movement.
- Observe standard precautions, and follow the general guidelines in Appendix A. Positively identify the patient, and label the appropriate tubes with the corresponding patient demographics, date, and time of collection. Perform a venipuncture.
- Remove the needle and apply direct pressure with dry gauze to stop bleeding.

- Observe/assess venipuncture site for bleeding or hematoma formation and secure gauze with adhesive bandage.
- Promptly transport the specimen to the laboratory for processing and analysis.

Filter Paper Test (Neonate)

- Obtain kit and cleanse heel with antiseptic. Observe standard precautions, and follow the general guidelines in Appendix A. Use gauze to dry the stick area completely. Perform heel stick, gently squeeze infant's heel, and touch filter paper to the puncture site. Completely fill the circles on the filter paper, saturating the filter paper with blood. Apply pressure to the heel stick with a gauze pad to stop the bleeding. Allow the filter paper to dry thoroughly, label the specimen, and promptly transport it to the laboratory. Alternatively, if a specimen collection kit is used, follow instructions for labeling and mailing to the testing laboratory.

POST-TEST:

- A report of the results will be sent to the requesting health-care provider (HCP), who will discuss the results with the patient.
- Reinforce information given by the patient's HCP regarding further testing, treatment, or referral to another HCP. Answer any questions or address any concerns voiced by the patient or family.
- Depending on the results of this procedure, additional testing may be performed to evaluate or monitor progression of the disease process and determine the need for a change in therapy. Evaluate test results in relation to the patient's symptoms and other tests performed.

RELATED MONOGRAPHS:

- Related tests include albumin, antibodies antithyroglobulin, biopsy thyroid, copper, PTH, protein, RAIU, thyroglobulin, TSI, TBII, thyroid scan, T_4, free T_4, T_3, free T_3, and US thyroid.
- Refer to the Endocrine System table at the end of the book for related tests by body system.

T

Thyroid-Stimulating Immunoglobulins

SYNONYM/ACRONYM: Thyrotropin receptor antibodies, TSI.

COMMON USE: To differentiate between antibodies that stimulate or inhibit thyroid hormone production related to disorders such as Graves' disease.

SPECIMEN: Serum (1 mL) collected in a red-top tube.

REFERENCE VALUE: (Method: Animal cell transfection with luciferase marker) Less than 130% of basal activity.

DESCRIPTION: There are two functional types of thyroid receptor immunoglobulins: *thyroid-stimulating immunoglobulin (TSI)* and *thyroid-binding inhibitory immunoglobulin (TBII)*. TSI reacts with the receptors, activates intracellular enzymes, and promotes epithelial cell activity that operates outside the feedback regulation for thyroid-stimulating hormone (TSH); TBII blocks the action of TSH and is believed to cause certain types of hyperthyroidism (see monograph titled "Thyroid-Binding Inhibitory Immunoglobulin"). These antibodies were formerly known as *long-acting thyroid stimulators.* High levels in pregnancy may have some predictive value for neonatal thyrotoxicosis. A positive result indicates that the antibodies are stimulating (TSI); a negative result indicates that the antibodies are blocking (TBII). TSI testing measures thyroid receptor immunoglobulin levels in the evaluation of thyroid disease.

INDICATIONS

- Follow-up to positive TBII assay in differentiating antibody stimulation from neutral or suppressing activity

- Monitor hyperthyroid patients at risk for relapse or remission

POTENTIAL DIAGNOSIS

Increased in
- Graves' disease *(this form of hyperthyroidism has an autoimmune component; the antibodies stimulate release of thyroid hormones outside the feedback loop that regulates TSH levels)*

Decreased in: N/A

CRITICAL FINDINGS: N/A

INTERFERING FACTORS
- Lithium may cause false-positive TBII results.

NURSING IMPLICATIONS AND PROCEDURE

PRETEST:
- Positively identify the patient using at least two unique identifiers before providing care, treatment, or services.
- *Patient Teaching:* Inform the patient this test can assist in assessing thyroid gland function.
- Obtain a history of the patient's complaints, including a list of known allergens, especially allergies or sensitivities to latex.

- Obtain a history of the patient's endocrine system, symptoms, and results of previously performed laboratory tests and diagnostic and surgical procedures.
- Obtain a list of the patient's current medications, including herbs, nutritional supplements, and nutraceuticals (see Appendix F).
- Review the procedure with the patient. Inform the patient that specimen collection takes approximately 5 to 10 min. Address concerns about pain and explain that there may be some discomfort during the venipuncture.
- *Sensitivity to social and cultural issues,* as well as concern for modesty, is important in providing psychological support before, during, and after the procedure.
- There are no food, fluid, or medication restrictions unless by medical direction.

INTRATEST:

- If the patient has a history of allergic reaction to latex, avoid the use of equipment containing latex.
- Instruct the patient to cooperate fully and to follow directions. Direct the patient to breathe normally and to avoid unnecessary movement.
- Observe standard precautions, and follow the general guidelines in Appendix A. Positively identify the patient, and label the appropriate tubes with the corresponding patient demographics, date, and time of collection. Perform a venipuncture.

- Remove the needle and apply direct pressure with dry gauze to stop bleeding. Observe/assess venipuncture site for bleeding or hematoma formation and secure gauze with adhesive bandage.
- Promptly transport the specimen to the laboratory for processing and analysis.

POST-TEST:

- A report of the results will be sent to the requesting health-care provider (HCP), who will discuss the results with the patient.
- Reinforce information given by the patient's HCP regarding further testing, treatment, or referral to another HCP. Answer any questions or address any concerns voiced by the patient or family.
- Depending on the results of this procedure, additional testing may be performed to evaluate or monitor progression of the disease process and determine the need for a change in therapy. Evaluate test results in relation to the patient's symptoms and other tests performed.

RELATED MONOGRAPHS:

- Related tests include albumin, antibodies antithyroglobulin, biopsy thyroid, copper, PTH, protein, RAIU, thyroglobulin, TBII, thyroid scan, TSH, T_4, free T_4, T_3, free T_3, and US thyroid.
- Refer to the Endocrine System table at the end of the book for related tests by body system.

Thyroxine-Binding Globulin

SYNONYM/ACRONYM: TBG.

COMMON USE: To evaluate thyroid hormone levels related to deficiency or excess to assist in diagnosing disorders such as hyperthyroidism and hypothyroidism.

SPECIMEN: Serum (1 mL) collected in a red- or tiger-top tube.

REFERENCE VALUE: (Method: Immunochemiluminometric assay [ICMA])

Age	Conventional Units	SI Units (Conventional Units × 10)
0–1 wk	3–8 mg/dL	30–80 mg/L
1–12 mo	1.6–3.6 mg/dL	16–36 mg/L
14–19 yr	1.2–2.5 mg/dL	12–25 mg/L
Greater than 20 yr	1.3–3.3 mg/dL	13–33 mg/L
Pregnancy, third trimester	4.7–5.9 mg/dL	47–59 mg/L
Oral contraceptives	1.5–5.5 mg/dL	15–55 mg/L

DESCRIPTION: Thyroxine-binding globulin (TBG) is the predominant protein carrier for circulating thyroxine (T_4) and triiodothyronine (T_3). T_4-binding prealbumin and T_4-binding albumin are the other transport proteins. Conditions that affect TBG levels and binding capacity also affect free T_3 and free T_4 levels.

INDICATIONS
• Differentiate elevated T_4 due to hyperthyroidism from increased TBG binding in euthyroid patients
• Evaluate hypothyroid patients
• Identify deficiency or excess of TBG due to hereditary abnormality

POTENTIAL DIAGNOSIS

Increased in
• Acute intermittent porphyria *(pathophysiology is unclear)*
• Estrogen therapy *(TBG is increased in the presence of exogenous or endogenous estrogens)*
• Genetically high TBG (rare)
• Hyperthyroidism *(related to increased levels of total thyroxine available for binding)*
• Infectious hepatitis and other liver diseases *(pathophysiology is unclear)*
• Neonates
• Pregnancy *(TBG is increased in the presence of exogenous or endogenous estrogens)*

Decreased in
• Acromegaly
• Chronic hepatic disease *(related to general decrease in protein synthesis)*
• Genetically low TBG
• Major illness *(related to general decrease in protein synthesis)*
• Marked hypoproteinemia, malnutrition *(related to general decrease in protein synthesis)*
• Nephrotic syndrome *(related to general increase in protein loss)*
• Ovarian hypofunction *(TBG is decreased in the absence of estrogens)*
• Surgical stress *(related to general decrease in protein synthesis)*
• Testosterone-producing tumors *(TBG is decreased in the presence of testosterone)*

CRITICAL FINDINGS: N/A

INTERFERING FACTORS
• Drugs and hormones that may increase TBG levels include estrogens, oral contraceptives, perphenazine, and tamoxifen.
• Drugs that may decrease TBG levels include anabolic steroids, androgens, asparaginase, corticosteroids, corticotropin, danazol, phenytoin, and propranolol.

NURSING IMPLICATIONS AND PROCEDURE

PRETEST:

- Positively identify the patient using at least two unique identifiers before providing care, treatment, or services.
- *Patient Teaching:* Inform the patient this test can assist in assessing thyroid gland function.
- Obtain a history of the patient's complaints, including a list of known allergens, especially allergies or sensitivities to latex.
- Obtain a history of the patient's endocrine system, symptoms, and results of previously performed laboratory tests and diagnostic and surgical procedures.
- Obtain a list of the patient's current medications, including herbs, nutritional supplements, and nutraceuticals (see Appendix F).
- Review the procedure with the patient. Inform the patient that specimen collection takes approximately 5 to 10 min. Address concerns about pain and explain that there may be some discomfort during the venipuncture.
- *Sensitivity to social and cultural issues,* as well as concern for modesty, is important in providing psychological support before, during, and after the procedure.
- There are no food, fluid, or medication restrictions unless by medical direction.

INTRATEST:

- If the patient has a history of allergic reaction to latex, avoid the use of equipment containing latex.
- Instruct the patient to cooperate fully and to follow directions. Direct the

patient to breathe normally and to avoid unnecessary movement.
- Observe standard precautions, and follow the general guidelines in Appendix A. Positively identify the patient, and label the appropriate tubes with the corresponding patient demographics, date, and time of collection. Perform a venipuncture.
- Remove the needle and apply direct pressure with dry gauze to stop bleeding. Observe/assess venipuncture site for bleeding or hematoma formation and secure gauze with adhesive bandage.
- Promptly transport the specimen to the laboratory for processing and analysis.

POST-TEST:

- A report of the results will be sent to the requesting health-care provider (HCP), who will discuss the results with the patient.
- Reinforce information given by the patient's HCP regarding further testing, treatment, or referral to another HCP. Answer any questions or address any concerns voiced by the patient or family.
- Depending on the results of this procedure, additional testing may be performed to evaluate or monitor progression of the disease process and determine the need for a change in therapy. Evaluate test results in relation to the patient's symptoms and other tests performed.

RELATED MONOGRAPHS:

- Related tests include antibodies antithyroglobulin, thyroglobulin, TBII, thyroid scan, TSH, TSI, T_3, free T_3, T_4, free T_4, and US thyroid.
- Refer to the Endocrine System table at the end of the book for related tests by body system.

T

Thyroxine, Free

SYNONYM/ACRONYM: Free T_4, FT_4.

COMMON USE: A complementary laboratory test in evaluating thyroid hormones levels related to deficiency or excess to assist in diagnosing hyperthyroidism and hypothyroidism.

SPECIMEN: Serum (1 mL) collected in a red- or tiger-top tube. Plasma (1 mL) collected in a green-top (heparin) tube is also acceptable.

REFERENCE VALUE: (Method: Immunoassay)

Age	Conventional Units	SI Units (Conventional Units × 12.9)
Newborn	0.8–2.8 ng/dL	10–36 pmol/L
1–12 mo	0.8–2.0 ng/dL	10–26 pmol/L
1–18 yr	0.8–1.7 ng/dL	10–22 pmol/L
Adult–older adult	0.8–1.5 ng/dL	10–19 pmol/L

DESCRIPTION: Thyroxine (T_4) is a hormone produced and secreted by the thyroid gland. Newborns are commonly tested for decreased T_4 levels by a filter paper method (see monograph titled "Thyroxine, Total"). Most T_4 in the serum (99.97%) is bound to thyroxine-binding globulin (TBG), prealbumin, and albumin. The remainder (0.03%) circulates as unbound or free T_4, which is the physiologically active form. Levels of free T_4 are proportional to levels of total T_4. The advantage of measuring free T_4 instead of total T_4 is that, unlike total T_4 measurements, free T_4 levels are not affected by fluctuations in TBG levels; as a result, free T_4 levels are considered the most accurate indicator of T_4 and its thyrometabolic activity. Free T_4 measurements are useful in evaluating thyroid disease when thyroid-stimulating hormone (TSH) levels alone provide insufficient information. Free T_4 and TSH levels are inversely proportional. Measurement of free T_4 is also recommended during treatment for hyperthyroidism until symptoms have abated and levels have decreased into the normal range.

INDICATIONS
- Evaluate signs of hypothyroidism or hyperthyroidism
- Monitor response to therapy for hypothyroidism or hyperthyroidism

POTENTIAL DIAGNOSIS

Increased in
- Hyperthyroidism *(thyroxine is produced independently of stimulation by TSH)*

- Hypothyroidism treated with T$_4$ *(laboratory tests do not distinguish between endogenous and exogenous sources)*

Decreased in
- Hypothyroidism *(thyroid hormones are not produced in sufficient quantities regardless of TSH levels)*
- Pregnancy (late)

CRITICAL FINDINGS: N/A

INTERFERING FACTORS
- Drugs that may increase free T$_4$ levels include acetylsalicylic acid, amiodarone, halofenate, heparin, iopanoic acid, levothyroxine, methimazole, and radiographic agents.
- Drugs that may decrease free T$_4$ levels include amiodarone, anabolic steroids, asparaginase, methadone, methimazole, oral contraceptives, and phenylbutazone.

NURSING IMPLICATIONS AND PROCEDURE

PRETEST:
▸ Positively identify the patient using at least two unique identifiers before providing care, treatment, or services.
▸ *Patient Teaching:* Inform the patient this test can assist in assessing thyroid gland function.
▸ Obtain a history of the patient's complaints, including a list of known allergens, especially allergies or sensitivities to latex.
▸ Obtain a history of the patient's endocrine system, symptoms, and results of previously performed laboratory tests and diagnostic and surgical procedures.
▸ Obtain a list of the patient's current medications, including herbs, nutritional supplements, and nutraceuticals (see Appendix F).
▸ Review the procedure with the patient. Inform the patient that specimen

collection takes approximately 5 to 10 min. Address concerns about pain and explain that there may be some discomfort during the venipuncture.
▸ *Sensitivity to social and cultural issues,* as well as concern for modesty, is important in providing psychological support before, during, and after the procedure.
▸ There are no food, fluid, or medication restrictions unless by medical direction.

INTRATEST:
▸ If the patient has a history of allergic reaction to latex, avoid the use of equipment containing latex.
▸ Instruct the patient to cooperate fully and to follow directions. Direct the patient to breathe normally and to avoid unnecessary movement.
▸ Observe standard precautions, and follow the general guidelines in Appendix A. Positively identify the patient, and label the appropriate tubes with the corresponding patient demographics, date, and time of collection. Perform a venipuncture.
▸ Remove the needle and apply direct pressure with dry gauze to stop bleeding. Observe/assess venipuncture site for bleeding or hematoma formation and secure gauze with adhesive bandage.
▸ Promptly transport the specimen to the laboratory for processing and analysis.

POST-TEST:
▸ A report of the results will be sent to the requesting health-care provider (HCP), who will discuss the results with the patient.
▸ Reinforce information given by the patient's HCP regarding further testing, treatment, or referral to another HCP. Answer any questions or address any concerns voiced by the patient or family.
▸ Depending on the results of this procedure, additional testing may be performed to evaluate or monitor progression of the disease process and determine the need for a change in therapy. Evaluate test results in relation to the patient's symptoms and other tests performed.

T

RELATED MONOGRAPHS:

▶ Related tests include albumin, antibodies antithyroglobulin, biopsy thyroid, copper, PTH, prealbumin, protein, RAIU, thyroglobulin, TBII, thyroid scan, TSH, TSI, T_4, T_3, free T_3, and US thyroid.

▶ Refer to the Endocrine System table at the end of the book for related tests by body system.

Thyroxine, Total

SYNONYM/ACRONYM: T_4.

COMMON USE: A first look at thyroid function and a tool to evaluate the effectiveness of therapeutic thyroid therapy.

SPECIMEN: Serum (1 mL) collected in a red- or tiger-top tube. Plasma (1 mL) collected in a green-top (heparin) tube is also acceptable.

REFERENCE VALUE: (Method: Immunoassay).

Age	Conventional Units	SI Units (Conventional Units × 12.9)
1–3 days	11.8–22.6 mcg/dL	152–292 nmol/L
1–2 wk	9.8–16.6 mcg/dL	126–214 nmol/L
1–4 mo	7.2–14.4 mcg/dL	93–186 nmol/L
5–12 mo	7.8–16.5 mcg/dL	101–213 nmol/L
1–5 yr	7.3–15.0 mcg/dL	94–194 nmol/L
5–10 yr	6.4–13.3 mcg/dL	83–172 nmol/L
10–15 yr	5.6–11.7 mcg/dL	72–151 nmol/L
Adult		
Male	4.6–10.5 mcg/dL	59–135 nmol/L
Female	5.5–11.0 mcg/dL	71–142 nmol/L
Pregnant female	5.5–16.0 mcg/dL	71–155 nmol/L
Over 60 yr	5.0–10.7 mcg/dL	65–138 nmol/L

DESCRIPTION: Thyroxine (T_4) is a hormone produced and secreted by the thyroid gland. Newborns are commonly tested for decreased T_4 levels by a filter paper method. Most T_4 in the serum (99.97%) is bound to thyroxine-binding globulin (TBG), prealbumin, and albumin. The remainder (0.03%) circulates as unbound or free T_4, which is the physiologically active form. Levels of free T_4 are proportional to levels of total T_4. The advantage of accurate indicator of T_4 and its thyrometabolic activity (see monograph titled "Thyroxine, Free").

INDICATIONS

- Evaluate signs of hypothyroidism or hyperthyroidism and neonatal screening for congenital hypothyroidism (required in all 50 states)
- Evaluate thyroid response to protein deficiency associated with severe illnesses
- Monitor response to therapy for hypothyroidism or hyperthyroidism

POTENTIAL DIAGNOSIS

Increased in

- Acute psychiatric illnesses *(pathophysiology is unknown, although there is a relationship between thyroid hormone levels and certain types of mental illness)*
- Excessive intake of iodine *(iodine is rapidly taken up by the body to form thyroxine)*
- Hepatitis *(related to decreased production of TBG by damaged liver cells)*
- Hyperthyroidism *(thyroxine is produced independently of stimulation by TSH)*
- Obesity
- Thyrotoxicosis due to Graves' disease *(thyroxine is produced independently of stimulation by TSH)*
- Thyrotoxicosis factitia *(laboratory tests do not distinguish between endogenous and exogenous sources)*

Decreased in

- Decreased TBG *(nephrotic syndrome, liver disease, gastrointestinal protein loss, malnutrition)*
- Hypothyroidism *(thyroid hormones are not produced in*

sufficient quantities regardless of TSH levels)
- Panhypopituitarism *(dysfunctional pituitary gland does not secrete enough thyrotropin to stimulate the thyroid to produce thyroxine)*
- Strenuous exercise

CRITICAL FINDINGS ✦

- *Hypothyroidism:* Less than 2.0 mcg/dL
- *Hyperthyroidism:* Greater than 20.0 mcg/dL

Note and immediately report to the health-care provider (HCP) any critically increased or decreased values and related symptoms.

At levels less than 2.0 mcg/dL, the patient is at risk for myxedema coma. Signs and symptoms of severe hypothyroidism include hypothermia, hypotension, bradycardia, hypoventilation, lethargy, and coma. Possible interventions include airway support, hourly monitoring for neurological function and blood pressure, and administration of IV thyroid hormone.

At levels greater than 20.0 mcg/dL, the patient is at risk for thyroid storm. Signs and symptoms of severe hyperthyroidism include hyperthermia, diaphoresis, vomiting, dehydration, and shock. Possible interventions include supportive treatment for shock, fluid and electrolyte replacement for dehydration, and administration of antithyroid drugs (propylthiouracil and Lugol's solution).

INTERFERING FACTORS

- Drugs that may increase T_4 levels include amiodarone, amphetamines, corticosteroids, ether, fluorouracil, glucocorticoids, halofenate, insulin, iobenzamic acid, iopanoic acid, ipodate, levarterenol, levodopa, levothyroxine, opiates, oral contraceptives, phenothiazine, and prostaglandins.

- Drugs, substances, and treatments that may decrease T_4 levels include acetylsalicylic acid, aminoglutethimide, aminosalicylic acid, amiodarone, anabolic steroids, anticonvulsants, asparaginase, barbiturates, carbimazole, chlorpromazine, chlorpropamide, cholestyramine, clofibrate, cobalt, colestipol, corticotropin, cortisone, cotrimoxazole, cytostatic therapy, danazol, dehydroepiandrosterone, dexamethasone, diazepam, diazo dyes (e.g., Evans blue), dinitrophenol, ethionamide, fenclofenac, halofenate, hydroxyphenylpyruvic acid, interferon alfa-2b, iothiouracil, iron, isotretinoin, liothyronine, lithium, lovastatin, methimazole, methylthiouracil, mitotane, norethindrone, penicillamine, penicillin, phenylacetic acid derivatives, phenylbutazone, potassium iodide, propylthiouracil, reserpine, salicylate, sodium nitroprusside, stanozolol, sulfonylureas, tetrachlorothyronine, tolbutamide, and triiodothyronine (T_3).

NURSING IMPLICATIONS AND PROCEDURE

PRETEST:

- Positively identify the patient using at least two unique identifiers before providing care, treatment, or services.
- *Patient Teaching:* Inform the patient this test can assist in assessing thyroid gland function.
- Obtain a history of the patient's complaints, including a list of known allergens, especially allergies or sensitivities to latex.
- Obtain a history of the patient's endocrine system, symptoms, and results of previously performed laboratory tests and diagnostic and surgical procedures.
- Obtain a list of the patient's current medications, including herbs, nutritional

supplements, and nutraceuticals (see Appendix F).
- Review the procedure with the patient. Inform the patient that specimen collection takes approximately 5 to 10 min. Address concerns about pain and explain that there may be some discomfort during the venipuncture.
- *Sensitivity to social and cultural issues,* as well as concern for modesty, is important in providing psychological support before, during, and after the procedure.
- There are no food, fluid, or medication restrictions unless by medical direction.

INTRATEST:

- If the patient has a history of allergic reaction to latex, avoid the use of equipment containing latex.
- Instruct the patient to cooperate fully and to follow directions. Direct the patient to breathe normally and to avoid unnecessary movement.
- Observe standard precautions, and follow the general guidelines in Appendix A. Positively identify the patient, and label the appropriate tubes with the corresponding patient demographics, date, and time of collection. Perform a venipuncture.
- Remove the needle and apply direct pressure with dry gauze to stop bleeding. Observe/assess venipuncture site for bleeding or hematoma formation and secure gauze with adhesive bandage.
- Promptly transport the specimen to the laboratory for processing and analysis.

POST-TEST:

- A report of the results will be sent to the requesting HCP, who will discuss the results with the patient.
- Reinforce information given by the patient's HCP regarding further testing, treatment, or referral to another HCP. Answer any questions or address any concerns voiced by the patient or family.
- Depending on the results of this procedure, additional testing may be performed to evaluate or monitor progression of the disease process and determine the need for a change in therapy. Evaluate test results in relation to the patient's symptoms and other tests performed.

T

▶ Related tests include albumin, antibodies antithyroglobulin, biopsy thyroid, copper, PTH, prealbumin, protein, RAIU, thyroglobulin, TBII, thyroid scan, TSH, TSI, free T_4, T_3, free T_3, and US thyroid.
▶ Refer to the Endocrine System table at the end of the book for related tests by body system.

Toxoplasma Antibody

SYNONYM/ACRONYM: Toxoplasmosis serology, toxoplasmosis titer.

COMMON USE: To assess for a past or present toxoplasmosis infection and to assess for the presence of antibodies.

SPECIMEN: Serum (1 mL) collected in a red-top tube.

REFERENCE VALUE: (Method: Indirect fluorescent antibody) Negative or less than a fourfold increase in titer.

DESCRIPTION: Toxoplasmosis is a severe, generalized granulomatous central nervous system disease caused by the protozoan *Toxoplasma gondii*. Transmission to humans occurs by ingesting undercooked meat or handling contaminated matter such as cat litter. Immunoglobulin (Ig) M antibodies develop approximately 5 days after infection and can remain elevated for 3 wk to several months. IgG antibodies develop 1 to 2 wk after infection and can remain elevated for months or years. *T. gondii* serology is part of the TORCH (*t*oxoplasmosis, *r*ubella, *c*ytomegalovirus, and *h*erpes simplex type 2) panel routinely performed on pregnant women. Fetal infection during the first trimester can cause spontaneous abortion or congenital defects. Immunocompromised individuals are also at high risk for serious complications if infected. The presence of IgM antibodies indicates acute or congenital infection; the presence of IgG antibodies indicates current or past infection.

INDICATIONS
- Assist in establishing a diagnosis of toxoplasmosis
- Document past exposure or immunity
- Serological screening during pregnancy

POTENTIAL DIAGNOSIS

Positive findings in
- *Toxoplasma* infection

CRITICAL FINDINGS: N/A

INTERFERING FACTORS: N/A

NURSING IMPLICATIONS AND PROCEDURE

PRETEST:

- Positively identify the patient using at least two unique identifiers before providing care, treatment, or services.
- *Patient Teaching:* Inform the patient this test can assist in assessing for toxoplasmosis infection.
- Obtain a history of the patient's complaints, including a list of known allergens, especially allergies or sensitivities to latex.
- Obtain a history of exposure.
- Obtain a history of the patient's immune and reproductive systems, a history of other potential sources of exposure, symptoms, and results of previously performed laboratory tests and diagnostic and surgical procedures.
- Obtain a list of the patient's current medications, including herbs, nutritional supplements, and nutraceuticals (see Appendix F).
- Review the procedure with the patient. Inform the patient that several tests may be necessary to confirm the diagnosis. Any individual positive result should be repeated in 3 wk to monitor a change in titer. Inform the patient that specimen collection takes approximately 5 to 10 min. Address concerns about pain and explain that there may be some discomfort during the venipuncture.
- *Sensitivity to social and cultural issues,* as well as concern for modesty, is important in providing psychological support before, during, and after the procedure.
- There are no food, fluid, or medication restrictions unless by medical direction.

INTRATEST:

- If the patient has a history of allergic reaction to latex, avoid the use of equipment containing latex.
- Instruct the patient to cooperate fully and to follow directions. Direct the patient to breathe normally and to avoid unnecessary movement.
- Observe standard precautions, and follow the general guidelines in Appendix A.

Positively identify the patient, and label the appropriate tubes with the corresponding patient demographics, date, and time of collection. Perform a venipuncture.
- Remove the needle and apply direct pressure with dry gauze to stop bleeding. Observe/assess venipuncture site for bleeding or hematoma formation and secure gauze with adhesive bandage.
- Promptly transport the specimen to the laboratory for processing and analysis.

POST-TEST:

- A report of the results will be sent to the requesting health-care provider (HCP), who will discuss the results with the patient.
- Recognize anxiety related to test results, and provide emotional support if results are positive and the patient is pregnant and/or immunocompromised. Discuss the implications of abnormal test results on the patient's lifestyle. Provide teaching and information regarding the clinical implications of the test results, as appropriate. Educate the patient regarding access to counseling services.
- Reinforce information given by the patient's HCP regarding further testing, treatment, or referral to another HCP. Instruct the patient in isolation precautions during time of communicability or contagion. Emphasize the need to return to have a convalescent blood sample taken in 3 wk. Answer any questions or address any concerns voiced by the patient or family.
- Depending on the results of this procedure, additional testing may be performed to evaluate or monitor progression of the disease process and determine the need for a change in therapy. Evaluate test results in relation to the patient's symptoms and other tests performed.

RELATED MONOGRAPHS:

- Related tests include CMV, fetal fibronectin, and rubella.
- Refer to the Immune and Reproductive systems tables at the end of the book for related tests by body system.

T

Transferrin

SYNONYM/ACRONYM: Siderophilin, TRF.

COMMON USE: To assess circulating iron levels related to dietary intake to assist in diagnosing disorders such as iron deficiency anemia or hemochromatosis.

SPECIMEN: Serum (1 mL) collected in a red- or tiger-top tube.

REFERENCE VALUE: (Method: Nephelometry)

Age	Conventional Units	SI Units (Conventional Units × 0.01)
Newborn	130–275 mg/dL	1.3–2.75 g/L
Adult		
Male	215–365 mg/dL	2.2–3.6 g/L
Female	250–380 mg/dL	2.5–3.8 g/L

DESCRIPTION: Transferrin is a glycoprotein formed in the liver. It transports circulating iron obtained from dietary intake and red blood cell breakdown. Transferrin carries 50% to 70% of the body's iron; normally it is approximately one-third saturated. Inadequate transferrin levels can lead to impaired hemoglobin synthesis and anemia. Transferrin is subject to diurnal variation, and it is responsible for the variation in levels of serum iron throughout the day. (See monograph titled "Iron-Binding Capacity [Total], Transferrin, and Iron Saturation.")

INDICATIONS
- Determine the iron-binding capacity of the blood
- Evaluate iron metabolism in iron-deficiency anemia
- Evaluate nutritional status
- Screen for hemochromatosis

POTENTIAL DIAGNOSIS

Increased in
- Estrogen therapy *(estrogen stimulates the liver to produce transferrin)*
- Iron-deficiency anemia *(the liver produces transferrin in response to decreased iron levels)*
- Pregnancy *(the liver produces transferrin in response to anemia of pregnancy)*

Decreased in
- Acute or chronic infection *(a negative acute-phase reactant protein whose levels decrease in response to inflammation)*
- Cancer (especially of the gastrointestinal tract) *(related to malnutrition)*
- Excessive protein loss from renal disease *(related to increased loss from damaged kidney)*
- Hepatic damage *(related to decreased synthesis in the liver)*
- Hereditary atransferrinemia
- Malnutrition *(related to a protein-deficient diet that does not*

provide the nutrients required for synthesis)

CRITICAL FINDINGS: N/A

INTERFERING FACTORS

- Drugs that may increase transferrin levels include carbamazepine, danazol, mestranol, and oral contraceptives.
- Drugs that may decrease transferrin levels include cortisone and dextran.
- Transferrin levels are subject to diurnal variation and should be collected in the morning, when levels are highest.
- Failure to follow dietary restrictions before the procedure may cause the procedure to be canceled or repeated.

NURSING IMPLICATIONS AND PROCEDURE

PRETEST:

- Positively identify the patient using at least two unique identifiers before providing care, treatment, or services.
- *Patient Teaching:* Inform the patient this test can assist in evaluating for anemia.
- Obtain a history of the patient's complaints, including a list of known allergens, especially allergies or sensitivities to latex.
- Obtain a history of the patient's hematopoietic system, symptoms, and results of previously performed laboratory tests and diagnostic and surgical procedures.
- Obtain a list of the patient's current medications, including herbs, nutritional supplements, and nutraceuticals (see Appendix F).
- Review the procedure with the patient. Inform the patient that specimen collection takes approximately 5 to 10 min. Address concerns about pain and explain that there may be some discomfort during the venipuncture.
- *Sensitivity to social and cultural issues,* as well as concern for modesty, is important in providing psychological support before, during, and after the procedure.
- Instruct the patient to fast for at least 12 hr before specimen collection.
- There are no fluid or medication restrictions unless by medical direction.

INTRATEST:

- Ensure that the patient has complied with dietary restrictions; ensure that food has been restricted for at least 12 hr prior to the procedure.
- If the patient has a history of allergic reaction to latex, avoid the use of equipment containing latex.
- Instruct the patient to cooperate fully and to follow directions. Direct the patient to breathe normally and to avoid unnecessary movement.
- Observe standard precautions, and follow the general guidelines in Appendix A. Positively identify the patient, and label the appropriate tubes with the corresponding patient demographics, date, and time of collection. Perform a venipuncture.
- Remove the needle and apply direct pressure with dry gauze to stop bleeding. Observe/assess venipuncture site for bleeding or hematoma formation and secure gauze with adhesive bandage.
- Promptly transport the specimen to the laboratory for processing and analysis.

POST-TEST:

- A report of the results will be sent to the requesting health-care provider (HCP), who will discuss the results with the patient.
- Instruct the patient to resume usual diet, as directed by the HCP.
- *Nutritional Considerations:* Educate the patient with abnormal iron values that numerous factors affect the absorption of iron, enhancing or decreasing absorption regardless of the original content of the iron-containing dietary source. Consumption of large amounts of alcohol damages the intestine and allows increased absorption of iron. A high intake of calcium and ascorbic acid also increases iron absorption.

T

Iron absorption after a meal is also increased by factors in meat, fish, or poultry. Iron absorption is decreased by the absence (gastric resection) or diminished presence (use of antacids) of gastric acid. Phytic acids from cereals; tannins from tea and coffee; oxalic acid from vegetables; and minerals such as copper, zinc, and manganese interfere with iron absorption.

▶ Reinforce information given by the patient's HCP regarding further testing, treatment, or referral to another HCP. Answer any questions or address any concerns voiced by the patient or family.

▶ Depending on the results of this procedure, additional testing may be performed to evaluate or monitor progression of the disease process and determine the need for a change in therapy. Evaluate test results in relation to the patient's symptoms and other tests performed.

RELATED MONOGRAPHS:

▶ Related tests include A/G, cancer antigens, CBC, CBC RBC count, CBC RBC indices, CBC RBC morphology, ferritin, iron/TIBC, prealbumin, and total protein.

▶ Refer to the Hematopoietic System table at the end of the book for related tests by body system.

Triglycerides

SYNONYM/ACRONYM: Trigs, TG.

COMMON USE: To evaluate triglyceride levels to assess cardiovascular disease risk and evaluate the effectiveness of therapeutic interventions.

SPECIMEN: Serum (1 mL) collected in a red- or tiger-top tube. Plasma (1 mL) collected in a green-top (heparin) tube is also acceptable.

REFERENCE VALUE: (Method: Spectrophotometry)

ATP III Classification	Conventional Units	SI Units (Conventional Units × 0.0113)
Normal	Less than 150 mg/dL	Less than 1.7 mmol/L
Borderline high	150–199 mg/dL	1.7–2.2 mmol/L
High	200–499 mg/dL	2.2–5.6 mmol/L
Very high	Greater than 500 mg/dL	Greater than 5.6 mmol/L

DESCRIPTION: Triglycerides (TGs) are a combination of three fatty acids and one glycerol molecule. They are necessary to provide energy for various metabolic processes. Excess triglycerides are stored in adipose tissue, and the fatty acids provide the raw materials needed for conversion to glucose (gluconeogenesis) or for direct use as an energy source. Although fatty acids originate in

T

the diet, many are also derived from unused glucose and amino acids that the liver converts into stored energy. Beyond triglyceride, total cholesterol, high-density lipoprotein (HDL), and low-density lipoprotein (LDL) cholesterol values, other important risk factors must be considered. The Framingham algorithm can assist in estimating the risk of developing coronary artery disease (CAD) within a 10-yr period. The National Cholesterol Education Program (NCEP) also provides important guidelines. The latest NCEP guidelines for target lipid levels, major risk factors, and therapeutic interventions are outlined in Adult Treatment Panel III (ATP III). Triglyceride levels vary by age, gender, weight, and race:

Levels increase with age.
Levels are higher in men than in women (among women, those who take oral contraceptives have levels that are 20 to 40 mg/dL higher than those who do not).
Levels are higher in overweight and obese people than in those with normal weight.
Levels in African Americans are approximately 10 to 20 mg/dL lower than in whites.

INDICATIONS

- Evaluate known or suspected disorders associated with altered triglyceride levels
- Identify hyperlipoproteinemia (hyperlipidemia) in patients with a family history of the disorder
- Monitor the response to drugs known to alter triglyceride levels
- Screen adults who are either over 40 yr or obese to estimate the risk for atherosclerotic cardiovascular disease

POTENTIAL DIAGNOSIS

Increased in

- Acute myocardial infarction *(elevated TG is identified as an independent risk factor in the development of CAD)*
- Alcoholism *(related to decreased breakdown of fats in the liver and increased blood levels)*
- Anorexia nervosa *(compensatory increase secondary to starvation)*
- Chronic ischemic heart disease *(elevated TG is identified as an independent risk factor in the development of CAD)*
- Cirrhosis *(increased TG blood levels related to decreased breakdown of fats in the liver)*
- Glycogen storage disease *(G6PD deficiency, e.g., von Gierke's disease, results in hepatic overproduction of very-low-density lipoprotein [VLDL] cholesterol, the TG-rich lipoprotein)*
- Gout *(TG is frequently elevated in patients with gout, possibly related to alterations in apolipoprotein E genotypes)*
- Hyperlipoproteinemia *(related to increase in transport proteins)*
- Hypertension *(associated with elevated TG, which is identified as an independent risk factor in the development of CAD)*
- Hypothyroidism *(significant relationship between elevated TG and decreased metabolism)*
- Impaired glucose tolerance *(increase in insulin stimulates production of TG by liver)*
- Metabolic syndrome *(syndrome consisting of obesity, high blood pressure, and insulin resistance)*
- Nephrotic syndrome *(related to absence or insufficient levels of lipoprotein lipase to remove circulating TG and to decreased catabolism of TG-rich VLDL lipoproteins)*

- Obesity *(significant and complex relationship between obesity and elevated TG)*
- Pancreatitis *(acute and chronic; related to effects on insulin production)*
- Pregnancy *(increased demand for production of hormones related to pregnancy)*
- Renal failure *(related to diabetes; elevated insulin levels stimulate production of TG by liver)*
- Respiratory distress syndrome *(related to artificial lung surfactant used for therapy)*
- Stress *(related to poor diet; effect of hormones secreted under stressful situations that affect glucose levels)*
- Syndrome X *(metabolic syndrome consisting of obesity, high blood pressure, and insulin resistance)*
- Werner's syndrome *(clinical features resemble syndrome X)*

Decreased in

- End-stage liver disease *(related to cessation of liver function that results in decreased production of TG and TG transport proteins)*
- Hyperthyroidism *(related to increased catabolism of VLDL transport proteins and general increase in metabolism)*
- Hypolipoproteinemia and abetalipoproteinemia *(related to decrease in transport proteins)*
- Intestinal lymphangiectasia
- Malabsorption disorders *(inadequate supply from dietary sources)*
- Malnutrition *(inadequate supply from dietary sources)*

CRITICAL FINDINGS: N/A

INTERFERING FACTORS

- Drugs that may increase triglyceride levels include acetylsalicylic acid, aldatense, atenolol, bisoprolol, β blockers, bendroflumethiazide, cholestyramine, conjugated estrogens, cyclosporine, estrogen/progestin therapy, estropipate, ethynodiol, etretinate, furosemide, glucocorticoids, hydrochlorothiazide, isotretinoin, labetalol, levonorgestrel, medroxyprogesterone, mepindolol, methyclothiazide, metoprolol, miconazole, mirtazapine, nadolol, nafarelin, oral contraceptives, oxprenolol, pindolol, prazosin, propranolol, tamoxifen, thiazides, ticlopidine, timolol, and tretinoin.
- Drugs and substances that may decrease triglyceride levels include anabolic steroids, ascorbic acid, beclobrate, bezafibrate, captopril, carvedilol, celiprolol, celiprolol, chenodiol, cholestyramine, cilazapril, ciprofibrate, clofibrate, colestipol, danazol, dextrothyroxine, doxazosin, enalapril, eptastatin (type IIb only), fenofibrate, flaxseed oil, fluvastatin, gemfibrozil, halofenate, insulin, levonorgestrel, levothyroxine, lifibrol, lovastatin, medroxyprogesterone, metformin, nafenopin, niacin, niceritrol, Norplant, pentoxifylline, pinacidil, pindolol, pravastatin, prazosin, probucol, simvastatin, and verapamil.
- Failure to follow dietary restrictions before the procedure may cause the procedure to be canceled or repeated.

NURSING IMPLICATIONS AND PROCEDURE

PRETEST:

▸ Positively identify the patient using at least two unique identifiers before providing care, treatment, or services.
▸ *Patient Teaching:* Inform the patient this test can assist in monitoring and evaluating lipid levels.
▸ Obtain a history of the patient's complaints, including a list of known

allergens, especially allergies or sensitivities to latex.

▶ Obtain a history of the patient's cardio-vascular system, symptoms, and results of previously performed labora-tory tests and diagnostic and surgical procedures.

▶ Obtain a list of the patient's current medications, including herbs, nutritional supplements, and nutraceuticals (see Appendix F).

▶ Review the procedure with the patient. Inform the patient that specimen collection takes approximately 5 to 10 min. Address concerns about pain and explain that there may be some discomfort during the venipuncture.

▶ *Sensitivity to social and cultural issues,* as well as concern for modesty, is impor-tant in providing psychological support before, during, and after the procedure.

▶ The patient should fast for 12 hr before specimen collection. Ideally, the patient should be on a stable diet for 3 wk and avoid alcohol consumption for 3 days before specimen collection. Protocols may vary among facilities.

▶ There are no medication restrictions unless by medical direction.

INTRATEST:

▶ Ensure that the patient has complied with dietary restrictions and other pre-testing preparations; assure that food has been restricted for at least 12 hr prior to the procedure.

▶ If the patient has a history of allergic reaction to latex, avoid the use of equipment containing latex.

▶ Instruct the patient to cooperate fully and to follow directions. Direct the patient to breathe normally and to avoid unnecessary movement.

▶ Observe standard precautions, and follow the general guidelines in Appendix A. Positively identify the patient, and label the appropriate tubes with the corresponding patient demo-graphics, date, and time of collection. Perform a venipuncture.

▶ Remove the needle and apply direct pressure with dry gauze to stop bleed-ing. Observe/assess venipuncture site for bleeding or hematoma formation and secure gauze with adhesive bandage.

▶ Promptly transport the specimen to the laboratory for processing and analysis.

POST-TEST:

▶ A report of the results will be sent to the requesting health-care provider (HCP), who will discuss the results with the patient.

▶ Instruct the patient to resume usual diet, as directed by the HCP.

▶ *Nutritional Considerations:* Increased triglyceride levels may be associated with atherosclerosis and CAD. The American Heart Association and National Heart, Lung, and Blood Institute (NHBLI) recommend nutritional therapy for individuals identified to be at high risk for developing CAD or indi-viduals who have specific risk factors and/or existing medical conditions (e.g., elevated LDL cholesterol levels, other lipid disorders, insulin-dependent diabetes, insulin resistance, or meta-bolic syndrome). If overweight, the patient should be encouraged to achieve a normal weight. The NHLBI's National Cholesterol Education Program (NCEP) revised its dietary guidelines for reducing CAD in 2001. Guidelines for the Therapeutic Lifestyle Changes (TLC) diet are outlined in the Third Report of the Expert Panel on Detection, Evaluation, and Treatment of High Blood Cholesterol in Adults (Adult Treatment Panel III [ATP III]). The TLC diet emphasizes a reduction in foods high in saturated fats and cholesterol. Red meats, eggs, and dairy products are the major sources of saturated fats and cholesterol. If triglycerides also are elevated, the patient should be advised to eliminate or reduce alcohol and sim-ple carbohydrates from the diet. The TLC approach also includes the use of plant stanols or sterols and increased dissolved fiber as an option for lower-ing LDL cholesterol levels; nutritional recommendations for daily total caloric intake; recommendations for allowable percentage of calories derived from fat (saturated and unsaturated), carbo-hydrates, protein, and cholesterol; as well as recommendations for daily expenditure of energy.

Nutritional Considerations: Overweight patients with high blood pressure should be encouraged to achieve a normal weight. Other changeable risk factors warranting patient education include strategies to safely decrease sodium intake, increase physical activity, decrease alcohol consumption, eliminate tobacco use, and decrease cholesterol levels.

Sensitivity to social and cultural issues: Numerous studies point to the increased prevalence of excess body weight in American children and adolescents. Experts estimate that obesity is present in 25% of the population ages 6 to 11 yr. The medical, social, and emotional consequences of excess body weight are significant. Special attention should be given to instructing the pediatric patient and caregiver regarding health risks and weight control.

Recognize anxiety related to test results, and be supportive of fear of shortened life expectancy. Discuss the implications of abnormal test results on the patient's lifestyle. Provide teaching and information regarding the clinical implications of the test results, as appropriate. Educate the patient regarding access to counseling services. Provide contact information, if desired, for the American Heart Association (www.americanheart.org) or the NHLBI (www.nhlbi.nih.gov).

Reinforce information given by the patient's HCP regarding further testing, treatment, or referral to another HCP. Answer any questions or address any concerns voiced by the patient or family.

Depending on the results of this procedure, additional testing may be performed to evaluate or monitor progression of the disease process and determine the need for a change in therapy. Evaluate test results in relation to the patient's symptoms and other tests performed.

RELATED MONOGRAPHS:

Related tests include antiarrhythmic drugs, apolipoprotein A and B, AST, atrial natriuretic peptide, blood gases, BNP, calcium (total and ionized), cholesterol (total, HDL, and LDL), CT cardiac scoring, C-reactive protein, CK and isoenzymes, echocardiography, glucose, glycated hemoglobin, Holter monitor, homocysteine, ketones, LDH and isoenzymes, lipoprotein electrophoresis, magnesium, MRI chest, myocardial infarct scan, myocardial perfusion heart scan, myoglobin, PET heart, potassium, and troponin.

Refer to the Cardiovascular System table at the end of the book for related tests by body system.

Triiodothyronine, Free

SYNONYM/ACRONYM: Free T_3, FT_3.

COMMON USE: A complementary adjunct to evaluate thyroid hormone levels primarily related to hyperthyroidism and to assess causes of hypothyroidism.

SPECIMEN: Serum (1 mL) collected in a red- or tiger-top tube.

REFERENCE VALUE: (Method: Immunoassay)

Age	Conventional Units	SI Units (Conventional Units × 0.01)
Children and adults	260–480 pg/dL	4.0–7.4 pmol/L
Pregnant women (4–9 mo gestation)	196–338 pg/dL	3.0–5.2 pmol/L

DESCRIPTION: Unlike the thyroid hormone thyroxine (T_4), most T_3 is converted enzymatically from T_4 in the tissues rather than being produced directly by the thyroid gland (see monograph titled "Thyroxine, Total"). Approximately one-third of T_4 is converted to T_3. Most T_3 in the serum (99.97%) is bound to thyroxine-binding globulin (TBG), prealbumin, and albumin. The remainder (0.03%) circulates as unbound or free T_3, which is the physiologically active form. Levels of free T_3 are proportional to levels of total T_3. The advantage of measuring free T_3 instead of total T_3 is that, unlike total T_3 measurements, free T_3 levels are not affected by fluctuations in TBG levels. T_3 is four to five times more biologically potent than T_4. This hormone, along with T_4, is responsible for maintaining a euthyroid state. Free T_3 measurements are rarely required, but they are indicated in the diagnosis of T_3 toxicosis and when certain drugs are being administered that interfere with the conversion of T_4 to T_3.

POTENTIAL DIAGNOSIS

Increased in
- High altitude
- Hyperthyroidism *(triiodothyronine is produced independently of stimulation by TSH)*
- T_3 toxicosis

Decreased in
- Hypothyroidism *(thyroid hormones are not produced in sufficient quantities regardless of TSH levels)*
- Malnutrition *(related to protein or iodine deficiency; iodine is needed for thyroid hormone synthesis and proteins are needed for transport)*
- Nonthyroidal chronic diseases
- Pregnancy (late)

CRITICAL FINDINGS: N/A

INTERFERING FACTORS
- Drugs that may increase free T_3 include acetylsalicylic acid, amiodarone, and levothyroxine.
- Drugs that may decrease free T_3 include amiodarone, methimazole, phenytoin, propranolol, and radiographic agents.

NURSING IMPLICATIONS AND PROCEDURE

PRETEST:
- Positively identify the patient using at least two unique identifiers before providing care, treatment, or services.
- *Patient Teaching:* Inform the patient this test can assist in assessing thyroid gland function.

INDICATIONS
- Adjunctive aid to thyroid-stimulating hormone (TSH) and free T_4 assessment
- Assist in the diagnosis of T_3 toxicosis

▶ Obtain a history of the patient's complaints, including a list of known allergens, especially allergies or sensitivities to latex.

▶ Obtain a history of the patient's endocrine system, symptoms, and results of previously performed laboratory tests and diagnostic and surgical procedures.

▶ Obtain a list of the patient's current medications, including herbs, nutritional supplements, and nutraceuticals (see Appendix F).

▶ Review the procedure with the patient. Inform the patient that specimen collection takes approximately 5 to 10 min. Address concerns about pain and explain that there may be some discomfort during the venipuncture.

▶ *Sensitivity to social and cultural issues,* as well as concern for modesty, is important in providing psychological support before, during, and after the procedure.

▶ There are no food, fluid, or medication restrictions unless by medical direction.

INTRATEST:

▶ If the patient has a history of allergic reaction to latex, avoid the use of equipment containing latex.

▶ Instruct the patient to cooperate fully and to follow directions. Direct the patient to breathe normally and to avoid unnecessary movement.

▶ Observe standard precautions, and follow the general guidelines in Appendix A. Positively identify the patient, and label the appropriate tubes with the corresponding patient demographics, date, and time of collection. Perform a venipuncture.

▶ Remove the needle and apply direct pressure with dry gauze to stop bleeding. Observe/assess venipuncture site for bleeding or hematoma formation and secure gauze with adhesive bandage.

▶ Promptly transport the specimen to the laboratory for processing and analysis.

POST-TEST:

▶ A report of the results will be sent to the requesting health-care provider (HCP), who will discuss the results with the patient.

▶ Reinforce information given by the patient's HCP regarding further testing, treatment, or referral to another HCP. Answer any questions or address any concerns voiced by the patient or family.

▶ Depending on the results of this procedure, additional testing may be performed to evaluate or monitor progression of the disease process and determine the need for a change in therapy. Evaluate test results in relation to the patient's symptoms and other tests performed.

RELATED MONOGRAPHS:

▶ Related tests include albumin, antibodies antithyroglobulin, biopsy thyroid, copper, PTH, prealbumin, protein, RAIU, thyroglobulin, TBII, thyroid scan, TSH, TSI, T_4, free T_4, T_3, and US thyroid.

▶ Refer to the Endocrine System table at the end of the book for related tests by body system.

Triiodothyronine, Total

SYNONYM/ACRONYM: T_3.

COMMON USE: To assist in evaluating thyroid function primarily related to diagnosing hyperthyroidism and monitoring the effectiveness of therapeutic interventions.

SPECIMEN: Serum (1 mL) collected in a red- or tiger-top tube. Plasma (1 mL) collected in a green-top (heparin) tube is also acceptable.

REFERENCE VALUE: (Method: Immunoassay)

Age	Conventional Units	SI Units (Conventional Units × 0.0154)
1–3 days	100–292 ng/dL	1.54–4.50 nmol/L
1–12 mo	105–245 ng/dL	1.62–3.77 nmol/L
1–5 yr	105–269 ng/dL	1.62–4.14 nmol/L
6–10 yr	94–241 ng/dL	1.45–3.71 nmol/L
16–20 yr	80–210 ng/dL	1.20–3.20 nmol/L
Adult	70–204 ng/dL	1.08–3.14 nmol/L
Older adult	40–181 ng/dL	0.62–2.79 nmol/L
Pregnant woman (last 4 mo gestation)	116–247 ng/dL	1.79–3.80 nmol/L

DESCRIPTION: Unlike the thyroid hormone thyroxine (T_4), most T_3 is converted enzymatically from T_4 in the tissues rather than being produced directly by the thyroid gland (see monograph titled "Thyroxine, Total"). Approximately one-third of T_4 is converted to T_3. Most T_3 in the serum (99.97%) is bound to thyroxine-binding globulin (TBG), prealbumin, and albumin. The remainder (0.03%) circulates as unbound or free T_3, which is the physiologically active form. Levels of free T_3 are proportional to levels of total T_3. The advantage of measuring free T_3 instead of total T_3 is that, unlike total T_3 measurements, free T_3 levels are not affected by fluctuations in TBG levels. T_3 is four to five times more biologically potent than T_4. This hormone, along with T_4, is responsible for maintaining a euthyroid state.

INDICATIONS

Adjunctive aid to thyroid-stimulating hormone (TSH) and free T_4 assessment.

POTENTIAL DIAGNOSIS

Increased in
- Conditions with increased TBG *(e.g., pregnancy and estrogen therapy)*
- Early thyroid failure
- Hyperthyroidism *(triiodothyronine is produced independently of stimulation by TSH)*
- Iodine-deficiency goiter
- T_3 toxicosis
- Thyrotoxicosis factitia *(laboratory tests do not distinguish between endogenous and exogenous sources)*
- Treated hyperthyroidism

Decreased in
- Acute and subacute nonthyroidal disease *(pathophysiology is unclear)*
- Conditions with decreased TBG *(TBG is the major transport protein)*
- Hypothyroidism *(thyroid hormones are not produced in sufficient quantities regardless of TSH levels)*
- Malnutrition *(related to insufficient protein sources to form albumin and TBG)*

T

CRITICAL FINDINGS: N/A

INTERFERING FACTORS

- Drugs that may increase total T_3 levels include amiodarone, amphetamine, benziodarone, clofibrate, fluorouracil, halofenate, insulin, levothyroxine, methadone, opiates, oral contraceptives, phenothiazine, phenytoin, prostaglandins, and T_3.
- Drugs that may decrease total T_3 levels include acetylsalicylic acid, amiodarone, anabolic steroids, asparaginase, carbamazepine, cholestyramine, clomiphene, colestipol, dexamethasone, fenclofenac, furosemide, glucocorticoids, hydrocortisone, interferon alfa-2b, iobenzamic acid, iopanoic acid, ipodate, isotretinoin, lithium, methimazole, netilmicin, oral contraceptives, penicillamine, phenylbutazone, phenytoin, potassium iodide, prednisone, propranolol, propylthiouracil, radiographic agents, sodium ipodate, salicylate, sulfonylureas, and tyropanoic acid.

NURSING IMPLICATIONS AND PROCEDURE

PRETEST:

- Positively identify the patient using at least two unique identifiers before providing care, treatment, or services.
- *Patient Teaching:* Inform the patient this test can assist in assessing thyroid gland function.
- Obtain a history of the patient's complaints, including a list of known allergens, especially allergies or sensitivities to latex.
- Obtain a history of the patient's endocrine system, symptoms, and results of previously performed laboratory tests and diagnostic and surgical procedures.
- Obtain a list of the patient's current medications, including herbs, nutritional supplements, and nutraceuticals (see Appendix F).

- Review the procedure with the patient. Inform the patient that specimen collection takes approximately 5 to 10 min. Address concerns about pain and explain that there may be some discomfort during the venipuncture.
- *Sensitivity to social and cultural issues,* as well as concern for modesty, is important in providing psychological support before, during, and after the procedure.
- There are no food, fluid, or medication restrictions unless by medical direction.

INTRATEST:

- If the patient has a history of allergic reaction to latex, avoid the use of equipment containing latex.
- Instruct the patient to cooperate fully and to follow directions. Direct the patient to breathe normally and to avoid unnecessary movement.
- Observe standard precautions, and follow the general guidelines in Appendix A. Positively identify the patient, and label the appropriate tubes with the corresponding patient demographics, date, and time of collection. Perform a venipuncture.
- Remove the needle and apply direct pressure with dry gauze to stop bleeding. Observe/assess venipuncture site for bleeding or hematoma formation and secure gauze with adhesive bandage.
- Promptly transport the specimen to the laboratory for processing and analysis.

POST-TEST:

- A report of the results will be sent to the requesting health-care provider (HCP), who will discuss the results with the patient.
- Reinforce information given by the patient's HCP regarding further testing, treatment, or referral to another HCP. Answer any questions or address any concerns voiced by the patient or family.
- Depending on the results of this procedure, additional testing may be performed to evaluate or monitor progression of the disease process and determine the need for a change in therapy. Evaluate test results in relation

to the patient's symptoms and other tests performed.

RELATED MONOGRAPHS:

▶ Related tests include albumin, antibodies antithyroglobulin, biopsy thyroid, copper,

PTH, prealbumin, protein, RAIU, thyroglobulin, TBII, thyroid scan, TSH, TSI, T_4, free T_4, free T_3, and US thyroid.
▶ Refer to the Endocrine System table at the end of the book for related tests by body system.

Troponins I and T

SYNONYM/ACRONYM: Cardiac troponin, cardiac troponin I (cTnI), cardiac troponin T (cTnT).

COMMON USE: To assist in evaluating myocardial muscle damage related to disorders such as myocardial infarction.

SPECIMEN: Serum (1 mL) collected in a red- or tiger-top tube. Plasma (1 mL) collected in a green-top (heparin) tube is also acceptable. Serial sampling is highly recommended. Care must be taken to use the same type of collection container if serial measurements are to be taken.

REFERENCE VALUE: (Method: Enzyme immunoassay)

Troponin I	Less than 0.35 ng/mL
Troponin T	Less than 0.20 mcg/L

DESCRIPTION: Troponin is a complex of three contractile proteins that regulate the interaction of actin and myosin. Troponin C is the calcium-binding subunit; it does not have a cardiac muscle–specific subunit. Troponin I and troponin T, however, do have cardiac muscle–specific subunits. They are detectable a few hours to 7 days after the

onset of symptoms of myocardial damage. Troponin I is thought to be a more specific marker of cardiac damage than troponin T. Cardiac troponin I begins to rise 2 to 6 hr after myocardial infarction (MI). It has a biphasic peak: It initially peaks at 15 to 24 hr after MI and then exhibits a lower peak after 60 to 80 hr. Cardiac troponin T levels rise 2 to 6 hr after MI and remain elevated. Both proteins return to the reference range 7 days after MI.

T

Timing for Appearance and Resolution of Serum/Plasma Cardiac Markers in Acute MI			
Cardiac Marker	Appearance (hr)	Peak (hr)	Resolution (days)
AST	6–8	24–48	3–4
CK (total)	4–6	24	2–3

Cardiac Marker	Appearance (hr)	Peak (hr)	Resolution (days)
CK-MB	4–6	15–20	2–3
LDH	12	24–48	10–14
Myoglobin	1–3	4–12	1
Troponin I	2–6	15–20	5–7

AST = aspartate aminotransferase; CK = creatine kinase; CK-MB = creatine kinase MB fraction; LDH = lactate dehydrogenase.

INDICATIONS

- Assist in establishing a diagnosis of MI
- Evaluate myocardial cell damage

POTENTIAL DIAGNOSIS

Increased in

Conditions that result in cardiac tissue damage; troponin is released from damaged tissue into the circulation.

- Acute MI
- Minor myocardial damage
- Myocardial damage after coronary artery bypass graft surgery or percutaneous transluminal coronary angioplasty
- Unstable angina pectoris

Decreased in: N/A

CRITICAL FINDINGS

- Troponin I: Greater than 0.5 ng/mL (initial sample only)

Note and immediately report to the health-care provider (HCP) increased results and related symptoms.

INTERFERING FACTORS: N/A

NURSING IMPLICATIONS AND PROCEDURE

PRETEST:

▸ Positively identify the patient using at least two unique identifiers before providing care, treatment, or services.

▸ *Patient Teaching:* Inform the patient this test can assist in evaluating heart damage.
▸ Obtain a history of the patient's complaints, including a list of known allergens, especially allergies or sensitivities to latex.
▸ Obtain a history of the patient's cardiovascular system, symptoms, and results of previously performed laboratory tests and diagnostic and surgical procedures.
▸ Obtain a list of the patient's current medications, including herbs, nutritional supplements, and nutraceuticals (see Appendix F).
▸ Review the procedure with the patient. Inform the patient that a number of samples will be collected. Collection at time of admission, 2 to 4 hr, 6 to 8 hr, and 12 hr after admission are the minimal recommendations. Additional samples may be requested. Inform the patient that specimen collection takes approximately 5 to 10 min. Address concerns about pain and explain that there may be some discomfort during the venipuncture.
▸ *Sensitivity to social and cultural issues,* as well as concern for modesty, is important in providing psychological support before, during, and after the procedure.
▸ There are no food, fluid, or medication restrictions unless by medical direction.

INTRATEST:

▸ If the patient has a history of allergic reaction to latex, avoid the use of equipment containing latex.
▸ Instruct the patient to cooperate fully and to follow directions. Direct the patient to breathe normally and to avoid unnecessary movement.

♦ Observe standard precautions, and follow the general guidelines in Appendix A. Positively identify the patient, and label the appropriate tubes with the corresponding patient demographics, date, and time of collection. Perform a venipuncture.

♦ Remove the needle and apply direct pressure with dry gauze to stop bleeding. Observe/assess venipuncture site for bleeding or hematoma formation and secure gauze with adhesive bandage.

♦ Promptly transport the specimen to the laboratory for processing and analysis.

POST-TEST:

♦ A report of the results will be sent to the requesting HCP, who will discuss the results with the patient.

♦ *Nutritional Considerations:* Increased troponin levels are associated with coronary artery disease (CAD). The American Heart Association and National Heart, Lung, and Blood Institute (NHBLI) recommend nutritional therapy for individuals identified to be at high risk for developing CAD or individuals who have specific risk factors and/or existing medical conditions (e.g., elevated LDL cholesterol levels, other lipid disorders, insulin-dependent diabetes, insulin resistance, or metabolic syndrome). If overweight, the patient should be encouraged to achieve a normal weight. The NHLBI's National Cholesterol Education Program (NCEP) revised its dietary guidelines for reducing CAD in 2001. Guidelines for the Therapeutic Lifestyle Changes (TLC) diet are outlined in the Third Report of the Expert Panel on Detection, Evaluation, and Treatment of High Blood Cholesterol in Adults (Adult Treatment Panel III [ATP III]). The TLC diet emphasizes a reduction in foods high in saturated fats and cholesterol. Red meats, eggs, and dairy products are the major sources of saturated fats and cholesterol. If triglycerides also are elevated, the patient should be advised to eliminate or reduce alcohol and simple carbohydrates from the diet. The TLC approach also includes the use of plant stanols or sterols and increased dissolved fiber as an option for lowering LDL cholesterol levels; nutritional recommendations for daily total caloric intake; recommendations for allowable percentage of calories derived from fat (saturated and unsaturated), carbohydrates, protein, and cholesterol; as well as recommendations for daily expenditure of energy.

♦ *Nutritional Considerations:* Overweight patients with high blood pressure should be encouraged to achieve a normal weight. Other changeable risk factors warranting patient education include strategies to safely decrease sodium intake, increase physical activity, decrease alcohol consumption, eliminate tobacco use, and decrease cholesterol levels.

♦ *Social and Cultural Considerations:* Numerous studies point to the prevalence of excess body weight in American children and adolescents. Experts estimate that obesity is present in 25% of the population ages 6 to 11 yr. The medical, social, and emotional consequences of excess body weight are significant. Special attention should be given to instructing the child and caregiver regarding health risks and weight-control education.

♦ Recognize anxiety related to test results, and be supportive of fear of shortened life expectancy. Discuss the implications of abnormal test results on the patient's lifestyle. Provide teaching and information regarding the clinical implications of the test results, as appropriate. Educate the patient regarding access to counseling services. Provide contact information, if desired, for the American Heart Association (www.americanheart.org) or the NHLBI (www.nhlbi.nih.gov).

♦ Reinforce information given by the patient's HCP regarding further testing, treatment, or referral to another HCP. Answer any questions or address any concerns voiced by the patient or family.

♦ Depending on the results of this procedure, additional testing may be performed to evaluate or monitor progression of the disease process and

T

determine the need for a change in therapy. Evaluate test results in relation to the patient's symptoms and other tests performed.

RELATED MONOGRAPHS:

▸ Related tests include antiarrhythmic drugs, apolipoprotein A and B, AST, ANP, blood pool imaging, BNP, calcium, ionized calcium, blood gases, cholesterol (total, HDL, and LDL), CRP, CT cardiac scoring, CK and isoenzymes, culture viral, echocardiography,

echocardiography transesophageal, ECG, exercise stress test, glucose, glycated hemoglobin, Holter monitor, homocysteine, ketones, LDH and isoenzymes, lipoprotein electrophoresis, magnesium, MRI chest, MI infarct scan, myocardial perfusion heart scan, myoglobin, pericardial fluid analysis, PET heart, potassium, and triglycerides.

▸ Refer to the Cardiovascular System table at the end of the book for related tests by body system.

Tuberculin Skin Tests

SYNONYM/ACRONYM: TB tine test, PPD, Mantoux skin test, QuantiFERON-TB Gold blood test (QFT-G).

COMMON USE: To evaluate for current or past tuberculin infection or exposure.

SPECIMEN: Whole blood (5 mL) collected in a green-top (LiHep or NaHep) tube.

REFERENCE VALUE: (Method: Intradermal skin test, enzyme-linked immunosorbent assay [ELISA] blood test) Negative.

DESCRIPTION: Tuberculin skin tests are done to determine past or present exposure to tuberculosis (TB). The multipuncture or tine test, a screening technique, uses either purified protein derivative (PPD) of tuberculin or old tuberculin. A positive response at the puncture site indicates cell-mediated immunity to the organism or a delayed hypersensitivity caused by interaction of the sensitized T lymphocytes. Verification of the patient's positive response to the multipuncture test is done with the more definitive Mantoux test using Aplisol or Tubersol

administered by intradermal injection. The Mantoux test is the test of choice in symptomatic patients. It is also used in some settings as a screening test. A negative result is judged if there is no sign of redness or induration at the site of the injection or if the zone of redness and induration is less than 5 mm in diameter. A positive result is evidenced by an area of erythema and induration at the injection site that is greater than 10 mm. A positive result does not distinguish between active and dormant infection. A positive response to

T

the Mantoux test is followed up with chest radiography and bacteriological sputum testing to confirm diagnosis. The QuantiFERON-TB Gold (QFT-G) blood test was approved by the U.S. Food and Drug Administration in 2005 for all applications in which the skin test is used. The blood test is a two-step procedure in which a sample of whole blood containing T lymphocytes from the patient is incubated with a reagent cocktail of peptides known to be present in individuals infected by *Myobacterium tuberculosis* but not found in the blood of previously vaccinated individuals or individuals who do not have the disease. The blood test offers the advantage of eliminating many of the false reactions encountered with skin testing, only a single patient visit is required, and results can be available within 24 hr.

INDICATIONS

• Evaluate cough, weight loss, fatigue, hemoptysis, and abnormal x-rays to determine if the cause of symptoms is TB
• Evaluate known or suspected exposure to TB, with or without symptoms, to determine if TB is present
• Evaluate patients with medical conditions placing them at risk for TB (e.g., AIDS, lymphoma, diabetes)
• Screen infants with the tine test at the time of first immunizations to determine TB exposure
• Screen populations at risk for developing TB (e.g., health-care providers [HCPs], nursing home residents, correctional facility personnel, prison inmates, and

residents of the inner city living in poor hygienic conditions)

POTENTIAL DIAGNOSIS

Positive findings in
• Pulmonary TB

CRITICAL FINDINGS

• Positive results

Note and immediately report to the HCP positive results and related symptoms.

INTERFERING FACTORS

Skin Test
• Drugs such as immunosuppressive agents or steroids can alter results.
• Diseases such as hematological cancers or sarcoidosis can alter results.
• Recent or present bacterial, fungal, or viral infections may affect results. False-positive results may be caused by the presence of nontuberculous mycobacteria or by serial testing.
• False-negative results can occur if sensitized T cells are temporarily decreased. False-negative results also can occur in the presence of bacterial infections, immunological deficiencies, immunosuppressive agents, live-virus vaccinations (e.g., measles, mumps, varicella, rubella), malnutrition, old age, overwhelming TB, renal failure, and active viral infections (e.g., chickenpox, measles, mumps).
• Improper storage of the tuberculin solution (e.g., with respect to temperature, exposure to light, and stability on opening) may affect the results.
• Improper technique when performing the intradermal injection (e.g., injecting into subcutaneous tissue) may cause false-negative results.
• Incorrect amount or dilution of antigen injected or delayed injection after drawing the antigen up

into the syringe may affect the results.

- Incorrect reading of the measurement of response or timing of the reading may interfere with results.
- ✷ It is not known whether the test has teratogenic effects or reproductive implications; the test should be administered to pregnant women only when clearly indicated.
- ✷ The test should not be administered to a patient with a previously positive tuberculin skin test because of the danger of severe reaction, including vesiculation, ulceration, and necrosis.
- The test does not distinguish between current and past infection.

Blood Test

- The QFT-G blood test has not been evaluated with patients who have impaired or altered immune function, have or are highly likely to develop TB, are younger than 17, are pregnant, or have diseases other than TB.

NURSING IMPLICATIONS AND PROCEDURE

PRETEST:

Blood and Skin Tests

- Positively identify the patient using at least two unique identifiers before providing care, treatment, or services.
- *Patient Teaching:* Inform the patient this test can assess for a tuberculin infection or exposure.
- Obtain a history of the patient's complaints, including a list of known allergens, especially allergies and sensitivities to latex.
- Obtain a history of the patient's immune and respiratory systems, symptoms, and results of previously performed laboratory tests and diagnostic and surgical procedures. Obtain a history of TB or TB exposure, signs and

symptoms indicating possible TB, and other skin tests or vaccinations and sensitivities.

- Obtain a list of the patient's current medications, including herbs, nutritional supplements, and nutraceuticals (see Appendix F).
- Review the procedure with the patient.

Skin Test

- Before beginning the test, ensure that the patient does not currently have TB and has not previously had a positive skin test. Do not administer the test if the patient has a skin rash or other eruptions at the test site. Inform the patient that the procedure takes approximately 5 min. Address concerns about pain and explain that a moderate amount of pain may be experienced when the intradermal injection is performed.
- Emphasize to the patient that the area should not be scratched or disturbed after the injection and before the reading.

Blood Test

- Inform the patient that specimen collection takes approximately 5 to 10 min. Address concerns about pain and explain that there may be some discomfort during the venipuncture.

Blood and Skin Tests

- *Sensitivity to social and cultural issues,* as well as concern for modesty, is important in providing psychological support before, during, and after the procedure.
- There are no food, fluid, or medication restrictions unless by medical direction.

INTRATEST:

Blood and Skin Tests

- If the patient has a history of allergic reaction to latex, avoid the use of equipment containing latex.
- Instruct the patient to cooperate fully and to follow directions. Direct the patient to breathe normally and to avoid unnecessary movement.
- Observe standard precautions, and follow the general guidelines in Appendix A. Positively identify the patient.

T

Skin Test

▶ Have epinephrine hydrochloride solution (1:1,000) available in the event of anaphylaxis.
▶ Cleanse the skin site on the lower anterior forearm with alcohol swabs and allow to air-dry.

Multipuncture Test

▶ Remove the cap covering the tines and stretch the forearm skin taut. Firmly press the device into the prepared site, hold it in place for 1 sec, and then remove it. Four punctures should be visible. Record the site, and remind the patient to return in 48 to 72 hr to have the test read. At the time of the reading, use a plastic ruler to measure the diameter of the largest indurated area, making sure the room is sufficiently lighted to perform the reading. A palpable induration greater than or equal to 2 mm at one or more of the punctures indicates a positive test result.

Mantoux (Intradermal) Test

▶ Prepare PPD or old tuberculin in a tuberculin syringe with a short, 26-gauge needle attached. Prepare the appropriate dilution and amount for the most commonly used intermediate strength (5 tuberculin units in 0.1 mL) or a first strength usually used for children (1 tuberculin unit in 0.1 mL). Inject the preparation intradermally at the prepared site as soon as it is drawn up into the syringe. When properly injected, a bleb or wheal 6 to 10 mm in diameter is formed within the layers of the skin. Record the site, and remind the patient to return in 48 to 72 hr to have the test read. At the time of the reading, use a plastic ruler to measure the diameter of the largest indurated area, making sure the room is sufficiently lighted to perform the reading. Palpate for thickening of the tissue; a positive result is indicated by a reaction of 5 mm or more with erythema and edema.

Blood Test

▶ Observe standard precautions, and follow the general guidelines in Appendix A. Positively identify the patient, and label the appropriate tubes with the corresponding patient demographics, date, and time of collection. Perform a venipuncture.
▶ Remove the needle and apply direct pressure with dry gauze to stop bleeding. Observe/assess venipuncture site for bleeding or hematoma formation and secure gauze with adhesive bandage.
▶ Promptly transport the specimen to the laboratory for processing and analysis.

POST-TEST:

▶ A report of the results will be sent to the requesting HCP, who will discuss the results with the patient.
▶ Recognize anxiety related to test results and be supportive of perceived loss of independence and fear of shortened life expectancy. Discuss the implications of abnormal test results on the patient's lifestyle. Provide teaching and information regarding the clinical implications of the test results, as appropriate. Counsel the patient, as appropriate, regarding the risk of transmission and proper prophylaxis, and reinforce the importance of strict adherence to the treatment regimen. Inform the patient that positive findings must be reported to local health department officials, who will question him or her regarding other persons who may have been exposed through contact. Educate the patient regarding access to counseling services.
▶ Reinforce information given by the patient's HCP regarding further testing, treatment, or referral to another HCP. Emphasize to the patient who receives skin testing of the need to return and have the test results read within the specified time frame of 48 to 72 hr after injection. Inform the patient that the effects from a positive response at the site can remain for 1 wk. Educate the patient that a positive result may put him or her at risk for infection related to impaired primary defenses, impaired gas exchange related to decrease in effective lung surface, and intolerance to activity related to an imbalance between oxygen supply and demand. Answer any questions or address any concerns voiced by the patient or family.

T

▶ Depending on the results of this procedure, additional testing may be performed to evaluate or monitor progression of the disease process and determine the need for a change in therapy. Evaluate test results in relation to the patient's symptoms and other tests performed.

RELATED MONOGRAPHS:

▶ Related tests include alveolar/arterial gradient, angiography pulmonary, biopsy lung, blood gases, bronchoscopy, calcium, carbon dioxide, chest x-ray, CBC WBC count and differential, CT thoracic, culture and smear mycobacteria, culture blood, culture sputum, cytology sputum, eosinophil count, ESR, gallium scan, Gram stain, lung perfusion scan, lung ventilation scan, mediastinoscopy, pleural fluid analysis, PFT, and zinc.

▶ Refer to the Immune and Respiratory systems tables at the end of the book for related tests by body system.

Tuning Fork Tests

SYNONYM/ACRONYM: Bing test, Rinne test, Schwabach test, Weber test.

COMMON USE: To assess for and determine type of hearing loss.

AREA OF APPLICATION: Ears.

CONTRAST: N/A.

DESCRIPTION: These noninvasive assessment procedures are done to distinguish conduction hearing loss from sensorineural hearing loss. They may be performed as part of the physical assessment examination and followed by hearing loss audiometry for confirmation of questionable results. The tuning fork tests described in this monograph are named for the four German otologists who described their use. Tuning fork tests are used less frequently by audiologists in favor of more sophisticated electronic methods, but presentation of the tuning fork test methodology is useful to illustrate the principles involved in electronic test methods.

A tuning fork is a bipronged metallic device that emits a clear tone at a particular pitch when it is set into vibration by holding the stem in the hand and striking one of the prongs or tines against a firm surface. The Bing test samples for conductive hearing loss by intermittently occluding and unblocking the opening of the ear canal while holding a vibrating tuning fork to the mastoid process behind the ear. The occlusion effect is absent in patients with conductive hearing loss and is present in patients with normal hearing or with sensorineural hearing loss. The Rinne test compares the patient's own hearing by bone conduction to his or her hearing by air conduction to determine whether hearing loss, if detected, is conductive or sensorineural. The Schwabach test compares the patient's level of bone conduction hearing to that of a presumed normal-hearing examiner. The Weber test has been modified by many audiologists for use with electronic equipment. When the test is administered, the patient is asked to tell the examiner the location of the tone heard (left ear, right ear, both ears, or midline) in order to determine whether the hearing loss is conductive, sensorineural, or mixed.

INDICATIONS

- Evaluate type of hearing loss (conductive or sensorineural)
- Screen for hearing loss as part of a routine physical examination and to determine the need for referral to an audiologist

POTENTIAL DIAGNOSIS

Normal findings in
- Normal air and bone conduction in both ears; no evidence of hearing loss
- Bing test: Pulsating sound that gets louder and softer when the opening to the ear canal is alternately opened and closed (*Note:* This result, observed in patients with normal hearing, is also observed in patients with sensorineural hearing loss.)
- Rinne test: Longer and louder tone heard by air conduction than by bone conduction (*Note:* This result, observed in patients with normal hearing, is also observed in

patients with sensorineural hearing loss.)
- Schwabach test: Same tone loudness heard equally long by the examiner and the patient
- Weber test: Same tone loudness heard equally in both ears

Abnormal findings in
- Conduction hearing loss related to or evidenced by:
  Impacted cerumen
  Obstruction of external ear canal *(presence of a foreign body)*
  Otitis externa *(infection in ear canal)*
  Otitis media *(poor eustachian tube function or infection)*
  Otitis media serus *(fluid in middle ear due to allergies or a cold)*
  Otosclerosis
  Bing test: No change in the loudness of the sound
  Rinne test: Tone louder or detected for a longer time than the air-conducted tone
  Schwabach test: Prolonged duration of tone when compared to that heard by the examiner
  Weber test: Lateralization of tone to one ear, indicating loss of hearing on that side (i.e., tone is heard in the poorer ear)
- Sensorineural hearing loss related to or evidenced by:
  Congenital damage or malformations of the inner ear
  Ménière's disease
  Ototoxic drugs *(aminoglycosides, e.g., gentamicin or tobramycin; salicylates, e.g., aspirin)*
  Presbyacusis *(gradual hearing loss experienced in advancing age)*
  Serious infections *(meningitis, measles, mumps, other viral, syphilis)*
  Trauma to the inner ear *(related to exposure to noise in excess of 90 dB or as a result of physical trauma)*
  Tumor *(e.g., acoustic neuroma, cerebellopontine angle tumor, meningioma)*
  Vascular disorders

Bing test: Pulsating sound that gets
louder and softer when the opening to
the ear canal is alternately opened
and closed

Rinne test: Tone heard louder by air
conduction

Schwabach test: Shortened duration of
tone when compared to that heard by
the examiner

Weber test: Lateralization of tone to one
ear indicating loss of hearing on the
other side (i.e., tone is heard in the
better ear)

CRITICAL FINDINGS: N/A

INTERFERING FACTORS

*Factors that may impair the
results of the examination*

• Poor technique in striking the
tuning fork or incorrect placement
can result in inaccurate results.

• Inability of the patient to understand how to identify responses or
unwillingness of the patient to
cooperate during the test can cause
inaccurate results.

• Hearing loss in the examiner can
affect results in those tests that
utilize hearing comparisons
between patient and examiner.

NURSING IMPLICATIONS AND PROCEDURE

PRETEST:

▶ Positively identify the patient using
at least two unique identifiers before
providing care, treatment, or services.

▶ *Patient Teaching:* Inform the patient this
procedure can assist in assessing for
hearing loss.

▶ Obtain a history of the patient's
complaints, including a list of known
allergens.

▶ Obtain a history of the patient's known
or suspected hearing loss, including
type and cause; ear conditions with
treatment regimens; ear surgery; and

other tests and procedures to assess
and diagnose auditory deficit.

▶ Obtain a history of the patient's
symptoms and results of previously
performed laboratory tests and diagnostic and surgical procedures.

▶ Obtain a list of the patient's current
medications, including herbs, nutritional
supplements, and nutraceuticals (see
Appendix F).

▶ Review the procedure with the patient.
Address concerns about pain and
explain that no discomfort will be experienced during the test. Inform the
patient that a health-care provider
(HCP) performs the test in a quiet,
darkened room, and that to evaluate
both ears, the test can take 5 to
10 min.

▶ Ensure that the external auditory canal
is clear of impacted cerumen.

▶ There are no food, fluid, or medication
restrictions unless by medical direction.

INTRATEST:

▶ Instruct the patient to cooperate fully
and to follow directions. Instruct the
patient to remain still throughout the
procedure because movement produces unreliable results.

▶ Seat the patient in a quiet environment
positioned such that the patient is
comfortable and is facing the examiner.
A tuning fork of 1,024 Hz is used
because it tests within the range of
human speech (400 to 5,000 Hz).

▶ *Bing test:* Tap the tuning fork handle
against the hand to start a light vibration. Hold the handle to the mastoid
process behind the ear while alternately
opening and closing the ear canal with
a finger. Ask the patient to report
whether he or she hears a change in
loudness or softness in sound. Record
the result as a positive Bing if the
patient reports a pulsating change in
sound. Record as a negative Bing if no
change in loudness is detected.

▶ *Rinne test:* Tap the tuning fork handle
against the hand to start a light vibration. Have the patient mask the ear not
being tested by moving a finger in and
out of the ear canal of that ear. Hold
the base of the vibrating tuning fork
with the thumb and forefinger of the

T

dominant hand and place it in contact with the patient's mastoid process (bone conduction). Ask the patient when the sound is no longer heard. Follow this with placement of the same vibrating tuning fork in front of the ear canal (air conduction) without touching the external part of the ear. Ask the patient which of the two has the loudest or longest tone. Repeat the test in the other ear. Record as Rinne positive if air conduction is heard longer and Rinne negative if bone conduction is heard longer.

- *Schwabach test:* Tap the tuning fork handle against the hand to start a light vibration. Hold the base of the tuning fork against one side of the patient's mastoid process and ask if the tone is heard. Have the patient mask the ear not being tested by moving a finger in and out of the ear canal of that ear. The examiner then places the tuning fork against the same side of his or her own mastoid process and listens for the tone. The tuning fork is alternated on the same side between the patient and examiner until the sound is no longer heard, noting whether the sound ceased to be heard by both the patient and the examiner at the same point in time. The procedure is repeated on the other ear. If the patient hears the tone for a longer or shorter time, count and note this in seconds.

- *Weber test:* Tap the tuning fork handle against the hand to start a light vibration. Hold the base of the vibrating tuning fork with the thumb and forefinger of the dominant hand and place it on the middle of the patient's forehead or at the vertex of the head. Ask the patient to determine if the sound is heard better and longer on one side than the other. Record as Weber right or left. If sound is heard equally, record as Weber negative.

POST-TEST:

- A report of the results will be sent to the requesting HCP, who will discuss the results with the patient.
- Recognize anxiety related to test results, and be supportive of impaired activity related to hearing loss and perceived loss of independence. Discuss the implications of abnormal test results on the patient's lifestyle. Provide teaching and information regarding the clinical implications of the test results, as appropriate. Educate the patient regarding access to counseling services. Provide contact information, if desired, for the American Speech-Language-Hearing Association (www.asha.org).
- Reinforce information given by the patient's HCP regarding further testing, treatment, or referral to another HCP. As appropriate, instruct the patient in the use, cleaning, and storing of a hearing aid. Answer any questions or address any concerns voiced by the patient or family.
- Depending on the results of this procedure, additional testing may be performed to evaluate or monitor progression of the disease process and determine the need for a change in therapy. Evaluate test results in relation to the patient's symptoms and other tests performed.

RELATED MONOGRAPHS:

- Related tests include antibiotic drugs, analgesic and antipyretic drugs, audiometry hearing loss, culture bacterial (ear), Gram stain, evoked brain potential studies for hearing loss, otoscopy, and spondee speech reception threshold.
- Refer to the Auditory System table at the end of the book for related tests by body system.

T

Ultrasound, Arterial Doppler, Carotid Studies

SYNONYM/ACRONYM: Carotid Doppler, carotid ultrasound, arterial ultrasound.

COMMON USE: To visualize and assess blood flow through the carotid arteries to assist in evaluating risk for stroke related to atherosclerosis.

AREA OF APPLICATION: Arteries.

CONTRAST: Done without contrast.

DESCRIPTION: Ultrasound (US) procedures are diagnostic, noninvasive, and relatively inexpensive. They take a short time to complete, do not use radiation, and cause no harm to the patient. Using the duplex scanning method, carotid US records sound waves to obtain information about the carotid arteries. The amplitude and waveform of the carotid pulse are measured, resulting in a two-dimensional image of the artery. Carotid arterial sites used for the studies include the common carotid, external carotid, and internal carotid. Blood flow direction, velocity, and the presence of flow disturbances can be readily assessed. The sound waves hit the moving red blood cells and are reflected back to the transducer, a flashlight-shaped device, pressed against the skin. The sound emitted by the equipment corresponds to the velocity of the blood flow through the vessel. The result is the visualization of the artery to assist in the diagnosis (i.e., presence, amount, location) of plaque causing vessel stenosis or atherosclerotic occlusion affecting the flow of blood to the brain. Depending on the degree of stenosis causing a reduction in vessel diameter, additional testing can be performed to determine the effect of stenosis on the hemodynamic status of the artery.

INDICATIONS

- Assist in the diagnosis of carotid artery occlusive disease, as evidenced by visualization of blood flow disruption
- Detect irregularities in the structure of the carotid arteries
- Detect plaque or stenosis of the carotid artery, as evidenced by turbulent blood flow or changes in Doppler signals indicating occlusion

POTENTIAL DIAGNOSIS

Normal findings in

- Normal blood flow through the carotid arteries with no evidence of occlusion or narrowing

Abnormal findings in

- Carotid artery occlusive disease (atherosclerosis)
- Plaque or stenosis of carotid artery
- Reduction in vessel diameter of more than 16%, indicating stenosis

CRITICAL FINDINGS: N/A

INTERFERING FACTORS

Factors that may impair clear imaging

- Attenuation of the sound waves by bony structures, which can impair clear imaging of the vessels.
- Incorrect placement of the transducer over the desired test site.
- Metallic objects (e.g., jewelry, body rings) within the examination field, which may inhibit organ visualization and cause unclear images.

U

• Inability of the patient to cooperate or remain still during the procedure because of age, significant pain, or mental status.

NURSING IMPLICATIONS AND PROCEDURE

PRETEST:

▶ Positively identify the patient using at least two unique identifiers before providing care, treatment, or services.

▶ *Patient Teaching:* Inform the patient this procedure can assist in assessing the carotid arteries in the neck.

▶ Obtain a history of the patient's complaints, including a list of known allergens, especially allergies or sensitivities to latex.

▶ Obtain a history of the patient's cardiovascular system, symptoms, and results of previously performed laboratory tests and diagnostic and surgical procedures.

▶ Note any recent procedures that can interfere with test results (i.e., barium or iodine-based contrast procedures, surgery, or biopsy). There should be 24 hr between administration of barium or iodine contrast medium and this test.

▶ Obtain a list of the patient's current medications, including anticoagulants, aspirin and other salicylates, herbs, nutritional supplements, and nutraceuticals (see Appendix F). Such products should be discontinued by medical direction for the appropriate number of days prior to a surgical procedure.

▶ Review the procedure with the patient. Address concerns about pain related to the procedure and explain that some pain may be experienced during the test, and there may be moments of discomfort. Inform the patient that the procedure is performed in a US department by a health-care provider (HCP) who specializes in this procedure, with support staff, and takes approximately 30 to 60 min.

▶ *Sensitivity to social and cultural issues,* as well as concern for modesty, is important in providing psychological support before, during, and after the procedure.

▶ Instruct the patient to remove jewelry and other metallic objects from the area to be examined.

▶ There are no food, fluid, or medication restrictions unless by medical direction.

INTRATEST:

▶ Ensure that the patient has removed all external metallic objects from the area to be examined prior to the procedure.

▶ Instruct the patient to void and change into the gown, robe, and foot coverings provided.

▶ Instruct the patient to cooperate fully and to follow directions. Ask the patient to remain still throughout the procedure because movement produces unreliable results.

▶ Observe standard precautions, and follow the general guidelines in Appendix A.

▶ Place the patient in the supine position on an examination table; other positions may be used during the examination.

▶ Expose the neck and drape the patient.

▶ Conductive gel is applied to the skin, and a Doppler transducer is moved over the skin to obtain images of the area of interest.

▶ Ask the patient to breathe normally during the examination. If necessary for better organ visualization, ask the patient to inhale deeply and hold his or her breath.

POST-TEST:

▶ A report of the results will be sent to the requesting HCP, who will discuss the results with the patient.

▶ When the study is completed, remove the gel from the skin.

▶ Instruct the patient to continue with diet, fluids, and medications, as directed by the HCP.

▶ *Nutritional Considerations:* Abnormal findings may be associated with cardiovascular disease. The American Heart Association and National Heart, Lung, and Blood Institute (NHBLI) recommend nutritional therapy for individuals identified to be at high risk for developing coronary artery disease (CAD) or individuals who have specific risk factors and/or existing medical conditions (e.g., elevated LDL cholesterol levels, other lipid disorders, insulin-dependent diabetes, insulin resistance, or metabolic syndrome). If overweight, the patient should be encouraged to achieve a normal weight. The NHLBI's National Cholesterol Education Program (NCEP) revised its dietary guidelines for reducing CAD in 2001. Guidelines for the Therapeutic Lifestyle Changes (TLC) diet are outlined in the Third Report of the Expert Panel on Detection, Evaluation, and Treatment of High Blood Cholesterol in Adults (Adult Treatment Panel III [ATP III]). The TLC diet emphasizes a reduction in foods high in saturated fats and cholesterol. Red meats, eggs, and dairy products are the major sources of saturated fats and cholesterol. If triglycerides also are elevated, the patient should be advised to eliminate or reduce alcohol and simple carbohydrates from the diet. The TLC approach also includes the use of plant stanols or sterols and increased dissolved fiber as an option for lowering LDL cholesterol levels; nutritional recommendations for daily total caloric intake; recommendations for allowable percentage of calories derived from fat (saturated and unsaturated), carbohydrates, protein, and cholesterol; as well as recommendations for daily expenditure of energy.

▶ *Nutritional Considerations:* Overweight patients with high blood pressure should be encouraged to achieve a normal weight. Other changeable risk factors warranting patient education include strategies to safely decrease sodium intake, increase physical activity, decrease alcohol consumption, eliminate tobacco use, and decrease cholesterol levels.

▶ *Social and Cultural Considerations:* Numerous studies point to the prevalence of excess body weight in American children and adolescents. Experts estimate that obesity is present in 25% of the population ages 6 to 11 yr. The medical, social, and emotional consequences of excess body weight are significant. Special attention should be given to instructing the child and caregiver regarding health risks and weight-control education.

▶ Recognize anxiety related to test results, and be supportive of fear of shortened life expectancy and perceived loss of independent function. Discuss the implications of abnormal test results on the patient's lifestyle. Provide teaching and information regarding the clinical implications of the test results, as appropriate. Educate the patient regarding access to counseling services. Provide contact information, if desired, for the American Heart Association (www.americanheart .org) or the NHLBI (www.nhlbi.nih.gov).

▶ Reinforce information given by the patient's HCP regarding further testing, treatment, or referral to another HCP. Answer any questions or address any concerns voiced by the patient or family.

▶ Instruct the patient in the use of any ordered medications. Explain the importance of adhering to the therapy regimen. As appropriate, instruct the patient in significant side effects and systemic reactions associated with the prescribed medication. Encourage him or her to review corresponding literature provided by a pharmacist.

▶ Depending on the results of this procedure, additional testing may be performed to evaluate or monitor progression of the disease process and determine the need for a change in therapy. Evaluate test results in relation to the patient's symptoms and other tests performed.

RELATED MONOGRAPHS:

▶ Related tests include angiography carotid, angiography coronary, antiarrhythmic drugs, apolipoprotein A & B, AST, blood gases, calcium, cholesterol (total, HDL, LDL), CT angiography, CT cardiac scoring, echocardiography, CRP, CK and isoenzymes, glucose, glycated hemoglobin, Holter monitor, homocysteine, ketones, LDH and isoenzymes, lipoprotein electrophoresis, magnesium, MRI angiography, MRI chest, myocardial infarction scan, myocardial perfusion heart scan, myoglobin, PET heart, triglycerides, and troponin.

▶ Refer to the Cardiovascular System table at the end of the book for related tests by body system.

Ultrasound, Arterial Doppler, Lower and Upper Extremity Studies

SYNONYM/ACRONYM: Doppler, arterial ultrasound, duplex scan.

COMMON USE: To visualize and assess blood flow through the arteries of the upper and lower extremities to assist in diagnosing disorders such as occlusion and aneurysm and evaluate for the presence of plaque and stenosis. This procedure can also be used to assess the effectiveness of therapeutic interventions such as arterial graphs and blood flow to transplanted organs.

AREA OF APPLICATION: Arteries of the lower and upper extremities.

CONTRAST: Done without contrast.

DESCRIPTION: Ultrasound (US) procedures are diagnostic, noninvasive, and relatively inexpensive. They take a short time to complete, do not use radiation, and cause no harm to the patient. Using the duplex scanning method, arterial leg US records sound waves to obtain information about the arteries of the lower extremities from the common femoral arteries and their branches as they extend into the calf area. The amplitude and waveform of the pulses are measured, resulting in a two-dimensional image of the artery. Blood flow direction, velocity, and the presence of flow disturbances can be readily assessed, and for diagnostic studies, the technique is done bilaterally. The sound waves hit the moving red blood cells and are reflected back to the transducer, a flashlight-shaped device, pressed against the skin. The sound that is emitted by the equipment corresponds to the velocity of the blood flow through the vessel. The result is the visualization of the artery to assist in the diagnosis (i.e., presence, amount, and location) of plaque causing vessel stenosis or occlusion and to help determine the cause of claudication. Arterial reconstruction and graft condition and patency can also be evaluated.

In arterial Doppler studies, arteriosclerotic disease of the peripheral vessels can be detected by slowly deflating blood pressure cuffs that are placed on an extremity such as the calf, ankle, or upper extremity. The systolic pressure of the various arteries of the extremities can be measured. The Doppler transducer can detect the first sign of blood flow through the cuffed artery, even the most minimal blood flow, as evidenced by a swishing noise. There is normally a reduction in systolic blood pressure from the arteries of the arms to the arteries of the legs; a reduction exceeding 20 mm Hg is indicative of occlusive disease (deep vein thrombosis) proximal to the area being tested. This procedure may also be used to monitor the patency of a graft, status of previous corrective

U

surgery, vascular status of the blood flow to a transplanted organ, blood flow to a mass, or the extent of vascular trauma.

INDICATIONS

- Aid in the diagnosis of small or large vessel arterial occlusive disease
- Aid in the diagnosis of spastic arterial disease, such as Raynaud's phenomenon
- Assist in the diagnosis of aneurysm, pseudoaneurysm, hematoma, arteriovenous malformation, or hemangioma
- Assist in the diagnosis of ischemia, arterial calcification, or plaques, as evidenced by visualization of blood flow disruption
- Detect irregularities in the structure of the arteries
- Detect plaque or stenosis of the lower extremity artery, as evidenced by turbulent blood flow or changes in Doppler signals indicating occlusion
- Determine the patency of a vascular graft, stent, or previous surgery
- Evaluate possible arterial trauma

POTENTIAL DIAGNOSIS

Normal findings in

- Normal blood flow through the lower extremity arteries with no evidence of vessel occlusion or narrowing
- Normal arterial systolic and diastolic Doppler signals
- Normal reduction in systolic blood pressure (i.e., less than 20 mm Hg) when compared to a normal extremity
- Normal ankle-to-brachial (AB) arterial blood pressure (ankle pressure divided by brachial pressure; normal AB pressure index is greater than 0.85)

Abnormal findings in

- AB pressure index less than 0.85, indicating significant arterial occlusive disease within the extremity
- Aneurysm
- Arterial calcification or plaques
- Embolic arterial occlusion
- Graft diameter reduction
- Hemangioma
- Hematoma
- Ischemia
- Large or small vessel occlusive disease
- Pseudoaneurysm
- Reduction in vessel diameter of more than 16%, indicating stenosis
- Spastic arterial occlusive disease, such as Raynaud's phenomenon

CRITICAL FINDINGS: N/A

INTERFERING FACTORS

This procedure is contraindicated for

- Patients with an open or draining lesion.

Factors that may impair the results of the examination

- Attenuation of the sound waves by bony structures, which can impair clear imaging of the vessels.
- Cold extremities, resulting in vasoconstriction, which can cause inaccurate measurements.
- Occlusion proximal to the site being studied, which would affect blood flow to the area.
- Cigarette smoking, because nicotine can cause constriction of the peripheral vessels.
- An abnormally large leg, making direct examination difficult.
- Incorrect placement of the transducer over the desired test site.
- Metallic objects (e.g., jewelry, body rings) within the examination field, which may inhibit organ visualization and cause unclear images.

• Inability of the patient to cooperate or remain still during the procedure because of age, significant pain, or mental status.

PRETEST:

▶ Positively identify the patient using at least two unique identifiers before providing care, treatment, or services.

▶ *Patient Teaching:* Inform the patient this procedure can assist in assessing blood flow to the upper and lower extremities.

▶ Obtain a history of the patient's complaints, including a list of known allergens, especially allergies or sensitivities to latex.

▶ Obtain a history of the patient's cardiovascular system, symptoms, and results of previously performed laboratory tests and diagnostic and surgical procedures.

▶ Report the presence of a lesion that is open or draining; maintain clean, dry dressing for the ulcer; protect the limb from trauma.

▶ Note any recent procedures that can interfere with test results (i.e., barium or iodine-based contrast procedures, surgery, or biopsy). There should be 24 hr between administration of barium or iodine contrast medium and this test.

▶ Obtain a list of the patient's current medications, including herbs, nutritional supplements, and nutraceuticals (see Appendix F).

▶ Review the procedure with the patient. Address concerns about pain related to the procedure and explain that some pain may be experienced during the test, and there may be moments of discomfort. Inform the patient that the procedure is performed in a US department by a health-care provider (HCP) specializing in this procedure, with support staff, and takes approximately 30 to 60 min.

▶ *Sensitivity to social and cultural issues,* as well as concern for modesty, is important in providing psychological support before, during, and after the procedure.

▶ Instruct the patient to remove jewelry and other metallic objects from the area to be examined.

▶ There are no food, fluid, or medication restrictions unless by medical direction.

INTRATEST:

▶ Ensure that the patient has removed all external metallic objects from the area to be examined prior to the procedure.

▶ Instruct the patient to void and change into the gown, robe, and foot coverings provided.

▶ Instruct the patient to cooperate fully and to follow directions. Ask the patient to remain still throughout the procedure because movement produces unreliable results.

▶ Observe standard precautions, and follow the general guidelines in Appendix A.

▶ Place the patient in the supine position on an examination table; other positions may be used during the examination.

▶ Expose the area of interest and drape the patient.

▶ Place blood pressure cuffs on the thigh, calf, and ankle.

▶ Apply conductive gel to the skin over the area distal to each of the cuffs to promote the passage of sound waves as a Doppler transducer is moved over the skin to obtain images of the area of interest.

▶ Inflate the thigh cuff to a level above the patient's systolic pressure found in the normal extremity.

▶ Place the Doppler transducer in the gel, distal to the inflated cuff, and slowly release the pressure in the cuff.

▶ When the swishing sound of blood flow is heard, record it at the highest point along the artery at which it is audible. The test is repeated at the calf and then the ankle.

POST-TEST:

▶ A report of the results will be sent to the requesting HCP, who will discuss the results with the patient.

▶ When the study is completed, remove the gel from the skin.

U

- Instruct the patient to continue diet, fluids, and medications, as directed by the HCP.
- *Nutritional Considerations:* A low-fat, low-cholesterol, and low-sodium diet should be consumed to reduce current disease processes and/or decrease risk of hypertension and coronary artery disease.
- Recognize anxiety related to test results, and be supportive of perceived loss of independent function. Discuss the implications of abnormal test results on the patient's lifestyle. Provide teaching and information regarding the clinical implications of the test results, as appropriate.
- Reinforce information given by the patient's HCP regarding further testing, treatment, or referral to another HCP. Answer any questions or address any concerns voiced by the patient or family.

- Depending on the results of this procedure, additional testing may be performed to evaluate or monitor progression of the disease process and determine the need for a change in therapy. Evaluate test results in relation to the patient's symptoms and other tests performed.

RELATED MONOGRAPHS:

- Related tests include alveolar/arterial ratio, angiography pulmonary, ANA, blood gases, CBC platelet count, CT angiography, D-Dimer, FDP, fibrinogen, lung perfusion scan, lung ventilation scan, MRI abdomen, MRI angiography, aPTT, plethysmography, PT/INR, US venous Doppler lower extremities, and venography lower extremity.
- Refer to the Cardiovascular System table at the end of the book for related tests by body system.

Ultrasound, A-scan

SYNONYM/ACRONYM: None.

COMMON USE: To assess for ocular tissue abnormality related to lens replacement in cataract surgery.

AREA OF APPLICATION: Eyes.

CONTRAST: N/A.

DESCRIPTION: Diagnostic techniques such as A-scan ultrasonography can be used to identify abnormal tissue. The A-scan employs a single-beam, linear sound wave to detect abnormalities by returning an echo when interference disrupts its straight path. When the sound wave is directed at lens vitreous, the normal homogeneous tissue does not return an echo; an opaque lens with a cataract will produce an echo. The returning waves produced by abnormal tissue are received by a microfilm that converts the sound energy into electrical impulses that are amplified and displayed on an oscilloscope as an ultrasonogram or echogram. The A-scan echo can be used to indicate the position of the cornea and retina. The A-scan is most commonly used to measure the axial length of the eye. This measurement is used to determine the power requirement for an intraocular lens used to replace the abnormal, opaque lens of the eye removed in cataract surgery. There are two different methods currently in use. The applanation method involves placement of an ultrasound (US) probe directly on the cornea. The immersion technique is more popular because it does not require direct contact and compression of the cornea. The immersion technique protects the cornea by placement of a fluid layer between the eye and the US probe. The accuracy of the immersion technique is thought to be greater than applanation because no corneal compression is caused by the immersion method. Therefore, the measured axial length achieved by immersion is closer to the true axial length of the cornea.

INDICATIONS

• Determination of power requirement for replacement intraocular lens in cataract surgery.

POTENTIAL DIAGNOSIS

Normal findings in
• Normal homogeneous ocular tissue

Abnormal findings in
• Cataract

CRITICAL FINDINGS: N/A

INTERFERING FACTORS

Factors that may impair the results of the examination
• Inability of the patient to cooperate and remain still during the

procedure may interfere with the test results.
• Rubbing or squeezing the eyes may affect results.
• Improper placement of the probe tip to the surface of the eye may produce inaccurate results.

NURSING IMPLICATIONS AND PROCEDURE

PRETEST:

▶ Positively identify the patient using at least two unique identifiers before providing care, treatment, or services.
▶ *Patient Teaching:* Inform the patient this procedure determines the strength of the lens that will be replaced during cataract surgery.
▶ Obtain a history of the patient's complaints, including a list of known allergens, especially topical anesthetic eyedrops.
▶ Obtain a history of the patient's known or suspected vision loss; changes in visual acuity, including type and cause; use of glasses or contact lenses; eye conditions with treatment regimens; eye surgery; and other tests and procedures to assess and diagnose visual deficit.
▶ Obtain a history of symptoms and results of previously performed laboratory tests and diagnostic and surgical procedures.
▶ Obtain a list of the patient's current medications, including herbs, nutritional supplements, and nutraceuticals (see Appendix F).
▶ Instruct the patient to remove contact lenses or glasses, as appropriate. Instruct the patient regarding the importance of keeping the eyes open for the test.
▶ Review the procedure with the patient. Explain that the patient will be requested to fixate the eyes during the procedure. Address concerns about pain and explain that no discomfort will be experienced during the test but that some discomfort may be experienced after the test when the numbness wears off from the anesthetic drops administered prior to the test. Inform

the patient that a health-care provider (HCP) performs the test in a quiet, darkened room and that evaluation of the eye upon which surgery is to be performed can take up 10 min.

▶ *Sensitivity to social and cultural issues,* as well as concern for modesty, is important in providing psychological support before, during, and after the procedure.

▶ There are no food, fluid, or medication restrictions unless by medical direction.

INTRATEST:

▶ Instruct the patient to cooperate fully and to follow directions. Ask the patient to remain still during the procedure because movement produces unreliable results.

▶ Seat the patient comfortably. Instruct the patient to look straight ahead, keeping the eyes open and unblinking.

▶ Instill topical anesthetic in each eye, as ordered, and provide time for it to work. Topical anesthetic drops are placed in the eye with the patient looking up and the solution directed at the six o'clock position of the sclera (white of the eye) near the limbus (gray, semi-transparent area of the eyeball where the cornea and sclera meet). Neither the dropper nor the bottle should touch the eyelashes.

▶ Ask the patient to place the chin in the chin rest and gently press the forehead against the support bar. When the US probe is properly positioned on the patient's surgical eye, a reading is automatically taken.

▶ Multiple measurements may be taken in order to ensure that a consistent and accurate reading has been achieved.

Variability between serial measurements is unavoidable using the applanation technique.

POST-TEST:

▶ A report of the results will be sent to the requesting HCP, who will discuss the results with the patient.

▶ Recognize anxiety related to test results, and be supportive of impaired activity related to vision loss, anticipated loss of driving privileges, or the possibility of requiring corrective lenses (self-image). Discuss the implications of test results on the patient's lifestyle. Reassure the patient regarding concerns related to the impending cataract surgery. Provide teaching and information regarding the clinical implications of the test results, as appropriate.

▶ Reinforce information given by the patient's HCP regarding further testing, treatment, or referral to another HCP. Answer any questions or address any concerns voiced by the patient or family.

▶ Depending on the results of this procedure, additional testing may be performed to evaluate or monitor progression of the disease process and determine the need for a change in therapy. Evaluate test results in relation to the patient's symptoms and other tests performed.

RELATED MONOGRAPHS:

▶ Related tests include refraction and slit-lamp biomicroscopy.

▶ Refer to the Ocular System table at the end of the book for related tests by body system.

Ultrasound, Biophysical Profile, Obstetric

SYNONYM/ACRONYM: BPP ultrasound, fetal age sonogram, gestational age sonogram, OB sonography, pregnancy ultrasound, pregnancy echo, pregnant uterus ultrasonography.

U

COMMON USE: To visualize and assess the fetus in utero to monitor fetal health related to growth, congenital abnormalities, distress, and demise. Also used to identify gender and multiple pregnancy and to obtain amniotic fluid for analysis.

AREA OF APPLICATION: Pelvis and abdominal region.

CONTRAST: Done without contrast.

DESCRIPTION: Ultrasound (US) procedures are diagnostic, noninvasive, and relatively inexpensive. They take a short time to complete, do not use radiation, and cause no harm to the patient. Obstetric US uses high-frequency waves of various intensities delivered by a transducer, a flashlight-shaped device, pressed against the skin or inserted into the vagina. The waves are bounced back, converted to electrical energy, amplified by the transducer, and displayed on a monitor to visualize the fetus and placenta. This procedure is done by a transabdominal or transvaginal approach, depending on when the procedure is performed (first trimester [transvaginal] vs. second trimester [transabdominal]). It is the safest method of examination to evaluate the uterus and determine fetal size, growth, and position; fetal structural abnormalities; ectopic pregnancy; placenta position and amount of amniotic fluid; and multiple gestation. Obstetric US is used to secure different types of information regarding the fetus, varying with the trimester during which the procedure is done. This procedure may also include a nonstress test (NST) in combination with Doppler monitoring of amniotic fluid volume, fetal heart, gross fetal movements, fetal muscle tone, and fetal respiratory movements to detect high-risk pregnancy. The procedure is indicated as a guide for amniocentesis, cordocentesis, fetoscopy, aspiration of multiple oocytes for in vitro fertilization, and other intrauterine interventional procedures. Because the pregnant uterus is filled with amniotic fluid, ultrasonography is an ideal method of evaluating the fetus and placenta; it is also the diagnostic examination of choice because no radiation is used and, in most cases, the accuracy is sufficient to make the diagnosis without any further imaging procedures.

The biophysical profile (BPP) considers five antepartum parameters measured to predict fetal wellness. The BPP is indicated in women with high-risk pregnancies to identify a fetus in distress or in jeopardy of demise. It includes fetal heart rate (FHR) measurement, fetal breathing movements, fetal body movements, fetal muscle tone, and amniotic fluid volume. Each of the five parameters is assigned a score of either 0 or 2, allowing a maximum or perfect score of 10. The NST is an external US monitoring of FHR performed either as part of the BPP or when one or more of the US procedures have abnormal results. The NST is interpreted as either reactive or nonreactive.

BPP Parameter	Normal: Score = 2	Abnormal: Score = 0
Fetal heart rate reactivity	Two or more movement-associated FHR accelerations of 15 or more beats/min above baseline, lasting 15 sec, in a 20-min interval	One or no movement-associated FHR accelerations of 15 or more beats/min above baseline in a 20-min interval
Fetal breathing movements	One or more breathing movements lasting 20–60 sec in a 30-min interval	Absent or no breathing movements lasting longer than 19 sec in a 30-min interval
Fetal body movements	Two or more discrete body or limb movements in a 30-min interval	Less than two discrete body or limb movements in a 30-min interval
Fetal muscle tone	One or more episodes of active limb extension and return to flexion (to include opening and closing of hand)	Absent movement, slow extension with partial return to flexion, partial opening of hand
Amniotic fluid volume	One or more pockets of fluid that are 2 cm or more in the vertical axis	No pockets of fluid or no pocket measuring at least 2 cm in the vertical axis

A contraction stress test (CST or oxytocin challenge test) may be requested in the event of an abnormal fetal heart rate in the BPP or NST. The CST is used to assess the fetus's ability to tolerate low oxygen levels as experienced during labor contractions. The CST includes external FHR monitoring by US and measurement of oxytocin (pitocin)-induced uterine contractions. Pressure changes during contractions are monitored on an external tocodynamometer. Results of the two tests are interpreted as negative or positive. A negative or normal finding is no late decelerations of FHR during three induced contractions over a 10-min period. A positive or abnormal finding is identified when frequent contractions of 90 sec or more occur and FHR decelerates beyond the time of the contractions. The amniotic fluid index (AFI) is another application of US used to estimate amniotic fluid volume. The abdomen is divided into four quadrants using the umbilicus to delineate upper and lower halves and linea nigra to delineate the left and right halves. The numbered score is determined by adding the sum in centimeters of fluid in pockets seen in each of the four quadrants. The score is interpreted in relation to gestational age. The median index is considered normal between 8 and 12 cm. Oligohydramnios (too little amniotic fluid) is associated with an index between 5 and 6 cm, and polyhydroamnios (too much amniotic luid) with an index between 18 and 22 cm.

INDICATIONS

- Detect blighted ovum (missed abortion), as evidenced by empty gestational sac
- Detect fetal death, as evidenced by absence of movement and fetal heart tones
- Detect fetal position before birth, such as breech or transverse presentations
- Detect tubal and other forms of ectopic pregnancy
- Determine and confirm pregnancy or multiple gestation by determining the number of gestational sacs in the first trimester
- Determine cause of bleeding, such as placenta previa or abruptio placentae
- Determine fetal effects of Rh incompatibility due to maternal sensitization
- Determine fetal gestational age by uterine size and measurements of crown-rump length, biparietal diameter, fetal extremities, head, and other parts of the anatomy at key phases of fetal development
- Determine fetal heart and body movements and detect high-risk pregnancy by monitoring fetal heart and respiratory movements in combination with Doppler US or real-time grayscale scanning
- Determine fetal structural anomalies, usually at the 20th week of gestation or later
- Determine the placental size, location, and site of implantation
- Differentiate a tumor (hydatidiform mole) from a normal pregnancy
- Guide the needle during amniocentesis and fetal transfusion

- Measure fetal gestational age and evaluate umbilical artery, uterine artery, and fetal aorta by Doppler examination to determine fetal intrauterine growth retardation
- Monitor placental growth and amniotic fluid volume

POTENTIAL DIAGNOSIS

Normal findings in

- Normal age, size, viability, position, and functional capacities of the fetus
- Normal placenta size, position, and structure; adequate volume of amniotic fluid
- BPP score of 8 to 10 is considered normal. Each of the fetal movements evaluated in the BPP is related to oxygen-dependent activities that originate from the central nervous system. Their presence is assumed to indicate normal brain function and absence of systemic hypoxia.

Abnormal findings in

- Abruptio placentae
- Adnexal torsion
- Cardiac abnormalities
- Ectopic pregnancy
- Fetal death
- Fetal hydrops
- Fetal malpresentation (breech, transverse)
- Hydrocephalus
- Intestinal atresia
- Myelomeningocele
- Multiple pregnancy
- Placenta previa
- Renal or skeletal defects
- BPP score between 4 and 6 is considered equivocal. Gestational age is important in determining intervals for retesting and/or a decision to deliver.

CRITICAL FINDINGS

- Abruptio placentae
- Adnexal torsion

- BPP score between 0 and 2 is abnormal and indicates the need for assessment and immediate delivery.
- Ectopic pregnancy
- Fetal death
- Placenta previa

It is essential that critical diagnoses be communicated immediately to the appropriate health-care provider (HCP). A listing of these diagnoses varies among facilities. Note and immediately report to the HCP abnormal results and related symptoms.

INTERFERING FACTORS

This procedure is contraindicated for
- Patients with latex allergy; use of the vaginal probe requires the probe to be covered with a condom-like sac, usually made from latex. Latex-free covers are available.

Factors that may impair clear imaging
- Incorrect placement of the transducer over the desired test site.
- Retained gas or barium from a previous radiological procedure.
- Dehydration, which can cause failure to demonstrate the boundaries between organs and tissue structures.
- Insufficiently full bladder, which fails to push the bowel from the pelvis and the uterus from the symphysis pubis, thereby prohibiting clear imaging of the pelvic organs in transabdominal imaging.
- Metallic objects (e.g., jewelry, body rings) within the examination field, which may inhibit organ visualization and cause unclear images.
- Improper adjustment of the US equipment to accommodate obese or thin patients, which can cause a poor-quality study.
- Patients who are very obese, who may exceed the weight limit for the equipment.

Factors that may result in incorrect values
- Absence of activity in a particular parameter of the BPP may be related to fetal sleep pattern; gestational age less than 33 wk or greater than 42 wk; maternal ingestion of glucose, nicotine, or alcohol; maternal administration of magnesium or medications; artificial or premature rupture of membranes; and/or labor.

Other considerations
- Inability of the patient to cooperate or remain still during the procedure because of significant pain or mental status may interfere with the test results.

NURSING IMPLICATIONS AND PROCEDURE

PRETEST:
- Positively identify the patient using at least two unique identifiers before providing care, treatment, or services.
- *Patient Teaching:* Inform the patient this procedure can assess abdomen and pelvic organ function.
- Obtain a history of the patient's complaints, including a list of known allergens, especially allergies or sensitivities to latex.
- Obtain a history of the patient's reproductive system, symptoms, and results of previously performed laboratory tests and diagnostic and surgical procedures.
- Note any recent procedures that can interfere with test results (i.e., barium procedures, surgery, or biopsy). There should be 24 hr between administration of barium and this test.
- Endoscopic retrograde cholangiopancreatography and colonoscopy, if ordered, should be scheduled after this procedure.
- Record the date of the last menstrual period. Obtain a history of menstrual dates, previous pregnancy, and treatment received for high-risk pregnancy.

- Obtain a list of the patient's current medications, including herbs, nutritional supplements, and nutraceuticals (see Appendix F).
- Review the procedure with the patient. Address concerns about pain related to the procedure and explain that some pain may be experienced during the test, and there may be moments of discomfort. Inform the patient the procedure is performed in a US department, usually by an HCP specializing in this procedure, and takes approximately 30 to 60 min.
- For the transvaginal approach, inform the patient that a sterile latex- or sheath-covered probe will be inserted into the vagina.
- *Sensitivity to social and cultural issues,* as well as concern for modesty, is important in providing psychological support before, during, and after the procedure.
- Instruct the patient receiving transabdominal US to drink five to six glasses of fluid 90 min before the procedure, and not to void, because the procedure requires a full bladder. Patients receiving transvaginal US only do not need to have a full bladder.
- Instruct the patient to remove jewelry and other metallic objects from the area to be examined prior to the procedure.
- There are no food or medication restrictions unless by medical direction. The test may be scheduled in relation to mealtime because fetal activity is highest 1 to 3 hr after the mother ingests a meal.

INTRATEST:

- Ensure that the patient has removed all external metallic objects from the area to be examined prior to the procedure.
- Ensure that the patient receiving transabdominal US drank five to six glasses of fluid and has not voided.
- Instruct the patient to change into the gown, robe, and foot coverings provided.
- Instruct the patient to cooperate fully and to follow directions. Ask the patient to remain still throughout the procedure because movement produces unreliable results.

- Observe standard precautions, and follow the general guidelines in Appendix A.
- Place the patient in the supine position on an examination table. The right- or left-side-up position may be used to allow gravity to reposition the liver, gas, and fluid to facilitate better organ visualization.
- Expose the abdominal area and drape the patient.
- *Transabdominal approach:* Conductive gel is applied to the skin, and a transducer is moved over the skin while the bladder is distended to obtain images of the area of interest.
- *Transvaginal approach:* A lubricated, covered probe is inserted into the vagina and moved to different levels to obtain images.
- Ask the patient to breathe normally during the examination. If necessary for better organ visualization, ask the patient to inhale deeply and hold her breath.

POST-TEST:

- A report of the results will be sent to the requesting HCP, who will discuss the results with the patient.
- Allow the patient to void, as needed.
- When the study is completed, remove the gel from the skin.
- Recognize anxiety related to test results. Discuss the implications of abnormal test results on the patient's lifestyle. Provide teaching and information regarding the clinical implications of the test results, as appropriate. Encourage the family to seek appropriate counseling if concerned with pregnancy termination and to seek genetic counseling if a chromosomal abnormality is determined. Decisions regarding elective abortion should take place in the presence of both parents. Provide a nonjudgmental, nonthreatening atmosphere for discussing the risks and difficulties of delivering and raising a developmentally challenged infant and for exploring other options (termination of pregnancy or adoption). It is also important to discuss problems the mother and father may experience (guilt, depression, anger) if fetal abnormalities are detected.

Reinforce information given by the patient's HCP regarding further testing, treatment, or referral to another HCP. Answer any questions or address any concerns voiced by the patient or family.

Depending on the results of this procedure, additional testing may be performed to evaluate or monitor progression of the disease process and determine the need for a change in therapy. Evaluate test results in relation to the patient's symptoms and other tests performed.

RELATED MONOGRAPHS:

Related tests include amniotic fluid analysis, biopsy chorionic villus, blood groups and antibodies, chromosome analysis, culture bacterial anal/genital, culture viral, fetal fibronectin, α_1-fetoprotein, hexosaminidase A and B, human chorionic gonadotropin, KUB, Kleihauer-Betke test, lecithin/sphingomyelin ratio, MRI abdomen, and prolactin.

Refer to the Reproductive System table at the end of the book for related tests by body system.

Ultrasound, Bladder

SYNONYM/ACRONYM: Bladder sonography.

COMMON USE: To visualize and assess the bladder to assist in diagnosing disorders such as retention, obstruction, distention, cancer, infection, bleeding, and inflammation.

AREA OF APPLICATION: Bladder.

CONTRAST: Done without contrast.

DESCRIPTION: Ultrasound (US) procedures are diagnostic, noninvasive, and relatively inexpensive. They take a short time to complete, do not use radiation, and cause no harm to the patient. Bladder US evaluates disorders of the bladder, such as masses or lesions. Bladder position, structure, and size are examined with the use of high-frequency waves of various intensities delivered by a transducer, a flashlight-shaped device, pressed against the skin. Methods for imaging include the transrectal, transurethral, and transvaginal approach. The waves are bounced back, converted to electrical energy, amplified by the transducer, and displayed on a monitor to evaluate the structure and position of the contents of the bladder. The examination is helpful for monitoring patient response to therapy for bladder disease. Bladder images can be included in ultrasonography of the kidneys, ureters, bladder, urethra, and gonads in diagnosing renal/neurological disorders. Bladder US may be the diagnostic examination of choice because no radiation is used and, in most cases, the accuracy is sufficient to make the diagnosis without any further imaging procedures.

U

INDICATIONS

• Assess residual urine after voiding to diagnose urinary tract obstruction causing overdistention
• Detect tumor of the bladder wall or pelvis, as evidenced by distorted position or changes in bladder contour
• Determine end-stage malignancy of the bladder caused by extension of a primary tumor of the ovary or other pelvic organ
• Evaluate the cause of urinary tract infection, urine retention, and flank pain
• Evaluate hematuria, urinary frequency, dysuria, and suprapubic pain
• Measure urinary bladder volume by transurethral or transvaginal approach

POTENTIAL DIAGNOSIS

Normal findings in

• Normal size, position, and contour of the bladder

Abnormal findings in

• Bladder diverticulum
• Cyst
• Cystitis
• Malignancy of the bladder
• Tumor
• Ureterocele
• Urinary tract obstruction

CRITICAL FINDINGS: N/A

INTERFERING FACTORS

This procedure is contraindicated for

• Patients with latex allergy; use of the vaginal probe requires the probe to be covered with a condom-like sac, usually made from latex. Latex-free covers are available.

Factors that may impair clear imaging

• Incorrect placement of the transducer over the desired test site.
• Retained gas or barium from a previous radiological procedure.
• Dehydration, which can cause failure to demonstrate the boundaries between organs and tissue structures.
• Insufficiently full bladder, which fails to push the bowel from the pelvis and the uterus from the symphysis pubis, thereby prohibiting clear imaging of the pelvic organs in transabdominal imaging.
• Metallic objects (e.g., jewelry, body rings) within the examination field, which may inhibit organ visualization and cause unclear images.

Other considerations

• Failure to follow pretesting preparations may cause the procedure to be canceled or repeated.
• Inability of the patient to cooperate or remain still during the procedure because of age, significant pain, or mental status, may interfere with the test results.

NURSING IMPLICATIONS AND PROCEDURE

PRETEST:

▶ Positively identify the patient using at least two unique identifiers before providing care, treatment, or services.
▶ *Patient Teaching:* Inform the patient this procedure can assist in assessing the bladder and pelvic organs.
▶ Obtain a history of the patient's complaints, including a list of known allergens, especially allergies or sensitivities to latex.
▶ Obtain a history of the patient's genitourinary system, symptoms, and results of previously performed laboratory tests and diagnostic and surgical procedures.
▶ Note any recent procedures that can interfere with test results (i.e., barium procedures, surgery, or biopsy). There should be 24 hr between administration of barium and this test.
▶ Endoscopic retrograde cholangiopancreatography, colonoscopy, and computed tomography of the abdomen, if ordered, should be scheduled after this procedure.
▶ Record the date of the last menstrual period and determine the possibility

U

of pregnancy in perimenopausal women.

▸ Obtain a list of the patient's current medications, including herbs, nutritional supplements, and nutraceuticals (see Appendix F).

▸ Review the procedure with the patient. Address concerns about pain related to the procedure. Explain to the patient that some pain may be experienced during the test, and there may be moments of discomfort. Inform the patient that the procedure is performed in a US department by a health-care provider (HCP), with support staff, and takes approximately 30 to 60 min.

▸ *Sensitivity to social and cultural issues,* as well as concern for modesty, is important in providing psychological support before, during, and after the procedure.

▸ Inform the patient for the transvaginal approach, that a sterile latex- or sheath-covered probe will be inserted into the vagina.

▸ Instruct the patient receiving transabdominal US to drink five to six glasses of fluid 90 min before the procedure, and not to void, because the procedure requires a full bladder. Patients receiving transvaginal US only do not need to have a full bladder.

▸ Instruct the patient to remove jewelry and other metallic objects from the area to be examined.

▸ There are no food, fluid, or medication restrictions unless by medical direction.

INTRATEST:

▸ Ensure that the patient has removed all external metallic objects from the area to be examined prior to the procedure.

▸ Ensure that the patient receiving transabdominal US drank five to six glasses of fluid and has not voided.

▸ Instruct the patient to change into the gown, robe, and foot coverings provided.

▸ Instruct the patient to cooperate fully and to follow directions. Instruct the patient to remain still throughout the procedure because movement produces unreliable results.

▸ Observe standard precautions, and follow the general guidelines in Appendix A.

▸ Place the patient in the supine position on an examination table. The right- or left-side-up positions may be used to allow

gravity to reposition the liver, gas, and fluid to facilitate better organ visualization.

▸ Expose the abdominal area and drape the patient.

▸ *Transabdominal approach:* Conductive gel is applied to the skin, and a transducer is moved over the skin while the bladder is distended to obtain images of the area of interest.

▸ *Transvaginal approach:* A covered and lubricated probe is inserted into the vagina and moved to different levels during scanning.

▸ Ask the patient to breathe normally during the examination. If necessary for better organ visualization, ask the patient to inhale deeply and hold his or her breath.

▸ If the patient is to be examined for residual urine volume, ask the patient to empty the bladder; repeat the procedure and calculate the volume.

POST-TEST:

▸ A report of the results will be sent to the requesting HCP, who will discuss the results with the patient.

▸ Allow the patient to void, as needed.

▸ When the study is completed, remove the gel from the skin.

▸ Recognize anxiety related to test results. Discuss the implications of abnormal test results on the patient's lifestyle. Provide teaching and information regarding the clinical implications of the test results, as appropriate.

▸ Reinforce information given by the patient's HCP regarding further testing, treatment, or referral to another HCP. Answer any questions or address any concerns voiced by the patient or family.

▸ Depending on the results of this procedure, additional testing may be performed to evaluate or monitor progression of the disease process and determine the need for a change in therapy. Evaluate test results in relation to the patient's symptoms and other tests performed.

RELATED MONOGRAPHS:

▸ Related tests include bladder cancer markers urine, CT pelvis, cystoscopy, IVP, KUB study, and MRI pelvis.

▸ Refer to the Genitourinary System table in the end of the book for related tests by body system.

U

Ultrasound, Breast

SYNONYM/ACRONYM: Mammographic ultrasound.

COMMON USE: Used in place of or in conjunction with mammography to assist in diagnosing disorders such as tumor, cancer, and cysts.

AREA OF APPLICATION: Breast.

CONTRAST: Done without contrast.

DESCRIPTION: Ultrasound (US) procedures are diagnostic, noninvasive, and relatively inexpensive. They take a short time to complete, do not use radiation, and cause no harm to the patient. When used in conjunction with mammography and clinical examination, breast US is indispensable in the diagnosis and management of benign and malignant process. Both breasts are usually examined during this procedure. The examination uses high-frequency waves of various intensities delivered by a transducer, a flashlight-shaped device, pressed against the skin. The waves are bounced back, converted to electrical energy, amplified by the transducer, and displayed on a monitor to determine the presence of palpable and nonpalpable masses and their size and structure. This procedure is useful in patients with an abnormal mass on a mammogram because it can determine whether the abnormality is cystic or solid; that is, it can differentiate between a palpable, fluid-filled cyst and a palpable, solid breast lesion (benign or malignant). It is especially useful in patients with dense breast tissue and in those with silicone prostheses, because the US beam easily penetrates in these situations, allowing routine examination that cannot be performed with x-ray mammography. The procedure can be done as an adjunct to mammography, or it can be done in place of mammography in patients who refuse x-ray exposure or those in whom it is contraindicated (e.g., pregnant women, women less than 25 yr). The procedure is indicated as a guide for biopsy and other interventional procedures and as a means of monitoring disease progression or the effects of treatment.

INDICATIONS
- Detect very small tumors in combination with mammography for diagnostic validation
- Determine the presence of nonpalpable abnormalities viewed on mammography of dense breast tissue and monitor changes in these abnormalities
- Differentiate among types of breast masses (e.g., cyst, solid tumor, other lesions) in dense breast tissue
- Evaluate palpable masses in young (less than age 25), pregnant, and lactating patients

U

- Guide interventional procedures such as cyst aspiration, large-needle core biopsy, fine-needle aspiration biopsy, abscess drainage, presurgical localization, and galactography
- Identify an abscess in a patient with mastitis

POTENTIAL DIAGNOSIS

Normal findings in
- Normal subcutaneous, mammary, and retromammary layers of tissue in both breasts; no evidence of pathological lesions (cyst or tumor) in either breast

Abnormal findings in
- Abscess
- Breast solid tumor, lesions
- Cancer (ductal carcinoma, infiltrating lobular carcinoma, medullary carcinoma, tubular carcinoma, and papillary carcinoma)
- Cystic breast disease
- Fibroadenoma
- Focal fibrosis
- Galactocele
- Hamartoma (fibroadenolipoma)
- Hematoma
- Papilloma
- Phyllodes tumor
- Radial scar

CRITICAL FINDINGS: N/A

INTERFERING FACTORS

Factors that may impair clear imaging:
- Incorrect placement of the transducer over the desired test site.
- Metallic objects (e.g., jewelry, body rings) within the examination field, which may inhibit organ visualization and cause unclear images.
- Excessively large breasts.
- Inability of the patient to cooperate or remain still during the procedure because of age, significant pain, or mental status.

NURSING IMPLICATIONS AND PROCEDURE

PRETEST:

▶ Positively identify the patient using at least two unique identifiers before providing care, treatment, or services.

▶ *Patient Teaching:* Inform the patient this procedure can assist in assessing the breast.

▶ Obtain a history of the patient's complaints, including a list of known allergens, especially allergies or sensitivities to latex.

▶ Obtain a history of the patient's reproductive system, symptoms, and results of previously performed laboratory tests and diagnostic and surgical procedures.

▶ Obtain a list of the patient's current medications, including herbs, nutritional supplements, and nutraceuticals (see Appendix F).

▶ Review the procedure with the patient. Address concerns about pain related to the procedure and explain that some pain may be experienced during the test, and there may be moments of discomfort. Inform the patient that the procedure is performed in a US department by a health-care provider (HCP) who specializes in this procedure, with support staff, and takes approximately 30 to 60 min.

▶ *Sensitivity to social and cultural issues,* as well as concern for modesty, is important in providing psychological support before, during, and after the procedure.

▶ Instruct the patient not to apply lotions, bath powder, or other substances to the chest and breast area before the examination.

▶ Instruct the patient to remove jewelry and other metallic objects from the area to be examined.

▶ There are no food, fluid, or medication restrictions unless by medical direction.

INTRATEST:

▶ Ensure that the patient has not applied lotions, bath powder, or other substances to the chest and breast area before the examination.

▶ Ensure that the patient has removed all external metallic objects from the area to be examined prior to the procedure.

U

- Instruct the patient to change into the gown and robe provided.
- Instruct the patient to cooperate fully and to follow directions. Instruct the patient to remain still throughout the procedure because movement produces unreliable results.
- Observe standard precautions, and follow the general guidelines in Appendix A.
- Place the patient in the supine position on an examination table. The right- and left-side-up positions are also used during the scan to facilitate better organ visualization.
- Expose the breast area and drape the patient.
- Conductive gel is applied to the skin and a transducer is moved over the skin to obtain images of the area of interest.
- Ask the patient to breathe normally during the examination. If necessary for better organ visualization, ask the patient to inhale deeply and hold her breath.

POST-TEST:

- A report of the results will be sent to the requesting HCP, who will discuss the results with the patient.
- When the study is completed, remove the gel from the skin.
- Recognize anxiety related to test results. Discuss the implications of abnormal test results on the patient's lifestyle. Provide teaching and information regarding the clinical implications of the test results, as appropriate. Educate the patient regarding access to counseling services. Provide contact information, if desired, for the American Cancer Society (www.cancer.org).
- Reinforce information given by the patient's HCP regarding further testing, treatment, or referral to another HCP. Decisions regarding the need for and frequency of breast self-examination, mammography, MRI breast, or other cancer screening procedures should be made after consultation between the patient and HCP. The most current guidelines for breast cancer screening of the general population as well as of individuals with increased risk are available from the American Cancer Society (www.cancer.org), the American College of Obstetricians and Gynecologists (ACOG) (www.acog.org), and the American College of Radiology (www.acr.org). Answer any questions or address any concerns voiced by the patient or family.
- Depending on the results of this procedure, additional testing may be performed to evaluate or monitor progression of the disease process and determine the need for a change in therapy. Evaluate test results in relation to the patient's symptoms and other tests performed.

RELATED MONOGRAPHS:

- Related tests include biopsy breast, cancer antigens, chest x-ray, CT thorax, ductograpy, mammogram, MRI breast, and stereotactic biopsy breast.
- Refer to the Reproductive System table at the end of the book for related tests by body system.

Ultrasound, Kidney

SYNONYM/ACRONYM: Renal ultrasound, renal sonography.

COMMON USE: To visualize and assess the kidneys to perform biopsies and assist in diagnosing disorders such as tumor, cancer, stones, and congenital anomalies. This procedure can also be used to evaluate therapeutic interventions such as transplants.

AREA OF APPLICATION: Kidney.

CONTRAST: Done without contrast.

DESCRIPTION: Ultrasound (US) procedures are diagnostic, noninvasive, and relatively inexpensive. They take a short time to complete, do not use radiation, and cause no harm to the patient. Renal US is used to evaluate renal system disorders. It is valuable for determining the internal components of renal masses (solid vs. cystic) and for evaluating other renal diseases, renal parenchyma, perirenal tissues, and obstruction. US uses high-frequency waves of various intensities delivered by a transducer, a flashlight-shaped device, pressed against the skin. The waves are bounced back, converted to electrical energy, amplified by the transducer, and displayed on a monitor to evaluate the structure, size, and position of the kidney. Renal US can be performed on the same day as a radionuclide scan or other radiological procedure and is especially valuable in patients who are in renal failure, have hypersensitivity to contrast medium, have a kidney that did not visualize on intravenous pyelography (IVP), or are pregnant. It does not rely on renal function or the injection of contrast medium to obtain a diagnosis. The procedure is indicated for evaluation after a kidney transplant and is used as a guide for biopsy and other interventional procedures, abscess drainage, and nephrostomy tube placement. Renal US may be the diagnostic examination of choice because no radiation is used and, in most cases, the accuracy is sufficient to make the diagnosis without any further imaging procedures.

INDICATIONS

- Aid in the diagnosis of the effect of chronic glomerulonephritis and end-stage chronic renal failure on the kidneys (e.g., decrease in size)
- Detect an accumulation of fluid in the kidney caused by backflow of urine, hemorrhage, or perirenal fluid
- Detect masses and differentiate between cysts or solid tumors, as evidenced by specific waveform patterns or absence of sound waves
- Determine the presence and location of renal or ureteral calculi and obstruction
- Determine the size, shape, and position of a nonfunctioning kidney to identify the cause
- Evaluate or plan therapy for renal tumors
- Evaluate renal transplantation for changes in kidney size
- Locate the site of and guide percutaneous renal biopsy, aspiration needle insertion, or nephrostomy tube insertion
- Monitor kidney development in children when renal disease has been diagnosed
- Provide the location and size of renal masses in patients who are unable to undergo IVP because of poor renal function or an allergy to iodinated contrast medium

POTENTIAL DIAGNOSIS

Normal findings in
- Absence of calculi, cysts, hydronephrosis, obstruction, or tumor

- Normal size, position, and shape of the kidneys and associated structures

Abnormal findings in
- Acute glomerulonephritis
- Acute pyelonephritis
- Congenital anomalies, such as absent, horseshoe, ectopic, or duplicated kidney
- Hydronephrosis
- Obstruction of ureters
- Perirenal abscess or hematoma
- Polycystic kidney
- Rejection of renal transplant
- Renal calculi
- Renal cysts, hypertrophy, or tumors
- Ureteral obstruction

CRITICAL FINDINGS: N/A

INTERFERING FACTORS

Factors that may impair clear imaging
- Attenuation of the sound waves by the ribs, which can impair clear imaging of the kidney.
- Incorrect placement of the transducer over the desired test site.
- Retained gas or barium from a previous radiological procedure.
- Metallic objects (e.g., jewelry, body rings) within the examination field, which may inhibit organ visualization and cause unclear images.

Other considerations
- Inability of the patient to cooperate or remain still during the procedure because of age, significant pain, or mental status may interfere with the test results.

NURSING IMPLICATIONS AND PROCEDURE

PRETEST:
- Positively identify the patient using at least two unique identifiers before providing care, treatment, or services.

- *Patient Teaching:* Inform the patient this procedure can assist in assessing kidney function.
- Obtain a history of the patient's complaints, including a list of known allergens, especially allergies or sensitivities to latex.
- Obtain a history of the patient's genitourinary system, symptoms, and results of previously performed laboratory tests and diagnostic and surgical procedures.
- Note any recent procedures that can interfere with test results (i.e., barium procedures, surgery, or biopsy). There should be 24 hr between administration of barium and this test.
- Endoscopic retrograde cholangiopancreatography, colonoscopy, and computed tomography of the abdomen, if ordered, should be scheduled after this procedure.
- Record the date of the last menstrual period and determine the possibility of pregnancy in perimenopausal women.
- Obtain a list of the patient's current medications, including herbs, nutritional supplements, and nutraceuticals (see Appendix F).
- Review the procedure with the patient. Address concerns about pain related to the procedure. Explain to the patient that some pain may be experienced during the test, and there may be moments of discomfort. Inform the patient that the procedure is performed in a US department, usually by a health-care provider (HCP), with support staff, and takes approximately 30 to 60 min.
- *Sensitivity to social and cultural issues,* as well as concern for modesty, is important in providing psychological support before, during, and after the procedure.
- Instruct the patient to remove jewelry and other metallic objects from the area to be examined.
- There are no food, fluid, or medication restrictions unless by medical direction.

INTRATEST:
- Ensure that the patient has removed all external metallic objects from the area to be examined prior to the procedure.

U

- Instruct the patient to void and change into the gown, robe, and foot coverings provided.
- Instruct the patient to cooperate fully and to follow directions. Instruct the patient to remain still throughout the procedure because movement produces unreliable results.
- Observe standard precautions, and follow the general guidelines in Appendix A.
- Place the patient in the supine position on an examination table. The right- or left-side-up positions may be used to allow gravity to reposition the liver, gas, and fluid to facilitate better organ visualization.
- Expose the abdominal and kidney area and drape the patient.
- Conductive gel is applied to the skin, and a transducer is moved over the skin to obtain images of the area of interest.
- Ask the patient to breathe normally during the examination. If necessary for better organ visualization, ask the patient to inhale deeply and hold his or her breath.

POST-TEST:

- A report of the results will be sent to the requesting HCP, who will discuss the results with the patient.
- When the study is completed, remove the gel from the skin.

- Recognize anxiety related to test results. Discuss the implications of abnormal test results on the patient's lifestyle. Provide teaching and information regarding the clinical implications of the test results, as appropriate.
- Reinforce information given by the patient's HCP regarding further testing, treatment, or referral to another HCP. Answer any questions or address any concerns voiced by the patient or family.
- Depending on the results of this procedure, additional testing may be performed to evaluate or monitor progression of the disease process and determine the need for a change in therapy. Evaluate test results in relation to the patient's symptoms and other tests performed.

RELATED MONOGRAPHS:

- Related tests include angiography renal, anti-glomerular basement membrane antibody, biopsy kidney, BUN, calculus kidney stone panel, CT abdomen, creatinine, creatinine clearance, cytology urine, erythropoeitin, group A streptococcal screen, IVP, KUB study, MRI abdomen, renogram, retrograde ureteropyelography, and UA.
- Refer to the Genitourinary System table at the end of the book for related tests by system.

Ultrasound, Liver and Biliary System

SYNONYM/ACRONYM: Gallbladder ultrasound, liver ultrasound, hepatobiliary sonography.

COMMON USE: To visualize and assess liver and gallbladder structure and function, assist in obtaining a biopsy, and diagnose disorders such as gallstones, cancer, tumors, cysts, and bleeding. Also used to evaluate the effectiveness of therapeutic interventions.

AREA OF APPLICATION: Liver, gallbladder, bile ducts.

CONTRAST: Done without contrast.

DESCRIPTION: Ultrasound (US) procedures are diagnostic, noninvasive, and relatively inexpensive. They take a short time to complete, do not use radiation, and cause no harm to the patient. Hepatobiliary US uses high-frequency waves of various intensities delivered by a transducer, a flashlight-shaped device, pressed against the skin. The waves are bounced back, converted to electrical energy, amplified by the transducer, and displayed on a monitor to evaluate the structure, size, and position of the liver and gallbladder in the right upper quadrant (RUQ) of the abdomen. The gallbladder and biliary system collect, store, concentrate, and transport bile to the intestines to aid in digestion. This procedure allows visualization of the gallbladder and bile ducts when the patient may have impaired liver function, and it is especially helpful when done on patients in whom gallstones cannot be visualized with oral or IV radiological studies. Liver US can be done in combination with a nuclear scan to obtain information about liver function and density differences in the liver. The procedure is indicated as a guide for biopsy and other interventional procedures. Hepatobiliary US may be the diagnostic examination of choice because no radiation is used and, in most cases, the accuracy is sufficient to make the diagnosis without any further imaging procedures.

INDICATIONS

- Detect cysts, polyps, hematoma, abscesses, hemangioma, adenoma, metastatic disease, hepatitis, or solid tumor of the liver or gallbladder, as evidenced by echoes specific to tissue density and sharply or poorly defined masses
- Detect gallstones or inflammation when oral cholecystography is inconclusive
- Detect hepatic lesions, as evidenced by density differences and echo-pattern changes
- Determine the cause of unexplained hepatomegaly and abnormal liver function tests
- Determine cause of unexplained RUQ pain
- Determine patency and diameter of the hepatic duct for dilation or obstruction
- Differentiate between obstructive and nonobstructive jaundice by determining the cause
- Evaluate response to therapy for tumor, as evidenced by a decrease in size of the organ
- Guide biopsy or tube placement
- Guide catheter placement into the gallbladder for stone dissolution and gallbladder fragmentation

POTENTIAL DIAGNOSIS

Normal findings in
- Normal size, position, and shape of the liver and gallbladder as well as patency of the cystic and common bile ducts

Abnormal findings in
- Biliary or hepatic duct obstruction/dilation
- Cirrhosis
- Gallbladder inflammation, stones, carcinoma, polyps
- Hematoma or trauma
- Hepatic tumors, metastasis, cysts, hemangioma, hepatitis
- Hepatocellular disease, adenoma
- Hepatomegaly
- Intrahepatic abscess
- Subphrenic abscesses

U

CRITICAL FINDINGS: N/A

INTERFERING FACTORS

Factors that may impair clear imaging

• Attenuation of the sound waves by the ribs, which can impair clear imaging of the right lobe of the liver.

• Incorrect placement of the transducer over the desired test site.

• Gas or feces in the gastrointestinal tract resulting from inadequate cleansing or failure to restrict food intake before the study.

• Retained barium from a previous radiological procedure.

• Metallic objects (e.g., jewelry, body rings) within the examination field, which may inhibit organ visualization and can produce unclear images.

• Inability of the patient to cooperate or remain still during the procedure because of age, significant pain, or mental status.

Other considerations

• Failure to follow dietary restrictions may cause the procedure to be canceled or repeated.

NURSING IMPLICATIONS AND PROCEDURE

PRETEST:

▸ Positively identify the patient using at least two unique identifiers before providing care, treatment, or services.

▸ *Patient Teaching:* Inform the patient this procedure can assist in assessing liver and biliary function.

▸ Obtain a history of the patient's complaints, including a list of known allergens, especially allergies or sensitivities to latex.

▸ Obtain a history of the patient's hepatobiliary system, symptoms, and results of previously performed laboratory tests and diagnostic and surgical procedures.

▸ Note any recent procedures that can interfere with test results (i.e., barium procedures, surgery, or biopsy). There should be 24 hr between administration of barium and this test.

▸ Endoscopic retrograde cholangiopancreatography, colonoscopy, and computed tomography of the abdomen, if ordered, should be scheduled after this procedure.

▸ Obtain a list of the patient's current medications, including herbs, nutritional supplements, and nutraceuticals (see Appendix F).

▸ Review the procedure with the patient. Address concerns about pain related to the procedure and explain that some pain may be experienced during the test, and there may be moments of discomfort. Inform the patient that the procedure is performed in a US department, usually by a health-care provider (HCP) who specializes in this procedure, with support staff, and takes approximately 30 to 60 min.

▸ *Sensitivity to social and cultural issues,* as well as concern for modesty, is important in providing psychological support before, during, and after the procedure.

▸ Instruct the patient to remove jewelry and other metallic objects from the area to be examined.

▸ The patient should fast and restrict fluids for 8 hr prior to the procedure. Protocols may vary among facilities.

INTRATEST:

▸ Ensure that food and fluids have been restricted for at least 8 hr prior to the procedure.

▸ Ensure that the patient has removed all external metallic objects from the area to be examined prior to the procedure.

▸ Instruct the patient to void and change into the gown, robe, and foot coverings provided.

▸ Instruct the patient to cooperate fully and to follow directions. Instruct the patient to remain still throughout the procedure because movement produces unreliable results.

U

- Observe standard precautions, and follow the general guidelines in Appendix A.
- Place the patient in the supine position on an examination table. The right- or left-side-up positions may be used to allow gravity to reposition the liver, gas, and fluid to facilitate better organ visualization.
- Expose the abdominal area and drape the patient.
- Conductive gel is applied to the skin, and a transducer is moved over the skin to obtain images of the area of interest.
- Ask the patient to breathe normally during the examination. If necessary for better organ visualization, ask the patient to inhale deeply and hold his or her breath.

POST-TEST:

- A report of the results will be sent to the requesting HCP, who will discuss the results with the patient.
- When the study is completed, remove the gel from the skin.
- Instruct the patient to resume usual diet and fluids, as directed by the HCP.
- Recognize anxiety related to test results. Discuss the implications of abnormal test results on the patient's lifestyle. Provide teaching and information regarding the clinical implications of the test results, as appropriate.
- Reinforce information given by the patient's HCP regarding further testing, treatment, or referral to another HCP. Answer any questions or address any concerns voiced by the patient or family.
- Depending on the results of this procedure, additional testing may be performed to evaluate or monitor progression of the disease process and determine the need for a change in therapy. Evaluate test results in relation to the patient's symptoms and other tests performed.

RELATED MONOGRAPHS:

- Related tests include ALP, ALT, AST, bilirubin, biopsy liver, cholangiography, colonoscopy, CT abdomen, endoscopy, ERCP, GGT, haptoglobin, hepatitis (A, B, C antigens and/or antibodies), hepatobiliary scan, laparoscopy abdominal, MRI abdomen, and radiofrequency ablation liver.
- Refer to the Hepatobiliary System table at the end of the book for related tests by body system.

Ultrasound, Lymph Nodes and Retroperitoneum

SYNONYM/ACRONYM: Lymph node sonography.

COMMON USE: To visualize and assess for lymph node enlargement related to disorders such as infection, abscess, tumor, and cancer. Also used as a tool to biopsy and evaluate the progress of therapeutic interventions.

AREA OF APPLICATION: Abdomen, pelvis, and retroperitoneum.

CONTRAST: Done without contrast.

U

DESCRIPTION: Ultrasound (US) procedures are diagnostic, noninvasive, and relatively inexpensive. They take a short time to complete, do not use radiation, and cause no harm to the patient. Lymph node US uses high-frequency waves of various intensities delivered by a transducer, a flashlight-shaped device, pressed against the skin. The waves are bounced back, converted to electrical energy, amplified by the transducer, and displayed on a monitor to evaluate the structure, size, and position of the lymph nodes to examine the retroperitoneum and surrounding tissues. This procedure is used for the evaluation of retroperitoneal pathology, usually lymph node enlargement. US is the preferred diagnostic method because this area is inaccessible to conventional radiography in diagnosing lymphadenopathy, although it can be used in combination with lymphangiography, magnetic resonance imaging, and computed tomography (CT) to confirm the diagnosis. The procedure may be used for monitoring the effect of radiation or chemotherapy on the lymph nodes. Lymph node US may be the diagnostic examination of choice because no radiation is used and, in most cases, the accuracy is sufficient to make the diagnosis without any further imaging procedures.

INDICATIONS
- Detect lymphoma
- Determine the location of enlarged nodes to plan radiation and other therapy
- Determine the size or enlargement of aortic and iliac lymph nodes

- Evaluate the effects of medical, radiation, or surgical therapy on the size of nodes or tumors, as evidenced by shrinkage or continued presence of the mass or nodes

POTENTIAL DIAGNOSIS

Normal findings in
- Normal retroperitoneal and intrapelvic node size of 1.5 cm in diameter

Abnormal findings in
- Infection or abscess
- Lymphoma
- Retroperitoneal tumor

CRITICAL FINDINGS: N/A

INTERFERING FACTORS

Factors that may impair clear imaging
- Incorrect placement of the transducer over the desired test site.
- Gas or feces in the gastrointestinal tract resulting from inadequate cleansing or failure to restrict food intake before the study.
- Retained barium from a previous radiological procedure.
- Dehydration, which can cause failure to demonstrate the boundaries between organs and tissue structures.
- Insufficiently full bladder, which fails to push the bowel from the pelvis and the uterus from the symphysis pubis, thereby prohibiting clear imaging of the pelvic organs in transabdominal imaging.
- Metallic objects (e.g., jewelry, or body rings) within the examination field which may inhibit organ visualization and cause unclear images.

Other considerations
- Failure to follow dietary/fluid instructions and other pretesting preparations may cause the procedure to be canceled or repeated.

U

- Inability of the patient to cooperate or remain still during the procedure because of age, significant pain, or mental status may interfere with the test results.

NURSING IMPLICATIONS AND PROCEDURE

PRETEST:

- Positively identify the patient using at least two unique identifiers before providing care, treatment, or services.
- *Patient Teaching:* Inform the patient this procedure can assist in assessing the lymph nodes and surrounding tissue.
- Obtain a history of the patient's complaints, including a list of known allergens, especially allergies or sensitivities to latex.
- Obtain a history of the patient's immune system, symptoms, and results of previously performed laboratory tests and diagnostic and surgical procedures.
- Note any recent procedures that can interfere with test results (i.e., barium procedures, surgery, or biopsy). There should be 24 hr between administration of barium and this test.
- Endoscopic retrograde cholangiopancreatography, colonoscopy, and CT of the abdomen, if ordered, should be scheduled after this procedure.
- Obtain a list of the patient's current medications, including herbs, nutritional supplements, and nutraceuticals (see Appendix F).
- Review the procedure with the patient. Address concerns about pain related to the procedure and explain that some pain may be experienced during the test, and there may be moments of discomfort. Inform the patient that the procedure is performed in a US department by a health-care provider (HCP) who specializes in this procedure, with support staff, and takes approximately 30 to 60 min.
- *Sensitivity to social and cultural issues,* as well as concern for modesty, is important in providing psychological support before, during, and after the procedure.

- Instruct the patient to remove jewelry and other metallic objects from the area to be examined.
- The patient should fast and restrict fluids for 8 hr prior to the procedure. Inform the patient that transabdominal US requires a full bladder. Protocols may vary among facilities.
- Instruct the patient to drink five to six glasses of fluid 90 min before the procedure, and not to void before the procedure.

INTRATEST:

- Ensure that food and fluids have been restricted for at least 8 hr prior to the procedure.
- Ensure that the patient receiving transabdominal US drank five to six glasses of fluid and has not voided.
- Ensure that the patient has removed all external metallic objects from the area to be examined prior to the procedure.
- Instruct the patient to change into the gown, robe, and foot coverings provided.
- Instruct the patient to cooperate fully and to follow directions. Ask the patient to remain still throughout the procedure because movement produces unreliable results.
- Observe standard precautions, and follow the general guidelines in Appendix A.
- Place the patient in the supine position on an examination table; other positions may be used during the examination.
- Expose the abdominal area and drape the patient.
- Conductive gel is applied to the skin, and a transducer is moved over the skin while the bladder is distended to obtain images of the area of interest.
- Ask the patient to breathe normally during the examination. If necessary for better organ visualization, ask the patient to inhale deeply and hold his or her breath.

POST-TEST:

- A report of the results will be sent to the requesting HCP, who will discuss the results with the patient.

U

- Allow the patient to void, as needed.
- When the study is completed, remove the gel from the skin.
- Instruct the patient to resume usual diet and fluids, as directed by the HCP.
- Recognize anxiety related to test results. Discuss the implications of abnormal test results on the patient's lifestyle. Provide teaching and information regarding the clinical implications of the test results, as appropriate.
- Reinforce information given by the patient's HCP regarding further testing, treatment, or referral to another HCP. Answer any questions or address any concerns voiced by the patient or family.
- Depending on the results of this procedure, additional testing may be

performed to evaluate or monitor progression of the disease process and determine the need for a change in therapy. Evaluate test results in relation to the patient's symptoms and other tests performed.

RELATED MONOGRAPHS:

- Related tests include angiography abdomen, biopsy bone marrow, biopsy lymph nodes, CBC, CBC hemoglobin, CBC RBC count, CBC RBC morphology and inclusions, CT abdomen, CT colonoscopy, ESR, gallium scan, KUB study, laparoscopy abdominal, lymphangiogram, and MRI abdomen.
- Refer to the Immune System table at the end of the book for related tests by body system.

Ultrasound, Pancreas

SYNONYM/ACRONYM: Pancreatic ultrasonography.

COMMON USE: To visualize and assess the pancreas to assist in diagnosing disorders such as tumor, cancer, obstruction, and cysts. Also used as a tool for biopsy and to evaluate the effectiveness of therapeutic interventions.

AREA OF APPLICATION: Pancreas and upper abdomen.

CONTRAST: Done without contrast.

DESCRIPTION: Ultrasound (US) procedures are diagnostic, noninvasive, and relatively inexpensive. They take a short time to complete, do not use radiation, and cause no harm to the patient. Pancreatic US uses high-frequency waves of various intensities delivered by a transducer, a flashlight-shaped device, pressed against the skin. The waves are bounced back, converted to electrical energy, amplified by the transducer,

and displayed on a monitor to determine the size, shape, and position of the pancreas; determine the presence of masses or other abnormalities of the pancreas; and examine the surrounding viscera. The procedure is indicated as a guide for biopsy, aspiration, and other interventional procedures. Pancreatic US may be the diagnostic examination of choice because no radiation is used and, in most

U

cases, the accuracy is sufficient to make the diagnosis without any further imaging procedures; however, it is usually done in combination with computed tomography (CT) or magnetic resonance imaging of the pancreas.

INDICATIONS
- Detect anatomic abnormalities as a consequence of pancreatitis
- Detect pancreatic cancer, as evidenced by a poorly defined mass or a mass in the head of the pancreas that obstructs the pancreatic duct
- Detect pancreatitis, as evidenced by pancreatic enlargement with increased echoes
- Detect pseudocysts, as evidenced by a well-defined mass with absence of echoes from the interior
- Monitor therapeutic response to tumor treatment
- Provide guidance for percutaneous aspiration and fine-needle biopsy of the pancreas

POTENTIAL DIAGNOSIS

Normal findings in
- Normal size, position, contour, and texture of the pancreas

Abnormal findings in
- Acute pancreatitis
- Calculi
- Pancreatic duct obstruction
- Pancreatic tumor
- Pseudocysts

CRITICAL FINDINGS: N/A

INTERFERING FACTORS

Factors that may impair clear imaging
- Attenuation of the sound waves by the ribs, which can impair clear imaging of the pancreas.

- Incorrect placement of the transducer over the desired test site.
- Gas or feces in the gastrointestinal (GI) tract resulting from inadequate cleansing or failure to restrict food intake before the study.
- Retained barium from a previous radiological procedure.
- Metallic objects (e.g., jewelry, body rings) within the examination field, which may inhibit organ visualization and cause unclear images.

Other considerations
- Failure to follow dietary and fluid restrictions and other pretesting preparations may cause the procedure to be canceled or repeated.
- Inability of the patient to cooperate or remain still during the procedure because of age, significant pain, or mental status may interfere with the test results.

NURSING IMPLICATIONS AND PROCEDURE

PRETEST:
- Positively identify the patient using at least two unique identifiers before providing care, treatment, or services.
- *Patient Teaching:* Inform the patient this procedure can assist in assessing pancreatic function.
- Obtain a history of the patient's complaints, including a list of known allergens, especially allergies or sensitivities to latex.
- Obtain a history of the patient's gastrointestinal system, symptoms, and results of previously performed laboratory tests and diagnostic and surgical procedures.
- Note any recent procedures that can interfere with test results (i.e., barium procedures, surgery, or biopsy). There should be 24 hr between administration of barium and this test.
- Endoscopic retrograde cholangiopancreatography, colonoscopy, and CT of the abdomen, if ordered, should be scheduled after this procedure.

▶ Record the date of the last menstrual period and determine the possibility of pregnancy in perimenopausal women.

▶ Obtain a list of the patient's current medications, including herbs, nutritional supplements, and nutraceuticals (see Appendix F).

▶ Review the procedure with the patient. Address concerns about pain related to the procedure and explain that some pain may be experienced during the test, and there may be moments of discomfort. Inform the patient that the procedure is performed in a US department, usually by a health-care provider (HCP) specializing in this procedure, with support staff, and takes approximately 30 to 60 min.

▶ *Sensitivity to social and cultural issues,* as well as concern for modesty, is important in providing psychological support before, during, and after the procedure.

▶ Instruct the patient to remove jewelry and other metallic objects from the area to be examined.

▶ The patient should fast and restrict fluids for 8 hr prior to the procedure. Protocols may vary among facilities.

INTRATEST:

▶ Ensure that food and fluids have been restricted for at least 8 hr prior to the procedure.

▶ Ensure that the patient has removed all external metallic objects from the area to be examined prior to the procedure.

▶ Instruct the patient to void and change into the gown, robe, and foot coverings provided.

▶ Instruct the patient to cooperate fully and to follow directions. Ask the patient to remain still throughout the procedure because movement produces unreliable results.

▶ Observe standard precautions, and follow the general guidelines in Appendix A.

▶ Place the patient in the supine position on an examination table. The right- or left-side-up position may be used to allow gravity to reposition the liver,

gas, and fluid to facilitate better organ visualization.

▶ Expose the abdominal area and drape the patient.

▶ Conductive gel is applied to the skin, and a transducer is moved over the skin to obtain images of the area of interest.

▶ Ask the patient to breathe normally during the examination. If necessary for better organ visualization, ask the patient to inhale deeply and hold his or her breath.

POST-TEST:

▶ A report of the results will be sent to the requesting HCP, who will discuss the results with the patient.

▶ When the study is completed, remove the gel from the skin.

▶ Instruct the patient to resume usual diet and fluids, as directed by the HCP.

▶ Recognize anxiety related to test results. Discuss the implications of abnormal test results on the patient's lifestyle. Provide teaching and information regarding the clinical implications of the test results, as appropriate.

▶ Reinforce information given by the patient's HCP regarding further testing, treatment, or referral to another HCP. Answer any questions or address any concerns voiced by the patient or family.

▶ Depending on the results of this procedure, additional testing may be needed to evaluate or monitor progression of the disease process and determine the need for a change in therapy. Evaluate test results in relation to the patient's symptoms and other tests performed.

RELATED MONOGRAPHS:

▶ Related tests include amylase, cancer antigens, CT abdomen, CT pancreas, C peptide, ERCP, KUB study, laparoscopy abdominal, lipase, MRI abdomen, MRI pancreas, and peritoneal fluid analysis.

▶ Refer to the Gastrointestinal System table at the end of the book for related tests by body system.

U

Ultrasound, Pelvis (Gynecologic, Nonobstetric)

SYNONYM/ACRONYM: Lower abdominal ultrasound, pelvic gynecologic (GYN) sonogram, pelvic sonography.

COMMON USE: To visualize and assess the pelvis for disorders such as uterine mass, tumor, cancer, cyst, and fibroids. This procedure can also be useful in evaluating ovulation and fallopian tube function related to fertility issues.

AREA OF APPLICATION: Pelvis and appendix region.

CONTRAST: Done without contrast.

DESCRIPTION: Ultrasound (US) procedures are diagnostic, noninvasive, and relatively inexpensive. They take a short time to complete, do not use radiation, and cause no harm to the patient. Gynecologic US uses high-frequency sound waves of various intensities delivered by a transducer, a flashlight-shaped device, pressed against the skin or inserted into the vagina. The waves are bounced back, converted to electrical energy, amplified by the transducer, and displayed on a monitor in order to determine the presence, size, and structure of masses and cysts and determine the position of an intrauterine contraceptive device (IUD); evaluate postmenopausal bleeding; and examine other abnormalities of the uterus, ovaries, fallopian tubes, and vagina.

This procedure is done by a transabdominal or transvaginal approach. The transabdominal approach provides a view of the pelvic organs posterior to the bladder. It requires a full bladder, thereby allowing a window for transmission of the US waves, pushing the uterus away from the pubic symphysis, pushing the bowel out of the pelvis, and acting as a reference for comparison in the evaluation of the internal structures of a mass or cyst being examined. The transvaginal approach focuses on the female reproductive organs and is often used to monitor ovulation over a period of days in patients undergoing fertility assessment. This approach is also used in obese patients or in patients with retroversion of the uterus because the sound waves are better able to reach the organ from the vaginal site. Transvaginal images are significantly more accurate compared to anterior transabdominal images in identifying paracervical, endometrial, and ovarian pathology, and the transvaginal approach does not require a full bladder. The procedure is indicated as a guide for biopsy and other interventional procedures. Pelvic US may be the diagnostic examination of choice because no radiation is used and, in most cases, the accuracy is sufficient to make the diagnosis without any further imaging procedures.

INDICATIONS

- Detect and monitor the treatment of pelvic inflammatory disease (PID) when done in combination with other laboratory tests
- Detect bleeding into the pelvis resulting from trauma to the area or ascites associated with tumor metastasis
- Detect masses in the pelvis and differentiate them from cysts or solid tumors, as evidenced by differences in sound-wave patterns
- Detect pelvic abscess or peritonitis caused by a ruptured appendix or diverticulitis
- Detect pregnancy, including ectopic pregnancy
- Detect the presence of ovarian cysts and malignancy and determine the type, if possible, as evidenced by size, outline, and change in position of other pelvic organs
- Evaluate the effectiveness of tumor therapy, as evidenced by a reduction in mass size
- Evaluate suspected fibroid tumor or bladder tumor
- Evaluate the thickness of the uterine wall
- Monitor placement and location of an IUD
- Monitor follicular size associated with fertility studies or to remove follicles for in vitro transplantation

POTENTIAL DIAGNOSIS

Normal findings in

- Normal size, position, location, and structure of pelvic organs (e.g., uterus, ovaries, fallopian tubes, vagina); IUD properly positioned within the uterine cavity

Abnormal findings in

- Abscess
- Adnexal torsion
- Appendicitis
- Ectopic pregnancy
- Endometrioma

- Fibroids (leiomyoma)
- Infection
- Nonovarian cyst
- Ovarian cysts
- Ovarian tumor
- Pelvic abscess
- Peritonitis
- PID
- Uterine tumor or adnexal tumor

CRITICAL FINDINGS

- Abscess
- Adnexal torsion
- Appendicitis
- Ectopic pregnancy
- Infection
- Tumor with significant mass effect

It is essential that critical diagnoses be communicated immediately to the appropriate health-care provider (HCP). A listing of these diagnoses varies among facilities. Note and immediately report to the HCP abnormal results and related symptoms.

INTERFERING FACTORS

This procedure is contraindicated for

- ✷ Patients with latex allergy; use of the vaginal probe requires the probe to be covered with a condom-like sac, usually made from latex. Latex-free covers are available.

Factors that may impair clear imaging

- Incorrect placement of the transducer over the desired test site.
- Gas or feces in the gastrointestinal tract resulting from inadequate cleansing or failure to restrict food intake before the study.
- Retained barium from a previous radiological procedure.
- Dehydration, which can cause failure to demonstrate the boundaries between organs and tissue structures.
- Insufficiently full bladder, which fails to push the bowel from the

U

pelvis and the uterus from the symphysis pubis, thereby prohibiting clear imaging of the pelvic organs in transabdominal imaging.
- Metallic objects (e.g., jewelry, body rings) within the examination field, which may inhibit organ visualization and cause unclear images.

Other considerations
- Failure to follow dietary/fluid instructions and other pretesting preparations may cause the procedure to be canceled or repeated.
- Inability of the patient to cooperate or remain still during the procedure because of age, significant pain, or mental status, may interfere with the test results.

NURSING IMPLICATIONS AND PROCEDURE

PRETEST:
- Positively identify the patient using at least two unique identifiers before providing care, treatment, or services.
- *Patient Teaching:* Inform the patient that this procedure can assist in assessing pelvic organ function.
- Obtain a history of the patient's complaints, including a list of known allergens, especially allergies or sensitivities to latex.
- Obtain a history of the patient's reproductive system, symptoms, and results of previously performed laboratory tests and diagnostic and surgical procedures.
- Note any recent procedures that can interfere with test results (i.e., barium procedures, surgery, or biopsy). There should be 24 hr between administration of barium and this test.
- Endoscopic retrograde cholangiopancreatography, colonoscopy, and computed tomography of the abdomen, if ordered, should be scheduled after this procedure.
- Record the date of the last menstrual period and determine the possibility of pregnancy in perimenopausal women.

- Obtain a list of the patient's current medications, including herbs, nutritional supplements, and nutraceuticals (see Appendix F).
- Review the procedure with the patient. Address concerns about pain related to the procedure and explain that some pain may be experienced during the test, and there may be moments of discomfort. Inform the patient that the procedure is performed in a US department by an HCP who specializes in this procedure, with support staff, and takes approximately 30 to 60 min.
- *Sensitivity to social and cultural issues,* as well as concern for modesty, is important in providing psychological support before, during, and after the procedure.
- Instruct the patient to remove jewelry and other metallic objects from the area to be examined.
- Instruct the patient that a latex or sterile sheath-covered probe will be inserted into the vagina for the transvaginal approach.
- The patient should fast and restrict fluids for 8 hr prior to the procedure. Protocols may vary among facilities.
- Instruct the patient receiving transabdominal US to drink three to five glasses of fluid 90 min before the examination and not to void, because the procedure requires a full bladder. Patients receiving transvaginal US only do not need to have a full bladder.

INTRATEST:
- Ensure that food and fluids have been restricted for at least 8 hr prior to the procedure.
- Ensure that the patient receiving transabdominal US drank three to five glasses of fluid and has not voided.
- Ensure that the patient has removed all external metallic objects from the area to be examined prior to the procedure.
- Instruct the patient to change into the gown, robe, and foot coverings provided. Remind her not to void before the procedure. Patients receiving transvaginal US do not need to have a full bladder.
- Instruct the patient to cooperate fully and to follow directions. Ask the patient to remain still throughout the procedure

U

because movement produces unreliable results.

- Observe standard precautions, and follow the general guidelines in Appendix A.
- Place the patient in the supine position on an examination table. The right- or left-side-up positions may be used to allow gravity to reposition the liver, gas, and fluid to facilitate better organ visualization.
- Expose the abdominal and pelvic area and drape the patient.
- *Transabdominal approach:* Conductive gel is applied to the skin, and a transducer is moved over the skin while the bladder is distended to obtain images of the area of interest.
- *Transvaginal approach:* A covered and lubricated probe is inserted into the vagina and moved to different levels. Images are obtained and recorded.
- Ask the patient to breathe normally during the examination. If necessary for better organ visualization, ask the patient to inhale deeply and hold her breath.

- Recognize anxiety related to test results. Discuss the implications of abnormal test results on the patient's lifestyle. Provide teaching and information regarding the clinical implications of the test results, as appropriate. Educate the patient regarding access to counseling services. Provide contact information, if desired, for the American Cancer Society (www.cancer.org).
- Reinforce information given by the patient's HCP regarding further testing, treatment, or referral to another HCP. Answer any questions or address any concerns voiced by the patient or family.
- Depending on the results of this procedure, additional testing may be needed to evaluate or monitor progression of the disease process and determine the need for a change in therapy. Evaluate test results in relation to the patient's symptoms and other tests performed.

POST-TEST:

- A report of the results will be sent to the requesting HCP, who will discuss the results with the patient.
- Allow the patient to void, as needed.
- When the study is completed, remove the gel from the skin.
- Instruct the patient to resume usual diet and fluids, as directed by the HCP.

RELATED MONOGRAPHS:

- Related tests include cancer antigens, colposcopy, CT abdomen, hysterosalpingography, KUB study, laparoscopy gynecologic, MRI abdomen, Pap smear, and PET pelvis.
- Refer to the Reproductive System table at the end of the book for related tests by body system.

Ultrasound, Prostate (Transrectal)

SYNONYM/ACRONYM: Prostate sonography.

COMMON USE: To visualize and assess the prostate gland as an adjunct of prostate-specific antigen (PSA) blood testing and examination to assist in diagnosing disorders such as tumor and cancer. Also used to assist in guiding biopsy of the prostate.

AREA OF APPLICATION: Prostate, seminal vesicles.

CONTRAST: Done without contrast.

U

DESCRIPTION: Ultrasound (US) procedures are diagnostic, non-invasive, and relatively inexpensive. They take a short time to complete, do not use radiation, and cause no harm to the patient. Prostate US is used for the evaluation of disorders of the prostate, especially in response to an elevated concentration of prostate-specific antigen (PSA) on a blood test and as a complement to a digital rectal examination. It uses high-frequency sound waves of various intensities delivered by a transducer, a candle-shaped device, which is lubricated, sheathed with a condom, and inserted a few inches into the rectum. The waves are bounced back, converted to electrical energy, amplified by the transducer, and displayed on a monitor to evaluate the structure, size, and position of the contents of the prostate (e.g., masses) as well as other prostate pathology. It aids in the diagnosis of prostatic cancer by evaluating palpable nodules and is useful as a guide to biopsy. This procedure can evaluate prostate tissue, the seminal vesicles, and surrounding perirectal tissue. It can also be used to stage carcinoma and to assist in radiation seed placement. The examination is helpful in monitoring patient response to therapy for prostatic disease. Micturition disorders can also be evaluated by this procedure. Prostate US may be the diagnostic examination of choice because no radiation is used and, in most cases, the accuracy is sufficient to make the diagnosis without any further imaging procedures.

INDICATIONS

- Aid in the diagnosis of micturition disorders
- Aid in prostate cancer diagnosis
- Assess prostatic calcifications
- Assist in guided needle biopsy of a suspected tumor
- Assist in radiation seed placement
- Determine prostatic cancer staging
- Detect prostatitis

POTENTIAL DIAGNOSIS

Normal findings in
- Normal size, consistency, and contour of the prostate gland

Abnormal findings in
- Benign prostatic hypertrophy or hyperplasia
- Micturition disorders
- Perirectal abscess
- Perirectal tumor
- Prostate abscess
- Prostate cancer
- Prostatitis
- Rectal tumor
- Seminal vesicle tumor

CRITICAL FINDINGS: N/A

INTERFERING FACTORS

This procedure is contraindicated for
- ◆ Patients with latex allergy; use of the rectal probe requires the probe to be covered with a condom, usually made from latex. Latex-free covers are available.

Factors that may impair clear imaging
- Attenuation of the sound waves by the pelvic bones, which can impair clear imaging of the prostate.
- Incorrect placement of the transducer over the desired test site.
- Gas or feces in the gastrointestinal tract resulting from inadequate cleansing or failure to restrict food intake before the study.

U

- Retained barium from a previous radiological procedure.
- Metallic objects (e.g., jewelry, body rings) within the examination field, which may inhibit organ visualization and cause unclear images.

Other considerations

- Failure to follow pretesting preparations may cause the procedure to be canceled or repeated.
- Inability of the patient to cooperate or remain still during the procedure because of age, significant pain, or mental status may interfere with the test results.

NURSING IMPLICATIONS AND PROCEDURE

PRETEST:

- Positively identify the patient using at least two unique identifiers before providing care, treatment, or services.
- *Patient Teaching:* Inform the patient this procedure can assist in evaluating the prostate gland.
- Obtain a history of the patient's complaints, including a list of known allergens, especially allergies or sensitivities to latex.
- Obtain a history of the patient's genitourinary system, symptoms, and results of previously performed laboratory tests and diagnostic and surgical procedures.
- Note any recent procedures that can interfere with test results (i.e., barium procedures, surgery, or biopsy). There should be 24 hr between administration of barium and this test.
- Colonoscopy and computed tomography of the abdomen, if ordered, should be scheduled after this procedure.
- Obtain a list of the patient's current medications, including herbs, nutritional supplements, and nutraceuticals (see Appendix F).
- Review the procedure with the patient. Address concerns about pain related to the procedure and explain that some pain may be experienced during the test, and there may be moments of discomfort. Inform the patient that the

procedure is performed in a US department by a health-care provider (HCP) who specializes in this procedure, with support staff, and takes approximately 30 to 60 min.

- Inform the patient that a sterile latex- or sheath-covered probe will be inserted into the rectum.
- *Sensitivity to social and cultural issues,* as well as concern for modesty, is important in providing psychological support before, during, and after the procedure.
- There are no food, fluid, or medication restrictions unless by medical direction.

INTRATEST:

- Instruct the patient to void and change into the gown, robe, and foot coverings provided.
- Instruct the patient to cooperate fully and to follow directions. Ask the patient to remain still throughout the procedure because movement produces unreliable results.
- Observe standard precautions, and follow the general guidelines in Appendix A.
- Place the patient on the examination table on his left side with his knees bent toward the chest; other positions may be used during the examination.
- Expose the rectal area and drape the patient.
- Cover the rectal probe with a lubricated condom and insert it into the rectum. Inform the patient that he may feel slight pressure as the transducer is inserted. Water may be introduced through the sheath surrounding the transducer.
- Ask the patient to breathe normally during the examination. If necessary for better organ visualization, ask the patient to inhale deeply and hold his breath.

POST-TEST:

- A report of the results will be sent to the requesting HCP, who will discuss the results with the patient.
- When the study is completed, remove the gel from the skin.
- *Nutritional Considerations*: There is growing evidence that inflammation and oxidation play key roles in the development of numerous diseases, including

prostate cancer. Research also indicates that diets containing dried beans, fresh fruits and vegetables, nuts, spices, whole grains, and smaller amounts of red meats can increase the amount of protective antioxidants. Regular exercise, especially in combination with a healthy diet, can bring about changes in the body's metabolism that decrease inflammation and oxidation.

▶ Recognize anxiety related to test results. Discuss the implications of abnormal test results on the patient's lifestyle. Provide teaching and information regarding the clinical implications of the test results, as appropriate. Educate the patient regarding access to counseling services. Provide contact information, if desired, for the National Cancer Institute (www.cancer.gov) or the Prostate Cancer Foundation (www.prostatecancerfoundation.org).

▶ Reinforce information given by the patient's HCP regarding further testing, treatment, or referral to another HCP. Answer any questions or address any concerns voiced by the patient or family. Decisions regarding the need for and frequency of routine PSA testing or other cancer screening procedures should be made after consultation between the patient and HCP. The most current guidelines for cervical cancer screening of the general population as well as of individuals with increased risk are available from the American Cancer Society (www.cancer.org) and the American Urological Association (www.aua.org).

▶ Depending on the results of this procedure, additional testing may be needed to evaluate or monitor progression of the disease process and determine the need for a change in therapy. Evaluate test results in relation to the patient's symptoms and other tests performed.

RELATED MONOGRAPHS:

▶ Related tests include biopsy prostate, CT pelvis, cystoscopy, cystourethrography voiding, IVP, KUB study, MRI pelvis, proctosigmoidoscopy, PSA, renogram, retrograde ureteropyelography, and semen analysis.

▶ Refer to the Genitourinary System table at the end of the book for related tests by body system.

Ultrasound, Scrotal

SYNONYM/ACRONYM: Scrotal sonography, ultrasound of the testes, testicular ultrasound.

COMMON USE: To visualize and assess scrotum structure and function to assist in diagnosing disorders such as tumor, cancer, pus, undescended testes, and inflammation.

AREA OF APPLICATION: Scrotum.

CONTRAST: Done without contrast.

DESCRIPTION: Ultrasound (US) procedures are diagnostic, noninvasive, and relatively inexpensive. They take a short time to complete, do not use radiation, and cause no harm to the patient. Scrotal US is used for the evaluation of disorders of the scrotum.

It is valuable in determining the internal components of masses (solid vs. cystic) and for the evaluation of the testicle, extratesticular and intrascrotal tissues, benign and malignant tumors, and other scrotal pathology. It uses high-frequency sound waves of various intensities delivered by a transducer, a flashlight-shaped device, which is pressed against the skin. The waves are bounced back, converted to electrical energy, amplified by the transducer, and displayed on a monitor to evaluate the structure, size, and position of the contents of the scrotum. Scrotal US can be performed before or after a radionuclide scan for further clarification of a testicular mass. Extratesticular lesions such as hydrocele, hematocele (blood in the scrotum), and pyocele (pus in the scrotum) can be identified, as can cryptorchidism (undescended testicles). Scrotal US may be the diagnostic examination of choice because no radiation is used and, in most cases, the accuracy is sufficient to make the diagnosis without any further imaging procedures.

INDICATIONS

- Aid in the diagnosis of a chronic inflammatory condition such as epididymitis
- Aid in the diagnosis of a mass and differentiate between a cyst and a solid tumor, as evidenced by specific waveform patterns or the absence of sound waves respectively
- Aid in the diagnosis of scrotal or testicular size, abnormality, or pathology
- Aid in the diagnosis of testicular torsion and associated testicular infarction
- Assist guided needle biopsy of a suspected testicle tumor

- Determine the cause of chronic scrotal swelling or pain
- Determine the presence of a hydrocele, pyocele, spermatocele, or hernia before surgery
- Evaluate the effectiveness of treatment for testicular infections
- Locate an undescended testicle

POTENTIAL DIAGNOSIS

Normal findings in

- Normal size, position, and shape of the scrotum and structure of the testes

Abnormal findings in

- Abscess
- Epididymal cyst
- Epididymitis
- Hematoma
- Hydrocele
- Infarction
- Microlithiasis
- Orchitis
- Pyocele
- Scrotal hernia
- Spermatocele
- Testicular torsion
- Tumor, benign or malignant
- Tunica albuginea cyst
- Undescended testicle (cryptorchidism)
- Varicocele

CRITICAL FINDINGS

- Testicular torsion

It is essential that critical diagnoses be communicated immediately to the appropriate health-care provider (HCP). A listing of these diagnoses varies among facilities. Note and immediately report to the HCP abnormal results and related symptoms.

INTERFERING FACTORS

Factors that may impair clear imaging

- Incorrect placement of the transducer over the desired test site.

- Metallic objects (e.g., jewelry, body rings) within the examination field, which may inhibit organ visualization and cause unclear images.
- Inability of the patient to cooperate or remain still during the procedure because of age, significant pain, or mental status.

NURSING IMPLICATIONS AND PROCEDURE

PRETEST:

- Positively identify the patient using at least two unique identifiers before providing care, treatment, or services.
- *Patient Teaching:* Inform the patient this procedure can assist in assessing the scrotum.
- Obtain a history of the patient's complaints, including a list of known allergens, especially allergies or sensitivities to latex.
- Obtain a history of the patient's reproductive system, symptoms, and results of previously performed laboratory tests and diagnostic and surgical procedures.
- Note any recent procedures that can interfere with test results (i.e., surgery or biopsy).
- Colonoscopy and computed tomography of the abdomen, if ordered, should be scheduled after this procedure.
- Obtain a list of the patient's current medications, including herbs, nutritional supplements, and nutraceuticals (see Appendix F).
- Review the procedure with the patient. Address concerns about pain related to the procedure and explain that some pain may be experienced during the test, and there may be moments of discomfort. Inform the patient that the procedure is performed in a US department, by an HCP who specializes in this procedure, with support staff, and takes approximately 30 to 60 min.
- *Sensitivity to social and cultural issues,* as well as concern for modesty, is important in providing psychological support before, during, and after the procedure.

- Instruct the patient to remove jewelry and other metallic objects from the area to be examined.
- There are no food, fluid, or medication restrictions unless by medical direction.

INTRATEST:

- Ensure that the patient has removed all external metallic objects from the area to be examined prior to the procedure.
- Instruct the patient to void and change into the gown, robe, and foot coverings provided.
- Instruct the patient to cooperate fully and to follow directions. Ask the patient to remain still throughout the procedure because movement produces unreliable results.
- Observe standard precautions, and follow the general guidelines in Appendix A.
- Place the patient in the supine position on an examination table; other positions may be used during the examination.
- Expose the abdomen/pelvic area and drape the patient.
- Lift the penis upward and gently tape it to the lower part of the abdomen. Elevate the scrotum with a rolled towel or sponge for immobilization.
- Conductive gel is applied to the skin, and a transducer is moved over the skin to obtain images of the area of interest.
- Ask the patient to breathe normally during the examination. If necessary for better organ visualization, ask the patient to inhale deeply and hold his breath.

POST-TEST:

- A report of the results will be sent to the requesting HCP, who will discuss the results with the patient.
- When the study is completed, remove the gel from the skin.
- Recognize anxiety related to test results. Discuss the implications of abnormal test results on the patient's lifestyle. Provide teaching and information regarding the clinical implications of the test results, as appropriate.
- Reinforce information given by the patient's HCP regarding further testing, treatment, or referral to another HCP. Answer any questions or address any concerns voiced by the patient or family.

- Depending on the results of this procedure, additional testing may be needed to evaluate or monitor progression of the disease process and determine the need for a change in therapy. Evaluate test results in relation to the patient's symptoms and other tests performed.

RELATED MONOGRAPHS:

- Related tests include AFP, CT pelvis, KUB study, MRI pelvis, and semen analysis.
- Refer to the Reproductive System table at the end of the book for related tests by body system.

Ultrasound, Spleen

SYNONYM/ACRONYM: Spleen ultrasonography.

COMMON USE: To visualize and assess the spleen for abscess, trauma, rupture, cancer, and tumor. Also used to evaluate the effectiveness of therapeutic interventions and assist with guided biopsy.

AREA OF APPLICATION: Spleen/left upper quadrant.

CONTRAST: Done without contrast.

DESCRIPTION: Ultrasound (US) procedures are diagnostic, noninvasive, and relatively inexpensive. They take a short time to complete, do not use radiation, and cause no harm to the patient. Spleen US uses high-frequency waves of various intensities delivered by a transducer, a flashlight-shaped device, pressed against the skin. The waves are bounced back, converted to electrical energy, amplified by the transducer, and displayed on a monitor to evaluate the structure, size, and position of the spleen. This test is valuable for determining the internal components of splenic masses (solid vs. cystic) and evaluating other splenic pathology, splenic trauma, and left upper quadrant perisplenic tissues. It can be performed to supplement a radionuclide scan or computed tomography (CT). It is especially valuable in patients who are in renal failure, are hypersensitive to contrast medium, or are pregnant, because it does not rely on adequate renal function or the injection of contrast medium to obtain a diagnosis. The procedure may also be used as a guide for biopsy, other interventional procedures, and abscess drainage. Spleen US may be the diagnostic examination of choice because no radiation is used and, in most cases, the accuracy is sufficient to make the diagnosis without any further imaging procedures.

INDICATIONS
- Detect the presence of a subphrenic abscess after splenectomy
- Detect splenic masses; differentiate between cysts or solid tumors (in combination with CT), as evidenced by specific waveform patterns or absence of sound waves respectively;

U

and determine whether they are intrasplenic or extrasplenic
- Determine late-stage sickle cell disease, as evidenced by decreased spleen size and presence of echoes
- Determine the presence of splenomegaly and assess the size and volume of the spleen in these cases, as evidenced by increased echoes and visibility of the spleen
- Differentiate spleen trauma from blood or fluid accumulation between the splenic capsule and parenchyma
- Evaluate the effect of medical or surgical therapy on the progression or resolution of splenic disease
- Evaluate the extent of abdominal trauma and spleen involvement, including enlargement or rupture, after a recent trauma
- Evaluate the spleen before splenectomy performed for thrombocytopenic purpura

POTENTIAL DIAGNOSIS

Normal findings in
- Normal size, position, and contour of the spleen and associated structures

Abnormal findings in
- Abscess
- Accessory or ectopic spleen
- Infection
- Lymphatic disease; lymph node enlargement
- Splenic calcifications
- Splenic masses, tumors, cysts, or infarction
- Splenic trauma
- Splenomegaly

CRITICAL FINDINGS: N/A

INTERFERING FACTORS

Factors that may impair clear imaging
- Attenuation of the sound waves by the ribs and an aerated left lung, which can impair clear imaging of the spleen.

- Masses near the testing site, which can displace the spleen and cause inaccurate results if confused with splenomegaly.
- Dehydration, which can cause failure to demonstrate the boundaries between organs and tissue structures.
- Incorrect placement of the transducer over the desired test site.
- Gas or feces in the gastrointestinal tract resulting from inadequate cleansing or failure to restrict food intake before the study.
- Retained barium from a previous radiological procedure.
- Metallic objects (e.g., jewelry, body rings) within the examination field, which may inhibit organ visualization and can produce unclear images.

Other considerations
- Failure to follow dietary restrictions and other pretesting preparations may cause the procedure to be canceled or repeated.
- Inability of the patient to cooperate or remain still during the procedure because of age, significant pain, or mental status may interfere with the test results.

NURSING IMPLICATIONS AND PROCEDURE

PRETEST:
- Positively identify the patient using at least two unique identifiers before providing care, treatment, or services.
- *Patient Teaching:* Inform the patient this procedure can assist in assessing the function of the spleen.
- Obtain a history of the patient's complaints, including a list of known allergens, especially allergies or sensitivities to latex.
- Obtain a history of the patient's hematopoietic system, symptoms, and results of previously performed laboratory tests and diagnostic and surgical procedures.
- Note any recent procedures that can interfere with test results (i.e., barium

procedures, surgery, or biopsy). There should be 24 hr between administration of barium and this test.

- Endoscopic retrograde cholangiopancreatography, colonoscopy, and CT of the abdomen, if ordered, should be scheduled after this procedure.
- Obtain a list of the patient's current medications, including herbs, nutritional supplements, and nutraceuticals (see Appendix F).
- Review the procedure with the patient. Address concerns about pain related to the procedure and explain that some pain may be experienced during the test, and there may be moments of discomfort. Inform the patient that the procedure is performed in a US department by a health-care provider (HCP) who specializes in this procedure, with support staff, and takes approximately 30 to 60 min.
- *Sensitivity to social and cultural issues,* as well as concern for modesty, is important in providing psychological support before, during, and after the procedure.
- Instruct the patient to remove jewelry and other metallic objects in the area to be examined.
- The patient should fast and restrict fluids for 8 hr prior to the procedure. Protocols may vary among facilities.

INTRATEST:

- Ensure that food and fluids have been restricted for at least 8 hr prior to the procedure.
- Ensure that the patient has removed all external metallic objects in the area prior to the procedure.
- Instruct the patient to void and change into the gown, robe, and foot coverings provided.
- Instruct the patient to cooperate fully and to follow directions. Ask the patient to remain still throughout the procedure because movement produces unreliable results.
- Observe standard precautions, and follow the general guidelines in Appendix A.
- Place the patient in the supine position on an examination table. The right- or left-side-up position may be used to allow gravity to reposition the liver, gas, and fluid to facilitate better organ visualization.
- Expose the abdominal area and drape the patient.
- Conductive gel is applied to the skin, and a transducer is moved over the skin to obtain images of the area of interest.
- Ask the patient to breathe normally during the examination. If necessary for better organ visualization, ask the patient to inhale deeply and hold his or her breath.

POST-TEST:

- A report of the results will be sent to the requesting HCP, who will discuss the results with the patient.
- When the study is completed, remove the gel from the skin.
- Instruct the patient to resume usual diet and fluids, as directed by the HCP.
- Recognize anxiety related to test results. Discuss the implications of abnormal test results on the patient's lifestyle. Provide teaching and information regarding the clinical implications of the test results, as appropriate.
- Reinforce information given by the patient's HCP regarding further testing, treatment, or referral to another HCP. Answer any questions or address any concerns voiced by the patient or family.
- Depending on the results of this procedure, additional testing may be performed to evaluate or monitor progression of the disease process and determine the need for a change in therapy. Evaluate test results in relation to the patient's symptoms and other tests performed.

RELATED MONOGRAPHS:

- Related tests include angiography abdomen, biopsy bone marrow, CBC platelet count, CBC WBC and differential, CT abdomen, KUB study, liver and spleen scan, MRI abdomen, sickle cell screen, and WBC scan.
- Refer to the Hematopoietic System table at the end of the book for related tests by body system.

U

Ultrasound, Thyroid and Parathyroid

SYNONYM/ACRONYM: Parathyroid sonography, thyroid echo, thyroid sonography.

COMMON USE: To visualize and assess the thyroid and parathyroid glands for tumor, cancer, and cyst. Also used to stage cancer, guide biopsies, and monitor the effectiveness of therapeutic interventions.

AREA OF APPLICATION: Anterior neck region, parathyroid, thyroid.

CONTRAST: Done without contrast.

DESCRIPTION: Ultrasound (US) procedures are diagnostic, noninvasive, and relatively inexpensive. They take a short time to complete, do not use radiation, and cause no harm to the patient. Thyroid and parathyroid US uses high-frequency sound waves of various intensities delivered by a transducer, a flashlight-shaped device, pressed against the skin. The waves are bounced back, converted to electrical energy, amplified by the transducer, and displayed on a monitor to determine the position, size, shape, weight, and presence of masses of the thyroid gland; enlargement of the parathyroid glands; and other abnormalities of the thyroid and parathyroid glands and surrounding tissues. The primary purpose of this procedure is to determine whether a nodule is a fluid-filled cyst (usually benign) or a solid tumor (possibly malignant). This procedure is useful in evaluating the glands' response to medical treatment or assessing the remaining tissue after surgical resection. The procedure may be indicated as a guide for biopsy, aspiration, or other interventional procedures. Thyroid and parathyroid US may be the diagnostic examination of choice because no radiation is used and, in most cases, the accuracy is sufficient to make the diagnosis without any further imaging procedures; it is clearly the procedure of choice when examining the glands of pregnant patients. This procedure is usually done in combination with nuclear medicine imaging procedures and computed tomography of the neck. Despite the advantages of the procedure, in some cases it may not detect small nodules and lesions (less than 1 cm), leading to false-negative findings.

INDICATIONS

- Assist in determining the presence of a tumor, as evidenced by an irregular border and shadowing at the distal edge, peripheral echoes, or high- and low-amplitude echoes, depending on the density of the tumor mass; and diagnosing tumor type (e.g., benign, adenoma, carcinoma)
- Assist in diagnosing the presence of a cyst, as evidenced by a smoothly outlined, echo-free amplitude except at the far borders of the mass
- Assist in diagnosis in the presence of a parathyroid enlargement indicating a tumor or hyperplasia, as evidenced by an echo pattern of lower amplitude than that for a thyroid tumor

U

- Determine the need for surgical biopsy of a tumor or fine-needle biopsy of a cyst
- Differentiate among a nodule, solid tumor, or fluid-filled cyst
- Evaluate the effect of a therapeutic regimen for a thyroid mass or Graves' disease by determining the size and weight of the gland
- Evaluate thyroid abnormalities during pregnancy

POTENTIAL DIAGNOSIS

Normal findings in

- Normal size, position, contour, and structure of the thyroid and parathyroid glands with uniform echo patterns throughout the glands; no evidence of tumor cysts or nodules in the glands

Abnormal findings in

- Glandular enlargement
- Goiter
- Graves' disease
- Parathyroid tumor or hyperplasia
- Thyroid cysts
- Thyroid tumors (benign or malignant)

CRITICAL FINDINGS: N/A

INTERFERING FACTORS

Factors that may impair clear imaging

- Attenuation of the sound waves by the ribs, which can impair clear imaging of the parathyroid.
- Incorrect placement of the transducer over the desired test site.
- Metallic objects (e.g., jewelry, body rings) within the examination field, which may inhibit organ visualization and cause unclear images.

Other considerations

- Nodules less than 1 cm in diameter may not be detected.
- Nonthyroid cysts may appear the same as thyroid cysts.
- Inability of the patient to cooperate or remain still during the procedure

because of age, significant pain, or mental status may interfere with the test results.

NURSING IMPLICATIONS AND PROCEDURE

PRETEST:

▶ Positively identify the patient using at least two unique identifiers before providing care, treatment, or services.
▶ *Patient Teaching:* Inform the patient this procedure can assist in assessing thyroid and parathyroid gland function.
▶ Obtain a history of the patient's complaints, including a list of known allergens, especially allergies or sensitivities to latex.
▶ Obtain a history of the patient's endocrine system, symptoms, and results of previously performed laboratory tests and diagnostic and surgical procedures.
▶ Note any recent procedures that can interfere with test results (i.e., barium procedures, surgery, or biopsy). There should be 24 hr between administration of barium and this test.
▶ Obtain a list of the patient's current medications, including herbs, nutritional supplements, and nutraceuticals (see Appendix F).
▶ Review the procedure with the patient. Address concerns about pain related to the procedure and explain that some pain may be experienced during the test, and there may be moments of discomfort. Inform the patient that the procedure is performed in a US department by a health-care provider (HCP), with support staff, and takes approximately 30 to 60 min.
▶ *Sensitivity to social and cultural issues,* as well as concern for modesty, is important in providing psychological support before, during, and after the procedure.
▶ Instruct the patient to remove jewelry and other metallic objects from the area to be examined.
▶ There are no food, fluid, or medication restrictions unless by medical direction.

INTRATEST:

▶ Ensure that the patient has removed all external metallic objects from the area to be examined prior to the procedure.

U

▶ Instruct the patient to void and change into the gown, robe, and foot coverings provided.

▶ Instruct the patient to cooperate fully and to follow directions. Ask the patient to remain still throughout the procedure because movement produces unreliable results.

▶ Observe standard precautions, and follow the general guidelines in Appendix A.

▶ Place the patient in the supine position on an examination table; other positions may be used during the examination.

▶ Expose the neck and chest area and drape the patient.

▶ Hyperextend the neck, and place a pillow under the patient's shoulders to maintain a comfortable position. (An alternative method of imaging includes the use of a bag filled with water or gel placed over the neck area.)

▶ Conductive gel is applied to the skin, and a transducer is moved over the skin to obtain images of the area of interest.

▶ Ask the patient to breathe normally during the examination. If necessary for better organ visualization, ask the patient to inhale deeply and hold his or her breath.

POST-TEST:

▶ A report of the results will be sent to the requesting HCP, who will discuss the results with the patient.

▶ When the study is completed, remove the gel from the skin.

▶ Recognize anxiety related to test results. Discuss the implications of abnormal test results on the patient's lifestyle. Provide teaching and information regarding the clinical implications of the test results, as appropriate.

▶ Reinforce information given by the patient's HCP regarding further testing, treatment, or referral to another HCP. Answer any questions or address any concerns voiced by the patient or family.

▶ Depending on the results of this procedure, additional testing may be performed to evaluate or monitor progression of the disease process and determine the need for a change in therapy. Evaluate test results in relation to the patient's symptoms and other tests performed.

RELATED MONOGRAPHS:

▶ Related tests include antibodies antithyroglobulin, biopsy thyroid, chest x-ray, CT thorax, MRI chest, PTH, parathyroid scan, radioactive iodine uptake, thyroid-binding inhibitory immunoglobulin, thyroglobulin, thyroid scan, TSH, thyroxine free, thyroxine total, triiodothyronine free, and triiodothyronine total.

▶ Refer to the Endocrine System table at the end of the book for related tests by body system.

Ultrasound, Venous Doppler, Extremity Studies

SYNONYM/ACRONYM: Venous duplex, venous sonogram, venous ultrasound.

COMMON USE: To assess venous blood flow in the upper and lower extremities to assist in diagnosing disorders such as deep vein thrombosis, venous insufficiency, causation of pulmonary embolism, varicose veins, and monitor the effects of therapeutic interventions.

AREA OF APPLICATION: Veins of the upper and lower extremities.

CONTRAST: Done without contrast.

U

DESCRIPTION: Ultrasound (US) procedures are diagnostic, noninvasive, and relatively inexpensive. They take a short time to complete, do not use radiation, and cause no harm to the patient. Peripheral venous Doppler US records sound waves to obtain information about the patency of the venous vasculature in the upper and lower extremities to identify narrowing or occlusions of the veins or arteries. In venous Doppler studies, the Doppler identifies moving red blood cells (RBCs) within the vein. The US beam is directed at the vein and through the Doppler transducer while the RBCs reflect the beam back to the transducer. The reflected sound waves or echoes are transformed by a computer into scans, graphs, or audible sounds. Blood flow direction, velocity, and the presence of flow disturbances can be readily assessed. The velocity of the blood flow is transformed as a "swishing" noise, audible through the audio speaker. If the vein is occluded, no swishing sound is heard.

For diagnostic studies, the procedure is done bilaterally. The sound emitted by the equipment corresponds to the velocity of the blood flow through the vessel occurring with spontaneous respirations. Changes in these sounds during respirations indicate the possibility of abnormal venous flow secondary to occlusive disease; the absence of sound indicates complete obstruction. Compression with a transducer augments a vessel for evaluation of thrombosis. Noncompressibility of the vessel indicates a thrombosis. Plethysmography may be performed to determine the filling time of calf veins to diagnose thrombotic disorder of a major vein and to identify incompetent valves in the venous system. An additional method used to evaluate incompetent valves is the Valsalva technique combined with venous duplex imaging.

INDICATIONS

- Aid in the diagnosis of venous occlusion secondary to thrombosis or thrombophlebitis
- Aid in the diagnosis of superficial thrombosis or deep vein thrombosis (DVT) leading to venous occlusion or obstruction, as evidenced by absence of venous flow, especially upon augmentation of the extremity; variations in flow during respirations; or failure of the veins to compress completely when the extremity is compressed
- Detect chronic venous insufficiency, as evidenced by reverse blood flow indicating incompetent valves
- Determine if further diagnostic procedures are needed to make or confirm a diagnosis
- Determine the source of emboli when pulmonary embolism is suspected or diagnosed
- Determine venous damage after trauma to the site
- Differentiate between primary and secondary varicose veins
- Evaluate the patency of the venous system in patients with a swollen, painful leg
- Monitor the effectiveness of therapeutic interventions

POTENTIAL DIAGNOSIS

Normal findings in

- Normal Doppler venous signal that occurs spontaneously with the patient's respiration
- Normal blood flow through the veins of the extremities with no evidence of vessel occlusion

U

Abnormal findings in
- Chronic venous insufficiency
- Primary varicose veins
- Recannulization in the area of an old thrombus
- Secondary varicose veins
- Superficial thrombosis or DVT
- Venous narrowing or occlusion secondary to thrombosis or thrombophlebitis
- Venous trauma

CRITICAL FINDINGS
- DVT

It is essential that critical diagnoses be communicated immediately to the appropriate health-care provider (HCP). A listing of these diagnoses varies among facilities. Note and immediately report to the HCP abnormal results and related symptoms.

INTERFERING FACTORS

This procedure is contraindicated for
- Patients with an open or draining lesion.

Factors that may impair clear imaging
- Attenuation of the sound waves by bony structures, which can impair clear imaging of the vessels.
- Cigarette smoking, because nicotine can cause constriction of the peripheral vessels.
- Incorrect placement of the transducer over the desired test site.
- Metallic objects (e.g., jewelry, body rings) within the examination field, which may inhibit organ visualization and cause unclear images.
- Cold extremities, resulting in vasoconstriction that can cause inaccurate measurements.
- Occlusion proximal to the site being studied, which would affect blood flow to the area.
- An abnormally large or swollen leg, making sonic penetration difficult.

- Incorrect positioning of the patient, which may produce poor visualization of the area to be examined.

Other considerations
- Inability of the patient to cooperate or remain still during the procedure because of age, significant pain, or mental status.

NURSING IMPLICATIONS AND PROCEDURE

PRETEST:

- Positively identify the patient using at least two unique identifiers before providing care, treatment, or services.
- *Patient Teaching:* Inform the patient this procedure can assist in assessing the veins.
- Obtain a history of the patient's complaints, including a list of known allergens, especially allergies or sensitivities to latex.
- Obtain a history of the patient's cardiovascular system, symptoms, and results of previously performed laboratory tests and diagnostic and surgical procedures.
- Report the presence of a lesion that is open or draining; maintain clean, dry dressing for the ulcer; protect the limb from trauma.
- Note any recent procedures that can interfere with test results (i.e., barium procedures, surgery, or biopsy). There should be 24 hr between administration of barium- or iodine-based contrast medium and this test.
- Endoscopic retrograde cholangiopancreatography, colonoscopy, and computed tomography of the abdomen, if ordered, should be scheduled after this procedure.
- Obtain a list of the patient's current medications, including herbs, nutritional supplements, and nutraceuticals (see Appendix F).
- Review the procedure with the patient. Address concerns about pain related to the procedure and explain that some pain may be experienced during the test, and there may be moments of discomfort. Inform the patient that the procedure is performed in a US department

by an HCP who specializes in this procedure, with support staff, and takes
approximately 30 to 60 min.
- *Sensitivity to social and cultural issues,*
as well as concern for modesty, is important in providing psychological support
before, during, and after the procedure.
- Instruct the patient to remove jewelry
and other metallic objects from the
area to be examined.
- There are no food, fluid, or medication
restrictions unless by medical direction.

INTRATEST:
- Ensure that the patient has removed all
external metallic objects from the area
to be examined prior to the procedure.
- Instruct the patient to void and change
into the gown, robe, and foot coverings
provided.
- Instruct the patient to cooperate fully
and to follow directions. Ask the patient
to remain still throughout the procedure
because movement produces unreliable results.
- Observe standard precautions, and follow the general guidelines in Appendix A.
- Place the patient in the supine position
on an examination table; other positions
may be used during the examination.
- Expose the area of interest and drape
the patient.
- Conductive gel is applied to the skin, and
a transducer is moved over the area to
obtain images of the area of interest.
Waveforms are visualized and recorded
with variations in respirations. Images with
and without compression are performed
proximally or distally to an obstruction to
obtain information about a venous occlusion or obstruction. The procedure can
be performed for both arms and legs to
obtain bilateral blood flow determination.
- Do not place the transducer on an
ulcer site when there is evidence of
venous stasis or ulcer.
- Ask the patient to breathe normally during the examination. If necessary for better organ visualization, ask the patient to
inhale deeply and hold his or her breath.

POST-TEST:
- A report of the results will be sent to
the requesting HCP, who will discuss
the results with the patient.

- When the study is completed, remove
the gel from the skin.
- Instruct the patient to continue diet,
fluids, and medications, as directed by
the HCP.
- *Nutritional Considerations:* Abnormal
findings may be associated with cardiovascular disease. The American Heart
Association and National Heart, Lung,
and Blood Institute (NHBLI) recommend
nutritional therapy for individuals identified to be at high risk for developing
coronary artery disease (CAD) or individuals who have specific risk factors and/
or existing medical conditions (e.g., elevated LDL cholesterol levels, other lipid
disorders, insulin-dependent diabetes,
insulin resistance, or metabolic syndrome). If overweight, the patient should
be encouraged to achieve a normal
weight. The NHLBI's National
Cholesterol Education Program (NCEP)
revised its dietary guidelines for reducing
CAD in 2001. Guidelines for the
Therapeutic Lifestyle Changes (TLC) diet
are outlined in the Third Report of the
Expert Panel on Detection, Evaluation,
and Treatment of High Blood
Cholesterol in Adults (Adult Treatment
Panel III [ATP III]). The TLC diet emphasizes a reduction in foods high in saturated fats and cholesterol. Red meats,
eggs, and dairy products are the major
sources of saturated fats and cholesterol.
If triglycerides also are elevated, the
patient should be advised to eliminate
or reduce alcohol and simple carbohydrates from the diet. The TLC approach
also includes the use of plant stanols or
sterols and increased dissolved fiber as
an option for lowering LDL cholesterol
levels; nutritional recommendations for
daily total caloric intake; recommendations for allowable percentage of calories derived from fat (saturated and
unsaturated), carbohydrates, protein,
and cholesterol; as well as recommendations for daily expenditure of energy.
- *Nutritional Considerations:* Overweight
patients with high blood pressure
should be encouraged to achieve a
normal weight. Other changeable risk
factors warranting patient education
include strategies to safely decrease
sodium intake, increase physical
activity, decrease alcohol consumption,

U

eliminate tobacco use, and decrease cholesterol levels.

Social and Cultural Considerations: Numerous studies point to the prevalence of excess body weight in American children and adolescents. Experts estimate that obesity is present in 25% of the population ages 6 to 11 yr. The medical, social, and emotional consequences of excess body weight are significant. Special attention should be given to instructing the child and caregiver regarding health risks and weight-control education.

◗ Recognize anxiety related to test results, and be supportive of fear of shortened life expectancy. Discuss the implications of abnormal test results on the patient's lifestyle. Provide teaching and information regarding the clinical implications of the test results, as appropriate. Educate the patient regarding access to counseling services. Provide contact information, if desired, for the American Heart Association (www.americanheart.org) or the NHLBI (www.nhlbi.nih.gov).

◗ Reinforce information given by the patient's HCP regarding further testing, treatment, or referral to another HCP. Answer any questions or address any concerns voiced by the patient or family.

◗ Depending on the results of this procedure, additional testing may be needed to evaluate or monitor progression of the disease process and determine the need for a change in therapy. Evaluate test results in relation to the patient's symptoms and other tests performed.

RELATED MONOGRAPHS:

◗ Related tests include alveolar/arterial ratio, angiography pulmonary, blood gases, CBC platelet count, CT angiography, D-dimer, FDP, fibrinogen, lung perfusion scan, lung ventilation scan, MRI abdomen, MRI angiography, aPTT, plethysmography, PT/INR, US arterial Doppler lower extremity studies, and venography lower extremities.

◗ Refer to the Cardiovascular System table at the end of the book for related tests by body system.

Upper Gastrointestinal and Small Bowel Series

SYNONYM/ACRONYM: Gastric radiography, stomach series, small bowel study, upper GI series, UGI.

COMMON USE: To assess the esophagus, stomach, and small bowel for disorders related to obstruction, perforation, weight loss, swallowing, pain, cancer, reflux disease, ulcers, and structural anomalies.

AREA OF APPLICATION: Esophagus, stomach, and small intestine.

CONTRAST: Barium sulfate.

DESCRIPTION: The upper gastrointestinal (GI) series is a radiological examination of the esophagus, stomach, and small intestine after ingestion of barium sulfate, which is a milkshake-like, radiopaque substance. A combination of x-ray and fluoroscopy techniques is used to record the study. Air may be instilled to provide double contrast and better visualization of the lumen of the esophagus, stomach, and duodenum. If perforation or obstruction is suspected, a water-soluble iodinated contrast medium is used. This test is especially useful in the evaluation of patients experiencing dysphagia, regurgitation, gastroesophageal reflux (GER), epigastric pain, hematemesis, melena, and unexplained weight loss. This test is also used to evaluate the results of gastric surgery, especially when an anastomotic leak is suspected. When a small bowel series is included, the test detects disorders of the jejunum and ileum. The patient's position is changed during the examination to allow visualization of the various structures and their function. The images are visualized on a fluoroscopic screen, recorded, and stored electronically or on x-ray film for review by a physician. Drugs such as glucagon may be given during an upper GI series to relax the GI tract; drugs such as metoclopramide (Reglan) may be given to accelerate the passage of the barium through the stomach and small intestine.

When the small bowel series is performed separately, the patient may be asked to drink several glasses of barium, or enteroclysis may be used to instill the barium. With enteroclysis, a catheter is passed through the nose or mouth and advanced past the pylorus and into the duodenum. Barium, followed by methylcellulose solution, is instilled via the catheter directly into the small bowel.

INDICATIONS
- Determine the cause of regurgitation or epigastric pain
- Determine the presence of neoplasms, ulcers, diverticula, obstruction, foreign body, and hiatal hernia
- Evaluate suspected GER, inflammatory process, congenital anomaly, motility disorder, or structural change
- Evaluate unexplained weight loss or anemia
- Identify and locate the origin of hematemesis

POTENTIAL DIAGNOSIS

Normal findings in
- Normal size, shape, position, and functioning of the esophagus, stomach, and small bowel

Abnormal findings in
- Achalasia
- Cancer of the esophagus
- Chalasis
- Congenital abnormalities
- Duodenal cancer, diverticula, and ulcers
- Esophageal diverticula, motility disorders, ulcers, varices, and inflammation
- Foreign body
- Gastric cancer, tumors, and ulcers
- Gastritis
- Hiatal hernia
- Perforation of the esophagus, stomach, or small bowel
- Polyps
- Small bowel tumors
- Strictures

CRITICAL FINDINGS
- Foreign body
- Perforated bowel
- Tumor with significant mass effect

It is essential that critical diagnoses be communicated immediately to the appropriate health-care provider (HCP). A listing of these diagnoses varies among facilities. Note and immediately report to the HCP abnormal results and related symptoms.

U

INTERFERING FACTORS

This procedure is contraindicated for

- Patients who are pregnant or suspected of being pregnant, unless the potential benefits of the procedure far outweigh the risks to the fetus and mother.
- Patients with an intestinal obstruction.
- Patients suspected of having upper GI perforation, in whom barium should not be used.

Factors that may impair clear imaging

- Inability of the patient to cooperate or remain still during the procedure because of age, significant pain, or mental status.
- Metallic objects (e.g., jewelry, body rings) within the examination field, which may inhibit organ visualization and cause unclear images.

Other considerations

- Failure to follow dietary restrictions before the procedure may cause the procedure to be canceled or repeated.
- Patients with swallowing problems may aspirate the barium, which could interfere with the procedure and cause patient complications.
- Possible constipation or partial bowel obstruction caused by retained barium in the small bowel or colon may affect test results.
- This procedure should be done after a kidney x-ray (IV pyelography) or computed tomography of the abdomen or pelvis.
- Consultation with a health-care provider (HCP) should occur before the procedure for radiation safety concerns regarding younger patients or patients who are lactating.
- Risks associated with radiation overexposure can result from frequent x-ray procedures. Personnel in the room with the patient should wear a protective lead apron, stand behind a shield, or leave the area while the examination is being done. Personnel working in the examination area should wear badges to record their level of radiation exposure.

NURSING IMPLICATIONS AND PROCEDURE

PRETEST:

- Positively identify the patient using at least two unique identifiers before providing care, treatment, or services.
- *Patient Teaching:* Inform the patient this procedure can assist in assessing the esophagus, stomach, and small intestine.
- Obtain a history of the patient's complaints, including a list of known allergens, especially allergies or sensitivities to latex, iodine, seafood, anesthetics, or contrast medium.
- Obtain a history of the patient's gastrointestinal system, symptoms, and results of previously performed laboratory tests and diagnostic and surgical procedures.
- Ensure that this procedure is performed before a barium swallow.
- Record the date of the last menstrual period and determine the possibility of pregnancy in perimenopausal women.
- Obtain a list of the patient's current medications, including anticoagulants, aspirin and other salicylates, herbs, nutritional supplements, and nutraceuticals, especially those known to affect coagulation (see Appendix F).
- Review the procedure with the patient. Address concerns about pain and explain that there may be moments of discomfort and some pain experienced during the procedure. Inform the patient that the procedure is usually performed in a radiology department by an HCP, with support staff, and takes approximately 30 to 60 min.
- *Sensitivity to social and cultural issues,* as well as concern for modesty, is important in providing psychological support before, during, and after the procedure.
- Explain to the patient that he or she will be asked to drink a milkshake-like solution that has an unpleasant chalky taste.
- Instruct the patient to remove jewelry and other metallic objects from the area to be examined prior to the procedure.

U

▶ Instruct the patient to fast and restrict fluids for 8 hr prior to the procedure. Protocols may vary among facilities.

INTRATEST:

▶ Ensure that the patient has complied with dietary and fluid restrictions for 8 hr prior to the procedure.

▶ Ensure that the patient has removed all external metallic objects from the area to be examined prior to the procedure.

▶ Have emergency equipment readily available.

▶ Instruct the patient to void prior to the procedure and to change into the gown, robe, and foot coverings provided.

▶ Instruct the patient to cooperate fully and to follow directions. Ask the patient to remain still throughout the procedure because movement produces unreliable results.

▶ Observe standard precautions, and follow the general guidelines in Appendix A.

Upper Gastrointestinal Series

▶ Place the patient on the x-ray table in a supine position, or ask the patient to stand in front of a fluoroscopy screen.

▶ Instruct the patient to take several swallows of the barium mixture through a straw while images are taken of the pharyngeal motion. An effervescent agent may also be administered to introduce air into the stomach.

Small Bowel Series

▶ If the small bowel is to be examined after the upper GI series, instruct the patient to drink an additional glass of barium while the small intestine is observed for passage of barium. Images are taken at 30- to 60-min intervals until the barium reaches the ileocecal valve. This process can last up to 5 hr, with follow-up images taken at 24 hr.

POST-TEST:

▶ A report of the examination will be sent to the requesting HCP, who will discuss the results with the patient.

▶ Instruct the patient to resume usual diet and fluids, as directed by the HCP.

▶ Monitor for reaction to iodinated contrast medium, including rash, urticaria,

tachycardia, hyperpnea, hypertension, palpitations, nausea, or vomiting, if iodine is used.

▶ Instruct the patient to immediately report symptoms such as fast heart rate, difficulty breathing, skin rash, itching, chest pain, persistent right shoulder pain, or abdominal pain. Immediately report symptoms to the appropriate HCP.

▶ Instruct the patient to take a mild laxative and increase fluid intake (four glasses) to aid in the elimination of barium unless contraindicated.

▶ Inform the patient that his or her stool will be white or light in color for 2 to 3 days. If the patient is unable to eliminate the barium, or if the stool does not return to normal color, the patient should notify the HCP.

▶ Recognize anxiety related to test results, and be supportive of perceived loss of independence and fear of shortened life expectancy. Discuss the implications of abnormal test results on the patient's lifestyle. Provide teaching and information regarding the clinical implications of the test results, as appropriate. Educate the patient regarding access to counseling services.

▶ Reinforce information given by the patient's HCP regarding further testing, treatment, or referral to another HCP. Answer any questions or address any concerns voiced by the patient or family.

▶ Depending on the results of this procedure, additional testing may be needed to evaluate or monitor progression of the disease process and determine the need for a change in therapy. Evaluate test results in relation to the patient's symptoms and other tests performed.

RELATED MONOGRAPHS:

▶ Related tests include barium enema, barium swallow, capsule endoscopy, CT abdomen, endoscopic retrograde cholangiopancreatography, esophageal manometry, fecal analysis, gastric acid stimulation test, gastric emptying scan, gastrin stimulation test, gastroesophageal reflux scan, *H. pylori* antibody, KUB study, MRI abdomen, and US pelvis.

▶ Refer to the Gastrointestinal System table at the end of the book for related tests by body system.

U

Urea Breath Test

SYNONYM/ACRONYM: PY test, C-14 urea breath test, breath test, pylori breath test, UBT.

COMMON USE: To assist in diagnosing a gastrointestinal infection and ulceration of the stomach or duodenum related to a *Helicobacter pylori* infection.

AREA OF APPLICATION: Stomach.

CONTRAST: Radioactive C-14 urea in capsule form.

DESCRIPTION: The C-14 urea breath test (UBT) is used to assist in the diagnosis of *Helicobacter pylori* infection. *H. pylori* is a bacteria that can infect the stomach lining. It has been implicated as the cause of many gastrointestinal conditions, including the development of duodenal and gastric ulcers. The UBT is a simple, noninvasive diagnostic nuclear medicine procedure that requires the patient to swallow a small amount of radiopharmaceutical C-14–labeled urea in a capsule with lukewarm water. In the presence of urease, an enzyme secreted by *H. pylori* in the gut, the urea in the capsule is broken down into nitrogen and C-14–labeled carbon dioxide (CO_2). The labeled CO_2 is absorbed through the stomach lining into the blood and excreted by the lungs. Breath samples are collected and trapped in a Mylar balloon. The C-14 urea is counted and quantitated with a liquid scintillation counter. The UBT can also be used to indicate the elimination of *H. pylori* infection after treatment with antibiotics. Other tests used to detect the presence of *H. pylori* include a blood *H. pylori* antibody test, a stool antigen test, and stomach biopsy.

INDICATIONS
- Aid in detection of *H. pylori* infection in the stomach
- Monitor eradication of *H. pylori* infection following treatment regimen
- Evaluation of new-onset dyspepsia

POTENTIAL DIAGNOSIS

Normal findings in
- Negative for *H. pylori*: Less than 50 dpm (disintegrations per minute)

Abnormal findings in
- Indeterminate for *H. pylori*: 50 to 199 dpm
- Positive for *H. pylori*: Greater than 200 dpm

CRITICAL FINDINGS: N/A

INTERFERING FACTORS

This procedure is contraindicated for
- Patients who are pregnant or suspected of being pregnant, unless the potential benefits of the procedure outweigh the risks to the fetus and the mother.

- Patients who have taken antibiotics, Pepto-Bismol, or bismuth in the past 30 days.
- Patients who have taken sucralfate in the past 14 days.
- Patients who have used a proton pump inhibitor within the past 14 days.

Other considerations
- Consultation with a health-care provider (HCP) should occur before the procedure for radiation safety concerns regarding younger patients or patients who are lactating.
- Failure to follow dietary restrictions and other pretesting preparations may cause the procedure to be canceled or repeated.
- Patients who have had resective gastric surgery have the potential for resultant bacterial overgrowth (non-*H. pylori* urease), which can cause a false-positive result.
- Achlorhydria can cause a false-positive result.

NURSING IMPLICATIONS AND PROCEDURE

PRETEST:
- Positively identify the patient using at least two unique identifiers before providing care, treatment, or services.
- *Patient Teaching:* Inform the patient this procedure can assist in diagnosing an infection of the stomach or intestine.
- Obtain a history of the patient's gastrointestinal system, symptoms, and results of previously performed laboratory tests and diagnostic and surgical procedures.
- Record the date of the last menstrual period and determine the possibility of pregnancy in premenopausal women.
- Obtain a list of the patient's current medications, including herbs, nutritional supplements, and nutraceuticals (see Appendix F).
- Review the procedure with the patient. Reassure the patient that the radionuclide poses no radioactive hazard and rarely produces side effects. Address concerns about pain and explain that there should be no discomfort during the procedure. Inform the patient that the procedure is done in the nuclear medicine department by technologists and support staff and usually takes approximately 30 to 60 min.
- *Sensitivity to social and cultural issues,* as well as concern for modesty, is important in providing psychological support before, during, and after the procedure.
- Instruct the patient to fast, restrict fluids, and, by medical direction, withhold medication for 6 hr prior to the procedure. Protocols may vary among facilities.

INTRATEST:
- Ensure the patient has complied with dietary and medication restrictions and pretesting preparations; assure that food, fluids, and medications have been restricted for at least 6 hr prior to the procedure.
- Instruct the patient to blow into a balloon prior to the start of the procedure to collect a sample of breath.
- Instruct the patient to swallow the C-14 capsule directly from a cup, followed by 20 mL of lukewarm water. Provide an additional 20 mL of lukewarm water for the patient to drink at 3 min after the dose.
- Breath samples are taken at different periods of time by instructing the patient to take in a deep breath and hold it for approximately 5 to 10 sec before exhaling through a straw into a Mylar balloon.
- Samples are counted on a liquid scintillation counter (LSC) and recorded in disintegrations per minute.

POST-TEST:
- A report of the examination will be sent to the requesting HCP, who will discuss the results with the patient.

- Instruct the patient to resume usual diet and medication, as directed by the HCP.
- Unless contraindicated, advise patient to drink increased amounts of fluids for 12 to 24 hr to eliminate the radionuclide from the body.
- If a woman who is breastfeeding must have a breathe test, she should not breastfeed the infant until the radionuclide has been eliminated. She should be instructed to express the milk and discard it during a 3-day period to prevent cessation of milk production.
- Recognize anxiety related to test results. Discuss the implications of abnormal test results on the patient's lifestyle. Provide teaching and information regarding the clinical implications of the test results, as appropriate.

- Reinforce information given by the patient's HCP regarding further testing, treatment, or referral to another HCP. Answer any questions or address any concerns voiced by the patient or family.
- Depending on the results of the procedure, additional testing may be performed to evaluate or monitor progression of the disease process and determine the need for change in therapy. Evaluate test results in relation to the patient's symptoms and other tests performed.

RELATED MONOGRAPHS:

- Related tests include EGD, gastric emptying scan, *H. pylori* antibody, KUB study, and UGI.
- See the Gastrointestinal System table at the end of the book for related tests by body system.

Urea Nitrogen, Blood

SYNONYM/ACRONYM: BUN.

COMMON USE: To assist in assessing for renal function and to assist in diagnosing disorders such as kidney failure and dehydration. Also used in monitoring the effectiveness of therapeutic interventions such as hemodialysis.

SPECIMEN: Serum (1 mL) collected in a red- or tiger-top tube. Plasma (1 mL) collected in a green-top (heparin) tube is also acceptable.

REFERENCE VALUE: (Method: Spectrophotometry)

Age	Conventional Units	SI Units (Conventional Units × 0.357)
Newborn–3 yr	5–17 mg/dL	1.8–6.0 mmol/L
4–13 yr	7–17 mg/dL	2.5–6.0 mmol/L
14 yr–adult	8–21 mg/dL	2.9–7.5 mmol/L
Adult older than 90 yr	10–31 mg/dL	3.6–11.1 mmol/L

DESCRIPTION: Urea is a nonprotein nitrogen compound formed in the liver from ammonia as an end product of protein metabolism. Urea diffuses freely into extracellular and intracellular fluid and is ultimately excreted by the kidneys. Blood urea nitrogen (BUN) levels reflect the balance between the production and excretion of urea. BUN and creatinine values are commonly evaluated together. The normal BUN/creatinine ratio is 15:1 to 24:1. (e.g., if a patient has a BUN of 15 mg/dL, the creatinine should be approximately 0.6 to 1.0 mg/dL). BUN is used in the following calculation to estimate serum osmolality:

$$(2 \times Na^+) + (glucose/18) + (BUN/2.8).$$

INDICATIONS
- Assess nutritional support
- Evaluate hemodialysis therapy
- Evaluate hydration
- Evaluate liver function
- Evaluate patients with lymphoma after chemotherapy (tumor lysis)
- Evaluate renal function
- Monitor the effects of drugs known to be nephrotoxic or hepatotoxic

POTENTIAL DIAGNOSIS

Increased in
- Acute renal failure (*related to decreased renal excretion*)
- Chronic glomerulonephritis (*related to decreased renal excretion*)
- Congestive heart failure (*related to decreased blood flow to the kidneys, decreased renal excretion, and accumulation in circulating blood*)
- Decreased renal perfusion (*reflects decreased renal excretion and increased blood levels*)

- Diabetes (*related to decreased renal excretion*)
- Excessive protein ingestion (*related to increased protein metabolism*)
- Gastrointestinal (GI) bleeding (*excessive blood protein in the GI tract and increased protein metabolism*)
- Hyperalimentation (*related to increased protein metabolism*)
- Hypovolemia (*related to decreased blood flow to the kidneys, decreased renal excretion, and accumulation in circulating blood*)
- Ketoacidosis (*dehydration from ketoacidosis correlates with decreased renal excretion of urea nitrogen*)
- Muscle wasting from starvation (*related to increased protein metabolism*)
- Neoplasms (*related to increased protein metabolism or to decreased renal excretion*)
- Nephrotoxic agents (*related to decreased renal excretion and accumulation in circulating blood*)
- Pyelonephritis (*related to decreased renal excretion*)
- Shock (*related to decreased blood flow to the kidneys, decreased renal excretion, and accumulation in circulating blood*)
- Urinary tract obstruction (*related to decreased renal excretion and accumulation in circulating blood*)

Decreased in
- Inadequate dietary protein (*urea nitrogen is a by-product of protein metabolism; less available protein is reflected in decreased BUN levels*)
- Low-protein/high-carbohydrate diet (*urea nitrogen is a by-product of protein metabolism; less

U

available protein is reflected in decreased BUN levels)

- Malabsorption syndromes *(urea nitrogen is a by-product of protein metabolism; less available protein is reflected in decreased BUN levels)*
- Pregnancy
- Severe liver disease *(BUN is synthesized in the liver, so liver damage results in decreased levels)*

CRITICAL FINDINGS ✦

- Greater than 100 mg/dL (nondialysis patients)

Note and immediately report to the health-care provider (HCP) any critically increased or decreased values and related symptoms.

A patient with a grossly elevated BUN may have signs and symptoms including acidemia, agitation, confusion, fatigue, nausea, vomiting, and coma. Possible interventions include treatment of the cause, administration of IV bicarbonate, a low-protein diet, hemodialysis, and caution with respect to prescribing and continuing nephrotoxic medications.

INTERFERING FACTORS

- Drugs, substances, and vitamins that may increase BUN levels include acetaminophen, alanine, aldatense, alkaline antacids, amphotericin B, antimony compounds, arsenicals, bacitracin, bismuth subsalicylate, capreomycin, carbenoxolone, carbutamide, cephalosporins, chloral hydrate, chloramphenicol, chlorthalidone, colistimethate, colistin, cotrimoxazole, dexamethasone, dextran, diclofenac, doxycycline, ethylene glycol, gentamicin, guanethidine, guanoxan, ibuprofen, ifosfamide, ipodate, kanamycin, mephenesin, metolazone, mitomycin, neomycin, phosphorus,

plicamycin, tertatolol, tetracycline, triamterene, triethylenemelamine, viomycin, and vitamin D.
- Drugs that may decrease BUN levels include acetohydroxamic acid, chloramphenicol, fluorides, paramethasone, phenothiazine, and streptomycin.

NURSING IMPLICATIONS AND PROCEDURE

PRETEST:

- Positively identify the patient using at least two unique identifiers before providing care, treatment, or services.
- *Patient Teaching:* Inform the patient this test can assist in assessing kidney function.
- Obtain a history of the patient's complaints, including a list of known allergens, especially allergies or sensitivities to latex.
- Obtain a history of the patient's genitourinary and hepatobiliary systems, symptoms, and results of previously performed laboratory tests and diagnostic and surgical procedures.
- Obtain a list of the patient's current medications, including herbs, nutritional supplements, and nutraceuticals (see Appendix F).
- Review the procedure with the patient. Inform the patient that specimen collection takes approximately 5 to 10 min. Address concerns about pain and explain that there may be some discomfort during the venipuncture.
- *Sensitivity to social and cultural issues,* as well as concern for modesty, is important in providing psychological support before, during, and after the procedure.
- There are no food, fluid, or medication restrictions unless by medical direction.

INTRATEST:

- If the patient has a history of allergic reaction to latex, avoid the use of equipment containing latex.

U

- Instruct the patient to cooperate fully and to follow directions. Direct the patient to breathe normally and to avoid unnecessary movement.
- Observe standard precautions, and follow the general guidelines in Appendix A. Positively identify the patient, and label the appropriate tubes with the corresponding patient demographics, date, and time of collection. Perform a venipuncture.
- Remove the needle and apply direct pressure with dry gauze to stop bleeding. Observe/assess venipuncture site for bleeding or hematoma formation and secure gauze with adhesive bandage.
- Promptly transport the specimen to the laboratory for processing and analysis.

POST-TEST:

- A report of the results will be sent to the requesting HCP, who will discuss the results with the patient.
- Monitor intake and output for fluid imbalance in renal dysfunction and dehydration.
- *Nutritional Considerations:* Nitrogen balance is commonly used as a nutritional assessment tool to indicate protein change. In healthy individuals, protein anabolism and catabolism are in equilibrium. During various disease states, nutritional intake decreases, resulting in a negative balance. During recovery from illness and with proper nutritional support, the nitrogen balance becomes positive. BUN is an important analyte to measure during administration of total parenteral nutrition (TPN). Educate the patient, as appropriate, in dietary adjustments required to maintain proper nitrogen balance. Inform the patient that the requesting HCP may prescribe TPN as part of the treatment plan.

- *Nutritional Considerations:* An elevated BUN can be caused by a high-protein diet or dehydration. Unless medically restricted, a healthy diet consisting of the five food groups of the food pyramid should be consumed daily. Water consumption should include six to eight 8-oz glasses of water per day, or water consumption equivalent to half of the body's weight in fluid ounces (32 fl oz = 1 qt; 34 fl oz = 1 L).
- Recognize anxiety related to test results. Discuss the implications of abnormal test results on the patient's lifestyle. Provide teaching and information regarding the clinical implications of the test results, as appropriate.
- Reinforce information given by the patient's HCP regarding further testing, treatment, or referral to another HCP. Answer any questions or address any concerns voiced by the patient or family.
- Depending on the results of this procedure, additional testing may be performed to evaluate or monitor progression of the disease process and determine the need for a change in therapy. Evaluate test results in relation to the patient's symptoms and other tests performed.

RELATED MONOGRAPHS:

- Related tests include anion gap, antibiotic drugs, biopsy kidney, calcium, calculus kidney stone panel, CT spleen, creatinine, creatinine clearance, cytology urine, cystoscopy, electrolytes, gallium scan, glucose, glycated hemoglobin, 5–HIAA, IVP, ketones, magnesium, microalbumin, osmolality, oxalate, phosphorus, protein total and fractions, renogram, US kidney, UA, urea nitrogen urine, and uric acid.
- Refer to the Genitourinary and Hepatobiliary systems tables at the end of the book for related tests by body system.

U

Urea Nitrogen, Urine

SYNONYM/ACRONYM: N/A.

COMMON USE: To assess renal function related to the progression of disorders such as diabetes, liver disease, and renal disease.

SPECIMEN: Urine (5 mL) from an unpreserved random or timed specimen collected in a clean plastic collection container.

REFERENCE VALUE: (Method: Spectrophotometry)

Conventional Units	SI Units (Conventional Units × 35.7)
12–20 g/24 hr	428–714 mmol/24 hr

DESCRIPTION: Urea is a nonprotein nitrogen compound formed in the liver from ammonia as an end product of protein metabolism. Urea diffuses freely into extracellular and intracellular fluid and is ultimately excreted by the kidneys. Urine urea nitrogen levels reflect the balance between the production and excretion of urea.

INDICATIONS

- Evaluate renal disease
- Predict the impact that other conditions, such as diabetes and liver disease, will have on the kidneys

POTENTIAL DIAGNOSIS

Increased in
- Diabetes *(related to increased protein metabolism)*
- Hyperthyroidism
- Increased dietary protein *(related to increased protein metabolism)*
- Postoperative period

Decreased in
- Liver disease *(BUN is synthesized in the liver, so liver damage results in decreased levels)*
- Low-protein/high-carbohydrate diet *(urea nitrogen is a by-product of protein metabolism; less available protein is reflected in decreased BUN levels)*
- Normal-growing pediatric patients *(increased demand for protein; less available protein is reflected in decreased BUN levels)*
- Pregnancy *(increased demand for protein; less available protein is reflected in decreased BUN levels)*
- Renal disease *(related to decreased renal excretion)*
- Toxemia *(related to hypertension and decreased renal excretion)*

CRITICAL FINDINGS: N/A

INTERFERING FACTORS

- Drugs that may increase urine urea nitrogen levels include alanine and glycine.
- Drugs that may decrease urine urea nitrogen levels include furosemide,

growth hormone, insulin, and testosterone.

• All urine voided for the timed collection period must be included in the collection or else falsely decreased values may be obtained. Compare output records with volume collected to verify that all voids were included in the collection.

NURSING IMPLICATIONS AND PROCEDURE

PRETEST:

▶ Positively identify the patient using at least two unique identifiers before providing care, treatment, or services.

▶ *Patient Teaching:* Inform the patient this test can assist in assessing kidney function.

▶ Obtain a history of the patient's complaints, including a list of known allergens, especially allergies or sensitivities to latex.

▶ Obtain a history of the patient's genitourinary and hepatobiliary systems, symptoms, and results of previously performed laboratory tests and diagnostic and surgical procedures.

▶ Obtain a list of the patient's current medications, including herbs, nutritional supplements, and nutraceuticals (see Appendix F).

▶ Review the procedure with the patient. Provide a nonmetallic urinal, bedpan, or toilet-mounted collection device. Address concerns about pain and explain that there should be no discomfort during the procedure.

▶ Usually a 24-hr time frame for urine collection is ordered. Inform the patient that all urine must be saved during that 24-hr period. Instruct the patient not to void directly into the laboratory collection container. Instruct the patient to avoid defecating in the collection device and to keep toilet tissue out of the collection device to prevent contamination of the specimen. Place a sign in the bathroom to remind the patient to save all urine.

▶ Instruct the patient to void all urine into the collection device and then to pour the urine into the laboratory collection container. Alternatively, the specimen can be left in the collection device for a health-care staff member to add to the laboratory collection container.

▶ *Sensitivity to social and cultural issues,* as well as concern for modesty, is important in providing psychological support before, during, and after the procedure.

▶ There are no food, fluid, or medication restrictions unless by medical direction.

INTRATEST:

▶ If the patient has a history of allergic reaction to latex, avoid the use of equipment containing latex.

▶ Instruct the patient to cooperate fully and to follow directions.

▶ Observe standard precautions, and follow the general guidelines in Appendix A. Positively identify the patient, and label the appropriate collection container with the corresponding patient demographics, date, and time of collection.

Random Specimen (Collect in Early Morning)

Clean-Catch Specimen

▶ Instruct the male patient to (1) thoroughly wash his hands, (2) cleanse the meatus, (3) void a small amount into the toilet, and (4) void directly into the specimen container.

▶ Instruct the female patient to (1) thoroughly wash her hands; (2) cleanse the labia from front to back; (3) while keeping the labia separated, void a small amount into the toilet; and (4) without interrupting the urine stream, void directly into the specimen container.

Indwelling Catheter

▶ Put on gloves. Empty drainage tube of urine. It may be necessary to clamp off the catheter for 15 to 30 min before specimen collection. Cleanse specimen port with antiseptic swab, and then aspirate 5 mL of urine with a 21- to 25-gauge needle and syringe. Transfer urine to a sterile container.

U

Timed Specimen

- Obtain a clean 3-L urine specimen container, toilet-mounted collection device, and plastic bag (for transport of the specimen container). The specimen must be refrigerated or kept on ice throughout the entire collection period. If an indwelling urinary catheter is in place, the drainage bag must be kept on ice.
- Begin the test between 6 and 8 a.m. if possible. Collect first voiding and discard. Record the time the specimen was discarded as the beginning of the timed collection period. The next morning, ask the patient to void at the same time the collection was started and add this last voiding to the container. Urinary output should be recorded throughout the collection time.
- If an indwelling catheter is in place, replace the tubing and container system at the start of the collection time. Keep the container system on ice during the collection period, or empty the urine into a larger container periodically during the collection period; monitor to ensure continued drainage, and conclude the test the next morning at the same hour the collection was begun.
- At the conclusion of the test, compare the quantity of urine with the urinary output record for the collection; if the specimen contains less than what was recorded as output, some urine may have been discarded, invalidating the test.
- Include on the collection container's label the amount of urine, test start and stop times, and ingestion of any medications that can affect test results.

General

- Promptly transport the specimen to the laboratory for processing and analysis.

POST-TEST:

- A report of the results will be sent to the requesting health-care provider (HCP), who will discuss the results with the patient.
- *Nutritional Considerations:* An elevated BUN can be caused by a high-protein diet or dehydration. Unless medically restricted, a healthy diet consisting of the five food groups of the food pyramid should be consumed daily. Water consumption should include six to eight 8-oz glasses of water per day, or water consumption equivalent to half of the body's weight in fluid ounces (32 fl oz = 1 qt; 34 fl oz = 1 L).
- Recognize anxiety related to test results. Discuss the implications of abnormal test results on the patient's lifestyle. Provide teaching and information regarding the clinical implications of the test results, as appropriate.
- Reinforce information given by the patient's HCP regarding further testing, treatment, or referral to another HCP. Answer any questions or address any concerns voiced by the patient or family.
- Depending on the results of this procedure, additional testing may be performed to evaluate or monitor progression of the disease process and determine the need for a change in therapy. Evaluate test results in relation to the patient's symptoms and other tests performed.

RELATED MONOGRAPHS:

- Related tests include anion gap, antibiotic drugs, biopsy kidney, BUN, calcium, calculus kidney stone panel, CT spleen, creatinine, creatinine clearance, cytology urine, cystoscopy, electrolytes, gallium scan, glucose, glycated hemoglobin, 5–HIAA, IVP, ketones, magnesium, microalbumin, osmolality, oxalate, phosphorus, protein total and fractions, renogram, US kidney, UA, and uric acid.
- Refer to the Genitourinary and Hepatobiliary systems tables at the end of the book for related tests by body system.

Urethrography, Retrograde

SYNONYM/ACRONYM: N/A.

COMMON USE: To assess urethral patency in order to evaluate the success of surgical interventions on patients who have urethral structures or other anomalies that interfere with urination.

AREA OF APPLICATION: Urethra.

CONTRAST: Radiopaque contrast medium.

DESCRIPTION: Retrograde urethrography is performed almost exclusively in male patients. It uses contrast medium, either injected or instilled via a catheter into the urethra, to visualize the membranous, bulbar, and penile portions, particularly after surgical repair of the urethra to assess the success of the surgery. The posterior portion of the urethra is visualized better when the procedure is performed with voiding cystourethrography. In women, it may be performed after surgical repair of the urethra to assess the success of the surgery and to assess structural abnormalities in conjunction with an evaluation for voiding dysfunction.

INDICATIONS
• Aid in the diagnosis of urethral strictures, lacerations, diverticula, and congenital anomalies

POTENTIAL DIAGNOSIS

Normal findings in
• Normal size, shape, and course of the membranous, bulbar, and penile portions of the urethra in male patients

• If the prostatic portion can be visualized, it also should appear normal

Abnormal findings in
• Congenital anomalies, such as urethral valves and perineal hypospadias
• False passages in the urethra
• Prostatic enlargement
• Tumors of the urethra
• Urethral calculi
• Urethral diverticula
• Urethral fistulas
• Urethral strictures and lacerations

CRITICAL FINDINGS: N/A

INTERFERING FACTORS

This procedure is contraindicated for
• Patients with allergies to shellfish or iodinated contrast medium. The contrast medium used may cause a life-threatening allergic reaction. Patients with a known hypersensitivity to the contrast medium may benefit from premedication with corticosteroids or the use of nonionic contrast medium.
• Patients who are pregnant or suspected of being pregnant, unless the potential benefits of the procedure far outweigh the risks to the fetus and mother.

U

- ❖ Elderly and other patients who are chronically dehydrated before the test, because of their risk of contrast-induced renal failure.
- ❖ Patients who are in renal failure.

Factors that may impair clear imaging
- Inability of the patient to cooperate or remain still during the procedure because of age, significant pain, or mental status.
- Metallic objects (e.g., jewelry, body rings) within the examination field, which may inhibit organ visualization and cause unclear images.

Other considerations
- Consultation with a health-care provider (HCP) should occur before the procedure for radiation safety concerns regarding younger patients or patients who are lactating.
- Risks associated with radiation overexposure can result from frequent x-ray procedures. Personnel in the room with the patient should wear a protective lead apron, stand behind a shield, or leave the area while the examination is being done. Personnel working in the examination area should wear badges to record their level of radiation exposure.

NURSING IMPLICATIONS AND PROCEDURE

PRETEST:
- Positively identify the patient using at least two unique identifiers before providing care, treatment, or services.

Patient Teaching: Inform the patient this procedure can assist in assessing the urethral patency.
- Obtain a history of the patient's complaints, including a list of known allergens, especially allergies or sensitivities to latex, iodine, seafood, anesthetics, or contrast medium.
- Obtain a history of the patient's genitourinary system, symptoms, and results of previously performed laboratory tests and diagnostic and surgical procedures.
- Ensure that this procedure is performed before an upper gastrointestinal study or barium swallow.
- Record the date of the last menstrual period and determine the possibility of pregnancy in perimenopausal women.
- Obtain a list of the patient's current medications, including herbs, nutritional supplements, and nutraceuticals (see Appendix F).
- Review the procedure with the patient. Address concerns about pain and explain that there may be moments of discomfort and some pain experienced during the procedure. Inform the patient that the procedure is performed in a cystoscopy room by an HCP, with support staff, and takes approximately 30 min.
- *Sensitivity to social and cultural issues,* as well as concern for modesty, is important in providing psychological support before, during, and after the procedure.
- Inform the patient that some pressure may be experienced when the catheter is inserted and contrast medium is instilled.
- Instruct the patient to remove jewelry and other metallic objects from the area to be examined prior to the procedure.
- There are no food or fluid restrictions unless by medical direction.
- *Make sure a written and informed consent has been signed prior to the procedure and before administering any medications.*

U

INTRATEST:

- Ensure the patient has removed all external metallic objects from the area to be examined prior to the procedure.
- Instruct the patient to void prior to the procedure and to change into the gown, robe, and foot coverings provided.
- Instruct the patient to cooperate fully and to follow directions. Ask the patient to lie still during the procedure because movement produces unclear images.
- Obtain and record the patient's baseline vital signs.
- Observe standard precautions, and follow the general guidelines in Appendix A.
- Place the patient on the table in a supine position.
- A single plain film is taken of the bladder and urethra.
- A catheter is filled with contrast medium to eliminate air pockets and is inserted until the balloon reaches the meatus. Inform the patient that the contrast medium may cause a temporary flushing of the face, a feeling of warmth, urticaria, headache, vomiting, or nausea.
- After three-fourths of the contrast medium is injected, another image is taken while the remainder of the contrast medium is injected.
- The procedure may be done on female patients using a double balloon to occlude the bladder neck from above and below the external meatus.

POST-TEST:

- A report of the examination will be sent to the requesting HCP, who will discuss the results with the patient.
- Instruct the patient to resume usual activities, as directed by the HCP.
- Monitor vital and neurological signs every 15 min until they return to preprocedure levels.
- Monitor fluid intake and urinary output for 24 hr after the procedure. Decreased urine output may indicate impending renal failure.
- Monitor for signs and symptoms of sepsis, including fever, chills, and severe pain in the kidney area.
- Instruct the patient to drink plenty of fluids to prevent stasis and to prevent the buildup of bacteria.
- Reinforce information given by the patient's HCP regarding further testing, treatment, or referral to another HCP. Answer any questions or address any concerns voiced by the patient or family.
- Depending on the results of this procedure, additional testing may be needed to evaluate or monitor progression of the disease process and determine the need for a change in therapy. Evaluate test results in relation to the patient's symptoms and other tests performed.

RELATED MONOGRAPHS:

- Related tests include CT abdomen, CT pelvis, cystometry, cystoscopy, IVP, MRI abdomen, PSA, renogram, retrograde ureteropyelography, urinalysis, and voiding cystourethrography.
- Refer to the Genitourinary System table at the end of the book for related tests by body system.

U

Uric Acid, Blood

SYNONYM/ACRONYM: Urate.

COMMON USE: To monitor uric acid levels during treatment for gout and evaluation of tissue destruction, liver damage, renal function, and monitor the effectiveness of therapeutic interventions.

SPECIMEN: Serum (1 mL) collected in a red- or tiger-top tube. Plasma (1 mL) collected in a green-top (heparin) tube is also acceptable.

REFERENCE VALUE: (Method: Spectrophotometry)

Age	Conventional Units	SI Units (Conventional Units × 0.059)
Child less than 12 yr	2.0–5.5 mg/dL	0.12–0.32 mmol/L
Adult younger than 60 yr		
Male	4.4–7.6 mg/dL	0.26–0.45 mmol/L
Female	2.3–6.6 mg/dL	0.14–0.39 mmol/L
Adult older than 60 yr		
Male	4.2–8.0 mg/dL	0.25–0.48 mmol/L
Female	3.5–7.3 mg/dL	0.21–0.43 mmol/L

DESCRIPTION: Uric acid is the end product of purine metabolism. Purines are important constituents of nucleic acids; purine turnover occurs continuously in the body, producing substantial amounts of uric acid even in the absence of purine intake from dietary sources such as organ meats (e.g., liver, thymus gland and/or pancreas [sweetbreads], kidney), legumes, and yeasts. Uric acid is filtered, absorbed, and secreted by the kidneys and is a common constituent of urine. Serum urate levels are affected by the amount of uric acid produced and by the efficiency of renal excretion. Values can vary based on diet, gender, body size, level of exercise, level of stress, and regularity in consumption of alcohol. Elevated uric acid levels can indicate conditions of critical cellular injury or destruction; hyperuricemia has an association with hypertension, hypertriglyceridemia, obesity, myocardial infarct, renal disease, and diabetes.

INDICATIONS
- Assist in the diagnosis of gout when there is a family history (autosomal dominant genetic disorder) or signs and symptoms of gout, indicated by elevated uric acid levels
- Determine the cause of known or suspected renal calculi
- Evaluate the extent of tissue destruction in infection, starvation, excessive exercise, malignancies, chemotherapy, or radiation therapy

U

- Evaluate possible liver damage in eclampsia, indicated by elevated uric acid levels
- Monitor the effects of drugs known to alter uric acid levels, either as a side effect or as a therapeutic effect

POTENTIAL DIAGNOSIS

Increased in

Conditions that result in high cellular turnover release nucleic acids into circulation, which are converted to uric acid by the liver.

- Acute tissue destruction as a result of starvation or excessive exercise *(related to cellular destruction)*
- Alcoholism
- Chemotherapy and radiation therapy *(related to high cellular turnover)*
- Chronic lead toxicity *(cellular destruction related to hemolysis)*
- Congestive heart failure *(related to cellular destruction)*
- Diabetes *(decreased renal excretion results in increased blood levels)*
- Down syndrome
- Eclampsia
- Excessive dietary purines *(purines are nucleic acid bases converted to uric acid by the liver)*
- Glucose-6-phosphate dehydrogenase deficiency *(cellular destruction related to hemolysis)*
- Gout *(usually related to excess dietary intake)*
- Hyperparathyroidism
- Hypertension *(related to effects on renal excretion)*
- Hypoparathyroidism *(related to disturbances in calcium and phosphorus homeostasis)*
- Lactic acidosis *(cellular destruction related to shock)*
- Lead poisoning *(cellular destruction related to hemolysis)*
- Lesch-Nyhan syndrome *(related to disorder of uric acid metabolism)*

- Multiple myeloma *(related to high cell turnover)*
- Pernicious anemia *(cellular destruction related to hemolysis)*
- Polycystic kidney disease *(related to decreased renal excretion, which results in increased blood levels)*
- Polycythemia *(related to increased cellular destruction)*
- Psoriasis
- Sickle cell anemia *(cellular destruction related to hemolysis)*
- Tumors *(related to high cell turnover)*
- Type III hyperlipidemia

Decreased in

- Fanconi's syndrome *(related to increased renal excretion)*
- Low-purine diet *(related to insufficient nutrients for liver to synthesize uric acid)*
- Severe liver disease *(uric acid synthesis occurs in the liver)*
- Wilson's disease *(affects normal liver function and is related to impaired tubular absorption)*

CRITICAL FINDINGS: N/A

INTERFERING FACTORS

- Drugs and substances that may increase uric acid levels include acetylsalicylic acid (low doses), aldatense, aminothiadiazole, anabolic steroids, antineoplastic agents, atenolol, azathioprine, azathymine, azauridine, chlorambucil, chlorthalidone, cisplatin, corn oil, cyclosporine, cyclothiazide, cytarabine, diapamide, diuretics, ethacrynic acid, ethambutol, ethoxzolamide, flumethiazide, hydrochlorothiazide, hydroflumethiazide, ibufenac, ibuprofen, levarterenol, mefruside, mercaptopurine, methicillin, methotrexate, methoxyflurane, methyclothiazide, mitomycin, morinamide, polythiazide, prednisone, pyrazinamide, quinethazone, salicylate, spironolactone, tacrolimus, theophylline, thiazide diuretics, thioguanine, thiotepa, triamterene, trichlormethiazide, vincristine, and warfarin.

- Drugs that may decrease uric acid levels include allopurinol, aspirin (high doses), azathioprine, benzbromaron, benziodarone, canola oil, chlorothiazide (given IV), chlorpromazine, chlorprothixene, cinchophen, clofibrate, corticosteroids, corticotropin, coumarin, dicumarol, enalapril, fenofibrate, flufenamic acid, guaifenesin, iodipamide, iodopyracet, iopanoic acid, ipodate, lisinopril, mefenamic acid, mersalyl, methotrexate, oxyphenbutazone, phenindione, phenolsulfonphthalein, probenecid, radiographic agents, seclazone, sulfinpyrazone, and verapamil.

NURSING IMPLICATIONS AND PROCEDURE

PRETEST:

- Positively identify the patient using at least two unique identifiers before providing care, treatment, or services.
- *Patient Teaching:* Inform the patient this test can assist in diagnosing gout and assessing kidney function.
- Obtain a history of the patient's complaints, including a list of known allergens, especially allergies or sensitivities to latex. Especially note pain and edema in joints and great toe (caused by precipitation of sodium urates), headache, fatigue, decreased urinary output, and hypertension.
- Obtain a history of the patient's genitourinary, hepatobiliary, and musculoskeletal systems; symptoms; and results of previously performed laboratory tests and diagnostic and surgical procedures.
- Obtain a list of the patient's current medications, including herbs, nutritional supplements, and nutraceuticals (see Appendix F).

- Review the procedure with the patient. Inform the patient that specimen collection takes approximately 5 to 10 min. Address concerns about pain and explain that there may be some discomfort during the venipuncture.
- *Sensitivity to social and cultural issues,* as well as concern for modesty, is important in providing psychological support before, during, and after the procedure.
- There are no food, fluid, or medication restrictions unless by medical direction.

INTRATEST:

- If the patient has a history of allergic reaction to latex, avoid the use of equipment containing latex.
- Instruct the patient to cooperate fully and to follow directions. Direct the patient to breathe normally and to avoid unnecessary movement.
- Observe standard precautions, and follow the general guidelines in Appendix A. Positively identify the patient, and label the appropriate tubes with the corresponding patient demographics, date, and time of collection. Perform a venipuncture.
- Remove the needle and apply direct pressure with dry gauze to stop bleeding. Observe/assess venipuncture site for bleeding or hematoma formation and secure gauze with adhesive bandage.
- Promptly transport the specimen to the laboratory for processing and analysis.

POST-TEST:

- A report of the results will be sent to the requesting health-care provider (HCP), who will discuss the results with the patient.
- *Nutritional Considerations:* Increased uric acid levels may be associated with the formation of kidney stones. Educate the patient, if appropriate, on the importance of drinking a sufficient amount of water when kidney stones are suspected.
- *Nutritional Considerations:* Increased uric acid levels may be associated with gout. Nutritional therapy may be appropriate for some patients identified as having gout. Educate the patient that foods high in oxalic acid include caffeinated beverages, raw

U

blackberries, gooseberries and plums, whole-wheat bread, beets, carrots, beans, rhubarb, spinach, dry cocoa, and Ovaltine. Foods high in purines include organ meats, which should be restricted. In other cases, the requesting HCP may not prescribe a low-purine or purine-restricted diet for treatment of gout because medications can control the condition easily and effectively.

▶ Recognize anxiety related to test results. Discuss the implications of abnormal test results on the patient's lifestyle. Provide teaching and information regarding the clinical implications of the test results, as appropriate.

▶ Reinforce information given by the patient's HCP regarding further testing, treatment, or referral to another HCP. Answer any questions or address any concerns voiced by the patient or family.

▶ Depending on the results of this procedure, additional testing may be performed to evaluate or monitor progression of the disease process and determine the need for a change in therapy. Evaluate test results in relation to the patient's symptoms and other tests performed.

RELATED MONOGRAPHS:

▶ Related tests include arthroscopy, biopsy bone marrow, calcium, calculus kidney stone panel, cholesterol, collagen cross-linked telopeptide, CBC, CBC RBC count, CBC RBC indices, CBC RBC morphology, creatinine, creatinine clearance, gastrin stimulation, G6PD, lactic acid, lead, PTH, parathyroid scan, phosphorus, sickle cell screen, synovial fluid analysis, UA, and uric acid urine.

▶ Refer to the Genitourinary, Hepatobiliary, and Musculoskeletal systems tables at the end of the book for related tests by body system.

Uric Acid, Urine

SYNONYM/ACRONYM: Urine urate.

COMMON USE: To assist in confirming a diagnosis of gout, assess renal function, evaluate for genetic defects related to uric acid levels, and monitor the effectiveness of therapeutic interventions.

SPECIMEN: Urine (5 mL) from a random or timed specimen collected in a clean plastic, unrefrigerated collection container. Sodium hydroxide preservative may be recommended to prevent precipitation of urates.

REFERENCE VALUE: (Method: Spectrophotometry)

Gender	Conventional Units*	SI Units (Conventional Units × 0.0059)
Male	250–800 mg/24 hr	1.48–4.72 mmol/24 hr
Female	250–750 mg/24 hr	1.48–4.43 mmol/24 hr

*Values reflect average purine diet.

U

DESCRIPTION: Uric acid is the end product of purine metabolism. Purines are important constituents of nucleic acids; purine turnover occurs continuously in the body, producing substantial amounts of uric acid even in the absence of purine intake from dietary sources such as organ meats (e.g., liver, thymus gland and/or pancreas [sweetbreads], kidney), legumes, and yeasts. Uric acid is filtered, absorbed, and secreted by the kidneys and is a common constituent of urine. The ratio of 24-hr urine uric acid to creatinine can be used as a test for detection of the Lesch-Nyhan syndrome, a disorder of uric acid metabolism associated with absence of the enzyme hypoxanthine-guanine phosphoribosyltransferase. The ratio in healthy patients is reported to range from 0.21 to 0.59. Patients with partial or complete enzyme deficiency can have ratios from 2.0 to 5.0.

INDICATIONS
- Compare urine and serum uric acid levels to provide an index of renal function
- Detect enzyme deficiencies and metabolic disturbances that affect the body's production of uric acid
- Monitor the response to therapy with uricosuric drugs
- Monitor urinary effects of disorders that cause hyperuricemia

POTENTIAL DIAGNOSIS

Increased in
- Disorders associated with impaired renal tubular absorption, such as Fanconi's syndrome and Wilson's disease
- Disorders of purine metabolism
- Excessive dietary intake of purines

- Gout
- Neoplastic disorders, such as leukemia, lymphosarcoma, and multiple myeloma *(related to increased cell turnover)*
- Pernicious anemia *(related to increased cell turnover)*
- Polycythemia vera *(related to increased cell turnover)*
- Renal calculus formation *(related to increased urinary excretion)*
- Sickle cell anemia *(related to increased cell turnover)*

Decreased in
- Chronic alcohol ingestion *(related to decreased excretion)*
- Hypertension *(related to decreased excretion)*
- Severe renal damage *(possibly resulting from chronic glomerulonephritis, collagen disorders, diabetic glomerulosclerosis, lactic acidosis, ketoacidosis, or alcohol abuse)*

CRITICAL FINDINGS: N/A

INTERFERING FACTORS
- Drugs that may increase urine uric acid levels include acetohexamide, ampicillin, ascorbic acid, azapropazone, benzbromarone, chlorpromazine, chlorprothixene, corticotropin, coumarin, dicumarol, ethyl biscoumacetate, iodipamide, iodopyracet, iopanoic acid, ipodate, mannose, merbarone, mercaptopurine, mersalyl, methotrexate, niacinamide, nifedipine, phenindione, phenolsulfonphthalein, phenylbutazone, phloridzin, probenecid, salicylates (long-term, large doses), seclazone, sulfinpyrazone, and verapamil.
- Drugs that may decrease urine uric acid levels include acetazolamide, allopurinol, angiotensin, benzbromarone, bumetanide, chlorothiazide, chlorthalidone, ethacrynic acid, ethambutol, ethoxzolamide, hydrochlorothiazide, levarterenol,

niacin, pyrazinoic acid, and thiazide diuretics.

- All urine voided for the timed collection period must be included in the collection or else falsely decreased values may be obtained. Compare output records with volume collected to verify that all voids were included in the collection.

NURSING IMPLICATIONS AND PROCEDURE

PRETEST:

- Positively identify the patient using at least two unique identifiers before providing care, treatment, or services.
- *Patient Teaching:* Inform the patient this test can assist in diagnosing gout and kidney disease.
- Obtain a history of the patient's complaints, including a list of known allergens, especially allergies or sensitivities to latex.
- Obtain a history of the patient's genitourinary system, symptoms, and results of previously performed laboratory tests and diagnostic and surgical procedures.
- Obtain a list of the patient's current medications, including herbs, nutritional supplements, and nutraceuticals (see Appendix F).
- Review the procedure with the patient. Provide a nonmetallic urinal, bedpan, or toilet-mounted collection device. Address concerns about pain and explain that there should be no discomfort during the procedure.
- Usually a 24-hr time frame for urine collection is ordered. Inform the patient that all urine must be saved during that 24-hr period. Instruct the patient not to void directly into the laboratory collection container. Instruct the patient to avoid defecating in the collection device and to keep toilet tissue out of the collection device to prevent contamination of the specimen. Place a sign in the bathroom to remind the patient to save all urine.

- Instruct the patient to void all urine into the collection device and then to pour the urine into the laboratory collection container. Alternatively, the specimen can be left in the collection device for a health-care staff member to add to the laboratory collection container.
- *Sensitivity to social and cultural issues,* as well as concern for modesty, is important in providing psychological support before, during, and after the procedure.
- There are no food, fluid, or medication restrictions unless by medical direction.

INTRATEST:

- If the patient has a history of allergic reaction to latex, avoid the use of equipment containing latex.
- Instruct the patient to cooperate fully and to follow directions.
- Observe standard precautions, and follow the general guidelines in Appendix A. Positively identify the patient, and label the appropriate collection containers with the corresponding patient demographics, date, and time of collection.

Random Specimen (Collect in Early Morning)
Clean-Catch Specimen
- Instruct the male patient to (1) thoroughly wash his hands, (2) cleanse the meatus, (3) void a small amount into the toilet, and (4) void directly into the specimen container.
- Instruct the female patient to (1) thoroughly wash her hands; (2) cleanse the labia from front to back; (3) while keeping the labia separated, void a small amount into the toilet; and (4) without interrupting the urine stream, void directly into the specimen container.

Indwelling Catheter
- Put on gloves. Empty drainage tube of urine. It may be necessary to clamp off the catheter for 15 to 30 min before specimen collection. Cleanse specimen port with antiseptic swab, and then aspirate 5 mL of urine with a 21- to 25-gauge needle and syringe. Transfer urine to a sterile container.

U

Timed Specimen

▶ Obtain a clean 3-L urine specimen container, toilet-mounted collection device, and plastic bag (for transport of the specimen container). The specimen must be refrigerated or kept on ice throughout the entire collection period. If an indwelling urinary catheter is in place, the drainage bag must be kept on ice.

▶ Begin the test between 6 and 8 a.m. if possible. Collect first voiding and discard. Record the time the specimen was discarded as the beginning of the timed collection period. The next morning, ask the patient to void at the same time the collection was started and add this last voiding to the container. Urinary output should be recorded throughout the collection time.

▶ If an indwelling catheter is in place, replace the tubing and container system at the start of the collection time. Keep the container system on ice during the collection period, or empty the urine into a larger container periodically during the collection period; monitor to ensure continued drainage, and conclude the test the next morning at the same hour the collection was begun.

▶ At the conclusion of the test, compare the quantity of urine with the urinary output record for the collection; if the specimen contains less than what was recorded as output, some urine may have been discarded, invalidating the test.

▶ Include on the collection container's label the amount of urine, test start and stop times, and any medications that can affect test results.

General

▶ Promptly transport the specimen to the laboratory for processing and analysis.

POST-TEST:

▶ A report of the results will be sent to the requesting health-care provider (HCP), who will discuss the results with the patient.

▶ Increased uric acid levels may be associated with the formation of kidney stones. Educate the patient, if appropriate, on the importance of drinking a sufficient amount of water when kidney stones are suspected.

▶ *Nutritional Considerations:* Increased uric acid levels may be associated with gout. Nutritional therapy may be appropriate for some patients identified as having gout. Educate the patient that foods high in oxalic acid include caffeinated beverages, raw blackberries, gooseberries and plums, whole-wheat bread, beets, carrots, beans, rhubarb, spinach, dry cocoa, and Ovaltine. Foods high in purines include organ meats, which should be restricted. In other cases, the requesting HCP may not prescribe a low-purine or purine-restricted diet for treatment of gout because medications can control the condition easily and effectively.

▶ Recognize anxiety related to test results. Discuss the implications of abnormal test results on the patient's lifestyle. Provide teaching and information regarding the clinical implications of the test results, as appropriate.

▶ Reinforce information given by the patient's HCP regarding further testing, treatment, or referral to another HCP. Answer any questions or address any concerns voiced by the patient or family.

▶ Depending on the results of this procedure, additional testing may be performed to evaluate or monitor progression of the disease process and determine the need for a change in therapy. Evaluate test results in relation to the patient's symptoms and other tests performed.

RELATED MONOGRAPHS:

▶ Related tests include arthroscopy, biopsy bone marrow, calcium, calculus kidney stone panel, cholesterol, collagen cross-linked telopeptide, CBC, CBC RBC count, CBC RBC indices, CBC RBC morphology, creatinine, creatinine clearance, gastrin stimulation, G6PD, lactic acid, lead, oxalate, PTH, parathyroid scan, phosphorus, sickle cell screen, synovial fluid analysis, UA, and uric acid blood.

▶ Refer to the Genitourinary System table at the end of the book for related tests by body system.

U

Urinalysis

SYNONYM/ACRONYM: UA.

COMMON USE: To screen urine for multiple substances such as infection, blood, sugar, bilirubin, urobilinogen, nitrates, and protein to assist in diagnosing disorders such as renal and liver disease as well as assess hydration status.

SPECIMEN: Urine (15 mL) from an unpreserved, random specimen collected in a clean plastic collection container.

REFERENCE VALUE: (Method: Macroscopic evaluation by dipstick and microscopic examination) Urinalysis comprises a battery of tests including a description of the color and appearance of urine; measurement of specific gravity and pH; and semiquantitative measurement of protein, glucose, ketones, urobilinogen, bilirubin, hemoglobin, nitrites, and leukocyte esterase. Urine sediment may also be examined for the presence of crystals, casts, renal epithelial cells, transitional epithelial cells, squamous epithelial cells, white blood cells (WBCs), red blood cells (RBCs), bacteria, yeast, sperm, and any other substances excreted in the urine that may have clinical significance. Examination of urine sediment is performed microscopically under high power, and results are reported as the number seen per high-power field (hpf). The color of normal urine ranges from light yellow to deep amber. The color depends on the patient's state of hydration (more concentrated samples are darker in color), diet, medication regimen, and exposure to other substances that may contribute to unusual color or odor. The appearance of normal urine is clear. Cloudiness is sometimes attributable to the presence of amorphous phosphates or urates as well as blood, WBCs, fat, or bacteria. Normal specific gravity is 1.001 to 1.029.

Dipstick

pH	5.0–9.0
Protein	Less than 20 mg/dL
Glucose	Negative
Ketones	Negative
Hemoglobin	Negative
Bilirubin	Negative
Urobilinogen	Up to 1 mg/dL
Nitrite	Negative
Leukocyte esterase	Negative
Specific gravity	1.001–1.029

Microscopic Examination

Red blood cells	Less than 5/hpf
White blood cells	Less than 5/hpf
Renal cells	None seen
Transitional cells	None seen
Squamous cells	Rare; usually no clinical significance
Casts	Rare hyaline; otherwise, none seen
Crystals in acid urine	Uric acid, calcium oxalate, amorphous urates
Crystals in alkaline urine	Triple phosphate, calcium phosphate, ammonium biurate, calcium carbonate, amorphous phosphates
Bacteria, yeast, parasites	None seen

DESCRIPTION: Routine urinalysis, one of the most widely ordered laboratory procedures, is used for basic screening purposes. It is a group of tests that evaluate the kidneys' ability to selectively excrete and reabsorb substances while maintaining proper water balance. The results can provide valuable information regarding the overall health of the patient and the patient's response to disease and treatment. The urine dipstick has a number of pads on it to indicate various biochemical markers. Urine pH is an indication of the kidneys' ability to help maintain balanced hydrogen ion concentration in the blood. Specific gravity is a reflection of the concentration ability of the kidneys. Urine protein is the most common indicator of renal disease, although there are conditions that can cause benign proteinuria. Glucose is used as an indicator of diabetes. The presence of ketones indicates impaired carbohydrate metabolism. Hemoglobin indicates the presence of blood, which is associated with renal disease. Bilirubin is used to assist in the detection of liver disorders. Urobilinogen indicates hepatic or hematopoietic conditions. Nitrites and leukocytes are used to test for bacteriuria and other sources of urinary tract infections (UTIs). Most laboratories have established criteria for the microscopic examination of urine based on patient population (e.g., pediatric, oncology, urology), unusual appearance, and biochemical reactions.

INDICATIONS

- Determine the presence of a genitourinary infection or abnormality
- Monitor the effects of physical or emotional stress
- Monitor fluid imbalances or treatment for fluid imbalances
- Monitor the response to drug therapy and evaluate undesired reactions to drugs that may impair renal function
- Provide screening as part of a general physical examination, especially on admission to a health-care facility or before surgery

POTENTIAL DIAGNOSIS

Unusual Color

Color	Presence of
Deep yellow	Riboflavin
Orange	Bilirubin, chrysophanic acid, phenazopiridine, santonin
Pink	Beet pigment, hemoglobin, myoglobin, porphyrin, rhubarb
Red	Beet pigment, hemoglobin, myoglobin, porphyrin, uroerythrin
Green	Oxidized bilirubin, Clorets (breath mint)
Blue	Diagnex, indican, methylene blue
Brown	Bilirubin, hematin, methemoglobin, metronidazole, nitrofurantoin, metabolites of rhubarb, senna
Black	Homogentisic acid, melanin
Smoky	Red blood cells

Test	Increased in	Decreased in
pH	Ingestion of citrus fruits	Ingestion of cranberries
	Vegetarian diets	High-protein diets
	Metabolic and respiratory alkalosis	Metabolic or respiratory acidosis
Protein	Benign proteinuria owing to stress, physical exercise, exposure to cold, or standing	N/A
	Diabetic nephropathy	
	Glomerulonephritis	
	Nephrosis	
	Toxemia of pregnancy	
Glucose	Diabetes	N/A
Ketones	Diabetes	N/A
	Fasting	
	Fever	
	High-protein diets	
	Isopropanol intoxication	
	Postanesthesia period	
	Starvation	
	Vomiting	
Hemoglobin	Diseases of the bladder	N/A
	Exercise (march hemoglobinuria)	
	Glomerulonephritis	
	Hemolytic anemia or other causes of hemolysis (e.g., drugs, parasites, transfusion reaction)	

(table continues on page 1316)

Test	Increased in	Decreased in
	Malignancy	
	Menstruation	
	Paroxysmal cold hemoglobinuria	
	Paroxysmal nocturnal hemoglobinuria	
	Pyelonephritis	
	Snake or spider bites	
	Trauma	
	Tuberculosis	
	Urinary tract infections	
	Urolithiasis	
Urobilinogen	Cirrhosis	Antibiotic therapy (suppresses normal intestinal flora)
	Heart failure	Obstruction of the bile duct
	Hemolytic anemia	
	Hepatitis	
	Infectious mononucleosis	
	Malaria	
	Pernicious anemia	
Bilirubin	Cirrhosis	N/A
	Hepatic tumor	
	Hepatitis	
Nitrites	Presence of nitrite-forming bacteria (e.g., *Citrobacter, Enterobacter, Escherichia coli, Klebsiella, Proteus, Pseudomonas, Salmonella, and some* species of *Staphylococcus*)	N/A
Leukocyte esterase	Bacterial infection	N/A
	Calculus formation	
	Fungal or parasitic infection	
	Glomerulonephritis	
	Interstitial nephritis	
	Tumor	
Specific gravity	Adrenal insufficiency	Diuresis
	Congestive heart failure	Excess IV fluids
	Dehydration	Excess hydration
	Diabetes	Hypothermia
	Diarrhea	Impaired renal concentrating ability
	Fever	
	Proteinuria	
	Sweating	
	Vomiting	
	Water restriction	
	X-ray dyes	

U

Formed Elements in Urine Sediment

Cellular Elements

- Clue cells (cell wall of the bacteria causes adhesion to epithelial cells) are present in nonspecific vaginitis caused by *Gardnerella vaginitis, Mobiluncus cortisii,* and *Mobiluncus mulieris.*
- RBCs are present in glomerulonephritis, lupus nephritis, focal glomerulonephritis, calculus, malignancy, infection, tuberculosis, infarction, renal vein thrombosis, trauma, hydronephrosis, polycystic kidney, urinary tract disease, prostatitis, pyelonephritis, appendicitis, salpingitis, diverticulitis, gout, scurvy, subacute bacterial endocarditis, infectious mononucleosis, hemoglobinopathies, coagulation disorders, heart failure, and malaria.
- Renal cells that have absorbed cholesterol and triglycerides are also known as *oval fat bodies.*
- Renal cells come from the lining of the collecting ducts, and increased numbers indicate acute tubular damage as seen in acute tubular necrosis, pyelonephritis, malignant nephrosclerosis, acute glomerulonephritis, acute drug or substance (salicylate, lead, or ethylene glycol) intoxication, or chemotherapy, resulting in desquamation, urolithiasis, and kidney transplant rejection.
- Squamous cells line the vagina and distal portion of the urethra. The presence of normal squamous epithelial cells in female urine is generally of no clinical significance. Abnormal cells with enlarged nuclei indicate the need for cytological studies to rule out malignancy.
- Transitional cells line the renal pelvis, ureter, bladder, and proximal portion of the urethra. Increased numbers are seen with infection, trauma, and malignancy.
- WBCs are present in acute UTI, tubulointerstitial nephritis, lupus nephritis, pyelonephritis, kidney transplant rejection, fever, and strenuous exercise.

Casts

- Granular casts are formed from protein or by the decomposition of cellular elements. They may be seen in renal disease, viral infections, or lead intoxication.
- Large numbers of hyaline casts may be seen in renal diseases, hypertension, congestive heart failure, or nephrotic syndrome and in more benign conditions such as fever, exposure to cold temperatures, exercise, or diuretic use.
- RBC casts may be found in acute glomerulonephritis, lupus nephritis, and subacute bacterial endocarditis.
- Waxy casts are seen in chronic renal failure or conditions such as kidney transplant rejection, in which there is renal stasis.
- WBC casts may be seen in lupus nephritis, acute glomerulonephritis, interstitial nephritis, and acute pyelonephritis.

Crystals

- Crystals found in freshly voided urine have more clinical significance than crystals seen in a urine sample that has been standing for more than 2 to 4 hr.
- Calcium oxalate crystals are found in ethylene glycol poisoning, urolithiasis, high dietary intake of oxalates, and Crohn's disease.
- Cystine crystals are seen in patients with cystinosis or cystinuria.
- Leucine or tyrosine crystals may be seen in patients with severe liver disease.
- Large numbers of uric acid crystals are seen in patients with urolithiasis,

U

gout, high dietary intake of foods rich in purines, or who are receiving chemotherapy (see monograph titled "Uric Acid, Urine").

CRITICAL FINDINGS ◈

Possible critical values are the presence of uric acid, cystine, leucine, or tyrosine crystals.

The combination of grossly elevated urine glucose and ketones is also considered significant.

Note and immediately report to the health-care provider (HCP) any critical values and related symptoms.

INTERFERING FACTORS

• Certain foods, such as onion, garlic, and asparagus, contain substances that may give urine an unusual odor. An ammonia-like odor may be produced by the presence of bacteria. Urine with a maple syrup–like odor may indicate a congenital metabolic defect (maple syrup urine disease).

• The various biochemical strips are subject to interference that may produce false-positive or false-negative results. Consult the laboratory for specific information regarding limitations of the method in use and a listing of interfering drugs.

• The dipstick method for protein detection is mostly sensitive to the presence of albumin; light-chain or Bence Jones proteins may not be detected by this method. Alkaline pH may produce false-positive protein results.

• Large amounts of ketones or ascorbic acid may produce false-negative or decreased color development on the glucose pad. Contamination of the collection container or specimen with chlorine, sodium hypochlorite, or peroxide may cause false-positive glucose results.

• False-positive ketone results may be produced in the presence of ascorbic acid, levodopa metabolites, valproic acid, phenazopyridine, phenylketones, or phthaleins.

• The hemoglobin pad may detect myoglobin, intact RBCs, and free hemoglobin. Contamination of the collection container or specimen with sodium hypochlorite or iodine may cause false-positive hemoglobin results. Negative or decreased hemoglobin results may occur in the presence of formalin, elevated protein, nitrite, ascorbic acid, or high specific gravity.

• False-negative nitrite results are common. Negative or decreased results may be seen in the presence of ascorbic acid and high specific gravity. Other causes of false-negative values relate to the amount of time the urine was in the bladder before voiding or the presence of pathogenic organisms that do not reduce nitrates to nitrites.

• False-positive leukocyte esterase reactions result from specimens contaminated by vaginal secretions. The presence of high glucose, protein, or ascorbic acid concentrations may cause false-negative results. Specimens with high specific gravity may also produce false-negative results. Patients with neutropenia (e.g., oncology patients) may also have false-negative results because they do not produce enough WBCs to exceed the sensitivity of the biochemical reaction.

• Specimens that cannot be delivered to the laboratory or tested within 1 hr should be refrigerated or should have a preservative added that is recommended by the laboratory. Specimens collected more than 2 hr before submission may be rejected for analysis.

- Because changes in the urine specimen occur over time, prompt and proper specimen processing, storage, and analysis are important to achieve accurate results.

Changes that may occur over time include:

Production of a stronger odor and an increase in pH (bacteria in the urine break urea down to ammonia)

A decrease in clarity (as bacterial growth proceeds or precipitates form)

A decrease in bilirubin and urobilinogen (oxidation to biliverdin and urobilin)

A decrease in ketones (lost through volatilization)

Decreased glucose (consumed by bacteria)

An increase in bacteria (growth over time)

Disintegration of casts, WBCs, and RBCs

An increase in nitrite (overgrowth of bacteria)

NURSING IMPLICATIONS AND PROCEDURE

PRETEST:

- Positively identify the patient using at least two unique identifiers before providing care, treatment, or services.
- *Patient Teaching:* Inform the patient this test can assist in assessing for disease, infection, and inflammation and evaluate for dehydration.
- Obtain a history of the patient's complaints, including a list of known allergens, especially allergies or sensitivities to latex.
- Obtain a history of the patient's endocrine, genitourinary, immune, hematopoietic, and hepatobiliary systems; symptoms; and results of previously performed laboratory tests and diagnostic and surgical procedures.
- Obtain a list of the patient's current medications, including herbs, nutritional

supplements, and nutraceuticals (see Appendix F).

- Review the procedure with the patient. If a catheterized specimen is to be collected, explain this procedure to the patient, and obtain a catheterization tray. Address concerns about pain and explain that there should be no discomfort during the procedure. Inform the patient that specimen collection takes approximately 5 to 10 min.
- *Sensitivity to social and cultural issues,* as well as concern for modesty, is important in providing psychological support before, during, and after the procedure.
- There are no food, fluid, or medication restrictions unless by medical direction.

INTRATEST:

- If the patient has a history of allergic reaction to latex, avoid the use of equipment containing latex.
- Instruct the patient to cooperate fully and to follow directions. Direct the patient to breathe normally and to avoid unnecessary movement.
- Observe standard precautions, and follow the general guidelines in Appendix A. Positively identify the patient, and label the appropriate collection container with the corresponding patient demographics, date, and time of collection.

Random Specimen (Collect in Early Morning)

Clean-Catch Specimen

- Instruct the male patient to (1) thoroughly wash his hands, (2) cleanse the meatus, (3) void a small amount into the toilet, and (4) void directly into the specimen container.
- Instruct the female patient to (1) thoroughly wash her hands; (2) cleanse the labia from front to back; (3) while keeping the labia separated, void a small amount into the toilet; and (4) without interrupting the urine stream, void directly into the specimen container.

Pediatric Urine Collector

- Put on gloves. Appropriately cleanse the genital area, and allow the area to dry. Remove the covering over the adhesive strips on the collector bag, and apply the bag over the genital area. Diaper the child. When specimen is obtained, place the entire collection bag in a sterile urine container.

Indwelling Catheter

▶ Put on gloves. Empty drainage tube of urine. It may be necessary to clamp off the catheter for 15 to 30 min before specimen collection. Cleanse specimen port with antiseptic swab, and then aspirate 5 mL of urine with a 21- to 25-gauge needle and syringe. Transfer urine to a sterile container.

Urinary Catheterization

▶ Place female patient in lithotomy position or male patient in supine position. Using sterile technique, open the straight urinary catheterization kit and perform urinary catheterization. Place the retained urine in a sterile specimen container.

Suprapubic Aspiration

▶ Place the patient in a supine position. Cleanse the area with antiseptic and drape with sterile drapes. A needle is inserted through the skin into the bladder. A syringe attached to the needle is used to aspirate the urine sample. The needle is then removed and a sterile dressing is applied to the site. Place the sterile sample in a sterile specimen container.

▶ Do not collect urine from the pouch from the patient with a urinary diversion (e.g., ileal conduit). Instead, perform catheterization through the stoma.

General

▶ Include on the collection container's label whether the specimen is clean catch or catheter and any medications that may interfere with test results.
▶ Promptly transport the specimen to the laboratory for processing and analysis.

POST-TEST:

▶ A report of the results will be sent to the requesting HCP, who will discuss the results with the patient.

▶ Instruct the patient to report symptoms such as pain related to tissue inflammation, pain or irritation during void, bladder spasms, or alterations in urinary elimination.
▶ Observe/assess for signs of inflammation if the specimen is obtained by suprapubic aspiration.
▶ Recognize anxiety related to test results. Discuss the implications of abnormal test results on the patient's lifestyle. Provide teaching and information regarding the clinical implications of the test results, as appropriate. Instruct the patient with a UTI, as appropriate, on the proper technique for wiping the perineal area (front to back) after a bowel movement. UTIs are more common in women who use diaphragm/spermicide contraception. These patients can be educated, as appropriate, in the proper insertion and removal of the contraceptive device to avoid recurrent UTIs.
▶ Reinforce information given by the patient's HCP regarding further testing, treatment, or referral to another HCP. Instruct the patient to begin antibiotic therapy, as prescribed, and instruct the patient in the importance of completing the entire course of antibiotic therapy even if symptoms are no longer present. Answer any questions or address any concerns voiced by the patient or family.
▶ Depending on the results of this procedure, additional testing may be performed to evaluate or monitor progression of the disease process and determine the need for a change in therapy. Evaluate test results in relation to the patient's symptoms and other tests performed.

RELATED MONOGRAPHS:

▶ Related tests include amino acids, angiography renal, antibodies, anti-glomerular basement membrane, biopsy bladder, biopsy kidney, bladder cancer marker, BUN, calcium, calculus kidney stone panel, CBC, creatinine, culture urine, cystometry, cystoscopy, cystourethrography voiding, cytology urine, electrolytes, glucose, glycated hemoglobin, IFE, IVP, ketones, KUB study, microalbumin, osmolality, oxalate, protein total, phosphorus, renogram, retrograde ureteropyelography, urea nitrogen

urine, and uric acid (blood and urine).
▶ Refer to the Endocrine, Genitourinary, Immune, Hematopoietic, and Hepatobiliary systems tables at the end of the book for related tests by body system.

Uterine Fibroid Embolization

SYNONYM/ACRONYM: UFE.

COMMON USE: A less invasive modality used to assist in treating fibroid tumors found in the uterine lining, heavy menstrual bleeding, and pelvic pain.

AREA OF APPLICATION: Uterus.

CONTRAST: IV iodine based.

DESCRIPTION: Uterine fibroid embolization (UFE) is a way of treating fibroid tumors of the uterus. Fibroid tumors, also known as myomas, are masses of fibrous and muscle tissue in the uterine wall that are benign but that may cause heavy menstrual bleeding, pain in the pelvic region, or pressure on the bladder or bowel. Using angiographic methods, a catheter is placed in each of the two uterine arteries, and small particles are injected to block the arterial branches that supply blood to the fibroids. The fibroid tissue dies, the mass shrinks, and the symptoms are relieved. This procedure, which is done under local anesthesia, is less invasive than open surgery done to remove uterine fibroids. Because the effects of uterine fibroid

embolization on fertility are not yet known, the ideal candidate is a premenopausal woman with symptoms from fibroid tumors who no longer wishes to become pregnant. This technique is an alternative for women who do not want to receive blood transfusions or do not wish to receive general anesthesia. This procedure may be used to halt severe bleeding following childbirth or caused by gynecological tumors.

INDICATIONS
• Treatment for anemia from chronic blood loss
• Treatment of fibroid tumors and tumor vascularity, for both single and multiple tumors
• Treatment of tumors in lieu of surgical resection

POTENTIAL DIAGNOSIS

Normal findings in
- Decrease in uterine bleeding
- Decrease of pelvic pain or fullness

Abnormal findings in
- No reduction in size of fibroid

CRITICAL FINDINGS: N/A

INTERFERING FACTORS

This procedure is contraindicated for

- ❄ Patients with allergies to shellfish or iodinated contrast medium. The contrast medium used may cause a life-threatening allergic reaction. Patients with a known hypersensitivity to contrast medium may benefit from premedication with corticosteroids or the use of nonionic contrast medium.
- Patients with bleeding disorders.
- Patients who are pregnant or suspected of being pregnant, unless the potential benefits of the procedure far outweigh the risks to the fetus and mother.
- Patients in whom cancer is a possibility or who have inflammation or infection in the pelvis.
- ❄ Elderly and other patients who are chronically dehydrated before the procedure, because of their risk of contrast-induced renal failure.
- ❄ Patients who are in renal failure.

Factors that may impair clear imaging

- Gas or feces in the gastrointestinal tract resulting from inadequate cleansing or failure to restrict food intake before the study.
- Retained barium from a previous radiological procedure.
- Metallic objects (e.g., jewelry, body rings) within the examination field, which may inhibit organ visualization and cause unclear images.

Other considerations
- Complications of the procedure include hemorrhage, infection at the insertion site, and cardiac arrhythmias.
- The procedure may be terminated if chest pain or severe cardiac arrhythmias occur.
- Inability of the patient to cooperate or remain still during the procedure because of age, significant pain, or mental status, may interfere with the test results.
- Failure to follow dietary restrictions before the procedure may cause the procedure to be canceled or repeated.
- Consultation with a health-care provider (HCP) should occur before the procedure for radiation safety concerns regarding younger patients or patients who are lactating.
- Risks associated with radiation overexposure can result from frequent x-ray procedures. Personnel in the room with the patient should wear a protective lead apron, stand behind a shield, or leave the area while the examination is being done. Personnel working in the examination area should wear badges to record their level of radiation exposure.
- A small percentage of women may pass a small piece of fibroid tissue after the procedure. Women with this problem may require a procedure called a D & C (dilatation and curettage).
- Some women may experience menopause shortly after the procedure.

NURSING IMPLICATIONS AND PROCEDURE

PRETEST:

▶ Positively identify the patient using at least two unique identifiers before providing care, treatment, or services.

- **Patient Teaching:** Inform the patient this procedure can assist in assessing and treating the uterus.
- Obtain a history of the patient's complaints, including a list of known allergens, especially allergies or sensitivities to latex, iodine, seafood, anesthetics, or contrast medium.
- Obtain a history of the patient's reproductive system, symptoms, and results of previously performed laboratory tests and diagnostic and surgical procedures.
- Note any recent procedures that can interfere with test results; include examinations utilizing barium- or iodine-based contrast medium.
- Record the date of the last menstrual period and determine the possibility of pregnancy in perimenopausal women.
- Obtain a list of the patient's current medications, including anticoagulants, aspirin and other salicylates, herbs, nutritional supplements, and nutraceuticals, especially those known to affect coagulation (see Appendix F). Such products should be discontinued by medical direction for the appropriate number of days prior to a surgical procedure. Note the last time and dose of medication taken.
- If contrast medium is scheduled to be used, patients receiving metformin (Glucophage) for non-insulin-dependent (type 2) diabetes should discontinue the drug on the day of the test and continue to withhold it for 48 hr after the test. Failure to do so may result in lactic acidosis.
- Review the procedure with the patient. Address concerns about pain and explain that there may be moments of discomfort and some pain experienced during the test. Explain that a sedative and/or anesthetic may be administered before the procedure to promote relaxation. Inform the patient that the procedure is performed in a radiology or vascular department by an HCP, with support staff, and takes approximately 30 to 120 min.
- **Sensitivity to social and cultural issues,** as well as concern for modesty, is important in providing psychological support before, during, and after the procedure.

- Explain that an IV line may be inserted to allow infusion of IV fluids, contrast medium, or sedatives. Usually normal saline is infused.
- Inform the patient that a burning and flushing sensation may be felt throughout the body during injection of the contrast medium. After injection of the contrast medium, the patient may experience an urge to cough, flushing, nausea, or a salty or metallic taste.
- Instruct the patient to remove jewelry and other metallic objects from the area to be examined prior to the procedure.
- Instruct the patient to fast and restrict fluids for 8 hr prior to the procedure. Instruct the patient to avoid taking anticoagulant medication or to reduce dosage as ordered prior to the procedure. Protocols may vary among facilities.
- *Make sure a written and informed consent has been signed prior to the procedure and before administering any medications.*
- This procedure may be terminated if chest pain, severe cardiac arrhythmias, or signs of a cerebrovascular accident occur.

INTRATEST:

- Ensure the patient has complied with dietary, fluid, and medication restrictions for 8 hr prior to the procedure.
- Ensure the patient has removed all external metallic objects from the area to be examined prior to the procedure.
- If the patient has a history of allergic reactions to any substance or drug, administer ordered prophylactic steroids or antihistamines before the procedure. Use nonionic contrast medium for the procedure.
- Have emergency equipment readily available.
- Instruct the patient to void prior to the procedure and to change into the gown, robe, and foot coverings provided.
- Instruct the patient to cooperate fully and to follow directions. Instruct the patient to remain still throughout the procedure because movement produces unreliable results.

▶ Record baseline vital signs and assess neurological status. Protocols may vary among facilities.

▶ Observe standard precautions, and follow the general guidelines in Appendix A.

▶ Establish an IV fluid line for the injection of emergency drugs and of sedatives.

▶ Administer an antianxiety agent, as ordered, if the patient has claustrophobia. Administer a sedative to an uncooperative adult, as ordered.

▶ Place electrocardiographic electrodes on the patient for cardiac monitoring. Establish baseline rhythm; determine if the patient has ventricular arrhythmias.

▶ Using a pen, mark the site of the patient's peripheral pulses before angiography; this allows for quicker and more consistent assessment of the pulses after the procedure.

▶ Place the patient in the supine position on an examination table. Cleanse the selected area, and cover with a sterile drape.

▶ The contrast medium is injected, and a rapid series of images is taken during and after the filling of the vessels to be examined. Delayed images may be taken to examine the vessels after a time and to monitor the venous phase of the procedure.

▶ Ask the patient to inhale deeply and hold her breath while the x-ray images are taken, and then to exhale after the images are taken.

▶ Instruct the patient to take slow, deep breaths if nausea occurs during the procedure. Monitor and administer an antiemetic agent if ordered. Ready an emesis basin for use.

▶ Particles are injected through the catheter to block the blood flow to the fibroids. The particles include polyvinyl alcohol, gelatin sponge (Gelfoam), and micospheres.

▶ The needle or catheter is removed, and a pressure dressing is applied over the puncture site.

▶ Monitor the patient for complications related to the procedure (e.g., allergic reaction, anaphylaxis, bronchospasm).

▶ Observe/assess the needle/catheter insertion site for bleeding, inflammation, or hematoma formation.

POST-TEST:

▶ A report of the examination will be sent to the requesting HCP, who will discuss the results with the patient.

▶ Instruct the patient to resume usual diet, fluids, medications, or activity, as directed by the HCP. Renal function should be assessed before metformin is resumed.

▶ Monitor vital signs and neurological status every 15 min for 1 hr, then every 2 hr for 4 hr, and then as ordered by the HCP. Take temperature every 4 hr for 24 hr. Monitor intake and output at least every 8 hr. Compare with baseline values. Notify the HCP if temperature is elevated. Protocols may vary among facilities.

▶ Observe for delayed allergic reactions, such as rash, urticaria, tachycardia, hyperpnea, hypertension, palpitations, nausea, or vomiting.

▶ Instruct the patient to immediately report symptoms such as fast heart rate, difficulty breathing, skin rash, itching, chest pain, persistent right shoulder pain, or abdominal pain. Immediately report symptoms to the appropriate HCP.

▶ Patients may experience pelvic cramps for several days after the procedure and possible mild nausea and fever.

▶ Assess extremities for signs of ischemia or absence of distal pulse caused by a catheter-induced thrombus.

▶ Instruct the patient in the care and assessment of the injection site.

▶ Instruct the patient to apply cold compresses to the puncture site as needed, to reduce discomfort or edema.

▶ Recognize anxiety related to test results, and be supportive of impaired activity related to genitourinary system. Discuss the implications of abnormal test results on the patient's lifestyle. Provide teaching and information regarding the clinical implications of the test results, as appropriate. Educate the patient regarding access to counseling services.

▶ Reinforce information given by the patient's HCP regarding further testing, treatment, or referral to another HCP. Answer any questions or address any concerns voiced by the patient or family.

U

Instruct the patient in the use of any ordered medications. Explain the importance of adhering to the therapy regimen. As appropriate, instruct the patient in significant side effects and systemic reactions associated with the prescribed medication. Encourage her to review corresponding literature provided by a pharmacist.

Depending on the results of this procedure, additional testing may be performed to evaluate or monitor progression of the disease process and determine the need for a change in therapy. Evaluate test results in relation to the patient's symptoms and other tests performed.

RELATED MONOGRAPHS:

Related tests include CBC, CT angiography, CT pelvis, hysterosalpingography, laparoscopy, MRA, MRI pelvis, PT/INR, and US pelvis.

Refer to the Reproductive System table at the end of the book for related tests by body system.

U

SYNONYM/ACRONYM: VMA.

COMMON USE: To assist in the diagnosis and follow up treatment of pheochromocytoma, neuroblastoma, and ganglioblastoma. This test can also be useful in evaluation and follow-up of hypertension.

SPECIMEN: Urine (25 mL) from a timed specimen collected in a clean plastic collection container with 6N hydrochloric acid as a preservative.

REFERENCE VALUE: (Method: High-pressure liquid chromatography)

Age	Conventional Units	SI Units (Conventional Units × 5.05)
3–6 yr	1.0–2.6 mg/24 hr	5–13 micromol/24 hr
7–10 yr	2.0–3.2 mg/24 hr	10–16 micromol/24 hr
11–16 yr	2.3–5.2 mg/24 hr	12–26 micromol/24 hr
17–83 yr	1.4–6.5 mg/24 hr	7–33 micromol/24 hr

DESCRIPTION: Vanillylmandelic acid (VMA) is a major metabolite of epinephrine and norepinephrine. It is elevated in conditions that also are marked by overproduction of catecholamines. Creatinine is usually measured simultaneously to ensure adequate collection and to calculate an excretion ratio of metabolite to creatinine.

INDICATIONS
• Assist in the diagnosis of neuroblastoma, ganglioneuroma, or pheochromocytoma
• Evaluate hypertension of unknown cause

POTENTIAL DIAGNOSIS

Increased in

Catecholamine-secreting tumors will cause an increase in VMA.
• Ganglioneuroma
• Hypertension secondary to pheochromocytoma
• Neuroblastoma
• Pheochromocytoma

Decreased in: N/A

CRITICAL FINDINGS: N/A

INTERFERING FACTORS
• Drugs that may increase VMA levels include ajmaline, chlorpromazine, glucagon, guaifenesin, guanethidine, isoproterenol, methyldopa, nitroglycerin, oxytetracycline, phenazopyridine, phenolsulfonphthalein, prochlorperazine, rauwolfia, reserpine, sulfobromophthalein, and syrosingopine.
• Drugs that may decrease VMA levels include brofaromine, guanethidine, guanfacine, imipramine, isocarboxazid, methyldopa, monoamine oxidase inhibitors, morphine, nialamide (in schizophrenics), and reserpine.
• Stress, hypoglycemia, hyperthyroidism, strenuous exercise, smoking, and drugs can produce elevated catecholamines.
• Recent radioactive scans within 1 wk of the test can interfere with test results.

- Failure to collect all urine and store 24-hr specimen properly will result in a falsely low result.
- Failure to follow dietary restrictions before the procedure may cause the procedure to be canceled or repeated.

NURSING IMPLICATIONS AND PROCEDURE

PRETEST:

▶ Positively identify the patient using at least two unique identifiers before providing care, treatment, or services.
▶ *Patient Teaching:* Inform the patient this test can assist in evaluating or the presence of tumors.
▶ Obtain a history of the patient's complaints, including a list of known allergens, especially allergies or sensitivities to latex.
▶ Obtain a history of the patient's endocrine system, symptoms, and results of previously performed laboratory tests and diagnostic and surgical procedures.
▶ Obtain a list of the patient's current medications, including herbs, nutritional supplements, and nutraceuticals (see Appendix F).
▶ Review the procedure with the patient. Provide a nonmetallic urinal, bedpan, or toilet-mounted collection device. Address concerns about pain and explain that there should be no discomfort during the procedure.
▶ *Sensitivity to social and cultural issues,* as well as concern for modesty, is important in providing psychological support before, during, and after the procedure.
▶ Usually a 24-hr time frame for urine collection is ordered. Inform the patient that all urine must be saved during that 24-hr period. Instruct the patient not to void directly into the laboratory collection container. Instruct the patient to avoid defecating in the collection device and to keep toilet tissue out of the collection device to prevent contamination of the specimen. Place a sign in the bathroom to remind the patient to save all urine.

▶ Instruct the patient to void all urine into the collection device and then to pour the urine into the laboratory collection container. Alternatively, the specimen can be left in the collection device for a health-care staff member to add to the laboratory collection container.
▶ There are no fluid restrictions unless by medical direction.
▶ Instruct the patient to abstain from smoking tobacco for 24 hr before testing.
▶ Inform the patient of the following dietary, medication, and activity restrictions in preparation for the test (protocols may vary among facilities):

The patient should not consume foods high in amines for 48 hr before testing (bananas, avocados, beer, aged cheese, chocolate, cocoa, coffee, fava beans, grains, tea, vanilla, walnuts, and red wine).

The patient should not consume foods or fluids high in caffeine for 48 hr before testing (coffee, tea, cocoa, and chocolate).

The patient should not consume any foods or fluids containing vanilla or licorice.

The patient should avoid self-prescribed medications (especially aspirin) and prescribed medications (especially pyridoxine, levodopa, amoxicillin, carbidopa, reserpine, and disulfiram) for 2 wk before testing and as directed.

The patient should avoid excessive exercise and stress during the 24-hr collection of urine.

INTRATEST:

▶ Ensure that the patient has complied with dietary, medication, and activity restrictions and pretesting preparations prior to the procedure.
▶ If the patient has a history of allergic reaction to latex, avoid the use of equipment containing latex.
▶ Instruct the patient to cooperate fully and to follow directions.
▶ Observe standard precautions, and follow the general guidelines in Appendix A. Positively identify the patient, and label the appropriate collection container with

the corresponding patient demographics, date, and time of collection.

Timed Specimen

▶ Obtain a clean 3-L urine specimen container, toilet-mounted collection device, and plastic bag (for transport of the specimen container). The specimen must be refrigerated or kept on ice throughout the entire collection period. If an indwelling urinary catheter is in place, the drainage bag must be kept on ice.

▶ Begin the test between 6 and 8 a.m. if possible. Collect first voiding and discard. Record the time the specimen was discarded as the beginning of the timed collection period. The next morning, ask the patient to void at the same time the collection was started and add this last voiding to the container. Urinary output should be recorded throughout the collection time.

▶ If an indwelling catheter is in place, replace the tubing and container system at the start of the collection time. Keep the container system on ice during the collection period, or empty the urine into a larger container periodically during the collection period; monitor to ensure continued drainage, and conclude the test the next morning at the same hour the collection was begun.

▶ At the conclusion of the test, compare the quantity of urine with the urinary output record for the collection; if the specimen contains less than what was recorded as output, some urine may have been discarded, invalidating the test.

▶ Include on the collection container's label the amount of urine, test start and stop times, and ingestion of any foods or medications that can affect test results.

▶ Promptly transport the specimen to the laboratory for processing and analysis.

POST-TEST:

▶ A report of the results will be sent to the requesting health-care provider (HCP), who will discuss the results with the patient.

▶ Instruct the patient to resume usual diet, fluids, medications, and activity, as directed by the HCP.

▶ *Nutritional Considerations:* Instruct the patient to avoid foods or drinks containing caffeine. Over-the-counter medications should be taken only under the advice of the patient's HCP.

▶ Recognize anxiety related to test results, and be supportive of fear of shortened life expectancy. Discuss the implications of abnormal test results on the patient's lifestyle. Provide teaching and information regarding the clinical implications of the test results, as appropriate. Educate the patient regarding access to counseling services.

▶ Reinforce information given by the patient's HCP regarding further testing, treatment, or referral to another HCP. Answer any questions or address any concerns voiced by the patient or family.

▶ Depending on the results of this procedure, additional testing may be performed to evaluate or monitor progression of the disease process and determine the need for a change in therapy. Evaluate test results in relation to the patient's symptoms and other tests performed.

RELATED MONOGRAPHS:

▶ Related tests include angiography adrenal, calcium, catecholamines, CT renal, homovanillic acid, metanephrines, and renin.

▶ Related to Endocrine System table at the end of the book for related tests by body system.

Varicella Antibodies

SYNONYM/ACRONYM: Varicella-zoster antibodies, chickenpox, VZ.

COMMON USE: To assist in diagnosing chickenpox or shingles related to a varicella-zoster infection and to assess for immunity.

SPECIMEN: Serum (1 mL) collected in a red-top tube.

REFERENCE VALUE: (Method: Indirect fluorescent antibody) Negative or less than a fourfold increase in titer.

DESCRIPTION: Varicella-zoster is a double-stranded DNA herpes virus that is responsible for two clinical syndromes: chickenpox and shingles. The incubation period is 2 to 3 wk, and it is highly contagious for about 2 wk beginning 2 days before a rash develops. It is transmitted in respiratory secretions. The primary exposure to the highly contagious virus usually occurs in susceptible school-age children. Adults without prior exposure and who become infected may have severe complications, including pneumonia. Neonatal infection from the mother is possible if exposure occurs during the last 3 wk of gestation. Shingles results when the presumably latent virus is reactivated. The presence of immunoglobulin (Ig) M antibodies indicates acute infection. The presence of IgG antibodies indicates current or past infection. A reactive varicella antibody result indicates immunity but does not protect an individual from shingles. There are also polymerase chain reaction methods that can detect varicella-zoster DNA in various specimen types.

INDICATIONS
- Determine susceptibility or immunity to chickenpox

POTENTIAL DIAGNOSIS

Positive findings in
- Varicella infection

Negative findings in: N/A

CRITICAL FINDINGS: N/A

INTERFERING FACTORS: N/A

NURSING IMPLICATIONS AND PROCEDURE

PRETEST:
- Positively identify the patient using at least two unique identifiers before providing care, treatment, or services.
- *Patient Teaching:* Inform the patient this test can assist in assessing for a viral infection or immunity.
- Obtain a history of the patient's complaints, including a list of known allergens, especially allergies or sensitivities to latex.
- Obtain a history of exposure to varicella.
- Obtain a history of the patient's immune and reproductive systems, symptoms, and results of previously performed laboratory tests and diagnostic and surgical procedures.

- Obtain a list of the patient's current medications, including herbs, nutritional supplements, and nutraceuticals (see Appendix F).
- Review the procedure with the patient. Inform the patient that several tests may be necessary to confirm diagnosis. Any individual positive result should be repeated in 7 to 14 days to monitor a change in titer. Inform the patient that specimen collection takes approximately 5 to 10 min. Address concerns about pain and explain that there may be some discomfort during the venipuncture.
- *Sensitivity to social and cultural issues,* as well as concern for modesty, is important in providing psychological support before, during, and after the procedure.
- There are no food, fluid, or medication restrictions unless by medical direction.

INTRATEST:

- If the patient has a history of allergic reaction to latex, avoid the use of equipment containing latex.
- Instruct the patient to cooperate fully and to follow directions. Direct the patient to breathe normally and to avoid unnecessary movement.
- Observe standard precautions, and follow the general guidelines in Appendix A. Positively identify the patient, and label the appropriate tube with the corresponding patient demographics, date, and time of collection. Perform a venipuncture; collect the specimen in a 5-mL red-top tube.
- Remove the needle and apply direct pressure with dry gauze to stop bleeding. Observe/assess venipuncture site for bleeding or hematoma formation and secure gauze with adhesive bandage.
- Promptly transport the specimen to the laboratory for processing and analysis.

POST-TEST:

- A report of the results will be sent to the requesting health-care provider (HCP), who will discuss the results with the patient.

- *Vaccination Considerations:* Record the date of last menstrual period and determine the possibility of pregnancy prior to administration of varicella vaccine to female varicella-nonimmune patients. Instruct patient not to become pregnant for 1 mo after being vaccinated with the varicella vaccine to protect any fetus from contracting the disease and having serious birth defects. Instruct on birth control methods to prevent pregnancy, if appropriate.
- Recognize anxiety related to test results, and provide emotional support if results are positive and the patient is pregnant. Inform the patient with shingles about access to pain management. Discuss the implications of abnormal test results on the patient's lifestyle. Provide teaching and information regarding the clinical implications of the test results, as appropriate. Educate the patient regarding access to counseling services.
- Reinforce information given by the patient's HCP regarding further testing, treatment, or referral to another HCP. Instruct the patient in isolation precautions during the time of communicability or contagion. Emphasize the need to return to have a convalescent blood sample taken in 7 to 14 days. Provide information regarding vaccine-preventable diseases where indicated (e.g., encephalitis, hepatitis A and B, human papillomavirus, influenza, measles, mumps, polio, rubella, smallpox, varicella, yellow fever). Answer any questions or address any concerns voiced by the patient or family.
- Depending on the results of this procedure, additional testing may be performed to evaluate or monitor progression of the disease process and determine the need for a change in therapy. Evaluate test results in relation to the patient's symptoms and other tests performed.

RELATED MONOGRAPHS:

- Refer to the Immune and Reproductive systems tables at the end of the book for related tests by body system.

Venography, Lower Extremity Studies

SYNONYM/ACRONYM: Lower limb venography, phlebography, venogram.

COMMON USE: To visualize and assess the venous vasculature in the lower extremities related to diagnosis of deep vein thrombosis and congenital anomalies.

AREA OF APPLICATION: Veins of the lower extremities.

CONTRAST: IV iodine based.

DESCRIPTION: Venography allows x-ray visualization of the venous vasculature system of the extremities after injection of an iodinated contrast medium. Lower extremity studies identify and locate thrombi within the venous system of the lower limbs. After injection of the contrast medium, x-ray images are taken at timed intervals. Usually both extremities are studied, and the unaffected side is used for comparison with the side suspected of having deep vein thrombosis (DVT) or other venous abnormalities, such as congenital malformations or incompetent valves. Thrombus formation usually occurs in the deep calf veins and at the venous junction and its valves. If DVT is not treated, it can lead to femoral and iliac venous occlusion, or the thrombus can become an embolus, causing a pulmonary embolism. Venography is accurate for thrombi in veins below the knee.

INDICATIONS
- Assess deep vein valvular competence
- Confirm a diagnosis of DVT
- Determine the cause of extremity swelling or pain
- Determine the source of emboli when pulmonary embolism is suspected or diagnosed
- Distinguish clot formation from venous obstruction
- Evaluate congenital venous malformations
- Locate a vein for arterial bypass graft surgery

POTENTIAL DIAGNOSIS

Normal findings in
No obstruction to flow and no filling defects after injection of radiopaque contrast medium; steady opacification of superficial and deep vasculature with no filling defects

Abnormal findings in
- Deep vein valvular incompetence
- DVT
- Pulmonary embolism
- Venous obstruction

CRITICAL FINDINGS
- DVT

It is essential that critical diagnoses be communicated immediately to the appropriate health-care provider (HCP). A listing of these diagnoses varies among facilities. Note and immediately report to the HCP abnormal results and related symptoms.

INTERFERING FACTORS

This procedure is contraindicated for

- Patients with allergies to shellfish or iodinated dye. The contrast medium used may cause a life-threatening allergic reaction. Patients with a known hypersensitivity to the contrast medium may benefit from premedication with corticosteroids or the use of non-ionic contrast medium.
- Patients who are pregnant or suspected of being pregnant, unless the potential benefits of the procedure far outweigh the risks to the fetus and mother.
- Elderly and other patients who are chronically dehydrated before the test, because of their risk of contrast-induced renal failure.
- Patients who are in renal failure.
- Patients with bleeding disorders.

Factors that may impair clear imaging

- Metallic objects (e.g., jewelry, body rings) within the examination field, which may inhibit organ visualization and cause unclear images.
- Movement of the leg being tested, excessive tourniquet constriction, insufficient injection of contrast medium, and delay between injection and the x-ray.
- Severe edema of the legs, making venous access impossible.

Other considerations

- Improper injection of the contrast medium that allows it to seep deep into the muscle tissue.
- Inability of the patient to cooperate or remain still during the procedure because of age, significant pain, or mental status, may interfere with the test results.
- Consultation with a HCP should occur before the procedure for radiation safety concerns regarding younger patients or patients who are lactating.
- Risks associated with radiation overexposure can result from frequent x-ray procedures. Personnel in the room with the patient should wear a protective lead apron, stand behind a shield, or leave the area while the examination is being done. Personnel working in the examination area should wear badges to record their level of radiation exposure.

NURSING IMPLICATIONS AND PROCEDURE

PRETEST:

- Positively identify the patient using at least two unique identifiers before providing care, treatment, or services.
- *Patient Teaching:* Inform the patient this procedure can assist in assessing the veins in the lower extremities.
- Obtain a history of the patient's complaints, including a list of known allergens, especially allergies or sensitivities to latex, iodine, seafood, contrast medium, anesthetics, and contrast medium.
- Note any recent procedures that can interfere with test results, including examinations using barium- or iodine-based contrast medium.
- Obtain a history of the patient's cardiovascular and respiratory systems, symptoms, and results of previously performed laboratory tests and diagnostic and surgical procedures.
- Record the date of the last menstrual period and determine the possibility of pregnancy in perimenopausal women.
- Obtain a list of the patient's current medications, including anticoagulants, aspirin and other salicylates, herbs, nutritional supplements, and nutraceuticals, especially those known to affect coagulation (see Appendix F). Such products should be discontinued by medical direction for the appropriate number of days prior to a surgical

procedure. Note the last time and dose of medication taken.

- Patients receiving metformin (Glucophage) for non-insulin-dependent (type 2) diabetes should discontinue the drug on the day of the test and continue to withhold it for 48 hr after the test. Failure to do so may result in lactic acidosis.
- Review the procedure with the patient. Address concerns about pain and explain to the patient that there may be moments of discomfort and some pain experienced during the procedure. Inform the patient that the procedure is usually performed in a radiology or vascular suite by an HCP, with support staff, and takes approximately 30 to 60 min.
- *Sensitivity to social and cultural issues,* as well as concern for modesty, is important in providing psychological support before, during, and after the procedure.
- Explain that an IV line may be inserted to allow infusion of IV fluids, contrast medium, or sedatives. Usually normal saline is infused.
- Inform the patient that a burning and flushing sensation may be felt throughout the body during injection of the contrast medium. After injection of the contrast medium, the patient may experience an urge to cough, flushing, nausea, or a salty or metallic taste.
- Instruct the patient to remove jewelry and other metallic objects from the area to be examined prior to the procedure.
- Instruct the patient to fast and restrict fluids for 8 hr prior to the procedure. Protocols may vary among facilities.
- *Make sure a written and informed consent has been signed prior to the procedure and before administering any medications.*
- This procedure may be terminated if chest pain, severe cardiac arrhythmias, or signs of a cerebrovascular accident occur.

INTRATEST:

- Ensure the patient has complied with dietary, fluid, and medication restrictions for 8 hr prior to the procedure.
- Ensure the patient has removed all external metallic objects from the area

to be examined prior to the procedure.
- If the patient has a history of allergic reactions to any substance or drug, administer ordered prophylactic steroids or antihistamines before the procedure. Use nonionic contrast medium for the procedure.
- Have emergency equipment readily available.
- Instruct the patient to void prior to the procedure and to change into the gown, robe, and foot coverings provided.
- Instruct the patient to cooperate fully and to follow directions. Ask the patient to remain still throughout the procedure because movement produces unreliable results.
- Record baseline vital signs, and continue to monitor throughout the procedure. Protocols may vary among facilities.
- Observe standard precautions, and follow the general guidelines in Appendix A.
- Establish an IV fluid line for the injection of emergency drugs and of sedatives.
- Administer an antianxiety agent, as ordered, if the patient has claustrophobia. Administer a sedative to a child or to an uncooperative adult, as ordered.
- Place electrocardiographic electrodes on the patient for cardiac monitoring. Establish baseline rhythm; determine if the patient has ventricular arrhythmias.
- Using a pen, mark the site of the patient's peripheral pulses before venography; this allows for quicker and more consistent assessment of the pulses after the procedure.
- Place the patient in the supine position on an examination table. Cleanse the selected area, and cover with a sterile drape.
- A local anesthetic is injected at the site, and a small incision is made or a needle inserted.
- The contrast medium is injected, and a rapid series of images is taken during and after the filling of the vessels to be examined.

- Instruct the patient to inhale deeply and hold his or her breath while the x-ray images are taken, and then to exhale.
- Instruct the patient to take slow, deep breaths if nausea occurs during the procedure.
- Monitor the patient for complications related to the procedure (e.g., allergic reaction, anaphylaxis, broncho-spasm).
- The needle or catheter is removed, and a pressure dressing is applied over the puncture site.
- Observe/assess the needle/catheter insertion site for bleeding, inflammation, or hematoma formation.

POST-TEST:

- A report of the examination will be sent to the requesting HCP, who will discuss the results with the patient.
- Instruct the patient to resume diet, fluids, and medications, as directed by the HCP. Renal function should be assessed before metformin is resumed.
- Monitor vital signs and neurological status every 15 min for 1 hr, then every 2 hr for 4 hr, and then as ordered by the HCP. Take temperature every 4 hr for 24 hr. Monitor intake and output at least every 8 hr. Compare with baseline values. Notify the HCP if temperature is elevated. Protocols may vary among facilities.
- Observe for delayed allergic reactions, such as rash, urticaria, tachycardia, hyperpnea, hypertension, palpitations, nausea, or vomiting.
- Instruct the patient to immediately report symptoms such as fast heart rate, difficulty breathing, skin rash, itching, chest pain, persistent right shoulder pain, or abdominal pain. Immediately report symptoms to the appropriate HCP.
- Assess extremities for signs of ischemia or absence of distal pulse

caused by a catheter-induced thrombus.
- Instruct the patient in the care and assessment of the site.
- Instruct the patient to apply cold compresses to the puncture site as needed to reduce discomfort or edema.
- Instruct the patient to maintain bed rest for 4 to 6 hr after the procedure or as ordered.
- Recognize anxiety related to test results, and be supportive of perceived loss of independent function. Discuss the implications of abnormal test results on the patient's lifestyle. Provide teaching and information regarding the clinical implications of the test results, as appropriate.
- Reinforce information given by the patient's HCP regarding further test-ing, treatment, or referral to another HCP. Answer any questions or address any concerns voiced by the patient or family.
- Depending on the results of this procedure, additional testing may be needed to evaluate or monitor progression of the disease process and determine the need for a change in therapy. Evaluate test results in relation to the patient's symptoms and other tests performed.

RELATED MONOGRAPHS:

- Related tests include alveolar/arterial gradient, angiography pulmonary, anti-bodies anticardiolipin, antithrombin III, blood gases, CT angiography, D-dimer, FDP, lactic acid, lung perfusion scan, lung ventilation scan, MRA, MRI abdomen, plethysmography, PT/INR, renogram, US peripheral Doppler, and US venous Doppler extremity studies.
- Refer to the Cardiovascular and Respiratory systems tables at the end of the book for related tests by body system.

Vertebroplasty

V

SYNONYM/ACRONYM: None.

COMMON USE: A minimally invasive procedure to treat the spine for disorders such as tumor, lesions, osteoporosis, vertebral compression, and pain.

AREA OF APPLICATION: Spine.

CONTRAST: None.

DESCRIPTION: Vertebroplasty is a minimally invasive, nonsurgical therapy used to repair a broken vertebra and to provide relief of pain related to vertebral compression in the spine that has been weakened by osteoporosis or tumoral lesions. Osteoporosis affects over 10 million women in the United States and accounts for over 700,000 vertebral fractures per year. This procedure is usually successful at alleviating the pain caused by a compression fracture less than 6 mo in duration with pain directly referable to the location of the fracture. Secondary benefits may include vertebra stabilization and reduction of the risk of further compression. This procedure is usually performed on an outpatient basis. The procedure involves injection of orthopedic cement mixture through a needle into a fracture site. Injection is visualized with guidance from radiological imaging. Vertebroplasty may be the preferred procedure when patients are too elderly or frail to tolerate open spinal surgery or if bones are too weak for surgical repair. Patients with a malignant tumor may benefit from vertebroplasty. Other possible applications include younger patients whose osteoporosis is caused by long-term steroid use or a metabolic disorder. This procedure is recommended after basic treatments such as bedrest and orthopedic braces have failed or when pain medication has been ineffective or caused the patient medical problems, including stomach ulcers.

INDICATIONS
- Assist in the detection of nonmalignant tumors before surgical resection.
- Repair of compression spinal fractures of varying ages. Fractures older than 6 mo will respond but at a slower rate. Fractures less than 4 wk old should be given a chance to heal without intervention unless they are associated with disabling pain or hospitalization.
- Repair of spinal problems due to tumors.

POTENTIAL DIAGNOSIS

Normal findings in
- Improvement in the ability to ambulate without pain
- Relief of back pain

Abnormal findings in
- Failure to reduce the patient's pain

- Failure to improve the patient's mobility

CRITICAL FINDINGS: N/A

INTERFERING FACTORS

This procedure is contraindicated for

- ◈ Patients with allergies to shellfish or iodinated dye. The contrast medium used may cause a life-threatening allergic reaction. Patients with a known hypersensitivity to the contrast medium may benefit from premedication with corticosteroids or the use of nonionic contrast medium.
- Pain that is primarily radicular in nature.
- Patients with bleeding disorders.
- Patients who are pregnant or suspected of being pregnant, unless the potential benefits of the procedure far outweigh the risks to the fetus and mother.
- Pain that is improving or that has been present and unchanged for years.
- Imaging procedures that suggest no fracture is present or that the fracture is remote from the patient's pain.

Factors that may impair clear imaging

- Gas or feces in the gastrointestinal tract resulting from inadequate cleansing or failure to restrict food intake before the study.
- Retained barium from a previous radiological procedure.
- Metallic objects (e.g., jewelry, body rings) within the examination field, which may inhibit organ visualization and cause unclear images.

Other considerations

- Complications of the procedure include hemorrhage, infection at the insertion site, and cardiac arrhythmias.

- The procedure may be terminated if chest pain, or severe cardiac arrhythmias occur.
- Inability of the patient to cooperate or remain still during the procedure because of age, significant pain, or mental status, may interfere with the test results.
- Failure to follow dietary restrictions before the procedure may cause the procedure to be canceled or repeated.
- Consultation with a health-care provider (HCP) should occur before the procedure for radiation safety concerns regarding younger patients or patients who are lactating.
- Risks associated with radiation overexposure can result from frequent x-ray procedures. Personnel in the room with the patient should wear a protective lead apron, stand behind a shield, or leave the area while the examination is being done. Personnel working in the examination area should wear badges to record their level of radiation exposure.

NURSING IMPLICATIONS AND PROCEDURE

PRETEST:

- Positively identify the patient using at least two unique identifiers before providing care, treatment, or services.
- *Patient Teaching:* Inform the patient this procedure can assist in improving spinal cord function.
- Obtain a history of the patient's complaints, including a list of known allergens, especially allergies or sensitivities to latex, iodine, seafood, contrast medium, anesthetics, or contrast medium.
- Note any recent procedures that can interfere with test results, including examinations using barium- or iodine-based contrast medium.

- Obtain a history of the patient's musculoskeletal system, symptoms, and results of previously performed laboratory tests and diagnostic and surgical procedures.
- Record the date of the last menstrual period and determine the possibility of pregnancy in perimenopausal women.
- Obtain a list of the patient's current medications, including anticoagulants, aspirin and other salicylates, herbs, nutritional supplements, and nutraceuticals, especially those known to affect coagulation (see Appendix F). Such products should be discontinued by medical direction for the appropriate number of days prior to a surgical procedure. Note the last time and dose of medication taken.
- Review the procedure with the patient. Address concerns about pain and explain that there may be moments of discomfort and some pain experienced during the test. Inform the patient that the procedure is usually performed in the radiology department by an HCP, with support staff, and takes approximately 30 to 90 min.
- *Sensitivity to social and cultural issues,* as well as concern for modesty, is important in providing psychological support before, during, and after the procedure.
- Explain that an IV line may be inserted to allow infusion of IV fluids, contrast medium, or sedatives. Usually normal saline is infused.
- Instruct the patient to remove jewelry and other metallic objects from the area to be examined prior to the procedure.
- Instruct the patient to fast and restrict fluids for 8 hr prior to the procedure. Protocols may vary among facilities.
- *Make sure a written and informed consent has been signed prior to the procedure and before administering any medications.*
- This procedure may be terminated if chest pain or severe cardiac arrhythmias occur.

INTRATEST:

- Ensure the patient has complied with dietary, fluid, and medication restrictions for 8 hr prior to the procedure.
- Ensure the patient has removed all external metallic objects from the area to be examined.
- If the patient has a history of allergic reactions to any substance or drug, administer ordered prophylactic steroids or antihistamines before the procedure. Use nonionic contrast medium for the procedure.
- Have emergency equipment readily available.
- Instruct the patient to void prior to the procedure and to change into the gown, robe, and foot coverings provided.
- Instruct the patient to cooperate fully and to follow directions. Ask the patient to remain still throughout the procedure because movement produces unreliable results.
- Record baseline vital signs, and continue to monitor throughout the procedure. Protocols may vary among facilities.
- Observe standard precautions, and follow the general guidelines in Appendix A.
- Establish an IV fluid line for the injection of emergency drugs and of sedatives.
- Administer an antianxiety agent, as ordered, if the patient has claustrophobia. Administer a sedative to a child or to an uncooperative adult, as ordered.
- Place electrocardiographic electrodes on the patient for cardiac monitoring. Establish baseline rhythm; determine if the patient has ventricular arrhythmias.
- Place the patient in the prone position on an examination table. Cleanse the selected area, and cover with a sterile drape.
- A local anesthetic is injected at the site, and a small incision is made or a needle inserted under fluoroscopy.
- Orthopedic cement is injected through the needle into the fracture.

- Ask the patient to inhale deeply and hold his or her breath while the images are taken, and then to exhale.
- Instruct the patient to take slow, deep breaths if nausea occurs during the procedure.
- Monitor the patient for complications related to the procedure (e.g., allergic reaction, anaphylaxis, broncho-spasm).
- The needle or catheter is removed, and a pressure dressing is applied over the puncture site.
- Observe/assess the needle/catheter insertion site for bleeding, inflammation, or hematoma formation.

POST-TEST:

- A report of the examination will be sent to the requesting HCP, who will discuss the results with the patient.
- Instruct the patient to resume usual diet, fluids, medications, or activity, as directed by the HCP. Renal function should be assessed before metformin is resumed.
- Monitor vital signs and neurological status every 15 min for 1 hr, then every 2 hr for 4 hr, and then as ordered by the HCP. Take temperature every 4 hr for 24 hr. Monitor intake and output at least every 8 hr. Compare with baseline values. Notify the HCP if temperature is elevated. Protocols may vary among facilities.
- Observe for delayed allergic reactions, such as rash, urticaria, tachycardia, hyperpnea, hypertension, palpitations, nausea, or vomiting.
- Instruct the patient to immediately report symptoms such as fast heart rate, difficulty breathing, skin rash, itching, chest pain, persistent right shoulder pain, or abdominal pain. Immediately report symptoms to the appropriate HCP.
- Instruct the patient and caregiver in the care and assessment of the site.
- Instruct the patient's caregiver to apply cold compresses to the puncture site as needed to reduce discomfort or edema.
- Instruct the patient to maintain bedrest for 4 to 6 hr after the procedure or as ordered.
- Recognize anxiety related to test results, and be supportive of impaired activity related to physical activity. Discuss the implications of abnormal test results on the patient's lifestyle. Provide teaching and information regarding the clinical implications of the test results, as appropriate.
- Reinforce information given by the patient's HCP regarding further testing, treatment, or referral to another HCP. Answer any questions or address any concerns voiced by the patient or family.
- Depending on the results of this procedure, additional testing may be performed to evaluate or monitor progression of the disease process and determine the need for a change in therapy. Evaluate test results in relation to the patient's symptoms and other tests performed.

RELATED MONOGRAPHS:

- Related tests include bone mineral densitometry, bone scan, CT spine, EMG, and MRI musculoskeletal.
- Refer to the Musculoskeletal System table at the end of the book for related tests by body system.

Visual Fields Test

SYNONYM/ACRONYM: Perimetry, VF.

COMMON USE: To assess visual field function related to the retina, optic nerve, and optic pathways to assist in diagnosing visual loss disorders such as brain tumors, macular degeneration, and diabetes.

AREA OF APPLICATION: Eyes.

CONTRAST: N/A.

DESCRIPTION: The visual field (VF) is the area within which objects can be seen by the eye as it fixes on a central point. The central field is an area extending 25° surrounding the fixation point. The peripheral field is the remainder of the area within which objects can be viewed. This test evaluates the central VF, except within the physiological blind spot, through systematic movement of the test object across a tangent screen. It tests the function of the retina, optic nerve, and optic pathways. VF testing may be performed manually by the examiner (confrontation VF examination) or by using partially or fully automated equipment (tangent screen, Goldman, Humphrey VF examination). In the manual VF test, the patient is asked to cover one eye and fix his or her gaze on the examiner. The examiner moves his or her hand out of the patient's VF and then gradually brings it back into the patient's VF. The patient signals the examiner when the hand comes back into view. The test is repeated on the other eye. The manual test is frequently used for screening because it is quick and simple. Tangent screen or Goldman testing is an automated method commonly used to create a map of the patient's VF and is described in greater detail in this monograph.

INDICATIONS
- Detect field vision loss and evaluate its progression or regression

POTENTIAL DIAGNOSIS

Normal findings in
- Normal central vision field will form a circle extending 25° superiorly, nasally, inferiorly, and temporally; 12° to 15° temporal to the central fixation point is a physiological blind spot, approximately 1.5° below the horizontal meridian. It is approximately 7.5° high and 5.5° wide. The patient should be able to see the test object throughout the entire central vision field except within the physiological blind spot.

Abnormal findings in
- Amblyopia
- Blepharochalasis
- Blurred vision
- Brain tumors
- Cerebrovascular accidents
- Choroidal nevus

- Diabetes with ophthalmic manifestations
- Glaucoma
- Headache
- Macular degeneration
- Macular drusen
- Nystagmus
- Optic neuritis or neuropathy
- Ptosis of eyelid
- Retinal detachment, hole, or tear
- Retinal exudates or hemorrhage
- Retinal occlusion of the artery or vein
- Retinitis pigmentosa
- Subjective visual disturbance
- Use of high-risk medications
- VF defect
- Vitreous traction syndrome

CRITICAL FINDINGS: N/A

INTERFERING FACTORS

Factors that may impair the results of the examination
- An uncooperative patient or a patient with severe vision loss who has difficulty seeing even a large vision screen may have test results that are invalid.
- Assess and make note of the patient's cooperation and reliability as good, fair, or poor, because it is difficult to evaluate factors such as general health, fatigue, or reaction time that affect test performance.

NURSING IMPLICATIONS AND PROCEDURE

PRETEST:
- Positively identify the patient using at least two unique identifiers before providing care, treatment, or services.
- *Patient Teaching:* Inform the patient this procedure assesses visual field function and vision loss.

- Obtain a history of the patient's complaints, including a list of known allergens.
- Obtain a history of the patient's known or suspected vision loss; changes in visual acuity, including type and cause; use of glasses or contact lenses; eye conditions with treatment regimens; eye surgery; and other tests and procedures to assess and diagnose visual deficit.
- Obtain a history of symptoms and results of previously performed laboratory tests and diagnostic and surgical procedures.
- Obtain a list of the patient's current medications, including herbs, nutritional supplements, and nutraceuticals (see Appendix F).
- Measurement of visual acuity with and without corrective lenses prior to testing is highly recommended. Instruct the patient to wear corrective lenses if appropriate and if worn to correct for distance vision. Instruct the patient regarding the importance of keeping the eyes open for the test.
- Review the procedure with the patient. Address concerns about pain and explain that no discomfort will be experienced during the test. Inform the patient that a health-care provider (HCP) performs the test in a quiet, darkened room and that to evaluate both eyes, the test can take up 30 min.
- *Sensitivity to social and cultural issues,* as well as concern for modesty, is important in providing psychological support before, during, and after the procedure.
- There are no food, fluid, or medication restrictions unless by medical direction.

INTRATEST:
- Instruct the patient to cooperate fully and to follow directions. Ask the patient to remain still during the procedure because movement produces unreliable results.
- Seat the patient 3 ft away from the tangent screen with the eye being tested directly in line with the central fixation tangent, usually a white disk,

on the screen. Cover the eye that is not being tested. Ask the patient to place the chin in the chin rest and gently press the forehead against the support bar. Reposition the patient as appropriate to ensure the eye(s) to be tested are properly aligned in front of the VF testing equipment. While the patient stares at the disk on the screen, the examiner moves an object toward the patient's visual field. The patient signals the examiner when the object enters his or her visual field. The patient's responses are recorded, and a map of the patient's VF, including areas of visual defect, can be drawn on paper manually or by a computer.

POST-TEST:

- A report of the results will be sent to the requesting HCP, who will discuss the results with the patient.
- Recognize anxiety related to test results, and be supportive of impaired activity related to vision loss, perceived loss of driving privileges, or the possibility of requiring corrective lenses (self-image). Discuss the implications of the test results on the patient's lifestyle. Provide contact information, if desired, for a general patient education Web site on the topic of eye care (e.g., www.allabout-vision.com). Provide contact information regarding vision aids, if desired, for ABLEDATA (sponsored by the National Institute on Disability and Rehabilitation Research [NIDRR], available at www.abledata.com). Information can also be obtained from the American Macular Degeneration

Foundation (www.macular.org), the Glaucoma Research Foundation (www.glaucoma.org), and the American Diabetes Association (www.diabetes.org).

- Reinforce information given by the patient's HCP regarding further testing, treatment, or referral to another HCP. Answer any questions or address any concerns voiced by the patient or family.
- Instruct the patient in the use of any ordered medications. Explain the importance of adhering to the therapy regimen. As appropriate, instruct the patient in significant side effects and systemic reactions associated with the prescribed medication. Encourage him or her to review corresponding literature provided by a pharmacist.
- Depending on the results of this procedure, additional testing may be performed to evaluate or monitor progression of the disease process and determine the need for a change in therapy. Evaluate test results in relation to the patient's symptoms and other tests performed.

RELATED MONOGRAPHS:

- Related tests include CT brain, EEG, evoked brain potentials, fluorescein angiography, fructosamine, fundus photography, glucagon, glucose, glycated hemoglobin, gonioscopy, insulin, intraocular pressure, microalbumin, plethysmography, PET brain, and slit-lamp biomicroscopy.
- Refer to the Ocular System table at the end of the book for related tests by body system.

Vitamin B$_{12}$

SYNONYM/ACRONYM: Cyanocobalamin.

COMMON USE: To assess vitamin B$_{12}$ levels to assist in diagnosing disorders such as pernicious anemia and malabsorption syndromes.

SPECIMEN: Serum (1 mL) collected in a red- or tiger-top tube.

REFERENCE VALUE: (Method: Immunochemiluminescent assay)

Age	Conventional Units	SI Units (Conventional Units × 0.738)
Newborn–11 mo	160–1,300 pg/mL	118–959 pmol/L
Adult	200–900 pg/mL	148–664 pmol/L

DESCRIPTION: Vitamin B$_{12}$ has a ringed crystalline structure that surrounds an atom of cobalt. It is essential in DNA synthesis, hematopoiesis, and central nervous system (CNS) integrity. It is derived solely from dietary intake. Animal products are the richest source of vitamin B$_{12}$. Its absorption depends on the presence of intrinsic factor. Circumstances that may result in a deficiency of this vitamin include the presence of stomach or intestinal disease as well as insufficient dietary intake of foods containing vitamin B$_{12}$. A significant increase in red blood cells (RBCs) mean corpuscular volume may be an important indicator of vitamin B$_{12}$ deficiency.

INDICATIONS

- Assist in the diagnosis of CNS disorders
- Assist in the diagnosis of megaloblastic anemia
- Evaluate alcoholism
- Evaluate malabsorption syndromes

POTENTIAL DIAGNOSIS

Increased in
Increases are noted in a number of conditions; pathophysiology is unclear.
- Chronic granulocytic leukemia
- Chronic obstructive pulmonary disease
- Chronic renal failure
- Diabetes
- Leukocytosis
- Liver cell damage (hepatitis, cirrhosis) *(stores in damaged hepatocytes are released into circulation; synthesis of transport proteins is diminished by liver damage)*
- Obesity
- Polycythemia vera
- Protein malnutrition *(lack of transport proteins increases circulating levels)*
- Severe congestive heart failure
- Some carcinomas

Decreased in
- Abnormalities of cobalamin transport or metabolism

- Bacterial overgrowth *(vitamin is consumed and utilized by the bacteria)*
- Crohn's disease *(related to poor absorption)*
- Dietary deficiency *(related to insufficient intake, e.g., in vegetarians)*
- Diphyllobothrium (fish tapeworm) infestation *(vitamin is consumed and utilized by the parasite)*
- Gastric or small intestine surgery *(related to dietary deficiency or poor absorption)*
- Hypochlorhydria *(related to ineffective digestion resulting in poor absorption)*
- Inflammatory bowel disease *(related to dietary deficiency or poor absorption)*
- Intestinal malabsorption
- Intrinsic factor deficiency *(required for proper vitamin B$_{12}$ absorption)*
- Late pregnancy *(related to dietary deficiency or poor absorption)*
- Pernicious anemia *(related to dietary deficiency or poor absorption)*

CRITICAL FINDINGS: N/A

INTERFERING FACTORS

- Drugs that may increase vitamin B$_{12}$ levels include chloral hydrate.
- Drugs that may decrease vitamin B$_{12}$ levels include alcohol, aminosalicylic acid, anticonvulsants, ascorbic acid, cholestyramine, cimetidine, colchicine, metformin, neomycin, oral contraceptives, ranitidine, and triamterene.
- Hemolysis or exposure of the specimen to light invalidates results.
- Specimen collection soon after blood transfusion can falsely increase vitamin B$_{12}$ levels.
- Failure to follow dietary restrictions before the procedure may cause

the procedure to be canceled or repeated.

NURSING IMPLICATIONS AND PROCEDURE

PRETEST:

- Positively identify the patient using at least two unique identifiers before providing care, treatment, or services.
- *Patient Teaching:* Inform the patient this test can assist in diagnosing a vitamin toxicity or deficiency.
- Obtain a history of the patient's complaints, including a list of known allergens, especially allergies or sensitivities to latex.
- Obtain a history of the patient's gastrointestinal and hematopoietic systems, symptoms, and results of previously performed laboratory tests and diagnostic and surgical procedures.
- Obtain a list of the patient's current medications, including herbs, nutritional supplements, and nutraceuticals (see Appendix F).
- Review the procedure with the patient. Inform the patient that specimen collection takes approximately 5 to 10 min. Address concerns about pain and explain that there may be some discomfort during the venipuncture.
- *Sensitivity to social and cultural issues,* as well as concern for modesty, is important in providing psychological support before, during, and after the procedure.
- Instruct the patient to fast for at least 12 hr before specimen collection. Protocols may vary among facilities.
- There are no fluid or medication restrictions unless by medical direction.

INTRATEST:

- Ensure that the patient has complied with dietary restrictions; assure that food has been restricted for at least 12 hr prior to the procedure.
- If the patient has a history of allergic reaction to latex, avoid the use of equipment containing latex.
- Instruct the patient to cooperate fully and to follow directions. Direct the patient to breathe normally and to avoid unnecessary movement.

- Observe standard precautions, and follow the general guidelines in Appendix A. Positively identify the patient, and label the appropriate tubes with the corresponding patient demographics, date, and time of collection. Perform a venipuncture. Protect the specimen from light.
- Remove the needle and apply direct pressure with dry gauze to stop bleeding. Observe/assess venipuncture site for bleeding or hematoma formation and secure gauze with adhesive bandage.
- Promptly transport the specimen to the laboratory for processing and analysis.

POST-TEST:

- A report of the results will be sent to the requesting health-care provider (HCP), who will discuss the results with the patient.
- Instruct the patient to resume usual diet, as directed by the HCP.
- *Nutritional Considerations:* Instruct the patient with vitamin B_{12} deficiency, as appropriate, in the use of vitamin supplements. Inform the patient, as appropriate, that the best dietary sources of

vitamin B_{12} are meats, fish, poultry, eggs, and milk.
- Reinforce information given by the patient's HCP regarding further testing, treatment, or referral to another HCP. Answer any questions or address any concerns voiced by the patient or family.
- Depending on the results of this procedure, additional testing may be performed to evaluate or monitor progression of the disease process and determine the need for a change in therapy. Evaluate test results in relation to the patient's symptoms and other tests performed.

RELATED MONOGRAPHS:

- Related tests include CBC, CBC RBC count, CBC RBC indices, CBC RBC morphology, CBC WBC count and differential, folate, gastric acid stimulation, gastrin stimulation, homocysteine, and intrinsic factor antibodies.
- Refer to the Gastrointestinal and Hematopoietic systems tables at the end of the book for related tests by body system.

Vitamin D

SYNONYM/ACRONYM: Cholecalciferol, vitamin D 1,25-dihydroxy.

COMMON USE: To assess vitamin D levels to assist in diagnosing disorders such as vitamin toxicity, malabsorption, and vitamin deficiency.

SPECIMEN: Serum (1 mL) collected in a red-top tube. Plasma (1 mL) collected in a green-top (heparin) tube is also acceptable.

REFERENCE VALUE: (Method: High-performance liquid chromatography)

Form	Conventional Units	SI Units (Conventional Units × 2.496)
Vitamin D 25-dihydroxy	20–100 ng/mL	49.92–249.6 nmol/L
Vitamin D 1,25-dihydroxy	15–60 pg/mL	37.4–149.8 pmol/L

V

DESCRIPTION: Vitamin D is a group of interrelated sterols that have hormonal activity in multiple organs and tissues of the body, including the kidneys, liver, skin, and bones. There are two metabolically active forms of vitamin D: vitamin D 25-dihydroxy and vitamin D 1,25-dihydroxy. Ergocalciferol (vitamin D_2) is formed when ergosterol in plants is exposed to sunlight. Ergocalciferol is absorbed by the stomach and intestine when orally ingested. Cholecalciferol (vitamin D_3) is formed when the skin is exposed to sunlight or ultraviolet light. Vitamins D_2 and D_3 enter the bloodstream after absorption. Vitamin D_3 is converted to vitamin D 25-dihydroxy by the liver and is the major circulating form of the vitamin. Vitamin D_2 is converted to vitamin D 1,25-dihydroxy (calcitriol) by the kidneys and is the more biologically active form. Vitamin D acts with parathyroid hormone and calcitonin to regulate calcium metabolism and osteoblast function. The effects of vitamin D deficiency have been studied for many years, and continued research indicates a link between vitamin D deficiency and the development of diseases such as heart failure, stroke, hypertension, cancer, autism, multiple sclerosis, type 2 diabetes, systemic lupus erythematosus, depression, and immune function. Adequate dietary intake sufficient to maintain bone health and normal calcium metabolism in adults age 19 to 50 yr is 5 mcg/day (200 IU/day) and in adults age 51 to 70 yr is 10 mcg/day (400 IU/day).

INDICATIONS
- Differential diagnosis of disorders of calcium and phosphorus metabolism
- Evaluate deficiency or suspected toxicity
- Investigate bone diseases
- Investigate malabsorption

POTENTIAL DIAGNOSIS

Increased in
- Endogenous vitamin D intoxication *(in conditions such as sarcoidosis, cat scratch disease, and some lymphomas, extrarenal conversion of 25-dihydroxy to 1,25-dihydroxy vitamin D occurs with a corresponding abnormal elevation of calcium)*
- Exogenous vitamin D intoxication

Decreased in
- Bowel resection *(related to lack of absorption)*
- Celiac disease *(related to lack of absorption)*
- Inflammatory bowel disease *(related to lack of absorption)*
- Malabsorption *(related to lack of absorption)*
- Osteomalacia *(related to dietary insufficiency)*
- Pancreatic insufficiency *(lack of digestive enzymes to metabolize fat-soluble vitamin D; malabsorption)*
- Rickets *(related to dietary insufficiency)*
- Thyrotoxicosis *(possibly related to increased calcium loss through sweat, urine, or feces with corresponding decrease in vitamin D levels)*

CRITICAL FINDINGS ◈
Vitamin toxicity can be as significant as problems brought about by vitamin deficiencies. The potential for

toxicity is especially important to consider with respect to fat-soluble vitamins, which are not eliminated from the body as quickly as water-soluble vitamins and can accumulate in the body. Most cases of toxicity are brought about by oversupplementing and can be avoided by consulting a qualified nutritionist for recommended daily dietary and supplemental allowances. Signs and symptoms of vitamin D toxicity include nausea, loss of appetite, vomiting, polyuria, muscle weakness, and constipation.

INTERFERING FACTORS
• Drugs that may increase vitamin D levels include pravastatin.

NURSING IMPLICATIONS AND PROCEDURE

PRETEST:
▶ Positively identify the patient using at least two unique identifiers before providing care, treatment, or services.
▶ *Patient Teaching:* Inform the patient this test can assist in diagnosing vitamin toxicity or deficiency.
▶ Obtain a history of the patient's complaints, including a list of known allergens, especially allergies or sensitivities to latex.
▶ Obtain a history of the patient's gastrointestinal and musculoskeletal systems, symptoms, and results of previously performed laboratory tests and diagnostic and surgical procedures.
▶ Obtain a list of the patient's current medications, including herbs, nutritional supplements, and nutraceuticals (see Appendix F).
▶ Review the procedure with the patient. Inform the patient that specimen collection takes approximately 5 to 10 min. Address concerns about pain and explain that there may be some discomfort during the venipuncture.
▶ *Sensitivity to social and cultural issues,* as well as concern for modesty, is important

in providing psychological support before, during, and after the procedure.
▶ There are no food, fluid, or medication restrictions unless by medical direction.

INTRATEST:
▶ If the patient has a history of allergic reaction to latex, avoid the use of equipment containing latex.
▶ Instruct the patient to cooperate fully and to follow directions. Direct the patient to breathe normally and to avoid unnecessary movement.
▶ Observe standard precautions, and follow the general guidelines in Appendix A. Positively identify the patient, and label the appropriate tubes with the corresponding patient demographics, date, and time of collection. Perform a venipuncture.
▶ Remove the needle and apply direct pressure with dry gauze to stop bleeding. Observe/assess venipuncture site for bleeding or hematoma formation and secure gauze with adhesive bandage.
▶ Promptly transport the specimen to the laboratory for processing and analysis.

POST-TEST:
▶ A report of the results will be sent to the requesting health-care provider (HCP), who will discuss the results with the patient.
▶ *Nutritional Considerations:* Educate the patient with vitamin D deficiency, as appropriate, that the main dietary sources of vitamin D are fortified dairy foods and cod liver oil. Explain to the patient that vitamin D is also synthesized by the body, in the skin, and is activated by sunlight.
▶ Reinforce information given by the patient's HCP regarding further testing, treatment, or referral to another HCP. Answer any questions or address any concerns voiced by the patient or family.
▶ Depending on the results of this procedure, additional testing may be performed to evaluate or monitor progression of the disease process and determine the need for a change in therapy. Evaluate test results in relation to the patient's symptoms and other tests performed.

V

RELATED MONOGRAPHS:

▶ Related tests include amylase, ANCA, biopsy intestinal, calcium, capsule endoscopy, colonoscopy, fecal analysis, fecal fat, antibodies gliadin antibodies, kidney stone panel, laparoscopy

abdominal, lipase, osteocalcin, oxalate, phosphorus, and proctosigmoidoscopy.
▶ Refer to the Gastrointestinal and Musculoskeletal systems tables at the end of the book for related tests by body system.

Vitamin E

SYNONYM/ACRONYM: Tocopherol.

COMMON USE: To assess vitamin E levels to assist in diagnosing vitamin toxicity, malabsorption, neuromuscular disorders, and vitamin deficiency.

SPECIMEN: Serum (1 mL) collected in a red- or tiger-top tube.

REFERENCE VALUE: (Method: High-performance liquid chromatography)

Age	Conventional Units	SI Units (Conventional Units × 23.22)
1–12 yr	0.3–0.9 mg/dL	7–21 micromol/L
13–19 yr	0.6–1.0 mg/dL	14–23 micromol/L
Adult	0.5–1.8 mg/dL	12–42 micromol/L

DESCRIPTION: Vitamin E is a powerful fat-soluble antioxidant that prevents the oxidation of unsaturated fatty acids, which can combine with polysaccharides to form deposits in tissue. For this reason, vitamin E is believed to reduce the risk of coronary artery disease. Vitamin E reserves in lung tissue provide a barrier against air pollution and protect red blood cell (RBC) membrane integrity from oxidation. Oxidation of fatty acids in RBC membranes can result in irreversible membrane damage and hemolysis. Studies are in progress to confirm the suspicion that oxidation also contributes to the formation of cataracts and macular degeneration of the retina. Because vitamin E is found in a wide variety of foods, a deficiency secondary to inadequate dietary intake is rare. Alpha-tocopherol appears to be the most plentiful and important form of eight vitamin E antioxidants; there are four tocopherols (alpha-, beta-, gamma-, and delta-) and four tocotrienols (alpha-, beta-, gamma-, and delta-). The recommended dietary allowance for adults is 15 mg (22.4 IU).

V

INDICATIONS

- Evaluate neuromuscular disorders in premature infants and adults
- Evaluate patients with malabsorption disorders
- Evaluate suspected hemolytic anemia in premature infants and adults
- Monitor patients on long-term parenteral nutrition

POTENTIAL DIAGNOSIS

Increased in

- Obstructive liver disease *(related to malabsorption associated with obstructive liver disease)*
- Vitamin E intoxication *(related to excessive intake)*

Decreased in

- Abetalipoproteinemia *(rare inherited disorder of fat metabolism evidenced by poor absorption of fat and fat-soluble vitamin E)*
- Hemolytic anemia *(related to deficiency of vitamin E, an important antioxidant that protects RBC cell membranes from weakening)*
- Malabsorption disorders, such as biliary atresia, cirrhosis, cystic fibrosis, chronic pancreatitis, pancreatic carcinoma, and chronic cholestasis

CRITICAL FINDINGS ❖

Vitamin toxicity can be as significant as problems brought about by vitamin deficiencies. The potential for toxicity is especially important to consider with respect to fat-soluble vitamins, which are not eliminated from the body as quickly as water-soluble vitamins and can accumulate in the body. Most cases of toxicity are brought about by oversupplementing and can be avoided by consulting a qualified nutritionist for recommended daily dietary and supplemental allowances. *Note*: Excessive supplementation of vitamin E (greater than 60 times the recommended dietary allowance over a period of 1 yr or longer) can result in excessive bleeding, delayed healing of wounds, and depression.

INTERFERING FACTORS

- Drugs that may increase vitamin E levels include anticonvulsants (in women).
- Drugs that may decrease vitamin E levels include anticonvulsants (in men).
- Exposure of the specimen to light decreases vitamin E levels, resulting in a falsely low result.

NURSING IMPLICATIONS AND PROCEDURE

PRETEST:

- Positively identify the patient using at least two unique identifiers before providing care, treatment, or services.
- *Patient Teaching:* Inform the patient this lab test can assist in evaluating vitamin toxicity or deficiency.
- Obtain a history of the patient's complaints, including a list of known allergens, especially allergies or sensitivities to latex.
- Obtain a history of the patient's cardiovascular, gastrointestinal, hematopoietic, and hepatobiliary systems; symptoms; and results of previously performed laboratory tests and diagnostic and surgical procedures.
- Obtain a list of the patient's current medications, including herbs, nutritional supplements, and nutraceuticals (see Appendix F).
- Review the procedure with the patient. Inform the patient that specimen collection takes approximately 5 to 10 min. Address concerns about pain and explain that there may be some discomfort during the venipuncture.
- *Sensitivity to social and cultural issues,* as well as concern for modesty, is important in providing psychological support before, during, and after the procedure.

▶ There are no food, fluid, or medication restrictions unless by medical direction.

▶ If the patient has a history of allergic reaction to latex, avoid the use of equipment containing latex.

▶ Instruct the patient to cooperate fully and to follow directions. Direct the patient to breathe normally and to avoid unnecessary movement.

▶ Observe standard precautions, and follow the general guidelines in Appendix A.

▶ Positively identify the patient, and label the appropriate tubes with the corresponding patient demographics, date, and time of collection. Perform a venipuncture.

▶ Remove the needle and apply direct pressure with dry gauze to stop bleeding. Observe/assess venipuncture site for bleeding or hematoma formation and secure gauze with adhesive bandage.

▶ Promptly transport the specimen to the laboratory for processing and analysis.

POST-TEST:

▶ A report of the results will be sent to the requesting health-care provider (HCP), who will discuss the results with the patient.

▶ *Nutritional Considerations:* Educate the patient with a vitamin E deficiency, if appropriate, that the main dietary sources of vitamin E are vegetable oils, whole grains, wheat germ, milk, eggs, meats, fish, and green leafy vegetables. Vitamin E is fairly stable at most cooking temperatures (except frying) and when exposed to acidic foods.

▶ Reinforce information given by the patient's HCP regarding further testing, treatment, or referral to another HCP. Answer any questions or address any concerns voiced by the patient or family.

▶ Depending on the results of this procedure, additional testing may be performed to evaluate or monitor progression of the disease process and determine the need for a change in therapy. Evaluate test results in relation to the patient's symptoms and other tests performed.

RELATED MONOGRAPHS:

▶ Related tests include amylase, antibodies gliadin, biopsy bone marrow, biopsy intestinal, capsule endoscopy, colonoscopy, complement, CBC, CBC hematocrit, CBC hemoglobin, CBC RBC count, CBC RBC indices, CBC RBC morphology, Coomb's antiglobulin direct and indirect, fecal analysis, fecal fat, Ham's test, Hgb electrophoresis, laparoscopy abdominal, lipase, osmotic fragility, and proctosigmoidoscopy.

▶ Refer to the Cardiovascular, Gastrointestinal, Hematopoietic, and Hepatobiliary systems tables at the end of the book for related tests by body system.

Vitamin K

SYNONYM/ACRONYM: Phylloquinone, phytonadione.

COMMON USE: Assessment of vitamin K levels to assist in diagnosing bleeding disorders where etiology is unknown, identify vitamin toxicity, and evaluate symptoms related to chronic antibiotic use.

SPECIMEN: Serum (1 mL) collected in a red-top tube.

REFERENCE VALUE: (Method: High-performance liquid chromatography)

V

Conventional Units	SI Units (Conventional Units × 2.22)
0.13–1.19 ng/mL	0.29–2.64 nmol/L

DESCRIPTION: Vitamin K is one of the fat-soluble vitamins. It is essential for the formation of prothrombin; factors VII, IX, and X; and proteins C and S. Vitamin K also works with vitamin D in synthesizing bone protein and regulating calcium levels (see monograph titled "Vitamin D.") Vitamin K levels are not often requested, but vitamin K is often prescribed as a medication. Approximately one-half of the body's vitamin K is produced by intestinal bacteria; the other half is obtained from dietary sources. There are three forms of vitamin K: vitamin K_1, or phylloquinone, which is found in foods; vitamin K_2, or menaquinone, which is synthesized by intestinal bacteria; and vitamin K_3, or menadione, which is the synthetic, water-soluble, pharmaceutical form of the vitamin. Vitamin K_3 is two to three times more potent than the naturally occurring forms.

INDICATIONS

Evaluation of bleeding of unknown cause (e.g., frequent nosebleeds, bruising).

POTENTIAL DIAGNOSIS

Increased in
• Excessive administration of vitamin K

Decreased in
• Antibiotic therapy *(related to decreased intestinal flora)*
• Chronic fat malabsorption *(related to lack of digestive enzymes and poor absorption)*

• Cystic fibrosis *(related to lack of digestive enzymes and poor absorption)*
• Diarrhea (in infants) *(related to increased loss in feces)*
• Gastrointestinal disease *(related to malabsorption)*
• Hemorrhagic disease of the newborn *(newborns normally have low levels of vitamin K; neonates at risk are those who are not given a prophylactic vitamin K shot at birth or those receiving nutrition strictly from breast milk, which has less vitamin K than cow's milk)*
• Hypoprothrombinemia *(related to insufficient levels of prothrombin, a vitamin K–dependent protein)*
• Liver disease *(interferes with storage of vitamin K)*
• Obstructive jaundice *(related to insufficient levels of bile salts required for absorption of vitamin K)*
• Pancreatic disease *(related to insufficient levels of enzymes to metabolize vitamin K)*

CRITICAL FINDINGS ✦

Vitamin toxicity can be as significant as problems brought about by vitamin deficiencies. The potential for toxicity is especially important to consider with respect to fat-soluble vitamins, which are not eliminated from the body as quickly as water-soluble vitamins and can accumulate in the body. The naturally occurring forms, vitamins K_1 and K_2, do not cause toxicity. Signs and symptoms of vitamin K_3 toxicity include bleeding and jaundice. Possible interventions include withholding the source.

INTERFERING FACTORS

- Drugs and substances that may decrease vitamin K levels include antibiotics, cholestyramine, coumarin, mineral oil, and warfarin.

NURSING IMPLICATIONS AND PROCEDURE

PRETEST:

▶ Positively identify the patient using at least two unique identifiers before providing care, treatment, or services.

▶ *Patient Teaching:* Inform the patient this test can assist in evaluating vitamin toxicity or deficiency.

▶ Obtain a history of the patient's complaints, including a list of known allergens, especially allergies or sensitivities to latex.

▶ Obtain a history of the patient's hematopoietic and hepatobiliary systems, symptoms, and results of previously performed laboratory tests and diagnostic and surgical procedures.

▶ Obtain a list of the patient's current medications, including herbs, nutritional supplements, and nutraceuticals (see Appendix F).

▶ Review the procedure with the patient. Inform the patient that specimen collection takes approximately 5 to 10 min. Address concerns about pain and explain that there may be some discomfort during the venipuncture.

▶ *Sensitivity to social and cultural issues,* as well as concern for modesty, is important in providing psychological support before, during, and after the procedure.

▶ There are no food, fluid, or medication restrictions unless by medical direction.

INTRATEST:

▶ If the patient has a history of allergic reaction to latex, avoid the use of equipment containing latex.

▶ Instruct the patient to cooperate fully and to follow directions. Direct the patient to breathe normally and to avoid unnecessary movement.

▶ Observe standard precautions, and follow the general guidelines in Appendix A. Positively identify the patient, and label the appropriate tubes with the corresponding patient demographics, date, and time of collection. Perform a venipuncture.

▶ Remove the needle and apply direct pressure with dry gauze to stop bleeding. Observe/assess venipuncture site for bleeding or hematoma formation and secure gauze with adhesive bandage.

▶ Promptly transport the specimen to the laboratory for processing and analysis.

POST-TEST:

▶ A report of the results will be sent to the requesting health-care provider (HCP), who will discuss the results with the patient.

▶ *Nutritional Considerations:* Inform the patient with a vitamin K deficiency, as appropriate, that the main dietary sources of vitamin K are cabbage, cauliflower, spinach and other green leafy vegetables, pork, liver, soybeans, and vegetable oils.

▶ Instruct the patient to report bleeding from any areas of the skin or mucous membranes.

▶ Inform the patient of the importance of taking precautions against bleeding or bruising, including the use of a soft bristle toothbrush, use of an electric razor, avoidance of constipation, avoidance of aspirin products, and avoidance of intramuscular injections.

▶ Reinforce information given by the patient's HCP regarding further testing, treatment, or referral to another HCP. Answer any questions or address any concerns voiced by the patient or family.

▶ Depending on the results of this procedure, additional testing may be performed to evaluate or monitor progression of the disease process and determine the need for a change in therapy. Evaluate test results in relation to the patient's symptoms and other tests performed.

RELATED MONOGRAPHS:

▶ Related tests include ALT, antithrombin III, AST, bilirubin, chloride sweat, CBC, fecal analysis, fecal fat, GGT, and PT/INR.

▶ Refer to the Hematopoietic and Hepatobiliary systems tables at the end of the book for related tests by body system.

Vitamins A, B₁, B₆, and C

SYNONYM/ACRONYM: Vitamin A: retinol, carotene; vitamin B₁: thiamine; vitamin B₆: niacin, pyroxidine, P-5′-P, pyridoxyl-5-phosphate; vitamin C: ascorbic acid.

COMMON USE: To assess vitamin deficiency or toxicity to assist in diagnosing nutritional disorders such as malabsorption; disorders that affect vision, skin, and bones; and other diseases.

SPECIMEN: Serum (1 mL) collected in a red-top tube each for vitamins A and C; plasma (1 mL) collected in a lavender-top (EDTA) tube each for vitamins B₁ and B₆.

REFERENCE VALUE: (Method: High-performance liquid chromatography)

Vitamin	Age	Conventional Units	SI Units
Vitamin A			*(Conventional Units × 0.0349)*
	1–6 yr	20–43 mcg/dL	0.70–1.50 micromol/L
	7–12 yr	26–49 mcg/dL	0.91–1.71 micromol/L
	13–19 yr	26–72 mcg/dL	0.91–2.51 micromol/L
	Adult	30–120 mcg/dL	1.05–4.19 micromol/L
Vitamin B₁			*(Conventional Units × 29.6)*
		0.21–0.43 mcg/dL	6.2–12.8 micromol/L
Vitamin B₆			*(Conversion Factor × 4.046)*
		5–30 ng/mL	20–121 nmol/L
Vitamin C			*(Conventional Units × 56.78)*
		0.6–1.9 mg/dL	34.1–107.9 micromol/L

DESCRIPTION: Vitamin assays are used in the measurement of nutritional status. Low levels indicate inadequate oral intake, poor nutritional status, or malabsorption problems. High levels indicate excessive intake, vitamin intoxication, or absorption problems. Vitamin A is a fat-soluble nutrient that promotes normal vision and prevents night blindness; contributes to growth of bone, teeth, and soft tissues; supports thyroxine formation; maintains epithelial cell membranes, skin, and mucous membranes; and acts as an anti-infection agent. Vitamins B₁, B₆, and C are water soluble. Vitamin B₁ acts as an enzyme and plays an important role in the Krebs cycle. Vitamin B$_6$ is important in heme synthesis and functions as a coenzyme in amino acid metabolism and glycogenolysis. It includes pyridoxine, pyridoxal, and pyridoxamine. Vitamin C promotes collagen synthesis, maintains capillary strength, facilitates release of iron from ferritin to form hemoglobin, and functions in the stress response.

INDICATIONS

Vitamin A
* Assist in the diagnosis of night blindness
* Evaluate skin disorders
* Investigate suspected vitamin A deficiency

Vitamin B$_1$
* Investigate suspected beriberi
* Monitor the effects of chronic alcoholism

Vitamin B$_6$
* Investigate suspected malabsorption or malnutrition
* Investigate suspected vitamin B$_6$ deficiency

Vitamin C
* Investigate suspected metabolic or malabsorptive disorders
* Investigate suspected scurvy

POTENTIAL DIAGNOSIS

Increased in
* Vitamin A:
  Chronic kidney disease
  Idiopathic hypercalcemia in infants
  Vitamin A toxicity

Decreased in
* Vitamin A:
  Abetalipoproteinemia (related to poor absorption)
  Carcinoid syndrome (related to poor absorption)

Chronic infections (vitamin A deficiency decreases ability to fight infection)
Cystic fibrosis (related to poor absorption)
Disseminated tuberculosis (related to poor absorption)
Hypothyroidism (condition decreases ability of beta carotene to convert to vitamin A)
Infantile blindness (related to dietary deficiency)
Liver, gastrointestinal (GI), or pancreatic disease (related to malabsorption or poor absorption)
Night blindness (related to chronic dietary deficiency or lack of absorption)
Protein malnutrition (related to dietary deficiency)
Sterility and teratogenesis (related to dietary deficiency)
Zinc deficiency (zinc is required for generation of vitamin A transport proteins)

* Vitamin B$_1$:
  Alcoholism (related to dietary deficiency)
  Carcinoid syndrome (related to dietary deficiency or lack of absorption)
  Hartnup's disease (related to dietary deficiency)
  Pellagra (related to dietary deficiency)

* Vitamin B$_6$ (this vitamin is involved in many essential functions, such as nucleic acid synthesis, enzyme activation, antibody production, electrolyte balance, and RBC formation; deficiencies result in a variety of conditions):
  Alcoholism (related to dietary deficiency)
  Asthma
  Carpal tunnel syndrome
  Gestational diabetes
  Lactation (related to dietary deficiency and/or increased demand)
  Malabsorption
  Malnutrition
  Neonatal seizures
  Normal pregnancies (related to dietary deficiency and/or increased demand)
  Occupational exposure to hydrazine compounds (enzymatic pathways are

altered by hydralazines in a manner that increases excretion of vitamin B_6)
Pellagra *(related to dietary deficiency)*
Pre-eclamptic edema
Renal dialysis
Uremia

- Vitamin C:
  Alcoholism *(related to dietary deficiency)*
  Anemia *(related to dietary deficiency)*
  Cancer *(related to dietary deficiency or lack of absorption)*
  Hemodialysis *(vitamin C is lost during the treatment)*
  Hyperthyroidism *(related to dietary deficiency and/or increased demand)*
  Malabsorption
  Pregnancy *(related to dietary deficiency and/or increased demand)*
  Rheumatoid disease
  Scurvy *(related to dietary deficiency or lack of absorption)*

CRITICAL FINDINGS

Vitamin toxicity can be as significant as problems brought about by vitamin deficiencies. The potential for toxicity is especially important to consider with respect to fat-soluble vitamins (A, D, E, and K), which are not eliminated from the body as quickly as water-soluble vitamins and can accumulate in the body. Most cases of toxicity are brought about by oversupplementing and can be avoided by consulting a qualified nutritionist for recommended daily dietary and supplemental allowances. Signs and symptoms of vitamin A toxicity may include headache, blurred vision, bone pain, joint pain, dry skin, and loss of appetite.

INTERFERING FACTORS

- Drugs and substances that may increase vitamin A levels include alcohol (moderate intake), oral contraceptives, and probucol.
- Drugs and substances that may decrease vitamin A levels include alcohol (chronic intake, alcoholism), allopurinol, cholestyramine, colestipol, mineral oil, and neomycin.
- Drugs that may decrease vitamin B_1 levels include glibenclamide, isoniazid, and valproic acid.
- Drugs that may decrease vitamin B_6 levels include amiodarone, anticonvulsants, cycloserine, disulfiram, ethanol, hydralazine, isoniazid, levodopa, oral contraceptives, penicillamine, pyrazinoic acid, and theophylline.
- Drugs and substances that may decrease vitamin C levels include acetylsalicylic acid, aminopyrine, barbiturates, estrogens, heavy metals, oral contraceptives, nitrosamines, and paraldehyde.
- Chronic tobacco smoking decreases vitamin C levels.
- Various diseases may affect vitamin levels (see Potential Diagnosis section).
- Diets high in freshwater fish and tea, which are thiamine antagonists, may cause decreased vitamin B_1 levels.
- Long-term hyperalimentation may result in decreased vitamin levels.
- Exposure of the specimen to light decreases vitamin levels, resulting in a falsely low results.

NURSING IMPLICATIONS AND PROCEDURE

PRETEST:

- Positively identify the patient using at least two unique identifiers before providing care, treatment, or services.
- *Patient Teaching:* Inform the patient this test can assist in evaluating vitamin toxicity or deficiency.
- Obtain a history of the patient's complaints, including a list of known allergens, especially allergies or sensitivities to latex.

- Obtain a history of the patient's gastrointestinal, genitourinary, hepatobiliary, immune, and musculoskeletal systems; symptoms; and results of previously performed laboratory tests and diagnostic and surgical procedures.
- Obtain a list of the patient's current medications, including herbs, nutritional supplements, and nutraceuticals (see Appendix F).
- Review the procedure with the patient. Inform the patient that specimen collection takes approximately 5 to 10 min. Address concerns about pain and explain that there may be some discomfort during the venipuncture.
- *Sensitivity to social and cultural issues,* as well as concern for modesty, is important in providing psychological support before, during, and after the procedure.
- Instruct the patient to fast for at least 12 hr before specimen collection for vitamin A.
- There are no fluid or medication restrictions unless by medical direction.

INTRATEST:

- Ensure that the patient has complied with dietary restrictions; assure that food has been restricted for at least 12 hr prior to the vitamin A test.
- If the patient has a history of allergic reaction to latex, avoid the use of equipment containing latex.
- Instruct the patient to cooperate fully and to follow directions. Direct the patient to breathe normally and to avoid unnecessary movement.
- Observe standard precautions, and follow the general guidelines in Appendix A. Positively identify the patient, and label the appropriate tubes with the corresponding patient demographics, date, and time of collection. Perform a venipuncture.
- Remove the needle and apply direct pressure with dry gauze to stop bleeding. Observe/assess venipuncture site for bleeding or hematoma formation and secure gauze with adhesive bandage.
- Promptly transport the specimen to the laboratory for processing and analysis.

POST-TEST:

- A report of the results will be sent to the requesting health-care provider (HCP), who will discuss the results with the patient.
- *Nutritional Considerations:* Educate the patient with a specific vitamin deficiency, as appropriate, regarding dietary sources of these vitamins. Advise the patient to ask a nutritionist to develop a diet plan recommended for his or her specific needs.

Vitamin A
- The main source of vitamin A comes from carotene, a yellow pigment noticeable in most fruits and vegetables, especially carrots, sweet potatoes, squash, apricots, and cantaloupe. It is also present in spinach, collards, broccoli, and cabbage. This vitamin is fairly stable at most cooking temperatures, but it is destroyed easily by light and oxidation.

Vitamin B₁
- Vitamin B₁ is the most stable with respect to the effects of environmental factors. It is found in meats, coffee, peanuts, and legumes. The body is also capable of making some vitamin B₁ by converting the amino acid tryptophan to niacin.

Vitamin B₆
- Good sources of vitamin B₆ include meats (especially beef and pork), whole grains, wheat germ, legumes (beans, peas, lentils), potatoes, oatmeal, and bananas. As with other water-soluble vitamins, it is best preserved by rapid cooking, although it is relatively stable at most cooking temperatures (except frying) and when exposed to acidic foods. This vitamin is destroyed rapidly by light and alkalis.

Vitamin C
- Citrus fruits are excellent dietary sources of vitamin C. Other good sources are green and red peppers, tomatoes, white potatoes, cabbage, broccoli, chard, kale, turnip greens, asparagus, berries, melons, pineapple, and guava. Vitamin C is destroyed by exposure to air, light, heat, or alkalis. Boiling water before cooking eliminates dissolved oxygen that destroys vitamin C in the process

of boiling. Vegetables should be crisp and cooked as quickly as possible.

General

▶ Reinforce information given by the patient's HCP regarding further testing, treatment, or referral to another HCP. Answer any questions or address any concerns voiced by the patient or family.

▶ Depending on the results of this procedure, additional testing may be performed to evaluate or monitor progression of the disease process and determine the need for a change in therapy. Evaluate test results in relation to the patient's symptoms and other tests performed.

RELATED MONOGRAPHS:

▶ Related tests include amylase, BUN, chloride sweat, CBC, creatinine, lipase, prealbumin, TSH, FT_4, and zinc.

▶ Refer to the Gastrointestinal, Genitourinary, Hepatobiliary, Immune, and Musculoskeletal systems tables at the end of the book for related tests by body system.

White Blood Cell Scan

SYNONYM/ACRONYM: Infection scintigraphy, inflammatory scan, labeled autologous leukocytes, labeled leukocyte scan, WBC imaging.

COMMON USE: To assist in identification of abscess, infection, and inflammation of the bone, bowel, wound, and skin.

AREA OF APPLICATION: Whole body.

CONTRAST: IV radionuclide combined with white blood cells.

DESCRIPTION: Because white blood cells (WBCs) naturally accumulate in areas of inflammation, the WBC scan uses radiolabeled WBCs to help determine the site of an acute infection or confirm the presence or absence of infection or inflammation at a suspected site. A gamma camera detects the radiation emitted from the injected radionuclide, and a representative image of the radionuclide distribution is obtained and recorded or stored electronically. Because of its better image resolution and greater specificity for acute infections, the WBC scan has replaced scanning with gallium-67 citrate (Ga-67). Some chronic infections associated with pulmonary disease, however, may be better imaged with Ga-67. The WBC scan is especially helpful in detecting postoperative infection sites and in documenting lack of residual infection after a course of therapy.

INDICATIONS

- Aid in the diagnosis of infectious or inflammatory diseases
- Differentiate infectious from noninfectious process
- Evaluate the effects of treatment
- Evaluate inflammatory bowel disease (IBD)
- Evaluate patients with fever of unknown origin

- Evaluate postsurgical sites and wound infections
- Evaluate suspected infection of an orthopedic prosthesis
- Evaluate suspected osteomyelitis

POTENTIAL DIAGNOSIS

Normal findings in
- No focal localization of the radionuclide, along with some slight localization of the radionuclide within the reticuloendothelial system (liver, spleen, and bone marrow)

Abnormal findings in
- Abscess
- Arthritis
- Infection
- Inflammation
- IBD
- Osteomyelitis

CRITICAL FINDINGS: N/A

INTERFERING FACTORS

This procedure is contraindicated for
- Patients who are pregnant or suspected of being pregnant, unless the potential benefits of the procedure far outweigh the risks to the fetus and mother.

Factors that may impair clear imaging
- Inability of the patient to cooperate or remain still during the procedure because of age, significant pain, or mental status.

W

- Retained barium from a previous radiological procedure, which may inhibit visualization of an abdominal lesion.
- Metallic objects (e.g., jewelry, body rings) within the examination field, which may inhibit organ visualization and cause unclear images.
- Other nuclear scans done within 48 hr and Ga-67 scans within 4 wk before the procedure.
- Lesions smaller than 1 to 2 cm, which may not be detectable.
- A distended bladder, which may obscure pelvic detail.

Other considerations

- Improper injection of the radionuclide that allows the tracer to seep deep into the muscle tissue produces erroneous hot spots.
- Patients with a low WBC count may need donor WBCs to complete the radionuclide labeling process; otherwise, Ga-67 scanning should be performed instead.
- False-negative images may be a result of hemodialysis, hyperglycemia, hyperalimentation, steroid therapy, and antibiotic therapy.
- The presence of multiple myeloma or thyroid cancer can result in a false-negative scan for bone abnormalities.
- Consultation with a health-care provider (HCP) should occur before the procedure for radiation safety concerns regarding younger patients or patients who are lactating.
- Risks associated with radiation overexposure can result from frequent x-ray or radionuclide procedures. Personnel working in the examination area should wear badges to record their level of radiation exposure.

NURSING IMPLICATIONS AND PROCEDURE

PRETEST:

- Positively identify the patient using at least two unique identifiers before providing care, treatment, or services.
- *Patient Teaching:* Inform the patient this test can assist in assessing for the presence of infection or inflammation.
- Obtain a history of the patient's complaints, including a list of known allergens, especially allergies or sensitivities to latex, iodine, seafood, contrast medium, or anesthetics.
- Obtain a history of the patient's immune system, symptoms, and results of previously performed laboratory tests and diagnostic and surgical procedures.
- Note any recent procedures that can interfere with test results, including barium examinations.
- Record the date of the last menstrual period and determine the possibility of pregnancy in perimenopausal women.
- Obtain a list of the patient's current medications, including anticoagulant therapy, aspirin and other salicylates, herbs, nutritional supplements, and nutraceuticals (see Appendix F). Note the last time and dose of medication taken.
- Review the procedure with the patient. Address concerns about pain related to the procedure and explain that some pain may be experienced during the test, and there may be moments of discomfort. Reassure the patient that the radionuclide poses no radioactive hazard and rarely produces side effects. Inform the patient that the procedure is performed in a nuclear medicine department by an HCP. It usually takes approximately 1 to 6 hr, and delayed images are needed 24 hr later. The patient may leave the department and return later to undergo delayed imaging.

Sensitivity to social and cultural issues, as well as concern for modesty, is important in providing psychological support before, during, and after the procedure.

▶ Instruct the patient to remove jewelry and other metallic objects from the area to be examined.

▶ There are no dietary or medication restrictions prior to the procedure, unless by medical direction.

▶ *Make sure a written and informed consent has been signed prior to the procedure and before administering any medications.*

INTRATEST:

▶ Ensure the patient has removed all external metallic objects prior to the procedure.

▶ If the patient has a history of allergic reactions to any substance or drug, administer ordered prophylactic steroids or antihistamines before the procedure.

▶ Have emergency equipment readily available.

▶ Instruct the patient to void prior to the procedure and to change into the gown, robe, and foot coverings provided.

▶ Observe standard precautions, and follow the general guidelines in Appendix A.

▶ Administer sedative to a child or to an uncooperative adult, as ordered.

▶ On the day of the test, draw a 50- to 80-mL sample of blood for separating the WBCs from the blood and an in vitro process of labeling with radionuclide.

▶ IV radionuclide-labeled autologous WBCs are administered.

▶ Images are recorded 1 to 6 hr postinjection depending on the radionuclide used. Delayed images may be required at 24 hr after the injection.

▶ Remove the needle or catheter and apply a pressure dressing over the puncture site.

▶ Observe/assess the needle/catheter insertion site for bleeding, inflammation, or hematoma formation.

▶ If abdominal abscess or infection is suspected, laxatives or enemas may be ordered before delayed imaging.

POST-TEST:

▶ A report of the results will be sent to the requesting HCP, who will discuss the results with the patient.

▶ Unless contraindicated, advise patient to drink increased amounts of fluids for 24 to 48 hr to eliminate the radionuclide from the body. Inform the patient that radionuclide is eliminated from the body within 6 to 24 hr.

▶ No other radionuclide tests should be scheduled for 24 to 48 hr after this procedure.

▶ Observe/assess the needle/catheter insertion site for bleeding, inflammation, or hematoma formation.

▶ Instruct the patient in the care and assessment of the injection site.

▶ If a woman who is breastfeeding must have a nuclear scan, she should not breastfeed the infant until the radionuclide has been eliminated. This could take as long as 3 days. She should be instructed to express the milk and discard it during the 3-day period to prevent cessation of milk production.

▶ Instruct the patient to immediately flush the toilet and to meticulously wash hands with soap and water after each voiding for 24 hr after the procedure.

▶ Instruct all caregivers to wear gloves when discarding urine for 24 hr after the procedure. Wash gloved hands with soap and water before removing gloves. Then wash hands after the gloves are removed.

▶ Recognize anxiety related to test results, and be supportive of perceived loss of independent function. Discuss the implications of abnormal test results on the patient's lifestyle. Provide teaching and information regarding the clinical implications of the test results, as appropriate.

▶ Reinforce information given by the patient's HCP regarding further testing, treatment, or referral to another HCP. Answer any questions or address any concerns voiced by the patient or family.

▶ Depending on the results of this procedure, additional testing may be needed to evaluate or monitor

progression of the disease process and determine the need for a change in therapy. Evaluate test results in relation to the patient's symptoms and other tests performed.

RELATED MONOGRAPHS:

▶ Related tests include angiography pulmonary, bone scan, colonoscopy, CBC, CBC WBC count and differential, CT abdomen, CT pelvis, CT spine, culture (blood, skin, wound), ESR, fecal analysis, gallium scan, GI blood loss scan, KUB, MRI musculoskeletal, MRI pelvis, MRI spine, proctosigmoidoscopy, radiography bone, US abdomen, US pelvis, and vitamin D.

▶ Refer to the Immune System table at the end of the book for related tests by body system.

Zinc

SYNONYM/ACRONYM: Zn.

COMMON USE: To assist in assessing for vitamin deficiency or toxicity, monitor therapeutic interventions, and assist in diagnosing disorders such as acrodermatitis enteropathica.

SPECIMEN: Serum (1 mL) collected in a trace element-free, royal blue-top tube.

REFERENCE VALUE: (Method: Atomic absorption spectrophotometry)

Age	Conventional Units	SI Units (Conventional Units × 0.153)
Newborn–6 mo	26–141 mcg/dL	4.0–21.6 micromol/L
6–11 mo	29–131 mcg/dL	4.5–20.1 micromol/L
1–4 yr	31–115 mcg/dL	4.8–17.6 micromol/L
4–5 yr	48–119 mcg/dL	7.4–18.2 micromol/L
6–9 yr	48–129 mcg/dL	7.3–19.7 micromol/L
10–13 yr	25–148 mcg/dL	3.9–22.7 micromol/L
14–17 yr	46–130 mcg/dL	7.1–19.9 micromol/L
Adult	70–120 mcg/dL	10.7–18.4 micromol/L

DESCRIPTION: Zinc is found in all body tissues, but the highest concentrations are found in the eye, bone, and male reproductive organs. Zinc is involved in RNA and DNA synthesis and is essential in the process of tissue repair. It is also required for the formation of collagen and the production of active vitamin A (for the visual pigment rhodopsin). Zinc also functions as a chelating agent to protect the body from lead and cadmium poisoning. Zinc is absorbed from the small intestine. Its absorption and excretion seem to be through the same sites as those for iron and copper. The body does not store zinc as it does copper and iron. Untreated zinc deficiency in infants may result in a condition called acrodermatitis enteropathica. Symptoms include growth retardation, diarrhea, impaired wound healing, and frequent infections. Adolescents and adults with zinc deficiency exhibit similar adverse effects on growth, sexual development, and immune function, as well as altered taste and smell, emotional instability, impaired adaptation to darkness, impaired night vision, tremors, and a bullous, pustular rash over the extremities.

INDICATIONS

- Assist in confirming acrodermatitis enteropathica
- Evaluate nutritional deficiency
- Evaluate possible toxicity
- Monitor replacement therapy in individuals with identified deficiencies
- Monitor therapy of individuals with Wilson's disease

Z

POTENTIAL DIAGNOSIS

Increased in

Zinc is contained in and secreted by numerous types of cells in the body. Damaged cells release zinc into circulation and increase blood levels.

- Anemia *(related to competitive relationship with copper; copper deficiency is associated with decreased production of red blood cells)*

Decreased in

This trace metal is an essential component of enzymes that participate in protein and carbohydrate metabolism. It is involved in DNA replication, insulin storage, carbon dioxide gas exchange, cellular immunity and healing, promotion of body growth, and sexual maturity. Deficiencies result in a variety of conditions.

- Acrodermatitis enteropathica *(congenital abnormality that affects zinc uptake and results in zinc deficiency)*
- AIDS
- Acute infections
- Acute stress
- Burns
- Cirrhosis
- Conditions that decrease albumin *(related to lack of available transport proteins)*
- Diabetes
- Long-term total parenteral nutrition
- Malabsorption
- Myocardial infarction
- Nephrotic syndrome
- Nutritional deficiency
- Pregnancy *(related to increased uptake by fetus; related to excessive levels of iron and folic acid prescribed during pregnancy and which interfere with absorption)*
- Pulmonary tuberculosis

CRITICAL FINDINGS: N/A

INTERFERING FACTORS

- Drugs that may increase zinc levels include auranofin, chlorthalidone, corticotropin, oral contraceptives, and penicillamine.
- Drugs that may decrease zinc levels include anticonvulsants, cisplatin, citrates, corticosteroids, estrogens, interferon, oral contraceptives, and prednisone.

NURSING IMPLICATIONS AND PROCEDURE

PRETEST:

- Positively identify the patient using at least two unique identifiers before providing care, treatment, or services.
- *Patient Teaching:* Inform the patient this test can assist in evaluating for disorders associated with abnormal zinc levels and monitor response to therapy.
- Obtain a history of the patient's complaints, including a list of known allergens, especially allergies or sensitivities to latex.
- Obtain a history of the patient's gastrointestinal, hepatobiliary, immune, and musculoskeletal systems; symptoms; and results of previously performed laboratory tests and diagnostic and surgical procedures.
- Obtain a list of the patient's current medications, including herbs, nutritional supplements, and nutraceuticals (see Appendix F).
- Review the procedure with the patient. Inform the patient that specimen collection takes approximately 5 to 10 min. Address concerns about pain and explain that there may be some discomfort during the venipuncture.
- *Sensitivity to social and cultural issues,* as well as concern for modesty, is important in providing psychological support before, during, and after the procedure.
- There are no food, fluid, or medication restrictions unless by medical direction.

INTRATEST:

▶ If the patient has a history of allergic reaction to latex, avoid the use of equipment containing latex.

▶ Instruct the patient to cooperate fully and to follow directions. Direct the patient to breathe normally and to avoid unnecessary movement.

▶ Observe standard precautions, and follow the general guidelines in Appendix A. Positively identify the patient, and label the appropriate tube with the corresponding patient demographics, date, and time of collection. Perform a venipuncture.

▶ Remove the needle and apply direct pressure with dry gauze to stop bleeding. Observe/assess venipuncture site for bleeding or hematoma formation and secure gauze with adhesive bandage.

▶ Promptly transport the specimen to the laboratory for processing and analysis.

POST-TEST:

▶ A report of the results will be sent to the requesting health-care provider (HCP), who will discuss the results with the patient.

▶ *Nutritional Considerations:* Topical or oral supplementation may be ordered for patients with zinc deficiency. Dietary sources high in zinc include shellfish,

red meat, wheat germ, and processed foods such as canned pork and beans and canned chili. Patients should be informed that phytates (from whole grains, coffee, cocoa, or tea) bind zinc and prevent it from being absorbed. Decreases in zinc also can be induced by increased intake of iron, copper, or manganese. Vitamin and mineral supplements with a greater than 3:1 iron/zinc ratio inhibit zinc absorption.

▶ Reinforce information given by the patient's HCP regarding further testing, treatment, or referral to another HCP. Answer any questions or address any concerns voiced by the patient or family.

▶ Depending on the results of this procedure, additional testing may be performed to evaluate or monitor progression of the disease process and determine the need for a change in therapy. Evaluate test results in relation to the patient's symptoms and other tests performed.

RELATED MONOGRAPHS:

▶ Related tests include albumin, CBC, CBC WBC and differential, copper, iron, and vitamin A.

▶ Refer to the Gastrointestinal, Immune, Hepatobiliary, and Musculoskeletal systems tables at the end of the book for related tests by body system.

System Tables

Auditory System

Laboratory Tests Associated With the Auditory System

Antibiotic drugs—aminoglycosides: amikacin, gentamicin, tobramycin; tricyclic
  glycopeptide: vancomycin, 102–106
Culture, bacterial, anal/genital, ear, eye, skin, and wound, 548–554
Zinc, 1361–1363

Diagnostic Tests Associated With the Auditory System

Audiometry hearing loss, 172–176
Computed tomography, brain, 463–467
Evoked brain potentials, 660–664
Magnetic resonance imaging, brain,
  924–928

Otoscopy, 995–997
Spondee speech reception threshold,
  1182–1185
Tuning fork tests,
  1237–1240

Cardiovascular System

Laboratory Tests Associated With the Cardiovascular System

Alveolar/arterial gradient, 32–35
Anion gap, 93–95
Antiarrhythmic drugs, 96–102
Apolipoprotein A and B, 157–161
Aspartate aminotransferase, 167–171
Atrial natriuretic peptide, 172
Blood gases, 250–261
B-type natriuretic peptide, 283–286
Calcium, blood, 290–294
Calcium, ionized, 295–298
Carbon dioxide, 312–315
Chloride, blood, 339–343
Cholesterol, HDL and LDL, 359–363
Cholesterol, total, 364–368
Complete blood count, 401–409
Complete blood count, hematocrit,
  409–414
Complete blood count, hemoglobin,
  414–420
Complete blood count, RBC count,
  426–432
C-reactive protein, 524–526
Creatine kinase and isoenzymes, 526–530
D-Dimer, 598–600
Digoxin, 96–102

Disopyramide, 96–102
Erythrocyte sedimentation rate,
  646–649
Fibrin degradation products, 686–689
Flecainide, 96–102
Homocysteine and methylmalonic acid,
  788–791
International normalized ratio (INR),
  1108–1112
Lactate dehydrogenase and iso-
  enzymes, 861–862
Lactic acid, 862–865
Lidocaine, 96–102
Lipoprotein electrophoresis, 886–887
Magnesium, blood, 910–913
Myoglobin, 980–983
Pericardial fluid analysis, 1022–1025
Potassium, blood, 1072–1077
Procainamide, 96–102
Prothrombin time and INR, 1108–1112
Quinidine, 96–102
Sodium, blood, 1175–1178
Triglycerides, 1221–1225
Troponins I and T, 1230–1233
Vitamin E, 1347–1349

Diagnostic Tests Associated With the Cardiovascular System

Endocrine System

Laboratory Tests Associated With the Endocrine System

(table continues on page 1366)

SYS

Laboratory Tests Associated With the Endocrine System

Insulin and insulin response to glucose, 829–832
Insulin antibodies, 832–834
Ketones, blood and urine, 852–855
Lactic acid, 862–865
Luteinizing hormone, 901–903
Magnesium, blood, 910–913
Magnesium, urine, 913–916
Metanephrines, 960–962
Metyrapone stimulation, 516–520
Glucagon, 730–734
Microalbumin, 965–968
Osmolality, blood and urine, 987–990
Parathyroid hormone, 1010–1013
Phosphorus, blood, 1030–1033
Phosphorus, urine, 1033–1036
Potassium, blood, 1072–1077
Potassium, urine, 1077–1081
Prealbumin, 1081–1083
Progesterone, 1087–1090

Prolactin, 1090–1093
Renin, 1140–1144
Sodium, blood, 1175–1178
Sodium, urine, 1179–1182
Testosterone, total, 1196–1199
Thyroglobulin, 1199–1201
Thyroid-binding inhibitory immunoglobulin, 1201
Thyroid-stimulating hormone, 1205–1207
Thyroid-stimulating immunoglobulins, 1208–1209
Thyroxine-binding globulin, 1209–1211
Thyroxine, free, 1212–1214
Thyroxine, total, 1214–1217
Triiodothyronine, free, 1225–1227
Triiodothyronine, total, 1227–1230
Urinalysis, 1313–1320
Vanillylmandelic acid, urine, 1326–1327

Diagnostic Tests Associated With the Endocrine System

Adrenal gland scan, 5–7
Angiography, adrenal, 71–75
Computed tomography, pituitary, 486–490
Lymphangiography, 906–909
Magnetic resonance imaging, pancreas, 939–943

Magnetic resonance imaging, pituitary, 947–950
Parathyroid scan, 1013–1015
Radioactive iodine uptake, 1124–1127
Sialography, 1167–1169
Thyroid scan, 1202–1205
Ultrasound, thyroid and parathyroid, 1284–1286

Gastrointestinal System

Laboratory Tests Associated With the Gastrointestinal System

Albumin and albumin/globulin ratio, 17–20
Amylase, 59–63
Antibodies, antineutrophilic cytoplasmic, 113–115
Antibodies, gliadin (immunoglobulin G and immunoglobulin A), 128–131

Biopsy, intestinal, 214–217
Calcium, blood, 290–294
Calcium, ionized, 295–298
Cancer antigens, 304–308
Cholesterol, total, 364–368
Complete blood count, 401–409

Laboratory Tests Associated With the Gastrointestinal System

Diagnostic Tests Associated With the Gastrointestinal System

SYS

Genitourinary System

Laboratory Tests Associated With the Genitourinary System

Acetaminophen, 63–66
Acid phosphatase, prostatic, 4
Albumin and albumin/globulin ratio, 17–20
Aldosterone, 21–25
Amikacin, 102–106
Amino acid screen, blood, 38–42
Amino acid screen, urine, 43–48
Anion gap, 93–95
Antiarrhythmic drugs, 96–102
Antibiotic drugs, 102–106
Antibodies, anti-glomerular basement membrane, 109–111
Antibodies, antineutrophic cytoplasmic, 113–115
Anticonvulsant drugs, 131–137
Antidepressant drugs, 139–143
Antidiuretic hormone, 143–146
Antipsychotic drugs, 146–150
β_2-Microglobulin, blood and urine, 177–180
Biopsy, bladder, 191–194
Biopsy, kidney, 217–220
Biopsy, prostate, 235–240
Bladder cancer markers, urine, 246–248
Blood gases, 250–261
Calcium, blood, 290–294
Calcium, ionized, 295–298
Calcium, urine, 298–302
Calculus, kidney stone panel, 303–304
Carbon dioxide, 312–315
Chloride, blood, 339–343
Complete blood count, 401–409
Complete blood count, hematocrit, 409–414
Complete blood count, hemoglobin, 414–420
Complete blood count, RBC count, 426–432

Creatinine, blood, 531–535
Creatinine, urine, and creatinine clearance, urine, 535–540
Culture, bacterial, urine, 569–572
Culture, viral, 574–577
Cyclosporine, 823–826
Cytology, urine, 593–595
Erythropoietin, 650–652
Gentamicin, 102–106
Gram stain, 753–756
Lithium, 146–150
Magnesium, blood, 910–913
Magnesium, urine, 913–916
Methotrexate, 823–826
Microalbumin, 965–968
Osmolality, blood and urine, 987–990
Oxalate, urine, 999–1002
Phosphorus, blood, 1030–1033
Phosphorus, urine, 1033–1036
Potassium, blood, 1072–1077
Potassium, urine, 1077–1081
Prostate-specific antigen, 1093–1095
Protein, urine: total quantitative and fractions, 1104–1107
Renin, 1140–1144
Salicylate, 63–66
Sodium, blood, 1175–1178
Sodium, urine, 1179–1182
Tobramycin, 102–106
Urea nitrogen, blood, 1296–1299
Urea nitrogen, urine, 1300–1302
Uric acid, blood, 1306–1309
Uric acid, urine, 1309–1312
Urinalysis, 1313–1320
Vancomycin, 102–106
Vitamins A, B_1, B_6, and C, 1352–1356

Diagnostic Tests Associated With the Genitourinary System

Angiography, renal, 88–92
Computed tomography, pelvis, 482–486
Computed tomography, renal, 491–495
Cystometry, 520–523

Cystoscopy, 581–584
Cystourethrography, voiding, 585–588
Electromyography, pelvic floor sphincter, 635–637

Diagnostic Tests Associated With the Genitourinary System

Hematopoietic System

Laboratory Tests Associated With the Hematopoietic System

(table continues on page 1370)

Laboratory Tests Associated With the Hematopoietic System

Methemoglobin, 963–965
Osmotic fragility, 991
Partial thromboplastin time, activated, 1016–1019
Plasminogen, 1036–1039
Platelet antibodies, 1039–1041
Porphyrins, urine, 1051–1054
Protein C, 1099–1101
Protein S, 1102–1104
Prothrombin time and INR, 1108–1112

Pyruvate kinase, 1123
Red blood cell cholinesterase, 1134–1136
Reticulocyte count, 1148–1150
Sickle cell screen, 1170–1172
Transferrin, 1219–1221
Urinalysis, 1313–1321
Vitamin B$_{12}$, 1342–1344
Vitamin E, 1347–1349
Vitamin K, 1349–1352

Diagnostic Tests Associated With the Hematopoietic System

Computed tomography, spleen, 499–503
Liver and spleen scan, 887–890
Ultrasound, spleen, 1281–1283

Hepatobiliary System

Laboratory Tests Associated With the Hepatobiliary System

Acetaminophen, 63–66
Acetylsalicylic acid, 63–66
Alanine aminotransferase, 14–16
Albumin, 17–20
Aldolase, 20
Alkaline phosphatase and isoenzymes, 25–29
Amino acid, blood, 38–42
Amino acid, urine, 43–48
Amitriptyline, 139–143
Ammonia, 51–53
Amylase, 59–63
Antibodies, antimitochondrial and antismooth muscle, 111–113
Antibodies, antineutrophilic cytoplasmic, 113–115
α_1-Antitrypsin and α_1-antitrypsin phenotyping, 153–156
Aspartate aminotransferase, 167–171
Bilirubin and bilirubin fractions, 187–191
Biopsy, liver, 220–223
Calcium, blood, 290–294
Calcium, ionized, 295–298
Carbamazepine, 131–137

Ceruloplasmin, 332–333
Cholesterol, total, 364–368
Coagulation factors, 374–381
Complete blood count, 401–409
Complete blood count, hematocrit, 409–414
Complete blood count, hemoglobin, 414–420
Complete blood count, RBC count, 426–432
Complete blood count, RBC morphology and inclusions, 436–441
Copper, 513–516
Desipramine, 139–143
Diazepam, 139–143
Doxepin, 139–143
Ethosuximide, 131–137
Fibrinogen, 689–692
δ-Glutamyltransferase, 711–713
Haloperidol, 146–150
Haptoglobin, 762–764
Hepatitis A antibody, 771–772
Hepatitis B antigen and antibody, 773–775
Hepatitis C antibody, 776–778

Laboratory Tests Associated With the Hepatobiliary System

Diagnostic Tests Associated With the Hepatobiliary System

Immune System

Laboratory Tests Associated With the Immune System

(table continues on page 1372)

Laboratory Tests Associated With the Immune System

Laboratory Tests Associated With the Immune System

Diagnostic Tests Associated With the Immune System

Musculoskeletal System

Laboratory Tests Associated With the Musculoskeletal System

(table continues on page 1374)

Laboratory Tests Associated With the Musculoskeletal System

Diagnostic Tests Associated With the Musculoskeletal System

Nutritional Considerations

Laboratory Tests With Nutritional Considerations

Ocular System

Laboratory Tests Associated With the Ocular System

Laboratory Tests Associated With the Ocular System

Anticonvulsant drugs: carbamazepine, ethosuximide, phenobarbital, phenytoin, primidone, valproic acid, 131–137
C-peptide, 521–523
Culture, bacterial, anal/genital, ear, eye, skin, and wound, 548–554
Fructosamine, 702–704

Glucagon, 730–734
Glucose, 734–739
Glycated hemoglobin A_{1C}, 748–750
Insulin and insulin response to glucose, 829–832
Microalbumin, 965–968
Rheumatoid factor, 1155–1157
Vitamins A, B_1, B_6, and C, 1352–1356

Diagnostic Tests Associated With the Ocular System

Color perception test, 391–393
Computed tomography, brain, 463–467
Evoked brain potentials, 660–664
Fluorescein angiography, 692–695
Fundus photography, 704–707
Gonioscopy, 751–753
Intraocular muscle function, 835–837
Intraocular pressure, 837–840

Magnetic resonance imaging, brain, 924–928
Nerve fiber analysis, 984–986
Pachymetry, 1003–1004
Plethysmography, 1041–1046
Refraction, 1136–1139
Schirmer test, 1162–1164
Slit-lamp biomicroscopy, 1172–1175
Ultrasound, A-scan, 1247–1249
Visual fields test, 1339–1341

Reproductive System

Laboratory Tests Associated With the Reproductive System

Acid phosphatase, prostatic, 4
Amino acid screen, blood, 38–42
Amino acid screen, urine, 43–48
Amniotic fluid analysis, 54–59
Antibodies, antisperm, 120–122
Antibodies, cardiolipin, immunoglobulin G, and immunoglobulin M, 126–128
Biopsy, breast, 203–207
Biopsy, cervical, 207–210
Biopsy, chorionic villus, 211–214
Cancer antigens, 304–308
Chlamydia group antibody, Ig, 337–339
Chromosome analysis, blood, 368–371
Collagen cross-linked N-telopeptide, 384–387
Culture, bacterial, anal/genital, 548–554
Culture, viral, 574–577

Cytomegalovirus, immunoglobulin G, and immunoglobulin M, 595–597
Estradiol, 659–660
Fern test, 54–59
Fetal fibronectin, 677–679
α_1-Fetoprotein, 679–683
Follicle-stimulating hormone, 699–701
Gram stain, 753–756
Her-2/neu oncoprotein, 203–207
Hexosaminidase A and B, 783–785
Human chorionic gonadotropin, 795–798
Human immunodeficiency virus type 1 and type 2 antibodies, 798–801
Human papillomavirus, 1005–1009
Inhibin-A, 679–683
Ki67, 203–207
Kleihauer-Betke test, 858–860
Lecithin/sphingomyelin ratio, 878–881
Lupus anticoagulant antibodies, 898–900

(table continues on page 1376)

Laboratory Tests Associated With the Reproductive System

Luteinizing hormone, 901–903
Magnesium, blood, 910–913
P53, 203–207
Papanicolaou smear, 1005–1009
Placental alpha microglobulin-1
   protein, 54–59
Proliferating cell nuclear antigen,
   203–207
Progesterone, 1087–1090

Prolactin, 1090–1093
Rubella antibodies, 1157–1159
S-phase fraction, 203–207
Semen analysis, 1164–1167
Syphilis serology, 1193–1195
Testosterone, total, 1196–1199
Toxoplasma antibody, 1217–1218
Urinalysis, 1313–1320
Varicella antibodies, 1329–1330

Diagnostic Tests Associated With the Reproductive System

Colposcopy, 393–396
Computed tomography, pelvis,
   482–486
Contraction stress test, 1251
Ductography, 607–610
Fetoscopy, 684–686
Hysterosalpingography, 809–812
Hysteroscopy, 812–814
Laparoscopy, gynecologic,
   871–875
Magnetic resonance imaging, breast,
   928–931

Mammography, 950–953
Nonstress test, 1249–1255
Positron emission tomography,
   FDG, 1059–1063
Stereotactic biopsy, breast, 1185–1188
Ultrasound, biophysical profile,
   obstetric, 1249–1255
Ultrasound, breast, 1258–1260
Ultrasound, pelvic, gynecologic,
   1272–1275
Ultrasound, scrotal, 1278–1281
Uterine fibroid embolization, 1321–1325

Respiratory System

Laboratory Tests Associated With the Respiratory System

Allergen-specific immunoglobulin E,
   29–31
Alveolar/arterial gradient and arterial/
   alveolar oxygen ratio, 32–35
Angiotensin-converting enzyme, 92–93
Anion gap, 93–95
Antibodies, anti-glomerular basement
   membrane, 109–111
α_1-Antitrypsin and α_1-antitrypsin
   phenotyping, 153–156
Biopsy, lung, 224–228
Blood gases, 250–261
Carbon dioxide, 312–315
Carboxyhemoglobin, 316–318
Chloride, blood, 339–343
Chloride, sweat, 343–348
Cold agglutinin titer, 381–383

Complete blood count, 401–409
Complete blood count, hematocrit,
   409–414
Complete blood count, hemoglobin,
   414–421
Complete blood count, RBC count,
   426–432
Complete blood count, RBC indices,
   432–435
Complete blood count, WBC count and
   differential, 441–449
Culture and smear, mycobacteria,
   543–548
Culture, bacterial, sputum, 558–562
Culture, bacterial, throat, 566–568
Culture, viral, 574–577
Cytology, sputum, 588–592

SYS

Laboratory Tests Associated With the Respiratory System

D-Dimer, 598–600
Eosinophil count, 641–644
Erythrocyte sedimentation rate,
  646–649
Fecal fat, 671–674
Gram stain, 753–756
Group A streptococcal screen, 756–758
Hypersensitivity pneumonitis,
  serology, 808

Immunoglobulin E, 817–819
Lactic acid, 862–865
Lecithin/sphingomyelin ratio,
  878–881
Methemoglobin, 963–965
Pleural fluid analysis, 1046–1051
Potassium, blood, 1072–1077
Rapid streptococcal screen, 756–758
Tuberculin skin tests, 1233–1237

SYS

Diagnostic Tests Associated With the Respiratory System

Angiography, pulmonary,
  84–88
Bronchoscopy, 279–283
Chest x-ray, 334–336
Computed tomography, thoracic,
  504–508
Endoscopy, sinus, 640–641
Lung perfusion scan, 891–894
Lung ventilation scan,
  894–897

Magnetic resonance imaging, chest,
  932–935
Mediastinoscopy, 957–960
Plethysmography, 1041–1046
Positron emission tomography, heart,
  1064–1068
Pulmonary function studies, 1114–1120
Pulse oximetry, 1120–1122
Venography, lower extremity
  studies, 1331–1334

Therapeutic Drug Monitoring and Toxicology

Laboratory Tests Associated With Therapeutic Drug Monitoring and Toxicology

Acetaminophen, 63–66
Acetylsalicylic acid, 63–66
Albumin, 17–20
Alcohol, ethyl, 603–607
Amikacin, 102–106
Amitriptyline, 139–143
Amphetamines, 603–607
Cannabinoids, 603–607
Carbamazepine, 131–137
Cocaine, 603–607
Cyclosporine, 823–826
Desipramine, 139–143
Diazepam, 603–607
Digoxin, 96–102

Disopyramide, 96–102
Doxepin, 139–143
Ethanol, 603–607
Ethosuximide, 131–137
Flecainide, 96–102
Gentamicin, 102–106
Haloperidol, 146–150
Imipramine, 139–143
Lead, 876–877
Lidocaine, 96–102
Lithium, 146–150
Methotrexate, 823–826
Nortriptyline, 139–143
Opiates, 603–607

(table continues on page 1378)

Laboratory Tests Associated With Therapeutic Drug Monitoring and Toxicology

SYS

Patient Preparation and Specimen Collection

PATIENT PREPARATION BEFORE DIAGNOSTIC AND LABORATORY PROCEDURES

The first step in any laboratory or diagnostic procedure is patient preparation or patient teaching before the performance of the procedure. This pretesting explanation to the patient or caregiver follows essentially the same pattern for all sites and types of studies and includes the following:

- *Statement of the purpose of the study.* The level of detail provided to patients about the test purpose depends on numerous factors and should be individualized appropriately in each particular setting.
- *Description of the procedure, including site and method.* It is a good idea to explain to the patient that you will be wearing gloves throughout the procedure. The explanation should help the patient understand that the use of gloves is standard practice established for his or her protection as well as yours. Many institutions require hand washing at the beginning and end of each specimen collection encounter and between each patient.
- *Description of the sensations, including discomfort and pain, that the patient may experience during the specimen collection procedure.* Address concerns about pain related to the procedure and suggest breathing or visualization techniques to promote relaxation. For pediatric patients, a doll may be used to "show" the procedure. Where appropriate, the use of sedative or anesthetizing agents may assist in allaying anxiety the patient may experience related to anticipation of pain associated with the procedure. Sensitivity to cultural and social issues, as well as concern for modesty, is important in providing psychological support.
- *Instruction regarding pretesting preparations related to diet, liquids, medications, and activity as well as any restrictions regarding diet, liquids, medications, activity, known allergies, therapies, or other procedures that might affect test results.* To increase patient compliance, the instructions should include an explanation of why strict adherence to the instructions is required.
- *Recognition of anxiety related to test results.* Provide a compassionate, reassuring environment. Be prepared to educate the patient regarding access to the appropriate counseling services. Encourage the patient to ask questions and verbalize his or her concerns.

Specific collection techniques and patient preparation vary by site, study required, and level of invasiveness. These techniques are described in the individual monographs.

- It is essential that the patient be positively and properly identified before providing care, treatment, or services. Specimens should always be labeled with the patient's name, date of birth (or some other unique identifier), date collected, time collected, and initials of the person collecting the sample.
- Orders should be completed accurately and submitted per laboratory policy.

BLOOD SPECIMENS

Most laboratory tests that require a blood specimen use venous blood. Venous blood can be collected directly from the vein or by way of capillary puncture. Capillary blood can be obtained from the fingertips or earlobes of adults and

APP

small children. Capillary blood can also be obtained from the heels of infants. The circumstances in which the capillary method is selected over direct venipuncture include cases in which:

• The patient has poor veins.
• The patient has small veins.
• The patient has a limited number of available veins.
• The patient has significant anxiety about the venipuncture procedure.

Venous blood also can be obtained from vascular access devices, such as heparin locks and central venous catheters. Examples of central venous catheters include the triple-lumen subclavian, Hickman, and Groshong catheters.

Fetal blood samples can be obtained, when warranted, by a qualified healthcare provider (HCP) from the scalp or from the umbilical cord.

Arterial blood can be collected from the radial, brachial, or femoral artery if blood gas analysis is requested.

Some general guidelines should be followed in the procurement and handling of blood specimens:

• The practice of an overnight fast before specimen collection is a general recommendation. Reference ranges are often based on fasting populations to provide some level of standardization for comparison. Some test results are dramatically affected by foods, however, and fasting is a pretest requirement. The presence of lipids in the blood also may interfere with the test method; fasting eliminates this potential source of error, especially if the patient already has elevated lipid levels. The laboratory should always be consulted if there is a question whether fasting is a requirement or a recommendation.
• Gloves and any other additional personal protective equipment indicated by the patient's condition should always be worn during the specimen collection process. Appendix G provides a more detailed description of standard precautions.
• Stress can cause variations in some test results. A sleeping patient should be gently awakened and allowed the opportunity to become oriented before collection site selection. Comatose or unconscious patients should be greeted in the same gentle manner because, although they are unable to respond, they may be capable of hearing and understanding. Anticipate instances in which patient cooperation may be an issue. Enlist a second person to assist with specimen collection to ensure a safe, quality collection experience for all involved.
• Localized activity such as the application of a tourniquet or clenching the hand to assist in visualizing the vein can cause variations in some test results. It is important to be aware of affected studies before specimen collection.
• Hemoconcentration may cause variations in some test results. The tourniquet should never be left in place for longer than 1 min.
• Previous puncture sites should be avoided when accessing a blood vessel by any means to reduce the potential for infection.
• Specimens should never be collected above an IV line because of the potential for dilution when the specimen and the IV solution combine in the collection container, falsely decreasing the result. It is also possible that substances in the IV solution could contaminate the specimen and result in falsely elevated test results.

- Changes in posture from supine to erect or long-term maintenance of a supine posture causes variations in some test results. It is important to be aware of this effect when results are interpreted and compared with previous values.
- Collection times for therapeutic drug (peak and trough) or other specific monitoring (e.g., chemotherapy, glucose, insulin, or potassium) should be documented carefully in relation to the time of medication administration. It is essential that this information be communicated clearly and accurately to avoid misunderstanding of the dose time in relation to the collection time. Miscommunication between the individual administering the medication and the individual collecting the specimen is the most frequent cause of subtherapeutic levels, toxic levels, and misleading information used in the calculation of future therapies.
- The laboratory should be consulted regarding minimum specimen collection requirements when multiple tube types or samples are required. The amount of serum or plasma collected can be estimated using assumptions of packed cell volume or hematocrit. The packed cell volume of a healthy woman is usually 38% to 44% of the total blood volume. If a full 5-mL red-top tube is collected, and the hematocrit is 38% to 44%, approximately 2.8 to 3.1 mL, or $[5 - (5 \times 0.44)]$ to $[5 - (5 \times 0.38)]$, of the total blood volume should be serum. Factors that invalidate estimation include conditions such as anemia, polycythemia, dehydration, and overhydration.
- The laboratory should be consulted regarding the preferred specimen container before specimen collection. Specific analytes may vary in concentration depending on whether the sample is serum or plasma. It is strongly recommended that when serial measurements are to be carried out, the same type of collection container be used so that fluctuations in values caused by variations in specimen type are not misinterpreted as changes in clinical status. Consultation regarding collection containers is also important because some laboratory methods are optimized for a specific specimen type (serum versus plasma). Also, preservatives present in collection containers, such as sodium fluoride, may exhibit a chemical interference with test reagents that can cause underestimation or overestimation of measured values. Other preservatives, such as EDTA, can block the analyte of interest in the sample from participating in the test reaction, invalidating test results. Finally, it is possible that some high-throughput, robotic equipment systems require specific and standardized collection containers.
- Prompt and proper specimen processing, storage, and analysis are important to achieve accurate results. Specimens collected in containers with solid or liquid preservatives or with gel separators should be mixed by inverting the tube 10 times immediately after the tube has been filled. Handle the specimen gently to avoid hemolysis. Specimens should always be transported to the laboratory as quickly as possible after collection.

Results that are evaluated outside the entire context of the preparatory, collection, and handling process may be interpreted erroneously if consideration is not given to the above-listed general guidelines.

Site Selection

Capillary Puncture: Assess the selected area. It should be free of lesions and calluses, there should be no edema, and the site should feel warm. If the site feels cool or appears pale or cyanotic, warm compresses can be applied over 3 to 5 min to dilate the capillaries. For fingersticks, the central, fleshy, distal portions of the third or fourth fingers are the preferred collection sites (Fig. A–1). For neonatal heel sticks, the medial and lateral surfaces of the plantar area are preferred to avoid direct puncture of the heel bone, which could result in osteomyelitis (Fig. A–2).

Venipuncture of Arm: Assess the arm for visibly accessible veins. The selected area should not be burned or scarred, have a tattoo, or have hematoma present. Even after the tourniquet is applied, not all patients have a prominent median cubital, cephalic, or basilic vein. Both arms should be observed because some

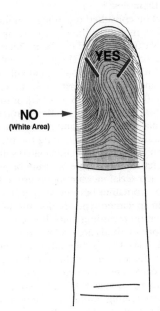

YES

NO →
(White Area)

Figure A–1 Site selection. Capillary puncture of the finger.

CALCANEUS BONE

YES

N O

YES

Figure A–2 Site selection. Capillary puncture of the heel.

patients have accessible veins in one arm and not the other. The median cubital vein in the antecubital fossa is the preferred venipuncture site. The patient may be able to provide the best information regarding venous access if he or she has had previous venipuncture experience (Fig. A–3). Alternative techniques to increase visibility of veins may include warming the arm, allowing the arm to dangle downward for a minute or two, tapping the antecubital area with the index finger, or massaging the arm upward from wrist to elbow. The condition of the vein also should be assessed before venipuncture. Sclerotic (hard, scarred) veins or veins in which phlebitis previously occurred should be avoided. Arms with a functioning hemodialysis access site should not be used. The arm on the affected side of a mastectomy should be avoided. In the case of a double mastectomy, the requesting HCP should be consulted before specimen collection.

Venipuncture of Hand and Wrist: If no veins in the arms are available, hands and wrists should be examined as described for the arm (see Fig. A–3). Consideration should be given to the venipuncture equipment selected because the veins in these areas are much smaller. Pediatric-sized collection containers and needles with a larger gauge may be more appropriate.

Venipuncture of Legs and Feet: The veins in the legs and feet can be accessed as with sites located on the arm, hand, or wrist. These extremities should be used only on the approval of the requesting HCP because veins in these locations are more prone to infection and formation of blood clots, especially in patients with diabetes, cardiac disease, and bleeding disorders.

Radial Arterial Puncture: The radial artery is the artery of choice for obtaining arterial blood gas specimens because it is close to the surface of the wrist and does not require a deep puncture. Its easy access also allows for more effective

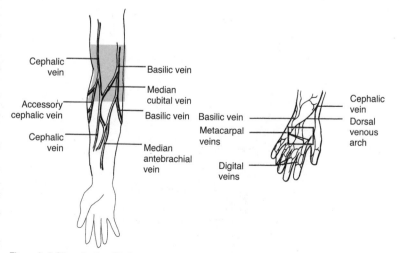

Figure A–3 Site selection. Venipuncture arm/hand.

compression after the needle has been removed. The nearby ulnar artery can provide sufficient collateral circulation to the hand during specimen collection and postcollection compression (Fig. A–4).

Percutaneous Umbilical Cord Sampling: The blood is aspirated from the umbilical cord under the guidance of ultrasonography and using a 20- or 22-gauge spinal needle inserted through the mother's abdomen.

Postnatal Umbilical Cord Sampling: The blood is aspirated from the umbilical cord using a 20- or 22-gauge needle and transferred to the appropriate collection container.

Fetal Scalp Sampling: The requesting HCP makes a puncture in the fetal scalp using a microblade, and the specimen is collected in a long capillary tube. The tube is usually capped on both ends immediately after specimen collection.

Locks and Catheters: These devices are sometimes inserted to provide a means for the administration of fluids or medications and to obtain blood specimens without the need for frequent venipuncture. The device first should be assessed for patency. The need for heparinization, irrigation, or clot removal depends on the type of device in use and the institution-specific or HCP-specific protocols in effect. Use sterile technique because these devices provide direct access to the patient's bloodstream. When IV fluids are being administered via a device at the time of specimen collection, blood should be obtained from the opposite side of the body. If this is not possible, the flow should be stopped for 5 min before specimen collection. The first 5 mL of blood collected should be discarded.

Selection of Blood Collection Equipment
In many cases when a blood sample is required, serum is the specimen type of choice. Plasma may be frequently substituted, however. Specimen processing is

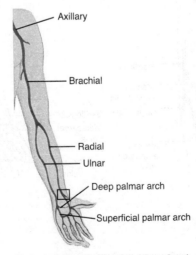

Figure A–4 Site selection. Arterial arm/hand.

more rapid for plasma samples than serum samples because the anticoagulated sample does not need to clot before centrifugation. Plasma samples also require less centrifugation time to achieve adequate separation. Consult with the testing laboratory regarding recommended specimen types. The basic blood collection tubes are shown on the inside cover of this book. Consider latex allergy when selecting the collection equipment appropriate for each patient. Equipment used in specimen collection includes:

- Gloves and other personal protective equipment depending on the situation
- Tourniquet
- Materials to cleanse or disinfect the collection site (alcohol preparations [70% alcohol], povidone-iodine solution [Betadine], or green soap are the most commonly used materials)
- Gauze (to wipe collection site dry after cleansing)
- Sterile lancet (capillary puncture)
- Syringe and needle (arterial puncture or venipuncture)
- Vial of heparin and syringe or heparin unit dose
- Sterile normal saline in 50-mL syringe (for indwelling devices such as Groshong catheter)
- Sterile cap or hub (for indwelling devices when the cap or hub will be replaced after specimen procurement)
- Needle and holder for vacuumized collection tube system (arterial puncture or venipuncture)
- Butterfly or winged infusion set (venipuncture)
- Collection container (vacuumized collection tube, capillary tube, or Microtainer)
- Bandage (to cover puncture site after specimen collection)

Collection Procedure

The procedures outlined here are basic in description. A phlebotomy or other text should be consulted for specific details regarding specimen collection and complications encountered during various types of blood collection. Positively identify the patient using at least two unique identifiers before providing care, treatment, or services. Label the appropriate tubes with the corresponding patient demographics, date, and time of collection before the specimen is collected. Obtain a history of the patient's complaints, including a list of known allergens, especially allergies or sensitivities to latex.

Capillary: Place the patient in a comfortable position either sitting or lying down. Positively identify the patient using at least two unique identifiers before providing care, treatment, or services. Label the appropriate tubes with the corresponding patient demographics, date, and time of collection before the specimen is collected. Assess whether the patient has allergies to the disinfectant or to latex if latex gloves or tourniquet will be used in the collection procedure. Use gloved hands to select the collection site as described in the site selection section. Cleanse the skin with the appropriate disinfectant and dry the area. Pull the skin tight by the thumb and index finger of the nondominant hand on either side of the puncture site and move them in opposite directions. Puncture the skin with a sterile lancet to a depth of approximately 2 mm, using a quick, firm motion. Wipe the first drop of blood away using the gauze. If flow is poor, the site should not be squeezed or the specimen may become contaminated with tissue fluid. Do not allow the collection container to touch the puncture site. Collect the sample in the capillary tube or Microtainer. The capillary tube should be held in a horizontal position to avoid the introduction of air bubbles into the sample. Microtainer tubes should be held in a downward-slanted direction to facilitate the flow of blood into the capillary scoop of the collection device. If a smear is required, allow a drop of blood to fall onto a clean microscope slide. Gently spread the drop across the slide using the edge of another slide. Apply slight pressure to the puncture site with a clean piece of gauze until bleeding stops, and then apply a bandage. Safely dispose of the sharps. Transport properly labeled specimens immediately to the laboratory.

Venipuncture Using a Syringe or Vacuumized Needle and Holder System: Place the patient in a comfortable position either sitting or lying down. Positively identify the patient using at least two unique identifiers before providing care, treatment, or services. Label the appropriate tubes with the corresponding patient demographics, date, and time of collection before the specimen is collected. Assess whether the patient has allergies to the disinfectant or to latex if latex gloves or tourniquet will be used in the collection procedure. Use gloved hands to select the collection site as described in the Site Selection section. Locate the vein visually, then by palpation using the index finger. The thumb should not be used because it has a pulse beat and may cause confusion in site selection or in differentiating a vein from an artery. Select the appropriate collection materials (needle size, butterfly, syringe, collection container size) on the basis of the vein size, vein depth, appearance of the collection site, patient's age, and anticipated level of cooperation. Cleanse the skin with the appropriate disinfectant and dry the area. Select the appropriate collection tubes. If blood cultures are to be collected, disinfect the top of the collection containers as directed by the testing laboratory. Be sure to have extra tubes within easy reach in case the vacuum in a collection tube is lost and a substitute is required. Apply the tourniquet 3 to 4 in. above the selected collection site. Remove the sterile needle cap, and inspect the tip of the needle for defects. Pull the skin tight by placing the thumb of the nondominant hand 1 or 2 in. below the puncture site and moving the thumb in the opposite direction. The thumb is placed below the puncture site to help avoid an accidental needle stick if the patient moves suddenly. Ensure that the needle is bevel up and held at an angle of approximately 15° to 30° (depending on the depth of the vein) (Fig. A–5).

Puncture the skin with smooth, firm motion using a sterile needle held by the dominant hand. A reduction in pressure is achieved when the needle has penetrated the vein successfully. Be sure to release the tourniquet within 1 min of application. Fill the vacuumized collection containers in the prescribed order of draw for the studies ordered. Tubes with anticoagulants can be gently mixed with the free nondominant hand as they are filled. When the required containers have been filled, withdraw the needle and apply pressure to the collection site until the bleeding stops. In most cases, a piece of gauze can be placed on the collection site and the arm bent upward to hold it in place while attention is given to disposing of the sharps safely. In cases in which a syringe is used, the barrel of the syringe should be gently pulled back during specimen collection and gently pushed in during the transfer to collection tubes. The vacuum in the collection container should not be allowed to suck the sample into the container, but rather the speed of entry should be controlled by the

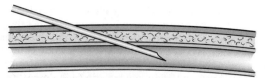

Figure A–5 Venipuncture needle placement at insertion.

pressure applied to the barrel. The blood should gently roll down the side of the tube to prevent hemolysis. Transport properly labeled specimens immediately to the laboratory.

Radial Artery Puncture: Place the patient in a comfortable position either sitting or lying down. Positively identify the patient using at least two unique identifiers before providing care, treatment, or services. Label the appropriate tubes with the corresponding patient demographics, date, and time of collection before the specimen is collected. Assess whether the patient has allergies to the disinfectant or to latex if latex gloves or tourniquet will be used in the collection procedure. Assess if the patient has an allergy to local anesthetics, and inform the HCP accordingly. Glove the hands, and select the collection site as described in the site selection section. Ensure that the patient has adequate collateral circulation to the hand if thrombosis of the radial artery occurs after arterial puncture by performing an Allen test before puncture. The Allen test is performed by occlusion of the ulnar and radial arteries on the palmar surface of the wrist with two fingers. The thumb should not be used to locate these arteries because it has a pulse. Compress both arteries, and ask the patient to open and close the fist several times until the palm turns pale. Release pressure only on the ulnar artery. Color should return to the palm within 5 sec if the ulnar artery is functioning. If color returns above the wrist, the Allen test is positive. The Allen test also should be performed on the opposite hand. The wrist to which color is restored fastest has better circulation and should be selected as the site for blood gas collection. Be sure to explain to the patient that an arterial puncture is painful. The site may be anesthetized with 1% to 2% lidocaine (Xylocaine) before puncture. The index finger of the nondominant hand is placed over the site where the needle will enter the artery, not the site where the needle will penetrate the skin. The specimen is collected in an air-free heparinized syringe, which is held like a dart in the dominant hand and inserted slowly, bevel up, about 5 to 10 mm below the palpating finger at a 45° to 60° angle. When blood enters the needle hub, arterial pressure should cause blood to pump into the syringe. When enough specimen has been collected, the needle is withdrawn from the arm, and pressure is applied to the collection site for a minimum of 5 to 10 min. Immediately after the needle has been withdrawn safely from the arm, the exposed end of the syringe should be stoppered.

Samples should be gently and well mixed to ensure proper mixing of the heparin with the sample. The heparin prevents formation of small clots that result in rejection of the sample. The tightly capped sample should be placed in an ice slurry immediately after collection. Information on the specimen label should be protected from water in the ice slurry by first placing the specimen in a protective plastic bag. Transport properly labeled specimens immediately to the laboratory.

APP

Indwelling Devices: Positively identify the patient using at least two unique identifiers before providing care, treatment, or services. Label the appropriate tubes with the corresponding patient demographics, date, and time of collection before the specimen is collected. Indwelling devices are either heparinized or irrigated after specimen collection. Before specimen collection, prepare the heparin in a syringe, if required. Allow the heparin (unit dose or prepared solution in the syringe) to equilibrate at room temperature during specimen collection. Cleanse the catheter cap or hub with povidone-iodine and 70% alcohol over 2 min. Using sterile gloves, remove the cap and attach a 5- or 10-mL syringe to the connector. Withdraw 5 mL of blood to be discarded. Clamp the catheter. (The Groshong catheter does not require clamping because it has a special valve that eliminates the need for clamping.) Attach another 5- or 10-mL syringe and begin collecting blood for transfer to the collection tubes. After the required specimen has been withdrawn, the device is heparinized by slowly injecting the heparin into the cap or hub of the device. Clamp the device 2 in. from the cap, remove the needle, and unclamp the device. Attach a new sterile cap or hub if the old one has been discarded. Groshong catheters are irrigated rather than heparinized. Irrigation of a Groshong catheter is accomplished by gently injecting 20 to 30 mL of sterile normal saline through the cap with moderate force. Remove the needle using some positive pressure (pressing down on the plunger) to prevent the solution from backing up into the syringe. Transport properly labeled specimens immediately to the laboratory.

Order of Draw for Glass or Plastic Tubes (Reflects Current CLSI [formerly NCCLS] Guideline: Recommended Order of Draw, H3-A6, [Vol 27, No 26])
Note: Always follow your facility's protocol for order of draw.

- First—Blood culture and other tests requiring sterile specimen (yellow or yellow/black stopper); blood culture bottle first, followed by sodium polyethanol sulfonate (SPS) tube for acid-fast bacilli specimens.
- Second—Coagulation studies (light blue [sodium citrate] stopper); sodium citrate forms calcium salts to remove calcium, and this prevents specimen clotting. *Note:* When using a winged blood or vacutainer collection set and the blue-top tube is the first tube drawn, a nonadditive red-top or coagulation discard tube should be collected first and discarded. The amount of blood in the discard tube needs to be sufficient to fill the winged collection set tubing's "dead space" or fill one-quarter of the discard tube. This is done to ensure complete filling of the blue-top tube. The blue-top tube to be used for testing must be filled to ensure the proper ratio of blood to additive in the test specimen blue-top tube.
- Third—Plain or nonadditive (red or red/gray [gel] stopper); red/gray-top serum separator tube (SST) contains a gel separator and clot activator. SSTs are not appropriate for all testing requiring a serum specimen. They are generally unacceptable for therapeutic drug monitoring and serology studies. The laboratory should be consulted if there are questions regarding the use of SSTs.
- Fourth—Additive tubes in the following order:

   Green stopper: Tube contains sodium heparin or lithium heparin anticoagulant (heparin inactivates thrombin and thromboplastin, and this prevents specimen clotting). For ammonia levels, use sodium or lithium heparin. For lithium levels, use sodium heparin.

Lavender stopper:Tube contains K_3 EDTA (tripotassium EDTA forms calcium salts to remove calcium from the sample, and this prevents specimen clotting while preserving the integrity of the red blood cell wall).

Gray stopper: Tube contains potassium oxalate/sodium fluoride (the potassium oxalate acts as an anticoagulant, and the sodium fluoride prevents glycolysis).

URINE SPECIMENS

The patient should be informed that improper collection, storage, and transport are the primary reasons for specimen rejection and subsequent requests for recollection. If the specimen is to be collected at home, it should be collected in a clean plastic container (preferably a container from the testing laboratory). Many studies require refrigeration after collection. If the collection container includes a preservative, the patient should be made aware of the contents and advised as to what the precaution labels mean (caution labels such as caustic, corrosive, acid, and base should be affixed to the container as appropriate). When a preservative or fixative is included in the container, the patient should be advised not to remove it. The patient also should be told not to void directly into the container. The patient should be given a collection device, if indicated, and instructed to void into the collection device. The specimen should be carefully transferred into the collection container. Urinary output should be recorded throughout the collection time if the specimen is being collected over a specified time interval. Some laboratories provide preprinted collection instructions tailored to their methods. The specimen should be transported promptly to the laboratory after collection.

Wear gloves and any other additional personal protective equipment indicated by the patient's condition. See Appendix G for a more detailed description of standard precautions. Assess whether the patient has allergies to the disinfectant or anesthetic, or to latex if latex gloves or catheter will be used in the procedure.

Random: These samples are mainly used for routine screening and can be collected at any time of the day. The patient should be instructed to void either directly into the collection container (if there is no preservative) or into a collection device for transfer into the specimen container.

First Morning: Urine on rising in the morning is very concentrated. These specimens are indicated when screening for substances that may not be detectable in a more dilute random sample. These specimens are also necessary for testing conditions such as orthostatic proteinuria, in which levels vary with changes in posture.

Second Void: In some cases, it is desirable to test freshly produced urine to evaluate the patient's current status, as with glucose and ketones. Explain to the patient that he or she should first void and then drink a glass of water. The patient should be instructed to wait 30 min and then void either directly into the collection container or into a collection device for transfer into the collection container.

Clean Catch: These midstream specimens are generally used for microbiological or cytological studies. They also may be requested for routine urinalysis to provide a specimen that is least contaminated with urethral cells, microorganisms, mucus, or other substances that may affect the interpretation of results.

Instruct the male patient first to wash hands thoroughly, then cleanse the meatus, void a small amount into the toilet, and void either directly into the specimen container or into a collection device for transfer into the specimen container. Instruct the female patient first to wash hands thoroughly, and then to cleanse the labia from front to back. While keeping the labia separated, the patient should void a small amount into the toilet, and then, without interrupting the urine stream, void either directly into the specimen container or into a collection device for transfer into the specimen container.

Catheterized Random or Clean Catch: "Straight catheterization" is indicated when the patient is unable to void, when the patient is unable to prepare properly for clean-catch specimen collection, or when the patient has an indwelling catheter in place from which a urine sample may be obtained. Before collecting a specimen from the catheter, observe the drainage tube to ensure that it is empty, and then clamp the tube distal to the collection port 15 min before specimen collection. Cleanse the port with an antiseptic swab such as 70% alcohol and allow the port to dry. Use a needle and syringe (sterile if indicated) to withdraw the required amount of specimen. Unclamp the tube.

Timed: To quantify substances in urine, 24-hr urine collections are used. They are also used to measure substances whose level of excretion varies over time. The use of preservatives and the handling of specimens during the timed collection may be subject to variability among laboratories. The testing laboratory should be consulted regarding specific instructions before starting the test. Many times the specimen must be refrigerated or kept on ice throughout the entire collection period. Explain to the patient that it is crucial for *all* urine to be included in the collection. Urinary output should be recorded throughout the collection time if the specimen is being collected over a specified time interval. The test should begin between 6 and 8 a.m. if possible. Instruct the patient to collect the first void of the day and discard it. The start time of the collection period begins at the time the first voided specimen was discarded and should be recorded along with the date on the collection container. The patient should be instructed to void at the same time the following morning and to add this last voiding to the container. This is the end time of the collection and should be recorded along with the date on the container. For patients who are in the hospital, the urinary output should be compared with the volume measured in the completed collection container. Discrepancies between the two volumes indicate that a collection might have been discarded. A creatinine level often is requested along with the study of interest to evaluate the completeness of the collection.

Catheterized Timed: Instructions for this type of collection are basically the same as those for timed specimen collection. The test should begin by changing the tubing and drainage bag. If a preservative is required, it can be placed directly in the drainage bag, or the specimen can be removed at frequent intervals (every 2 hr) and transferred to the collection container to which the preservative has been added. The drainage bag must be kept on ice or emptied periodically into the collection container during the entire collection period if indicated by the testing laboratory. The tubing should be monitored throughout the collection period to ensure continued drainage.

Suprapubic Aspiration: This procedure is performed by inserting a needle directly into the bladder. Because the bladder is normally sterile, the urine collected should also be free from any contamination caused by the presence of microorganisms. Place the patient in a supine position. Cleanse the area with antiseptic and drape with sterile drapes. A local anesthetic may be administered before insertion of the needle. A needle is inserted through the skin into the bladder. A syringe attached to the needle is used to aspirate the urine sample. The needle is then removed and a sterile dressing is applied to the site. Place the sterile sample in a sterile specimen container. The site must be observed for signs of inflammation or infection.

Pediatric: Specimen collection can be achieved by any of the above-described methods using collection devices specifically designed for pediatric patients. Appropriately cleanse the genital area and allow the area to dry. For a random collection, remove the covering of the adhesive strips on the collector bag and apply over the genital area. Diaper the child. When the specimen is obtained, place the entire collection bag in the specimen container (use a sterile container as appropriate for the requested study). Some laboratories may have specific preferences for the submission of urine specimens for culture. Consult the laboratory before collection to avoid specimen rejection.

BODY FLUID, STOOL, AND TISSUE

Wear gloves and any other additional personal protective equipment indicated by the patient's condition. See Appendix G for a more detailed description of standard precautions. Assess whether the patient has allergies to the disinfectant or anesthetic or to latex if latex gloves will be used in the procedure.

Specific collection techniques vary by site, study required, and level of invasiveness. These techniques are described in the individual monographs.

DIAGNOSTIC TESTING

Wear gloves and any other additional personal protective equipment indicated by the patient's condition. See Appendix G for a more detailed description of standard precautions. Assess whether the patient has allergies to the disinfectant, anesthetic, contrast material, or medications or to latex if latex gloves, catheter, or tourniquet will be used in the procedure.

A sleeping patient should be gently awakened and allowed the opportunity to become oriented before preparation for the selected study. Comatose or unconscious patients should be greeted in the same gentle manner because, although they are unable to respond, they may be capable of hearing and understanding. Anticipate instances in which patient cooperation may be an issue. Enlist a second person to help with preparing the patient for the procedure to ensure a safe, quality testing experience for all involved.

Specific techniques and patient preparation vary by site, study required, and level of invasiveness. These techniques are described in the individual monographs.

APP

Appendix B

Potential Nursing Diagnoses Associated With Laboratory and Diagnostic Testing

PRETEST PHASE

Anxiety related to undiagnosed health problems

Anxiety related to perceived threat to health status

Anxiety and fear related to anticipated diagnostic results

Anxiety and fear related to perception of diagnostic procedure as frightening or embarrassing

Powerlessness related to unfamiliar procedure, equipment, environment, or personnel

Knowledge deficit related to lack of information or possible misinterpretation of information provided about the procedure

Knowledge deficit related to informed consent, legal implications of testing

Potential for noncompliance with test protocols related to inability to understand or follow instructions

Potential for noncompliance with test protocols related to presence of high anxiety, confusion, or denial

Potential for noncompliance with test protocols related to lack of knowledge or appropriate instruction

Potential for noncompliance with test protocols related to confusion, weakness, and other individual factors

INTRATEST PHASE

Risk for injury related to developmental age, psychological factors, and test procedures

Risk for infection or allergic reaction related to altered immune function, history of chronic illness, allergens, or infectious agent

Risk for latex allergy response associated with test equipment

Pain, nausea, vomiting, or diarrhea related to laboratory and diagnostic procedures

Injury, actual or risk for, related to invasive procedure associated with laboratory or diagnostic testing

Risk for infection related to invasive procedures

Risk for bleeding associated with altered bleeding tendencies related to invasive procedures

Fatigue related to diagnostic procedure

Anxiety and fear related to arterial puncture or venipuncture

Risk for injury, bleeding, hematoma, or infection related to arterial puncture or venipuncture

Pain related to arterial puncture or venipuncture

Risk for impaired skin integrity

Potential impairment of gas exchange associated with test procedure

POST-TEST PHASE

Knowledge deficit related to significance of test results and potential need for further testing

Knowledge deficit related to test outcome deviation that may necessitate medication or lifestyle alterations

Anxiety and fear related to test outcome that may necessitate medication or lifestyle alterations

Ineffective coping related to test outcome and potential for other interventional techniques or procedures

Anticipatory grieving related to test outcome

Anticipatory or actual grieving related to perceived loss of health or threat of death associated with diagnostic outcome

Decisional conflict related to test outcome and potential for interventional procedures

Potential alteration in tissue perfusion: cerebral, cardiopulmonary, or peripheral

Knowledge deficit related to care after procedure

Potential for caregiver strain or interrupted family process related to laboratory or diagnostic results

Self-image disturbance related to altered ability to perform activities of daily living due to diagnostic findings

1392

Guidelines for Age-Specific Communication

Effective communication between the health-care provider and the patient is influenced by the patient's cognitive abilities, sensory development or deprivation, level of stress, and environment. Effective communication with individuals at any stage of life is possible if one recognizes that it is essential to employ age-specific communication techniques based on an understanding of the continuum of human development as highlighted here.

INFANT (BIRTH TO 1 YR)

Physical
Rapid gains in height and weight
Gradual shift from reflexive movements to intentional actions

Motor and Sensory
Responds to light and sound
Progresses to raising and turning head, bringing hand to mouth, rolling over, sitting upright, and standing

Cognitive
Learns by imitation
Progresses to recognize familiar objects and people
Advances to speaking three or four words

Psychosocial
Significant persons are parents or primary caregivers
Develops sense of trust and security if needs are met
May show fear of strangers
May exhibit separation anxiety

Interventions
Keep a parent or primary caregiver in view
Involve significant persons in care if appropriate
Provide consistency in health-care staff to limit the number of strangers
Face the infant when providing care
Use soothing nonverbal communication, such as holding, rocking, and cuddling
Assess immunizations
Maintain safety and keep crib side rails up at all times

TODDLER (1 TO 4 YR)

Physical
Learning bladder and bowel control
Temporary teeth erupt
Physiological systems mature

Motor and Sensory
Developing a higher level of manual dexterity (builds towers with blocks)
Progresses to walking, jumping, and climbing
Loves to experiment

Cognitive
Has a short attention span
Understands simple directions and requests

Psychosocial
Significant persons are parents
Asserts independence
Understands ownership
Attached to security objects
Knows own gender
Plays simple games

Interventions
Face the toddler during interactions
Give one direction at a time
Tie words to action (toddlers learn by example)
Use firm, direct approach; avoid harsh/excited words or actions
Use distraction techniques
Use soothing nonverbal communication, such as rocking, cuddling, and holding
Communicate through play (dolls, puppets, music)
Prepare shortly before a procedure

Allow choices when possible

Encourage mother or parent to stay with the child as appropriate

Encourage parents to participate in care as appropriate

Maintain safety and keep crib side rails up at all times

CHILD (5 TO 12 YR)

Physical

Growth is slow and regular

Permanent teeth erupt

Pubescent changes start

May experience growing pains

May experience fatigue

Motor and Sensory

Skips and hops

Dresses and undresses independently

Throws and catches a ball

Uses common utensils and tools

Draws, paints, and likes quiet as well as active games

Cognitive

Major cognitive skill is communication

Understands numbers and can count

Constructs sentences and asks questions

Capable of logical thinking and can reason

Takes pride in accomplishments

Develops increased attention span

Psychosocial

Significant persons are parents, siblings, peers, teachers (prefers friends to family)

Increases independence and begins to assert self (may be physically aggressive)

Masters new tasks and acquires new skills

Behavior can be modified by rewards and punishment

Works hard to be successful

Interventions

Clearly define and reinforce behavior limits

Tell jokes and play games with rules

Check for special words used to identify parents, body parts, or body functions

Explain procedures in advance using correct terminology

Use dolls or puppets for explanations when performing procedures

Provide privacy

Involve whenever possible

Allow to have some control

Promote independence

Praise for good behavior

Acknowledge fear, pain, or family separation

ADOLESCENT (13 TO 18 YR)

Physical

Growth in skeletal size is rapid

Reproductive system matures

Vital signs approximate those of an adult

Motor and Sensory

Easily fatigued

May need more rest and sleep in early adolescence

Awkwardness in gross motor activity

Demonstrates improving fine motor skills

Cognitive

Increased ability to use abstract thought and logic

Able to handle hypothetical situations and thoughts

Shows growth in self-esteem but is challenged by bouts of insecurity

Avoids asking questions for fear of appearing unintelligent

Psychosocial

Develops sexual identity

Shows interest in and confusion with own development

Develops concern with physical appearance

Establishes critical need for privacy

Values belonging to peer group

Perceives self as invincible

Identity is threatened by hospitalization

Interventions

Likes to be treated like an adult

Do not talk to others about the patient in front of him or her

Do not ask questions about drugs, sex, or use of tobacco in front of parents

Provide information about routines and therapy

Provide privacy

Supplement information with rationale

Encourage questions

Allow to maintain control

Involve in decision making and care

Allow for expression of fear, such as fear of bodily injury and loss of control

ADULT (19 TO 65 YEARS)

Physical

Reaches physical and sexual maturity

Prone to health problems related to an inability to cope with new responsibilities

Health-care needs related to preventive medicine

Adjustment to menopause (women) and sexual dysfunction (men) in middle adulthood

Motor and Sensory

Skills are fully developed

Cognitive

Focuses on time constraints and want to learn only what is practical for him or her

May be dual caregivers (i.e., parents and children)

Psychosocial

Experiences emotional stress secondary to mate selection, vocational selection, assuming occupational roles, marriage, childbearing, financial pressure, and independence

Interventions

Involve family in patient's care and education

Explain benefits of adhering to treatment plan

Be honest and supportive

Respect personal values

Provide privacy

Keep a hopeful attitude

Focus on strengths, and not limitations

Recognize that unknown factors may affect behavior

Encourage patient to ask questions and talk about concerns

Provide information and support to make health-care decisions

GERIATRIC (65 AND OLDER)

Physical

Ages gradually and individually

Experiences decreased tolerance to heat/cold

Encounters declining cardiac and renal function

Experiences skeletal changes (bones become more prominent, shrinkage in vertebral disks, stiff joints)

Becomes subject to increased susceptibility to infection and to high blood pressure

Undergoes skin changes

Motor and Sensory

Experiences decrease in mobility, visual acuity, ability to respond to stimuli, hearing, and motor skills

Cognitive

Experiences decrease in memory, slowing of mental functions, slowness in learning, and drop in performance

Psychosocial

Encounters lifestyle changes secondary to children leaving home, children providing grandchildren, re-establishing a relationship as a couple, and retirement/hobbies

Develops increased concern for health and financial security

Accepts concept of own mortality

Faces decreased authority and autonomy

Experiences depression related to decreased physical, motor, and cognitive abilities

Interventions

Explain instructions well to patient and family

Ask questions to verify understanding

Review important points repeatedly

Keep room clutter-free and call bell within reach

APP

Control room temperature for comfort
Consider additional lighting at night
Watch for signs of drug toxicity
Give respect and provide privacy
Focus on strengths, and not limitations
Avoid assuming loss of abilities
Seek information as necessary to deal with impairments

Include patient in conversation/activity to prevent social isolation
Encourage to talk about feelings
Use humor and stay positive
Provide information and support regarding end-of-life decisions
Provide teaching for safety
Provide teaching for medications and test preparations

APP

Appendix D

Transfusion Reactions: Laboratory Findings and Potential Nursing Interventions

These reactions are mainly associated with the transfusion of leuko-reduced packed red blood cells.

CATEGORIES:

I. Acute (Less Than 24 hr) Immune-Mediated Transfusion Reactions
   a. ABO and non-ABO acute hemolytic
   b. Febrile nonhemolytic
   c. Urticarial/allergic reaction
   d. Anaphylactic reaction

II. Acute (Less Than 24 hr) Non–Immune-Mediated Transfusion Reactions
   a. Transfusion-related acute lung injury
   b. Circulatory overload
   c. Metabolic complications
   d. Hypothermia
   e. Hypotension associated with angiotensin-converting enzyme inhibition
   f. Embolism (air and particulate)
   g. Nonimmune hemolysis

III. Delayed (Greater Than 24 hr) Immune-Mediated Transfusion Reactions
   a. Hemolytic
   b. Alloimmunization to red blood cell, white blood cell, platelet, and protein antigens
   c. Graft versus host

IV. Delayed (Greater Than 24 hr) Non–Immune-Mediated Transfusion Reactions
   a. Iron overload

I. Acute Immune-Mediated Transfusion Reactions	
a. ABO and non-ABO	Dramatic, severe, and can be fatal; incidence of acute hemolytic is 1:38,000 to 1:70,000 units; result of reaction between antibodies in the patient's plasma and the corresponding antigen being present on the donor's cells; severity affected by amount of patient antibody present, quantity of antigen on transfused cells, volume of blood transfused
Symptoms	Fever, chills, hypotension, tachycardia, nausea, vomiting, lower back pain, hemoglobinuria, renal failure with oliguria, flushing, generalized bleeding, pain or oozing at the infusion site
Laboratory findings	Positive DAT; elevated: indirect bilirubin (5 to 7 hr post-transfusion), LDH, BUN, creatinine, PT, aPTT; decreased: anti-A and anti-B titers, haptoglobin; hemoglobinemia; hemoglobinuria; hypofibrinogenemia; thrombocytopenia; positive urinary hemosiderin; presence of spherocytes and RBC fragments on peripheral smear

(table continues on page 1398)

I. Acute Immune-Mediated Transfusion Reactions (continued)

Treatment	Immediately stop transfusion, maintain renal flow at greater than 100 mL/hr by use of osmotic and diuretic agents (e.g., Lasix, furosemide); monitor for development of DIC (uncontrolled bleeding, decreasing platelet count, prolonged PT/PTT); future transfusion with O-negative packed cells
b. Febrile nonhemolytic	Most common type of transfusion reaction; incidence is 1:200 to 1:17 (0.5% to 6.0%); repeat occurrences are uncommon; result of antileukocyte, antiplatelet, or anti-HLA antibodies
Symptoms	Fever, chills, headache, vomiting
Laboratory findings	Negative DAT, transient leukopenia
Treatment	Immediately stop transfusion; administer antipyretics (steroids in severe cases); transfuse with leukocyte-reduced blood after two documented febrile nonhemolytic reactions
c. Urticarial/allergic reaction	Second most common type of reaction; incidence is 1:100 to 1:33 (1% to 3%); histamine-mediated reaction of allergen + IgE fixed on mast cells
Symptoms	Local erythema, hives, itching, usually no fever
Laboratory findings	Negative DAT
Treatment	Immediately stop transfusion; keep line open; administer antihistamines (e.g., diphenhydramine 25–50 mg); resume transfusion when symptoms subside; for future transfusions, premedicate with antihistamines
d. Anaphylactic reaction	Occurs rapidly with 10 mL or less; 1 in 700 individuals are IgA deficient and 25% have anti-IgA antibodies that will react to donor's plasma proteins; incidence is 1:20,000 to 1:50,000
Symptoms	Hypotension, urticaria, flushing, substernal pain, abdominal cramping, laryngeal edema, bronchospasm, circulatory collapse, anxiety
Laboratory findings	Negative DAT, presence of IgG class anti-IgA antibodies or undetectable level of IgA
Treatment	Treat for anaphylaxis with epinephrine, steroid therapy as needed, oxygen therapy as needed, Trendelenburg position, fluids; for future transfusions, premedicate with antihistamines and transfuse with IgA-deficient donor blood or autologous blood

---

II. Acute Non–Immune-Mediated Transfusion Reactions

a. Transfusion-related acute lung injury	Incidence of reaction to anti-WBC antibodies in donated whole blood–derived platelets, 1:432; in plasma-containing blood component, 1:2,000; in blood component, 1:5,000; fresh frozen plasma, 1:7,900
Symptoms	Hypoxemia, respiratory failure, hypotension, fever
Laboratory findings	Positive WBC antibody screen (donor or recipient), incompatible WBC crossmatch
Treatment	Supportive care until recovered; implicated donors should be deferred from future donation
b. Circulatory overload	Incidence is less than 1%; result of volume overload
Symptoms	Dyspnea, orthopnea, cough, tachycardia, hypertension, headache
Laboratory findings	N/A
Treatment	Upright posture, oxygen, diuretic, administer blood slowly, phlebotomy (250-mL increments)
c. Metabolic complications	Hypocalcemia resulting from rapid massive infusion of citrate; incidence is dependent on clinical setting
Symptoms	Paresthesia, tetany, arrhythmia
Laboratory findings	Elevated ionized calcium level, prolonged Q-T interval on ECG
Treatment	Slow calcium infusion, oral calcium supplement for mild symptoms; monitor ionized calcium levels (severe symptoms)
d. Hypothermia	Result of rapid infusion of cold blood
Symptoms	Cardiac arrhythmia
Laboratory findings	N/A
Treatment	Utilize blood warmer
e. Hypotension associated with ACE inhibition	Patients on ACE inhibitors receiving leukocyte-reduced packed cells have experienced hypotension (believed to be the result of an interaction between the ACE inhibitor and the kinin/prekallikrein system); incidence is dependent on the clinical setting
Symptoms	Flushing, hypotension
Laboratory findings	Positive DAT, hemolyzed intra- or post-transfusion specimen
Treatment	Avoid bedside leukocyte filtration

(table continues on page 1400)

APP

II. Acute Non–Immune-Mediated Transfusion Reactions (continued)

f. *Embolism (air and particulate)*	Result of air infusion via line; incidence is rare
Symptoms	Sudden shortness of breath, acute cyanosis, pain, cough, hypotension, cardiac arrhythmia
Laboratory findings	N/A
Treatment	Position patient on left side with legs elevated above head and chest
g. *Nonimmune hemolysis*	Result of physical or chemical destruction of RBCs (e.g., heating, freezing, hemolytic drug, solution added to blood); incidence is rare
Symptoms	Hemoglobinuria
Laboratory findings	Positive plasma-free hemoglobin, positive DAT, obvious hemolysis in unit containing the blood
Treatment	Identify and eliminate cause

III. Delayed Immune-Mediated Transfusion Reactions

a. *Hemolytic*	Anamnestic immune response to RBC antigens; incidence is 1:11,000 to 1:50,000
Symptoms	Fever, anemia, mild jaundice
Laboratory findings	Positive antibody screen, urinary hemosiderin, and DAT; increased LDH, bilirubin
Treatment	Identify antibody and transfuse compatible blood as needed
b. *Alloimmunization to RBC, WBC, platelet, and protein antigens*	Immune response to RBC, WBC, or platelet antigens; incidence is 1:100
Symptoms	Delayed hemolytic reaction
Laboratory findings	Positive antibody screen and DAT
Treatment	Avoid unnecessary transfusions; give leukocyte-reduced blood if transfusion is necessary
c. *Graft versus host*	Donor lymphocytes attack recipient's host tissue; incidence is rare
Symptoms	Erythroderma, maculopapular rash, anorexia, nausea, vomiting, diarrhea, hepatitis, pancytopenia, fever
Laboratory findings	Abnormal skin biopsy, incompatible HLA typing
Treatment	Methotrexate, corticosteroids; transfuse with irradiated blood products

IV. Delayed Non–Immune-Mediated Transfusion Reactions

a. Iron overload	Result of chronic transfusions (greater than 100)
Symptoms	Symptoms associated with diabetes, cirrhosis, cardiomyopathy
Laboratory findings	Increased iron levels
Treatment	Desferrioxamine

ACE = angiotensin-converting enzyme; BUN = blood urea nitrogen; DAT = (Coombs') direct antiglobulin test; DIC = disseminated intravascular coagulation; ECG = electrocardiogram; HLA = human leukocyte antigen; Ig = immunoglobulin; LDH = lactate dehydrogenase; N/A = not applicable; PT = prothrombin time; PTT = partial thromboplastin time; RBC = red blood cell; WBC = white blood cell.

Introduction to CLIA

The acronym *CLIA* stands for Clinical Laboratory Improvement Amendments. In 1988, Congress passed CLIA in order to establish quality standards that would apply to laboratory testing nationwide. The standards ensure that, regardless of location, all clinical testing on human specimens is performed with accuracy, reliability, and timeliness. In 1992, CLIA's final regulations distinguished between levels of test complexity. Three categories were established: waived complexity, moderate complexity (includes the subcategory of Provider-Performed Microscopy [PPM]), and high complexity testing. Permission to perform clinical laboratory testing in any or all categories requires the laboratory director to submit an application to enroll in the CLIA program, pay the applicable fee, and meet quality requirements that correspond to the type of certificate that is obtained. The 10–1–04 edition of 42 CFR Ch. IV, Part 493, the most current version of CLIA regulations, is the source used to write this introduction (available at wwwn.cdc.gov/clia/pdf/42cfr493_2004.pdf).

A Certificate of Waiver (COW) obtained by the appropriate health-care provider (HCP) allows qualified nursing or other health-care personnel to perform procedures classified as waived testing in an HCP's office or in a hospital nursing unit. Waived testing includes tests that are cleared by the U.S. Food and Drug Administration (FDA) for home use, have manufacturers' instructions to follow, and pose no harm to the patient if testing is performed incorrectly. The testing process utilizes controls. Examples of waived testing include dipstick urinalysis, fecal occult blood, ovulation testing, urine pregnancy tests, erythrocyte sedimentation rate (nonautomated), hemoglobin (copper sulfate method), blood glucose (on glucose meters cleared by the FDA), spun hematocrit, and hemoglobin by single analyte instruments that are self-contained with direct measurement and readout.

In addition to waived testing, PPM testing can be performed in an HCP's office. A PPM certificate obtained by a physician or midlevel practitioner allows the practitioner to perform PPM testing on specimens obtained during the patient's office visit. A midlevel practitioner can perform this type of testing under the direct supervision of a physician or in independent practice if authorized by the state. A microscope is utilized to view the specimens during the patient's office visit. PPM tests are performed on specimens in situations in which the accuracy of the findings would be compromised if a delay in testing were to occur. The testing process has no available controls. Examples of PPM testing include urine sediment examinations; potassium hydroxide preparations; pinworm examinations; fern tests; nasal smears for granulocytes; fecal leukocyte examinations; qualitative semen analysis (limited to determining the presence or absence of sperm and detection of motility); postcoital direct; qualitative examinations of vaginal or cervical mucus; and wet-mount testing for the presence or absence of bacteria, fungi, parasites, and cellular elements.

Hospital and reference laboratories perform tests of moderate and high complexity. The laboratory director must obtain the corresponding CLIA certificate and have personnel qualified to perform tests of moderate and high complexity.

Effects of Natural Products on Laboratory Values

The use of natural products has increased significantly, but to date, their preparation is unregulated. Their actions can affect normal and abnormal physiological processes as well as interact with prescription medications. Their presence in the body, alone or in combination with over-the-counter products or prescription medications, may physiologically affect the intended target or cause analytical interference in such a way that the test result is affected. For this reason, it is important to note their use. The natural products listed here are contraindicated or are recommended for use with caution in patients with body system disorders or patients taking medications for these disorders. The requesting health-care provider (HCP) and laboratory should be advised if the patient is regularly using these products so that their potential effects can be taken into consideration when reviewing results.

This list is not all-inclusive. Questions regarding the potential benefits and contraindications of natural products should be referred to the appropriate HCP. As a general recommendation, natural products and nutraceuticals are contraindicated during pregnancy and lactation.

NATURAL PRODUCTS THAT MAY AFFECT CARDIOVASCULAR DISORDERS OR INTERACT WITH THERAPEUTICS (INCLUDING HYPERTENSION AND HYPOTENSION)

Natural Products
Adonis
Aloe
Bromelain
Buckthorn
Cascara
Chinese rhubarb
Coleus
Dong quai
Elder
Ephedra
Ergot
Frangula
Garlic
Ginseng
Goldenseal
Green tea (with caffeine)
Henbane
Horsetail
Lily of the valley
Ma-huang
Reishi
Senna
Squill
Tylophora
Valerian
Yohimbe bark

NATURAL PRODUCTS AND NUTRACEUTICALS THAT MAY AFFECT ENDOCRINE DISORDERS OR INTERACT WITH THERAPEUTICS

Natural Products
Bilberry
Bitter melon
Bladderwrack
Blupleurum
Bugleweed
Echinacea
Ephedra
Fenugreek
Garcinia
Garlic
Ginseng
Goat's rue
Green tea (with caffeine)
Guggul
Licorice
Marshmallow
Olive leaf
Psyllium
Tylophora

Minerals
Chromium

APP

Nutraceuticals
Dehydroepiandrosterone
a-Lipoic acid
Para-aminobenzoic acid
Thyroid extract

NATURAL PRODUCTS AND NUTRACEUTICALS THAT MAY AFFECT GASTROINTESTINAL DISORDERS OR INTERACT WITH THERAPEUTICS

Natural Products
Bromelain
Cascara
Chinese rhubarb
Dandelion
Psyllium
Senna

Nutraceuticals
Betaine hydrochloride

NATURAL PRODUCTS AND NUTRACEUTICALS THAT MAY AFFECT GENITOURINARY DISORDERS OR INTERACT WITH THERAPEUTICS

Natural Products
Aloe
Arabinoxylane
Bladderwrack
Buckthorn
Cascara
Chinese rhubarb
Dandelion
Echinacea
Ephedra
Ergot
Frangula
Ginseng
Guarana
Horse chestnut
Horsetail
Licorice
Parsley oil (high doses)
Saw palmetto
Senna
Stinging nettle
White oak
White willow

Nutraceuticals
Creatine
Modified citrus pectin

NATURAL PRODUCTS AND NUTRACEUTICALS THAT MAY AFFECT BLEEDING DISORDERS OR INTERACT WITH THERAPEUTICS

Natural Products
Arnica
Astragalus
Bilberry
Bromelian
Cat's claw
Cayenne
Coleus
Cordyceps
Devil's claw
Dong quai
Evening primrose
Feverfew
Garlic
Ginger
Gingko
Ginseng
Grape seed
Green tea (with caffeine)
Guggui
Horse chestnut
Papaya
Red clover
Red yeast rice
Reishi
Turmeric
White willow

Nutraceuticals
Docosahexaenoic acid (DHA)
Fish oils (the omega-3 fatty acids: EPA and DHA)

NATURAL PRODUCTS AND NUTRACEUTICALS THAT MAY AFFECT HEPATOBILIARY DISORDERS OR INTERACT WITH THERAPEUTICS

Natural Products
Alkanet
Alpine ragwort

Coltsfoot
Comfrey
Dusty miller
Forget-me-not
Germander
Groundsel
Olive leaf
Parsley oil (large doses)
Pennyroyal
Peppermint
Ragwort
Red yeast rice
Sweet clover
White oak
White willow

Nutraceuticals
Creatine

NATURAL PRODUCTS AND AMINO ACIDS THAT MAY AFFECT IMMUNE DISORDERS OR INTERACT WITH THERAPEUTICS

Natural Products
Astragalus
Black cohosh

Echinacea
Saw palmetto

Amino Acids
Arginine

NATURAL PRODUCTS THAT MAY AFFECT RESPIRATORY DISORDERS OR INTERACT WITH THERAPEUTICS

Natural Products
Artichoke
Cayenne
Chamomile
Cordyceps
Echinacea
Feverfew
Garlic
Peppermint oil
White willow

Standard and Universal Precautions

Recommendations for Isolation Precautions in Hospitals*

RATIONALE FOR ISOLATION PRECAUTIONS IN HOSPITALS

Transmission of infection within a hospital requires three elements: a source of infecting microorganisms, a susceptible host, and a means of transmission for the microorganism.

Source

Human sources of the infecting microorganisms in hospitals may be patients, personnel, or, on occasion, visitors, and may include persons with acute disease, persons in the incubation period of a disease, persons who are colonized by an infectious agent but have no apparent disease, or persons who are chronic carriers of an infectious agent. Other sources of infecting microorganisms can be the patient's own endogenous flora, which may be difficult to control, and inanimate environmental objects that have become contaminated, including equipment and medications.

Host

Resistance among persons to pathogenic microorganisms varies greatly. Some persons may be immune to infection or may be able to resist colonization by an infectious agent; others exposed to the same agent may establish a commensal relationship with the infecting microorganism and become asymptomatic carriers; still others may develop clinical disease. Host factors such as age; underlying diseases; certain treatments with antimicrobials, corticosteroids, or other immunosuppressive agents; irradiation; and breaks in the first line of defense mechanisms caused by such factors as surgical operations, anesthesia, and indwelling urinary and central venous catheters (urinary catheters and central venous catheters) may render patients more susceptible to infection.

Transmission

The classic definition of *transmission* is an appraisal of how classes of pathogens cause infection. Simply stated, microorganisms are transmitted in hospitals by several routes, and the same microorganism may be transmitted by more than one route. There are three common modes of transmission: contact, droplet, and airborne. Within this context, health-care providers need to differentiate between nosocomial infection and health-care-associated infection (HAI). The term *nosocomial infection* refers to those infections that are acquired in a hospital. Whereas an HAI can be acquired from delivery of care in multiple settings including, hospitals, long-term care, ambulatory care, or home care. The difference between the two terms is that in nosocomial infections we know the infection was acquired in the hospital. With HAI we know that the infection was acquired somewhere along the health-care path, we are just not sure exactly when or where. An example would be an individual who moves from home care, to acute care, to long-term care. Additional modes of transmission

*SOURCE: Adapted from http://www.cdc.gov/ncidod/dhqp/gl_isolation.html.

are common vehicle and vectorborne, which will be discussed briefly for the purpose of this guideline as neither play a significant role in the typical nosocomial or HAI infections.

1. *Contact transmission*, the most important and frequent mode of transmission of nosocomial or HAI infections, is divided into two subgroups: direct-contact transmission and indirect-contact transmission.

   1a. *Direct-contact transmission* involves a direct body surface-to-body surface contact and physical transfer of microorganisms between a susceptible host and an infected or colonized person. In the health-care setting this occurs most frequently between patient and health-care personnel through a mucous membrane crack or ungloved patient contact with infected/infested skin. Examples of such contacts can include turning a patient, giving a patient a bath, or performing other patient-care activities that require direct contact. Direct-contact transmission also can occur between two patients, with one serving as the source of the infectious microorganisms and the other as a susceptible host.

   1b. *Indirect-contact transmission* involves contact of a susceptible host with a contaminated intermediate object, usually inanimate, such as contaminated instruments, toys, needles, dressings, or shared patient care devices such as glucose monitoring machines. For children, those inanimate objects can even include toys. Other sources are insufficient hand hygiene, or gloves that are not changed between patients, as well as soiled clothing such as uniforms or laboratory coats have been found to be a source for indirect-contact transmission. Multi-drug resistant organisms (MDRO) are a special concern in health-care settings. Transmission usually occurs patient-to-patient by the hands of health-care workers.

2. *Droplet transmission*, theoretically, is a form of contact transmission. However, the mechanism of transfer of the pathogen to the host is quite distinct from either direct—or indirect-contact transmission. Therefore, droplet transmission is considered a separate route of transmission in this guideline. Historically droplet size is defined as being 5 µm or greater. Droplets are generated from the source person primarily during coughing, sneezing, and talking, and during the performance of certain procedures such as suctioning and bronchoscopy. Transmission occurs when droplets containing microorganisms generated from the infected person are propelled a short distance through the air and deposited on the host's conjunctivae, nasal mucosa, or mouth. The general rule of thumb has been that droplets will travel approximately 3 ft from the source to the host. However studies suggest that droplets from organisms such as smallpox, and severe acute respiratory distress syndrome (SARS) can travel a distance of 6 ft or more from source to host. Therefore the suggested distance of 3 ft is considered to be a recommendation rather a mandate. As a result distance should not be the only criteria used to decide whether or not the use of a mask is appropriate. Because droplets do not remain suspended in the air, special air handling and ventilation are not required to prevent droplet transmission; that is, droplet transmission must not be confused with airborne transmission.

3. *Airborne transmission* occurs by dissemination of either airborne droplet nuclei (small-particle residue [5 µm or smaller in size] of evaporated droplets containing microorganisms that remain suspended in the air for long periods of time) or dust particles containing the infectious

agent. Microorganisms carried in this manner can be dispersed widely by air currents and may become inhaled by a susceptible host within the same room or over a longer distance from the source patient, depending on environmental factors; therefore, special air handling and ventilation such as an airborne infection isolation room are required to prevent airborne transmission. Microorganisms transmitted by airborne transmission include *Mycobacterium tuberculosis, Aspergillus spp.,* and the rubeola and varicella viruses.

4. *Common vehicle transmission* applies to microorganisms transmitted by contaminated items such as food, water, medications, devices, and equipment.
5. *Vectorborne transmission* occurs when vectors such as mosquitoes, flies, rats, and other vermin transmit microorganisms; this route of transmission is of less significance in hospitals in the United States than in other regions of the world.

Isolation precautions are designed to prevent transmission of microorganisms by these routes in hospitals. Because agent and host factors are more difficult to control, interruption of transfer of microorganisms is directed primarily at transmission. This goal can be more readily achieved by having an infection control nurse assist in the implementation of policies at the unit level; adequate staff with minimal use of outside staff; clinical laboratory support to promptly report important organisms or outbreak concerns; implementation of a culture of safety within the organization; adherence of health-care workers to recommended infection control guidelines; surveillance for HAIs; and continuing education of health-care workers, patients, and families. The recommendations presented in this guideline are based on this concept.

Placing a patient on isolation precautions, however, often presents certain disadvantages to the hospital, patients, personnel, and visitors. Isolation precautions may require specialized equipment and environmental modifications that add to the cost of hospitalization. Isolation precautions may make frequent visits by nurses, physicians, and other personnel inconvenient, and they may make it more difficult for personnel to give the prompt and frequent care that sometimes is required. The use of a multi-patient room for one patient uses valuable space that otherwise might accommodate several patients. Moreover, forced solitude deprives the patient of normal social relationships and may be psychologically harmful, especially to children. These disadvantages, however, must be weighed against the hospital's mission to prevent the spread of serious and epidemiologically important microorganisms in the hospital.

FUNDAMENTALS OF ISOLATION PRECAUTIONS

A variety of infection control measures are used for decreasing the risk of transmission of microorganisms in hospitals. These measures make up the fundamentals of isolation precautions. Examples of Personal Protective Equipment (PPE) used in infection control include gloves, gowns, masks, goggles, and shoe covers.

Hand Hygiene and Gloving

Hand hygiene is frequently called the single most important measure to reduce the risks of transmitting organisms from one person to another or from one site to another on the same patient. The concept of hand hygiene includes hand washing, or in the absence of visible soiling, the use of approved alcohol-based products for hand disinfecting. The scientific rationale, indications, methods, and products for hand washing are delineated in other publications.

Hand washing, or the use of alcohol-based products should be completed as promptly and thoroughly as possible between patient contacts and after contact with blood, body fluids, secretions, and excretions. Hand hygiene should also occur after contact with equipment or articles contaminated by blood, fluids, secretions, or excretions. Such hygiene is an important component of infection control and isolation precautions. In addition to hand hygiene, gloves play a key role in reducing the risks of microorganism transmission. The effectiveness of hand hygiene can be reduced by health-care workers wearing artificial nails as they can harbor pathogenic organisms. It is recommended that health-care workers who provide direct patient care be restricted from wearing these nails.

Gloves are worn for three important reasons in hospitals. First, gloves are worn to provide a protective barrier and to prevent gross contamination of the hands when touching blood, body fluids, secretions, excretions, mucous membranes, and nonintact skin; the wearing of gloves in specified circumstances to reduce the risk of exposures to bloodborne pathogens is mandated by the Occupational Safety and Health Administration (OSHA) bloodborne pathogens final rule. Second, gloves are worn to reduce the likelihood that microorganisms present on the hands of personnel will be transmitted to patients during invasive or other patient-care procedures that involve touching a patient's mucous membranes and nonintact skin. Third, gloves are worn to reduce the likelihood that hands of personnel contaminated with microorganisms from a patient or a fomite can transmit these microorganisms to another patient. In this situation, gloves must be changed between patient contacts and hands washed after gloves are removed.

Wearing gloves does not replace the need for hand hygiene, because gloves may have small, inapparent defects or may be torn during use, and hands can become contaminated during removal of gloves. Changing gloves is recommended when provision of care requires touching equipment that is moved from room to room. Failure to change gloves between patient contacts is an infection control hazard.

Patient Placement

Appropriate patient placement is a significant component of isolation precautions. A private room is important to prevent direct- or indirect-contact transmission when the source patient has poor hygienic habits, contaminates the environment, or cannot be expected to assist in maintaining infection control precautions to limit transmission of microorganisms (e.g., infants, children, and patients with altered mental status). When possible, a patient with highly transmissible or epidemiologically important microorganisms is placed in a private room with hand washing and toilet facilities to reduce opportunities for transmission of microorganisms.

When a private room is not available, an infected patient is placed with an appropriate roommate. Patients infected by the same microorganism usually can share a room, provided they are not infected with other potentially transmissible microorganisms and the likelihood of reinfection with the same organism is minimal. Such sharing of rooms, also referred to as cohorting patients, is useful especially during outbreaks or when there is a shortage of private rooms. When a private room is not available and cohorting is not achievable or recommended, it is very important to consider the epidemiology and mode of transmission of the infecting pathogen and the patient population being served in determining patient placement. Under these circumstances, consultation with infection control professionals is advised before patient placement. Moreover, when an infected patient shares a room with a noninfected patient, it also is important that patients, personnel, and visitors take precautions to prevent the spread of infection and that room-mates are selected carefully.

Guidelines for construction, equipment, air handling, and ventilation for isolation rooms are delineated in other publications. A private room with appropriate air handling and ventilation is particularly important for reducing the risk of transmission of microorganisms from a source patient to susceptible patients and other persons in hospitals when the microorganism is spread by airborne transmission. Some hospitals use an isolation room with an anteroom as an extra measure of precaution to prevent airborne transmission. Adequate data regarding the need for an anteroom, however, is not available. Ventilation recommendations for isolation rooms housing patients with pulmonary tuber-culosis have been delineated in other Centers for Disease Control and Prevention (CDC) guidelines.

Transport of Infected Patients

Limiting the movement and transport of patients infected with virulent or epidemiologically important microorganisms and ensuring that such patients leave their rooms only for essential purposes reduces opportunities for trans-mission of microorganisms in hospitals. When patient transport is necessary, it is important that (1) appropriate barriers (e.g., masks, impervious dressings) are worn or used by the patient to reduce the opportunity for transmission of pertinent microorganisms to other patients, personnel, and visitors and to reduce contamination of the environment; (2) personnel in the area to which the patient is to be taken are notified of the impending arrival of the patient and of the precautions to be used to reduce the risk of transmission of infec-tious microorganisms; and (3) patients are informed of ways by which they can assist in preventing the transmission of their infectious microorganisms to others.

Masks, Respiratory Protection, Eye Protection, Face Shields

Various types of masks, goggles, and face shields are worn alone or in combi-nation to provide barrier protection. A mask that covers both the nose and the mouth, and goggles or a face shield are worn by hospital personnel during procedures and patient-care activities that are likely to generate splashes or sprays of blood, body fluids, secretions, or excretions to provide protection of the mucous membranes of the eyes, nose, and mouth from contact transmis-sion of pathogens. The use of masks also protects the patient from exposure to organisms from health-care workers during sterile procedures, and protects health-care workers and others from exposure to coughing patients. The wear-ing of masks, eye protection, and face shields in specified circumstances to reduce the risk of exposures to bloodborne pathogens is mandated by the OSHA bloodborne pathogens final rule. A surgical mask generally is worn by hospital personnel to provide protection against spread of infectious large-particle droplets that are transmitted by close contact and generally travel only short distances (up to 3 ft) from infected patients who are coughing or sneezing.

An area of major concern and controversy over the last several years has been the role and selection of respiratory protection equipment and the implications of a respiratory protection program for prevention of transmission of tuberculosis in hospitals. Traditionally, although the efficacy was not proven, a surgical mask was worn for isolation precautions in hospitals when patients were known or suspected to be infected with pathogens spread by the airborne route of transmission. In 1990, however, the CDC tuberculosis guidelines stated that surgical masks may not be effective in preventing the inhalation of droplet nuclei and recommended the use of disposable particulate respirators, despite the fact that the efficacy of particulate respirators in protecting persons from the inhalation of *M. tuberculosis* had not been demonstrated. By definition, particulate respirators included dust-mist (DM), dust-fume-mist (DFM), or high-efficiency particulate air (HEPA) filter respirators certified by the CDC National Institute for Occupational Safety and Health (NIOSH); because the generic term "particulate respirator" was used in the 1990 guidelines, the implication was that any of these respirators provided sufficient protection.

In 1993, a draft revision of the CDC tuberculosis guidelines outlined performance criteria for respirators and stated that some DM or DFM respirators might not meet these criteria. After review of public comments, the guidelines were finalized in October 1994, with the draft respirator criteria unchanged. At that time, the only class of respirators that were known to consistently meet or exceed the performance criteria outlined in the 1994 tuberculosis guidelines and that were certified by NIOSH (as required by OSHA) were HEPA filter respirators. Subsequently, NIOSH revised the testing and certification requirements for all types of air-purifying respirators, including those used for tuberculosis control. The new rule, effective in July 1995, provides a broader range of certified respirators that meet the performance criteria recommended by the CDC in the 1994 tuberculosis guidelines. NIOSH has indicated that the N95 (N category at 95% efficiency) meets the CDC performance criteria for a tuberculosis respirator. Current recommendations encourage health-care care workers to undergo fit-testing. The goal of fit-testing is to ensure that the health-care worker's respirator (N95 mask) fits well during job performance. The frequency of fit-testing has not been specified. Generally fit-testing should be repeated when there is a change in facial features, a change in mask model or sizing, and for any condition effecting the health-care worker's respiratory function. During testing, it is important to assess theses salient points, mask positioning and fit across the nose, cheeks, and chin, with room for eye protection, and room to talk. Additional information on the evolution of respirator recommendations, regulations to protect hospital personnel, and the role of various federal agencies in respiratory protection for hospital personnel has been published.

Gowns and Protective Apparel

Various types of gowns and protective apparel are worn to provide barrier protection and to reduce opportunities for transmission of microorganisms in hospitals. Gowns are worn to prevent contamination of clothing and to protect the skin of personnel from blood and body fluid exposures. Gowns, especially treated to make them impermeable to liquids, leg coverings, boots, or shoe covers provide greater protection to the skin when splashes or large quantities of infective material are present or anticipated. Gowns should cover the arms, torso, and legs to mid-thigh providing complete coverage of these areas. Remove gowns cautiously to prevent contamination of clothing. Gowns and all other PPE should be removed and discarded prior to leaving the patients room. The wearing of gowns and protective apparel under specified circumstances to reduce the risk of exposures to bloodborne pathogens is mandated by the OSHA bloodborne pathogens final rule. (Categories IB/IC)

Gowns are also worn by personnel during the care of patients infected with epidemiologically important microorganisms to reduce the opportunity for transmission of pathogens from patients or items in their environment to other patients or environments; when gowns are worn for this purpose, they are removed before leaving the patient's environment and hands are washed. Adequate data regarding the efficacy of gowns for this purpose, however, are not available.

Patient-Care Equipment and Articles

Many factors determine whether special handling and disposal of used patient-care equipment and articles are prudent or required, including the likelihood of contamination with infective material; the ability to cut, stick, or otherwise cause injury (needles, scalpels, and other sharp instruments [sharps]); the severity of the associated disease; and the environmental stability of the pathogens involved. Some used articles are enclosed in containers or bags to prevent inadvertent exposures to patients, personnel, and visitors and to prevent contamination of the environment. Used sharps are placed in puncture-resistant containers; other articles are placed in a bag. One bag is adequate if the bag is sturdy and the article can be placed in the bag without contaminating the outside of the bag; otherwise, two bags are used.

The scientific rationale, indications, methods, products, and equipment for reprocessing patient-care equipment are delineated in other publications. Contaminated, reusable critical medical devices or patient-care equipment (i.e., equipment that enters normally sterile tissue or through which blood flows) or semicritical medical devices or patient-care equipment (i.e., equipment that touches mucous membranes) are sterilized or disinfected (reprocessed) after use to reduce the risk of transmission of microorganisms to other patients; the type of reprocessing is determined by the article and its intended use, the manufacturer's recommendations, hospital policy, and any applicable guidelines and regulations.

Noncritical equipment (i.e., equipment that touches intact skin) contaminated with blood, body fluids, secretions, or excretions is cleaned and disinfected after use, according to hospital policy. Contaminated disposable (single-use) patient-care equipment is handled and transported in a manner that reduces the risk of transmission of microorganisms and decreases environmental contamination in the hospital; the equipment is disposed of according to hospital policy and applicable regulations.

Linen and Laundry

Although soiled linen may be contaminated with pathogenic microorganisms, the risk of disease transmission is negligible if it is handled, transported, and laundered in a manner that avoids transfer of microorganisms to patients, personnel, and environments. Rather than rigid rules and regulations, hygienic and common sense storage and processing of clean and soiled linen are recommended. The methods for handling, transporting, and laundering of soiled linen are determined by hospital policy and any applicable regulations.

Dishes, Glasses, Cups, and Eating Utensils

No special precautions are needed for dishes, glasses, cups, or eating utensils. Either disposable or reusable dishes and utensils can be used for patients on isolation precautions. The combination of hot water and detergents used in hospital dishwashers is sufficient to decontaminate dishes, glasses, cups, and eating utensils.

Routine and Terminal Cleaning

The room, or cubicle, and bedside equipment of patients on Transmission-Based Precautions are cleaned using the same procedures used for patients on Standard Precautions, unless the infecting microorganism(s) and the amount of environmental contamination indicates special cleaning. In addition to thorough cleaning, adequate disinfection of bedside equipment and environmental surfaces (e.g., bedrails, bedside tables, carts, commodes, doorknobs, faucet handles) is indicated for certain pathogens, especially enterococci, which can survive in the inanimate environment for prolonged periods of time. Patients admitted to hospital rooms that previously were occupied by patients infected or colonized with such pathogens are at increased risk of infection from contaminated environmental surfaces and bedside equipment if they have not been cleaned and disinfected adequately. The methods, thoroughness, and frequency of cleaning and the products used are determined by hospital policy.

APP

HOSPITAL INFECTION CONTROL PRACTICES ADVISORY COMMITTEE (HICPAC) ISOLATION PRECAUTIONS

There are two tiers of HICPAC isolation precautions, first Standard Precautions, and second Transmission-Based Precautions. In the first, and most important, tier are those precautions designed for the care of all patients in hospitals, regardless of their diagnosis or presumed infection status. Implementation of these "Standard Precautions" is the primary strategy for successful nosocomial infection control. In the second tier are precautions designed only for the care of specified patients. These additional "Transmission-Based Precautions" are for patients known or suspected to be infected by epidemiologically important pathogens spread by airborne or droplet transmission or by contact with dry skin or contaminated surfaces.

Standard Precautions

Standard Precautions synthesize the major features of Universal Precautions (UP), and Body Substance Isolation (BSI) under the premise that transmissible infections agents can be contained in multiple care situations and apply to all patients receiving care in any health-care setting, regardless of their diagnosis or presumed infection status. Standard Precautions apply to (1) blood; (2) all body fluids, secretions, and excretions except sweat, regardless of whether they contain visible blood; (3) nonintact skin; and (4) mucous membranes. Standard Precautions are designed to reduce the risk of transmission of microorganisms from both recognized and unrecognized sources of infection in hospitals. Basic Standard Precautions include the use of gown, mask, gloves, and goggles or face shield as appropriate. Three new recommendations focused on patient protection have been added to Standard Precaution guidelines, (1) Respiratory Hygiene/Cough Etiquette, (2) mask use for catheter insertion/ injection (spinal, epidural), and (3) safe injection practices.

Respiratory Hygiene/Cough Etiquette was developed as a response to SARS focusing on patients and family members who enter the health-care setting with undiagnosed respiratory symptoms including cough, congestion, runny nose, and productive secretions. There are five basic goals associated with Respiratory Hygiene/Cough Etiquette: (1) to educate interceding staff, family, patients, and visitors when a high-risk patient enters the health-care setting with regard to description of respiratory symptoms, the importance of reporting symptoms, description of the types and use of PPE, (2) to communicate information regarding respiratory hygiene and cough etiquette via posted instructions in appropriate languages, (3) to enforce source control measures (covering mouth when coughing or sneezing, proper disposal of contaminated tissues, appropriate use of surgical masks by the coughing individual), (4) to enforce effective hand hygiene, and (5) to maintain a distance of 3 to 6 ft or more from source person if PPE is not being used.

Protection with mask use during spinal procedures (epidural injection or catheter placement), is recommended to prevent contamination from oropharyngeal droplets causing infection. The October 2005 HICPAC concluded that there is sufficient evidence to support this recommended change in practice.

Safe injection focuses on preventing pathogen outbreaks from ineffective infection control practice. Conceptually, emphasis is placed on aseptic technique with use of sterile single-use needles and syringes, use of disposable needles, use of single rather than multiple dose vials, and prevention of contamination of injection devices and medication. Emphasis is placed on the training and retraining of aseptic technique and infection control practices.

Transmission-Based Precautions

Transmission-Based Precautions are designed for patients documented or suspected to be infected with highly transmissible or epidemiologically important pathogens for which additional precautions beyond Standard Precautions are needed to interrupt transmission in hospitals. There are three types of Transmission-Based Precautions: Airborne Precautions (or Airborne Infection Isolation Precautions [AIIR]), Droplet Precautions, and Contact Precautions. They may be combined for diseases that have multiple routes of transmission. When used either singularly or in combination, they are to be used in addition to Standard Precautions.

Airborne Precautions are designed to reduce the risk of airborne transmission of infectious agents. Airborne transmission occurs by dissemination of either airborne droplet nuclei (small-particle residue [5 μm or smaller in size] of evaporated droplets that may remain suspended in the air for long periods of time) or dust particles containing the infectious agent. Microorganisms carried in this manner can be dispersed widely by air currents and may become inhaled by or deposited on a susceptible host within the same room or over a longer distance from the source patient, depending on environmental factors; therefore, special air handling and ventilation are required to prevent airborne transmission. Airborne Precautions apply to patients known or suspected to be infected with epidemiologically important pathogens that can be transmitted by the airborne route.

Droplet Precautions are designed to reduce the risk of droplet transmission of infectious agents. Droplet transmission involves contact of the conjunctivae or the mucous membranes of the nose or mouth of a susceptible person with large-particle droplets (larger than 5 μm in size) containing microorganisms generated from a person who has a clinical disease or who is a carrier of the microorganism. Droplets are generated from the source person primarily during coughing, sneezing, or talking and during the performance of certain procedures such as suctioning and bronchoscopy. Transmission via large-particle droplets requires close contact between source and recipient persons because droplets do not remain suspended in the air and generally travel only short distances. General rule of thumb has been that droplets will carry through the air a distance of usually 3 or fewer feet. However, evidence suggests that some droplets such as chickenpox or SARS can carry as far as 6 ft from their source. Therefore the suggested distance of 3 ft should be considered an example of how far a droplet can carry from the source to the host rather than an exact measurement. Because droplets do not remain suspended in the air, special air handling and ventilation are not required to prevent droplet transmission. Droplet Precautions apply to any patient known or suspected to be infected with epidemiologically important pathogens that can be transmitted by infectious droplets.

Contact Precautions are designed to reduce the risk of transmission of epidemiologically important microorganisms by direct or indirect contact. Contact precautions also apply in the presence of fecal incontinence, excessive wound drainage, and any other body secretions that may indicate a contamination/transmission risk. Direct-contact transmission involves skin-to-skin contact and physical transfer of microorganisms to a susceptible host from an infected or colonized person, such as occurs when personnel turn patients, bathe patients, or perform other patient-care activities that require physical contact. Direct-contact transmission also can occur between two patients (e.g., by hand contact), with one serving as the source of infectious microorganisms and the other as a susceptible host. Indirect-contact transmission involves contact of a susceptible host with a contaminated intermediate object, usually inanimate, in the patient's environment. Contact Precautions apply to specified patients known or suspected to be infected or colonized (presence of microorganism in or on patient but without clinical signs and symptoms of infection) with epidemiologically important microorganisms than can be transmitted by direct or indirect contact.

EMPIRIC USE OF AIRBORNE, DROPLET, OR CONTACT PRECAUTIONS

In many instances, the risk of nosocomial transmission of infection may be highest before a definitive diagnosis can be made and before precautions based on that diagnosis can be implemented. The routine use of Standard Precautions for all patients should reduce greatly this risk for conditions other than those requiring Airborne, Droplet, or Contact Precautions. Although it is not possible to prospectively identify all patients needing these enhanced precautions, certain clinical syndromes and conditions carry a sufficiently high risk to warrant the empiric addition of enhanced precautions (Transmission-Based Precautions) while a definitive diagnosis is pursued and test recommendations are to institute Transmission-Based Precautions in these instances until test results are obtained.

The organisms listed under the column "Potential Pathogens" are not intended to represent the complete or even most likely diagnoses, but rather possible etiologic agents that require additional precautions beyond Standard Precautions until they can be ruled out. Infection control professionals are encouraged to modify or adapt this table according to local conditions. To ensure that appropriate empiric precautions are always implemented, hospitals must have systems in place to evaluate patients routinely, according to these criteria as part of their preadmission and admission care.

IMMUNOCOMPROMISED PATIENTS

Immunocompromised patients vary in their susceptibility to nosocomial infections, depending on the severity and duration of immunosuppression. They generally are at increased risk for bacterial, fungal, parasitic, and viral infections from both endogenous and exogenous sources. The use of Standard Precautions for all patients and Transmission-Based Precautions for specified patients, as recommended in this guideline, should reduce the acquisition by these patients of institutionally acquired bacteria from other patients and environments. A new prevention strategy called Protective Environment has been designed to protect this type of patient, (specifically hematiopoietic stem cell patients) by decreasing environmental exposure risk in the days immediately after transplant.

It is beyond the scope of this guideline to address the various measures that may be used for immunocompromised patients to delay or prevent acquisition of potential pathogens during temporary periods of neutropenia. Rather, the primary objective of this guideline is to prevent transmission of pathogens from infected or colonized patients in hospitals. Users of this guideline, however, are referred to the "Guideline for Prevention of Nosocomial Pneumonia" (95, 96) for the HICPAC recommendations for prevention of nosocomial aspergillosis and Legionnaires' disease in immunocompromised patients.

RECOMMENDATIONS

The recommendations presented below are categorized as follows:

Category IA. Strongly recommended for all hospitals and strongly supported by well-designed experimental or epidemiological studies.

Category IB. Strongly recommended for all hospitals and reviewed as effective by experts in the field and a consensus of HICPAC based on strong rationale and suggestive evidence, even though definitive scientific studies have not been done.

Category IC. Mandated for implementation in health-care settings by state or federal standards/regulation.

Category II. Suggested for implementation in many hospitals. Recommendations may be supported by suggestive clinical or epidemiological studies, a strong theoretical rationale, or definitive studies applicable to some, but not all, hospitals.

No recommendation; unresolved issue. Practices for which insufficient evidence or consensus regarding efficacy exists.

The recommendations are limited to the topic of isolation precautions. Therefore, they must be supplemented by hospital policies and procedures for other aspects of infection and environmental control, occupational health, administrative and legal issues, and other issues beyond the scope of this guideline.

1. **Administrative Control**
   a. Education

      Ensure transmission prevention is incorporated into organizational objectives and occupational safety programs with development of appropriate policies and procedures. Transmission prevention strategies should be supported fiscally, with human resource including infection control staff and programs, laboratory resources for surveillance, and investigation. The presence of HAIs should provide some direction for staffing and decontamination decisions with the assistance of infection control in design, detection strategies, and monitoring of performance measures. (Categories IA/IB/IC/II)

      Develop a system to ensure that hospital patients, personnel, and visitors are educated about use of precautions and their responsibility for adherence to them. (Category IB/IC)

   b. Adherence to Precautions

      Periodically evaluate adherence to precautions, and use findings to direct improvements. (Category IB)

2. **Standard Precautions**

   Implementation of Standard Precautions is based on the assumption that all patients are a potential source of transmissible infection. Adherence to state and federal law in provision of protection for health-care personnel is required. (Category IC)

   a. Hand Hygiene

      (1) Perform hand hygiene after touching blood, body fluids, secretions, excretions, nonintact skin, and contaminated items; immediately after gloves are removed; prior to direct patient contact; between patient contacts; and when otherwise indicated to prevent transfer of microorganisms to other patients or environments. Hand hygiene may be necessary between tasks or procedures on the same patient to prevent cross contamination of different body sites. Wash hands with an antimicrobial soap, or plain (nonantimicrobial) soap and water when visibly soiled. An alcohol-based hand rub may be used in the absence of visible soiling or after soiling has been removed with plain (nonantimicrobial) soap and water. Artificial nails or extenders are not to be worn by individuals providing direct patient contact. (Categories IA/IB/IC/II)

      (2) Use a plain (nonantimicrobial) soap for routine hand washing. (Category IB)

      (3) Use an antimicrobial agent or a waterless antiseptic agent for specific circumstances (e.g., control of outbreaks or hyperendemic infections), as defined by the infection control program. (Category IB) (See Contact Precautions for additional recommendations on using antimicrobial and antiseptic agents.)

   b. Gloves

      Wear gloves (clean, nonsterile gloves are adequate) when touching blood, body fluids, secretions, excretions, and contaminated items. Put on clean gloves just before touching mucous membranes and nonintact skin. Change gloves between tasks and procedures on the same patient after contact with material that may contain a high concentration of microorganisms. Remove gloves promptly after use, before touching noncontaminated items and environmental surfaces, and before going to another patient, and wash hands immediately to avoid transfer of microorganisms to other patients or environments. (Category IB)

c. Mask, Eye Protection, Face Shield

Wear a mask and eye protection or a face shield to protect mucous membranes of the eyes, nose, and mouth during procedures and patient-care activities that are likely to generate splashes or sprays of blood, body fluids, secretions, and excretions. (Category IB)

d. Gown

Wear a gown (a clean, nonsterile gown is adequate) to protect skin and to prevent soiling of clothing during procedures and patient-care activities that are likely to generate splashes or sprays of blood, body fluids, secretions, or excretions. Select a gown that is appropriate for the activity and amount of fluid likely to be encountered. Remove a soiled gown as promptly as possible, and wash hands to avoid transfer of microorganisms to other patients or environments. (Category IB)

e. Patient-Care Equipment

Handle used patient-care equipment soiled with blood, body fluids, secretions, and excretions in a manner that prevents skin and mucous membrane exposures, contamination of clothing, and transfer of microorganisms to other patients and environments. Ensure that reusable equipment is not used for the care of another patient until it has been cleaned and reprocessed appropriately. Ensure that single-use items are discarded properly. (Category IB)

f. Environmental Control

Ensure that the hospital has adequate procedures for the routine care, cleaning, and disinfection of environmental surfaces, beds, bedrails, bedside equipment, and other frequently touched surfaces, and ensure that these procedures are being followed. (Category IB)

g. Linen

Handle, transport, and process used linen soiled with blood, body fluids, secretions, and excretions in a manner that prevents skin and mucous membrane exposures and contamination of clothing, and that avoids transfer of microorganisms to other patients and environments. (Category IB)

h. Occupational Health and Bloodborne Pathogens

(1) Take care to prevent injuries when using needles, scalpels, and other sharp instruments or devices; when handling sharp instruments after procedures; when cleaning used instruments; and when disposing of used needles. Never recap used needles, or otherwise manipulate them using both hands, or use any other technique that involves directing the point of a needle toward any part of the body; rather, use either a one-handed "scoop" technique or a mechanical device designed for holding the needle sheath. Do not remove used needles from disposable syringes by hand, and do not bend, break, or otherwise manipulate used needles by hand. Place used disposable syringes and needles, scalpel blades, and other sharp items in appropriate puncture-resistant containers, which are located as close as practical to the area in which the items were used, and place reusable syringes and needles in a puncture-resistant container for transport to the reprocessing area. (Category IB)

(2) Use mouthpieces, resuscitation bags, or other ventilation devices as an alternative to mouth-to-mouth resuscitation methods in areas where the need for resuscitation is predictable. (Category IB)

i. Patient Placement

Place a patient who contaminates the environment or who does not (or cannot be expected to) assist in maintaining appropriate hygiene or environmental control in a private room. If a private room is not available, consult with infection control professionals regarding patient placement or other alternatives. (Category IB)

3. **Airborne Precautions**

In addition to Standard Precautions, use Airborne Precautions, or the equivalent, for patients known or suspected to be infected with microorganisms transmitted by airborne droplet nuclei (small-particle residue [5 µm or smaller in size] of evaporated droplets containing microorganisms that remain suspended in the air and that can be dispersed widely by air currents within a room or over a long distance). (Category IB)

a. Patient Placement

Place the patient in a private room that has (1) monitored negative air pressure in relation to the surrounding areas, (2) 6 to 12 air changes per hour, and (3) appropriate discharge of air outdoors or monitored high-efficiency filtration of room air before the air is circulated to other areas in the hospital. Keep the room door closed and the patient in the room. When a private room is not available, place the patient in a room with a patient who has active infection with the same microorganism, unless otherwise recommended, but with no other infection. When a private room is not available and cohorting is not desirable, consultation with infection control professionals is advised before patient placement. (Category IB)

b. Respiratory Protection

Wear respiratory protection (N95 respirator) when entering the room of a patient with known or suspected infectious pulmonary tuberculosis. Susceptible persons should not enter the room of patients known or suspected to have measles (rubeola) or varicella (chickenpox) if other immune caregivers are available. If susceptible persons must enter the room of a patient known or suspected to have measles (rubeola) or varicella, they should wear respiratory protection (N95 respirator). Persons immune to measles (rubeola) or varicella need not wear respiratory protection. (Category IB)

c. Patient Transport

Limit the movement and transport of the patient from the room to essential purposes only. If transport or movement is necessary, minimize patient dispersal of droplet nuclei by placing a surgical mask on the patient, if possible. (Category IB)

d. Additional Precautions for Preventing Transmission of Tuberculosis: Consult the Centers for Disease Control and Prevention's "Guidelines for Preventing the Transmission of Tuberculosis in Health-Care Facilities" for additional prevention strategies.

4. **Droplet Precautions**

In addition to Standard Precautions, use Droplet Precautions, or the equivalent, for a patient known or suspected to be infected with microorganisms transmitted by droplets (large-particle droplets [larger than 5 μm in size] that can be generated by the patient during coughing, sneezing, talking, or the performance of procedures). (Category IB)

a. Patient Placement

Place the patient in a private room. When a private room is not available, place the patient in a room with a patient(s) who has active infection with the same microorganism but with no other infection (cohorting). When a private room is not available and cohorting is not achievable, maintain spatial separation of at least 3 ft between the infected patient and other patients and visitors. Special air handling and ventilation are not necessary, and the door may remain open. (Category IB)

b. Mask

In addition to wearing a mask as outlined under Standard Precautions, wear a mask when working within 3 ft of the patient. (Logistically, some hospitals may want to implement the wearing of a mask to enter the room.) (Category IB)

c. Patient Transport

Limit the movement and transport of the patient from the room to essential purposes only. If transport or movement is necessary, minimize patient dispersal of droplets by masking the patient, if possible. (Category IB)

5. **Contact Precautions**

In addition to Standard Precautions, use Contact Precautions, or the equivalent, for specified patients known or suspected to be infected or colonized with epidemiologically important microorganisms that can be transmitted by direct contact with the patient (hand or skin-to-skin contact that occurs when performing patient-care activities that require touching the patient's dry skin) or indirect contact (touching) with environmental surfaces or patient-care items in the patient's environment. (Category IB)

a. Patient Placement

Place the patient in a private room. When a private room is not available, place the patient in a room with a patient(s) who has active infection with the same microorganism but with no other infection (cohorting). When a private room is not available and cohorting is not achievable, consider the epidemiology of the microorganism and the patient population when determining patient placement. Consultation with infection control professionals is advised before patient placement. (Category IB)

b. Gloves and Hand Hygiene

In addition to wearing gloves as outlined under Standard Precautions, wear gloves (clean, nonsterile gloves are adequate) when entering the room. During the course of providing care for a patient, change gloves after having contact with infective material that may contain high concentrations of microorganisms (fecal material and wound drainage). Remove gloves before leaving the patient's room and wash hands immediately with an antimicrobial agent or a waterless antiseptic agent. After glove removal and hand washing, do not touch potentially contaminated environmental surfaces or items in the patient's room to avoid transfer of microorganisms to other patients or environments. (Category IB)

c. Gown

In addition to wearing a gown as outlined under Standard Precautions, wear a gown (a clean, nonsterile gown is adequate) when entering the room if you anticipate that your clothing will have substantial contact with the patient, environmental surfaces, or items in the patient's room, or if the patient is incontinent or has diarrhea, an ileostomy, a colostomy, or wound drainage not contained by a dressing. Remove the gown before leaving the patient's environment. After gown removal, ensure that clothing does not contact potentially contaminated environmental surfaces to avoid transfer of microorganisms to other patients or environments. (Category IB)

d. Patient Transport

Limit the movement and transport of the patient from the room to essential purposes only. If the patient is transported out of the room, ensure that precautions are maintained to minimize the risk of transmission of microorganisms to other patients and contamination of environmental surfaces or equipment. (Category IB)

e. Patient-Care Equipment

When possible, dedicate the use of noncritical patient-care equipment to a single patient (or cohort of patients infected or colonized with the pathogen requiring precautions) to avoid sharing between patients. If use of common equipment or items is unavoidable, then adequately clean and disinfect them before use for another patient. (Category IB)

f. Additional Precautions for Preventing the Spread of Vancomycin Resistance

Consult the HICPAC report on preventing the spread of vancomycin resistance for additional prevention strategies.

Revision to OSHA's Bloodborne Pathogens Standard*

TECHNICAL BACKGROUND AND SUMMARY

Background

The Occupational Safety and Health Administration (OSHA) published the Occupational Exposure to Bloodborne Pathogens standard in 1991 because of a significant health risk associated with exposure to viruses and other microorganisms that cause bloodborne diseases. Of primary concern are HIV and the hepatitis B and hepatitis C viruses.

The standard sets forth requirements for employers with workers exposed to blood or other potentially infectious materials. In order to reduce or eliminate the hazards of occupational exposure, an employer must implement an exposure control plan for the worksite with details on employee protection measures. The plan must also describe how an employer will use a combination of engineering and work practice controls, ensure the use of personal protective clothing and equipment, provide training, medical surveillance, hepatitis B vaccinations, and signs and labels, among other provisions. Engineering controls are the primary means of eliminating or minimizing

---

*SOURCE: Adapted from http://www.osha.gov/needlesticks/needlefact.html.

employee exposure and include the use of safer medical devices, such as needleless devices, shielded needle devices, and plastic capillary tubes.

Nearly 20 years have passed since the bloodborne pathogens standard was published. Since then, many different medical devices have been developed to reduce the risk of needlesticks and other sharps injuries. These devices replace sharps with non-needle devices or incorporate safety features designed to reduce injury. Despite these advances in technology, needlesticks and other sharps injuries continue to be of concern due to the high frequency of their occurrence and the severity of the health effects.

The Centers for Disease Control and Prevention estimate that health-care workers sustain nearly 600,000 percutaneous injuries annually involving contaminated sharps. In response to both the continued concern over such exposures and the technological developments which can increase employee protection, Congress passed the ***Needlestick Safety and Prevention Act*** directing OSHA to revise the bloodborne pathogens standard to establish in greater detail requirements that employers identify and make use of effective and safer medical devices. That revision was published on January 18, 2001, and became effective April 18, 2001.

SUMMARY

The revision to OSHA's bloodborne pathogens standard added new requirements for employers, including additions to the exposure control plan and keeping a sharps injury log. It does not impose new requirements for employers to protect workers from sharps injuries; the original standard already required employers to adopt engineering and work practice controls that would eliminate or minimize employee exposure from hazards associated with bloodborne pathogens.

The revision does, however, specify in greater detail the engineering controls, such as safer medical devices, which must be used to reduce or eliminate worker exposure.

EXPOSURE CONTROL PLAN

The revision includes new requirements regarding the employer's Exposure Control Plan, including an annual review and update to reflect changes in technology that eliminate or reduce exposure to bloodborne pathogens. The employer must:

- take into account innovations in medical procedure and technological developments that reduce the risk of exposure (e.g., newly available medical devices designed to reduce needlesticks); and
- document consideration and use of appropriate, commercially available, and effective safer devices (e.g., describe the devices identified as candidates for use, the method(s) used to evaluate those devices, and justification for the eventual selection).

No one medical device is considered appropriate or effective for all circumstances.

Employers must select devices that, based on reasonable judgment:

- will not jeopardize patient or employee safety or be medically inadvisable; and
- will make an exposure incident involving a contaminated sharp less likely to occur.

EMPLOYEE INPUT

Employers must solicit input from non-managerial employees responsible for direct patient care regarding the identification, evaluation, and selection of effective engineering controls, including safer medical devices. Employees selected should represent the range of exposure situations encountered in the workplace, such as those in geriatric, pediatric, or nuclear medicine, and others involved in direct care of patients.

OSHA will check for compliance with this provision during inspections by questioning a representative number of employees to determine if and how their input was requested.

Documentation of Employee Input

Employers are required to document, in the Exposure Control Plan, how they received input from employees. This obligation can be met by:

- listing the employees involved and describing the process by which input was requested; or
- presenting other documentation, including references to the minutes of meetings, copies of documents used to request employee participation, or records of responses received from employees.

RECORDKEEPING

Employers who have employees who are occupationally exposed to blood or other potentially infectious materials, and who are required to maintain a log of occupational injuries and illnesses under existing recordkeeping rules, must also maintain a sharps injury log. That log will be maintained in a manner that protects the privacy of employees. At a minimum, the log will contain the following:

- The type and brand of device involved in the incident
- Location of the incident (e.g., department or work area)
- Description of the incident

The sharps injury log may include additional information as long as an employee's privacy is protected. The format of the log can be determined by the employer.

MODIFICATION OF DEFINITIONS

The revision to the bloodborne pathogens standard includes modification of definitions relating to engineering controls. Two terms have been added to the standard, while the description of an existing term has been amended.

Engineering Controls

Engineering Controls include all control measures that isolate or remove a hazard from the workplace, such as sharps disposal containers and self-sheathing needles. The original bloodborne pathogens standard was not specific regarding the applicability of various engineering controls (other than the above examples) in the health-care setting. The revision now specifies that "safer medical devices, such as sharps with engineered sharps injury protections and needleless systems" constitute an effective engineering control, and must be used where feasible.

Sharps With Engineered Sharps Injury Protections

This is a new term which includes non-needle sharps or needle devices containing built-in safety features that are used for collecting fluids or administering medications or other fluids, or other procedures involving the risk of sharps injury. This description covers a broad array of devices, including:

- syringes with a sliding sheath that shields the attached needle after use;
- needles that retract into a syringe after use;
- shielded or retracting catheters; and
- intravenous (IV) medication delivery systems that use a catheter port with a needle housed in a protective covering.

Needleless Systems

This is a new term defined as devices which provide an alternative to needles for various procedures to reduce the risk of injury involving contaminated sharps. Examples include:

- IV medication systems which administer medication or fluids through a catheter port using non-needle connections; and
- jet injection systems which deliver liquid medication beneath the skin or through a muscle.

Laboratory Critical Findings

Monograph Title	Critical Finding
Therapeutic Drugs	
Analgesic and Antipyretic Drugs	
Acetaminophen	Greater than 150 mcg/mL (4 hr postingestion); greater than 50 mcg/mL (12 hr postingestion)
Acetylsalicylic acid	Greater than 50 mg/dL
Antiarrhythmic Drugs	
Digoxin	Greater than 2.5 ng/mL
Disopyramide	Greater than 7 mcg/mL
Flecainide	Greater than 1 mcg/mL
Lidocaine	Greater than 6 mcg/mL
Procainamide	Greater than 12 mcg/mL; procainamide + N-acetyl procainamide: greater than 30 mcg/mL
Quinidine	Greater than 8 mcg/mL
Antibiotic Drugs	
Aminoglycosides: Amikacin	Peak greater than 30 mcg/mL, trough greater than 8 mcg/mL
Aminoglycosides: Gentamicin	Peak greater than 12 mcg/mL, trough greater than 2 mcg/mL
Aminoglycosides: Tobramycin	Peak greater than 12 mcg/mL, trough greater than 2 mcg/mL
Tricyclic Glycopeptide: Vancomycin	Peak greater than 80 mcg/mL, trough greater than 20 mcg/mL
Anticonvulsant Drugs	
Carbamazepine	Greater than 20 mcg/mL
Ethosuximide	Greater than 200 mcg/mL
Phenobarbital	Greater than 60 mcg/mL
Phenytoin	Greater than 40 mcg/mL
Primidone	Greater than 24 mcg/mL
Valproic Acid	Greater than 200 mcg/mL
Antidepressant Drugs (Cyclic)	
Amitriptyline	Greater than 500 ng/mL
Nortriptyline	Greater than 500 ng/mL; combined amitriptyline and nortriptyline: greater than 500 ng/mL
Doxepin and Desmethyldoxepin	Greater than 500 ng/mL
Imipramine and Desipramine	Greater than 500 ng/mL
Antipsychotic Drugs and Antimanic Drugs	
Haloperidol	Greater than 42 ng/mL
Lithium	Greater than 2 mEq/L

(table continues on page 1426)

Monograph Title	Critical Finding
Immunosuppressants	
Cyclosporine	Greater than 400 ng/mL
Methotrexate	Greater than 1.00 micromol/L after 48 hr with high-dose therapy; greater than 0.02 micromol/L after 48 hr with low-dose therapy
Alphabetical Listing	
Bilirubin and Bilirubin Fractions	Total bilirubin: greater than 15 mg/dL
Biopsies	Assessment of clear margins after tissue excision; classification or grading of tumor; identification of malignancy
Biopsy, Chorionic Villus	Identification of abnormalities in chorionic villus tissue
Bleeding Time	Greater than 14 min
Blood Gases	pH less than 7.20 or greater than 7.60; HCO_3 less than 10 or greater than 40 mmol/L; Pco_2 less than 20 or greater than 67 mm Hg; Po_2 less than 45 mm Hg
Blood Groups and Antibodies	Note and immediately report to the health-care provider any signs and symptoms associated with a blood transfusion reaction
Calcium, Blood	Less than 7 mg/dL or greater than 12 mg/dL
Calcium, Ionized	Less than 3.2 mg/dL or greater than 6.2 mg/dL
Carbon Dioxide	Less than 15 mmol/L or greater than 40 mmol/L
Carboxyhemoglobin	30%–40%: dizziness, muscle weakness, vision problems, confusion, increased heart rate, increased breathing rate; 50%–60%: loss of consciousness, coma; greater than 60%: death
Cerebrospinal Fluid Analysis	Positive Gram stain, India ink preparation, or culture; presence of malignant cells or blasts; elevated WBC count; glucose less than 37 mg/dL or greater than 440 mg/dL
Chloride, Blood	Less than 80 mEq/L or greater than 115 mEq/L
Chloride, Sweat	20 yr or younger: greater than 60 mEq/L considered diagnostic of cystic fibrosis; older than 20 years: greater than 70 mEq/L considered diagnostic of cystic fibrosis
Complete Blood Count, Hematocrit	Less than 18% or greater than 54%
Complete Blood Count, Hemoglobin	Less than 6.0 g/dL or greater than 18.0 g/dL
Complete Blood Count, Platelet Count	Less than 50,000/mm³; greater than 1,000,000/mm³

Complete Blood Count, RBC Morphology and Inclusions	The presence of abnormal cells, other morphological characteristics, or cellular inclusions may signify a potentially life-threatening or serious health condition and should be investigated. Examples are the presence of sickle cells, moderate numbers of spherocytes, marked schistocytosis, oval macrocytes, basophilic stippling, nucleated RBCs (if the patient is not an infant), or malarial organisms
Complete Blood Count, WBC Count and Differential	Less than 2.5 WBC $\times$ 10^3/mm^3 or 2,500 WBC/mm^3; greater than 30.0 WBC $\times$ 10^3/mm^3 or 30,000 WBC/mm^3
Creatinine, Blood	Potential critical value is greater than 7.4 mg/dL (nondialysis patient)
Creatinine, Urine, and Creatinine Clearance, Urine	Degree of impairment—marked: less than 28 mL/min/1.73 m^2
Cultures	Positive for acid-fast bacillus, *Campylobacter, Clostridium difficile, Corynebacterium diphtheriae, Escherichia coli O157:H7,* influenza, *Legionella, Listeria,* methicillin-resistant *Staphylococcus aureus*, respiratory syncytial virus, rotavirus, *Salmonella, Shigella*, vancomycin-resistant enterococcus, varicella, *Vibrio,* and *Yersinia.* Positive findings in any sterile body fluid such as amniotic fluid, blood, pericardial fluid, peritoneal fluid, pleural fluid. Lists of specific organisms may vary by facility; specific organisms are required to be reported to local, state, and national departments of health.
Fibrinogen	Less than 80 mg/dL
Glucose	Less than 40 mg/dL; greater than 400 mg/dL
Gram Stain	Any positive results in blood, cerebrospinal fluid, or any body cavity fluid
Iron	Serious toxicity: greater than 400 mcg/dL; lethal: greater than 1,000 mcg/dL
Ketones, Blood and Urine	Strongly positive test results for ketones
Lactic Acid	Greater than or equal to 31 mg/dL
Lead	Levels greater than 30 mcg/dL indicate significant exposure; levels greater than 60 mcg/dL require chelation therapy
Lecithin/Sphingomyelin Ratio	An L/S ratio less than 1.5:1 is predictive of respiratory distress syndrome at the time of delivery

(table continues on page 1428)

Monograph Title	Critical Finding
Magnesium, Blood	Less than 1.2 mg/dL; greater than 4.9 mg/dL
Methemoglobin	Signs of central nervous system depression can occur at levels greater than 45%; death may occur at levels greater than 70%
Osmolality, Blood	Less than 265 mOsm/kg; greater than 320 mOsm/kg
Phosphorus, Blood	Values less than 1.0 mg/dL may have significant effects on the neuromuscular, gastrointestinal, cardiopulmonary, and skeletal systems
Potassium, Blood	Less than 2.5 mEq/L; greater than 6.5 mEq/L
Prothrombin Time and International Normalized Ratio	PT greater than 27 sec; INR greater than 5
Pseudocholinesterase and Dibucaine Number	A positive result indicates that the patient is at risk for prolonged or unrecoverable apnea related to the inability to metabolize succinylcholine
Rubella Antibodies	A nonimmune status in pregnant patients may present significant health consequences for the developing fetus if the mother is exposed to an infected individual
Sodium, Blood	Less than 120 mEq/L; greater than 160 mEq/L
Thyroxine, Total	Less than 2.0 mcg/dL; greater than 20.0 mcg/dL
Troponin I	Greater than 0.5 ng/mL (initial sample only)
Tuberculin Skin Tests	Positive results
Urea Nitrogen, Blood	Greater than 100 mg/dL (nondialysis patients)
Urinalysis	Presence of uric acid, cystine, leucine, or tyrosine crystals; the combination of grossly elevated urine glucose and ketones is also considered significant
Vitamins D, E, K	Vitamin toxicity can be as significant as problems brought about by vitamin deficiencies. The potential for toxicity is especially important to consider with respect to fat-soluble vitamins, which are not eliminated from the body as quickly as water-soluble vitamins and can accumulate in the body.

Appendix I

Diagnostic Critical Findings

Monograph Title	Critical Finding
Angiography, Abdomen	Abscess; aneurysm
Angiography, Coronary	Aneurysm; aortic dissection
Angiography, Pulmonary	Pulmonary embolism
Chest X-Ray	Foreign body; malposition of tube, line, or post-operative device (pacemaker); pneumonia; pneumoperitoneum; pneumothorax; spine fracture
Computed Tomography, Abdomen	Abscess; acute gastrointestinal (GI) bleed; aortic aneurysm; appendicitis; aortic dissection; bowel perforation; bowel obstruction; mesenteric torsion; significant solid organ laceration; tumor with significant mass effect; visceral injury
Computed Tomography, Angiography	Brain or spinal cord ischemia; emboli; hemorrhage; leaking aortic aneurysm; occlusion; tumor with significant mass effect
Computed Tomography, Brain	Abscess; acute hemorrhage; aneurysm; infarction; infection; tumor with significant mass effect
Computed Tomography, Pelvis	Ectopic pregnancy; tumor with significant mass effect
Computed Tomography, Spine	Cord compression; fracture; tumor with significant mass effect
Computed Tomography, Spleen	Abscess; hemorrhage; laceration
Computed Tomography, Thoracic	Aortic aneurysm; aortic dissection; pneumothorax; pulmonary embolism
Echocardiography	Aneurysm; infection; obstruction; tumor with significant mass effect
Echocardiography, Transesophageal	Aneurysm; aortic dissection
Electrocardiogram	Acute changes in ST elevation may indicate acute myocardial infarction or pericarditis; bradycardia (less than 40 beats per min); premature ventricular contractions greater than three in a row, pauses greater than 3 sec, or identified blocks; tachycardia (greater than 120 beats per min), supraventricular tachycardia, and ventricular tachycardia
Electroencephalography	Abscess; brain death; head injury; hemorrhage; intracranial hemorrhage
Esophagogastroduodenoscopy	Presence and location of acute GI bleed
Gastrointestinal Blood Loss Scan	Acute GI bleed
Kidney, Ureter, and Bladder Study	Bowel obstruction; ischemic bowel; visceral injury

(table continues on page 1430)

Monograph Title	Critical Finding
Laparoscopy, Abdominal	Appendicitis
Laparoscopy, Gynecologic	Ectopic pregnancy; foreign body; tumor with significant mass effect
Liver and Spleen Scan	Visceral injury
Lung Perfusion Scan	Pulmonary embolism
Lung Ventilation Scan	Pulmonary embolism
Magnetic Resonance Angiography	Aortic aneurysm; aortic dissection; occlusion; tumor with significant mass effect; vertebral artery dissection
Magnetic Resonance Imaging, Abdomen	Acute GI bleed; aortic aneurysm; infection; tumor with significant mass effect
Magnetic Resonance Imaging, Brain	Abscess; cerebral aneurysm; cerebral infarct; hydrocephalus; skull fracture or contusion; tumor with significant mass effect
Magnetic Resonance Imaging, Chest	Aortic aneurysm; aortic dissection; tumor with significant mass effect
Plethysmography	Deep vein thrombosis
Positron Emission Tomography, Brain	Aneurysm; cerebrovascular accident; tumor with significant mass effect
Ultrasound, Biophysical Profile, Obstetric	Abruptio placentae; adnexal torsion; biophysical profile score between 0 and 2 is abnormal and indicates the need for assessment and immediate delivery; ectopic pregnancy; fetal death; placenta previa
Ultrasound, Pelvis (Gynecologic, Nonobstetric)	Abscess; adnexal torsion; appendicitis; ectopic pregnancy; infection; tumor with significant mass effect
Ultrasound, Scrotal	Testicular torsion
Ultrasound, Venous Doppler, Extremity Studies	Deep vein thrombosis
Upper Gastrointestinal and Small Bowel Series	Foreign body; perforated bowel; tumor with significant mass effect
Venography, Lower Extremity Studies	Deep vein valvular incompetence; deep vein thrombosis; pulmonary embolism; venous obstruction

APP

Bibliography

2000 Test Catalog. Mayo Medical Laboratory, Rochester, MN, 1999.

AABB Technical Manual, ed 15. American Association of Blood Banks, Bethesda, MD, 2005.

Abbott Axsym System CK-MB: Abbott Laboratories Product Literature. Abbott Laboratories, Chicago, 1999.

Abbott Axsym System Troponin I: Abbott Laboratories Product Literature. Abbott Laboratories, Chicago, 1997.

Abrams, C: ADH-associated pathologies. Med Lab Obs 32:24, 2000.

Abramson, N, and Melton, B: Leukocytosis: Basics of clinical assessment. Am Fam Physician 62:2053, 2000.

Alder, A, and Carlton, C: Introduction to Radiologic Sciences and Patient Care, ed 4. Elsevier Science Health Science, St. Louis, MO, 2007.

Aetna Clinical Policy Bulletins: Urea Breath Testing for *H. pylori* Infection, 2006. Available at www.aetna.com/cpb/medical/data/100_199/0177.html (accessed 7/11/08).

Ahmed, A: Autoantibody detection in autoimmune diseases. Advance for Administrators of the Laboratory Oct:68, 1998.

Albareda, M, et al: Influence of endogenous insulin on C-peptide levels in subjects with type 2 diabetes. Diabetes Res Clin Pract 68:202, 2004. Available at www.ncbi.nlm.nih.gov/pubmed/15936461 (accessed 9/3/09).

Alexander, D: Pseudocholinesterase Deficiency. Available at http://emedicine.medscape.com/article/247019-overview (accessed 7/11/08).

Alter, J: New Molecular Tests Can Predict the Return of Prostate Cancer. Available at www.ezinearticles.com/?New-Molecular-Tests-Can-Predict-The-Return-of-Prostate-Cancer&id=350579 (accessed 7/27/09).

Alter, M, et al: Testing for Viral Hepatitis. Abbott Diagnostics Educational Services, Chicago, 1992.

American Academy of Pediatrics, Screening for Elevated Blood Levels. Available at www.aappolicy.aappublications.org/cgi/content/full/pediatrics;101/6/1072 (accessed 12/13/09).

American Cancer Society: Guidelines for the Early Detection of Cancer. Available at www.cancer.org (accessed 7/27/09).

American Diabetes Association: Clinical practice recommendations 1998. Diabetes Care 21:S23, 1998.

American Heart Association: Step 1, Step 2 and TLC Diets. Available at www.americanheart.org/presenter.jhtml?identifier=4764 (accessed 8/1/10).

———. Classification of Functional Capacity and Objective Assessment. Available at http://americanheart.org/presenter.jhtml?identifier=4569 (accessed 8/12/09).

American Society for Clinical Laboratory Science. Role of the clinical laboratory in response to an expanding geriatric population. Available at www.ascls.org/position/ExpandingGeriatric.asp (accessed 6/29/10).

———. Type, Degree and Configuration of Hearing Loss. Available at www.asha.org/public/hearing/disorders/types.htm (accessed 6/14/09).

American Speech-Language-Hearing Association. Guidelines for Audiologic Assessment of Children from Birth to 5 Years of Age. Available at www.asha.org/docs/pdf/GL2004-00002.pdf (accessed 7/22/08).

Andolina, V, Lille, S, and Willison, K: Mammographic Imaging, a Practical Guide, ed 2. Lippincott Williams & Wilkins, Baltimore, 2001.

Angelini, D. Update on non-obstetric surgical conditions in pregnancy: Pancreatitis. Available at www.medscape.com/viewarticle/452759_4 (accessed 7/7/10).

Appleyard, M, et al: A randomized trial comparing wireless capsule endoscopy with push enteroscopy for the detection of small-bowel lesions. Gastroenterology 119:1431, 2000.

Arky, R, et al (eds): Physician's Desk Reference, ed 50. Medical Economics Company, Montvale, NJ, 1996.

Arthritis: Sarcoidosis. Available at www.arthritis.webmd.com/arthritis-sarcoidosis (accessed 6/6/09).

ARUP Laboratories: Receptor Blocking and Receptor Modulating Reference Ranges. Available at www.aruplab.com/guides/ug/tests.jsp (accessed 5/30/09).

BIB

1431

Assessing Coagulation. Available at www.anaesthetist.com/icu/organs/blood/coag.htm (accessed 11/30/09).

Ballard Medical Products: Kimberly-Clark PYtest C-Urea Breath Test. Available at www.kchealthcare.com (accessed 7/22/08).

Ballinger, P, and Frank, E: Merrill's Atlas of Radiographic Positions and Radiologic Procedures, ed 10. Mosby, St. Louis, MO, 2003.

Banez, E, Triplett, DA, and Koepke, J: Laboratory monitoring of heparin therapy—the effect of different salts of heparin on the activated partial thromboplastin time. Am J Clin Pathol 74:569, 1980.

Barclay, L, and Vega, C: Transfusion Related Acute Lung Injury Defined. Available at www.medscape.com (accessed 9/8/07).

Bard, BTA: Product Literature. Bard Diagnostic Sciences, Redmond, WA, 1996.

Baskin, L, and Hsu, R: Laboratory evaluation of proteinuria. Med Lab Obs 31:30, 1999.

Baurmash, HD: Submandibular salivary stones: current management modalities. J Oral Maxillofac Surg 62:369, 2004.

Becton Dickinson: Understanding Additives: Heparin. Available at www.bd.com/vacutainer/labnotes/2004winterspring/additives_heparin.asp (accessed 7/22/08).

Beers, M, and Porter, R: The Merck Manual, ed 18. Merck Sharp & Dohme Research Laboratories, Rahway, NJ, 2006.

Ben-Yoseph, Y, et al: Maternal serum hexosaminidase A in pregnancy: Effects of gestational age and fetal genotype. Am J Med Genet 29:891. Available at www3.inetrscience.wiley.com/journal/110519641 (accessed 11/19/09).

Berkow, R, et al (eds): The Merck Manual of Diagnosis and Treatment, ed 17. Merck Sharp & Dohme Research Laboratories, Rahway, NJ, 1999.

Beutler, E, et al (eds): Williams Hematology, ed 7. McGraw-Hill, New York, 2005.

Biochemistry of Neurotransmitters. Available at www.themedicalbiochemistrypage.org/nerves.html (accessed 1/17/06).

Biou, D, et al: Cerebrospinal fluid protein concentrations in children: Age related values in patients without disorders of the central nervous system. Clinical Chemistry 46:399, 2000.

Bishop, ML, Duben-Engelkirk, JL, and Fody, EP: Clinical Chemistry Principles, Procedures, Correlations, ed 5. Lippincott Williams & Wilkins, Philadelphia, 2005.

Bladder cancer and biochemical assays. Clinical Laboratory Strategies 5:3, 2000.

Blocki, F: Vitamin D Deficiency. Advance for Administrators of the Laboratory 18:1, 2009.

Boddie, D, et al: Isoenzyme analysis of hyperamylasaemia associated with ruptured abdominal aortic aneurysms. J R Coll Surg Edinb 43:306, 1998. Available at www.rcsed.ac.uk/journal/vol435/4350004.htm (accessed 7/15/09).

Bodor, G: New gold standard in cardiac markers. Advance for Administrators of the Laboratory Jul: 43, 1998.

Borazanci, E: Interpreting Abnormal PT, aPTT times, 2009. Available at www.lib.sh.lsuhsc.edu/am_rpt/media/files/09242009.pdf (accessed 11/12/09).

Bouma, B, and Meijers, J: Role of blood coagulation factor XI in downregulation of fibrinolysis. Curr Opin Hematol 7:266, 2000.

Bounameaux, H, et al: D-dimer testing in suspected venous thromboembolism—An update. QJM 90:437, 1997.

Boyd, R, and Hoerl, B: Basic Medical Microbiology. Little, Brown, Boston, 1977.

Braunstein, G: HCG Testing Volume I: A Clinical Guide for the Testing of Human Chorionic Gonadotropin. Abbott Diagnostics Educational Services, Chicago, 1993.

———. HCG Testing Volume II: Answers to Frequently Asked Questions About HCG Testing. Abbott Diagnostics Educational Services, Chicago, 1991.

Brigden, M: Clinical utility of the erythrocyte sedimentation rate. Am Fam Physician 30:5, 1999.

Bringing homocysteine into your lab. Clinical Laboratory Strategies 3:1, 1998.

Broun, R, et al: Excessive zinc ingestion: A reversible cause of sideroblastic anemia and bone marrow depression. JAMA 264: 1441: 1998. Available at www.faqs.org/abstracts/health/ excessive-zinc-ingestion-a-reversible -cause-of-sideroblastic-anemia-and-bone -marrow-depression.html (accessed 8/8/09).

Burtis, C, and Ashwood, E (eds): Tietz Textbook of Clinical Chemistry, ed 2. WB Saunders, Philadelphia, 1994.

Calgary Laboratory Services: Blood Collection Tubes, Order of Draw, 2003. Available at www.calgarylabservices .com (accessed 3/6/05).

Calvo, M, and Park Y: Changing phosphorus content of the U.S. diet: Potential for adverse effects on bone. J Nutr 126: 1168S, 1996.

Carlton, R, and Alder A: Principles of Radiographic Imaging, ed 4. Delmar Thomson, Clifton Park, NY, 2006.

Carpinito, G: Product technology brief: Enzyme immunoassay for bladder cancer. Clinical Laboratory Products Apr:32, 1999.

Castellone, D: Coagulation: The good, the bad and the unacceptable. Advance for Medical Laboratory Professionals Nov:53, 1999.

Cavanaugh, B: Nurses' Manual of Laboratory and Diagnostic Tests, ed 4. FA Davis, Philadelphia, 2003.

Centers for Medicare and Medicaid Services: CLIA Program: Clinical Laboratory Improvement Amendments, March 24, 2005. Available at www.cms .hhs.gov/clia/ (accessed 4/3/05).

Centre for Digestive Diseases: Urea Breath Test, 2003. Available at www.cdd.com.au/html/hospital/ procedures/procedure%20descriptions/ urea%20breath%20test.html (accessed 7/22/08).

Cevik, I, et al: Short-term effect of digital rectal exam on serum prostate-specific antigen levels: A prospective study. Eur Urol 29:403, 1996. Available at www.ncbi.nlm.nih.gov/pubmed/ 8791045 (accessed 7/22/08).

Chernecky, C, and Berger, B: Laboratory Tests and Diagnostic Procedures, ed 2. WB Saunders, Philadelphia, 1997.

Christenson, R: The basics of bone. Clinical Laboratory News May:10, 1998.

————. Biochemical cardiac markers present and future. MLO Med Lab Obs 31:26, 1999.

Ciesla, B: Targeting the thalassemias. Advance for Medical Laboratory Professionals Apr:12, 2000.

CLR: Table of critical limits, 2009–2010. Available at www.clr-online.com (accessed 7/31/10).

Colombraro, G: Pediatrics: Core Content at a Glance. Lippincott–Raven, Philadelphia, 1998.

Constantinescu, M, and Hilman, B: The sweat test for quantitation of electrolytes. Lab Med 27:472, 1996.

Contraction Stress Test. Available at www .webmd.com/baby/contraction-stress-test (accessed 7/22/08).

Corbett, J: Laboratory Tests and Diagnostic Procedures with Nursing Diagnosis, ed 7. Prentice-Hall Health, Upper Saddle River, NJ, 2007.

Cornforth, T: Hysteroscopy FAQ. Available at http://womenshealth.about.com/cs/ surgery/a/hysteroscopyqa.htm (accessed 12/3/09).

Corning Clinical Laboratories. The 1996/1997 Reference Manual. Corning Clinical Laboratories, Teterboro, NJ, 1996.

Cramer, DA: Homocysteine vs cholesterol: Competing views or a unifying explanation of arteriosclerotic cardiovascular disease. Laboratory Medicine 29:410, 1998.

Cunningham, V: A review of disseminated intravascular coagulation. Med Lab Obs 31:42, 1999.

D'Alessandro, S, et al: Changes in human parotid salivary protein and sialic acid levels during pregnancy. Archives of Oral Biology 34(10):829, 1989.

D'Amico, et al: Preoperative PSA velocity and the risk of death from prostate cancer after radical prostatectomy. NEJM 351:2, 2004.

Davidsohn, I, and Henry, J (eds): Todd-Sanford: Clinical Diagnosis by Laboratory Methods, ed 15. WB Saunders, Philadelphia, 1994.

Department of Health and Human Services, Office of Disease Prevention and Health Promotion: Healthy People 2000. Available at www.healthypeople .gov (accessed 8/01/10).

Dictionary. Available at www.biology -online.org.

BIB

DiLeo, G: Amniotic Fluid and the Biophysical Profile. Available at www.gynob.com/biopamfl.htm (accessed 7/22/08).

DiPiro, J, et al: Pharmacotherapy: A Pathophysiologic Approach. McGraw-Hill, New York, 2008.

Disorders of Neuromuscular Transmission. Available at www.merck.com/mmpe/print/sec16/ch223/ch223b.html (accessed 7/22/08).

Dooley WC: Breast ductoscopy and the evolution of the intra-ductal approach to breast cancer. Breast J 15:90.

Doshi, M: Blood Gas and Electrolyte Regulation. Colorado Association for Continuing Medical Laboratory Education, Denver, 1997.

Drug Cutoff Concentrations. Available at www.workplace.samhsa.gov/DrugTesting/Level_1_Pages/OMB_extension.aspx (accessed 11/24/09).

Drugs Causing Thrombocytopenia or Low Platelet Count. Available at www.medicineworld.org/physicians/hematology/thrombocytopenia.html (accessed 8/13/09).

Dubin, D: Rapid Interpretation of EKGs. C.O.V.E.R. Publishing, Tampa, FL, 1989.

Dutton, AG, Norcutt, TA, and Torres, L: Basic Medical Techniques and Patient Care in Imaging Technology, ed 6. Lippincott, Williams & Wilkins, Philadelphia, 2003.

Eastman, G, Wald, C, and Crossin, J: Getting Started in Clinical Radiology. Thieme Medical Publishers, New York, 2006.

Eby, C: Warfarin dosing. Should labs offer pharmacogenetic testing? Clinical Laboratory News June:10, 2009.

Eikelboom, W, and Weitz, JI: Selective factor Xa inhibition. Lancet 372:6, 2008. Available at www.medscape.com/viewarticle/456874_2 (accessed 11/18/09).

eMedicine: Microscopic polyangiitis, 2003. Available at www.emedicine.com/med/topic2931.htm (accessed 7/22/08).

Estimating Coronary Heart Disease (CHD): Risk Using Framingham Heart Study Prediction Score Sheets. Available at www.nhlbi.nih.gov/about/framingham/riskabs.htm (accessed 7/22/08).

Falk, RA, and Miller, S: Clinical evaluation of osteoporosis. Advance for Administrators of the Laboratory May:57, 1999.

First blood test for congestive heart failure wins FDA clearance. Clinical Laboratory Strategies 5:1, 2000.

Fischbach, F: A Manual of Laboratory and Diagnostic Tests, ed 7. Lippincott Williams & Wilkins, Philadelphia, 2004.

———. Nurses' Quick Reference to Common Laboratory and Diagnostic Tests, ed 4. Lippincott-Raven, Philadelphia, 2005.

Foley, K: Beta-2 microglobulin: A facultative marker. Advance for Medical Laboratory Professionals Sept:13, 2008.

Gantzer, M: The value of urinalysis: An old method continues to prove its worth. Clinical Laboratory News Jan:14, 1998.

Gearhart, P: Biophysical Profile, Ultrasound. Last updated October 17, 2008. Available at http://emedicine.medscape.com/article/405454-overview (accessed 7/22/08).

Geriatric Laboratory Values. Available at http://www.ascp.com/education/meetings/upload/labvalues.pdf (accessed 6/29/10).

Gerson, M: Cardiac Nuclear Medicine, ed 3. McGraw-Hill, New York, 1997.

Gill, K: Abdominal Ultrasound: A Practioner's Guide. WB Saunders, Philadelphia, 2001.

The Gleason System. Available at http://www.phoenix5.org/Infolink/GleasonGrading.html (accessed 8/2/10).

Goldenberg, W: Myasthenia Gravis. Available at http://emedicine.medscape.com/article/793136-overview (accessed 6/1/09).

Goldfarb, D, et al: Age related changes in tissue levels of prostatic acid phosphatase and prostate specific antigen. Available at www.ncbi.nlm.nih/pubmed/2430115 (accessed 6/29/10).

Golish, J: Diagnostic Procedure Handbook with Key Word Index. Lexi-Company, Cleveland, OH, 1992.

Green, R: Macrocytic and marrow failure anemias. Lab Med 30:595, 1999.

Gregersen, P: Tracking Down RA Genes. Available at www.arthritis.org/research/researchupdate/04march_april/tracking.asp (accessed 7/22/08).

Gruenwald, J, Brendler, T, and Jaenicke, C (eds): PDR for Herbal Medicines, ed 2. Thomson Medical Economics, Montvale, NJ, 2000.

Gunderman, R: Essential Radiology, ed 2. Thieme Medical Publishers, New York, 2006.

Guyton, JR, et al: Relationship of plasma lipoprotein Lp(a) levels to race and to apolipoprotein B. Arteriosclerosis 5:265, 1985. Abstract available at www.ncbi.nlm.nih.gov/pubmed/3158297 (accessed 7/9/09).

Hautmann, S, et al: Supersensitive prostate-specific antigen (PSA) in serum of women with benign breast disease or breast cancer. Anticancer Res 20:2151, 2000. Available at www.ncbi.nlm.nih.gov/pubmed/10928169 (accessed 7/22/08).

Hearing Assessment. Available at www.asha.org/public/hearing/testing/assess.htm (accessed 7/22/08).

Hennerici, M, and Neiserberg-Heusler, D: Vascular Diagnosis with Ultrasound. Thieme Medical Publishers, New York, 1998.

Hermans, C: The Blood Coagulation Cascade Revisited: Clinician's Perspectives. Available at www.siz.be/public/file/siztalks/02_Heremans%20Expose%20Godinne%20Intensive%20Care%2027102006.pdf (accessed 11/30/09).

Hicks, J, and Boeckx, R: Pediatric Clinical Chemistry. WB Saunders, Philadelphia, 1984.

Hoeltke, L: Phlebotomy: The Clinical Laboratory Manual Series. Delmar Thomson Learning, Albany, NY, 1995.

Hopfer Deglin, J, and Hazard Vallerand, A: Davis's Drug Guide for Nurses. FA Davis, Philadelphia, 2005.

Hopper, K: The Modern Coagulation cascade and Coagulation Abnormalities Associated with Sepsis. 50th Congresso Nazionale Multisala SCIVAC, 2005. Available at www.ivis.org/proceedings/scivac/2005/Hopper1_en.pdf?LA=1 (accessed 11/29/09).

Howard, V: Age-Specific Guidelines. Champlain Valley Physicians Hospital Medical Center, Plattsburgh, NY, 2000.

HPV Vaccine Information for Young Women. Available at www.cdc.gov/std/hpv/stdfact-hpv-vaccine-young-women.htm (accessed 8/23/09).

hs-CRP: Detecting the Inflammation of Silent Atherosclerosis. Dade Behring, Newark, NJ, 1999.

hs-CRP to Improve Cardiac Risk Assessment. Dade Behring, Newark, NJ, 1999.

Hughes, V: How Does Jaundice Affect Breast Feeding? Available at www.ameda.com.au/17346.pdf (accessed 12/2/09).

Ikanomova, K: Inflammation and metabolic syndrome. Turk J Endocrinol Metab 3:85, 2004.

Importance of Urinalysis: Lab Notes. Becton Dickinson Vacutainer Systems, Franklin Lakes, NJ, 1996.

Indman, P: Hysteroscopy. Available at www.gynalternatives.com/hsc.htm (accessed 12/5/09).

Inoue, S: Leukocytosis. Available at http://emedicine.medscape.com/article/956278-overview (accessed 7/23/08).

International Medicine Clinic Research Consortium: Effect of digital rectal examination on serum prostate antigen in a primary care setting. Arch Intern Med 155:389, 1995. Available at http://archinte.ama-assn.org/cgi/content/abstract/155/4/389 (accessed 7/23/08).

International Warfarin Pharmacogenetics Consortium: Estimation of the warfarin dose with clinical and pharmacogenetic data. NEJM 360:753, 2009.

Interpretations of Decreased Visual Acuity. Available at http://fpnotebook.com/eye/sx/dcrsdvsacty.htm (accessed 6/17/09).

Izbicki, G, et al: Transfusion-related leukocytosis in critically ill patients. Critical Care Medicine 32:439, 2004. Available at www.ccmjournal.com (accessed 8/19/07).

Jacobs, DS, DeMott, WR, and Oxley, DK: Laboratory Test Handbook, ed 5. Lexi-Comp, Hudson, OH, 2001.

Jaffe, M, and McVan, B: Davis's Laboratory and Diagnostic Test Handbook. FA Davis, Philadelphia, 1997.

Jhang, J: Abnormal Basic Coagulation Testing. Available at www.pathology.columbia.edu/education/residency/coag.pdf (accessed 10/31/09).

Johns Hopkins Prostate Bulletin. Available at www.hopkinsprostate.com (accessed 4/20/06).

Jones, P: Newborn screening: What's new? Lab Med 39:737, 2008.

BIB

Kandarian, P: ThinPrep imaging follows ThinPrep PAP to market. Clinical Laboratory Products May:37, 2000.

Kaplan, L, and Sawin, C: Laboratory Support for the Diagnosis and Monitoring of Thyroid Disease. National Academy of Clinical Biochemistry, Washington, DC, 1996.

Kee, J: Laboratory and Diagnostic Tests with Nursing Implications, ed 5. Appleton & Lange, Stamford, CT, 1999.

King, D: New methods facilitating Down's syndrome screening. Advance for Laboratory Professionals May:8, 2000.

Kirschner, C, et al: Current Procedural Terminology 2001. AMA Press, Chicago, 2000.

Koepke, J: Update on reticulocyte counting. Lab Med 30:339, 1999.

Kraus, L, and Kraus, A: Carbamoylation of amino acids and proteins in uremia. Kidney Int 59:5102, 2001. Available at www.nature.com/ki/journal/v59/n78s/full/4492325a.html (accessed 7/7/09).

Lab Corp: Laboratory testing information, 2010. Available at www.labcorp.com (accessed 8/2/10).

Lab Tests Online. Available at Labtestsonline.org (accessed 8/2/10).

Landicho, H: Product technology brief: Urine assay quantitates bladder tumor antigen. Clinical Laboratory Products May:46, 2000.

LaValle, J, et al: Natural Therapeutics Pocket Guide. Lexi-Comp, Hudson, OH, 2000.

Lee Y, et al: SIADH associated with Guillain-Barré syndrome. J Nephrol 23:630, 2004.

Lehman, C: Saunders Manual of Clinical Laboratory Science. WB Saunders, Philadelphia, 1998.

Leukopenia. Available at www.wikipedia.org (accessed 8/20/07).

Lewandrowski, KB, et al: Cyst fluid analysis in the differential diagnosis of pancreatic cysts. A comparison of pseudocysts, serous cystadenomas, mucinous cystic neoplasms, and mucinous cystadeno-carcinoma. Ann Surg 217:41, 1993. Available at www.ncbi.nlm.nih.gov (accessed 5/16/06).

Lewis, B, and Swain, P: Capsule endoscopy in the evaluation of patients with suspected small intestinal bleeding, a blinded analysis: The results of the first clinical trial. Gastrointest Endosc 53:AB70, 2001.

Lewis, S, et al: Medical Surgical Nursing Assessment and Management of Clinical Problems, ed 6. Mosby, Philadelphia, 2003.

Liquid Rho (D) Human IVIG for Hemolytic Disease in Newborns. Available at http://rhophylac.com/includes/pdf/PI%20Information%20Chart.pdf (accessed 8/31/10).

Liu, N, and Garon, J: A new generation of thyroid testing. Advance for Administrators of the Laboratory Nov:29, 1999.

Lott, J: Clinical laboratory testing in hepatobiliary diseases. Advance for Medical Laboratory Professionals Jan:24, 2000.

Lutz, C, and Przytulski, K: Nutrition and Diet Therapy. FA Davis, Philadelphia, 1997.

Maher, K: Against the grain: A celiac disease review. Med Lab Obs 40:22, 2008.

Malarkey, L, and McMorrow, M: Nurses's Manual of Laboratory Tests and Diagnostic Procedures, ed 2. WB Saunders, Philadelphia, 2000.

Marking time with bone markers: New tests aid in managing osteoporosis. Clinical Laboratory Strategies Jul:3, 1998.

Martin, F, and Clark, J: Introduction to Audiology, ed 8. Pearson Education, Boston, MA, 2003.

Masood, H: Menopause, hormones, and osteoporosis. Advance for Administrators of the Laboratory Feb:64, 2000.

Massey, L: Error free urinalysis. Advance for Medical Laboratory Professionals Mar:19, 2000.

McCall, R, and Tankersly, C: Phlebotomy Essentials, ed 4. JB Lippincott, Philadelphia, 2007.

McEvoy, G, et al (eds): American Hospital Formulary Service: AHFS Drug Information. American Society of Hospital Pharmacists, Bethesda, MD, 1991.

McMorrow, ME, and Malarkey, L: Laboratory and Diagnostic Tests: A Pocket Guide. WB Saunders, Philadelphia, 1998.

Medscape: Regular Cola Consumption Linked to Lower Bone Density in Women, 2003. Available at www.medscape.com/viewarticle/461898 (accessed 7/23/08).

Meredith, J, and Rosenthal, N: Differential diagnosis of microcytic anemias. Lab Med 30:538, 1999.

Merck Manual of Geriatrics. App I, Laboratory values. Available at www .merck.com/mkgr/mmg/appndxs/app1 .jsp (accessed 7/29/10).

———. Type, Degree and Configuration of Hearing Loss. Available at www.asha .org/public/hearing/disorders/types. htm (accessed 6/14/09).

Metzger, B, and Coustan, D: Summary and recommendations of the Fourth International Workshop-Conference on Gestational Diabetes Mellitus. Diabetes Care 21:B161, 1998.

Miale, J: Laboratory Medicine, ed 5. Mosby, St. Louis, MO, 1997.

Miller, S: Preventing and detecting neural tube defects. Med Lab Obs 31:32, 1999.

Montgomery, J: Improvements in prostate cancer detection. Advance for Administrators of the Laboratory Oct:66, 1999.

Morris, E, and Liberman, L: Breast MRI: Diagnosis and Intervention. Springer, New York, 2005.

Morris, R: New Highly Specific Autoantibody Markers in RA. Present Status and Future Prospects. International Rheumatology Network. Available at www.rdlinc.com/pdf/ articles/AutoantibodiesRA-DrMorris -10-5-06_4.pdf (accessed 7/23/08).

Moving toward a more precise definition of myocardial infarction. Clinical Laboratory Strategies 5:1, 2000.

MRI Registry Review Program. Medical Imaging Consultants, West Patterson, NJ, 1999.

Myasthenia Gravis Foundation of America: Patient Education Materials. Available at www.myasthenia.org/pe_informational -materials.cfm (accessed 7/23/08).

Nageotte MP, Casal D, Senyei AE: Fetal fibronectin in patients at increased risk for premature birth. Am J Obstet Gynecol 170:20, 1994.

Nakagawa, S, et al: Human hexosaminidase isoenzymes. Assay of platelet activity for heterozygote identification during preg- nancy. Clin Chim Acta 88:2492 1978. Available at www.researchprofiles .collexis.com/einstein/pubDetail .asp?t=pm&id=699320 (accessed 11/19/09).

National Institute of Neurological Disorders and Stroke: Myasthenia Gravis Fact Sheet. Available at www .ninds.nih.gov/disorders/myasthenia _gravis/detail_myasthenia_gravis.htm (accessed 7/23/08).

NCCN Practice Guidelines in Oncology: Her2 Testing: Summary for Breast Cancer Patients, V.1.2007. Available at http://nccn.org/patients/fact_sheet.asp (accessed 7/23/08).

NCEP Issues Major New Cholesterol Guidelines. National Institutes of Health, Bethesda, MD, 2001.

Neonatal Handbook. Available at www.netsvic.org.au/nets/handbook/ index.cfm?doc_id=460 (accessed 6/29/10).

Nester, E, et al: Microbiology: Molecules, Microbes, and Man. Holt, Reinhart, & Winston, New York, 1973.

A new era in newborn screening. Clinical Laboratory Strategies 5:1, 2000.

New thyroid testing guidelines. Clinical Laboratory Strategies 6:2, 2001.

New York Heart Association Classification (for CHF). Available at www.hcoa.org/ hcoacme/chf-cme/chf00070.htm (accessed 8/12/09).

The next evolution in chest pain evalua- tion. Clinical Laboratory Strategies 4:1, 1999.

Nitowsky, H, et al: Human hexosamini- dase isoenzymes. IV. Effects of oral contraceptive steroids on serum hexosaminidase activity. Am J Obstet Gynecol 134:642, 1979. Available at www.researchprofiles.collexis.com/ einstein/pubDetail.asp?t=pm&id= 463955 (accessed 11/19/09).

Olds, SB, et al: Maternal Newborn Nursing, ed 7. Prentice Hall, Upper Saddle River, NJ, 2003.

Omar, S, et al: Late-onset neutropenia in very low birth weight infants. Pediatrics 106:e55, 2000. Available at www.pediatrics.aappublications.com (accessed 8/19/07).

Pagana, K, and Pagana, T: Diagnostic Testing and Nursing Implications: A Case Study Approach, ed 5. Mosby, Philadelphia, 1999.

Palkuti, H: International Normalized Ratio (INR): Clinical Significance and Applications. BioData Corporation, Horsham, PA, 1995.

BIB

Peaceman AM, et al: Fetal fibronectin as a predictor of preterm birth in patients with symptoms: A multicenter trial. Am J Obstet Gynecol 177:13, 1997.

Peart, O: Appleton & Lange Review for Mammography, McGraw-Hill, New York, 2002.

Peter, J: Use and Interpretation of Tests in Clinical Immunology, ed 8. Specialty Labs, Santa Monica, CA, 1991.

———. Use and Interpretation of Tests in Infectious Disease, ed 4. Specialty Labs, Santa Monica, CA, 1996.

Peter, J, and Reyes, H: Use and Interpretation of Tests in Allergy and Immunology. Specialty Labs, Santa Monica, CA, 1992.

Peterson, P, and Cornacchia, M: Anemia: Pathophysiology, clinical features, and laboratory evaluation. Lab Med 30:463, 1999.

Petros, P: Thyrotoxicosis and pregnancy. PloS Med 2:e370, 2005. Available at www.ncbi.nlm.nih.gov/pmc/articles/PMC1322287/ (accessed 7/11/09).

Petrillo, M, and Sanger, S: Emotionalized Care of Hospitalized Children: An Environmental Approach, ed 2. JB Lippincott, Philadelphia, 1980.

Phlebotomy Pages: New order of draw, 2003–2005. Available at www.phlebotomypages.com/new_draw.htm (accessed 7/23/08).

Plaut, D: Detection of colon cancer. Advance for Administrators of the Laboratory 17:10, 2008.

Pokorski, R: Laboratory values in the elderly. J Ins Med 22(2):117, 1990.

Prechota, W, and Staszewski, A: Reference ranges of lipids and apolipoproteins in pregnancy. Eur J Obstet Gynecol Reprod Biol 45:27, 1992. Available at www.ncbi.nlm.nih.gov/pubmed/1618359 (accessed 7/9/09).

Pregnancy and pancreatitis. Available at http://pregnancyandpancreatitis.blogspot.com (accessed 7/7/10).

Prostate-Specific Antigen Best Practice Statement 2009 Update. Available at www.auanet.org/content/guidelines-and-quality-care/clinical.../psa09.pdf (accessed 7/27/09).

Quanta Lite CCP IgG ELISA package insert. Available at www.inovadx.com/Products/di_files/708790.html (accessed 7/23/08).

Quest Diagnostics, Test Menu. Available at www.questdiagnostics.com (accessed 8/1/10).

Quinley, ED: Immunohematology Principles and Practice, ed 2. Lippincott-Raven, Philadelphia, 1998.

Quinn, D, et al: D-dimers in the diagnosis of pulmonary embolism. Am J Respir Crit Care Med 159:1445, 1999.

Reber, G, et al: Comparison of two rapid D-dimer assays for the exclusion of venous thromboembolism. Blood Coagul Fibrinolysis 9:387, 1998.

Re-examining the ADA criteria for diagnosing diabetes. Clinical Laboratory Strategies Mar:3, 2000.

Remaley, A, Woods, JJ, and Glickman, JW: Point of care testing of parathyroid hormone during the surgical treatment of hyperparathyroidism. Med Lab Obs 31:20, 1999.

Renne, T, and Gailani, R: Role of factor XII in hemostasis and thrombosis: Clinical implications. Expert Rev Cardiovasc Ther 5:733, 2007.

Riddel, J, et al: Theories of blood coagulation. J Pediatr Oncol Nurs 24:123: 2007. Available at www.aphon.org/files/public/theories_of_coag.pdf (accessed 12/5/09).

Ringel, M: Bladder tumor markers: Where do they fit in disease management? Clinical Laboratory News May:18, 1998.

Rodak, B: Diagnostic Hematology. WB Saunders, Philadelphia, 1995.

Rowlett, R: SI units for clinical data. In How Many? A Dictionary of Units of Measurement. University of North Carolina, Chapel Hill, 2001. Available at www.unc.edu/~rowlett/units/scales/clinical_data.html (accessed 7/20/08).

Rubaltelli, F, et al.: Transcutaneous bilirubin measurement: A multicenter evaluation of a new device. Pediatrics 107:1264, 2000. Available at http://pediatrics.org (accessed 7/23/08).

Runge, V: Contrast-Enhanced Clinical Magnetic Resonance Imaging. University Press of Kentucky, Lexington, 1996.

Sainato, D: C-reactive protein and cardiovascular disease. Clinical Laboratory News Jun:1, 2000.

Salonen, J, et al: Serum copper and the risk of acute myocardial infarction: A prospective study in men in eastern Finland. Am J Epidemiol 134:268, 1991. Available at www.age.oxfordjournals .org/cgi/content/abstract/134/3/268 (accessed 8/14/09).

Sandrick, K: Teasing out the value of new C-reactive protein test. CAP Today 14:43, 2000.

Savage, G, Charrier, M, and Vanhannen, L: Bioavailability of soluble oxalate from tea and the effect of consuming milk with the tea. Eur J Clin Nutr 57:415, 2003.

Schull, P: Illustrated Guide to Diagnostic Tests, ed 2. Springhouse Publishing, Springhouse, PA, 1998.

Seeram, E: Computed Tomography: Physical Principles, Clinical Application, and Quality Control, ed 2. WB Saunders, Philadelphia, 2001.

Shackett, P: Nuclear Medicine Technology—Procedures and Quick Reference. Lippincott Williams & Wilkins, Philadelphia, 2000.

Sharp, P, et al: Practical Nuclear Medicine, ed 2. Oxford Medical Publications, New York, 1998.

Shimeld, LA: Essentials of Diagnostic Microbiology. Delmar Thomson Learning, Albany, NY, 1999.

Snopek, A: Fundamentals of Special Radiographic Procedures, ed. 5. Saunders-Elsevier, St. Louis, MO, 2006.

Society of Nuclear Medicine: Procedure Guidelines for C-14 Urea Breath Test, 2001. Available at http://interactive .snm.org/docs/pg_ch07_0403.pdf (accessed 7/23/08).

Soldin, S, Brugnara, C, and Hicks, JM: Pediatric Reference Ranges, ed 3. AACC Press, Washington, DC, 1999.

Soloway, M, et al: Use of a new tumor marker, urinary NMP22, in the detection of occult or rapidly recurring transitional cell carcinoma of the urinary tract following surgical treatment. J Urol 156:363, 1996.

Spruill, W, Wade, W, and Cobb, H: Estimating glomerular filtration rate with a modification of diet in renal disease equation: Implications for pharmacy. Am J Health-Syst Pharm 64:652, 2007. Available at www .medscape.com/viewarticle/555611 (accessed 7/23/08).

Stein, H, Slatt, B, and Stein, R: The Ophthalmic Assistant: A Guide for Ophthalmic Personnel, ed 6. Mosby, St. Louis, MO, 1994.

Steine-Martin, EA, Lotspeich-Steininger, CA, and Koepke, JA: Clinical Hematology: Principles, Procedures, Correlations. Lippincott-Raven, Philadelphia, 1998.

Strasinger, S: Urinalysis and Body Fluids, ed 5. FA Davis, Philadelphia, 2008.

Strasinger, S, and Di Lorenzo, M: Phlebotomy Workbook for the Multiskilled Healthcare Professional. FA Davis, Philadelphia, 1996.

Sutton, I: Monitoring anticoagulation therapy. Advance for Medical Laboratory Professionals Jan:10, 2000.

Tamul, K: Determining fetal-maternal hemorrhage with flow cytometry. Advance for Laboratory Professionals June:18, 2000.

Tervaert, J: Infections in primary vasculitides. Cleve Clin J Med 69:SI124, 2002.

Testing Services for Hereditary Motor Sensory Neuropathy. Athena Diagnostics, Worcester, MA, 2000.

Thelan, L, et al: Critical Care Nursing: Diagnosis and Management, ed 3. Mosby, St. Louis, MO, 1998.

Thomas, DV, and Wolinski, AP: Submandibular Calculus on Conventional Sialography. Available at www.eurorad.org/case.php?id=1446 (accessed 12/3/09).

Thrombocytopenia—Drug Induced. Available at www2.hmc.psu.edu/ healthinfo/hie/1/000556.htm (accessed 8/13/09).

Tietz, N: Clinical Guide to Laboratory Tests. AACC Press, Washington, DC, 1995.

Tilkian, S, Boudreau Conover, M, and Tilkian, AG: Clinical and Nursing Implications of Laboratory Tests, ed 5. Mosby, St. Louis, MO, 1995.

TNM Staging System. Available at http:// prostateinfo.com/patients/tests/ staging.asp (accessed 7/23/08).

Torry, R, et al: Localization and characterization of antithrombin in human kidneys. J Histochem Cytochem 47:313, 1999.

Transcutaneous Bilirubin Measurement is as Effective as Laboratory Serum Bilirubin Measurements at Detecting Hyperbilirubinemia. Available at www .med.umich.edu/pediatrics/ebm/cats/ bili.htm (accessed 7/23/08).

BIB

Tressler, K: Clinical Laboratory and Diagnostic Tests: Significance and Nursing Implications, ed 3. Appleton & Lange, Norwalk, CT, 1995.

Twiname, BG, and Boyd, S: Student Nurse Handbook: Difficult Concepts Made Easy. Appleton & Lange, Stamford, CT, 1995.

Understanding Gleason Grading. Available at www.phoenix5.org/Infolink/GleasonGrading.html (accessed 7/22/08).

U.S. Food and Drug Administration: Information for Healthcare Professionals Gadolinium-Based Contrast Agents for Magnetic Resonance Imaging (marketed as Magnevist, MultiHance, Omniscan, OptiMARK, Prohance). Available at www.fda.gov/cder/drug/infosheets/hcp/gcca_200705.htm (accessed 7/23/08).

Using FISH for prenatal diagnosis. Clinical Laboratory Strategies Mar:2, 2000.

Uzunlar, H, Eroglu, A, and Bostan, H: Thoracic epidural anesthesia combined with remifentanil-propofol without muscle relaxants in a myasthenic gravis patient for abdominal surgery. Internet Journal of Anesthesiology 9:1, 2005. Available at www.ispub.com/ostia/index.php?xmlFilePath=journals/ija/vol9n1/thoracic.xml (accessed 7/23/08).

Van Dyne, R: Diagnosing common bleeding disorders. Advance for the Administrators of the Laboratory Oct:74, 1998.

Van Leeuwen, A, and Perry, E: Basic Principles of Chemistry: Techniques Using Alternate Measurements. Colorado Association for Continuing Medical Laboratory Education, Denver, 2000.

Venes, D (ed): Taber's Cyclopedic Medical Dictionary, ed 20. FA Davis, Philadelphia, 2005.

Vitros Chemistry System Test Methodology Manual. Ortho-Clinical Diagnostics, Rochester, NY, 1999.

Von Schulthess, G: Clinical Positron Emission Tomography. Lippincott Williams & Wilkins, Philadelphia, 2001.

Warell, D, Cox, TM, and Firth, JD (eds): Oxford Textbook of Medicine. Oxford University Press, New York, 2005.

Wasserman, M, et al: Utility of fever, white blood cells, and differential count in predicting bacterial infections in the elderly. J Am Geriatr Soc 37:537, 1989.

WebMD: Hysteroscopy. Available at www.webmd.com/infertility-and-reproduction/guide/hysteroscopy (accessed 12/3/09)

———. Hysteroscopy for Dysfunctional Uterine Bleeding. Available at http://women.webmd.com/hysteroscopy-20795 (accessed 12/3/09)

———. Web MD Health Topics, 2005. Available at www.webmd.com (accessed 8/2/10).

Wentz, P: Chelation therapy: Conventional treatments. Advance for Administrators of the Laboratory May:74, 2000.

———. Homocyst(e)ine, the bad amino acid. Advance for the Laboratory May:71, 1999.

———. Megaloblastic anemias: Laboratory screening and confirmation. Advance for Administrators of the Laboratory Nov:57, 1999.

Widman, FK, and Ittani, CA: An Introduction to Clinical Immunology and Serology. FA Davis, Philadelphia, 1998.

Wikipedia: LEEP procedure. Available at http://en.wikipedia.org/wiki/Loop_electrical_excision_procedure (accessed 7/2/08).

Wilk, A, and van Venrooj, W: The Use of Anti-cyclic Citrullinated Peptide (anti-CCP) Antibodies in RA. Available at www.rheumatology.org/publications/hotline/1003anticcp.asp (accessed 7/23/08).

Wilson, D: Nurses' Guide to Understanding Laboratory and Diagnostic Tests. Lippincott Williams & Wilkins, Philadelphia, 1999.

Winter, W: Evaluating calcium disorders. Advance for Administrators of the Laboratory Jul:30, 2000.

———. Real-time monitoring of diabetes. Clinical Laboratory News June:12, 2000.

Wolf, P: Cardiac infarction markers: Do we need another one? ASCP Spring Teleconferences, Chicago, 1999.

Wong, D, and Hess, C: Wong and Whaley's Clinical Manual of Pediatric Nursing, ed 5. Mosby, St. Louis, MO, 2000.

World Health Organization: Blood Lead Levels in Children. Available at www.euro.who.int/Document/EHI/ENHIS_FactSheet_4_5.pdf (accessed 12/13/09).

Wright, M, and Dearing, L: The role of HLA testing in autoimmune disease. Advance for Administrators of the Laboratory Apr:81, 2000.

Wu, J: Prostate cancer progress. Advance for Administrators of the Laboratory Jul:25, 1998.

Yamamoto, D, et al. A utility of ductography and fiberoptic ductoscopy for patients with nipple discharge. Breast Cancer Res Treat 70:103, 2001.

Yeomans, E, et al: Umbilical cord pH, P_{CO_2}, and bicarbonate following uncomplicated term vaginal deliveries. Am J Obstet Gynecol 151:798, 1985.

Young, D: Effects of Drugs on Clinical Laboratory Tests, ed 5. AACC Press, Washington, DC, 2000.

Young, D, and Friedman, R: Effects of Disease on Clinical Laboratory Tests, ed 4. AACC Press, Washington, DC, 2001.

Yu, H, and Berkel, H: Prostate-specific antigen (PSA) in women. J La State Med Soc 151:209, 1999. Available at http://www.ncbi.nlm.nih.gov/pubmed/ 10234897?ordinalpos=1&itool;= EntrezSystem2.PEntrez.Pubmed .Pubmed_ResultsPanel.Pubmed _RVDocSum (accessed 7/23/08).

BIB

Index

IND

IND

IND

IND

IND

IND

IND

IND

IND

IND

IND

IND

IND

IND

IND

IND

IND

IND

IND

IND

IND

IND

IND

IND

IND

IND

IND

IND

IND

IND

IND

IND

IND

IND

IND

IND

IND

IND

IND

IND

IND

IND

IND

IND

IND

IND

IND

IND

IND

IND

IND

IND

IND

IND